NSCA's Essentials of Personal Training

SECOND EDITION

National Strength and Conditioning Association

Jared W. Coburn, PhD, CSCS,*D, FNSCA
California State University, Fullerton

Moh H. Malek, PhD, CSCS,*D, NSCA-CPT,*D, FNSCA
Wayne State University, Detroit

Editors

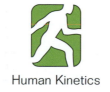

Human Kinetics

Library of Congress Cataloging-in-Publication Data

NSCA's essentials of personal training / Jared W. Coburn and Moh H. Malek, editors. -- 2nd ed.
   p. cm.
 Includes bibliographical references and index.
 ISBN-13: 978-0-7360-8415-4 (hard cover)
 ISBN-10: 0-7360-8415-0 (hard cover)
 1. Personal trainers. 2. Physical education and training. 3. Muscle strength. 4. Physical fitness--Physiological aspects. I. Coburn, Jared W. II. Malek, Moh H. III. National Strength & Conditioning Association (U.S.)
 GV428.7.N73 2012
 613.7'1--dc22

                2011004875

ISBN: 978-0-7360-8415-4

The Web addresses cited in this text were current as of February 2011, unless otherwise noted.

Acquisitions Editors: Michael S. Bahrke, PhD, and Roger W. Earle; **Developmental Editor:** Christine M. Drews; **Assistant Editors:** Brendan Shea and Steven Calderwood; **Copyeditor:** Joyce Sexton; **Indexer:** Betty Frizzell; **Permissions Manager:** Dalene Reeder; **Graphic Designer:** Nancy Rasmus; **Graphic Artist:** Kathleen Boudreau-Fuoss; **Cover Designer:** Keith Blomberg; **Photographs (interior):** © Human Kinetics, unless otherwise noted; **Photo Asset Manager:** Laura Fitch; **Visual Production Assistant:** Joyce Brumfield; **Photo Production Manager:** Jason Allen; **Art Manager:** Kelly Hendren; **Associate Art Manager:** Alan. L. Wilborn; **Art Style Development:** Joanne Brummett; **Illustrations:** © Human Kinetics; **Printer:** Walsworth

Photos on pages 341, 436, 448, 453, 455, and 456 courtesy of Stacy Peterson of Acceleration Sports, San Diego.

Printed in the United States of America   10 9 8

The paper in this book was manufactured using responsible forestry methods.

Human Kinetics
Website: www.HumanKinetics.com

United States: Human Kinetics
P.O. Box 5076
Champaign, IL 61825-5076
800-747-4457
e-mail: humank@hkusa.com

Canada: Human Kinetics
475 Devonshire Road Unit 100
Windsor, ON N8Y 2L5
800-465-7301 (in Canada only)
e-mail: info@hkcanada.com

Europe: Human Kinetics
107 Bradford Road
Stanningley
Leeds LS28 6AT, United Kingdom
+44 (0) 113 255 5665
e-mail: hk@hkeurope.com

Australia: Human Kinetics
57A Price Avenue
Lower Mitcham, South Australia 5062
08 8372 0999
e-mail: info@hkaustralia.com

New Zealand: Human Kinetics
P.O. Box 80
Mitcham Shopping Centre, South Australia 5062
0800 222 062
e-mail: info@hknewzealand.com

E4877

Contents

Contributors

Travis W. Beck, PhD
University of Oklahoma, Norman

David T. Beine, MS, ATC, LAT
Milwaukee School of Engineering

Lee E. Brown, EdD, CSCS,*D, FNSCA, FACSM
California State University, Fullerton

Jared W. Coburn, PhD, CSCS,*D, FNSCA, FACSM
California State University, Fullerton

Joel T. Cramer, PhD, CSCS,*D, NSCA-CPT,*D, FNSCA, FACSM, FISSN
Oklahoma State University, Stillwater

Kyle T. Ebersole, PhD, LAT
University of Wisconsin-Milwaukee

Tammy K. Evetovich, PhD, CSCS, FACSM
Wayne State College, Wayne, NE

Avery D. Faigenbaum, EdD, CSCS,*D, FNSCA, FACSM
The College of New Jersey, Ewing, NJ

Ryan Fiddler, MS
Oklahoma State University, Stillwater

Sean P. Flanagan, PhD, ATC, CSCS,*D
California State University, Northridge

John F. Graham, MS, CSCS,*D, FNSCA
Lehigh Valley Health Network, Allentown/
Bethlehem, PA

G. Gregory Haff, PhD, CSCS,*D, FNSCA
Edith Cowan University, Western Australia

Erin E. Haff, MA
Edith Cowan University, Western Australia

Patrick S. Hagerman, EdD, CSCS, NSCA-CPT, FNSCA
Axia College at University of Phoenix

Bradley D. Hatfield, PhD, FACSM, FNAK
University of Maryland, College Park

Allen Hedrick, MA, CSCS,*D, RSCC,*D, FNSCA
Colorado State University-Pueblo

David L. Herbert, JD
David L. Herbert & Associates, Attorneys and
Counselors at Law, Canton, OH

Kristi R. Hinnerichs, PhD, ATC, CSCS,*D
Wayne State College, Wayne, NE

Phil Kaplan, MS, NSCA-CPT
Phil Kaplan's Fitness, Sunrise, FL

Tom P. LaFontaine, PhD, CSCS, NSCA-CPT, FACSM, FAACVPR
Optimus: The Center for Health, Columbia, MO

Moh H. Malek, PhD, CSCS,*D, NSCA-CPT,*D, FNSCA, FACSM
Wayne State University, Detroit

Robert Mamula, CSCS
University of California, San Diego

John P. McCarthy, PhD, PT, CSCS,*D, FNSCA, FACSM
University of Alabama at Birmingham

Kevin Messey, MS, ATC, CSCS
University of California, San Diego

David R. Pearson, PhD, CSCS*D, FNSCA
Ball State University, Muncie, IN

Stacy Peterson, MA, CSCS, FACSM
Acceleration Sports, San Diego

Sharon Rana, PhD, CSCS
Ohio University, Athens, OH

Peter Ronai, MS, CSCS,*D, NSCA-CPT,*D
Sacred Heart University, Fairfield, CT

Jane L.P. Roy, PhD, CSCS
University of Alabama at Birmingham

Eric D. Ryan, PhD, CSCS, NSCA-CPT
University of North Carolina at Chapel Hill

Douglas B. Smith, PhD
Oklahoma State University, Stillwater

Paul Sorace, MS, CSCS,*D
Hackensack University Medical Center, New
Jersey

Marie Spano, MS, RD, CSCS, CSSD, FISSN
Spano Sports Nutrition Consulting, Atlanta, GA

Shinya Takahashi, PhD, CSCS, NSCA-CPT
University of Nebraska-Lincoln

N. Travis Triplett, PhD, CSCS,*D, FNSCA
Appalachian State University, Boone, NC

Vanessa van den Heuvel Yang, MS, ATC
University of California, San Diego

Joseph P. Weir, PhD, FNSCA, FACSM
Des Moines University, Des Moines, IA

Wayne L. Westcott, PhD, CSCS
Quincy College, Quincy, MA

Jason B. White, PhD
Ohio University, Athens, OH

William C. Whiting, PhD, CSCS, FACSM
California State University, Northridge

Contributors to the Previous Edition

Anthony A. Abbott, EdD, CSCS,*D, NSCA-CPT,*D, FNSCA, FACSM

Thomas R. Baechle, EdD, CSCS,*D, retired; NSCA-CPT,*D, retired

Lee E. Brown, EdD, CSCS,*D, FNSCA, FACSM

Jared W. Coburn, PhD, CSCS,*D, FNSCA, FACSM

Matthew J. Comeau, PhD, ATC, LAT, CSCS

Joel T. Cramer, PhD, CSCS,*D, NSCA-CPT,*D, FNSCA, FACSM, FISSN

J. Henry "Hank" Drought, MS, CSCS,*D, NSCA-CPT,*D

Roger W. Earle, MA, CSCS,*D, NSCA-CPT,*D

JoAnn Eickhoff-Shemek, PhD, FACSM, FAWHP

Todd Ellenbecker, PT, MS, SCS, OCS, CSCS

Avery D. Faigenbaum, EdD, CSCS,*D, FNSCA, FACSM

John F. Graham, MS, CSCS,*D, FNSCA

Mike Greenwood, PhD, FNSCA, FISSN, FACSM, CSCS,*D

Patrick S. Hagerman, EdD, CSCS, NSCA-CPT, FNSCA

Everett Harman, PhD, CSCS, NSCA-CPT

Bradley D. Hatfield, PhD, FACSM, FNAK

Allen Hedrick, MA, CSCS,*D, RSCC,*D, FNSCA

Susan L. Heinrich, MS

Carlos E. Jiménez, MD, NSCA-CPT

Phil Kaplan, MS, NSCA-CPT

John A.C. Kordich, MEd, CSCS,*D, NSCA-CPT,*D, FNSCA

Len Kravitz, PhD

Tom P. LaFontaine, PhD, CSCS, NSCA-CPT, FACSM, FAACVPR

David R. Pearson, PhD, CSCS*D, FNSCA

David H. Potach, PT, MS, CSCS,*D, NSCA-CPT,*D

Kristin J. Reimers, MS, RD

Torrey Smith, MA, CSCS,*D, NSCA-CPT,*D

N. Travis Triplett, PhD, CSCS,*D, FNSCA

Christine L. Vega, MPH, RD, CSCS,*D, NSCA-CPT,*D

Robert Watine, MD

Joseph P. Weir, PhD, FNSCA, FACSM

Wayne L. Westcott, PhD, CSCS

Mark A. Williams, PhD, FACSM, FAACVPR

Preface

NSCA's Essentials of Personal Training is the most complete and authoritative book on the theory and practice of personal training. As with the first edition, the second edition will serve as the primary resource for individuals preparing for the NSCA-Certified Personal Trainer (NSCA-CPT) exam.

The authors of the book include college and university professors, researchers, personal trainers, athletic trainers, physical therapists, and nutritionists. The book presents state-of-the-art information regarding applied aspects of personal training while also providing the scientific principles that guide this practice. The content of the textbook has been designed to present the knowledge, skills, and abilities (KSAs) required by a personal trainer. These KSAs are presented in 13 content areas that are presented in six sections of the textbook. They are as follows:

- Part I: Exercise sciences. The first part of the book contains foundational exercise science–related information about anatomy, physiology, bioenergetics, biomechanics, training adaptations, exercise psychology, motivation and goal setting, and general nutrition guidelines.

- Part II: Initial consultation and evaluation. This section includes detailed guidelines about assessing a client, selecting and administering fitness tests, and interpreting the results based on descriptive and normative data.

- Part III: Exercise technique. The chapters in this part of the book describe proper exercise technique and instructional approaches for flexibility; body-weight, free weight, and machine resistance exercises; and cardiovascular activities. In addition, targeted muscles and common performance errors are identified.

- Part IV: Program design. The focus of this section is the complex process of designing safe, effective, and goal-specific resistance, aerobic, plyometric, and speed training programs.

- Part V: Clients with unique needs. This part of the book describes a variety of clients who have special needs and limitations (e.g., prepubescents, pregnant women, the elderly, and athletes) or physical conditions (e.g., obesity, hyperlipidemia, diabetes, hypertension, low back pain, heart disease, epilepsy). This section details how to modify an exercise program; identify exercise contraindications; and when, how, and to whom to refer a client with a condition beyond the personal trainer's scope of practice.

- Part VI: Safety and legal issues. The last section provides guidelines on the design and layout of commercial and home fitness facilities, basic exercise equipment maintenance, and important legal issues a personal trainer should understand and be aware of.

NSCA's Essentials of Personal Training contains features and elements that personal trainers will find helpful:

- More than 220 full-color photographs that clearly illustrate and accurately depict proper exercise technique

- Chapter objectives and key points

- Sidebars with practical explanations and applications

- Testing protocols and norms for assessing clients

- Over 120 chapter questions that can be used to help prepare for the NSCA-Certified Personal Trainer exam

- A comprehensive glossary of frequently used terms and concepts that are bolded in the text

NSCA's Essentials of Personal Training is the most comprehensive reference available for personal trainers and other fitness professionals. As an exam preparation tool, it is unmatched in its scope and relevance to the NSCA-Certified Personal Trainer examination.

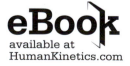
eBook available at HumanKinetics.com

Updates to the Second Edition

The second edition of *NSCA's Essentials of Personal Training* updates and expands on the information presented in the first edition. Every effort has been made to present the latest scientific and practical information of interest to personal trainers. Updates in this edition include the following:

- The incorporation of the latest research from exercise science throughout
- New and revised chapter questions to help readers prepare for the NSCA-CPT exam
- Updated information regarding the structure and function of the muscular, skeletal, and cardiorespiratory and other systems (chapters 1 and 2)
- New and revised figures and tables throughout the book
- Expanded and updated information regarding proper nutrition for the personal training client (chapter 7)
- Updated information regarding client screening and testing based on the latest guidelines from prominent exercise science organizations (chapters 9, 10, and 11)
- Revised or rewritten chapters on exercise prescription and technique for flexibility training, resistance training, aerobic endurance exercise, and plyometric and speed training (chapters 12-17)
- A rewritten chapter on resistance training program design, providing the latest information on the application of periodization of training (chapter 15)
- Revised, expanded, and updated information regarding the application of nutrition principles to clients with metabolic concerns (chapter 19)
- New information regarding injuries, rehabilitation, and clients with cardiovascular, respiratory, and orthopedic conditions (chapters 20 and 21)
- New guidelines for determining training loads for clients who are athletes (chapter 23)

Instructor Resources

In addition to the updated content, this edition also contains newly created instructor resources available online at www.humankinetics.com/NSCAsEssentialsofPersonalTraining:

- *Instructor guide.* The instructor guide, written by Brad Schoenfeld, contains chapter summaries; sample lecture outlines; ideas for assignments, lab activities, and class projects; ideas for discussion or essay topics; additional suggested readings, including websites; and tips for presenting important key concepts.
- *Image bank.* This comprehensive resource provides figures, tables, and photos from the textbook for incorporation into lectures and presentations.

Whether used for learning the essentials of personal training, for preparing for a certification exam, or as a reference by professionals, *NSCA's Essentials of Personal Training, Second Edition,* will help practitioners and the scientific community better understand how to develop and administer safe and effective personal training programs.

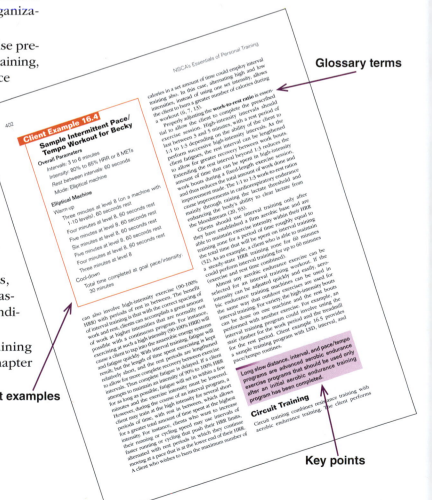

Glossary terms

Client examples

Key points

Sidebars that highlight applied content

Exercise Psychology for the Personal Trainer

Minimizing Procrastination

The 14th-century philosopher Jean Buridan told the story of a mule that starved to death trying to decide between two equidistant bales of hay. The bales of hay were equally desirable, so the mule could not decide which way to go. The fable presents a valuable analogy for human indecision. Health and fitness are attributes desired by everyone, but only a disappointing margin of our population manages to commit to and maintain an exercise lifestyle. If people believe they have too many options that they must decide between—diets, devices, or personal trainers—the decision-making process itself often leads to stagnation. Personal trainers have to think beyond the personal training session and toward influencing clients to exercise not only today, or next week, but for the long haul. When a client procrastinates, he or she is weighing options, left in a frozen state of indecision, trying to decide if the perceived pain will outweigh the potential benefit.

Identifying False Beliefs

Because quick fixes are so often positioned as solutions, many clients have allowed flawed and misleading information into their belief systems. If, for example, a client believes that weight loss can be achieved only by severely restricting food intake, he or she is going to block out the personal trainer's suggestions of a more appropriate caloric intake. Further, many people have been conditioned to believe that exercise is not for them or that their bodies will not respond to exercise as the bodies of others do. "No pain, no gain" is another flawed belief. This belief increases a person's tendency to overtrain, which can sabotage the potential for results.

Practical Motivational Techniques

1. Have the client use an exercise log or journal to document baseline measurements and the details of each workout. Teach the client not only to use the journal as a report card for exercise sessions, but also to record emotions, meals, and perspectives on progress.

2. Begin clients with exercise sessions that involve familiar activities. Lack of familiarity with an exercise mode can frustrate clients and lead to a lack of desire to continue exercising.

3. Whenever possible, offer choices. Keep the client involved in decisions, but offer choices that are equally beneficial. Rather than having the client question whether he or she should exercise at all today, change the decision: "Would you rather do your warm-up on the elliptical climber or the exercise bike today?"

4. Provide feedback often. Look for small achievements. The personal trainer can notice and comment on increases in aerobic capacity, increases in strength, and decreases in body fat while providing exercise assistance. If, for example, the client moves up 5 pounds (2.5 kg) in a specific resistance training exercise, make it clear that progress is taking place.

5. Model the appropriate behavior by acting as a role model and set an example of an exercise commitment.

6. Prepare the client for periods during which momentum may be disrupted. If the client understands that even the most dedicated individuals have exercise lapses, those lapses are less likely to result in program abandonment. One of the best things a personal trainer can do for clients is to act as a role model and set an example of an exercise commitment.

7. Use social support resources. The personal trainer can check on a client's moods, responses, and adherence by tactful use of telephone contact. If possible, conversations with family members regarding resources or motivational information. If possible, e-mail correspondence, and mailing of education, desired outcome and course of action can all contribute to motivation and adherence by providing a stronger support network at home.

8. Let the past go. If a client feels as if he or she failed to obtain the benefits of an exercise in the past, focus instead on future goals.

9. Substitute a "do your best" outlook for a "be perfect" attitude. Clients who strive are guaranteed to hit a point of perceived failure. Teach clients to understand that effort and commitment is the equivalent of excellence.

10. Agree on a motivational affirmation and have the client write it down.

NSCA's Essentials of Personal Training

Conclusion

Typically the personal trainer has the challenge of working with clients who have a broad spectrum of fitness or exercise capabilities. To gather baseline assessments, the personal trainer may test for a variety of fitness parameters such as HR, BP, body composition, cardiovascular endurance, muscular strength, muscular endurance, and flexibility and then make comparisons to established sets of descriptive or normative data. The resulting conclusions can then form the basis for the client's exercise prescription.

Study Questions

1. A 40-year-old female client's resting blood pressure was 115/72 during the initial assessment. When measuring her blood pressure one month later, to what level of mercury (Hg) should the bladder be inflated?

   A. 115 mm
   B. 125 mm
   C. 135 mm
   D. 150 mm

2. All of the following skinfold sites are appropriate for performing a three-site skinfold for a 45-year-old male client EXCEPT

   A. chest.
   B. suprailium.
   C. abdomen.
   D. thigh.

3. Calculate the estimated $\dot{V}O_2$max value for a 38-year-old male client who weighs 88 kg and ran 1.5 miles in 13:30.

   A. 34.5 ml · kg^{-1} · min^{-1}
   B. 36.2 ml · kg^{-1} · min^{-1}
   C. 39.9 ml · kg^{-1} · min^{-1}
   D. 41.5 ml · kg^{-1} · min^{-1}

4. Which of the following is an assessment of local muscular endurance for a 38-year-old female client?

   A. bench press 35 pounds at 60 beats/min until failure
   B. 12-minute run/walk
   C. Åstrand-Ryhming cycle ergometer test
   D. YMCA step test

Applied Knowledge Question

A 28-year-old female recently hired a personal trainer. Her fitness evaluation indicated the following information:

Height: 66 inches
Weight: 150 pounds
Resting heart rate: 75 beats/min
Resting BP: 128/82
Body fat: 20%
$\dot{V}O_2$max: 26 ml · kg^{-1} · min^{-1}
1RM bench press: 140 pounds
1RM leg press: 310 pounds
Partial curl-up test (1 minute): 25

Which of the fitness evaluation results is below average for this client and should be given attention when setting goals? How do you know this to be true?

Learning aids at the end of each chapter include study questions, an applied knowledge question, and references

---

Fast Leg Drill

Intensity level: High
Equipment: None
Purpose: Move lower extremities at a faster speed than during normal running

Beginning position: Perform at a walk, beginning with right foot.

Movement: After the third step, perform a fast sequence of the following motions: dorsiflexed and great toe extended as in butt kicker; bring right knee forward as if foot; flex hip so that thigh is parallel to ground, then unfold leg and drive foot to ground. Repeat every third step.

Advanced variations: (1) ankling for three steps, then fast leg motion one step, focusing on one leg at a time; (2) ankling for three steps, then fast leg motion one step, alternating legs; (3) ankling for two steps, then fast leg motion one step, focusing on one leg at a time; (4) straight-leg bounding for three steps, then fast leg motion one step, focusing on one leg at a time; (5) straight-leg bounding for two steps, then fast leg one step, alternating legs; (6) straight-leg bounding one step, then fast leg one step, focusing on one leg at a time; (7) continuous fast leg for distance.

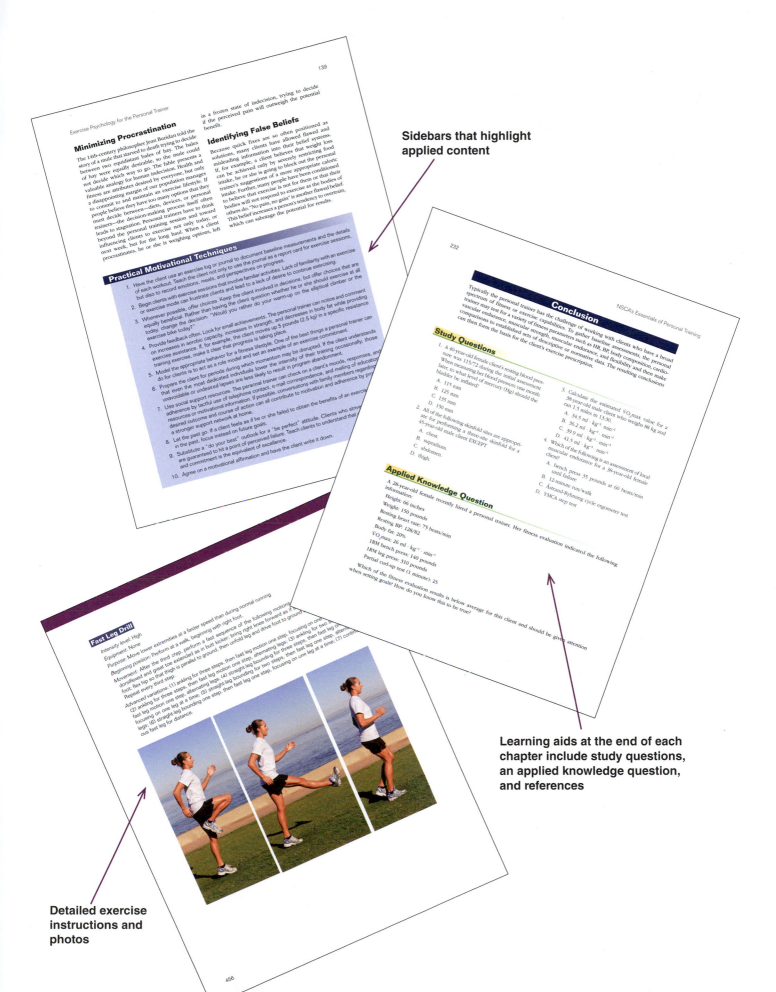

Detailed exercise instructions and photos

Acknowledgments

First, we would like to thank the authors of the various chapters of this book. Their willingness to accommodate the many revisions and recommendations provided over the past several years is greatly appreciated. We are confident that their expertise has made this a strong book that will contribute in a positive way to the practice of personal training. In addition, we are thankful for the helpful chapter reviews we received from Jay Dawes, Kristy Richardson, Travis Triplett, and Carrie White.

We would also like to thank the staff at Human Kinetics for the many hours they have spent bringing the book to completion. In particular, we would like to thank Chris Drews and Brendan Shea for their extraordinary help, patience, and attention to detail.

The staff at NSCA has been instrumental in assuring that the book is up to date, checked for accuracy, and that it will meet the needs of those who will turn to it for expert guidance and information. In particular, we are thankful to Torrey Smith and Keith Cinea. We are also grateful to past NSCA president Lee Brown for asking us to edit this book in the first place.

Last but not least, we would like to thank our families. This includes our parents, the late Darrel and Mary Coburn and Frida Malek; our wives Tamara Coburn and Bridget Malek; and children Dara and Jansen Coburn.

Credits

Figures 1.1, 4.5, 4.6, 4.7, 4.8, 4.10, 4.13, and 4.16 Reprinted, by permission, from NSCA, 2008, Biomechanics of resistance exercise, by E. Harman. In *Essentials of strength training and conditioning,* 3rd ed., edited by T. Baechle and R. Earle (Champaign, IL: Human Kinetics), 68, 69, 69, 70, 76, 73, and 81.

Figures 1.2, 1.3, 1.4, 2.5, 2.6, 2.7, 2.10, and 2.11 Reprinted, by permission, from NSCA, 2008, Structure and function of the muscular, neuromuscular, cardiovascular, and respiratory systems, by G.R. Hunter and R.T. Harris. In *Essentials of strength training and conditioning,* 3rd ed., edited by T. Baechle and R. Earle (Champaign, IL: Human Kinetics), 5, 5, 6, 15, 14, 15, 17, and 18

Figures 1.5, 1.6, 1.7, 1.8, 2.1, 2.8, 2.13, 3.1, 6.2, 6.4, 6.5, 6.6, 6.7 and Tables 6.2 and 6.4 Adapted, by permission, from J.H. Wilmore, D.L. Costill, and W.L. Kenney, 2008, *Physiology of sport and exercise,* 4th ed. (Champaign, IL: Human Kinetics), 32, 80, 81, 95, 140, 139, 148, 50, 172, 230, 226, 228, 285, 237, 415 and 103 and 239.

Figure 1.9 Reprinted from R. Behnke, 2006, *Kinetic anatomy,* 2nd ed. (Champaign, IL: Human Kinetics), 5.

Figures 1.10a, 4.1, 21.3, 21.12, and 21.13 Reprinted, by permission, from J. Watkins, 2010, *Structure and function of the musculoskeletal system,* 2nd ed. (Champaign, IL: Human Kinetics), 8, 25, 122, 193, and 312.

Figure 1.10b Reprinted from L. Cartwright and W. Pitney, 2011, *Fundamentals of athletic training,* 3rd ed. (Champaign, IL: Human Kinetics), 34.

Figures 2.2, 2.3, and 6.3 Reprinted, by permission, from S.K. Powers and E.T. Howley, 2004, *Exercise physiology: Theory and application to fitness and performance,* 5th ed. (New York: McGraw-Hill Companies), 205, 206, and 97. © The McGraw-Hill Companies.

Figures 2.4, 4.11, 4.12, and 4.14 Adapted, by permission, from W.C Whiting and S. Rugg, 2006, *Dynatomy: Dynamic human anatomy* (Champaign, IL: Human Kinetics, Inc.), 15, 76, 77, and 123.

Figure 2.9 Reprinted, by permission, from P.O. Åstrand et al., 2003, *Textbook of work physiology: Physiological bases of exercise,* 4th ed. (Champaign, IL: Human Kinetics), 136.

Figures 3.2, 3.3, 3.4, 3.5, 3.6, 3.7, 3.8, 3.9 Reprinted, by permission, from NSCA, 2008, Bioenergetics of exercise and training, by J.T. Cramer. In *Essentials of strength training and conditioning,* 3rd ed., edited by T. Baechle and R. Earle (Champaign, IL: Human Kinetics), 25, 26, 28, 29, 30, 31, 35, 36.

Figure 4.2 Reprinted, by permission, from E.A. Harman, M. Johnson, and P.N. Frykman, 1992, "A movement oriented approach to exercise prescription," *NSCA Journal* 14(1): 47-54.

Figures 4.3, 4.4, 4.9 Adapted, by permission, from W.C. Whiting and R.F. Zernicke, 1998, *Biomechanics of musculoskeletal injury* (Champaign, IL: Human Kinetics), 108, 109, 67.

Figure 4.15 Reprinted, by permission, from NSCA, 2000, Biomechanics of resistance exercise, by E. Harman. In *Essentials of strength training and conditioning,* 2nd ed., edited by T. Baechle and R. Earle (Champaign, IL: Human Kinetics), 43.

Figures 5.1 and 5.2 Reprinted, by permission, from NSCA, 2008, Adaptations to anaerobic training programs, by N.A. Ratamess. In *Essentials of strength training and conditioning,* 3rd ed., edited by T. Baechle and R. Earle (Champaign, IL: Human Kinetics), 97, 152.

Figure 6.1 Reprinted, by permission, from J. Hoffman, 2002, *Physiological aspects of sport training and performance* (Champaign, IL: Human Kinetics), 50.

Figure 8.1 Adapted, by permission, D.E. Sherwood and D.J. Selder, 1979, "Cardiorespiratory health, reaction time, and aging," *Medicine and Science in Sports* 11: 186-189.

Figure 8.2 Reprinted from *Neurobiology of Aging,* Vol. 11, R.E. Dustman et al., "Age and fitness effects on EEG, ERPs, visual sensitivity, and cognition," pp. 193-200, Copyright 1990, with permission from Elsevier Science.

Figure 9.1 Reprinted, by permission, from ACSM, 2010, *ACSM's guidelines for exercise testing and prescription,* 8th ed. (Philadelphia, PA: Lippincott, Williams, and Wilkins), 24.

Figure 9.2 Reprinted, by permission, from T. Olds and K. Norton, 1999, *Pre-exercise and health screening guide* (Champaign, IL: Human Kinetics), 29.

PAR-Q Form From Physical Activity Readiness Questionnaire (PAR-Q) © 2002. Reprinted with permission for the Canadian Society for Exercise Physiology. http://www.csep.ca/forms.asp

Health Risk Analysis Form B. Sharkey and S. Gaskill, 2007, *Fitness and health,* 7th ed. (Champaign, IL: Human Kinetics), 64-68; Data for Life Expectancy from CDC, 2010, National Vital Statistics Reports.

YMCA Cycle Ergometer Test Adapted, by permission, from American College of Sports Medicine, 2010, *ACSM's resource manual for guidelines for exercise testing and prescription,* 6th ed. Philadelphia: Lippincott Williams & Wilkins

Tables 11.3 and 11.9 Reprinted, by permission, from V. Heyward, 2010, *Advanced fitness and exercise prescription,* 6th ed. (Champaign, IL: Human Kinetics), 32 and 204.

Table 11.10 Reprinted, by permission, from V. Heyward and D. Wagner, 2004, *Applied body composition assessment,* 2nd ed. (Champaign, IL: Human Kinetics), 9.

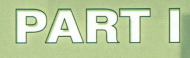

Exercise Sciences

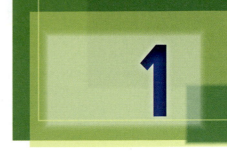

Structure and Function of the Muscular, Nervous, and Skeletal Systems

Jared W. Coburn, PhD, and Moh H. Malek, PhD

After completing this chapter, you will be able to

- describe the structure and function of skeletal muscle;
- list and explain the steps in the sliding filament theory of muscle action;
- explain the concept of muscle fiber types and how it applies to exercise performance;
- describe the structure and function of the nervous system as it applies to the control of skeletal muscle; and
- explain the role of exercise in bone health, as well as the function of tendons and ligaments in physical activity.

Physical activity occurs due to the combined and coordinated efforts of the muscular, nervous, and skeletal systems. The nervous system is responsible for initiating and modifying the activation of muscles. The muscles produce movement by generating forces to rotate bones around joints. This chapter explores the basic structure and function of these systems as they apply to the practice of personal training.

The Muscular System

Muscles generate force when they are activated. This is referred to as a *muscle contraction* or *muscle action*. Of the three types of muscle—smooth, cardiac, and skeletal—it is the third type that attaches to bones, causing them to rotate around joints. It is this function of skeletal muscles that allows us to run, jump, and lift and throw things. The function of muscle is dictated by its structure.

Gross Anatomy of Skeletal Muscle

The system of skeletal muscles is illustrated in figure 1.1. Each skeletal muscle (e.g., deltoid, pectoralis major, gastrocnemius) is surrounded by a layer of connective tissue referred to as **epimysium.** A muscle is further divided into bundles of **muscle**

fibers. A bundle of muscle fibers is called a **fasciculus** or **fascicle.** Each fasciculus is surrounded by connective tissue called **perimysium.** Within a fasciculus, each muscle fiber is surrounded and separated from adjacent fibers by a layer of connective tissue referred to as **endomysium.** Together, these connective tissues help transmit the force of muscle action to the bone via another connective tissue structure, the tendon. Figure 1.2 illustrates these connective tissue structures and their relationship to the muscle.

Microscopic Anatomy of Skeletal Muscle

Each muscle fiber is a cell, with many of the same structural components as other cells (figure 1.3). For example, each muscle fiber is surrounded by a plasma membrane, referred to as the *sarcolemma*. The sarcolemma encloses the contents of the cell, regulates the passage of materials such as glucose into and out of the cell, and receives and conducts stimuli in the form of electrical impulses or **action**

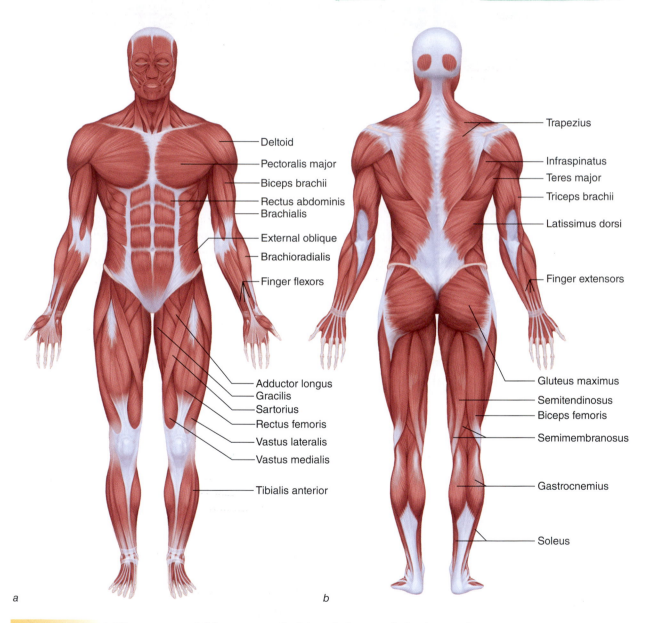

a   b

FIGURE 1.1   (a) Front view and (b) rear view of adult male human skeletal musculature.

Reprinted by permission from NSCA 2008.

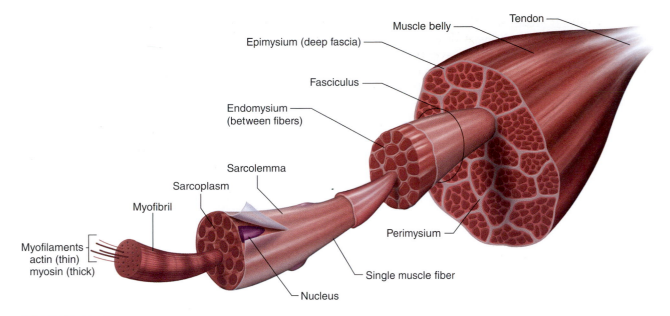

FIGURE 1.2 The gross structure of skeletal muscle. The whole muscle, the fasciculus, and individual muscle fibers are surrounded by the connective tissues epimysium, perimysium, and endomysium, respectively.
Reprinted by permission from NSCA 2008.

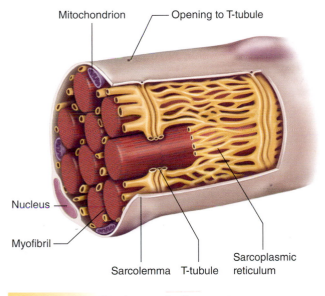

FIGURE 1.3 Single muscle fiber anatomy.
Reprinted by permission from NSCA 2008.

tance training and aerobic endurance training are discussed in chapters 5 and 6, respectively.

Within the boundary of the sarcolemma, but outside the nuclei, is the cytoplasm, referred to as *sarcoplasm in muscle*. This watery solution contains the cell's energy sources, such as adenosine triphosphate (ATP) (the only direct source of energy for muscle actions), phosphocreatine, glycogen, and fat droplets. Also suspended within the sarcoplasm are organelles. These include **mitochondria** (singular is *mitochondrion*), which are the sites of aerobic ATP production within the cell and thus of great importance for aerobic exercise performance. Another important organelle is the **sarcoplasmic reticulum.** This organelle stores calcium and regulates the muscle action process by altering the intracellular calcium concentration. Specifically, the sarcoplasmic reticulum releases calcium into the sarcoplasm of the cell when an action potential passes to the interior of the cell via structures called *transverse tubules* or *T-tubules*. The T-tubules are channels that form from openings in the sarcolemma of the muscle cell.

> A muscle fiber is a cell that is specialized to contract and generate force (tension).

Myofibril

Each muscle cell contains columnar protein structures that run parallel to the length of the muscle fiber. These structures are known as **myofibrils**

potentials. Skeletal muscle cells are multinucleated, meaning they possess more than one nucleus. In fact, skeletal muscle cells possess many nuclei as a result of the embryonic fusion of singly nucleated cells during development. The nuclei contain the genetic material, or DNA, of the cell, and are largely responsible for initiating the processes associated with adaptations to exercise, such as muscle cell enlargement or hypertrophy. Adaptations to resis-

(figure 1.4). Each myofibril is a bundle of **myofila-ments,** which primarily consist of **myosin** (thick) and **actin** (thin) filaments. The myosin and actin filaments are arranged in a regular pattern along the length of the myofibril, giving it a striated, or striped, appearance.

Myosin filaments are formed from the aggregation of myosin molecules. Each myosin molecule consists of a head, neck, and tail. The head is capable of attaching to and pulling on the actin filament. Energy from the splitting, or hydrolysis, of ATP is used to perform this power stroke, an important step in the

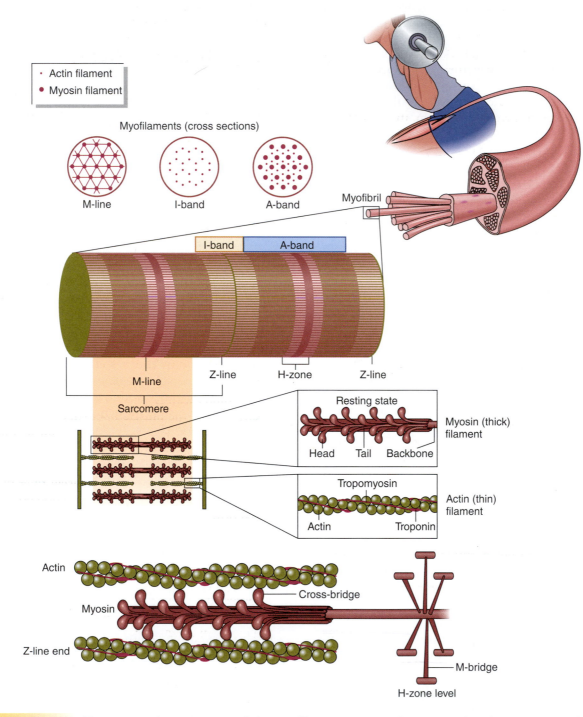

FIGURE 1.4   The structural arrangement of the myofilaments actin and myosin within the sarcomere, the basic functional unit of skeletal muscle.

Reprinted by permission from NSCA 2008.

process of muscle activation. The neck structure connects the head to the tail. The middle of the myosin filament is oriented in a tail-to-tail fashion, such that the head portions project outward from the ends of the filament (figure 1.4). The protein titin acts to maintain the position of the myosin filament relative to actin.

Each actin filament is formed from individual globular or G-actin proteins (figure 1.4). Each G-actin has a binding site for a myosin head. The G-actin proteins assemble into strands of filamentous, or F-actin. Associated with the actin filament are two other protein structures: **tropomyosin** and **troponin.** Collectively, tropomyosin and troponin are considered regulatory proteins as they regulate the interaction of myosin and actin, the contractile proteins. Tropomyosin is a rod-like protein that spans the length of seven G-actin proteins along the length of the actin filament. When the muscle cell is at rest, tropomyosin lies over the myosin binding sites on actin. Each end of a tropomyosin filament is attached to troponin. When bound to calcium, troponin causes the movement of tropomyosin away from the myosin binding sites on actin. This allows the myosin head to attach and pull on actin, a critical step in the muscle activation process. The protein nebulin acts to ensure the correct length of the actin filaments.

Sarcomere

The **sarcomere** is the basic contractile unit of muscle (figure 1.4). It extends from one Z-line to an adjacent Z-line. The A-band is determined by the width of a myosin filament. It is the A-band that provides the dark striation of skeletal muscle. Actin filaments are anchored at one end to the Z-line. They extend inward to the center of the sarcomere. The area of the A-band that contains myosin, but not actin, is the H-zone. In the middle of the H-zone is a dark line called the *M-line*. The M-line helps align adjacent myosin filaments. The I-band spans the distance between the ends of adjacent myosin filaments. As such, each I-band lies partly in each of two sarcomeres. The I-bands are less dense than the A-bands, and thus they are responsible for giving skeletal muscle its light striation.

> The basic functional and contractile unit of skeletal muscle is the sarcomere.

Neuromuscular Junction

In order to contract, muscle fibers must normally receive a stimulus from the nervous system. This communication between the nervous and muscle

systems occurs at a specialized region referred to as the *neuromuscular junction* (figure 1.5*a*). Each muscle fiber has a single neuromuscular junction, located at the approximate center of the length of the cell. Structures at the neuromuscular junction include the axon terminal of the neuron; a specialized region of the muscle cell membrane called the *motor endplate*; and the space between the axon terminal and motor endplate, referred to as the *synaptic cleft* or *neuromuscular cleft*.

Sliding Filament Theory

Although the exact details are still being determined, the sliding filament theory is still the most widely accepted theory of muscle action (9). This theory states that a muscle shortens or lengthens when the filaments (actin and myosin) slide past each other, without the filaments themselves changing in length. The following steps detail the series of events that occur during muscle action:

1. An action potential passes along the length of a neuron, leading to the release of the excitatory neurotransmitter acetylcholine (ACh) at the neuromuscular junction. When the neuron is at rest, ACh is stored in the axon terminal of the neuron within structures called *synaptic vesicles*. It is the action potential that leads to the release of stored ACh into the synaptic cleft between the axon terminal of the neuron and the muscle fiber.

2. The ACh migrates across the synaptic cleft and binds with ACh receptors on the motor endplate of the muscle fiber (figure 1.5*a*).

3. This leads to the generation of an action potential along the sarcolemma of the muscle fiber. In addition, this action potential will travel to the interior of the muscle fiber via T-tubules. The movement of the action potential down the T-tubule triggers the release of stored calcium from the sarcoplasmic reticulum (figure 1.5*b*).

4. Once released into the sarcoplasm, the calcium migrates to, and binds with, troponin molecules located along the length of the actin filaments (figure 1.5*c*).

5. The binding of calcium to troponin causes a conformational change in the shape of troponin. Because tropomyosin is attached to troponin, this moves tropomyosin such that binding sites on actin are exposed to the myosin head.

6. When a muscle is in a rested state, the myosin head is actually "energized"; that is, it is storing

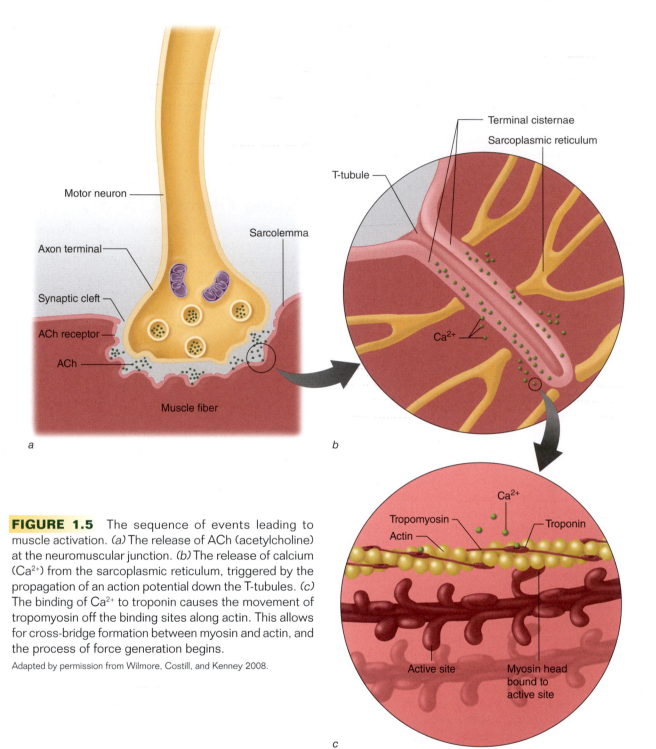

FIGURE 1.5 The sequence of events leading to muscle activation. (a) The release of ACh (acetylcholine) at the neuromuscular junction. (b) The release of calcium (Ca²⁺) from the sarcoplasmic reticulum, triggered by the propagation of an action potential down the T-tubules. (c) The binding of Ca²⁺ to troponin causes the movement of tropomyosin off the binding sites along actin. This allows for cross-bridge formation between myosin and actin, and the process of force generation begins.

Adapted by permission from Wilmore, Costill, and Kenney 2008.

the energy released from the breakdown of ATP to adenosine diphosphate (ADP) and inorganic phosphate (P_i). When the binding sites on actin are exposed to the myosin head, it is able to attach, forming a cross-bridge, and attempt to pull the actin filament toward the center of the sarcomere. Whether it is successful at pulling and thus shortening the muscle

depends on the amount of force generated by the cross-bridges that are pulling and the external force that opposes the cross-bridges.

7. After pulling on the actin filament, the myosin head is now in a lower energy state. In order to cause detachment from the actin filament, as well as to energize the head, a fresh ATP molecule must be bound. Once it is bound,

the myosin head detaches from actin, and the enzyme myosin **adenosine triphosphatase (ATPase)** causes the splitting of the ATP molecule. This once again energizes the myosin head. If the binding sites on actin are still exposed, the myosin head may once again form a cross-bridge with actin, again attempting to pull toward the center of the sarcomere. This process will continue provided that the muscle fiber is being stimulated to contract by its motor neuron.

> According to the sliding filament theory, a muscle shortens or lengthens because the actin and myosin filaments slide past each other, without the filaments themselves changing length.

Types of Muscle Actions

It is important to recognize that when stimulated, muscle fibers always attempt to shorten. That is, the cross-bridges always attempt to pull actin toward the center of the sarcomere, which would cause shortening of the sarcomere and thus the muscle. However, muscles are typically contracting against some type of external resistance, such as a barbell or dumbbell, which may be acting in opposition to the muscle force. If the amount of force produced by a muscle is greater than the external resistance acting in the opposite direction, a **concentric muscle action** will result. During a concentric muscle action, the resistance is overcome and the muscle shortens. If the amount of force produced by a muscle is less than an opposing external resistance, the muscle will lengthen even as it attempts to shorten. This lengthening muscle action is known as an **eccentric muscle action.** Lastly, if the muscle force is equal and opposite to that of an external resistance, an **isometric (static) muscle action** results. In this case, the muscle neither shortens nor lengthens, but remains the same length.

During the performance of resistance training exercises, the concentric phase is perceived by the exerciser as more difficult than the eccentric phase. For example, during performance of the bench press, lifting the barbell upward off the chest (concentric actions of the pectoralis major, anterior deltoid, and triceps brachii muscles) is more difficult than lowering the barbell to the chest (eccentric actions of the same muscles). This sometimes leads to the erroneous perception that the eccentric phase is less important than the concentric phase. However, there is evidence (3, 8) that an emphasis on both the concentric and eccentric action phases is important in order to maximize the benefits of resistance training.

Delayed-Onset Muscle Soreness (DOMS) and Eccentric Muscle Actions

It is not uncommon to experience muscular pain and discomfort 24 to 48 hours after beginning an exercise program or performing novel exercises. This delayed-onset muscle soreness (DOMS) was originally believed to be the result of lactic acid accumulation. However, recent research suggests that it likely results from some combination of connective and muscle tissue damage followed by an inflammatory reaction that activates pain receptors (2). This damage is primarily caused by eccentric muscle actions and resulting micro-tears in connective and muscle tissues. The pain that results may last for days, reducing range of motion, strength, and the ability to produce force quickly (2, 13). Strategies to combat the pain and performance decrements resulting from DOMS have included nutritional supplements, massage, ice, and ultrasound (1, 2). It appears, however, that exercise itself may be the best means of decreasing pain associated with DOMS, although its analgesic effects are temporary (2).

Muscle Fiber Types

While all muscle fibers are designed to contract and produce force, all fibers are not alike when it comes to contractile performance and basic physiological characteristics. For example, muscle fibers from the same muscle may differ in the force they produce, the time they take to reach peak force, their preference for aerobic versus anaerobic metabolism, and fatigability. This has led to the concept of muscle fiber typing. That is, muscle fibers may be classified into "types" based on different characteristics of interest. To determine muscle fiber type, a muscle biopsy must be performed. This technique involves the removal of a small amount of muscle via insertion of a muscle biopsy needle through an incision in the muscle. Following removal of the muscle tissue, it may be quickly frozen and then processed. While many types of analyses may be performed, determination of the biochemical and contractile properties of the muscle fibers is likely of greatest practical significance to the personal trainer.

One biochemical property of muscle fibers is the ability to produce ATP aerobically, a characteristic called *oxidative capacity* since oxygen is necessary for aerobic metabolism. Fibers that have large and numerous mitochondria, and that are surrounded by an ample supply of capillaries to deliver blood and oxygen, are considered oxidative fibers. In addition, these fibers possess a large amount of **myoglobin,** which delivers oxygen from the muscle cell membrane to the mitochondria, enhancing aerobic capacity and lessening the reliance on anaerobic ATP production.

As explained previously, the enzyme myosin ATPase is responsible for splitting ATP, thus making energy available for muscle action. Several forms of myosin ATPase exist, and these differ in the rate at which they split ATP. Fibers with a myosin ATPase form that has high ATPase activity will have a high rate of shortening due to the rapid availability of energy from ATP to support the muscle action process. The opposite is true with fibers demonstrating low ATPase activity. This concept that the type of myosin ATPase affects maximal shortening velocity of a muscle fiber provides us with a link between the biochemical (type of myosin ATPase) and contractile (shortening velocity) characteristics of muscle.

In addition to maximal shortening velocity, two other contractile characteristics of muscle are maximal force production and fiber efficiency. For example, fibers may differ in the amount of force they produce relative to their size (cross-sectional area). This is referred to as *specific tension*. Fibers may also be described based on efficiency. An efficient fiber is able to produce more work with a given expenditure of ATP.

Differences in the biochemical and contractile properties of muscle fibers have led physiologists to classify muscle fibers into types. It is generally agreed that one type of slow fiber and two types of fast fibers exist. Slow fibers have alternatively been referred to as **type I,** *slow oxidative (SO),* or *slow-twitch* fibers. As can be inferred from the name, these fibers have high oxidative capacity and are fatigue resistant, but they contract and relax slowly. The two types of fast fibers are known as **type IIa,** *fast oxidative glycolytic (FOG),* and **type IIx,** *fast glycolytic (FG),* fibers. Both fast fiber types are large and powerful, with moderate to high anaerobic metabolic capability. The primary distinction between the two is that FOG fibers have moderate oxidative and anaerobic capacity, providing them with some fatigue resistance in comparison to the purely anaerobic and highly fatigable FG fibers.

It should be acknowledged, however, that the characteristics by which fibers are categorized into types lie on a continuum rather than being discrete categories. For example, at what point does a fiber have enough mitochondria to be classified as an oxidative fiber? From a practical standpoint, muscle

fibers will adapt based on the physiological stress placed on them. For example, both type I and type II fibers will increase in size in response to regular resistance training. More will be said about adaptations to resistance and aerobic endurance training in chapters 5 and 6, respectively.

The Nervous System

While skeletal muscles produce the force that allows us to move and exercise, it is the nervous system that directs and controls the voluntary movement.

Organization of the Nervous System

Anatomically, the entire nervous system can be divided into the central nervous system and peripheral nervous system (figure 1.6). The central nervous system consists of the brain and spinal cord. As its name implies, the peripheral nervous system lies outside the central nervous system. The peripheral nervous system functions to relay nerve impulses from the central nervous system to the periphery (to skeletal muscles, for example) or from the periphery back to the central nervous system. The nervous system may also be thought of as having somatic (voluntary) and autonomic (involuntary) functions. The somatic nervous system is responsible for activating skeletal muscles, for example the rhythmic actions of the quadriceps femoris muscles during cycling. The autonomic nervous system controls involuntary functions such as contraction of the

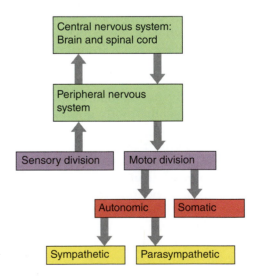

FIGURE 1.6 Organization of the central and peripheral branches of the nervous system.

Adapted by permission from Wilmore, Costill, and Kenney 2008.

heart and smooth muscle in blood vessels, as well as glands.

Neurons

The most basic unit of the nervous system is the nerve cell, or neuron. The neurons that conduct impulses from the central nervous system to the muscles are known as *motor neurons* or *efferent neurons*. It is these motor signals that cause skeletal muscles to contract. The neurons responsible for carrying impulses from the periphery toward the central nervous system are called the *sensory* or *afferent neurons*. Sensory neurons relay impulses from the periphery to the central nervous system regarding such information as tension, stretch, movement, and pain. The site of communication between two neurons or a neuron and a gland or muscle cell is known as a *synapse*. For example, the synapse

between a motor neuron and a skeletal muscle fiber is called the *neuromuscular junction*, as discussed earlier in this chapter.

The structure of a typical motor neuron is presented in figure 1.7. Dendrites are projections from the neuron cell body. The dendrites serve to receive excitatory or inhibitory signals (or both) from other neurons. Both the dendrites and the cell body of a motor neuron are located in the anterior gray horn of the spinal cord. If sufficiently excited, a neuron will transmit an action potential down its axon, away from the cell body. The axon extends outward from the spinal cord and may innervate a muscle that is a relatively great distance away from the spine. In the case of a motor neuron that activates skeletal muscle, the action potential causes the release of ACh at the neuromuscular junction. This leads to the process of muscle action discussed earlier (see "Sliding Filament Theory").

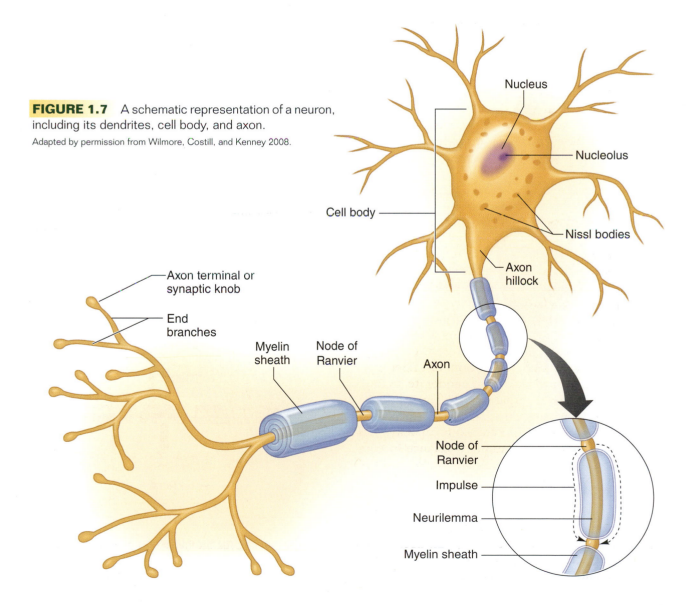

FIGURE 1.7 A schematic representation of a neuron, including its dendrites, cell body, and axon.

Adapted by permission from Wilmore, Costill, and Kenney 2008.

In addition to motor neurons, there are a variety of sensory neurons that convey information from the periphery, such as from the muscles and joints, back to the central nervous system. Two sensory structures with particular significance to exercise training are the **muscle spindle** and the **Golgi tendon organ (GTO).**

Muscle Spindle

As its name implies, the muscle spindle is a spindle-shaped sensory organ, meaning that it is thicker in the middle and tapered at either end. It is a stretch receptor that is widely dispersed throughout most skeletal muscles. Muscle spindles are specialized to sense changes in muscle length, particularly when the muscle changes length rapidly. Each muscle spindle is enclosed within a capsule (figure 1.8) and lies parallel to extrafusal fibers (ordinary skeletal muscle fibers). The muscle spindle contains specialized muscle fibers called *intrafusal fibers*. These intrafusal fibers have contractile proteins at each end (actin and myosin) and a central region that is wrapped by sensory nerve endings. Because the intrafusal fibers of the muscle spindle lie parallel to the extrafusal muscle fibers, a stretching force applied to the muscle will stretch both intrafusal and extrafusal muscle fibers. This will cause a sensory discharge from the muscle spindle that is carried toward the spinal cord. This leads to a motor response, activation of the muscle that was initially

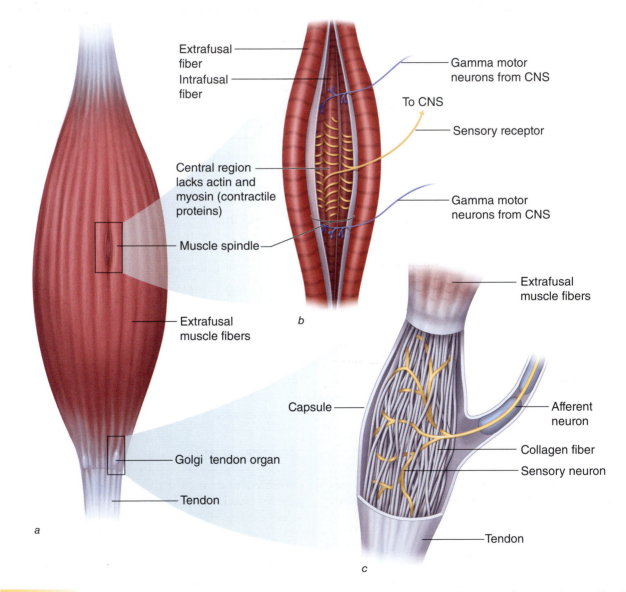

FIGURE 1.8   (a) The location of a muscle spindle within a skeletal muscle. (b) Structure of a muscle spindle. (c) Structure of a Golgi tendon organ.

Adapted by permission from Wilmore, Costill, and Kenney 2008.

stretched. This reflex is known as the **myotatic** or **stretch reflex.** From a practical standpoint, static stretching exercises are typically done in such a way as to avoid activation of the muscle spindles. Moving slowly into a stretched position avoids activation of the muscle spindle. This is important because muscles are most easily stretched when they are relaxed. There are other times, however, when activation of the muscle spindle is desired during training. For example, plyometric exercises are performed by rapidly stretching a muscle, and this is followed immediately by a concentric action of the same muscle. This rapid stretch of the muscle will activate the stretch reflex, leading to a more powerful concentric action.

Golgi Tendon Organ

The Golgi tendon organ is located at the junction of the muscle and the tendon that attaches the muscle to the bone (figure 1.8). It appears to play a role in protecting the muscle from injury. The Golgi tendon organ is deformed when the muscle is activated. If the force of the muscle action is great enough, it will cause the Golgi tendon organ to convey sensory information to the spinal cord, which will lead to relaxation of the acting muscle and stimulation of the antagonist muscle. This protective reflex presumably prevents injury to the muscle and joint due to a potentially excessive force of muscle action.

The Motor Unit

A motor neuron and the muscle fibers it innervates is known as a **motor unit.** All fibers in a given motor unit are of the same fiber type. Indeed, it is the motor neuron that gives the fibers their metabolic and contractile characteristics. Motor units may vary in the number of fibers innervated. For example, motor units in small muscles, such as the hand, have relatively few fibers. Larger muscles, such as those in the thigh, contain a large number of fibers per motor unit.

> All fibers of a single motor unit are of the same muscle fiber type. The different muscle fiber types have distinct anatomical and physiological characteristics, which determine their functional capacities.

Gradation of Force

It is possible for the nervous system to vary the force produced by a muscle over a wide range of intensities. For example, individuals may be able to curl a 10-pound dumbbell but can also work their way up the dumbbell rack to curl a 60-pound dumbbell with maximal effort. In the simplest sense, there are two mechanisms that the nervous system may use to vary, or grade, force production to accomplish these tasks. One method is to vary the number of motor units, and thus muscle fibers, that are activated. This is known as *motor unit recruitment.* The second method is to increase the firing rate of motor units already activated, a process known as *rate coding.*

When a light weight is lifted, a relatively small number of motor units are activated. As the resistance increases, that is, as a heavier dumbbell is lifted, more motor units can be added, or "recruited," to the active pool of motor units, and thus force is increased due to the increased number of muscle fibers contracting. Recruitment of all motor units would thus require the lifting of maximal or near-maximal weights at maximal intensity. It is also important to understand that there is a specific order in which motor units are recruited. This has been referred to as the *size principle of motor unit recruitment* (7). The first motor units recruited are the smaller type I motor units. These motor units have a lower threshold for being activated and thus are recruited even during low-force muscle actions. The next motor units recruited are the type IIa motor units, followed by the type IIx motor units. These type II motor units are larger than the type I motor units, and they have a higher threshold that must be reached before they are activated. It appears that most people are unable to activate all of their motor units but are able to recruit more motor units with training (10).

It is also possible to increase muscle force production by increasing the firing rate of already activated motor units (12). If a muscle is stimulated to contract before it has a chance to relax from a previous stimulus, it will produce greater force. Evidence suggests that well-trained weightlifters, even among older adults, have higher maximal motor unit discharge rates than untrained individuals (11).

The Skeletal System

Movement and exercise are possible because skeletal muscles attach to bones, which are in turn connected at joints. The pulling of muscles on bones causes the bones to rotate. It is this combined functioning of muscles, bones, and joints that allows us to lift weights, run on a treadmill, and participate in a cycling class. Figure 1.9 shows the structure of a long bone. In addition to providing a system of bony levers, the skeleton performs a number of other important anatomical and physiological functions.

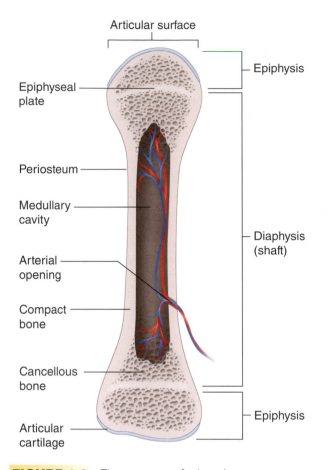

FIGURE 1.9   The anatomy of a long bone.
Reprinted from Behnke 2006.

For example, bones are the primary storage site for minerals, such as calcium and phosphorus. They are also the location for blood cell formation, and they serve to protect internal organs and the spinal cord.

Organization of the Skeletal System

The typical person has 206 bones that make up the skeletal system (figure 1.10). The bones can be divided into two anatomical divisions: the **axial skeleton** and the **appendicular skeleton.** The axial skeleton consists primarily of the skull, vertebral column, sternum, and ribs. These bones protect important internal organs, such as the brain, heart, and lungs, but also offer sites for skeletal muscle attachments. The appendicular skeleton includes the bones of the upper and lower limbs. The rotations of these bones around joints are responsible for most of the movements associated with exercise, such as lifting, running, throwing, kicking, and striking.

Osteoporosis and Exercise

Bone is a complex, living, and dynamic tissue. It is constantly undergoing a process called *remodeling*, in which bone-destroying cells called *osteoclasts* break down bone while other cells, called *osteoblasts*, stimulate bone synthesis. The two types, or categories, of bone are cortical (compact) bone and cancellous (trabecular) bone. Cortical bone is hard and dense and is found primarily in the outer layers of the shafts of long bones, such as the arms and legs. Cancellous bone, also called *spongy bone*, is much less dense than cortical bone and is found in the interior area of long bones, the vertebrae, and the head of the femur. It is the site of hematopoiesis, the synthesis of blood cells. Calcium and phosphorus are two important minerals that help form the body's bones.

Osteoporosis, literally meaning "porous bones," is a condition in which the bones become weak and brittle. In this weakened condition, they are more susceptible to breaking, particularly in the spine and hip. Along with proper nutrition, including adequate calcium intake, exercise is an important component of bone health. According to Wolff's law, bone will adapt in response to stresses placed on it. For example, weight-bearing exercises, such as running, have been shown to lead to increases in bone mineral density (5). Resistance training is also effective at increasing bone mineral density (4), with eccentric loading being an especially potent stimulus for bone growth (6, 14). This information has obvious implications for personal trainers, who should incorporate weight-bearing exercises like walking or running (or both) into a comprehensive resistance training program, along with an emphasis on eccentric loading, when training their clients.

> Like muscle, bone adapts to exercise by increasing in mass and strength. Weight-bearing exercises and resistance training are the best forms of exercise for increasing bone mineral density.

Tendons and Ligaments

Associated with the skeletal system are two other connective tissues, tendons and ligaments. Tendons were discussed earlier in the chapter as a connective tissue that attaches muscle to bone. Tendons are well suited for withstanding the tensile forces produced when muscles pull on bones. They are primarily formed from the inelastic protein collagen. Ligaments connect bones to other bones. Ligaments are formed from collagen as well, but they also contain an elastic protein called *elastin*. This affords liga-

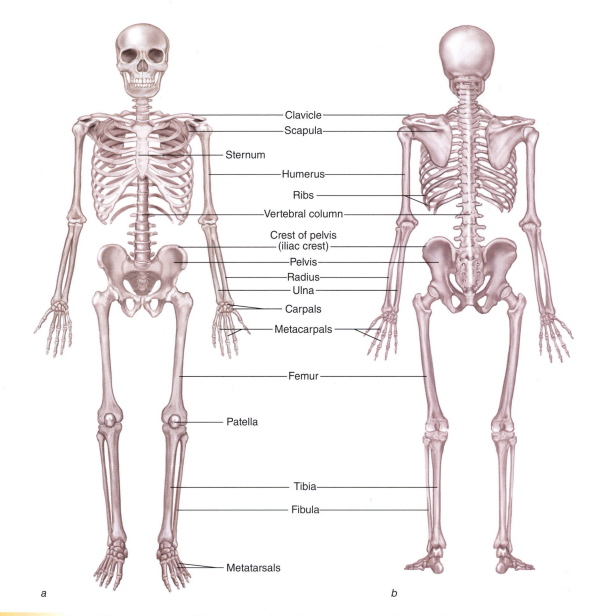

FIGURE 1.10 (a) Front view and (b) rear view of an adult male human skeleton.

a: Reprinted by permission from Watkins 2010. b: Reprinted by permission from Cartwright and Pitney 2011.

ments some ability to stretch, thus allowing for a balance between stabilizing a joint and permitting some mobility.

Conclusion

In the simplest sense, exercise involves nervous system activation of muscles, which in turn pull on bones and their associated connective tissues. Personal trainers should have an intimate understanding of the structure and function of these tissues to appreciate how they work during exercise. This knowledge will help the personal trainer conduct safe and effective exercise programs and will provide a foundation for understanding the specific adaptations that occur with repeated bouts of varied types of physical activity.

Study Questions

1. Aerobic ATP production within the cell occurs in which of the following cellular organelles?

    A. mitochondria

    B. sarcoplasmic reticulum

    C. myofibril

    D. T-tubule

2. Which of the following is the thick myofilament?

    A. actin

    B. troponin

    C. myosin

    D. tropomyosin

3. Which of the following types of muscle action occurs when the muscle lengthens despite attempting to shorten?

    A. concentric

    B. eccentric

    C. isometric

    D. isokinetic

4. Which of the following muscle fiber types has moderate oxidative and anaerobic capacity?

    A. SO

    B. FOG

    C. FG

    D. slow-twitch

5. Which of the following branches of the nervous system is responsible for activating skeletal muscles?

    A. sensory

    B. autonomic

    C. afferent

    D. somatic

Applied Knowledge Question

What advice would you give a client who is interested in knowing how to exercise to avoid osteoporosis?

References

1. Beck, T.W., T.J. Housh, G.O. Johnson, R.J. Schmidt, D.J. Housh, J.W. Coburn, M.H. Malek, and M. Mielke. 2007. Effects of a protease supplement on eccentric exercise-induced markers of delayed-onset muscle soreness and muscle damage. *Journal of Strength and Conditioning Research* 21: 661-667.

2. Cheung, K., P. Hume, and L. Maxwell. 2003. Delayed onset muscle soreness: Treatment strategies and performance factors. *Sports Medicine (Auckland)* 33: 145-164.

3. Colliander, E.B., and P.A. Tesch. 1990. Effects of eccentric and concentric muscle actions in resistance training. *Acta Physiologica Scandinavica* 140: 31-39.

4. Conroy, B.P., W.J. Kraemer, C.M. Maresh, S.J. Fleck, M.H. Stone, A.C. Fry, P.D. Miller, and G.P. Dalsky. 1993. Bone mineral density in elite junior Olympic weightlifters. *Medicine and Science in Sports and Exercise* 25: 1103-1109.

5. Duncan, C.S., C.J. Blimkie, C.T. Cowell, S.T. Burke, J.N. Briody, and R. Howman-Giles. 2002. Bone mineral density in adolescent female athletes: Relationship to exercise type and muscle strength. *Medicine and Science in Sports and Exercise* 34: 286-294.

6. Hawkins, S.A., E.T. Schroeder, R.A. Wiswell, S.V. Jaque, T.J. Marcell, and K. Costa. 1999. Eccentric muscle action increases site-specific osteogenic response. *Medicine and Science in Sports and Exercise* 31: 1287-1292.

7. Henneman, E., G. Somjen, and D.O. Carpenter. 1965. Functional significance of cell size in spinal motoneurons. *Journal of Neurophysiology* 28: 560-580.

8. Higbie, E.J., K.J. Cureton, G.L. Warren 3rd, and B.M. Prior. 1996. Effects of concentric and eccentric training on muscle strength, cross-sectional area, and neural activation. *Journal of Applied Physiology* 81: 2173-2181.

9. Huxley, H.E. 1969. The mechanism of muscular contraction. *Science (New York)* 164: 1356-1365.

10. Knight, C.A., and G. Kamen. 2001. Adaptations in muscular activation of the knee extensor muscles with strength training in young and older adults. *Journal of Electromyography and Kinesiology* 11: 405-412.

11. Leong, B., G. Kamen, C. Patten, and J.R. Burke. 1999. Maximal motor unit discharge rates in the quadriceps muscles of older weight lifters. *Medicine and Science in Sports and Exercise* 31: 1638-1644.

12. Milner-Brown, H.S., R.B. Stein, and R. Yemm. 1973. Changes in firing rate of human motor units during linearly changing voluntary contractions. *Journal of Physiology* 230: 371-390.

13. Nguyen, D., L.E. Brown, J.W. Coburn, D.A. Judelson, A.D. Eurich, A.V. Khamoui, and B.P. Uribe. 2009. Effect of delayed-onset muscle soreness on elbow flexion strength and rate of velocity development. *Journal of Strength and Conditioning Research* 23: 1282-1286.

14. Schroeder, E.T., S.A. Hawkins, and S.V. Jaque. 2004. Musculoskeletal adaptations to 16 weeks of eccentric progressive resistance training in young women. *Journal of Strength and Conditioning Research* 18: 227-235.

Cardiorespiratory System and Gas Exchange

Moh H. Malek, PhD

After completing this chapter, you will be able to

- describe the anatomical and physiological characteristics of the cardiovascular system,

- describe the electrical conduction system of the heart and the basic electrocardiogram,

- describe the mechanisms that control the circulation of blood throughout the body,

- describe the anatomical and physiological characteristics of the respiratory system,

- explain the exchange of gases between the lungs and the blood, and

- understand the mechanisms that control respiration.

The cardiovascular and respiratory systems work in unison to provide oxygen and nutrients to the body under various perturbations such as exercise. In addition, these two systems are instrumental in clearing metabolic by-products from the muscle. This chapter summarizes the structure and function of both systems.

The cardiovascular system transports nutrients and removes metabolic waste products while helping to maintain the environment for all the body's functions. The blood transports oxygen from the lungs to the tissues for use in cellular metabolism and transports carbon dioxide from the tissues to the lungs, where it is removed from the body.

Cardiovascular Anatomy and Physiology

Before discussing the cardiovascular system and gas exchange, it is important to briefly discuss the characteristics of blood, which is involved in transporting oxygen, nutrients, and metabolic by-products throughout the body. Whole blood can be separated into plasma, leukocytes and platelets, and erythrocytes, which compose approximately 55%, <1%, and 45% of whole blood, respectively (see figure 2.1). In addition, the normal pH range of arterial blood is approximately 7.4, and deviations from this number can be influenced by factors such as exercise, stress, or disease. It should be noted, however, that physiological tolerance for changes in pH for arterial blood and muscle are between 6.9

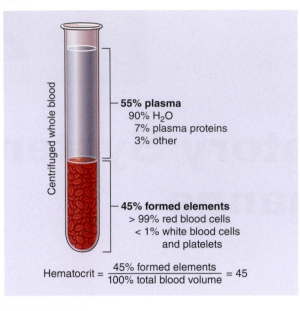

Chapter 2

FIGURE 2.1 The various components of whole blood after it has been centrifuged.

Adapted by permission from Wilmore, Costill, and Kenney 2008.

and 7.5 and 6.63 and 7.10, respectively. Nevertheless, the pH is regulated by buffers such as bicarbonate, ventilation, and kidney function.

Oxygen Transport

Oxygen is dissolved in the blood as well as carried via hemoglobin. Since oxygen dissolved in the blood accounts for a very small percentage (0.3 ml O_2 per 100 ml of blood or around 2%), we will focus on hemoglobin (4). Hemoglobin is an iron-containing protein within the red blood cells that has the capacity to bind between one and four oxygen molecules. Each gram of hemoglobin, therefore, can carry approximately 1.39 ml of oxygen. In addition, healthy blood has approximately 15 g of hemoglobin per 100 ml. Therefore, the capacity of healthy blood to carry oxygen approximates 20.8 ml of oxygen per 100 ml of blood (20.8 ml O_2/100 ml of blood = ~[15 g of Hb/100 ml] × [1.39 ml of O_2]) (3). The average healthy adult who is not anemic has around 5.0 L of blood volume, which accounts for close to 7% of his or her body weight.

Oxygen–Hemoglobin Dissociation Curve

Now that we have an understanding of how oxygen is carried in the blood, it is important to discuss the oxygen–hemoglobin dissociation curve. This curve illustrates the saturation of hemoglobin at various partial pressures. Partial pressure is essentially the pressure exerted by one gas in a mixture of gasses and is calculated as the product of total pressure of a gas mixture and the percent concentration of the specific gas. For example, normal atmospheric pressure is 760 mmHg, whereas the percent concentration of oxygen in the atmosphere is 20.93%. Therefore, the partial pressure of oxygen at sea level is approximately 159 mmHg (760 mmHg × [20.93/100]). As shown in figure 2.2, the relationship between partial pressure of oxygen and oxygen saturation is sigmoidal (S-shaped) as opposed to linear (direct). This is, in part, due to cooperative binding, which means that as oxygen binds to hemoglobin it facilitates subsequent binding of oxygen molecules (2). That is, binding of the first oxygen molecule to hemoglobin increases hemoglobin's affinity for oxygen such that the fourth oxygen molecule binds to hemoglobin at a much higher affinity than the first oxygen molecule. Therefore, as the oxygen partial pressure increases, hemoglobin becomes saturated, but this saturation begins to plateau. Typically, at around 60 mmHg, the curve beings to become relatively flat, with approximately 90% of hemoglobin saturated with oxygen. The subsequent increase from 60 mmHg to 100 mmHg results in an increase to 98% of hemoglobin saturated with oxygen.

Factors Influencing the Oxygen–Hemoglobin Curve

Various factors can, however, influence the oxygen–hemoglobin curve, thus shifting the curve to the

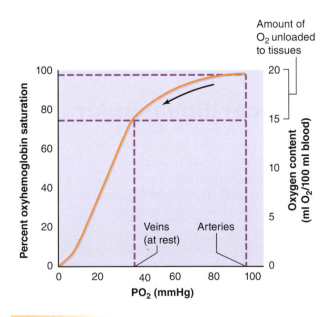

FIGURE 2.2 Oxyhemoglobin dissociation curve.

Reprinted, by permission, from S.K. Powers and E.T. Howley, 2004, *Exercise physiology: Theory and application to fitness and performance*, 5th ed. (New York: McGraw-Hill Companies), 205. With permission from The McGraw-Hill Companies.

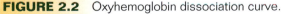

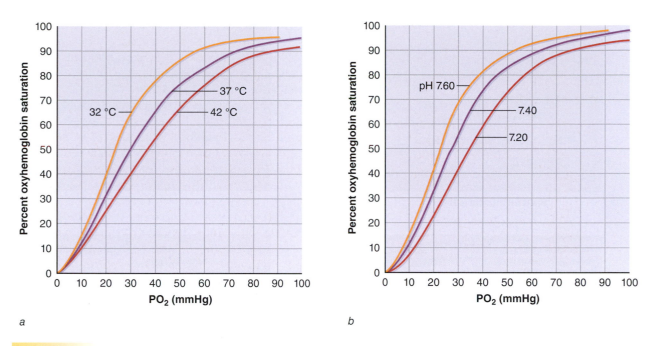

FIGURE 2.3 Shifts in the oxyhemoglobin curve with (a) changes in core body temperature and (b) changes in blood pH concentrations.

Reprinted, by permission, from S.K. Powers and E.T. Howley, 2004, *Exercise physiology: Theory and application to fitness and performance*, 5th ed. (New York: McGraw-Hill), 206. ©The McGraw-Hill Companies.

right or left. For example, a decrease in core body temperature results in shifting the curve toward the left, whereas an increase in temperature results in shifting the curve toward the right (figure 2.3*a*). Another factor that can cause a leftward or rightward shift in the curve is arterial blood acidity. As shown in figure 2.3*b*, blood with low pH (acidic) results in the curve shifting right, whereas blood with high pH (alkalosis) results in the curve shifting left. To apply the oxygen–hemoglobin dissociation curve to a practical setting, consider exercise. Typically, exercise will increase core body temperature, which shifts the curve toward the right; thus, oxygen is released at a higher partial pressure so that it can be used by the working muscles rather than staying bound to hemoglobin.

Cardiac Morphology

The heart is composed of cardiac muscle, which unlike skeletal muscle is mononucleated, contains four chambers (right atrium, left atrium, right ventricle, and left ventricle), and is under involuntary neural control (1) (figure 2.4). That is, the heart has its own internal pacemaker, and therefore the heart beats automatically. The electrical conduction system of the heart begins with the sinoatrial (SA) node, which is the primary intrinsic pacemaker of the heart. The SA node generates an electrical impulse that spreads across the **atrium** to the atrioventricu-

lar (AV) node (figure 2.5). From there, the impulse continues to spread down through the left and right bundle branches into the Purkinje system. The Purkinje system is a series of fibers that surround the **ventricles,** which then stimulate ventricular contraction. Note that the impulse from the SA node spreads very quickly (~0.08 m/s) across both atria and then slows through the AV node, allowing for a time delay between excitation of the atria and ventricles so the filling can occur. When the impulse reaches the Purkinje fiber, the result is ventricular contraction. The entire time to complete the impulse (SA node → AV node → Purkinje fibers → contraction of ventricles) is approximately 0.2 seconds (1).

As shown in figure 2.6 on page 21, venous blood (deoxygenated) returns to the right atrium via the superior and inferior vena cava and is delivered to the right ventricle. The superior vena cava returns deoxygenated blood from the head and upper extremities, whereas the inferior vena cava returns deoxygenated blood from the trunk and lower extremity. From there, the deoxygenated blood is delivered to the lung by the pulmonary artery where gas exchange occurs. That is, the deoxygenated blood is loaded with oxygen while the metabolic by-products are removed. The oxygenated blood now returns to the left atrium via the pulmonary vein and is delivered to the left ventricle. At this point, the oxygen-rich blood is ready to be delivered throughout the body via the aorta and thereafter to organs and tissues through miles of vasculature.

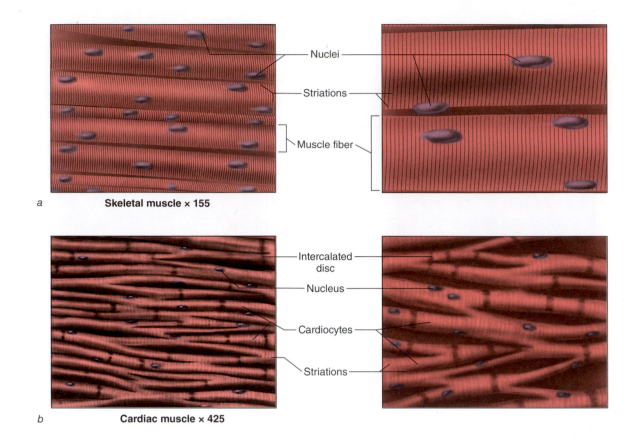

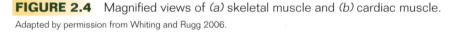

FIGURE 2.4   Magnified views of (a) skeletal muscle and (b) cardiac muscle.

Adapted by permission from Whiting and Rugg 2006.

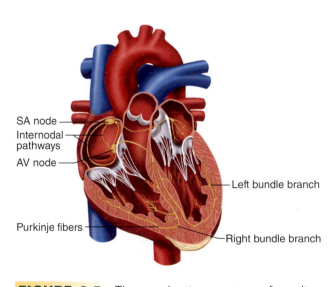

FIGURE 2.5   The conduction system of cardiac muscle.

Reprinted by permission from NSCA 2008.

The circulation of the heart and lungs (central circulation) and that of the rest of the body (peripheral circulation) form a single closed-circuit system with two components: an arterial system, which carries blood away from the heart, and a venous system, which returns blood toward the heart.

Electrocardiogram

A way to record the electrical activity of the heart at the surface of the body is to place 10 to 12 electrodes on the chest. The electrical impulses generated by the heart (discussed earlier) are detected by the surface electrodes and are presented as distinct patterns called the *electrocardiogram (ECG)*. The ECG has three distinct components: (1) P-wave, (2) QRS complex, and (3) T-wave (1). As shown in figure 2.7, the P-wave represents atrial depolarization, occurring when the impulse travels from the SA node to the AV node. The QRS complex reflects ventricular depolarization and occurs when the impulse continues from the AV node to the Purkinje fibers that

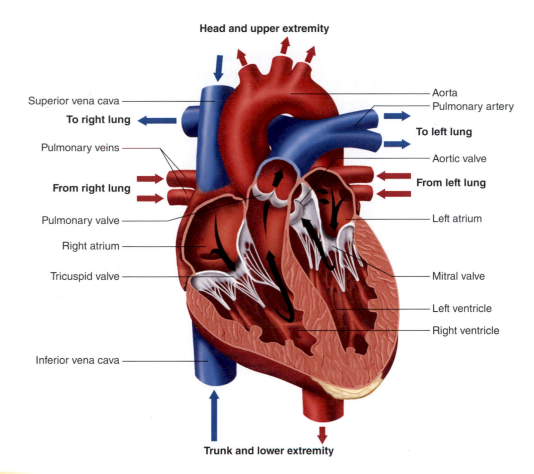

FIGURE 2.6   Structure of the human heart and corresponding blood flow pathway.

Reprinted by permission from NSCA 2008.

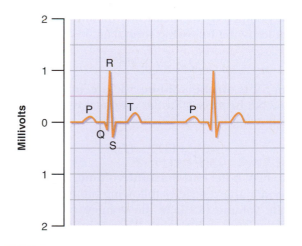

FIGURE 2.7   The various phases of the resting electrocardiogram.

Reprinted by permission from NSCA 2008.

are throughout the ventricles. The T-wave represents electrical recovery (repolarization) of the ventricles. Note that atrial repolarization does occur but cannot be seen since it takes place during the QRS complex.

Typically, ECGs are obtained during incremental exercise tests in a clinical setting to examine the heart under stress.

Circulation

The circulation system is composed of arteries, which carry blood away from the heart toward the tissues and organs, and veins, which carry blood from the tissues and organs back to the heart, with one exception—the pulmonary veins (mentioned earlier) carry oxygenated blood from the lungs to the heart. For the systemic circulation, arteries are typically a high-pressure system, ranging from around 100 mmHg in the aorta to approximately 60 mmHg in the arterioles. The veins are characterized by very low pressure relative to the arteries. Due to this low-pressure system, veins have one-way valves and smooth muscle bands that continue moving venous blood toward the heart as we move or contract muscles in our extremities (figure 2.8).

The resistance of the entire systemic circulation is called the **total peripheral resistance.** As blood

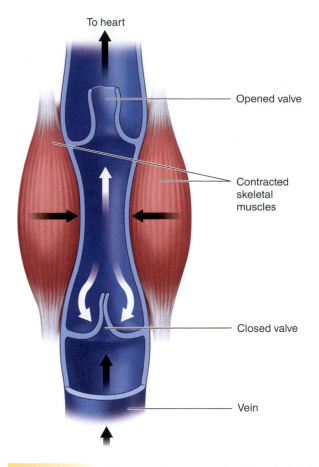

FIGURE 2.8 The muscle pump. As the skeletal muscles contract, they squeeze the veins in the legs and assist in the return of blood to the heart. Valves within the veins ensure the unidirectional flow of blood back to the heart.

Adapted by permission from Wilmore, Costill, and Kenney 2008.

vessels constrict, peripheral resistance increases, whereas with dilation peripheral resistance decreases. Note, however, that many factors can influence constriction or dilation of vessels, such as type of exercise, **sympathetic nervous system** stimulation, local muscle tissue metabolism, and environmental stressors (i.e., heat or cold). For example, during exercise the sympathetic nervous system stimulates arterial vasodilation, which then increases blood flow to the working muscles. As shown in figure 2.9, during exercise, blood is redistributed from other organs to the muscles used for that particular exercise.

Cardiac Cycle

The cardiac cycle consists of the events that occur from the start of one heartbeat to the start of another heartbeat. The cardiac cycle, therefore, is composed of periods of relaxation (called *diastole*)

and contraction (called *systole*). The diastolic phase allows for the heart to fill with blood. **Systolic blood pressure (SBP)** is the pressure exerted against the arterial walls as blood is forcefully ejected during ventricular contraction (systole). Simultaneous measurement of SBP and heart rate (HR) is useful in describing the work of the heart and can provide an indirect estimation of myocardial oxygen uptake. This estimate of the work of the heart, referred to as the **rate–pressure product (RPP)**, or *double product*, is obtained with the following equation (1):

$$RPP = SBP \times HR \qquad \textbf{(2.1)}$$

Conversely, **diastolic blood pressure (DBP)** is the pressure exerted against the arterial walls when no blood is being forcefully ejected through the vessels (diastole). It provides an indication of peripheral resistance or vascular stiffness, tending to decrease with vasodilation and increase with vasoconstriction. In addition, the **mean arterial pressure (MAP)** is the mean blood pressure throughout the cardiac cycle, but should not be mistaken for the average of the systolic and diastolic pressures. The mean arterial pressure is typically estimated with the following equation:

$$MAP = DBP + [.333 \times (SBP - DBP)] \qquad \textbf{(2.2)}$$

Cardiac Output

Cardiac output ($\dot{Q}$) is defined as the amount of blood pumped by the heart in 1 minute and is represented by the following formula:

$$\dot{Q} = SV \times HR \qquad \textbf{(2.3)}$$

where SV is **stroke volume**, the amount of blood ejected per heartbeat. Stroke volume is estimated by the following formula:

$$SV = EDV - ESV \qquad \textbf{(2.4)}$$

where EDV is the **end-diastolic volume**, the volume of blood in the ventricles following filling. The end-systolic volume (ESV) is the volume of blood in ventricles after contraction. Therefore, the cardiac output is estimated as

$$\dot{Q} = (EDV - ESV) \times HR. \qquad \textbf{(2.5)}$$

The Frank-Starling principle indicates that the more the left ventricle is stretched, the more forceful the contraction and thus the greater volume of blood leaving the ventricle. This principle is thus based on the length–tension relationship. An increase in preload (EDV) is directly influenced by

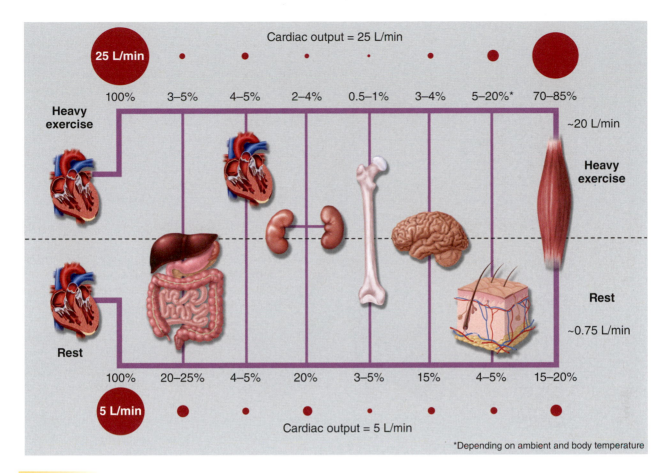

Cardiac output = 25 L/min

25 L/min

	100%	3–5%	4–5%	2–4%	0.5–1%	3–4%	5–20%*	70–85%

Heavy exercise

~20 L/min

Heavy exercise

Rest

~0.75 L/min

Rest

	100%	20–25%	4–5%	20%	3–5%	15%	4–5%	15–20%

5 L/min

Cardiac output = 5 L/min

*Depending on ambient and body temperature

FIGURE 2.9 Redistribution of blood from a resting to a heavy exercise state.

Reprinted by permission from Åstrand et al. 2003.

the heart volume and **venous return** of blood to the heart.

Respiratory System

The primary function of the respiratory system is the basic exchange of oxygen and carbon dioxide. This section discusses the anatomy and physiology of the lungs as well as gas exchange.

Structure

As air passes through the nose, the nasal cavities perform three distinct functions, which include warming, humidifying, and purifying the air. Air is then distributed to the lungs via the trachea, bronchi, and bronchioles. The trachea is then divided into the left and right bronchi, and each division thereafter is an additional generation. There are approximately 23 generations, finally ending with the alveoli where gas exchange occurs (figure 2.10) (1).

Inspiration is an active process that involves the diaphragm and external intercostal muscles (figure

2.11). Contraction of the diaphragm results in expansion of the thorax and thus lowers air pressure in the lungs. Since gases move from an area of high pressure to one of low pressure, air moves into the lungs. Note, however, that during exercise, other muscles (scalene, sternocleidomastoid, pectoralis major and minor) are involved in inspiration. Expiration, at rest, is a passive response and involves no muscles, because the external intercostal muscles and the diaphragm relax, resulting in increased pressure in the lungs and exhalation of air. During exercise, however, the internal intercostal and abdominal muscles are involved to facilitate movement of air in and out of the lungs.

Lung Volumes

Spirometry is a method used in either clinical or research settings to examine static lung volumes. Figure 2.12 shows the various lung volumes that can be measured while the individual is breathing through the spirometer. In addition, there are descriptions of lung capacities that are combinations of various lung volumes.

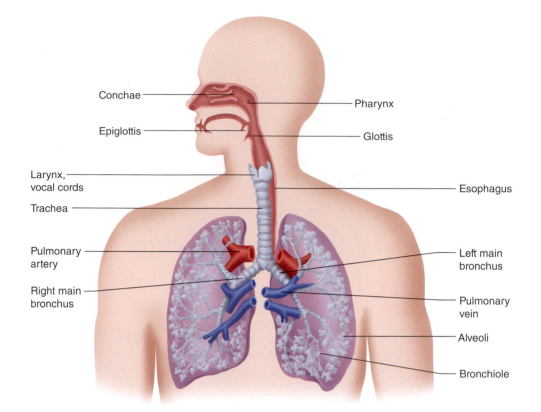

Conchae

Epiglottis

Larynx, vocal cords

Trachea

Pulmonary artery

Right main bronchus

Pharynx

Glottis

Esophagus

Left main bronchus

Pulmonary vein

Alveoli

Bronchiole

FIGURE 2.10 The respiratory system.

Reprinted by permission from NSCA 2008.

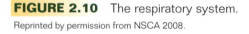

Expiration

Inspiration

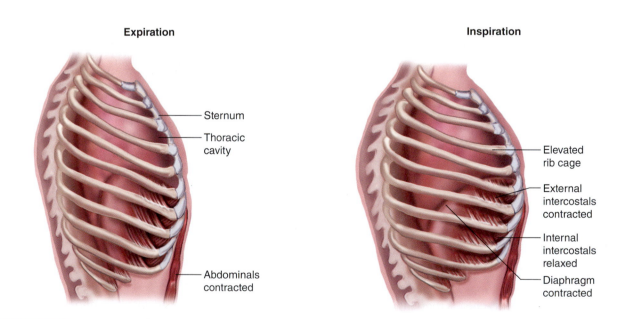

Sternum

Thoracic cavity

Abdominals contracted

Elevated rib cage

External intercostals contracted

Internal intercostals relaxed

Diaphragm contracted

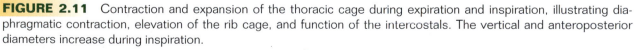

FIGURE 2.11 Contraction and expansion of the thoracic cage during expiration and inspiration, illustrating diaphragmatic contraction, elevation of the rib cage, and function of the intercostals. The vertical and anteroposterior diameters increase during inspiration.

Reprinted by permission from NSCA 2008.

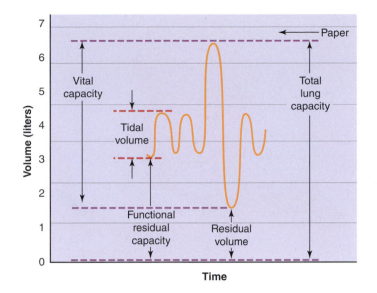

FIGURE 2.12 Various pulmonary function indices from basic spirometry.

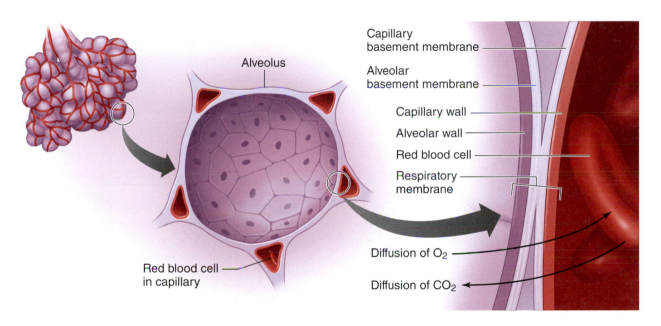

FIGURE 2.13 The anatomy of the respiratory membrane, showing the exchange of oxygen and carbon dioxide between an alveolus and pulmonary capillary blood.
Based on Wilmore, Costill, and Kenney 2008 (5).

Gas Exchange

The alveolus is covered with capillaries, which are the smallest unit of blood vessels within the body and are the site of gas exchange. The movement of gas such as oxygen or carbon dioxide across a cell membrane is called *diffusion* (figure 2.13). Diffusion occurs when there is a concentration gradient, that is, a greater concentration of a gas on one side of the membrane. As mentioned previously, gas moves from an area of high concentration to one of low concentration. At the tissue level, oxygen is used by cells and carbon dioxide is produced. The partial pressures of oxygen and carbon dioxide are different both within the tissue and within the arterial blood. As illustrated in figure 2.14, inspired oxygen has a partial pressure of 159 mmHg; however, as it reaches the alveoli the partial pressure is reduced to 100 mmHg due to various factors such as humidifying of the air in the respiratory tract. The partial pressure

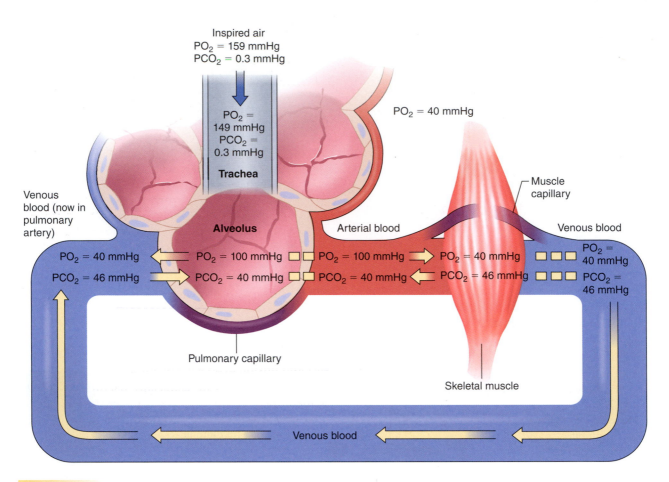

FIGURE 2.14   Alveolus and gas exchange.

From E. Fox, R. Bowers, and M. Foss, 1993, *The physiological basis for exercise and sport*, 5th ed. (Dubuque, IA: Wm. C. Brown). Reprinted with permission of McGraw-Hill companies.

of oxygen and carbon dioxide in the venous blood is approximately 40 and 46 mmHg, respectively. Based on the pressure gradients, gas exchange occurs and thereafter the blood is rich with oxygen (100 mmHg), with a concomitant reduction in carbon dioxide (see figure 2.14). Now the oxygen-loaded blood is delivered to the tissue (i.e., working muscle). Similar to gas exchange in the alveolus, gas exchange in the tissue follows the pressure gradient. Thus, oxygen diffuses into the tissue, whereas carbon dioxide diffuses out of the tissue (see figure 2.14). The deoxygenated blood (venous blood) is then returned to the alveolus, and the cycle of gas exchange is repeated.

> **With ventilation, oxygen diffuses from the alveoli into the pulmonary blood, and carbon dioxide diffuses from the blood into the alveoli.**

Oxygen Uptake

Oxygen uptake ($\dot{V}O_2$) is the amount of oxygen used by the tissues of the body. Note that the term *oxygen*

consumption is used interchangeably with *oxygen uptake;* however, traditionally the term *oxygen consumption* is used when the amount of oxygen used by the tissue is directly measured. Typically, $\dot{V}O_2$ in exercise physiology is measured at the mouth using a metabolic cart. $\dot{V}O_2$ is primarily related to the ability of the heart and circulatory system to transport oxygen via blood to the tissues and the ability of the tissues to extract oxygen. The formula that represents $\dot{V}O_2$ is the Fick equation (equation 2.6):

$$\dot{V}O_2 = \dot{Q} \times a\text{–}\bar{v}O_2 \qquad \textbf{(2.6)}$$

$$\dot{V}O_2 = (HR \times SV) \times a\text{–}\bar{v}O_2 \qquad \textbf{(2.6.1)}$$

$$\dot{V}O_2 = (HR) \times (EDV - ESV) \times a\text{–}\bar{v}O_2 \quad \textbf{(2.6.2)}$$

where $\dot{V}O_2$ is the product of cardiac output ($\dot{Q}$, equation 2.3) and a–$\bar{v}O_2$ difference. The a–$\bar{v}O_2$ difference is the arterial oxygen content minus the venous oxygen content in milliliters of O_2 per 100 ml of blood. This difference helps us know the amount of oxygen that has been extracted from the transported blood for use in exercise. As shown in

TABLE 2.1   Relationship Between Exercise Intensity and Oxygen Extraction

Exercise intensity	Arterial side	Venous return	Extraction
Rest	20 ml O_2/100 ml blood	14 ml O_2/100 ml blood	6 ml O_2/100 ml blood
Moderate	20 ml O_2/100 ml blood	10 ml O_2/100 ml blood	10 ml O_2/100 ml blood
High	20 ml O_2/100 ml blood	4 ml O_2/100 ml blood	16 ml O_2/100 ml blood

table 2.1, oxygen extraction a–$\bar{v}O_2$ increases with exercise intensity. The following is an example of calculating $\dot{V}O_2$:

$$\dot{V}O_2 = (HR \times SV) \times a\text{–}\bar{v}O_2$$

$$\dot{V}O_2 = (80 \text{ beats/min} \times 65 \text{ ml blood/beat}) \times$$
$$(6 \text{ ml } O_2 \text{ ml/100 ml blood})$$

$$\dot{V}O_2 = 312 \text{ ml } O_2/\text{min}$$

This value is in absolute terms (ml O_2/min), but can also be expressed relative to the individual's body mass (ml · kg^{-1} · min^{-1}).

$$\dot{V}O_2 = (312 \text{ ml } O_2/\text{min}) / 75.0 \text{ kg}$$

$$\dot{V}O_2 = 4.16 \text{ ml · kg}^{-1} \text{ · min}^{-1}$$

Maximal oxygen uptake ($\dot{V}O_2$max) is described as the highest amount of oxygen that can be used at the cellular level for the entire body. $\dot{V}O_2$max (or $\dot{V}O_2$peak) has been found to correlate well with the degree of physical conditioning and is recognized as the most accepted measure of cardiorespiratory fitness. Resting $\dot{V}O_2$ is typically estimated at 3.5 ml · kg^{-1} · min^{-1}, whereas $\dot{V}O_2$max has been reported close to 80 ml · kg^{-1} · min^{-1} in elite endurance athletes.

Conclusion

Knowledge of the cardiovascular and respiratory systems facilitates understanding of gas exchange at rest and during exercise. The information presented in this chapter can be especially useful because it is incumbent upon personal trainers to explain to clients the underlying physiology related to the conditioning program they are performing.

Study Questions

1. Which of the following is the correct sequence of structures that the blood travels through?

   A. superior vena cava, right atrium, left atrium, left ventricle, aorta

   B. inferior vena cava, right atrium, right ventricle, pulmonary vein, left atrium

   C. pulmonary vein, pulmonary artery, left ventricle, left atrium, aorta

   D. superior vena cava, aorta, left atrium, right ventricle

2. Which of the following are components of the Fick equation for oxygen uptake ($\dot{V}O_2$)?

   I. heart rate

   II. systolic pressure

   III. stroke volume

   IV. diastolic pressure

   A. I and III only

   B. I and IV only

   C. II and III only

   D. II and IV only

3. Gas exchange in the lungs occurs at which of the following sites?

   A. capillary wall

   B. basement membrane

   C. bronchi

   D. alveoli

4. Cardiac output ($\dot{Q}$) is a product of stroke volume (SV) and heart rate (HR). Which of the following equations represents stroke volume?

   A. $\dot{V}O_2$ – HR

   B. $\dot{V}O_2$ – SV

   C. EDV – HR

   D. EDV – ESV

5. The heart's conduction pathway begins at which of the following sites?

   A. AV node

   B. Purkinje fibers

   C. right ventrical

   D. SA node

Applied Knowledge Question

A 25-year-old, 170-pound (77.11 kg) male has been using a treadmill for his aerobic endurance workouts. His exercise heart rate is 160 beats/min, his stroke volume is 100 ml per beat, and he has an a–$\bar{v}O_2$ of 13 ml O_2 ml/100 ml blood. What is the absolute and relative $\dot{V}O_2$ of this individual during treadmill exercise?

References

1. Guyton, A.C., and J.E. Hall. 2006. *Textbook of Medical Physiology.* Philadelphia: Elsevier Saunders.

2. Nelson, D.L. and M.M. Cox. 2008. *Lehninger Principles of Biochemistry.* New York: W.H. Freeman.

3. Wagner, P.D. 1996. Determinants of maximal oxygen transport and utilization. *Annual Review of Physiology* 58: 21-50.

4. West, J.B. 2008. *Respiratory Physiology: The Essentials.* Philadelphia: Wolters Kluwer Health/Lippincott Williams & Wilkins. p. ix.

5. Wilmore, J.H., D.L. Costill, and W.L. Kenney 2008. *Physiology of Sport and Exercise,* 4th ed. Champaign, IL: Human Kinetics.

Bioenergetics

N. Travis Triplett, PhD

After completing this chapter, you will be able to

- understand the basic terminology of bioenergetics and metabolism related to exercise and training;

- discuss the central role of adenosine triphosphate in muscular activity;

- explain the basic energy systems present in the human body and the ability of each to supply energy for various activities;

- discuss the effects of training on the bioenergetics of skeletal muscle;

- recognize the substrates used by each energy system and discuss patterns of substrate use with various types of activities; and

- develop training programs that demonstrate an understanding of human bioenergetics and metabolism, especially the metabolic specificity of training.

To properly and effectively design exercise and training programs, a personal trainer must have knowledge of the production and use of energy in biological systems. After defining essential bioenergetics terminology, including the role of adenosine triphosphate (ATP), this chapter deals with the three basic energy systems that are used to replenish ATP in human skeletal muscle. Then we look at how substrates, or substances that come mainly from the foods we eat, are used for various types of activities, including specifics on how each type of substrate is broken down for energy production and how the main substrate, muscle glycogen, is replenished. Finally we discuss the metabolic specificity of training, which relates to the limitations of each energy system and the contribution of each energy system to physical activity.

Essential Terminology

The ability or capacity to perform physical work requires energy. In the human body, the conversion of chemical energy to mechanical energy is necessary for movement to occur. **Bioenergetics,** or the flow of energy in a biological system, primarily concerns the conversion of food—or large carbohydrate, protein, and fat molecules that contain chemical energy—into biologically usable forms of

The author would like to acknowledge the contributions of Drs. Michael Conley and Michael Stone to this chapter. Much of the content is directly attributed to Dr. Conley's work in the second edition and Dr. Stone's work in the first edition of *Essentials of Strength Training and Conditioning.*

energy. The breakdown of chemical bonds in these molecules releases the energy necessary to perform physical activity.

The process of breaking down large molecules into smaller molecules, such as the breakdown of carbohydrates into glucose, is generally accompanied by the release of energy and is termed **catabolic.** The synthesis of larger molecules from smaller molecules can be accomplished using the energy released from catabolic reactions. This building-up process is termed **anabolic,** and an example is the formation of proteins from amino acids. The human body is in a constant state of anabolism and catabolism, which is defined as *metabolism,* or the total of all the catabolic and anabolic reactions in the body. Energy obtained from catabolic reactions is used to drive anabolic reactions through an intermediate molecule, **adenosine triphosphate (ATP).** Without an adequate supply of ATP, muscular activity and muscle growth would not be possible. Thus, when designing training programs, personal trainers should have a basic understanding of how exercise affects ATP use and resynthesis.

Adenosine triphosphate is composed of adenine, a nitrogen-containing base; ribose, a five-carbon sugar (adenine and ribose together are called *adenosine*); and three phosphate groups (figure 3.1). The removal of one phosphate group yields adenosine diphosphate (ADP); removal of a second phosphate group yields adenosine monophosphate (AMP). Adenosine triphosphate is classified as a high-energy molecule because it stores large amounts of energy in the chemical bonds of the two terminal phosphate groups. The breaking of these chemical bonds releases energy to power various reactions in the body. Because muscle cells store ATP only in limited amounts and activity requires a constant supply of ATP to provide the energy needed for muscle actions, ATP-producing processes must also occur in the cell.

Energy Systems

Three energy systems exist in the human body to replenish ATP:

- Phosphagen system (an anaerobic process, i.e., one that occurs in the absence of oxygen)
- Glycolysis (two types: fast glycolysis and slow glycolysis; both are also anaerobic)
- Oxidative system (an aerobic process, i.e., one that requires oxygen)

Of the three main food components (carbohydrates, fats, and proteins), only carbohydrates can be metabolized for energy without the direct involvement of oxygen (6).

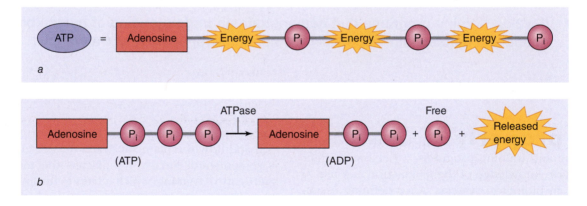

FIGURE 3.1   (a) The structure of an ATP (adenosine triphosphate) molecule, showing the high-energy phosphate bonds. (b) When the third phosphate on the ATP molecule is separated from adenosine by the action of adenosine triphosphatase (ATPase), energy is released.

Adapted by permission from Wilmore, Costill and Kenney 2008.

Composition of Adenosine Triphosphate

- Adenine (a nitrogen-containing base)
- Ribose (a five-carbon or pentose sugar)
- Three phosphate groups

Together called *adenosine*

Together called *triphosphate*

Energy stored in the chemical bonds of ATP is used to power muscular activity. The replenishment of ATP in human skeletal muscle is accomplished by three basic energy systems: (1) phosphagen, (2) glycolytic, and (3) oxidative.

Phosphagen System

The **phosphagen system** is the primary source of ATP for short-term, high-intensity activities (e.g., jumping and sprinting) but is active at the start of all types of exercise regardless of intensity (6). For instance, even during the first few seconds of an easy 5K jog or a moderate-intensity spinning class, the energy for the muscular activity is derived primarily from the phosphagen system. This energy system relies on the chemical reactions of ATP and creatine phosphate, both phosphagens, which involve the enzymes myosin adenosine triphosphatase (ATPase) and creatine kinase. Myosin ATPase increases the rate of breakdown of ATP to form ADP and inorganic phosphate (P_i) and releases energy, all of which is a catabolic reaction. Creatine kinase increases the rate of synthesis of ATP from creatine phosphate and ADP by supplying a phosphate group that combines with ADP to form ATP, which is an anabolic reaction.

These reactions provide energy at a high rate; however, because ATP and creatine phosphate are stored in the muscle in small amounts, the phosphagen system cannot supply enough energy for continuous, long-duration activities (7). Generally, type II (fast-twitch) muscle fibers contain greater concentrations of phosphagens than type I (slow-twitch) fibers (22).

Creatine kinase activity primarily regulates the breakdown of creatine phosphate. An increase in the muscle cell concentration of ADP promotes creatine kinase activity; an increase in ATP concentration inhibits it (33). At the beginning of exercise, ATP is broken down to ADP, releasing energy for muscular actions. This increase in ADP concentration activates creatine kinase to promote the formation of ATP from the breakdown of creatine phosphate. Creatine kinase activity remains elevated if exercise continues at a high intensity. If exercise is discontinued, or continues at an intensity low enough to allow glycolysis or the oxidative system to supply an adequate amount of ATP for the muscle cells' energy demands, the muscle cell concentration of ATP will likely increase. This increase in ATP then results in a decrease in creatine kinase activity.

Glycolysis

Glycolysis is the breakdown of carbohydrates, either **glycogen** stored in the muscle or glucose delivered in the blood, to produce ATP (6). The ATP provided by glycolysis supplements the phosphagen system initially and then becomes the primary source of ATP for high-intensity muscular activity that lasts up to about 2 minutes, such as keeping a good volley going in a rigorous game of racquetball or running 600 to 800 m. The process of glycolysis involves many enzymes controlling a series of chemical reactions (figure 3.2). The enzymes for glycolysis are located in the cytoplasm of the cells (the sarcoplasm in muscle cells).

As seen in figure 3.2, the process of glycolysis may occur in one of two ways, termed fast glycolysis and slow glycolysis. Fast glycolysis has commonly been called *anaerobic glycolysis,* and slow glycolysis has been termed *aerobic glycolysis,* as a result of the ultimate fate of the pyruvate. However, because glycolysis itself does not depend on oxygen, *these terms are not an accurate way of describing the process* (6). During fast glycolysis, the end product, **pyruvate,** is converted to lactate, providing energy (ATP) at a faster rate than with slow glycolysis, in which pyruvate is transported to the mitochondria for energy production through the oxidative system. The fate of the end products is controlled by the energy demands within the cell. If energy must be supplied at a high rate, such as during resistance training, fast glycolysis is primarily used. If the energy demand is not as high and oxygen is present in sufficient quantities in the cell, for example at the beginning of a low-intensity dance aerobics class, slow glycolysis is activated. Another by-product of interest is reduced nicotinamide adenine dinucleotide (NADH), which goes to the electron transport system for further ATP production (*reduced* refers to the added hydrogen).

The net reaction for fast glycolysis may be summarized as follows:

$$\text{Glucose} + 2P_i + 2ADP \rightarrow$$
$$2\text{lactate} + 2ATP + H_2O \qquad \textbf{(3.1)}$$

The net reaction for slow glycolysis may be summarized as follows:

$$\text{Glucose} + 2P_i + 2ADP + 2NAD^+ \rightarrow$$
$$2\text{pyruvate} + 2ATP + 2NADH + 2H_2O \qquad \textbf{(3.2)}$$

Energy Yield of Glycolysis

Glycolysis produces a net of two molecules of ATP from one molecule of glucose. However, if glycogen (the stored form of glucose) is used, there is a net production of three ATPs because the reaction of phosphorylating (adding a phosphate group to)

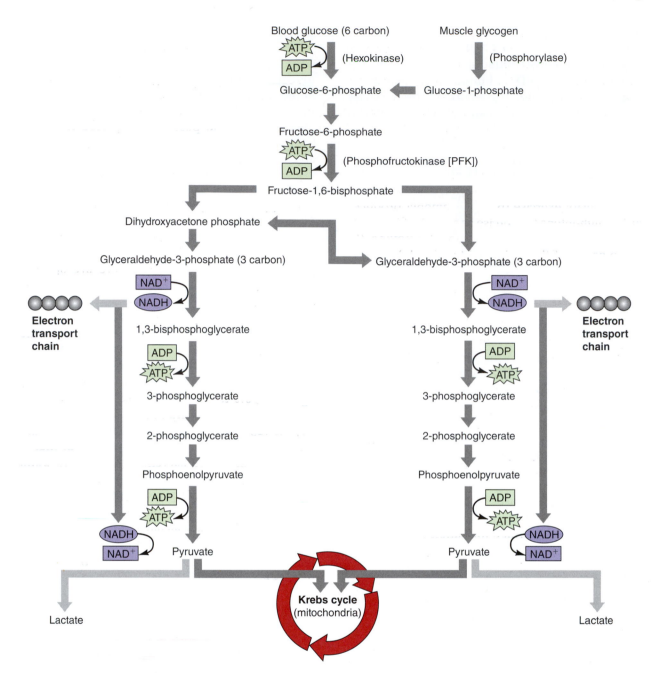

FIGURE 3.2   Glycolysis. ATP = adenosine triphosphate; ADP = adenosine diphosphate; NAD⁺, NADH = nicotinamide adenine dinucleotide.

Reprinted by permission from NSCA 2008.

glucose, which requires one ATP, is bypassed (6) (see figure 3.2).

Glycolysis Regulation

Glycolysis is stimulated during intense muscular activity by ADP, P_i, ammonia, and a slight decrease in pH and is strongly stimulated by AMP (6, 18). It is inhibited by the markedly lowered pH that may be observed during periods of inadequate oxygen supply and by increased levels of ATP, creatine phosphate, citrate, and free fatty acids (6, 18) that are usually present at rest. The phosphorylation of glucose by hexokinase (see figure 3.2) primarily controls glycolysis; but we must also consider the rate of glycogen breakdown to glucose, which is controlled by phosphorylase (figure 3.2), in the regulation of glycolysis (6, 34). In other words, if glycogen is not being broken down into glucose quickly enough and the supply of free glucose has already been depleted, glycolysis will be slowed.

Another important consideration in the regulation of any series of reactions is the **rate-limiting step,** that is, the slowest reaction in the series. The rate-limiting step in glycolysis is the conversion of fructose-6-phosphate to fructose-1,6-biphosphate (see figure 3.2), a reaction controlled by the enzyme phosphofructokinase (PFK). Thus the activity of PFK is the primary factor in the regulation of the rate of glycolysis. Activation of the phosphagen energy system stimulates glycolysis (by stimulating PFK) to contribute to the energy production of high-intensity exercise (6, 45). Ammonia produced during high-intensity exercise as a result of increased AMP or amino acid deamination (removing the amino group of the amino acid molecule) can also stimulate PFK.

Lactic Acid and Blood Lactate

Fast glycolysis occurs during periods of reduced oxygen availability in the muscle cells and results in the formation of the end-product **lactate,** which can be converted to lactic acid. Muscular fatigue experienced during exercise has been associated with high muscle tissue concentrations of lactic acid (25), but the fatigue is more likely a result of decreased tissue pH from many sources of acid, including the intermediates of glycolysis (35).

As pH decreases (becomes more acidic), it is believed to inhibit glycolytic reactions and directly interfere with muscle action, possibly by inhibiting calcium binding to troponin or by interfering with actin–myosin cross-bridge formation (44). Also, the decrease in pH levels inhibits the enzyme activity of the cell's energy systems (1). The overall effect is a decrease in available energy and muscle action force during exercise. Lactate is often used as an energy substrate, especially in type I and cardiac muscle fibers (28). It is also used in **gluconeogenesis,** the formation of glucose, during extended exercise and recovery (4, 28). The clearance of lactate from the blood indicates a person's ability to recover. Lactate can be cleared by oxidation within the muscle fiber in which it was produced, or it can be transported in the blood to other muscle fibers to be oxidized (28). Lactate can also be transported in the blood to the liver, where it is converted to glucose. This process is referred to as the **Cori cycle** and is depicted in figure 3.3.

Normally there is a low concentration of lactate in blood and muscle. The reported normal range of lactate concentration in blood is 0.5 to 2.2 mmol/L at rest (14, 30). Lactate production increases with increasing exercise intensity (1, 14, 37) and appears to depend on muscle fiber type. The higher rate of lactate production by type II muscle fibers may

reflect a concentration or activity of glycolytic enzymes that is higher than that of type I muscle fibers (10).

Gollnick, Bayly, and Hodgson (14) have reported that blood lactate concentrations normally return to preexercise values within an hour after activity. Light activity during the postexercise period has been shown to increase lactate clearance rates, and aerobically trained (14) and anaerobically trained (31, 32) individuals have faster lactate clearance rates than untrained people. Peak blood lactate concentrations occur approximately 5 minutes after the cessation of exercise, a delay frequently attributed to the time required to transport lactate from the tissue to the blood (14, 24).

It is widely accepted that there are specific inflection points in the lactate accumulation curve (figure 3.4) as exercise intensity increases (6, 35). The exercise intensity or relative intensity at which blood lactate begins an abrupt increase above the baseline concentration has been termed the **lactate threshold (LT)** (48). The LT represents an increasing reliance on anaerobic mechanisms. The LT typically begins at 50% to 60% of maximal oxygen uptake in untrained subjects and at 70% to 80% in trained subjects (13, 15, 23). A second increase in the rate of lactate accumulation has been noted at higher relative intensities of exercise. This second point of inflection, termed the **onset of blood lactate accumulation (OBLA),** generally occurs when the concentration of blood lactate is near 4 mmol/L (41, 43). The breaks in the lactate accumulation curve may correspond to the points at which intermediate and large motor units are recruited during increasing exercise intensities (23). The muscle cells associated with large motor units are typically type II fibers,

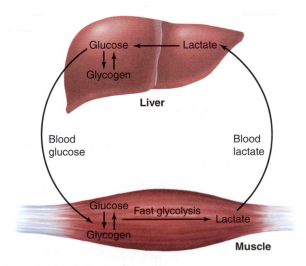

FIGURE 3.3 The Cori cycle.

Reprinted by permission from NSCA 2008.

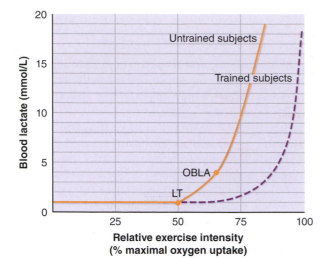

FIGURE 3.4 Lactate threshold (LT) and onset of blood lactate accumulation (OBLA).

Reprinted by permission from NSCA 2008.

which are particularly suited for anaerobic metabolism and lactate production.

It has been suggested that training at intensities near or above the LT or OBLA changes the LT and OBLA so that lactate accumulation occurs later at a higher exercise intensity (9). This shift probably occurs as a result of several factors but, in particular, as a result of the increased mitochondrial content that allows for greater production of ATP through aerobic mechanisms. The shift allows the individual to perform at higher percentages of maximal oxygen uptake without as much lactate accumulation in the blood (6, 23).

Oxidative (Aerobic) System

The **oxidative system,** the primary source of ATP at rest and during aerobic activities, uses primarily carbohydrates and fats as substrates (6). Clients who are walking on a treadmill, doing water aerobics, or participating in a yoga class are relying primarily on the oxidative system. Protein is normally not metabolized significantly except during long-term starvation and long bouts (>90 minutes) of exercise (8, 27). At rest, approximately 70% of the ATP produced is derived from fats and 30% from carbohydrates. Following the onset of activity, as the intensity of the exercise increases, there is a shift in substrate preference from fats to carbohydrates. During high-intensity aerobic exercise, almost 100% of the energy is derived from carbohydrates if an adequate supply is available. However, during prolonged, submaximal, steady-state work there is a gradual shift from carbohydrates back to fats and protein as energy substrates (6).

Glucose and Glycogen Oxidation

The oxidative metabolism of blood glucose and muscle glycogen begins with glycolysis. If oxygen is present in sufficient quantities, then the end product of glycolysis, pyruvate, is not converted to lactate but is transported to the mitochondria, which are specialized organelles within the cell. When pyruvate enters the mitochondria, it is converted to acetyl-CoA (CoA stands for coenzyme A) and can then enter the **Krebs cycle** for further ATP production. Also transported there are two molecules of NADH produced during the glycolytic reactions. The Krebs cycle, another series of reactions, produces two ATPs indirectly from guanine triphosphate (GTP) for each molecule of glucose (figure 3.5). Also produced in the Krebs cycle from one molecule of glucose are an additional six molecules of NADH and two molecules of reduced flavin adenine dinucleotide ($FADH_2$). The number of ATPs and amount of NADH and $FADH_2$ are different if fat or protein enters the Krebs cycle, although all of these substrates must be converted to acetyl-CoA before entering the Krebs cycle.

These molecules transport hydrogen atoms to the **electron transport chain (ETC)** to be used to produce ATP from ADP (6). The ETC uses the NADH and $FADH_2$ molecules to rephosphorylate ADP to ATP (figure 3.6). The hydrogen atoms are passed down the chain, a series of electron carriers known as *cytochromes*, to form a concentration gradient of protons to provide energy for ATP production, with oxygen serving as the final electron acceptor (resulting in the formation of water). Because NADH and $FADH_2$ enter the ETC at different sites, they differ in their ability to produce ATP. One molecule of NADH can produce three molecules of ATP, whereas one molecule of $FADH_2$ can produce only two molecules of ATP. The production of ATP during this process is referred to as *oxidative phosphorylation*. The oxidative system, beginning with glycolysis, results in the production of approximately 38 ATPs from the degradation of one glucose molecule (6). Table 3.1 summarizes the ATP yield of these processes.

Fat Oxidation

Fats can also be used by the oxidative energy system. Triglycerides stored in fat cells can be broken down by an enzyme known as *hormone-sensitive lipase.* This enzyme releases free fatty acids from the fat cells into the blood, where they can circulate and enter muscle fibers (6, 19). Additionally, limited quantities of triglycerides are stored within the muscle, along with a form of hormone-sensitive lipase, to serve as a source of free fatty acids within the muscle (6, 11). Free fatty acids enter the mitochondria, where they undergo **beta oxidation,** a

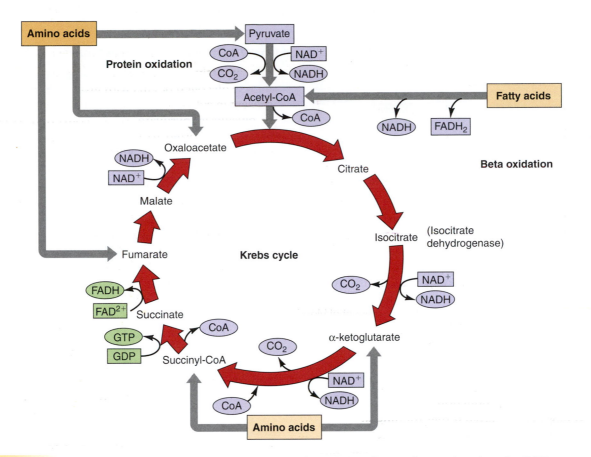

FIGURE 3.5 The Krebs cycle. CoA = coenzyme A; FAD^{2+}, $FADH_2$ = flavin adenine dinucleotide; GDP = guanine diphosphate; GTP = guanine triphosphate; NAD^+, NADH = nicotinamide adenine dinucleotide.

Reprinted by permission from NSCA 2008.

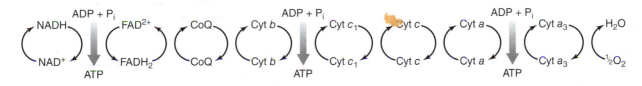

FIGURE 3.6 The electron transport chain. CoQ = coenzyme Q; Cyt = cytochrome; ATP = adenosine triphosphate; ADP = adenosine diphosphate; P_i = inorganic phosphate; NADH, NAD^+ = nicotinamide adenine dinucleotide; $FADH_2$, FAD^{2+} = flavin adenine dinucleotide; H_2O = water; O_2 = oxygen.

Reprinted by permission from NSCA 2008.

TABLE 3.1   Total Energy Yield From the Oxidation of One Glucose Molecule

Process	ATP production
SLOW GLYCOLYSIS	
Substrate-level phosphorylation	4
Oxidative phosphorylation: 2 NADH (3 ATP each)	6
KREBS CYCLE (TWO ROTATIONS THROUGH THE KREBS CYCLE PER GLUCOSE)	
Substrate-level phosphorylation	2
Oxidative phosphorylation: 8 NADH (3 ATP each)	24
Via GTP: 2 $FADH_2$ (2 ATP each)	4
Total	**40***

*Glycolysis consumes 2 ATP (if starting with glucose), so net ATP production is 40 – 2 = 38. This figure may also be reported as 36 ATP depending on which shuttle system is used to transport the NADH to the mitochondria. ATP = adenosine triphosphate; NADH = nicotinamide adenine dinucleotide; GTP = guanine triphosphate; $FADH_2$ = flavin adenine dinucleotide.

TABLE 3.2   Total Energy Yield From the Oxidation of One (18-Carbon) Triglyceride Molecule

Process	ATP production
One molecule of glycerol	22
18-CARBON FATTY ACID METABOLISM*	
147 ATP per fatty acid × three fatty acids per triglyceride molecule	441
Total	**463**

*Other triglycerides that contain different amounts of carbons will yield more or less ATP. ATP = adenosine triphosphate.

series of reactions in which the free fatty acids are broken down, resulting in the formation of acetyl-CoA and hydrogen atoms (figure 3.5). The acetyl-CoA enters the Krebs cycle directly, and the hydrogen atoms are carried by NADH and $FADH_2$ to the ETC (6). An example of the ATP produced from a typical triglyceride molecule is shown in table 3.2.

Protein Oxidation

Although not a significant source of energy for most activities, protein can be broken down into its constituent amino acids by various metabolic processes. These amino acids can then be converted into glucose (in a process known as *gluconeogenesis*), pyruvate, or various Krebs cycle intermediates to produce ATP (figure 3.5). The contribution of amino acids to the production of ATP has been estimated to be minimal during short-term exercise but may amount to 3% to 18% of the energy requirements during prolonged activity (5, 42). The major amino acids that are oxidized in skeletal muscle appear to be the branched-chain amino acids (leucine, isoleucine, and valine), although alanine, aspartate, and glutamate may also be used (16). The nitrogen-containing waste products of amino acid breakdown are eliminated through the formation of urea and small amounts of ammonia, which end up in the urine. The elimination of ammonia is important because ammonia is toxic and is associated with fatigue (6).

Oxidative (Aerobic) System Regulation

The rate-limiting step in the Krebs cycle (see figure 3.5) is the conversion of isocitrate to α-ketoglutarate,

a reaction controlled by the enzyme isocitrate dehydrogenase. Isocitrate dehydrogenase is stimulated by ADP and normally inhibited by ATP. The reactions that produce NADH or $FADH_2$ also influence the regulation of the Krebs cycle. If NAD^+ and FAD^{2+} are not available in sufficient quantities to accept hydrogen, the rate of the Krebs cycle is reduced. Also, when GTP accumulates, the concentration of succinyl CoA increases, which inhibits the initial reaction (oxaloacetate + acetyl-CoA → citrate + CoA) of the Krebs cycle. The ETC is inhibited by ATP and stimulated by ADP (6). Figure 3.7 presents a simplified overview of the metabolism of fat, carbohydrate, and protein.

All three energy systems are active at a given time; however, the extent to which each is used depends primarily on the intensity of the activity and secondarily on its duration.

Energy Production and Capacity

The phosphagen, glycolytic, and oxidative energy systems differ in their ability to supply energy for activities of various intensities and durations (tables 3.3 and 3.4). Exercise intensity is defined as a level of muscular activity that can be quantified in terms of power output, with *power* defined as the amount of physical work performed for a particular duration of time.

Activities such as performing resistance training and performing a serve in tennis that are high in intensity, and thus have a high power output, require rapidly supplied energy and rely almost entirely on the energy supplied by the phosphagen system.

TABLE 3.3   Rankings of Rate and Capacity of Adenosine Triphosphate (ATP) Production

System	Rate of ATP production	Capacity of ATP production
Phosphagen	1	5
Fast glycolysis	2	4
Slow glycolysis	3	3
Oxidation of carbohydrate	4	2
Oxidation of fat and protein	5	1

1 = fastest or greatest; 5 = slowest or least; ATP = adenosine triphosphate.

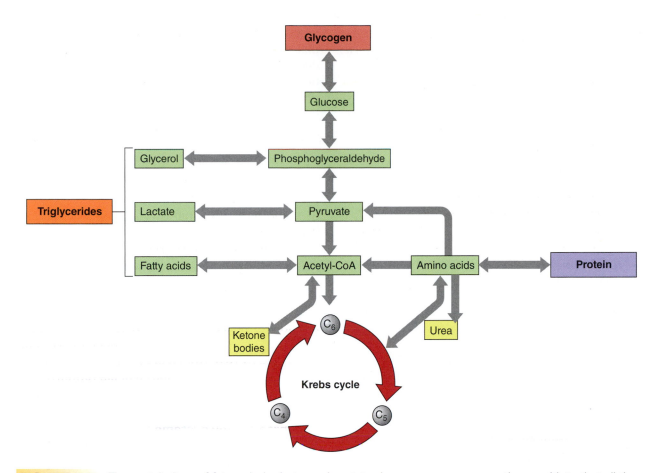

FIGURE 3.7 The metabolism of fat, carbohydrate, and protein share some common pathways. Note that all three are reduced to acetyl-CoA and enter the Krebs cycle.

Reprinted by permission from NSCA 2008.

TABLE 3.4 Effect of Event Duration on Primary Energy System Used

Duration of event	Intensity of event	Primary energy system(s)
0 to 6 s	Very intense	Phosphagen
6 to 30 s	Intense	Phosphagen and fast glycolysis
30 s to 2 min	Heavy	Fast glycolysis
2 to 3 min	Moderate	Fast glycolysis and oxidative system
>3 min	Light	Oxidative system

Activities that are of lower intensity but longer duration, such as a 10-mile (16 km) bike ride or swimming laps in the pool for an hour, require a large energy supply and rely on the energy supplied by the oxidative energy system (table 3.3). The primary source of energy for activities between these two extremes differs depending on the intensity and duration of the event (table 3.4). In general, short, high-intensity activities (e.g., jumping or kicking and punching moves in cardio kickboxing) rely on the phosphagen energy system and fast glycolysis. As the intensity decreases and the duration increases, the emphasis gradually shifts to slow glycolysis and the oxidative energy system (6, 38).

The duration of the activity also influences which energy system is used. Specific exercises within a prescribed program can range in duration from approximately 5 seconds (e.g., one set of bench press at 90% of the 1RM [1-repetition maximum]) to more than an hour (e.g., low-intensity, extended-duration treadmill walking). If an individual makes a best effort (an effort that results in the best possible performance for a given activity), the time considerations shown in table 3.4 are reasonable (6, 36, 44, 46).

At no time, during either exercise or rest, does any single energy system provide the complete supply of energy. During exercise, the degree to which anaerobic and oxidative systems contribute to the energy being produced is determined primarily by the exercise intensity and secondarily by exercise duration (6, 38).

In general, there is an inverse relationship between the relative rate and total amount of ATP that a given energy system can produce. As a result, the phosphagen energy system primarily supplies ATP for high-intensity activities of short duration (e.g., sprinting across a football field), the glycolytic system for moderate- to high-intensity activities of short to medium duration (e.g., running once around a track), and the oxidative system for low-intensity activities of long duration (e.g., completing a 20-mile [32 km] bike ride).

> The phosphagen energy system primarily supplies ATP for high-intensity activities of short duration, the glycolytic system for moderate- to high-intensity activities of short to medium duration, and the oxidative system for low-intensity activities of long duration.

Metabolic Specificity of Training

Appropriate exercise intensities and rest intervals can permit the "selection" of specific energy systems during training for specific athletic events or training goals (e.g., to improve short-term endurance) (6). Few sports or physical activities require maximal sustained-effort exercise to exhaustion or near exhaustion. Most sports and training activities (such as football, cardio kickboxing, spinning, and resistance training) are intermittent in nature and therefore produce metabolic profiles that are very similar to that for a series of high-intensity, constant- or near-constant-effort exercise bouts interspersed with rest periods. In this type of exercise, the power output (a measure of exercise intensity) produced during each exercise bout is much greater than the maximal power output that can be sustained using aerobic energy sources. Chapters 15, 16, and 17 discuss training methods that allow appropriate metabolic systems to be stressed.

Substrate Depletion and Repletion

Energy substrates—molecules that provide starting materials for bioenergetic reactions, including phosphagens (ATP and creatine phosphate), glucose, glycogen, lactate, free fatty acids, and amino acids—can be selectively depleted during the performance of activities of various intensities and durations. Subsequently, the amount of energy that can be produced by the bioenergetic systems decreases. Fatigue experienced during many activities is frequently associated with the depletion of phosphagens (13, 18) and glycogen (6, 20, 27, 36); the depletion of substrates such as free fatty acids, lactate, and amino acids typically does not occur to the extent that performance is limited. Consequently, the depletion and repletion pattern of phosphagens and glycogen following physical activity is important in exercise bioenergetics.

Phosphagens

Fatigue during exercise appears to be at least partially related to the decrease in phosphagens. Phosphagen concentrations in muscle are more rapidly depleted as a result of high-intensity anaerobic exercise than of aerobic exercise (13, 18). Creatine phosphate can decrease markedly (50% to 70%) during the first stage (5-30 seconds) of high-intensity exercise and can be almost eliminated as a result of very intense exercise to exhaustion (17, 21, 29). Muscle ATP concentrations do not decrease by more than about 60% from initial values, however, even during very intense exercise (17). It is also important to note that dynamic muscle actions, such as a complete repetition of a weight training exercise, use more metabolic energy and typically deplete phosphagens to a greater extent than do isometric muscle actions, such as arm wrestling, in which there is no visible shortening of the muscle (3).

Postexercise phosphagen repletion can occur in a relatively short period; complete resynthesis of ATP appears to occur within 3 to 5 minutes, and complete creatine phosphate resynthesis can occur within 8 minutes (18). Repletion of phosphagens occurs largely as a result of aerobic metabolism, although fast glycolysis can contribute to ATP resynthesis after high-intensity exercise (24).

Glycogen

Limited stores of glycogen are available for exercise. Approximately 300 to 400 g of glycogen is stored in the body's total muscle, and about 70 to 100 g is stored in the liver (40). Resting concentrations of liver and muscle glycogen can be influenced by training and dietary manipulations (12, 40). Research suggests that both anaerobic training, including sprinting and resistance training (2) and typical aerobic endurance training can increase resting muscle glycogen concentration.

The rate of glycogen depletion is related to exercise intensity (40). Muscle glycogen is a more important energy source than is liver glycogen during moderate- and high-intensity exercise; liver glycogen appears to be more important during low-intensity exercise, and its contribution to metabolic processes increases with duration of exercise. Increases in relative exercise intensity of maximal oxygen uptake result in increases in the rate of muscle **glycogenolysis,** which increases available glycogen for the glycolysis pathway (6, 36). At relative intensities of exercise above 60% of maximal oxygen uptake, muscle glycogen becomes an increasingly important energy substrate; and the entire glycogen content of some muscle cells can become depleted during exercise (39).

Very high-intensity, intermittent exercise, such as resistance training or half-court basketball, can cause substantial depletion of muscle glycogen (decreases of 20% to 60%) with relatively few sets of exercise (low total workloads) (26, 36, 44). Although phosphagens may be the primary limiting factor during resistance exercise with few repetitions or few sets, muscle glycogen may become the limiting factor for resistance training with many total sets and larger total amounts of work (36). This type of exercise could cause selective muscle fiber glycogen depletion (more depletion in type II fibers) that can also limit performance (36). As with other types of dynamic exercise, the rate of muscle glycogenolysis during resistance exercise depends on intensity. However, it appears that equal amounts of total work produce equal amounts of glycogen depletion, regardless of relative exercise intensity (36).

Repletion of muscle glycogen during recovery is related to postexercise carbohydrate ingestion. Repletion appears to be optimal if 0.7 to 3.0 g of carbohydrate per kilogram of body weight is ingested every 2 hours following exercise (12, 40). Muscle glycogen may be completely replenished within 24 hours, provided sufficient carbohydrate is ingested (12, 40). However, if the exercise has a high eccentric component (associated with exercise-induced muscle damage), more time may be required to completely replenish muscle glycogen.

Oxygen Uptake and the Aerobic and Anaerobic Contributions to Exercise

Oxygen uptake (or consumption) is a measure of a person's ability to take in and use oxygen. The higher the oxygen uptake, the more fit the person is thought to be. During low-intensity exercise with a constant power output, oxygen uptake increases for the first few minutes until a steady state of uptake (oxygen demand equals oxygen consumption) is

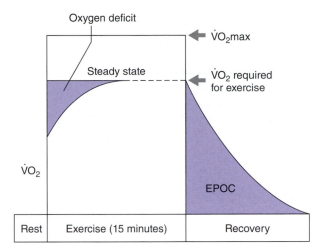

FIGURE 3.8 Low-intensity, steady-state exercise metabolism: 75% of maximal oxygen uptake ($\dot{V}O_2$max). EPOC = excess postexercise oxygen consumption; $\dot{V}O_2$ = oxygen uptake.

Reprinted by permission from NSCA 2008.

reached (figure 3.8) (6). At the start of the exercise bout, however, some of the energy must be supplied through anaerobic mechanisms (47). This anaerobic contribution to the total energy cost of exercise is termed the **oxygen deficit.** After exercise, oxygen uptake remains above preexercise levels for a period of time that varies according to the intensity and length of the exercise. Postexercise oxygen uptake has been termed the **oxygen debt,** or the **excess postexercise oxygen consumption (EPOC).** The EPOC is the oxygen uptake above resting values used to restore the body to the preexercise condition. There are only small to moderate relationships between the oxygen deficit and the EPOC; the oxygen deficit may influence the size of the EPOC, but the two are not equal (6).

Anaerobic mechanisms provide much of the energy for work if the exercise intensity is above the maximal oxygen uptake that a person can attain (figure 3.9). For instance, if a client who was not used to that type of activity jumped right into an advanced spinning class, most of the energy would be supplied by anaerobic mechanisms. Generally, as the contribution of anaerobic mechanisms supporting the exercise increases, the exercise duration decreases (6, 15).

Practical Application of Energy Systems

The concept of energy systems can seem very abstract; but with only a basic understanding of

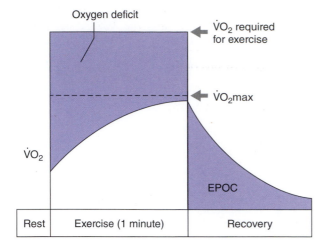

FIGURE 3.9 High-intensity, non-steady-state exercise metabolism (80% of maximum power output). The required $\dot{V}O_2$ here is the oxygen uptake that would be required to sustain the exercise if such an uptake were possible to attain. Because it is not, the oxygen deficit lasts for the duration of the exercise. EPOC = excess postexercise oxygen consumption; $\dot{V}O_2$max = maximal oxygen uptake.

Reprinted by permission from NSCA 2008.

the general time frames of energy system use, one can determine the primary energy system that will be taxed in various types of exercise or activities. The main thing to remember is that the higher the exercise intensity, the shorter the amount of time the exercise can be performed and the greater the reliance on the fastest ATP-producing energy systems, which also have the least capacity. The opposite is also true; the lower the exercise intensity, the longer that exercise can be performed, and the greater the reliance on the slower ATP-producing energy

systems. In this case, ATP can be produced as long as the body has a good supply of muscle glycogen and fatty acids. When assessing clients' needs, it is important to consider their training goals from the energy system perspective so that exercise selection and the manner of performing those exercises can be optimized. Rest periods between sets and exercises also factor into this because longer rest periods allow for more complete ATP resynthesis from the phosphagen system. For example, if a client wants to improve his or her ability to get to the first base marker in the company softball game, repeat activities that stress the phosphagen system are suggested (sprints, intervals on the bike, exercises to improve leg strength, and overall lower body power exercises). If the client wants to train for a 20-mile (32 km) hike in the Alps, activities that stress the oxidative system are best, such as work on almost any cardio equipment for extended periods of time.

Conclusion

One can design more productive training programs through an understanding of how energy is produced during various types of exercise and how energy production can be modified by specific training regimens. Which energy system is used to supply energy for muscular action is determined primarily by the intensity and secondarily by the duration of exercise. Metabolic responses and the subsequent training adaptations are largely regulated by those characteristics (e.g., intensity and duration) and form the basis of metabolic specificity of exercise and training. This principle of specificity allows for enhanced physical adaptation and program results through the implementation of precise training programs.

Study Questions

1. Which of the following describes the process of fast glycolysis?

   I. a breakdown of glycogen

   II. its end product is converted to lactate

   III. a breakdown of glucose

   IV. its end product is sent to the Krebs cycle

   A. I, II, and III only

   B. I, II, and IV only

   C. II, III, and IV only

   D. I, III ,and IV only

2. Which of the following describes what a client would be doing to allow the oxidative system to contribute the greatest *percentage* toward total ATP production?

   A. sitting quietly

   B. walking

   C. jogging

   D. sprinting

3. Which of the following energy systems is capable of producing the greatest amount (capacity) of ATP?

   A. phosphagen

   B. fast glycolysis

   C. slow glycolysis

   D. oxidative

4. Which of the following energy systems is capable of producing ATP at the greatest rate?

   A. phosphagen

   B. fast glycolysis

   C. slow glycolysis

   D. oxidative

Applied Knowledge Question

Fill in the chart to describe the changes in the sources of energy to produce ATP as a client participates in a maximum treadmill test. Write *Most* if it is the primary source of energy during the activity. Write *Least* if it is the least-used source of energy during the activity.

Activity	Carbohydrate	Fat
While the client is sitting in a chair listening to the personal trainer		
The first few seconds of the treadmill test		
During a stage when the client reached steady state		
At the end of the test as the client reaches maximum		

References

1. Barany, M., and C. Arus. 1990. Lactic acid production in intact muscle, as followed by 13C and 1H nuclear magnetic resonance. In: *Human Muscle Power,* N.L. Jones, N. McCartney, and A.J. McComas, eds. Champaign, IL: Human Kinetics. pp. 153-164.

2. Boobis, I., C. Williams, and S.N. Wooten. 1983. Influence of sprint training on muscle metabolism during brief maximal exercise in man. *Journal of Physiology* 342: 36-37P.

3. Bridges, C.R., B.J. Clark III, R.L. Hammond, and L.W. Stephenson. 1991. Skeletal muscle bioenergetics during frequency-dependent fatigue. *American Journal of Physiology* 29: C643-C651.

4. Brooks, G.A. 1986. The lactate shuttle during exercise and recovery. *Medicine and Science in Sports and Exercise* 18: 360-368.

5. Brooks, G.A. 1987. Amino acid and protein metabolism during exercise and recovery. *Medicine and Science in Sports and Exercise* 19: S150-S156.

6. Brooks, G.A., T.D. Fahey, and K.M. Baldwin. 2005. *Exercise Physiology: Human Bioenergetics and Its Applications,* 4th ed. New York: Wiley.

7. Cerretelli, P., D. Rennie, and D. Pendergast. 1980. Kinetics of metabolic transients during exercise. *International Journal of Sports Medicine* 55: 178-180.

8. Dohm, G.L., R.T. Williams, G.J. Kasperek, and R.J. VanRij. 1982. Increased excretion of urea and N-methylhistidine by rats and humans after a bout of exercise. *Journal of Applied Physiology* 52: 27-33.

9. Donovan, C.M., and G.A. Brooks. 1983. Endurance training affects lactate clearance, not lactate production. *American Journal of Physiology* 244: E83-E92.

10. Dudley, G.A., and R. Terjung. 1985. Influence of aerobic metabolism on IMP accumulation in fast-twitch muscle. *American Journal of Physiology* 248: C37-C42.

11. DuFax, B., G. Assmann, and W. Hollman. 1982. Plasma lipoproteins and physical activity: A review. *International Journal of Sports Medicine* 3: 123-136.

12. Friedman, J.E., P.D. Neufer, and L.G. Dohm. 1991. Regulation of glycogen synthesis following exercise. *Sports Medicine* 11 (4): 232-243.

13. Gollnick, P.D., and W.M. Bayly. 1986. Biochemical training adaptations and maximal power. In: *Human Muscle Power,* N.L. Jones, N. McCartney, and A.J. McComas, eds. Champaign, IL: Human Kinetics. pp. 255-267.

14. Gollnick, P.D., W.M. Bayly, and D.R. Hodgson. 1986. Exercise intensity, training diet and lactate concentration in muscle and blood. *Medicine and Science in Sports and Exercise* 18: 334-340.

15. Gollnick, P.D., and L. Hermansen. 1982. Significance of skeletal muscle oxidative enzyme enhancement with endurance training. *Clinical Physiology* 2: 1-12.

16. Graham, T.E., J.W.E. Rush, and D.A. Maclean. 1995. Skeletal muscle amino acid metabolism and ammonia production during exercise. In: *Exercise Metabolism,* M. Hargreaves, ed. Champaign, IL: Human Kinetics. pp. 41-72.

17. Hirvonen, J., S. Ruhunen, H. Rusko, and M. Harkonen. 1987. Breakdown of high-energy phosphate compounds and lactate accumulation during short submaximal exercise. *European Journal of Applied Physiology* 56: 253-259.

18. Hultman, E., and H. Sjoholm. 1986. Biochemical causes of fatigue. In: *Human Muscle Power,* N.L. Jones, N. McCartney, and A.J. McComas, eds. Champaign, IL: Human Kinetics. pp. 215-235.

19. Hurley, B.F., D.R. Seals, J.M. Hagberg, A.C. Goldberg, S.M. Ostrove, J.O. Holloszy, W.G. Wiest, and A.P. Goldberg. 1984. Strength training and lipoprotein lipid profiles: Increased HDL cholesterol in body builders versus powerlifters and effects of androgen use. *Journal of the American Medical Association* 252: 507-513.

20. Jacobs, I., P. Kaiser, and P. Tesch. 1981. Muscle strength and fatigue after selective glycogen depletion in human skeletal muscle fibers. *European Journal of Applied Physiology* 46: 47-53.

21. Jacobs, I., P.A. Tesch, O. Bar-Or, J. Karlsson, and R. Dotow. 1983. Lactate in human skeletal muscle after 10 and 30 s of supramaximal exercise. *Journal of Applied Physiology* 55: 365-367.

22. Jansson, E., C. Sylven, and E. Nordevang. 1982. Myoglobin in the quadriceps femoris muscle of competitive cyclists and in untrained men. *Acta Physiologica Scandinavica* 114: 627-629.

23. Jones, N., and R. Ehrsam. 1982. The anaerobic threshold. In: *Exercise and Sport Sciences Review,* vol. 10, R.L. Terjung, ed. Philadelphia: Franklin Press. pp. 49-83.

24. Juel, C. 1988. Intracellular pH recovery and lactate efflux in mouse soleus muscles stimulated in vitro: The involvement of sodium/proton exchange and a lactate carrier. *Acta Physiologica Scandinavica* 132: 363-371.

25. Kreisberg, R.A. 1980. Lactate homeostasis and lactic acidosis. *Annals of Internal Medicine* 92 (2): 227-237.

26. Lambert, C.P., M.G. Flynn, J.B. Boone, T.J. Michaud, and J. Rodriguez-Zayas. 1991. Effects of carbohydrate feeding on multiple-bout resistance exercise. *Journal of Applied Sports Science Research* 5 (4): 192-197.

27. Lemon, P.W., and J.P. Mullin. 1980. Effect of initial muscle glycogen levels on protein catabolism during exercise. *Journal of Applied Physiology: Respiration in Environmental Exercise Physiology* 48: 624-629.

28. Mazzeo, R.S., G.A. Brooks, D.A. Schoeller, and T.F. Budinger. 1986. Disposal of blood [1-13C] lactate in humans during rest and exercise. *Journal of Applied Physiology* 60 (10): 232-241.

29. McCartney, N., L.L. Spriet, G.J.F. Heigenhauser, J.M. Kowalchuk, J.R. Sutton, and N.L. Jones. 1986. Muscle power and metabolism in maximal intermittent exercise. *Journal of Applied Physiology* 60: 1164-1169.

30. McGee, D.S., T.C. Jesse, M.H. Stone, and D. Blessing. 1992. Leg and hip endurance adaptations to three different weight-training programs. *Journal of Applied Sports Science Research* 6 (2): 92-95.

31. McMillan, J.L., M.H. Stone, J. Sartin, R. Keith, D. Marple, C. Brown, and R.D. Lewis. 1993. 20-hour physiological responses to a single weight-training session. *Journal of Strength and Conditioning Research* 7 (1): 9-21.

32. Pierce, K., R. Rozenek, M. Stone, and D. Blessing. 1987. The effects of weight training on plasma cortisol, lactate, heart rate, anxiety and perceived exertion (abstract). *Journal of Applied Sports Science Research* 1 (3): 58.

33. Poortmans, J.R. 1984. Protein turnover and amino acid oxidation during and after exercise. *Medicine and Science in Sports and Exercise* 17: 130-147.

34. Richter, E.A., H. Galbo, and N.J. Christensen. 1981. Control of exercise-induced muscular glycogenolysis by adrenal medullary hormones in rats. *Journal of Applied Physiology* 50: 21-26.

35. Roberts, R.A., F. Ghiasvand, and D. Parker. 2004. Biochemistry of exercise-induced metabolic acidosis. *American Journal of Physiology: Regulatory, Integrative, and Comparative Physiology* 287 (3): R502-516.

36. Roberts, R.A., D.R. Pearson, D.L. Costill, W.J. Fink, D.D. Pascoe, M.A. Benedict, C.P. Lambert, and J.J. Zachweija. 1992. Muscle glycogenolysis during differing intensities of weight-resistance exercise. *Journal of Applied Physiology* 70 (4): 1700-1706.

37. Rozenek, R., L. Rosenau, P. Rosenau, and M.H. Stone. 1993. The effect of intensity on heart rate and blood lactate response to resistance exercise. *Journal of Strength and Conditioning Research* 7 (1): 51-54.

38. Sahlin, K., M. Tonkonogi, and K. Soderlund. 1998. Energy supply and muscle fatigue in humans. *Acta Physiologica Scandinavica* 162 (3): 261-266.

39. Saltin, B., and P.D. Gollnick. 1983. Skeletal muscle adaptability: Significance for metabolism and performance. In: *Handbook of Physiology,* L.D. Peachey, R.H. Adrian, and S.R. Geiger, eds. Baltimore: Williams & Wilkins. pp. 540-555.

40. Sherman, W.M., and G.S. Wimer. 1991. Insufficient carbohydrate during training: Does it impair performance? *International Journal of Sports Nutrition* 1 (1): 28-44.

41. Sjodin, B., and I. Jacobs. 1981. Onset of blood lactate accumulation and marathon running performance. *International Journal of Sports Medicine* 2: 23-26.

42. Smith, S.A., S.J. Montain, R.P. Matott, G.P. Zientara, F.A. Jolesz, and R.A. Fielding. 1998. Creatine supplementation and age influence muscle metabolism during exercise. *Journal of Applied Physiology* 85: 1349-1356.

43. Tanaka, K., Y. Matsuura, S. Kumagai, A. Matsuzuka, K. Hirakoba, and K. Asano. 1983. Relationships of anaerobic threshold and onset of blood lactate accumulation with endurance performance. *European Journal of Applied Physiology* 52: 51-56.

44. Tesch, P. 1980. Muscle fatigue in man, with special reference to lactate accumulation during short intense exercise. *Acta Physiologica Scandinavica* 480: 1-40.

45. Tesch, P.A., B. Colliander, and P. Kaiser. 1986. Muscle metabolism during intense, heavy resistance exercise. *European Journal of Applied Physiology* 55: 362-366.

46. Tesch, P.A., L.L. Ploutz-Snyder, L. Ystrom, M.J. Castro, and G.A. Dudley. 1998. Skeletal muscle glycogen loss evoked by resistance exercise. *Journal of Strength and Conditioning Research* 12: 67-73.

47. Warren, B.J., M.H. Stone, J.T. Kearney, S.J. Fleck, G.D. Wilson, and W.J. Kraemer. 1992. The effects of short-term overwork on performance measures and blood metabolites in elite junior weightlifters. *International Journal of Sports Medicine* 13 (5): 372-376.

48. Yoshida, I. 1984. Effect of dietary modifications on lactate threshold and onset of blood lactate accumulation during incremental exercise. *European Journal of Applied Physiology* 53: 200-205.

Biomechanics

William C. Whiting, PhD, and Sean P. Flanagan, PhD

After completing this chapter, you will be able to

- describe human movements using appropriate anatomical and mechanical terminology,

- apply mechanical concepts to human movement problems,

- understand the factors contributing to human strength and power,

- determine the muscle actions involved in movement tasks, and

- analyze biomechanical aspects of resistance exercises.

Success as a personal trainer requires expertise in a number of scientific subdisciplines. Among these are functional anatomy and biomechanics. In designing exercise programs for performance enhancement and injury prevention, personal trainers must understand human anatomy from a functional perspective and be able to apply biomechanical principles to meet their clients' goals.

Functional anatomy is the study of how body systems cooperate to perform certain tasks (32). Muscles do not always work according to their anatomical classification (35). For example, the quadriceps muscle group is anatomically defined as a knee extensor. However, these muscles actually control movement during the eccentric, or "down," phase of the squat—even though the knee is flexing. To design effective exercise interventions, it is necessary to know which muscles are active during which activities and match them with the appropriate exercises.

Biomechanics is a field of study that applies mechanical principles to understand the function of living organisms and systems. With respect to human movement, several areas of biomechanics are relevant, including movement mechanics, fluid mechanics, material mechanics, and joint mechanics. While fluid, material, and joint mechanics have important applications to human movement and are mentioned briefly, the focus of this chapter is on movement mechanics and applicable mechanical concepts.

Understanding these concepts is essential in selecting effective exercises. In the first part of the chapter, we define mechanical terms and concepts in an unambiguous way; these definitions may differ from the everyday meanings of the terms. Although the human body *acts like* a mechanical system during movement, the second part of this chapter examines how our biological structure creates unique mechanical properties. The third part of the chapter combines knowledge of mechanics and anatomy, detailing a formula for determining which muscles are active during a movement. In the last section, the biomechanics of resistance exercise is explored.

Chapter 4

Mechanical Foundations

Mechanics is the branch of physics that deals with the effects of forces and energy on bodies. This section on mechanical foundations focuses on mechanical terminology and concepts that are relevant to human movements involved in strength and conditioning programs.

Mechanical Terminology and Principles

As with every specialized area of study, biomechanics has its own vocabulary. Many of the terms defined and applied here have specific meanings, sometimes different from the meanings of the terms as used by the lay public. Terms such as *strength*, *work*, *power*, and *energy* have common meanings that may differ from scientific definitions and may incorrectly be used interchangeably. The chapter defines each of these terms, along with others.

In biomechanics, for example, the term *body* refers to any collection of matter. Thus in mechanical terms, *body* may refer to the entire human body, a limb segment (e.g., a thigh or forearm), or some other collection of matter (e.g., a piece of chalk). Mechanically speaking, there are two basic types of movement: (1) **linear motion,** in which a body moves in a straight line **(rectilinear motion)** or along a curved path **(curvilinear motion)** and (2) **angular motion** (also **rotational motion)** in which a body rotates about a fixed line known as the **axis of rotation** (also **fulcrum** or **pivot).** Many human movements (e.g., running, jumping, throwing) involve a combination of linear and angular motion in what is called **general motion.** It is often useful to think about these movements occurring in an anatomical plane, that is, in the **frontal, sagittal,** or **transverse plane** (figure 4.1). Major movements of the joints are presented in figure 4.2, and we will refer to them throughout the chapter.

The study of movement from a descriptive perspective *without* regard to the underlying forces is termed **kinematics.** Kinematic assessment involves the spatial and timing characteristics of movement using five primary variables: (1) timing, or temporal, measures (e.g., an athlete took 0.8 seconds to lift the barbell); (2) position or location (e.g., a client held his or her arm in 90° of abduction); (3) displacement (e.g., a trainee moved his or her elbow through 60° of flexion); (4) velocity (e.g., a volleyball player extended his or her knee at 600°/s while jumping); and (5) **acceleration,** or change in velocity per unit time (e.g., gravity accelerated a jumper's body toward the ground at 9.81 m/s^2).

In contrast to kinematics, movement assessment *with* respect to the forces involved is called **kinetics.** Forces can be thought of as the causes of motion. Human movement happens as a result of mechanical factors that produce and control movement from the inside (internal forces such as muscle forces) or affect the body from the outside (external forces such as gravity). Many of the mechanical measures (e.g., force, torque) presented in the next sections are kinetic variables.

Units of Measure

Before we explore specific mechanical measures, a few notes are needed on units of measure. Internationally, the standard system of unit measures is Le Système International d'Unités (SI system) (19). In the United States and elsewhere, a traditional (also

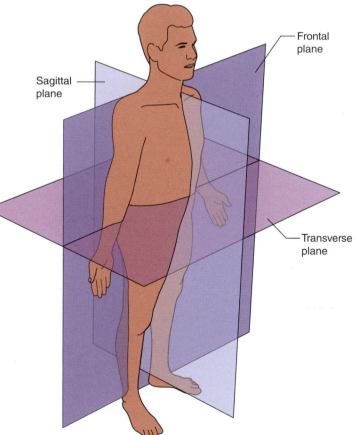

Sagittal plane

Frontal plane

Transverse plane

FIGURE 4.1 The three major planes of the human body in the **anatomical position.**

Reprinted by permission from Watkins 2010.

Wrist—sagittal
Flexion
Exercise: wrist curl
Sport: basketball free throw

Extension
Exercise: wrist extension
Sport: racquetball backhand

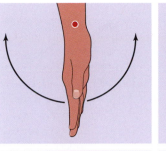

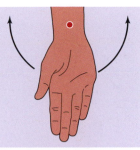

Wrist—frontal
Ulnar deviation
Exercise: specific wrist curl
Sport: baseball bat swing

Radial deviation
Exercise: specific wrist curl
Sport: golf backswing

Elbow—sagittal
Flexion
Exercise: biceps curl
Sport: bowling

Extension
Exercise: triceps pushdown
Sport: shot put

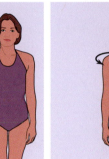

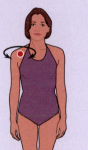

Shoulder—sagittal
Flexion
Exercise: front shoulder raise
Sport: boxing uppercut punch

Extension
Exercise: neutral-grip seated row
Sport: freestyle swimming stroke

Shoulder—frontal
Adduction
Exercise: wide-grip lat pulldown
Sport: swimming breast stroke

Abduction
Exercise: wide-grip shoulder press
Sport: springboard diving

Shoulder—transverse
Internal rotation
Exercise: arm wrestle movement (with dumbbell or cable)
Sport: baseball pitch

External rotation
Exercise: reverse arm wrestle movement
Sport: karate block

Shoulder—transverse
(upper arm to 90° to trunk)
Horizontal adduction
Exercise: dumbbell chest fly
Sport: tennis forehand

Horizontal abduction
Exercise: bent-over lateral raise
Sport: tennis backhand

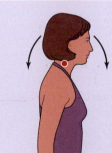

Neck—sagittal
Flexion
Exercise: neck machine
Sport: somersault

Extension
Exercise: dynamic back bridge
Sport: back flip

Neck—transverse
Left rotation
Exercise: manual resistance
Sport: wrestling movement

Right rotation
Exercise: manual resistance
Sport: wrestling movement

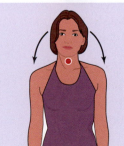

Neck—frontal
Left lateral flexion
Exercise: neck machine
Sport: slalom skiing

Right lateral flexion
Exercise: neck machine
Sport: slalom skiing

(continued)

FIGURE 4.2 Major body movements. Planes of movement are relative to the body in the anatomical position. The list includes common exercises that provide resistance to the movements and related physical activities.

Reprinted by permission from Harman and Johnson 1992.

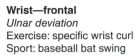

Trunk—sagittal
Flexion
Exercise: sit-up
Sport: javelin throw
follow-through

Extension
Exercise: stiff-leg deadlift
Sport: back flip

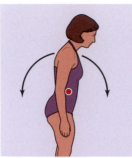

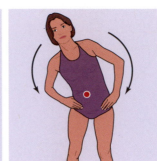

Trunk—frontal
Left lateral flexion
Exercise: medicine ball
overhead hook throw
Sport: gymnastics side aerial

Right lateral flexion
Exercise: side bend
Sport: basketball hook shot

Trunk—transverse
Left rotation
Exercise: medicine ball side
toss
Sport: baseball batting

Right rotation
Exercise: torso machine
Sport: golf swing

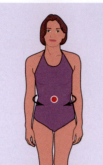

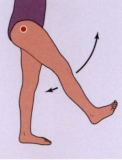

Hip—sagittal
Flexion
Exercise: leg raise
Sport: American football punt

Extension
Exercise: back squat
Sport: long jump take-off

Hip—frontal
Adduction
Exercise: standing
adduction machine
Sport: soccer side step

Abduction
Exercise: standing
abduction machine
Sport: rollerblading

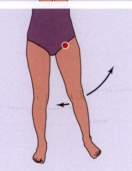

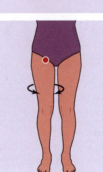

Hip—transverse
Internal rotation
Exercise: resisted internal rotation
Sport: basketball pivot movement

External rotation
Exercise: resisted external rotation
Sport: figure skating turn

Hip—transverse
(upper leg to 90° to trunk)
Horizontal adduction
Exercise: adduction machine
Sport: karate in-sweep

Horizontal abduction
Exercise: seated abduction
machine
Sport: wrestling escape

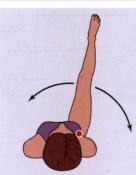

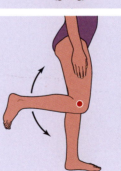

Knee—sagittal
Flexion
Exercise: leg (knee) curl
Sport: diving tuck

Extension
Exercise: leg (knee) extension
Sport: volleyball block

Ankle—sagittal
Dorsiflexion
Exercise: toe raise
Sport: running

Plantar flexion
Exercise: calf (heel) raise
Sport: high jump

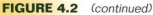

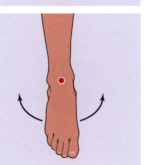

Ankle (subtalar)—frontal
Inversion
Exercise: resisted inversion
Sport: soccer dribbling

Eversion
Exercise: resisted eversion
Sport: speed skating

FIGURE 4.2 *(continued)*

TABLE 4.1 Units of Measure and Conversions

Quantity	SI (International) unit	Conversion multiplier	Traditional (British) unit	Conversion multiplier	SI (International) unit
Distance	meter	× 3.28 =	foot	× 0.3048 =	meter
Angle	radian	× 57.3 =	degree	× 0.0175 =	radian
Velocity	meters/second	× 2.24 =	miles/hour	× 0.447 =	meters/second
Force	newton	× 0.225 =	pound	× 4.45 =	newton
Force	kilogram (kgf)	× 2.205 =	pound	× 0.4535 =	kilogram (kgf)
Work, energy	joule	× 0.738 =	foot-pound	× 1.356 =	joule
Power	watt	× 0.0013 =	horsepower	× 745.7 =	watt
Torque	newton-meter	× 0.738 =	foot-pound	× 1.356 =	newton-meter

known as Imperial, British, or English) system is sometimes used. Standard units of measure in each of these systems, along with conversion factors, are presented in table 4.1.

We highlight one particular unit of measure, the kilogram, which can be a source of confusion. The potential confusion arises from the relation between mass (a quantity of matter) and weight (a measure of the effect of gravity on a mass). In the SI system, kilogram (kg) is the unit of mass, with weight measured in newtons (N) of force. Kilogram is also used, however, in some contexts as a unit of force (rather than mass). In the weight room, for example, barbell plates are commonly identified as 10 kg, 20 kg, and so on. In this context, kilogram (kg) is used as a unit measure of force. Thus, the term *kilogram* is used as both a unit of mass (quantity of matter, or kgm) and a unit of force (kg plates in a weight room, or kgf).

Force

Force, a fundamental element in human movement mechanics, is defined as a mechanical action or effect applied to a body that tends to produce acceleration. Many forces are relevant to personal trainers as they work with clients. These include *internal forces* acting inside the body (e.g., muscle, tendon, ligament) and *external forces,* those acting from the outside (e.g., gravity, **friction**, air resistance). The standard SI unit of force is the newton (N). The traditional system measures force in pounds (lb). One pound equals 4.45 N.

The effect of forces in producing, controlling, or altering human movement depends on the combined effect of seven force-related factors (33):

- Magnitude (how much force is produced or applied)
- Location (where on a body or structure the force is applied)
- Direction (where the force is directed)
- Duration (during a single force application, how long the force is applied)
- Frequency (how many times the force is applied in a given time period)
- Variability (if the magnitude of the force is constant or changing over the application period)
- Rate (how quickly the force is produced or applied)

Force is a fundamental mechanical element in human movement, with forces acting both internally and externally upon the body in motion

Newton's Laws of Motion

Mechanical analysis of human movement is based largely on the work of Sir Isaac Newton (1642-1727). Most notably, Newton's three laws of motion form the foundation for classical mechanics and provide the rules that govern the physics of human movement. Newton's laws of motion are as follows:

- First law of motion: A body at rest or in motion tends to remain at rest or in motion unless acted upon by an outside force.
- Second law of motion: A net force (ΣF) acting on a body produces an acceleration (*a*) proportional to the force according to the equation

$$\Sigma F = m \times a \qquad (4.1)$$

(where *m* = mass). In other words, force equals mass times acceleration.

- Third law of motion: For every action there is an equal and opposite reaction.

Newton's laws of motion apply to all human movements. The first law of motion essentially dictates that forces are required to start, stop, or modify body movements. When a jumper leaves the ground, for example, a force (gravity) acts to slow the upward movement until the jumper reaches his or her peak, and then continues to act in accelerating the jumper's body toward the ground for landing.

Newton's second law of motion is seen in a lifting task (e.g., deadlift). The individual must exert enough force to overcome the force of gravity and accelerate the barbell upward. The equation $F = m \times a$ can be used to determine the magnitude of bar acceleration. A greater force (F) will produce a proportionally greater acceleration (a).

Newton's third law of motion says that every force produces an equal and opposite reaction force. In running, for example, at each foot contact, the foot exerts a force on the ground. The ground equally and oppositely reacts against the runner's foot to produce what is termed a *ground reaction force*. The magnitude and direction of the ground reaction force determine the runner's acceleration.

Momentum and Impulse

Momentum characterizes a body's "quantity of motion." In general, the larger the body and the faster it is moving, the greater its momentum. In mechanical terms, *linear momentum* is calculated as the product of mass (m) and velocity (v). Increasing either a body's size (mass) or velocity increases its linear momentum. Similarly, *angular momentum* is the product of moment of inertia (I) and **angular velocity** (ω), where I is the resistance to a change in a body's state of angular motion. The magnitude of the moment of inertia depends on two factors: (1) body mass and (2) the distribution of the mass relative to the axis of rotation. The effect of mass distribution can be seen in the swinging of a softball bat. The resistance to rotation is greatest when the bat is swung with hands at the handle end of the bat. If the batter "chokes up" on the bat by sliding his or her hands up the handle toward the barrel, it will be easier to swing—even though the mass is the same—because more of the bat's mass is closer to the rotational axis (the hands). Similarly, turning the bat over and swinging it with hands on the barrel would be even easier because most of the bat's mass is located close to the hands.

From a performance perspective, the principle of momentum *transfer* is essential. *Transfer of momentum* is the mechanism by which momentum is transferred from one body to another. In a throwing motion, for example, a softball pitcher transfers momentum sequentially from the legs and torso to the upper arm, to the forearm, and eventually to the hand and the ball at pitch release. Another example of momentum transfer can be seen when someone "cheats" during a maximal bicep curl exercise. By rocking his or her body prior to the actual elbow flexion, the person can transfer momentum to the barbell and allow more weight to be curled than would be possible in the absence of prior body movement.

To change (either increase or decrease) momentum, a mechanical *impulse* must be applied. Impulse is the product of force (F) multiplied by time (t). Thus, increasing the amount of applied force or the time of force application results in a greater change in momentum.

Torque

As described earlier, force is the mechanical agent responsible for linear movements. For angular motion, the analogous mechanical agent is termed **torque** (T), or **moment of force** (M, usually shortened to "moment"), and is defined as the effect of a force that tends to cause rotation or twisting about an axis. Despite the fact that there is a technical difference between the two terms (i.e., *moment* typically refers to the rotational or bending action of a force; *torque* refers to the twisting action of a force), the two terms often are used interchangeably. For simplicity and brevity, we will use the term *torque* throughout this chapter.

The turning effects of torques are evident throughout the human musculoskeletal system. At the knee, for example, the quadriceps muscle group creates a torque that tends to extend the joint. The hamstring muscle group generates a torque that tends to flex the knee. The flexor torque created by the hamstrings is illustrated in figure 4.3b.

> **Torque creates an angular acceleration similar to the way force creates a linear acceleration.**

The magnitude of torque (T) is calculated as the mathematical product of force (F) times moment arm (d):

$$T = F \times d \qquad \textbf{(4.2)}$$

The **moment arm** is defined as the perpendicular distance (d) from the fulcrum (axis) to the **line of force action**. The standard unit of torque, or moment, arises from the product of the two component terms: force in newtons (N) and moment arm in meters (m). Thus, the unit of torque is the newton-meter (N·m). In the traditional (British) system, torque is measured in foot-pounds (ft-lb).

Careful consideration of the torque equation (4.2) reveals several concepts that are important for human movement mechanics. First, the magnitude of the torque depends on two variables (F and d).

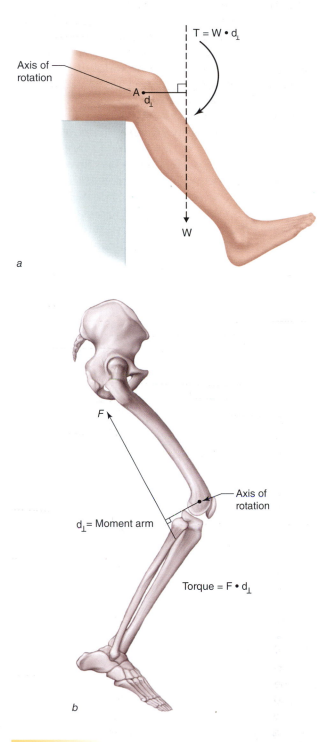

$$T = W \cdot d_{\perp}$$

Axis of rotation

A

$d_{\perp}$

W

a

F

$d_{\perp}$ = Moment arm

Axis of rotation

Torque = $F \cdot d_{\perp}$

b

FIGURE 4.3 (a) Torque calculation at the knee when the line of force action is perpendicular. (b) Torque calculation when the force is not perpendicular involves using trigonometric functions.

Adapted by permission from Whiting and Zernicke 1998.

To increase torque, one can increase either the force or the moment arm or both. Conversely, to decrease torque, one can decrease the force, decrease the moment arm, or both.

A second torque-related concept involves instances when a force is applied *through* the axis of rotation. In this case, the moment arm is zero and no torque is produced. At human joints, this leads to a situation in which body tissues (e.g., bone) can be subjected to high forces, but with no torque created. Compressive forces acting through the center of a vertebral body, for example, will create no vertebral rotation but may subject the vertebral body to increased risk of injury (22).

A third torque-related concept arises from the fact that in most human movement situations, more than one torque is being applied. The resulting movement of a body subjected to multiple torques is based on the *net torque* (also *net moment*), which is simply the mathematical sum of all the component torques. An example of net torque is shown in figure 4.4. In this example, the person is holding his arm in 90°

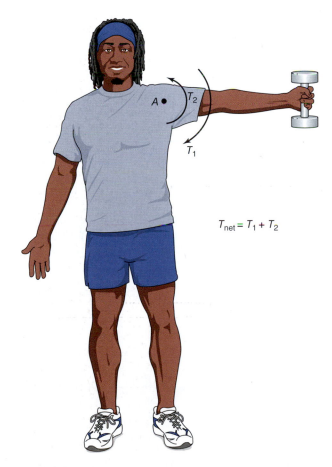

A

T_2

T_1

$$T_{net} = T_1 + T_2$$

FIGURE 4.4 Net torque calculated as the sum of all component moments acting about a joint axis.

Adapted by permission from Whiting and Zernicke 1998.

of abduction. Gravity, acting on both the arm and dumbbell, creates a torque (T_1) about the glenohumeral axis that tends to adduct the arm. If T_1 was the only torque, the arm would adduct under the effect of gravity. To maintain the arm in the abducted position, the abductor muscles (e.g., middle deltoid, supraspinatus) need to create an equal and opposite torque to oppose the torque created by gravity. This counterbalancing torque (T_2) created by the abductors in this example tends to abduct the arm.

The shoulder movement that results depends on the relative magnitudes of these two torques (T_1 and T_2). Adding the torques creates a net torque at the joint. If T_1 and T_2 are equal in magnitude (but opposite in direction), the net torque is zero and the arm maintains its abducted position (i.e., no movement occurs). If the gravitational torque (T_1) is greater than that created by the abductors (T_2), the net torque favors gravity and the arm will adduct. If the torque created by the abductors (T_2) exceeds the gravitational torque (T_1), the net torque favors the muscle action and the arm will further abduct.

The relevance of torque-related concepts is of critical importance to the assessment of human movements and the design of exercise programs. This topic will be discussed in further detail later in the chapter.

> Joint motions are produced and controlled by the net effect of internal (muscle) torques and external torques created by forces such as gravity.

Lever Systems

With an understanding of the concept of torque, one can visualize joint motion typically resulting from the body's anatomical structures acting as a system of mechanical levers. A **lever** is defined as a rigid structure, fixed at a single point (*fulcrum* or *axis*), to which two forces are applied (figure 4.5). In terms of human movement, the rigid structure is a bone moving about its axis of rotation. One of the forces (F_A) is commonly termed the *applied force* (also *effort force*) and is produced by active muscle. The other force (F_R), referred to as the *resistance force* (also *load*), is produced by the weight being lifted (i.e., gravity) or another external force being applied (e.g., friction, elastic band).

These three lever system components (F_A, F_R, fulcrum) can be spatially arranged in three different configurations. Each of these unique configurations is termed a *lever class*. In a **first-class lever,** the fulcrum is located between the two forces (figure 4.6). A **second-class lever** has F_R located between the fulcrum and F_A (figure 4.7). In a **third-class lever,** F_A lies between the fulcrum and F_R (figure 4.8). Joints in the human body are predominantly third-class levers, with some first-class levers and relatively few second-class levers.

The distances between components are irrelevant in terms of defining the lever class. However, the distances between components are critically important in determining the mechanical function of a joint. To help illustrate this, we introduce the concept of **mechanical advantage,** which is defined as the ratio $F_R : F_A$ (or alternatively as the ratio [F_A moment arm : F_R moment arm]). If the mechanical advantage is equal to 1, the moment arms of the resistance force and applied force are equal, and neither force has an advantage. If the mechanical advantage is less than 1, the resistance force is at an advantage and the applied force will need to be greater than the resistance force to overcome the resistance. Conversely, if the mechanical advantage is greater than 1, the applied force has an advantage over the resistive force. For first-class levers, the

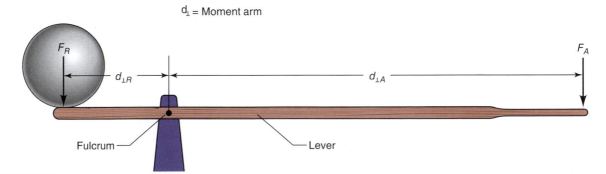

$d_\perp$ = Moment arm

FIGURE 4.5 A lever. Force exerted perpendicular to the lever at one contact point is resisted by another force at a different contact point. F_A = force applied to the lever; $d_{\perp A}$ = moment arm of the applied force; F_R = force resisting the lever's rotation; $d_{\perp R}$ = moment arm of the resistive force.

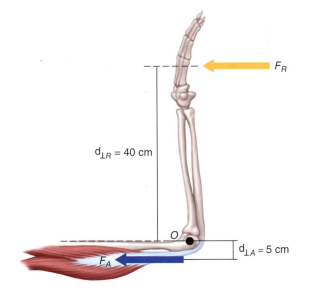

$d_{\perp R} = 40$ cm

F_R

O

$d_{\perp A} = 5$ cm

F_A

FIGURE 4.6 A first-class lever (the forearm): extending the elbow against resistance.

Reprinted by permission from NSCA 2008.

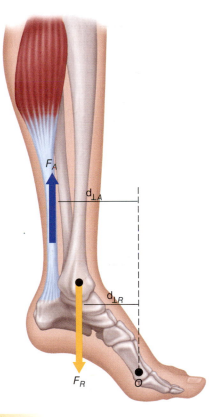

F_A

$d_{\perp A}$

$d_{\perp R}$

F_R

O

FIGURE 4.7 A second-class lever: the foot during plantar flexion against resistance, as when one is standing up on the toes. F_A = muscle force; F_R= resistive force; $d_{\perp A}$ = moment arm of the muscle force; $d_{\perp R}$ = moment arm of the resistive force. When the body is raised, the ball of the foot, being the point about which the foot rotates, is the fulcrum (O). Because $d_{\perp A}$ is greater than $d_{\perp R}$, F_A is less than F_R.

Reprinted by permission from NSCA 2008.

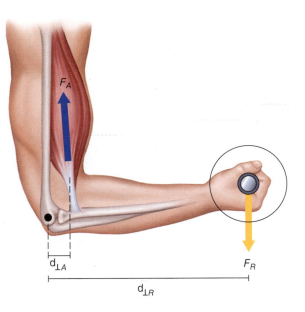

F_A

$d_{\perp A}$

$d_{\perp R}$

F_R

FIGURE 4.8 A third-class lever: the forearm during the arm curl exercise. F_A = muscle force; F_R = resistive force; $d_{\perp A}$ = moment arm of the muscle force; $d_{\perp R}$ = moment arm of the resistive force. Because $d_{\perp A}$ is much smaller than $d_{\perp R}$, F_A must be much greater than F_R.

Reprinted by permission from NSCA 2008.

force with the longer moment arm will have the mechanical advantage. For second-class levers, the applied force always has the mechanical advantage. For third-class levers, the resistance force always has the mechanical advantage.

Work

Work is a term with multiple meanings, ranging from a place of employment (e.g., "I'm going to work tomorrow") to physical effort ("I'm working really hard") to energy expenditure ("I worked off 300 calories while cycling"). Mechanically, however, work has a specific definition related to how much force is applied and how far an object moves. Mechanical **work** (*W*) is defined as the product of force (*F*) times the distance (*d*) through which an object moves:

$$W = F \times d$$ (4.3)

The standard unit of work is the joule (1 J = 1 N·m). A person performing a bench press, for example, who lifts 800 N (~180 pounds) through a distance of 0.5 m (~20 inches) has performed 400 J of mechanical work (figure 4.9).

In a free-weight exercise, the vertical displacement can be measured by the difference in the bar's highest point and its lowest point during each repetition (e.g., d_{AB} in figure 4.9). For a weight stack

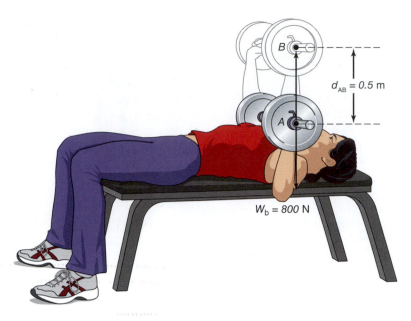

FIGURE 4.9   Calculation of work during resistance exercise.
Reprinted by permission from Whiting and Zernicke 2008.

machine, the high and low points of the stack can be used to measure the vertical displacement.

In addition to the weight being lifted, consideration should be given to the portion of the person's body weight that is being moved, or lifted. In a squat, for example, the lower extremities are lifting both the barbell and a large portion of the person's own body weight with each repetition. With a leg press machine, the structure and geometry of the device dictate how much of a client's body weight is involved. If a client is pushing horizontally to lift a weight stack, little of his or her body weight is involved. In contrast, in an inclined sled-type leg press device, the amount of body weight being lifted during the lift varies with the degree of sled inclination.

Power

Mechanical work alone does not always completely describe the mechanics of a particular movement. In the bench press example presented in the previous section, the exerciser performed 400 J of work during each up phase. In a set of 10 repetitions bench pressing the 800 N weight, the person performs 400 J of work each rep. If the first rep takes 1 second and the last rep takes 2 seconds, there clearly is a mechanical difference between the lifts, despite the fact that the work is the same (400 J) for the two reps. The difference is not in the amount of work performed, but in the rate at which the work is performed. The rate of work, termed mechanical

power (P), is calculated as the amount of work (W) divided by the time (t) needed to do the work:

$$P = W / t \qquad \textbf{(4.4)}$$

The standard unit of power is the watt (1 W = 1 J/s). In the bench press example, the up phase of the first rep would have a power of 400 W (400 J / 1 s), while the last rep would have a lower power of 200 W (400 J / 2 s). In the traditional (British) system, power is measured in *horsepower* (hp), where 1 hp = 550 ft-lb/s.

Power may also be calculated as the product of force (F) and velocity (v):

$$P = F \times v \qquad \textbf{(4.5)}$$

Many high-speed movement tasks (e.g., jumping, throwing) require high power output. To produce powerful movements and to train for power, a person must generate high forces while moving at a high rate of speed (i.e., high velocity). Many general fitness exercises, such as swimming, walking, and yoga, are performed at relatively slow speeds and therefore are not appropriate for enhancing power. "Explosive" exercises such as power cleans and snatches, martial arts kicking and punching, and various forms of jumping are much more conducive to power development.

As an interesting aside, it should be noted that the sport of *powerlifting,* despite its name, should be classified as a strength sport, and not a power sport. The three events in powerlifting competitions are the squat, bench press, and deadlift. At maximal levels, none of these lifts is performed quickly. Thus, while tremendous strength certainly is required for powerlifting success, the power output is two to three times lower than for the Olympic lifts (14).

Energy

Energy is another term with multiple meanings. A child, for example, may be very energetic, or a worker at the end of the day may have run out of energy. Mechanical energy, however (as is the case with mechanical work), has a specific meaning. **Mechanical energy** is defined as the ability, or capacity, to perform mechanical work. Of the many types of energy (e.g., chemical, nuclear, electromagnetic), mechanical energy is the form most commonly used in the description and assessment of human movement. Mechanical energy can be classified as either kinetic energy (energy of motion) or potential energy (energy of position or deformation). Consistent with the two forms of motion, there are two types of kinetic energy. *Linear kinetic energy* (LKE) is measured as

$$LKE = \tfrac{1}{2} \times m \times v^2 \qquad (4.6)$$

where m = mass and v = linear velocity. *Angular kinetic energy* (AKE) is defined as

$$AKE = \tfrac{1}{2} \times I \times \omega^2 \qquad (4.7)$$

where I = moment of inertia and ω = angular velocity. An important element of these two kinetic energy equations is the squaring of the velocity terms (v and ω). A comparatively small increase in v and ω can result in a considerable increase in kinetic energy. For example, a runner who speeds up from 5 m/s to 6 m/s (a 20% increase) would increase his or her linear kinetic energy by 44%.

Potential energy can take two forms. The first form, potential energy of position, is termed *gravitational potential energy* and measures the potential to perform mechanical work as a function of a body's height above a reference level (usually the ground). Thus, a barbell held overhead with arms fully extended has more gravitational potential energy than the same barbell held at chest level.

The magnitude of gravitational potential energy (*PE*) is calculated as

$$PE = m \times g \times h \qquad (4.8)$$

where m equals mass, g equals gravitational acceleration (~9.81 m/s^2), and h equals height (in meters) above the reference level.

The second form of potential energy, termed *deformational* (also *strain*) *energy*, is energy stored within a body when it is deformed (i.e., stretched, compressed, bent, twisted). Examples of deformational energy include a stretched calcaneal (Achilles) tendon, a pole-vaulter's bent pole, and a compressed intervertebral disc. When the force that caused the deformation is removed, the body typically returns to its original (unloaded) shape or configuration and in doing so releases, or returns, some of the stored deformational energy. The stored energy is not totally returned, as some of it is lost as heat energy. Deformational energy storage and return is important in many movement tasks, as illustrated in the stretch–shortening cycle explained later in this chapter.

Mechanical and Movement Efficiency

In biomechanical terms, **efficiency** refers to how much mechanical output (work) can be produced with use of a given amount of metabolic input (energy). The ratio of mechanical output to metabolic input defines the efficiency of a movement task. Human skeletal muscle, for example, is only about 25% efficient. In practical terms, this means that only one-quarter of the metabolic energy involved in muscle activity goes toward performing mechanical work. The remaining three-quarters is converted to heat or used in energy recovery processes (9).

In addition to the relative inefficiency of muscle in performing mechanical work, several actions or conditions also contribute to movement inefficiency (32). These include

- muscular coactivation (**antagonist** muscle action that works against **agonist** muscle action on the opposite side of a joint),
- jerky movements (alternating changes of direction requiring metabolic energy to accelerate and decelerate limb segments),
- extraneous movements (excessive arm movements during running above and beyond those needed for balance),
- isometric actions (in isometric tasks, there is no displacement, and thus no mechanical work is produced), and
- excessive center of gravity excursions (metabolic energy required to raise and lower the body's center of gravity beyond that minimally required for a given task).

Biomechanics of Human Movement

The laws of mechanics govern the way we move. However, personal trainers need to appreciate that humans are biological beings and not machines.

Unique characteristics of the muscular system affect how we generate forces and torques. We begin this section by discussing the structure and function of muscle.

Muscle

Skeletal (striated) muscle makes up a substantial portion (40-45%) of body weight and performs many necessary functions (e.g., movement, protection, heat production). With regard to human movement, muscle generates the forces required to move limb segments at major joints and stabilize body regions. Understanding the roles of muscle is essential to the work of personal trainers.

Muscle tissue has four distinguishing characteristics: (1) *excitability,* the ability to respond to a stimulus; (2) *contractility,* the ability to generate a pulling force (also called *tension*); (3) *extensibility,* the ability to lengthen, or stretch; and (4) *elasticity,* the ability to return to its original length and shape when the force is removed. Absence or compromise of any of these properties affects muscle's ability to produce and control human movements.

Muscular action is largely under voluntary control, but may also be involved in reflex (e.g., rapid response to a painful stimulus) and stereotypical (e.g., automatic nonreflex actions such as walking) movements.

Muscle Architecture

Muscle tissue is composed of structural elements that can generate force (*contractile components*), as well as other structures (e.g., connective tissue) that cannot produce force (*noncontractile components*) but are nonetheless important to the proper physiological and mechanical function of muscle. The hierarchical structure of muscle is depicted in figure 1.1 on page 4 of chapter 1, with a single muscle fiber shown in figure 1.2 on page 5. The functional unit for force production within the myofibril is the sarcomere (figure 1.3, p. 5).

The fibers within muscle are arranged in a variety of ways (figure 4.10). In some muscles (e.g., biceps brachii, semitendinosus), the muscle fibers run parallel to a line between the muscle's origin and insertion (line of pull). These muscles are categorized as *fusiform.* In other muscles, the fibers are arranged at an angle (normally <30°) to the line of pull. This angle is termed the **pennation angle.** A unipennate muscle such as the semimembranosus has a single set of fibers, all with the same line of pull. Bipennate muscles such as the rectus femoris have two sets of fibers with different angles. Multipennate muscles (e.g., deltoid) have many sets of fibers acting at a variety of angles. Other muscles, such as the pectoralis major and latissimus dorsi, have a radiating fiber arrangement.

Pennation proves advantageous by allowing more muscle fibers to be packed into a given volume and increasing force production potential by providing a greater functional cross-sectional area than nonpennate muscles. Resistance training cannot change a muscle's architecture. Understanding structural differences, however, can help personal trainers recognize a muscle's function and potential for injury. The quadriceps group, for example, is designed for force production, whereas the hamstring group is better suited for rapid shortening. These design differences place the two-joint hamstrings (composed of the semitendinosus, semimembranosus, and biceps femoris long head) at greater injury risk than the primarily one-joint quadriceps (composed of the vastus medialis, vastus lateralis, and vastus intermedius) during explosive, high-power tasks such as sprinting and jumping.

Types of Muscle Action

The forces generated by muscle are resisted by external forces such as weights, cables, bands, and resistance machines. The net torque created by internal (muscle) and external (resistance) forces dictates the resultant joint motion. If the net torque is zero, the muscle action is isometric, and there is no joint movement. If the torque produced by muscle is greater than that created by the external forces, the muscle action is concentric (active muscle shortening). Conversely, if the torque created by the external resistance exceeds that produced by the muscles, the muscle action is eccentric (active muscle lengthening).

The type of muscle action determines the type of mechanical work produced. Positive work occurs if the muscular force and the displacement are in the same direction. During positive work, energy is generated by the muscles and transferred to the segments (26) by **concentric muscle actions.** In contrast, negative work occurs if the muscular force and displacement are in opposite directions. During negative work, energy is transferred to the muscles from segments. This energy is being absorbed by the muscles through **eccentric muscle actions.** During **isometric muscle actions,** there is no joint movement and, by definition, no work. However, these muscle actions are important in the transfer of energy between segments. In cycling, for example, if one is pedaling with toe clips, there is little to no movement of the ankle joint, but the gastrocnemius and soleus are producing high forces. These muscular forces transfer energy

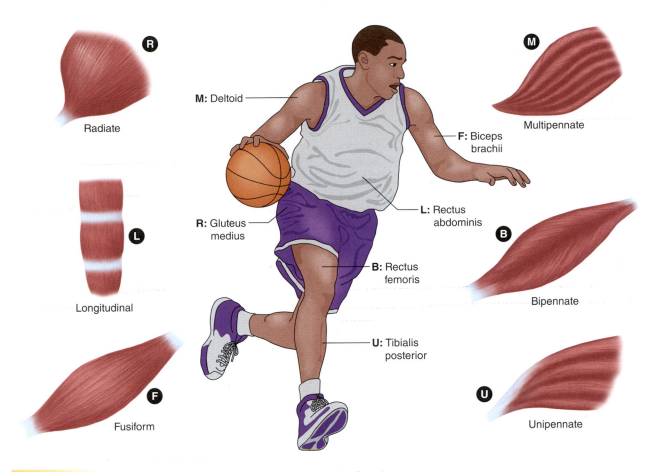

FIGURE 4.10 Muscle fiber arrangements and an example of each.

generated by the gluteals and quadriceps to the pedal (13).

> The type of muscle action (isometric, concentric, eccentric) is an important factor in the production and control of joint motion, and in the transfer of energy between body segments during movements.

Length-Tension

The contractile component (actin-myosin) of muscle generates force. The elements of the noncontractile component (e.g., connective tissue sheaths, tendon, titin proteins) also contribute to the overall force profile of the musculotendinous unit. The combined effect of all the muscle's structural elements is reflected in the *length–tension* relation, which basically says that the force produced by the musculotendinous unit is determined, in part, by the muscle's length. A schematic length–tension curve is shown in figure 4.11.

The inverted-U–shaped *active component* represents the contribution of the sarcomeres in producing force. If a sarcomere is too short, there is (1) complete overlap between the actin filaments, (2) myosin filament pressure against the Z-lines, and (3) diminished capacity for myosin binding, all resulting in reduced force production. As the sarcomere lengthens, it reaches a range of optimal filament

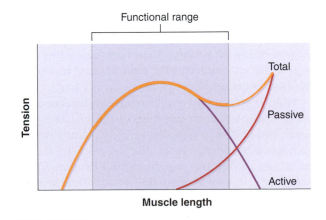

FIGURE 4.11 Length–tension relationship of skeletal muscle.

overlap and maximum force production. As the sarcomere further lengthens, actin-filament overlap decreases and force production drops.

The noncontractile component does not contribute to the muscle's force profile until the muscle is stretched past its resting length, as reflected in the right side of the length–tension curve (figure 4.11). In this portion of the curve, the passive, noncontractile elements want to recoil and thus produce resistive tension. The musculotendinous unit's total force production is reflected by the summation of the active contractile and passive noncontractile components.

Clearly there is a limit to the length a muscle can attain, dictated by the range of motion of the joints the muscle crosses. This results in a *functional range* of muscle length as shown in figure 4.11.

Application of the length–tension relation is readily seen in the following example comparing a calf raise exercise in a standing position to one in a seated position. The gastrocnemius (GA) crosses (i.e., has action at) two joints as a knee flexor and an ankle plantarflexor. In a standing position, the GA assumes a lengthened position and can generate substantially more force than when the knee is flexed in the seated calf raise and the GA is shortened. In the seated calf raise, with the GA's role diminished due to its shorter length, greater demand is placed on the single-joint soleus.

Force-Velocity

In addition to its length, a muscle's ability to generate force depends on its velocity, or speed, of contraction. Each point on a *force–velocity* curve (figure 4.12) represents the maximal force the muscle can produce at the given velocity when the muscle is maximally activated. During concentric muscle actions, faster muscle velocities are associated with lower force production. During isometric muscle actions, more force is produced than at any concentric speed. Eccentrically, muscles are capable of generating more force than they can either concentrically or isometrically, and appear to be less affected by movement speed.

The force–velocity relationship can be illustrated using a simple bicep curl exercise. With no weight in hand, elbow flexion happens quickly. As successively heavier weights are held, the velocity of flexion decreases. When the weight cannot be moved, the exerciser is at, or very near, his or her isometric maximum. At even higher weights, the muscles cannot lift the weight or even hold it in a set position. They can only control elbow extension in eccentric action consistent with higher forces found in the eccentric portion of the force–velocity curve.

The larger forces generated with eccentric muscle action form the basis for "negative" training. When negatives are performed, either the resistance is increased during the lowering phase or some form of assistance is given during the raising phase. This type of training is an effective means of increasing strength and hypertrophy (16).

Fiber Type and Specific Tension

The maximum force production capability of a muscle is proportional to its cross-sectional area. Theoretically, multiplying the cross-sectional area (cm^2) by the force of contraction per unit area (N/cm^2) would yield the force (N) of the muscle. The force of contraction per unit area is known as *specific tension* (20). Research on isolated motor units has shown that fast-twitch muscle fibers have a higher specific tension ($22\ N/cm^2$) than slow-twitch muscle fibers ($15\ N/cm^2$) (5). Whole muscles have highly variable specific tensions (21). This finding is not surprising, considering that whole muscles in humans have a mix of fiber types. Based on current evidence, muscles that are predominantly fast-twitch will have only a slightly higher specific tension than muscles that are predominantly slow-twitch (20). However, fast-twitch fibers tend to be larger than slow-twitch fibers, so the absolute tension they can develop is greater.

Recruitment

Both intramuscular and intermuscular coordination play a role in the maximum amount of force a muscle can produce. Intramuscularly, or within a muscle, force can be increased by (1) increasing

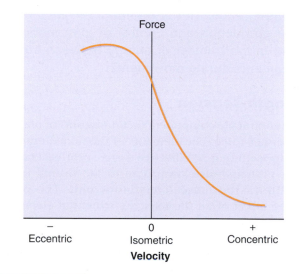
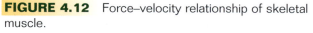

FIGURE 4.12   Force–velocity relationship of skeletal muscle.

Reprinted by permission from Whiting and Rugg 2005.

the firing frequency of the motor unit, (2) increasing the number of motor units recruited, and (3) recruiting progressively larger motor units. Intermuscularly, or among more than one muscle, force can be increased by increasing the activation of the agonists and synergists, decreasing the activation of antagonists, or both. During the first few weeks of training, much of the improvement in strength gains is attributed to these neural adaptations (23), because the increase in strength gains exceeds the increase in muscle fiber size.

Personal trainers need to be cognizant of this fact. A client may be greatly encouraged by large, initial increases in strength but become discouraged with the slower rate of improvement that follows. In addition to providing encouragement, the personal trainer should educate the client about how the slower gains due to hypertrophy will result in enhanced strength and improved physical appearance.

Time History of Activation

Muscular force development is not instantaneous; it takes time. Maximal muscle force can take up to 0.5 seconds to develop (31). If an activity lasts less than 0.5 seconds, maximal muscular force will not be attained. In such instances, the rate of force development (RFD) is an important quality in determining performance. *Rate of force development* can be defined as the time rate of change of force, or the ratio of the change in force over the change in time. Rate of force development should not be confused with power. Force can be quickly developed isometrically, for example, yet power would be zero since there is no muscle length change. The RFD can be improved with resistance exercise (31).

Another means of enhancing RFD is through use of the stretch–shortening cycle (SSC). The SSC requires an eccentric muscle action immediately followed by a concentric muscle action. Enhanced force production using the SSC has been attributed to storage of elastic energy and enhanced neural drive (6). During eccentric muscle action, the muscle is developing force, so the muscle does not commence concentric action with zero force. This can be thought of as "pre-forcing" the muscle (34).

This pre-forcing can be seen in the bench press or squat inside a squat rack, when it is harder to lift the bar from the bottom position if it is resting on the supports (with no muscle action). The lift is slightly easier if the muscles are tensed prior to lifting the bar (by holding it above the support, for example) because the muscles are pre-forced, and it is easier still if the bar is quickly reversed at the bottom position due to the combined effects of pre-forcing the muscle and the recoil of the elastic components of the muscle–tendon complex.

Moment Arms and Levers of the Human Body

Moment arms can vary considerably among individuals. For example, Bassett and colleagues demonstrated that the standard deviation of the moment arm of the supraspinatus was 52% of the mean (3). This fact may help explain why two people can have similar muscle sizes but different levels of strength. A person with a larger moment arm (tendinous insertions farther away from the joint) can produce more torque for the same level of muscular force. This principle is illustrated in figure 4.13.

Figure 4.13 also demonstrates another important point: Although the distances between a muscle and its tendinous insertions are fixed, the moment arms of that muscle change as a function of joint angle (1). By extension, the torque-producing capability of a muscle also changes as a function of joint angle. Greater torque can be produced at some points in the range of motion than at others.

Recall that there are three classifications of lever systems. The importance of classifying human joints by lever class goes beyond mere application of classical mechanics to anatomical structures. Each lever class has advantages and disadvantages with respect to human movement capabilities. For example, third-class levers in the human body (e.g., biceps brachii acting at the elbow joint) have the applied (muscle) force between the elbow joint axis (fulcrum) and the resistance force (e.g., dumbbell held in the hand). In this structural arrangement, the *mechanical advantage* (F_A moment arm / F_R moment arm) is much less than 1. In practical terms, this means that given its short moment arm, the muscle must generate a relatively high force to create flexion at the elbow. This apparent disadvantage of an anatomical third-class lever is offset by the joint's ability to increase the effective speed (velocity) of movement. During elbow extension, for example, a given angular displacement produces different linear displacements for points along the forearm and hand. Points farther away from the joint axis move a greater distance along the curved arc than do points closer to the axis. Since all points along the forearm move with the same *angular velocity,* the more distal points (e.g., dumbbell) have higher *linear velocities.* This movement advantage is used by baseball pitchers and volleyball spikers to generate high hand velocities prior to ball release and contact, respectively.

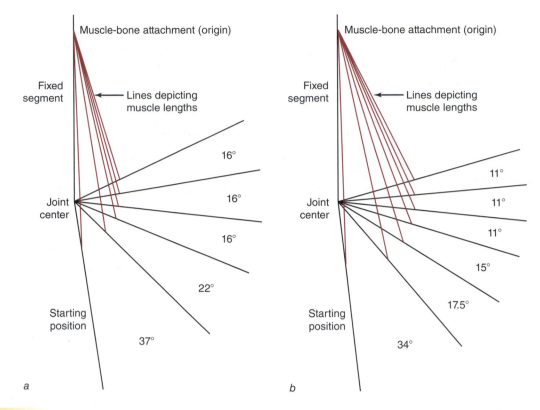

FIGURE 4.13 Changes in joint angle with equal increments of muscle shortening when the tendon is inserted *(a)* closer to and *(b)* farther from the joint center. Configuration *b* has a larger moment arm and thus greater torque for a given muscle force, but less rotation per unit of muscle contraction and thus slower movement speed.

Reprinted by permission from NSCA 2008.

Strength and Sticking Points

With respect to human performance, *strength* generally refers to the ability to exert force. Measurement of strength ranges from simple methods (e.g., how much weight a person can lift) to more complex methods available using technological advances such as force transducers, accelerometers, and **isokinetic** devices. Given the complexities of muscle force production, and given that force generation depends on the speed of muscle action and adaptations to resistance training (2, 11, 25), a more precise definition of strength is the maximal force that a muscle or muscle group can generate at a specified velocity (17). In practical terms, it is not always possible to measure velocity while measuring strength. In such cases, older and simpler methods are still used.

Expressing strength is usually limited to the amount that can be lifted through the weakest point in the range of motion, termed the *sticking point* (or *sticking region*). Determining the sticking point is difficult; it is not simply the point in the range or motion where the external resistance has the largest moment arm (8) because that may also be the same point in the range of motion where the muscle's moment arm is largest. Rather, the sticking point probably occurs where the external resistance has the greatest mechanical advantage compared to the muscle.

Kinematic and Kinetic Chains

In engineering, a series of linkages is referred to as a *kinematic* chain. If the two ends of the series are fixed, the chain is said to be *closed*. If the terminal end of one link is not fixed, the chain is said to be *open*. A functional consequence of a closed chain is that movement of one joint will cause every other joint to move in a predictable fashion. Open chains are not subject to these constraints: Movement at one joint will not necessarily cause movement at another joint.

In the mid-1950s, Steindler (28) suggested that the body operates as a *kinetic* chain. He described an open kinetic chain as "a combination in which the terminal joint is free" and a closed kinetic chain as one "in which the terminal joint meets some considerable external resistance which prohibits or restrains free movement." Steindler noted that a chain is only "strictly and absolutely closed" when no visible motion is produced, yet he believed it was acceptable to "apply the term in all situations in which the peripheral joint of the chain meets with overwhelming external resistance." This is often interpreted as the terminal segment (hand, foot) being fixed.

Note that Steindler used the term *kinetic* (forces), whereas engineers use the term *kinematic* (motion), yet they appear to be talking about the same thing. "Kinetic chain" is not used in engineering or robotics, because kinematic chain is the technically correct description. Yet the term *kinetic chain* is used more often in exercise publications, if not interchangeably with *kinematic chain*.

Steindler acknowledged that the chain is rarely "strictly and absolutely closed." This is apparent if we look at the physical description, yet his definition is still confusing because he never described "considerable" external resistance. For example, the squat and leg press are kinematically and kinetically similar (10), yet the terminal segment (foot) is fixed during the squat and moving during the leg press. Similarly, the bench press and push-up have similar muscle activation patterns throughout the range of motion (4) even when the resistance could hardly be characterized as "considerable."

One could garner more utility from the terms by looking at the functional consequences rather than physical descriptions of the motion. An open chain is one in which movement of one joint is independent of the other joints in the chain, while a closed chain is one in which movement of one joint causes the other joints in the chain to move in a predictable manner (20). Thus, an open chain movement usually involves a single joint moving (e.g., arm curl, leg curl) against some form of angular resistance. A closed chain movement involves multiple joints moving, usually against a linear resistance (e.g., bench press, squat).

The importance of recognizing a closed chain activity lies in the fact that the motions of multiple joints are coupled (36). For example, during standing in a weight-bearing position and performing a squat motion, flexion of the knee cannot occur without simultaneous flexion of the hip and dorsiflexion of the ankle. A limitation in the range of motion of any one of the joints will affect the range of motion of the entire exercise. Similarly, the torques at the joints are also coupled: As one lowers in the squat position and increases the flexion angles of the joints, all of the muscles in the chain increase their internal torques. Weakness at any one joint will consequently limit performance of the entire movement.

Caution is warranted in using the terms *open chain* and *closed chain*, since there is not universal agreement on how these terms are defined in the literature.

Muscular Control of Movement

One of the essential tasks faced by personal trainers in designing and prescribing exercise programs is identifying which specific muscles are active in producing and controlling movements at a particular joint. As discussed earlier, we know that muscles can act in three modes: isometric, concentric, and eccentric. The concentric muscle actions at major joints are listed in table 4.2. A fundamental skill necessary for personal trainers is to determine for a given joint movement (1) the specific muscles involved and (2) the type of muscle action.

The following muscle control formula provides a step-by-step algorithm for determining muscle involvement and action for any joint movement (32). The formula involves six steps:

Step 1: Identify the joint *movement* (e.g., abduction, flexion) or position.

Step 2: Identify the *effect of the external force* (e.g., gravity) on the joint movement or position by asking the question, "What movement would the external force produce in the absence of muscle action (i.e., if there were no active muscles)?"

Step 3: Identify the *type of muscle action* (concentric, eccentric, isometric) using the answers from step 1 (#1) and step 2 (#2) as follows:

a. If #1 and #2 are in the *opposite* direction, then the muscles are actively shortening in a *concentric action*. Speed of movement is not a factor.

b. If #1 and #2 are in the *same* direction, then ask "What is the speed of movement?"

 1. If the movement is *faster* than what the external force would produce by itself, then the muscles are actively shortening in a *concentric action*.

 2. If the movement is *slower* than what the external force would produce by itself, then the muscles are actively lengthening in an *eccentric action*.

c. If no movement is occurring yet the external force would produce movement if acting by itself, then the muscles are performing an *isometric action*.

TABLE 4.2 Muscle Action Table

I. Hip and knee joint muscle actions

HIP JOINT			
Extension	**Flexion**	**Abduction**	**Lateral rotation**
Gluteus maximus	Psoas major	Gluteus medius	Gluteus maximus
Semitendinosus	Iliacus	*Gluteus minimus*	Piriformis
Semimembranosus	Pectineus	*Tensor fasciae latae*	Gemellus superior
Biceps femoris long head	Rectus femoris	*Gluteus maximus, superior fibers*	Obturator internus
Adductor magnus, posterior fibers	*Adductor brevis*	*Psoas major*	Gemellus inferior
	Adductor longus	*Iliacus*	Obturator externus
	Adductor magnus, anterior upper fibers	*Sartorius*	Quadratus femoris
	Tensor fasciae latae		*Psoas major*
	Sartorius		*Iliacus*
			Sartorius

Adduction	**Medial rotation**
Pectineus	Gluteus minimus
Adductor brevis	*Tensor fasciae latae*
Adductor longus	*Pectineus*
Adductor magnus	*Adductor brevis*
Gracilis	*Adductor longus*
Gluteus maximus, inferior fibers	*Adductor magnus, anterior upper fibers*

KNEE JOINT			
Extension	**Flexion**	**Medial rotation***	**Lateral rotation**
Vastus medialis	Semimembranosus	Popliteus	Biceps femoris
Vastus intermedius	Semitendinosus	Semimembranosus	
Vastus lateralis	Biceps femoris	Semitendinosus	
Rectus femoris	*Sartorius*	*Sartorius*	
	Gracilis	*Gracilis*	
	Popliteus		
	Gastrocnemius		
	Plantaris		

II. Ankle and subtalar joint muscle actions

ANKLE JOINT		SUBTALAR JOINT	
Plantarflexion	**Dorsiflexion**	**Inversion**	**Eversion**
Gastrocnemius	Tibialis anterior	Tibialis anterior	Peroneus longus
Soleus	Extensor digitorum longus	Tibialis posterior	Peroneus brevis
Plantaris	Peroneus tertius	*Flexor hallucis longus*	Peroneus tertius
Tibialis posterior	Extensor hallucis longus	*Flexor digitorum longus*	Extensor digitorum longus
Flexor hallucis longus		*Gastrocnemius*	
Flexor digitorum longus		*Soleus*	
Peroneus longus		*Plantaris*	
Peroneus brevis			

III. Shoulder girdle and shoulder joint muscle actions

SHOULDER GIRDLE

Elevation	Depression	Retraction	Protraction
Levator scapula	Lower trapezius	Rhomboids	Pectoralis minor
Upper trapezius	Pectoralis minor	Middle trapezius	Serratus anterior
Rhomboids			

Upward rotation	Downward rotation		
Trapezius	Rhomboids		
Serratus anterior	Levator scapula		
	Pectoralis minor		

SHOULDER (GLENOHUMERAL) JOINT

Flexion	Extension	Adduction	Abduction
Pectoralis major, clavicular portion	Pectoralis major, sternal portion	Latissimus dorsi	Middle deltoid
Anterior deltoid	Latissimus dorsi	Teres major	Supraspinatus
Biceps brachii, short head	Teres major	Pectoralis major, sternal portion	Anterior deltoid
Coracobrachialis	*Posterior deltoid*		*Biceps brachii*
	Triceps brachii, long head		

Medial rotation	Lateral rotation	Horizontal flexion	Horizontal extension
Latissimus dorsi	Teres minor	Pectoralis major	Middle deltoid
Teres major	Infraspinatus	Anterior deltoid	Posterior deltoid
Subscapularis	*Posterior deltoid*	*Coracobrachialis*	Teres minor
Anterior deltoid		*Biceps brachii, short head*	Infraspinatus
Pectoralis major			*Teres major*
Biceps brachii, short head			*Latissimus dorsi*

IV. Elbow, radioulnar, and wrist joint muscle actions

ELBOW JOINT

Flexion	Extension	Radioulnar joint	
Biceps brachii	Triceps brachii	**Supination**	**Pronation**
Brachialis	*Anconeus*	Biceps brachii	Pronator teres
Brachioradialis		Supinator	Pronator quadratus
		*Brachioradialis***	*Brachioradialis***

WRIST JOINT

Flexion	Extension	Radial deviation (abduction	Ulnar deviation (adduction)
Flexor carpi radialis	Extensor carpi radialis longus	Flexor carpi radialis	Flexor carpi ulnaris
Flexor carpi ulnaris	Extensor carpi radialis brevis	Extensor carpi radialis longus	Extensor carpi ulnaris
Flexor digitorum superficialis	Extensor carpi ulnaris	Extensor carpi radialis brevis	
Flexor digitorum profundus	*Extensor indicis*		
Palmaris longus	*Extensor digiti minimi*		
	Extensor digitorum		

(continued)

TABLE 4.2 *(continued)*

V. Vertebral column muscles actions

VERTEBRAL COLUMN (THORACIC AND LUMBAR REGIONS)			
Flexion	**Lateral flexion**	**Rotation to the same side**	**Rotation to the opposite side**
Rectus abdominis	External oblique	Internal oblique	External oblique
External oblique	Internal oblique	Erector spinae group	Multifidus
Internal oblique	Quadratus lumborum		
Psoas major (lumbar region)	*Rectus abdominis*		
	Erector spinae group		
Extension			
Erector spinae group	Multifidus		

Nonitalicized muscles are considered prime movers. Italicized muscles represent assistant movers.
*Rotation can occur only when the knee is flexed.
**Brachioradialis functions to move the forearm to the mid or neutral position.

d. Movements *across gravity* (i.e., parallel to the ground) with no other external force acting are produced by a *concentric action*. When gravity cannot influence the joint movement in question, shortening (concentric) action is needed to pull the segment against its own inertia. The speed of movement is not a factor.

We have now identified the type of muscle action. Steps 4 through 6 identify which muscles are involved in producing or controlling the movement.

Step 4: Identify the *plane of movement* (frontal, sagittal, transverse) and the *axis of rotation*. The purpose of this step is to identify which side of the joint the muscles controlling the movement cross (e.g., flexors cross one side of a joint, while extensors cross the opposite side).

Step 5: Ask "On which side of the joint axis are muscles lengthening and on which side are they shortening during the movement?"

Step 6: Combine the information from steps 3 and 5 to *determine which muscles must be producing or controlling the movement*. For example, if a concentric (shortening) action is required (from step 3) and the muscles on the anterior side of the joint are shortening (from step 5), then the anterior muscles must be actively producing the movement. The information in table 4.2 allows us to name the specific muscles.

We now apply the muscle control formula to a biceps curl exercise. Consider the simple movement (figure 4.14) of elbow flexion as the person moves the joint from position *a* (elbow fully extended) to position *b* (elbow flexed).

Step 1: The movement is flexion.

Step 2: The external force (gravity) tends to extend the elbow.

Step 3: The movement (flexion) is opposite that created by the external force, so the muscles are actively shortening in *concentric action*.

Step 4: Movement occurs in the sagittal plane about an axis through the elbow joint.

Step 5: The muscles on the joint's anterior surface are shortening during the movement, while the muscles on the posterior side are lengthening.

Step 6: The muscle action is concentric (from step 3), and muscles on the anterior side of the joint are shortening (from step 5). Thus, the anterior muscles actively produce the movement. Information in table 4.2 identifies the biceps brachii, brachialis, and brachioradialis as the muscles responsible for the movement.

Now consider the reverse movement (figure 4.14) going from position *b* to position *a* as the elbow extends. The movement speed is slow (i.e., the movement happens more slowly than it would if the external force were acting by itself in the absence of any muscle action).

Step 1: The movement is extension.

Step 2: The external force (gravity) tends to extend the elbow.

Step 3: The movement (extension) is the same as that created by the external force, so we ask "What is the speed of movement?" The speed is slow, which dictates that the controlling muscles are actively lengthening in an *eccentric action*.

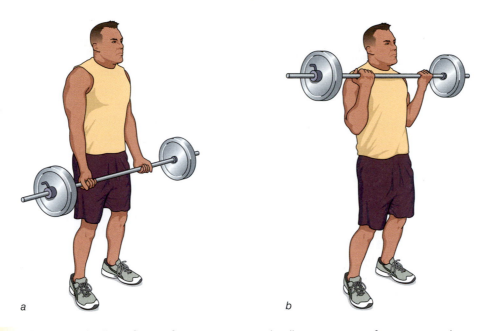

a   b

FIGURE 4.14   Biceps curl: elbow flexion from position *a* to *b*; elbow extension from position *b* to *a*.

Reprinted by permission from Whiting and Rugg 2005.

Step 4: Movement occurs in the sagittal plane about an axis through the elbow joint.

Step 5: The muscles on the anterior side are lengthening, while the muscles on the posterior side are shortening.

Step 6: The muscle action is eccentric (from step 3), and muscles on the anterior side are lengthening (from step 5). Thus the anterior muscles actively control the movement. Thus, the biceps brachii, brachialis, and brachioradialis are the muscles responsible for controlling the movement. In actions such as this, the muscles normally identified as elbow flexors (biceps, brachialis, brachioradialis) act eccentrically to control elbow extension.

If the elbow extension from position *b* to position *a* occurred quickly (i.e., faster than it would if gravity were acting alone), the muscle control formula would dictate concentric action of the elbow extensors (triceps brachii) as producing the rapid extension.

Space constraints preclude inclusion of more than one example here; however, more examples are described by Whiting and Rugg (32).

When prescribing and evaluating specific exercises, personal trainers should keep in mind that variations in lifting and movement technique can affect muscle recruitment. Consider a few examples:

■   To train the elbow flexors (biceps brachii, brachialis, brachioradialis), many exercises are available

(e.g., hammer curls, EZ-bar curls, supinated curls, reverse [pronated] curls). The three elbow flexors are not used equally in each exercise type, largely because forearm position affects the recruitment of the biceps brachii and brachioradialis. For example, hammer curls maximize brachioradialis involvement since the brachioradialis is strongest in midposition (between supination and pronation). Supinated curls target the biceps brachii because the biceps is the strongest supinator of the forearm and in supination is placed in an advantageous position. In contrast, the brachialis is the prime mover in a reverse curl since its insertion on the ulna means that its length and line of pull are unaffected by forearm position. Although the biceps brachii is involved in a reverse curl, the pronated forearm position places the biceps at an anatomical disadvantage to maximize its force contribution.

■   Comparing a flat bench press to an incline bench press shows that the muscle involvement of the pectoralis major differs. In a flat bench press, the primary shoulder motion is horizontal adduction, and the sternal portion of the pectoralis major plays a large role. In an incline bench press, shoulder motion is a combination of horizontal adduction and flexion; and as the incline increases, the sternal portion of the pectoralis major is less involved. The incline press targets the clavicular portion of the pectoralis major because it functions as both a horizontal adductor and flexor. Thus, at steeper inclines, the sternal portion of the pectoralis major becomes less involved, and less weight can be lifted.

■ In a narrow-stance squat, the primary muscle action is provided by the hip extensors. In a wide-stance squat, both the hip extensors and adductors are involved. With more muscle involvement in the wide stance, heavier weights can be lifted.

> Understanding which muscles are controlling a movement, and how modifying the exercise affects those muscles, is key in selecting appropriate exercises for a given goal.

Biomechanics of Resistance Exercise

Training to improve motor qualities (such as strength, power, or endurance) requires the application of a progressive overload over time. In many instances, the overload stimulus is provided by some sort of resistance to a particular set of movements. Resistance may be classified as one of three types: constant, variable, or accommodating. Because each type of resistance stresses the body in unique ways, the biomechanics of several different types of resistance are discussed next.

Constant-Resistance Devices

A constant resistive force does not change throughout the range of motion. Free weights and certain machines provide a constant-resistance force.

Free Weights

A free weight is any object that has a fixed mass and no constraints on its motion. By this definition, barbells, dumbbells, medicine balls, and a person's body (or parts of it) are all considered free weights. A free weight has a force (weight) acting on it by virtue of being in a gravitational field, which is constant and in the (vertical) direction of the gravity. Thus, the resistance to movement provided by a free weight depends on the direction of movement. In the vertical direction, the resistance provided by the free weight equals the sum of the product of the object's mass times its acceleration and the object's weight (mass times the acceleration due to gravity, -9.81 m/s^2). In all other directions, the resistance equals the product of mass times acceleration. This concept can be expressed as

$$F_R = ma + W \qquad \qquad \textbf{(4.9)}$$

Note that the object's weight, W, is equal to zero in all directions except the vertical.

To move (accelerate) a free weight, the force must be slightly greater than its weight; otherwise, the weight won't move. The greater the force above this threshold, the faster the weight moves. During a typical exercise repetition, a person starts in a static position (with zero velocity), performs some motion, reverses direction (at which point the velocity is zero), and returns back to the starting position (where the velocity is again zero). From this rather simple description, the velocity (and thus acceleration) clearly is not constant, but rather changes throughout the movement. However, if the movement speed is sufficiently slow, we tend to approximate the acceleration as zero and state that the resistance provided by free weights is constant and equal to its weight (mg).

Even if the external forces are constant throughout a movement, the internal forces will not be constant. The reason is that these forces produce torques that must be overcome by the body to move the limbs. Recall that torque is the product of force and its moment arm, and the moment arm is the perpendicular distance from the force to the axis of rotation. During single-joint movements (such as the arm curl in figure 4.15), the moment arm of the

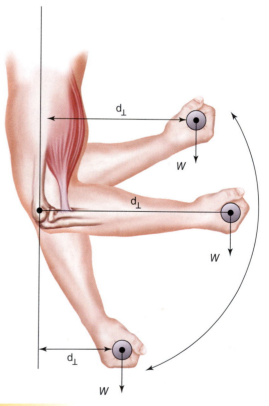

FIGURE 4.15 The horizontal distance ($d_\perp$) from the weight to the elbow changes throughout the curl movement, causing the torque exerted by the weight (W) of the object to change as well.

free weight is constantly changing throughout the range of motion. When the limb is in a horizontal position, the free weight's moment arm will be the greatest and will decrease in both directions until the weight is either directly above or below the joint. At this point, the moment arm will be zero, and consequently the torque will be zero.

One can apply this concept to change the resistance throughout the range of motion by modifying the exercise position. For example, when performing a leg curl or shoulder lateral raise in the standing position, the moment arm of the weight will be the greatest when the leg or arm is horizontal, which in these cases happens to be at roughly 90° of knee flexion or shoulder abduction, respectively. If the exercise is performed supine (for the leg curl) or side-lying (for the lateral raise), the moment arm of the weight is still greatest when the leg or arm is horizontal, but this is at the starting (neutral) position. Similarly, the forearm is horizontal at 90° of elbow flexion during the arm curl in the standing position, but is 90° minus the angle of the bench during the preacher curl. Using these concepts, the personal trainer can modify exercises to stress the musculature at different points in the range of motion.

During multijoint movements (such as the squat or bench press), the path of the bar may appear linear, but that linear motion is still produced by angular motion at the joints. The same principle applies: The resistance of a constant weight will be the greatest when the moment arm is the longest. For both the squat and bench press, the moment arm tends to be greatest during the lower part of the lift and decreases as the person moves toward the top of the lift. At the top, the moment arm is essentially zero and the skeletal system is supporting the weight with little muscle action needed.

During multijoint movements, technique variations can shift the demand from the muscles of one joint to another. For example, during the squat exercise, greater forward trunk inclination moves the weight in the anterior direction. This effectively increases the moment arm at the hips and ankles and decreases the moment arm at the knees. Consequently, the muscular demand on the hip extensors and plantarflexors will be greater and the demand on the knee extensors will be less in this position compared to a more upright position.

Certain mechanical constraints during the task should be appreciated as well (36). Because it is necessary to maintain balance throughout a lift such as the squat, the vertical projection of the combined center of mass of the bar and person must remain within the confines of the base of support created by the feet. If the bar is placed lower on the back, the exerciser has to lean forward to maintain balance. For the reasons just outlined, this increases demand on the hip extensors and plantarflexors and decreases demand on the knee extensors. Similarly, placing the bar in front of the shoulders (e.g., front squat) requires the exerciser to be more upright, increasing the demand on the knee extensors and decreasing the demand on the hip extensors and plantarflexors.

Even within the mechanical constraints of the task, variations in lifting technique can and do occur. In an attempt to lift more weight, clients may adopt subtle or not-so-subtle strategies to shift the demand from relatively weaker muscles to stronger ones. Many factors go into determining if these compensatory strategies are acceptable or not, and they are beyond the scope of this chapter. However, the personal trainer needs to be vigilant in spotting and correcting deviations that could result in injury.

Single- and multijoint movements can complement each other. For example, the demand on the quadriceps during a squat increases as the knee flexion angle increases; the demand is greater at the bottom of the lift where the knee flexion angle is largest and decreases to zero as the knee flexion angle approaches zero (i.e., fully extended knee). Conversely, during a seated knee extension exercise, since moment arm is the largest when the leg is horizontal, the demand on the quadriceps increases as the knee extends. Thus, performing both the squat and knee extension exercise would maximize the demand on the quadriceps throughout the full range of motion, and may be beneficial in certain situations (29). The same can be said for other combinations of single- and multijoint movements.

Machines

Unlike a free weight, a machine constrains the motion of the resistance in some way. The path of the resistance can be linear (as with a leg press or Smith machine) or angular (e.g., knee extension or knee curl machine). Although some devices allow pulleys to pivot in many directions, the direction of the resistance must still be in the direction of the cable, and such devices are classified as machines for the purposes of this chapter. A machine with a fixed resistance will constrain movement in some way, but the external resistance will not change. Examples include a pulldown machine using a single pulley, a Smith machine, or any device that uses a pulley with a lever and a fixed axis.

Variable-Resistance Devices

A variable resistive force will increase or decrease (or both) throughout the range of motion. Certain machines, elastic bands and tubes, and chains attached to the end of a barbell have this property of variable resistance.

Machines

A machine with variable resistance has a resistance that changes throughout the range of motion. Any machine that loads weight plates to the end of the lever varies its resistance due to the changing of the moment arm (similarly to a free weight attached to the end of a limb performing a single-joint exercise). The greatest resistance will occur when the lever is parallel to the floor. The greatest torque-producing capability of a muscle group does not necessarily occur when the distal segment is horizontal. In an effort to develop machines that match the human strength curve (i.e., the demand is greatest where the torque-producing capability is greatest and lower in other points in the range of motion), machines were developed that had a cam with a variable radius (figure 4.16). The goal of the variable cam was to adjust the moment arm of the weight stack throughout the range of motion, more closely mimicking the torque-producing capabilities of various muscle groups. Since everyone doesn't have identical strength curves for a given joint, this goal met with limited or no success (12, 15).

Elastic Resistance

The elastic properties of materials can also be used to provide variable resistance. Resistances in this category follow Hooke's law:

$$F_R = -kx \qquad \textbf{(4.10)}$$

Where k is the spring constant (i.e., a measure of the material's stiffness, or resistance to being stretched) and x is the distance the material has been stretched. Elastic tubing, elastic bands, coils, and springs all have elastic properties that provide resistance. The larger the k, the stiffer the material, with a larger force required to stretch it. The negative sign indicates that the resistance is directed opposite to the direction of the stretch. Unlike the resistance force with a free weight, the resistance force is not constant but increases proportionally with the distance the material is stretched beyond its resting length. Thus, resistance is minimal at the beginning of the exercise and increases as the movement is performed. It is important to remember that the resistance is related to the relative change in the original length of the material, and not the actual length to which the material stretched (27). For example, stretching a piece of tubing from its resting length to 0.5 m would result in different forces than

stretching that same piece of tubing from 0.5 m to 1 m. Even though the distance the material has been stretched is 0.5 m, the resistance would be larger in the second case.

Another characteristic of elastic materials that is often overlooked involves their fatigue properties (27). After repeated stretch cycles, a material will lose its ability to provide resistance. Fatigue-related changes happen based on the amount of deformation per stretch cycle and the number of cycles. Investigators found that the resistance provided by tubing and bands decreased between 5% and 6%, and between 9% and 12%, respectively, when deformed to 100% of their initial length for 501 cycles. At 200% deformation, the resistance provided by both tubes and bands decreased by 10% to 15%, with most of the decrease in resistance appearing during the first 50 repetitions (28). These results suggest that elastic materials should be replaced frequently to ensure consistent loading.

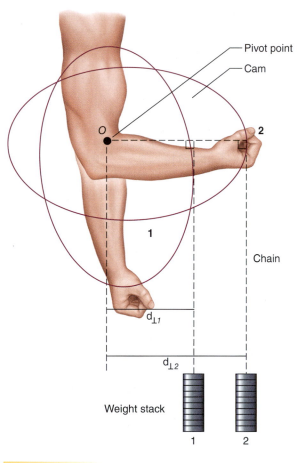

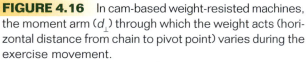

FIGURE 4.16 In cam-based weight-resisted machines, the moment arm ($d_\perp$) through which the weight acts (horizontal distance from chain to pivot point) varies during the exercise movement.

Incremental loading also may be problematic. Manufacturers often use color coding to indicate material resistance. Caution is warranted in interpreting color codes, as differences can be profound and can vary for bands and tubing. For example, the green band of one manufacturer provides almost twice the resistance of the yellow band, and the black band provides 1.5 times the resistance of the green band. For the same manufacturer, green tubing provides five times more resistance than yellow tubing, and black tubing provides 1.5 times the resistance of green tubing (27).

Chains

Recently, the practice of attaching heavy metal chains to a barbell has been implemented as a method of varying the resistance of a lift. The theory is that, during linear lifts such as the bench press or squat (without chains), the resistance is greatest at the bottom of the lift and gets progressively less as the bar moves to the top position (see earlier discussion). With chains attached to the bar, most of the chain's weight is on the floor at bottom of the lift. As the bar rises, more of the chain lifts off the floor, and greater resistance is provided as the lift progresses. Research on this practice is in its infancy, and more studies are needed to examine the mechanics of chain resistance.

Accommodating-Resistance Devices

An accommodating resistive force will vary depending on the force applied to it. In other words, accommodating resistances provide resistance that is proportional to the client's effort. Accommodating resistances include isokinetic dynamometers, flywheels, and fluid resistance.

Isokinetic Dynamometers

Isokinetic devices are designed to control movement speed to provide, at least nominally, constant angular velocity. (*Note:* The term *isokinetic* literally means "same force." Isokinetic devices, however, control the kinematic variable of angular velocity, and thus a more correct term would be "isokinematic." However, given the pervasive use of "isokinetic," we ignore the technical discrepancy and use "isokinetic" in this section.) With an isokinetic device, the limb moves at a predetermined speed, anywhere from 0°/s (isometric) up to 300°/s (eccentrically) and 500°/s (concentrically). When the movement of the limb exceeds the predetermined speed, the machine provides an equal and opposite force (torque) to maintain the specified angular velocity (24). This

force (torque) is what the exerciser exerts on the machine.

Flywheels

Flywheels require the exerciser to pull a cord, which in turn rotates a disk. Resistance is provided by the rotating disk with a mass located some distance away from the disk's axis of rotation. The flywheel's resistance increases as its angular acceleration increases. In other words, the harder one pulls on the cord, the greater the resistance to the motion provided by the flywheel (7). Additionally, the kinetic energy of the flywheel is stored (up to 80%, depending on the design). At the end of the pull, the cord will start rewinding, and the exerciser must resist it using eccentric muscle actions.

Fluid Resistance

Hydraulic and pneumatic devices that use some sort of piston to push or pull a fluid (liquid for hydraulic and gas for pneumatic) through a cylinder and movements performed under water have similar biomechanical properties. Fluid resistance follows the form

$$F_R \propto \rho\, A v^2. \qquad (4.11)$$

This means that the resistance force is proportional to the product of ρ, the fluid density, A, the surface area, and v^2, the square of the movement velocity. With machines, the density of the fluid and the cross-sectional area of the piston are inherent in the design of the equipment, and are thus fixed, so the resistance that the machine provides to the exerciser increases with the velocity of the movement. Note that this is not a linear relationship: Doubling the velocity will increase the resistance fourfold.

Performing Exercises in the Water

When someone exercises in water, a buoyant force acts in the upward direction, in opposition to gravity in the downward direction. When a person floats in water, the buoyant force and gravitational force cancel (i.e., the net vertical force is zero). When a person performs exercises in the shallow end of a pool, the buoyant force depends on how much of the body is submerged. The buoyant force is approximately 50% when the body is submerged up to the hip (level of the anterior superior iliac spine), but increases up to 90% when the body is submerged to the neck (at the level of C-7) (30).

This fact can be used to create exercises that are buoyancy supported, buoyancy assisted, or buoyancy resisted (31).

- Buoyancy-supported exercises occur parallel to the bottom of the pool. For example, while the exerciser is performing shoulder horizontal abduction and adduction when submerged up to the neck, the buoyant force helps support the arm and the resistance will mainly be in the direction of movement.
- Buoyancy-assisted movements occur in the direction of the buoyant force.
- Buoyancy-resisted movements occur in the opposite direction of the buoyant force.

While an exerciser is submerged up to the neck, the buoyant force assists with the performance of shoulder flexion. Conversely, the buoyant force has to be overcome when the person is reversing directions and performing shoulder extension. Some devices, such as aquatic dumbbells, increase the buoyant force. When used, they make buoyancy-assisted exercises easier and buoyancy-resisted exercises more difficult.

The resistance force provided by the water, called *drag,* follows the formula discussed previously for hydraulic machines (Equation 4.11). As with machines, the force is accommodating and proportional to the velocity squared. Additionally, the surface area, A, can be manipulated to increase or decrease the magnitude of the resistance. Consider

performing shoulder flexion and extension underwater. The surface area will be lower if the palm is facing toward the midline as opposed to facing anteriorly (figure 4.17), making the exercise easier. The exercise can be made more difficult if it is performed in the anatomical position using webbed gloves or paddles. Like resistive forces in hydraulic machines, the resistance force provided by water always acts in the direction opposite of the movement. Therefore, the muscle actions required to overcome the force will always be concentric.

> **Selection of the type of resistance—constant, variable, or accommodating—is an important factor in designing a safe and effective exercise program.**

Conclusion

Understanding basic biomechanical principles is important for knowing how exercises elicit desired training effects while minimizing the likelihood of injury. Personal trainers with a solid foundation in biomechanics are better prepared to establish training goals and prescribe exercise programs that are effective and efficient in improving the physical capabilities of their clients.

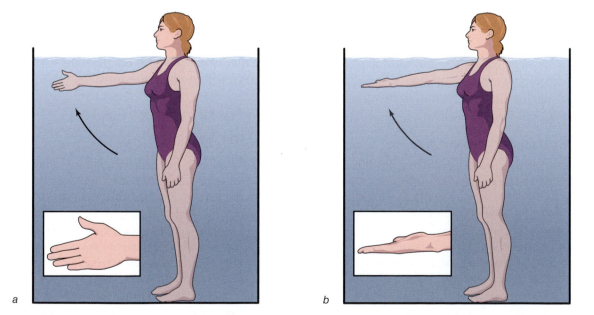

FIGURE 4.17 Shoulder flexion exercise in the water with *(a)* palm facing toward midline and *(b)* palm facing anteriorly.

Study Questions

1. Which of the following exercise modes requires the client to produce the most power?

    A. a 60 kg weight lifted in 1 second

    B. a 60 kg weight lifted in 0.1 seconds

    C. a 30 kg weight lifted in 1 second

    D. a 30 kg weight lifted in 0.1 seconds

2. Which of the following is the best example of an open chain exercise?

    A. standing barbell curl

    B. push-up

    C. squat

    D. pull-up

3. Which of the following changes will increase concentric force production?

    A. decreased rate coding

    B. decreased leverage over the joint range of motion

    C. increased contraction velocity

    D. increased physiological cross-sectional area

4. Which of the following best describes the muscular control of the downward movement phase of the squat exercise?

    A. the hip extensors, knee extensors, and ankle plantarflexors acting concentrically

    B. the hip flexors, knee flexors, and ankle dorsiflexors acting concentrically

    C. the hip extensors, knee extensors, and ankle plantarflexors acting eccentrically

    D. the hip flexors, knee flexors, and ankle dorsiflexors acting eccentrically

Applied Knowledge Question

Fill in the chart with examples of resistance training exercises and equipment for each type of external resistance that can be applied to the body.

Type of external resistance	Examples
Free weights	
Constant-resistance machines	
Variable-resistance machines	
Elastic materials	
Accommodating-resistance machines	

References

1. An, K.N., F.C. Hui, B.F. Morrey, R.L. Linscheid, and E.Y. Chao. 1981. Muscles across the elbow joint: A biomechanical analysis. *Journal of Biomechanics* 14 (10): 659-661.

2. Andersen, L.L., J.L. Andersen, S.P. Magnusson, C. Suetta, J.L. Madsen, L.R. Christensen, and P. Aagaard. 2005. Changes in the human muscle force-velocity relationship in response to resistance training and subsequent detraining. *Journal of Applied Physiology* 99 (1): 87-94.

3. Bassett, R.W., A.O. Browne, B.F. Morrey, and K.N. An. 1990. Glenohumeral muscle force and moment mechanics in a position of shoulder instability. *Journal of Biomechanics* 23 (5): 405-407.

4. Blackard, D.O., R.L. Jensen, and W.P. Ebben. 1999. Use of EMG analysis in challenging kinetic chain terminology. *Medicine and Science in Sports and Exercise* 31 (3): 443-448.

5. Bodine, S.C., R.R. Roy, E. Eldred, and V.R. Edgerton. 1987. Maximal force as a function of anatomical features of motor units in the cat tibialis anterior. *Journal of Neurophysiology* 57 (6): 1730-1745.

6. Bosco, C., J.H.T. Vitasalo, P.V. Komi, and P. Luhtanen. 1982. Combined effect of elastic energy and myoelectrical potentiation during stretch-shortening cycle exercise. *Acta Physiologica Scandinavica* 114 (4): 557-565.

7. Chiu, L.Z.F., and G.J. Salem. 2006. Comparison of joint kinetics during free weight and flywheel resistance exercise. *Journal of Strength and Conditioning Research* 20 (3): 555-562.

8. Elliott, B.C., G.J. Wilson, and G.K. Kerr. 1989. A biomechanical analysis of the sticking region in the bench press. *Medicine and Science in Sports and Exercise* 21 (4): 450-462.

9. Enoka, R.M. 1994. *Neuromechanical Basis of Human Movement.* Champaign, IL: Human Kinetics.

10. Escamilla, R.F., G.S. Fleisig, N.G. Zheng, S.W. Barrentine, K.E. Wilk, and J.R. Andrews. 1998. Biomechanics of the knee during closed kinetic chain and open kinetic chain exercises. *Medicine and Science in Sports and Exercise* 30 (4): 556-569.

11. Finni, T., S. Ikegawa, V. Lepola, and P.V. Komi. 2003. Comparison of force-velocity relationships of vastus lateralis muscle in isokinetic and in stretch-shortening cycle exercises. *Acta Physiologica Scandinavica* 177 (4): 483-491.

12. Folland, J., and B. Morris. 2008. Variable-cam resistance training machines: Do they match the angle-torque relationship in humans? *Journal of Sports Sciences* 26 (2): 163-169.

13. Fregly, B.J., and F.E. Zajac. 1996. A state-space analysis of mechanical energy generation, absorption, and transfer during pedaling. *Journal of Biomechanics* 29 (1): 81-90.

14. Garhammer, J., and T. McLaughlin. 1980. Power output as a function of load variation in olympic and power lifting. *Journal of Biomechanics* 13 (2): 198.

15. Harman, E. 1983. Resistive torque analysis of 5 nautilus exercise machines. *Medicine and Science in Sports and Exercise* 15 (2): 113.

16. Hather, B.M., P.A. Tesch, P. Buchanan, and G.A. Dudley. 1991. Influence of eccentric actions on skeletal-muscle adaptations to resistance training. *Acta Physiologica Scandinavica* 143 (2): 177-185.

17. Knuttgen, H., and W.J. Kraemer. 1987. Terminology and measurement in exercise performance. *Journal of Applied Sport Science Research* 1 (1): 1-10.

18. Lehmkuhl, L.D., and L.K. Smith. 1983. *Brunnstrom's Clinical Kinesiology.* Philadelphia: Davis.

19. Le Système International d' Unités. 2006. Sevres, France: Bureau International des Poids et Mesures.

20. Lieber, R.L. 1992. *Skeletal Muscle Structure and Function: Implications for Rehabilitation and Sports Medicine.* Baltimore: Williams & Wilkins.

21. Maganaris, C.N., V. Baltzopoulos, D. Ball, and A.J. Sargeant. 2001. In vivo specific tension of human skeletal muscle. *Journal of Applied Physiology* 90 (3): 865-872.

22. McGill, S.M. 2007. *Low Back Disorders: Evidence-Based Prevention and Rehabilitation.* Champaign, IL: Human Kinetics.

23. Moritani, T., and H.A. deVries. 1979. Neural factors versus hypertrophy in the time course of muscle strength gain. *American Journal of Physical Medicine & Rehabilitation* 58 (3): 115-130.

24. Perrin, D.H. 1993. *Isokinetic Exercise and Assessment.* Champaign, IL: Human Kinetics.

25. Perrine, J.J., and V.R. Edgerton. 1978. Muscle force-velocity and power-velocity relationships under isokinetic loading. *Medicine and Science in Sports and Exercise* 10 (3): 159-166.

26. Robertson, D.G.E., and D.A. Winter. 1980. Mechanical energy generation, absorption and transfer amongst segments during walking. *Journal of Biomechanics* 13 (10): 845-854.

27. Simoneau, G.G., S.M. Bereda, D.C. Sobush, and A.J. Starsky. 2001. Biomechanics of elastic resistance in therapeutic exercise programs. *Journal of Orthopaedic and Sports Physical Therapy* 31 (1): 16-24.

28. Steindler, A. 1973. *Kinesiology of the Human Body Under Normal and Pathologic Conditions.* Springfield, IL: Charles C Thomas.

29. Steinkamp, L.A., M.F. Dillingham, M.D. Markel, J.A. Hill, and K.R. Kaufman. 1993. Biomechanical considerations in patellofemoral joint rehabilitation. *American Journal of Sports Medicine* 21 (3): 438-444.

30. Thein, J.M., and L.T. Brody. 1998. Aquatic based rehabilitation and training for the elite athlete. *Journal of Orthopaedic and Sports Physical Therapy* 27 (1): 32-41.

31. Thorstensson, A., J. Karlsson, J.H.T. Vitasalo, P. Luhtanen, and P.V. Komi. 1976. Effect of strength training on EMG of human skeletal-muscle. *Acta Physiologica Scandinavica* 98 (2): 232-236.

32. Whiting, W.C., and S. Rugg. 2006. *Dynatomy: Dynamic Human Anatomy.* Champaign, IL: Human Kinetics.

33. Whiting, W.C., and R.F. Zernicke. 2008. *Biomechanics of Musculoskeletal Injury.* Champaign, IL: Human Kinetics.

34. Zajac, F.E. 1993. Muscle coordination of movement: A perspective. *Journal of Biomechanics* 26 (S1): 109-124.

35. Zajac, F.E., and M.E. Gordon. 1989. Determining muscle's force and action in multi-articular movement. *Exercise and Sport Sciences Reviews* 17: 187-230.

36. Zatsiorsky, V.M. 1998. *Kinematics of Human Motion.* Champaign, IL: Human Kinetics.

Resistance Training Adaptations

Joseph P. Weir, PhD, and Lee E. Brown, EdD

After completing this chapter, you will be able to

- describe the acute and chronic adaptations to resistance exercise,

- identify factors that affect the magnitude or rate of adaptations to resistance training,

- design resistance training programs that maximize the specific adaptations of interest,

- design resistance training programs that avoid overtraining, and

- understand the effects of detraining and know how to reduce them.

As clients embark on a resistance training program, their bodies respond in several notable ways. This chapter examines the physiological adaptations that occur with resistance training, both during acute bouts of training and over time. Personal trainers who understand these adaptations can design resistance training programs that will best meet clients' individual needs. Such personal trainers have a keen sense of how to train each physiological system with the client's personal goals in mind.

This chapter explains general adaptations that result from progressive overload. These include neurological, muscle and connective tissue, skeletal, metabolic, hormonal, cardiorespiratory, and body composition changes. As with all types of exercise training, resistance training is highly specific, so we examine particular areas of resistance training specificity. We also explain the impact of gender, age, and genetics on physiological adaptations. The final sections of the chapter deal with overtraining as an unwanted physiological response that must be prevented in the personal training setting, as well as the effects of detraining and how to avoid them.

Basic Adaptations to Resistance Training

In studying the adaptations to resistance training, it is useful to distinguish between acute and chronic adaptations. Acute adaptations, which are often referred to as "responses" to exercise, are the changes that occur in the body during and shortly after an exercise bout. As an example, fuel substrates in muscle such as creatine phosphate (CP) can become depleted during an exercise bout. In contrast, chronic adaptations are changes in the body that occur after repeated training bouts and persist long after a training session is over. For example, long-term resistance training results in increases in muscle mass, which largely drive the increase in force production capability of the muscle. Two subsequent sections of this chapter address the acute and chronic adaptations that typically occur with resistance training.

> Acute adaptations are changes that occur in the body during and shortly after an exercise bout. Chronic adaptations are changes in the body that occur after repeated training bouts and that persist long after a training session is over.

The key to inducing increases in muscle size and strength is to place the system under overload; that is, the neuromuscular system must experience a training stress that it is not accustomed to experiencing. The same holds true if one is considering adaptations in bone and connective tissue. Progressive overload results in the muscle's ability to handle heavier loads, and this indicates that a variety of physiological adaptations have occurred.

A large volume of literature describes the adaptations to resistance training overload. The rapidity with which overload increases the capacity for muscle to handle heavier loads at the start of a training program suggests that there is a dramatic increase in the activation of motor units during the initial phases of resistance training. Scientific studies have indicated that improvements in strength associated with the early stages of resistance training are primarily due to neurological adaptations. In addition, during this time the quality of muscle protein (e.g., myosin heavy chains and myosin adenosine triphosphatase [ATPase]) also changes to allow for more rapid and forceful contractile capabilities.

Although the ultimate magnitude of muscle size increases is primarily determined by genetic factors, numerous studies have established that resistance training leads to muscle hypertrophy. Hypertrophy of muscle fibers is usually not measurable until approximately 8 to 12 weeks after the initiation of the training program. The continued interplay of hypertrophic and neurological adaptations to resistance training continues with long-term training. The impact of long-term training on muscle hypertrophy remains less well studied, but the absolute magnitude of gains in muscle size and strength is lower as clients approach their genetic limits. Nevertheless, continued training over a client's life-time helps to improve quality of life and minimize the consequences of aging.

A variety of cellular adaptations occur with resistance training programs. These include changes in anaerobic enzyme quantity, changes in stored energy substrates (e.g., glycogen and phosphagens), increased myofibrillar protein content (i.e., increased actin and myosin proteins), and increased noncontractile muscle proteins. In addition, important changes occur within the central and peripheral nervous systems to help in the activation of motor units to produce specific force and power requirements. Furthermore, a variety of changes occur in other physiological systems (e.g., endocrine, immune, and cardiorespiratory) that support the neuromuscular adaptations to a resistance training program. All these adaptations support the neuromuscular improvements in force, velocity, and power capabilities in the body consequent to resistance training.

Acute Adaptations

The short-term changes that occur in the neuromuscular system during and immediately after a training session drive the chronic adaptations. This section presents an overview of the major acute responses to resistance exercise, specifically exploring responses involving the neurological, muscular, and endocrine systems. These acute responses are summarized in table 5.1.

TABLE 5.1 Acute Responses to Resistance Training

Variable	Acute response
NEUROLOGICAL RESPONSES	
EMG amplitude	Increases
Number of motor units recruited	Increases
MUSCULAR CHANGES	
Hydrogen ion concentration	Increases
Inorganic phosphate concentration	Increases
Ammonia levels	Increases
ATP concentration	No change or slight decrease
CP concentration	Decreases
Glycogen concentration	Decreases
ENDOCRINE CHANGES	
Epinephrine concentration	Increases
Cortisol concentration	Increases
Testosterone concentration	Increases
Growth hormone concentration	Increases

EMG = electromyogram; ATP = adenosine triphosphate; CP = creatine phosphate.

Neurological Changes

Resistance training, like all physical activity, requires activation of skeletal muscle. The process of skeletal muscle activation involves action potential generation on the muscle cell membrane (sarcolemma) via acetylcholine release from the alpha motor neuron that **innervates** (stimulates) a particular muscle cell. The action potential is manifested as a voltage change on the sarcolemma that can be recorded with either surface or intramuscular electrodes. The technique of recording these electrical events is referred to as *electromyography* (*EMG*). The size of an EMG signal varies as a function of muscle force output, but is also affected by other factors such as fatigue and muscle fiber composition (27). Much of what we know about neurological responses and adaptations to resistance training comes from studies using EMG.

Control of muscle force is accomplished by the interplay of two control factors: motor unit recruitment and rate coding (28). Motor unit **recruitment** simply refers to the process in which tasks that require more force involve the activation of more motor units. An individual performing a 100-pound (45 kg) bench press would need to turn on more motor units than would be required to perform a 50-pound (23 kg) bench press. **Rate coding** refers to control of motor unit firing rate (number of action potentials per unit of time). Within certain limits, the faster the firing rate, the more force is produced. Therefore, a motor unit that was activated at a rate of, say, 20 times per second during the 50-pound bench press may be firing at 30 times per second during the 100-pound bench press. As a general rule, small muscles (like those in the hands) that require very precise motor control achieve full recruitment at relatively low percentages of maximum force output (e.g., 50% of maximum), and after this point depend entirely on firing rate to increase force production. In contrast, large muscles like those in the quadriceps employ recruitment up to 90% of maximum or more, and maximum firing rates tend to be lower than for the small muscles (7). Therefore, one can generalize that small muscles depend more heavily on firing rate to control force output while large muscles tend to depend more heavily on recruitment.

During a typical set of resistance exercise using weights, a pool of motor units in the involved muscle is activated and each motor unit is firing at some rate. As the person progresses from one repetition to the next, the muscle begins to fatigue, and changes in recruitment and firing rate occur. It is likely that motor unit recruitment increases over time to compensate for the loss in force production capability of the previously activated motor units (97). In addition, motor units that were firing at low rates at the start of the set may have to fire at higher rates (rate coding) as the set progresses in response to the fatigue associated with the task. These changes are manifested in changes in the surface EMG signal. Specifically, the size of the surface EMG signal gets larger during a set of resistance training exercise (90). This reflects changes in motor unit recruitment and firing rate.

Motor unit recruitment is based on the **size principle** (29) (figure 5.1). In general, motor units that innervate slow-twitch motor units innervate fewer fibers than motor units that innervate fast-twitch fibers. In addition, both the muscle fiber size and alpha motor neuron diameters of slow-twitch motor units are smaller than those of their fast-twitch counterparts. The smaller neuron size of slow-twitch motor units results in a lower threshold for activation for these motor neurons. Therefore, they are recruited at low force levels. In contrast, large motor neurons, such as those that typically innervate fast-twitch muscle fibers, have higher recruitment thresholds and are recruited at higher force levels. As the force requirements of a task increase and more motor units are recruited, the nervous system recruits larger motor units (30).

One implication of the size principle is that to recruit high-threshold (fast-twitch) motor units, one must engage in tasks that require high force outputs. In addition, the terms *slow-twitch* and *fast-twitch* do not imply that the nervous system turns on slow-twitch motor units only during slow muscle actions and fast-twitch motor units only during fast muscle actions. Rather, motor unit recruitment follows the size principle and is therefore dependent on the force production requirements of a task, so

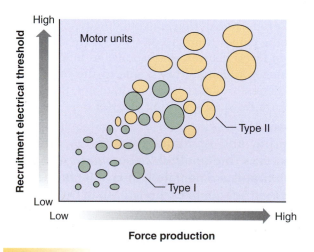

FIGURE 5.1 Graphic representation of the size principle.

Reprinted by permission from NSCA 2008.

that fast-twitch fibers are recruited even during slow (or isometric) muscle actions if the force demands are high enough.

> Recruitment of motor units for force production follows the size principle, meaning that smaller motor units are recruited at lower force levels and larger motor units are recruited at higher force levels.

Muscular Changes

As already noted, during a set of resistance exercise, muscles experience fatigue. While fatigue is a highly complex phenomenon, it is clear that the acute changes in muscle cells include accumulation of metabolites and depletion of fuel substrates (24). The factors involved are tied to the metabolic pathways that are primarily stressed during anaerobic activities (like resistance training), specifically the phosphagen system and glycolysis. Metabolites that accumulate include hydrogen ion (H^+, which results in a decrease in muscle pH), inorganic phosphate (P_i), and ammonia (86). All of these have been studied as potential causes of muscle fatigue.

As noted earlier, CP can become depleted during resistance exercise, reflecting the reliance on the phosphagen system during typical resistance training. Creatine phosphate is important for phosphorylation of adenosine diphosphate (ADP) to adenosine triphosphate (ATP) during high-intensity exercise, and depletion of CP likely leads to decreased power production. Although complete glycogen depletion is unlikely to occur with resistance training, glycogen breakdown is an important factor in the supply of energy for this type of training (84, 106). In fact, it has been estimated that over 80% of the ATP production during bodybuilding-type resistance training comes from glycolysis (79). Therefore, glycogen levels decrease in response to high-intensity resistance training. This points to the importance of adequate dietary carbohydrate for those who perform resistance training (46, 82).

> During and immediately after resistance exercise, metabolites accumulate and fuel substrates are depleted; thus, clients need to include adequate carbohydrate in their diets.

Endocrine Changes

Hormones are blood-borne molecules that are produced in glands called *endocrine glands*. There are two primary types of hormones: (1) protein and peptide hormones and (2) steroid hormones. Two examples of protein and peptide hormones are growth hormone and insulin. Steroid hormones are all derived from a common precursor (cholesterol) and include hormones such as testosterone (the primary male sex hormone) and estrogen (the primary female sex hormone).

Many hormones have effects on either the growth or the degradation of tissue such as muscle tissue. Anabolic hormones such as testosterone, growth hormone (GH), and insulin tend to stimulate growth processes in tissues, while catabolic hormones such as cortisol use tissue degradation to help maintain homeostasis of variables like blood glucose. The concentration of many of these hormones is affected by an acute bout of exercise. Indeed, changes in some hormone concentrations are needed to support the metabolic response to exercise. For example, exercise results in increases in concentrations of epinephrine. Epinephrine increases fat and carbohydrate breakdown by the cell so that more ATP will be available for muscle contraction. Epinephrine also has effects on the central nervous system, which may facilitate motor unit activation.

Other hormone concentrations are increased during a bout of resistance training. Acute increases in anabolic hormones may have little effect on a particular exercise bout, but they likely play an important role in stimulating adaptations to training. For example, testosterone and GH concentrations are elevated with resistance training in males (50, 71, 75, 76, 111). These hormones stimulate increases in skeletal muscle protein synthesis. Therefore, they are important for development of muscle mass. The cumulative effect of acute increases in testosterone and GH concentrations with repeated training sessions may contribute to the long-term accretion of muscle mass. Indeed, the repeated increases in anabolic hormone concentrations during multiple training bouts over time may be a more potent endocrine stimulus than any changes in chronic hormone concentrations (75).

The hormonal response to resistance exercise is dependent on the characteristics of the training bout. As a general rule, bouts that have higher volume and shorter rest periods elicit stronger endocrine responses than do bouts with lower volume and longer rest periods (14, 69, 75), although the differences between protocols may diminish with prolonged training (14). Similarly, large muscle mass exercises have a more powerful stimulus than do small muscle mass exercises (75). Other factors such as sex and age can affect the acute endocrine response. Males tend to have larger acute changes in anabolic hormone concentrations than do females (25). Similarly, elderly individuals tend to exhibit an attenuated anabolic hormonal response to training relative to younger individuals (25).

Chronic Adaptations

Chronic adaptations are long-term changes in the structure and function of the body as a consequence of exercise training. With respect to resistance training, the general adaptations that one sees following prolonged resistance training are increases in strength and muscle mass. Increases in strength are influenced by changes in neurological function as well as changes in muscle mass. In addition, changes in muscle enzyme and substrate concentrations may influence muscle endurance. These chronic adaptations are summarized in table 5.2.

Neurological Changes

It is a common observation that increases in strength occur rapidly during the early stages of a resistance training program and that they are larger than can be accounted for by changes in muscle size. These early strength gains are often attributed to so-called "neural factors" (96), and several studies have indicated that strength increases consequent to resistance training are influenced by increases in neural drive (29, 47, 60, 166). The assumption that neural factors are involved is based not only on the discrepancy between hypertrophic and strength increases early in a training program but also on increases in EMG amplitude measured during maximal contractions (47, 66, 96).

The influence of neural factors on strength gains is believed to be dominant in the early phases of a training program (one to two months), and thereafter strength increases are primarily mediated by hypertrophy (52, 108) (figure 5.2). Much of this effect is likely due to improvements in skill in performing the resistance exercises, especially in individuals who are using free weight exercises that require balance and efficiency of movement in order to be performed well. However, some evidence suggests that part of this effect is due to changes in motor unit recruitment and firing rate. With respect to motor unit recruitment, the argument is that many untrained individuals are unable to activate all the motor units that are available, and resistance training may result in an increase in the ability to activate high-threshold motor

units, leading to an increase in force production capability that is independent of muscle hypertrophy. We should note, however, that according to some studies, untrained individuals are able to recruit all available motor units (9, 92, 107). In addition, not all studies show an increase in EMG amplitude following resistance training programs (41, 127). Recent evidence suggests that resistance training can also increase maximal motor unit firing rates (102). This would increase muscle force production capability independent of hypertrophy.

In addition to changes in motor unit recruitment and firing rate, other neurological adaptations have

TABLE 5.2 Chronic Adaptations to Resistance Training

Variable	Chronic adaptation
MUSCLE PERFORMANCE	
Muscle strength	Increases
Muscle endurance	Increases
Muscle power	Increases
MUSCLE ENZYMES	
Phosphagen system enzyme concentrations	May increase
Phosphagen system enzyme absolute levels	Increase
Glycolytic enzyme concentrations	May increase
Glycolytic enzyme absolute levels	Increase
MUSCLE SUBSTRATES	
ATP concentration	May increase
ATP absolute levels	Increase
CP concentration	May increase
CP absolute levels	Increase
ATP and CP changes during exercise	Decrease
Lactate increase during exercise	Decreases
MUSCLE FIBER CHARACTERISTICS	
Type I CSA	Increases (<type II)
Type II CSA	Increases (>type I)
% Type IIa	Increases
% Type IIx	Decreases
% Type I	No change
BODY COMPOSITION	
% Fat	Likely decreases
Fat-free mass	Increases
Metabolic rate	Likely increases
NEUROLOGICAL CHANGES	
EMG amplitude during MVC	Likely increases
Motor unit recruitment	Likely increases
Motor unit firing rate	Increases
Cocontraction	Decreases
STRUCTURAL CHANGES	
Connective tissue strength	Likely increases
Bone density/mass	Likely increases

ATP = adenosine triphosphate; CP = creatine phosphate; CSA = cross-sectional area; EMG = electromyogram; MVC = maximal voluntary contraction.

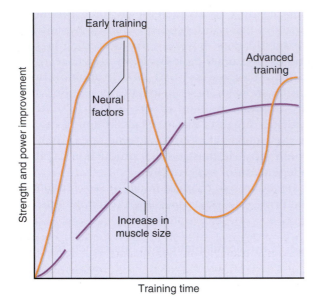

FIGURE 5.2 The contributions of neural factors and muscular size to improvements in strength. Neural factors include those related to improved skill, motor recruitment, and firing rate.

Reprinted by permission from NSCA 2008.

been reported in the literature. *Cocontraction* (or *coactivation*) refers to the simultaneous activation of an agonist and an antagonist during a motor task. As an example, during knee extension exercise, the quadriceps muscles are the agonists (prime movers) while the hamstrings serve as the antagonist. Several studies have shown significant cocontraction during isometric and isokinetic actions of the knee joint (99, 105, 128). Decreased cocontraction would decrease the antagonist torque that must be overcome by the agonist during a muscle action, thus enhancing the expression of strength. There appear to be decreases in cocontraction following isometric resistance training (17). Whether similar changes in cocontraction occur during dynamic exercise, such as with free weights, is unknown but appears likely. Other work has shown changes in motor neuron excitability (109) and increases in motor unit synchronization following resistance training (95). Neural factors have also been inferred from observations that unilateral resistance training results in increases in strength of the untrained limb (54, 126, 127), as well as from observations that isometric resistance training at one joint angle results in strength increases that are larger at the trained angle than at other joint angles (64, 119, 127).

Muscle Tissue Changes

Resistance training results in adaptations in muscles, tendons, and ligaments. The most obvious adapta-

tion in skeletal muscle is **hypertrophy,** that is, an increase in muscle size (cross-sectional area and volume). Resistance training results in an increase in cross-sectional area of both type I and type II muscle fibers. However, type II fibers typically show a greater degree of hypertrophy than type I fibers (33, 114) and also suffer from greater atrophy following detraining (57). The increase in cross-sectional area is attributed to an increase in both the size and number of myofibrils within a given muscle fiber. Thus resistance training causes an increase in protein synthesis (and/or a decrease in protein degradation), resulting in a greater number of actin and myosin filaments. The increase in myofibril number is possibly the result of "splitting" of existing myofibrils into separate "daughter" myofibrils (42). **Hyperplasia,** or the increase in number of muscle fibers, has not been definitively shown to occur in humans, but there is evidence for hyperplasia in animal models (4). The net result of an increase in muscle cross-sectional area, and the associated increase in actin and myosin filaments, is an increase in force and power production capability of the muscle.

> The primary adaptation of skeletal muscle to long-term resistance training is hypertrophy, or increased cross-sectional area of the muscle fiber, resulting in increased force and power production capability.

With respect to muscle fiber types, resistance training induces a fiber subtype shift from type IIx to type IIa muscle fibers (44, 114, 122). These subtype shifts are observable after just a few training sessions (112) and likely reflect a change in the myosin heavy-chain composition of the muscle cell. Therefore, resistance training alters not only the quantity of muscle tissue (hypertrophy) but also its quality. However, to date there is little evidence to suggest that resistance training can induce a shift from slow- to fast-twitch fibers or vice versa.

The hypertrophic response to resistance training is the net result of an increase in protein synthesis relative to protein breakdown in the muscle cell (120). Protein synthesis clearly increases following resistance training (19, 83). The extent of protein degradation is less clear; but it is probable that increased degradation occurs, since the hypertrophic response to resistance training is less than would be expected solely on the basis of the magnitude of the increased protein synthesis seen following resistance training bouts (19). The protein degradation may be a consequence of muscle damage that has occurred during training, and there is some speculation that the damage may be a stimulus for hypertrophy. In support of this notion, researchers have shown that training responses are enhanced when eccentric actions are included in the training, as occurs during typical resistance training (20, 53, 78), and eccentric actions are primarily implicated in the development of delayed onset muscle soreness and muscle damage.

In addition to increasing contractile protein content of skeletal muscle, resistance training appears to increase the content of cytoskeletal and structural proteins in skeletal muscle. These proteins help give cells shape and structural integrity. In skeletal muscle, they are also involved in force transmission from the myofibrils to the extracellular matrix and in the storage of elastic energy as occurs in stretch–shortening cycle activities. The study of adaptations in skeletal muscle cytoskeleton proteins to resistance training is newer and less developed than work on contractile protein changes. Nonetheless, there is clear evidence that the content of cytoskeletal proteins such as desmin increases in response to resistance training (101, 131). In addition, strength and power athletes have been shown to have higher levels of the protein titin, a large elastic structural protein, which may enhance elastic energy storage (91). Unfortunately, resistance training has not been shown to affect expression of the key protein dystrophin (101, 131).

Skeletal Changes

It is tempting to think of the skeletal system as an inert framework comprising simply a set of levers that muscles act upon to create movement. However, bone tissue is very much "alive" and is a dynamic tissue. In addition to its role in movement and protection, bone serves as a depot for important minerals, most notably calcium. **Osteoporosis** is the consequence of long-term net demineralization of bone. In recent years, resistance training has been studied for its possible influence on bone mineral density (BMD). Bone tissue is significantly affected by strain; that is, deformation (bending) of bone rapidly stimulates bone cells to begin activities that stimulate bone formation (6, 65). Therefore, it seems logical to examine the effects of resistance training on bone formation, especially in the context of osteoporosis. Because osteoporosis is mainly, though not exclusively, a condition associated with postmenopausal women, most research has focused on women. Specifically, researchers have focused on the effect of resistance training on the accumulation of bone tissue prior to menopause (peak bone mass is typically achieved prior to age 40 (6), as well as on the effect of resistance training on the decline in bone mass associated with aging and menopause. Menopause is particularly critical in the development of osteoporosis because hormones like estrogen, which facilitate bone formation, markedly decline after menopause. Accumulation of bone mass prior to menopause is considered important because the greater the bone mass prior to menopause, the less severe the consequences of loss of bone mass.

The research literature has shown quite clearly that, in cross-sectional studies, stronger women tend to have thicker and stronger bones. However, selection bias may influence such studies (3). Intervention studies are less clear as to whether resistance training programs result in increases in bone mass. Some of these studies show no significant effect of resistance training on bone tissue (10, 104), while others have shown that resistance training programs can positively affect bone tissue (87, 121). Differences between studies are influenced by factors such as length and characteristics (e.g., intensity, volume, type of exercises) of the training programs, small sample sizes, differences in the extent of bone demineralization prior to training, gender, and age. A recent meta-analysis has reported that high-intensity resistance training can significantly increase lumbar spine BMD but not BMD of the femoral neck in premenopausal women (89). Nonetheless, there is enough evidence in the literature to suggest that resistance training very likely has a positive effect on bone tissue (6). What has not been examined in depth is the effect of explosive and plyometric types of training on BMD. Both strain magnitude and strain rate affect the stimulus for bone formation (6), and these would be expected to be higher with explosive and plyometric training. In addition to the obvious effects of resistance training on muscle mass and strength, resistance training may lead to decreased risk for osteoporosis, fractures, and falls in later life.

> The greater the bone mass prior to menopause, the less severe are the consequences of loss of bone mass. Resistance training may lead to decreased risk for osteoporosis, fractures, and falls in later life.

Tendon and Ligament Changes

Tendons and ligaments can also undergo adaption following prolonged resistance training. These connective tissues, which are comprised primarily of bundles of fibrous collagen, have relatively few cells in their structure, so they do not require much blood, oxygen, or nutrients. Consequently, they also have poor vascular supplies, which increases the time it takes them to recover from injuries. One effect of acute loading during exercise may be to stimulate collagen turnover and net collagen production (80, 94). While research has consistently shown that tendons can adapt to the loads applied during training, there is little data so far on the specific effects of training on ligaments.

Recent research employing ultrasound and magnetic resonance imaging technology has found changes in tendon size and mechanical properties associated with physical activity. For example, one study showed that male distance runners have larger Achilles tendon cross-sectional areas than kayakers do (67), while another showed that elite fencers and badminton players have significantly greater patellar tendon cross-sectional areas (and thigh–muscle cross-sectional area and strength) in the lead leg than in the non-lead leg (23). Both fencing and badminton involve unilateral lunging motions that place high eccentric loads on the lead leg. Other research has suggested that the specific effects of physical activity on tendon size may vary according to sex. One study found that female distance runners do not exhibit greater cross-sectional area of either the Achilles or patellar tendons relative to female controls and that female runners have markedly lower tendon cross-sectional areas relative to male distance runners (129). The study's authors suggested that sex differences in tendon size might be due to endocrine differences between males and females because (a) estrogen and progesterone receptors are present in fibroblasts of ligaments and (b) estrogen has been shown to inhibit collagen synthesis. This interpretation is supported by data showing suppressed rates of collagen synthesis post-exercise in women taking oral contraceptives (51).

Longitudinal training studies have shown that resistance training can alter tendon mechanical properties. For example, tendon stiffness (amount of force per unit of tendon length change under load) has been shown to be increased following 12 weeks of heavy load (70% of 1-RM) leg extension exercise, but not with light load training. In addition, tendon cross-sectional area has been reported to increase with resistance training (67); however, other studies have not shown increases in tendon size (77). Further research is necessary to more clearly delineate the training variables (e.g., type, load, volume, frequency) that maximize the training benefits to tendons and determine how this affects injury risk and rehabilitation.

Metabolic Changes

Research has shown that chronic resistance training induces a variety of cellular changes that affect the metabolism of skeletal muscle. All studies of metabolic adaptations to resistance training are complicated by the fact that hypertrophy will dilute enzyme and substrate levels, so that changes in absolute levels may result in no change of relative levels (e.g., per unit of muscle mass). In addition, relative decreases in concentrations may simply reflect hypertrophy.

Resistance training primarily stresses anaerobic metabolism, and therefore one should expect that any enzymatic or substrate adaptations would involve anaerobic metabolism. Anaerobic metabolism is typically thought of as having two components: the phosphagen system and glycolysis. Studies conflict regarding increases in substrate and enzyme concentrations in either of these components. With respect to the phosphagen system, some studies have demonstrated that resistance training does not result in increased concentration of ATP or CP (118), while others have shown increases in these variables (85). Similarly, some data suggest that the enzymes involved in this system, creatine kinase and myokinase, are not found in higher concentrations following resistance training (117). However, other data do indicate that resistance training results in higher concentrations of these enzymes (22). Differences between studies likely reflect differences in training mode and volume and indicate the importance of designing programs to meet the specific needs of individual clients.

With respect to glycolytic activity, research has typically shown that key enzymes involved in the glycolytic pathway (e.g., phosphofructokinase, lactate dehydrogenase) are not found in higher concentrations following resistance training (69). However, these results may be specific to the type of resistance training performed, since bodybuilders who perform higher-volume training with shorter rest periods than powerlifters have glycolytic enzyme concentrations similar to those of aerobic endurance athletes such as swimmers (118). This suggests that high-volume resistance training may induce glycolytic enzymatic adaptations that increase muscle endurance.

For both the phosphagen and glycolytic adaptations to resistance training just described, it is important to note that although some studies indicate no change in the concentrations of key substrates and enzymes, the total volume of these substrates and enzymes in a given muscle will be higher due to the increase in total muscle mass. Therefore, the absolute muscle endurance will likely increase following resistance training. This is evident in an increased ability to perform additional repetitions of a resistance training exercise (12, 116).

Endocrine Changes

While resistance training can cause large changes in hormone concentrations during and after a bout of training (63), the long-term effects of resistance training on resting hormone concentrations are less clear. Also, understanding of these effects is complicated by the fact that overtraining can cause changes in hormone concentrations that are different from those seen during "normal" training situations. That said, some evidence suggests that prolonged resistance training results in chronically elevated testosterone concentrations (48, 76) that should facilitate an environment conducive to muscle growth. In contrast, other studies show no changes in resting testosterone concentrations (2, 49, 50). There does not appear to be a chronic training effect on resting GH concentrations (48, 50, 76). However, the cumulative effect of acute increases in GH in response to resistance training likely has a significant influence on long-term muscle hypertrophy.

Chronic resistance training may also affect the magnitude of the endocrine response and the sensitivity of tissues to a hormone. Research has shown that several training sessions are required before an increase in testosterone concentration is elicited by resistance exercise (76). Similarly, chronic resistance training alters the acute epinephrine response to bouts of exercise (45, 73). Chronic training may affect sensitivity by increasing the quantity of the receptors for the hormone on the target tissue (62). Through upregulation of hormone receptors, the effect of a given concentration of a hormone is amplified.

Cardiorespiratory Changes

Resistance training places a much different stress on the cardiorespiratory system than does cardiorespiratory endurance exercise such as running or cycling, and therefore the effects on the cardiorespiratory system are quite different. With respect to aerobic endurance performance, resistance training has not been shown to result in an increase in peak $\dot{V}O_2$ (55, 74, 88). This likely stems from the fact that while heart rate values are elevated during resistance training, the total metabolic demands are lower than are those associated with comparable heart rate values elicited during aerobic endurance exercise (21). Therefore there is little stimulus for increased peak $\dot{V}O_2$. This indicates that it is misleading to use target heart rate zones during resistance exercise as an indicator of cardiovascular fitness training.

Although resistance training programs do not typically improve maximal oxygen consumption to the extent seen with other modes of cardiovascular training (e.g., running, cycling), they augment the development of cardiovascular endurance performance and improve running efficiency while not causing any negative effects on the development of maximal oxygen consumption (55, 56, 100). Therefore, although resistance training does not directly increase peak $\dot{V}O_2$, it can serve as an important adjunct to cardiovascular training. Nonetheless, to achieve optimal results in increasing the cardiorespiratory endurance capabilities of a client requires aerobic endurance–specific training. Chapter 16 provides the details of such programs for achieving improvements in maximal oxygen consumption and discusses the effects of such training on strength gains.

> Increasing cardiorespiratory endurance capabilities requires aerobic endurance–specific training to achieve optimal results; however, resistance training can augment cardiovascular endurance performance and running efficiency by increasing muscle strength and power.

As noted previously, resistance training depends primarily on anaerobic metabolism to generate ATP for muscle actions. Therefore, it is not surprising that resistance training does not appear to improve skeletal muscle cellular aerobic function as assessed by oxidative enzyme activity and capillary density. However, it does induce increases in capillarization so that capillary supply is maintained in spite of increased muscle size (44). Both myoglobin concentration (117) and mitochondrial density (85) tend to decrease with resistance training. Both of these changes reflect the effects of hypertrophy and the lack of oxidative stress (and therefore stimulus) that occurs during resistance training.

Despite the lack of improvement in skeletal muscle cellular aerobic function, it is important to note that normal increases in muscle size (i.e., hypertrophy) with resistance training do not reduce muscle endurance. On the contrary, increases in muscle size and strength due to resistance training increase local muscle endurance (12, 116). That is, a hypertrophied muscle, with the corresponding increases in strength and volume of metabolic enzymes and substrates (but not necessarily a higher density), can do more work over time.

Body Composition Changes

A variety of models have been developed to quantify body composition. For the personal trainer, the model that best relates to the needs of clients is the two-component model, which segregates the body into fat mass and fat-free mass (FFM). The FFM is composed of tissues such as muscle, bone, and connective tissue. As noted previously, resistance training can affect all of these components, so it follows that a resistance training program inducing hypertrophy will directly affect body composition. That is, increases in FFM, independent of changes in fat mass, will decrease body fat percentage. According to several studies, resistance training increases FFM and decreases body fat percentage in men (13), women (26, 103), and persons who are elderly (58).

Resistance training may also affect the amount of fat mass in the body as a consequence of the direct effect of the training on energy consumption. Higher-volume training burns more calories than lower-volume training. In addition, resistance training elevates energy consumption during the recovery period between training sessions, further facilitating fat loss (110).

An added benefit of resistance training is that increases in FFM, especially muscle mass, may increase resting metabolic rate and total daily energy expenditure. This occurs because muscle tissue, unlike fat tissue, has a high metabolic rate. That is, since the normal resting energy requirements of muscle are high, clients with more muscle mass should burn more calories at rest and throughout the day. However, while some studies have shown that resistance exercise can increase resting metabolic rate (58, 103), others have not (13, 26). It is also unclear whether resistance training significantly increases total daily energy expenditure (103). Nonetheless, given the clear effect of resistance exercise on FFM and its possible effect on resting metabolic rate, resistance training should be a critical component of any comprehensive program to control body fat.

Factors That Influence Adaptations to Resistance Training

A variety of factors affect the adaptations to resistance training described in the previous sections. These include factors such as **specificity** (i.e., the ability of the body to make adaptations that uniquely enhance performance in activities that are most similar to the exercise stressor), sex, age, and genetics. These factors affect the magnitude and rate of long-term adaptations that occur in the body. The following subsections explore these topics.

Specificity

Exercise training has been shown to be highly specific. That is, the body adapts to exercise in such a way that it can perform optimally in relation to a particular type of exercise stressor, but not necessarily other types of exercise. For instance, distance running has little to no positive effect on bench press performance. However, specificity also influences resistance exercise adaptations. In terms of resistance exercises, the correlations between static and dynamic performance are poor (5). A variety of studies have examined the effect of one type of resistance training on performance of other types of resistance exercise. In general, strength increases are larger in modes of exercise like those used during training. For example, resistance training with weights results in much larger performance increases on the weights than are seen with isokinetic tests (125). Isometric exercise training has also been shown to have little to no effect on performance of free weight exercises that involve the same muscle groups. Thus, it appears that the effects of resistance training are specific to the muscle action mode in which the exercise was performed.

Resistance training adaptations are also specific with respect to the velocity with which muscle actions have been performed in training. That is, strength increases tend to be greater when individuals are tested in situations that involve muscle actions occurring at velocities similar to those experienced during training (8, 125). Further, plyometric-type training is more effective than relatively slow-velocity heavy resistance exercise in improving power production (122). Therefore, for people who are performing resistance exercise to improve athletic performance, the personal trainer should tailor the training program as much as possible so it involves types of muscle actions similar to those seen during the athletic competition. Likewise, although all clients will benefit from a well-rounded resistance training program, an older client desiring the strength and endurance to carry heavy bags of groceries long distances would benefit from walking with hand weights, and a client desiring the strength to do home improvement projects such as pounding fence posts or repairing a deck would benefit from pushing and pulling exercises.

Sex

Males and females respond to resistance training in much the same way, yet males and females show significant quantitative differences in strength, muscle mass, and hormone levels. With respect to muscle strength, much of the difference between the sexes is attributable to differences in body size and body composition. Specifically, men tend to be larger than women, and the associated differences in muscle mass contribute to strength differences. Similarly, women tend to have a higher percentage of body fat than men; therefore, most women have less muscle per pound of body weight. These differences in body size and body composition are largely driven by differences in hormone levels between men and women, most notably differences in testosterone and estrogen levels. For example, adult male athletes have approximately 10 times the testosterone concentration of comparable female athletes (16). Interestingly, sex-related differences in strength are larger in the upper body than in the lower body (11), which likely reflects sex differences in the distribution of muscle mass (93). That is, women and men tend to exhibit similar lower body strength, whereas men typically have much greater upper body strength than women.

When one looks at sex differences in strength on a per pound of fat-free mass basis, strength differences shrink (11, 130). When assessed per unit of muscle cross-sectional area, sex differences are negligible (59). Furthermore, muscle architecture characteristics are similar between males and females (1). Thus, it appears that the force production capability of a given amount of muscle is not affected by whether one is male or female.

> The force production capability of a given amount of muscle is not affected by a person's sex.

Age

The process of aging produces a variety of changes in all body systems. The neuromuscular system is no exception. Starting in the 30s, muscle mass appears to decline progressively with time (61). This loss of muscle mass is referred to as **sarcopenia.** In addition to the loss in muscle mass, some evidence suggests that muscle quality also declines with age (35). That is, for a given amount of muscle, the amount of force that can be generated by that muscle declines. Aging skeletal muscle experiences muscle loss more severely in the high-threshold fast-twitch motor units (81). Therefore, as individuals age, they have not only diminished ability to produce force but also diminished ability to produce force rapidly. These aging effects on skeletal muscle affect performance in physical tasks such as those required for everyday activities, and may be associated with the increased incidence of falls that occurs with age.

Fortunately, these deleterious effects of aging can be moderated or even reversed (over the short term) with a program of high-intensity resistance training. Numerous studies have shown that resistance training can increase muscle mass and strength in persons who are elderly (18, 31, 34). In addition, the training can result in significant improvements in muscle function in particular and also general motor performance (e.g., walking, stair climbing) (32). Strength gains can be dramatic (upward of 200% for knee extension strength), and increases in muscle size may occur in both type I and type II muscle fibers (34). Resistance training in people who are elderly also increases bone density (98). Chapter 18 presents a more comprehensive overview of resistance training in older adults.

> As individuals age they not only have diminished ability to produce force; they also have diminished ability to produce force rapidly.

Genetics

Information about the physiological variables mentioned in the previous sections collectively demonstrates that human beings do not pick their successful activities as much as the activities pick them. This is due at least in part to what each individual brings to the table when beginning a resistance training program. Several factors are beyond a person's capacity to change. That is, people are limited by their genetic potential. Relative percentage of type I and type II fibers limits hypertrophy and either explosive or aerobic endurance capabilities. Sex plays a role in hormonal expression, further placing a ceiling on hypertrophy and thereby strength. Age limits the available muscle mass and the propagation of action potentials, which together limit not only strength but also the speed of movement. A personal trainer cannot devise a program that will take a client beyond the client's genetic capabilities. However, the average untrained client can make much improvement within his or her genetic potential.

Overtraining

Although physical adaptations are best brought about by increases in training volume and intensity, at certain points in a training program, more is not better. Inappropriate levels of volume or intensity can lead to a phenomenon known as **overtraining.** As the term suggests, overtraining is a condition in which an individual trains too much, resulting in "staleness" and general fatigue. The overtraining condition does not enhance strength and power levels in the client but leads to decreased performance. A detailed discussion of the many aspects of resistance exercise overtraining (e.g., metabolic, neuromuscular, endocrine) as both a physical and a psychological phenomenon is beyond the scope of this chapter, and the reader is referred to other detailed reviews on the topic (36, 115). Because of the danger of overtraining, the toleration of and recovery from resistance exercise stress are crucial factors that must be monitored carefully in every resistance training program.

Overtraining in resistance exercise has received much less attention than aerobic endurance overtraining, as significantly fewer studies have been reported. These studies make it clear that what we have found to be markers of overtraining in aerobic endurance exercise are not always representative of overtraining in resistance exercise. It appears that the two primary types of overtraining in resistance exercise are too much intensity and too much volume (36). Yet each has been difficult to study. However, it is clear that resistance exercise overtraining can lead to decreases in neuromuscular performance (15, 37, 38, 39, 40). It is interesting to note that, at least in experimental situations, inducing an overtraining state requires a very severe exercise intervention but can be accomplished through repeated bouts of high-intensity exercise (~100% 1RM [1-repetition maximum]) with relatively low volume (37, 38, 39). Many overtraining syndromes are a function of the rate of progression—that is, attempting to do too much, too soon before the body's physiological adaptations can cope with the stress. This typically results in extreme soreness or injury.

Individuals may fall into either or both of two overtraining scenarios: (1) overtraining of a muscle group or (2) overtraining of the body. Both scenarios are common, and many people may experience both. Overtraining is most often a result of increasing the volume of the program at too rapid a pace. In addition, some people may maintain too many days at high intensity without varying their load or taking a rest. Effective program design includes increasing and decreasing the total volume of the workout and using the concepts of periodization to plan changes in volume, intensity, and recovery (115) (see chapter 23). The difficulty in dealing with real overtraining and the symptoms that may develop is that there is no 100% accurate measurement for the onset of overtraining: Generally, once symptoms develop, overtraining is certain and strength gains have stopped. Once symptoms have developed, the most effective cure is rest (36).

Some programs use short periods of overwork followed by rest or reduced training to achieve the benefits of a "rebound" or supercompensation in physical strength and power (36). This process of "overreaching" (see page 102) is best used only by elite athletes in conjunction with experienced coaches, and most clients would be best served by more moderate training regimens.

Detraining

Detraining refers to the physiological and performance adaptations that occur when an individual ceases an exercise training program. These changes are the exact opposite of what occurs during training programs, and the individual regresses toward his or her condition prior to starting the program. Specifically, muscle tissue loses mass (57, 113), and the changes in neurological function (e.g., recruitment, rate coding, cocontraction) that occurred with training dissipate (47). Thus, the muscle becomes weaker and less powerful. Skeletal muscle atrophy appears to occur faster in the fast-twitch muscle fibers (57).

There is relatively little research on the detraining process with resistance training as compared to the training process, so the rapidity of the detraining process is poorly understood. However, short-term detraining (14 days) appears to have little effect on muscle strength and explosive power in experienced resistance-trained athletes (57) and recreational strength trainers (72), suggesting that the effects are relatively slow. Extended detraining (32 weeks) did result in significant decreases in muscle strength in previously resistance-trained females, but values were still above pretraining levels (113). Detraining appears to affect different aspects of neuromuscular performance differently. For example, isometric strength performance

Symptoms of Overtraining From Resistance Exercise

- Plateau followed by decrease of strength gains
- Sleep disturbances
- Decrease in lean body mass (when not dieting)
- Decreased appetite
- A cold that just won't go away
- Persistent flu-like symptoms
- Loss of interest in the training program
- Mood changes
- Excessive muscle soreness

appears to decay more rapidly than other strength measures (72, 123, 124). Similarly, performance on anaerobic metabolic tests (e.g., Wingate test) is more severely affected by detraining than performance on strength and explosive power tests (72). The effects of detraining can be significantly reduced with the incorporation of just one to two training sessions per week (43); clients with unexpectedly busy or difficult schedules may maintain a certain level of strength by training once or twice a week.

Conclusion

Resistance training is a very potent physiological stimulus. It has substantive effects on almost every system in the body, including muscle, bone, nerve, hormones, and connective tissue. Although resistance training is not a panacea, its effects are almost universally positive; and personal trainers should encourage all clients to engage in a vigorous program of resistance training. Benefits include improved appearance, improved body composition, increased muscle strength and power, increased muscle endurance, and stronger bones and connective tissue. These changes can improve quality of life and may have significant health benefits, including the attenuation of the deleterious effects of sarcopenia during aging and possibly attenuation of the effects of osteoporosis. In addition, the increased muscle performance (strength, endurance, power) will likely improve the performance of activities of daily living, so that tasks like carrying groceries and changing a tire are more easily accomplished.

Study Questions

1. Which of the following is most likely to occur during muscular fatigue?

   I. motor unit recruitment increases

   II. rate coding increases

   III. muscle pH decreases

   IV. ATP stores increase

   A. I and II only

   B. II and IV only

   C. I and IV only

   D. II and III only

2. Which of the following is primarily responsible for activation of fast-twitch motor units?

   A. increased speed demands

   B. increased force demands

   C. decreased speed demands

   D. decreased force demands

3. Which of the following are the most influential training factors promoting increased hormonal responses?

   A. higher volume, shorter rest periods, smaller muscle mass exercises

   B. higher volume, longer rest periods, larger muscle mass exercises

   C. higher volume, shorter rest periods, larger muscle mass exercises

   D. lower volume, shorter rest periods, larger muscle mass exercises

4. Resistance exercise augments aerobic endurance performance by which of the following?

   A. increased $\dot{V}O_2$

   B. increased oxidative enzyme activity

   C. increased capillary density

   D. increased muscular strength and power

Applied Knowledge Question

Complete the following chart to describe two ways the body's systems adapt to chronic participation in a resistance training program.

System	Two adaptations
Nervous	
Muscular	
Skeletal	
Metabolic	
Hormonal	
Cardiorespiratory	

References

1. Abe, T., W.F. Brechue, S. Fujita, and J.B. Brown. 1998. Gender differences in FFM accumulation and architectural characteristics of muscle. *Medicine and Science in Sports and Exercise* 30 (7): 1066-1070.

2. Alen, M., A. Pakarinen, K. Hakkinen, and P.V. Komi. 1988. Responses of serum androgenic-anabolic and catabolic hormones to prolonged strength training. *International Journal of Sports Medicine* 9: 229-233.

3. American College of Sports Medicine. 1995. Position stand: Osteoporosis and exercise. *Medicine and Science in Sports and Exercise* 27: i-vii.

4. Antonio, J., and W.J. Gonyea. 1993. Skeletal muscle hyperplasia. *Medicine and Science in Sports and Exercise* 25 (12): 1333-1345.

5. Baker, D., G. Wilson, and B. Carlyon. 1994. Generality versus specificity: A comparison of dynamic and isometric measures of strength and speed-power. *European Journal of Applied Physiology* 68 (4): 350-355.

6. Barry, D.W., and W.M. Kohrt. 2008. Exercise and the preservation of bone health. *Journal of Cardiopulmonary Rehabilitation* 28: 153-162.

7. Basmajian, J.V., and C.J. DeLuca. 1985. *Muscles Alive: Their Functions Revealed by Electromyography,* 5th ed. Baltimore: Williams & Wilkins. p. 164.

8. Behm, D.G., and D.G. Sale. 1993. Intended rather than actual movement velocity determines velocity-specific training response. *Journal of Applied Physiology* 74 (1): 359-368.

9. Bellemare, F., J.J. Woods, R. Johansson, and B. Bigland-Ritchie. 1983. Motor unit discharge rates in maximal voluntary contractions of three human muscles. *Journal of Neurophysiology* 50: 1380-1392.

10. Bemben, D.A., N.L. Fetters, M.G. Bemben, N. Nabavi, and E.T. Koh. 2000. Musculoskeletal responses to high- and low-intensity resistance training in early postmenopausal women. *Medicine and Science in Sports and Exercise* 32 (11): 1949-1957.

11. Bishop, P., K. Cureton, and M. Collins. 1987. Sex difference in muscular strength in equally-trained men and women. *Ergonomics* 30 (4): 675-687.

12. Braith, R.W., J.E. Graves, S.H. Leggett, and M.L. Pollock. 1993. Effect of training on the relationship between maximal and submaximal strength. *Medicine and Science in Sports and Exercise* 25 (1): 132-138.

13. Broeder, C.E., K.A. Burrhus, L.S. Svanevik, and J.H. Wilmore. 1992. The effects of either high-intensity resistance or endurance training on resting metabolic rate. *American Journal of Clinical Nutrition* 55 (4): 802-810.

14. Buresh, R., K. Berg, and J. French. 2009. The effect of resistive exercise rest interval on hormonal response, strength, and hypertrophy with training. *Journal of Strength and Conditioning Research* 23: 62-71.

15. Callister, R., R.J. Callister, S.J. Fleck, and G.A. Dudley. 1990. Physiological and performance responses to overtraining in elite judo athletes. *Medicine and Science in Sports and Exercise* 22 (6): 816-824.

16. Cardinale, M., and M.H. Stone. 2006. Is testosterone influencing explosive performance? *Journal of Strength and Conditioning Research* 20: 103-107.

17. Carolan, B., and E. Cafarelli. 1992. Adaptations in coactivation after isometric resistance training. *Journal of Applied Physiology* 73 (3): 911-917.

18. Charette, S.L., L. McEvoy, G. Pyka, C. Snow-Harter, D. Guido, R.A. Wiswell, and R. Marcus. 1991. Muscle hypertrophy response to resistance training in older women. *Journal of Applied Physiology* 70: 1912-1916.

19. Chesley, A., J.D. MacDougall, M.A. Tarnopolsky, S.A. Atkinson, and K. Smith. 1992. Changes in human muscle protein synthesis after resistance exercise. *Journal of Applied Physiology* 73 (4): 1383-1388.

20. Colliander, E.B., and P.A. Tesch. 1990. Effects of eccentric and concentric muscle actions in resistance training. *Acta Physiologica Scandinavica* 140: 31-39.

21. Collins, M.A., K.J. Cureton, D.W. Hill, and C.A. Ray. 1991. Relationship between heart rate to oxygen uptake during weight lifting exercise. *Medicine and Science in Sports and Exercise* 23 (5): 636-640.

22. Costill, D.L., E.F. Coyle, W.F. Fink, G.R. Lesmes, and F.A. Witzman. 1979. Adaptations in skeletal muscle following strength training. *Journal of Applied Physiology* 46: 96-99.

23. Couppe, C., M. Kongsgaard, P. Aagaard, P. Hansen, J. Bojsen-Moller, M. Kjaer, and S.P. Magnusson. Habitual loading results in tendon hypertrophy and increased stiffness of the human patellar tendon. *Journal of Applied Physiology*, 105: 805-810, 2008.

24. Crewther, B., J. Cronin, and J. Keough. 2006. Possible stimuli for strength and power adaptation. Acute metabolic responses. *Sports Medicine* 36: 215-238.

25. Crewther, B., J. Keough, J. Cronin, and C. Cook. 2006. Possible stimuli for strength and power adaptation. Acute hormonal responses. *Sports Medicine* 36: 65-78.

26. Cullinen, K., and M. Caldwell. 1998. Weight training increases fat-free mass and strength in untrained young women. *Journal of the American Dietetic Association* 98 (4): 414-418.

27. DeLuca, C.J. 1997. The use of surface electromyography in biomechanics. *Journal of Applied Biomechanics* 13: 135-163.

28. Deschenes, M. 1989. Short review: Rate coding and motor unit recruitment patterns. *Journal of Applied Sport Science Research* 3 (2): 33-39.

29. Dons, B., K. Bollerup, F. Bonde-Peterson, and S. Hanacke. 1979. The effect of weight-lifting exercise related to muscle fiber composition and muscle cross-sectional area in humans. *European Journal of Applied Physiology* 40: 95-106.

30. Enoka, R.M. 1994. *Neuromechanical Basis of Kinesiology,* 2nd ed. Champaign, IL: Human Kinetics. p. 194.

31. Fiatarone, M.A., E.C. Marks, N.D. Ryan, C.N. Meredith, L.A. Lipsitz, and W.J. Evans. 1990. High-intensity strength training in nonagenarians. Effects on skeletal muscle. *Journal of the American Medical Association* 263: 3029-3034.

32. Fiatarone, M.A., E.R. O'Neill, N.D. Ryan, K.M. Clements, G.R. Solares, M.E. Nelson, S.B. Roberts, J.J. Kehayias, L.A. Lipsitz, and W.J. Evans. 1994. Exercise training and nutritional supplementation for physical frailty in very elderly people. *New England Journal of Medicine* 330 (25): 1769-1775.

33. Folland, J.P., and A.G. Williams. 2007. The adaptations to strength training. Morphological and neurological contributions to increased strength. *Sports Medicine* 37: 145-168.

34. Frontera, W.R., C.N. Meredith, K.P. O'Reilly, H.G. Knuttgen, and W.J. Evans. 1988. Strength conditioning in older men: Skeletal muscle hypertrophy and improved function. *Journal of Applied Physiology* 64: 1038-1044.

35. Frontera, W.R., D. Suh, L.S. Krivickas, V.A. Hughes, R. Goldstein, and R. Roubenoff. 2000. Skeletal muscle fiber quality in older men and women. *American Journal of Physiology* 279: C611-C616.

36. Fry, A.C., and W.J. Kraemer. 1997. Resistance exercise overtraining and overreaching. *Sports Medicine* 23 (2): 106-129.

37. Fry, A.C., J.M. Webber, L.W. Weiss, M.D. Fry, and Y. Li. 2000. Impaired performances with excessive high-intensity free-weight training. *Journal of Strength and Conditioning Research* 14 (1): 54-61.

38. Fry, A.C., W.J. Kraemer, F. Van Borselen, J.M. Lynch, J.L. Marsit, E.P. Roy, N.T. Triplett, and H.G. Knuttgen. 1994. Performance decrements with high-intensity resistance exercise overtraining. *Medicine and Science in Sports and Exercise* 26 (9): 1165-1173.

39. Fry, A.C., W.J. Kraemer, F. Van Borselen, J.M. Lynch, N.T. Triplett, L.P. Koziris, and S.J. Fleck. 1994. Catecholamine responses to short-term, high-intensity resistance exercise overtraining. *Journal of Applied Physiology* 77 (2): 941-946.

40. Fry, A.C., W.J. Kraemer, J.M. Lynch, N.T. Triplett, and L.P. Koziris. 1994. Does short-term near maximal intensity machine resistance training induce overtraining? *Journal of Strength and Conditioning Research* 8 (3): 188-191.

41. Garfinkel, S., and E. Cafarelli. 1992. Relative changes in maximal force, EMG, and muscle cross-sectional area after isometric training. *Medicine and Science in Sports and Exercise* 24: 1220-1227.

42. Goldspink, G. 1992. Cellular and molecular aspects of adaptation in skeletal muscle. In: *Strength and Power in Sport: The Encyclopedia of Sports Medicine,* P.V. Komi, ed. Oxford, England: Blackwell Scientific. pp. 211-229.

43. Graves, J.E., M.L. Pollock, S.H. Leggett, R.W. Braith, D.M. Carpenter, and L.E. Bishop. 1988. Effect of reduced training frequency on muscular strength. *International Journal of Sports Medicine* 9 (5): 316-319.

44. Green, H., C. Goreham, J. Ouyang, M. Bull-Burnett, and D. Ranney. 1999. Regulation of fiber size, oxidative potential, and capillarization in human muscle by resistance exercise. *American Journal of Physiology* 276 (2 Pt 2): R591-R596.

45. Guezennec, Y., L. Leger, F. Lhoste, M. Aymonod, and P.C. Pesquies. 1986. Hormone and metabolite response to weight-lifting training sessions. *International Journal of Sports Medicine* 7: 100-105.

46. Haff, G.G., M.H. Stone, B.J. Warren, R. Keith, R.L. Johnson, D.C. Nieman, F. Williams, and K.B. Kirksey. 1999. The effect of carbohydrate supplementation on multiple sessions and bouts of resistance exercise. *Journal of Strength and Conditioning Research* 13 (3): 111-117.

47. Häkkinen, K., A. Pakarinen, W.J. Kraemer, A. Häkkinen, H. Valkeinen, and M. Alen. 2001. Selective muscle hypertrophy, changes in EMG and force, and serum hormones during strength training in older women. *Journal of Applied Physiology* 91 (2): 569-580.

48. Häkkinen, K., A. Pakarinen, W.J. Kraemer, R.U. Newton, and M. Alen. 2000. Basal concentrations and acute responses of serum hormones and strength development during heavy resistance training in middle-aged and elderly men and women. *Journal of Gerontology* 55 (2): B95-B105.

49. Häkkinen, K., A. Parkarinen, M. Alen, H. Kauhanen, and P.V. Komi. 1988. Neuromuscular and hormonal adaptations in athletes to strength training in two years. *Journal of Applied Physiology* 65: 2406-2412.

50. Häkkinen, K., and P.V. Komi. 1983. Electromyographic changes during strength training and detraining. *Medicine and Science in Sports and Exercise* 15: 455-460.

51. Hansen, M., B.F. Miller, L. Holm, S. Doessing, S.G. Petersen, D. Skovgaard, J. Frystyk, A. Flyvbjerg, S. Koskinen, J. Pingel, M. Kjaer, and H. Langberg. Effect of oral contraceptives in vivo on collagen synthesis in tendon and muscle connective tissue in young women. *Journal of Applied Physiology,* 106: 1435-1443, 2009.

52. Harris, R.T., and G.A. Dudley. 2000. Neuromuscular anatomy and adaptations to conditioning. In: *Essentials of Strength Training and Conditioning,* T.R. Baechle and R.W. Earle, eds. Champaign, IL: Human Kinetics. pp. 15-23.

53. Hather, B.M., P.A. Tesch, P. Buchannon, and G.A. Dudley. 1991. Influence of eccentric actions on skeletal muscle adaptation to resistance training. *Acta Physiologica Scandinavica* 143: 177-185.

54. Hellebrandt, F.A., A.M. Parrish, and J.J. Houtz. 1947. Cross education: The influence of unilateral exercise on the contralateral limb. *Archives of Physical Medicine* 28: 76-85.

55. Hickson, R.C., B.A. Dvorak, E.M. Gorostiaga, T.T. Kurowski, and C. Foster. 1988. Potential for strength and endurance training to amplify endurance performance. *Journal of Applied Physiology* 65: 2285-2290.

56. Hoff, J., J. Helgerud, and U. Wisloff. 1999. Maximal strength training improves work economy in trained female cross-country skiers. *Medicine and Science in Sports and Exercise* 31 (6): 870-877.

57. Hortobagyi, T., J.A. Houmard, J.R. Stevenson, D.D. Fraser, R.A. Johns, and R.G. Israel. 1993. The effects of detraining in power athletes. *Medicine and Science in Sports and Exercise* 28 (8): 929-935.

58. Hunter, G.R., C.J. Wetzstein, D.A. Fields, A. Brown, and M.M. Bamman. 2000. Resistance training increases total energy expenditure and free-living physical activity in older adults. *Journal of Applied Physiology* 89 (3): 977-984.

59. Ikai, M., and A.H. Steinhaus. 1961. Some factors modifying the expression of human strength. *Journal of Applied Physiology* 16: 157-163.

60. Ikai, M., and T. Fukunaga. 1968. Calculation of muscle strength per unit cross-sectional area of human muscle by means of ultrasonic measurement. *Internationale Zeitschrift fur angewandte Physiologie, einschliesslich Arbeitsphysiologie* 26 (1): 26-32.

61. Imamura, K., H. Ashida, T. Ishikawawa, and M. Fujii. 1983. Human major psoas muscle and sacrospinalis muscle in relation to age: A study by computed tomography. *Journal of Gerontology* 38 (6): 678-681.

62. Inoue, K., S. Yamasaki, T. Fushiki, T. Kano, T. Moritani, K. Itoh, and E. Sugimoto. 1993. Rapid increase in the number of androgen receptors following electrical stimulation. *European Journal of Applied Physiology* 66 (2): 134-140.

63. Judelson, D.A., C.M. Maresh, L.M. Yamamoto, M.J. Farrell, L.E. Armstrong, W.J. Kraemer, J.S. Volek, B.A. Spiering, D.J. Casa, and J.M. Anderson. 2008. Effect of hydration state on resistance exercise-induced endocrine markers of anabolism, catabolism, and metabolism. *Journal of Applied Physiology* 105: 816-824.

64. Kitai, T.A., and D.G. Sale. 1989. Specificity of joint angle in isometric testing. *European Journal of Applied Physiology* 58: 744-748.

65. Kohrt, W.M., S.A. Bloomfield, K.D. Little, M.E. Nelson, and V.R. Yingling. 2004. American College of Sports Medicine position stand. Physical activity and bone health. *Medicine and Science in Sports and Exercise* 36: 1985-1996.

66. Komi, P.V., J.T. Viitasalo, R. Rauramaa, and V. Vihko. 1978. Effect of isometric strength training on mechanical, electrical, and metabolic aspects of muscle function. *European Journal of Applied Physiology* 40: 45-55.

67. Kongsgaard, M., P. Aagaard, M. Kjaer, and S.P. Magnusson. Structural Achilles tendon properties in athletes subjected to different exercise modes and in Achilles tendon rupture patients. *Journal of Applied Physiology,* 99: 1965-1971, 2005.

68. Kongsgaard, M., S. Reitelseder, T.G. Pedersen, L. Holm, P. Aagaard, M. Kjaer, and S.P. Magnusson. Region specific patellar tendon hypertrophy in humans flowing resistance training. *Acta Physiologica,* 191: 111-121, 2007.

69. Kraemer, W.J. 1992. Endocrine responses and adaptations to strength training. In: *Strength and Power in Sport: The Encyclopedia of Sports Medicine,* P.V. Komi, ed. Oxford, England: Blackwell Scientific. pp. 291-304.

70. Kraemer, W.J., and N.A. Ratamess. 2005. Hormonal responses and adaptations to resistance exercise and training. *Sports Medicine* 35: 339-361.

71. Kraemer, W.J., B.J. Noble, B. Culver, and R.V. Lewis. 1985. Changes in plasma proenkephalin peptide F and catecholamine levels during graded exercise in men. *Proceedings of the National Academy of Sciences* 82: 6349-6351.

72. Kraemer, W.J., J.F. Patton, S.E. Gordon, E.A. Harman, M.R. Deschenes, K. Reynolds, R.U. Newton, N.T. Triplett, and J.E. Dziados. 1995. Compatibility of high intensity strength and endurance training on hormonal and skeletal muscle adaptations. *Journal of Applied Physiology* 78 (3): 976-989.

73. Kraemer, W.J., K. Häkkinen, R.U. Newton, M. McCormick, B.C. Nindl, J.S. Volek, L.A. Gotshalk, S.J. Fleck, W.W. Campbell, S.E. Gordon, P.A. Farrell, and W.J. Evans. 1998. Acute hormonal responses to heavy resistance exercise in younger and older men. *European Journal of Applied Physiology* 77 (3): 206-211.

74. Kraemer, W.J., L.P. Koziris, N.A. Ratamess, K. Häkkinen, N.T. Triplett-McBride, A.C. Fry, S.E. Gordon, J.S. Volek, D.N. French, M.R. Rubin, A.L. Gomez, M.T. Sharman, J.M. Lynch, M. Izquierdo, R.U. Newton, and S.J. Fleck. 2002. Detraining produces minimal changes in physical performance and hormonal variables in recreationally strength-trained men. *Journal of Strength and Conditioning Research* 16 (3): 373-382.

75. Kraemer, W.J., R.S. Staron, F.C. Hagerman, R.S. Hikida, A.C. Fry, S.E. Gordon, B.C. Nindl, L.A. Gotshalk, J.S. Volek, J.O. Marx, R.U. Newton, and K. Häkkinen. 1998. The effects of short-term resistance training on endocrine function in men and women. *European Journal of Applied Physiology* 78 (1): 69-76.

76. Kraemer, W.J., S.J. Fleck, and W.J. Evans. 1996. Strength and power: Physiological mechanisms of adaptation. *Exercise and Sport Science Reviews* 24: 363-397.

77. Kubo, K., T. Ikebukuro, H. Yata, and N. Tsunoda. Time course of changes in muscle and tendon properties during strength training and detraining. *Journal of Strength and Conditioning Research*, 24: 322-331, 2010.

78. LaCerte, M., B.J. deLateur, A.P. Alquist, and K.A. Questad. 1992. Concentric versus combined concentric-eccentric isokinetic training programs: Effect on peak torque of human quadriceps femoris muscle. *Archives of Physical Medicine and Rehabilitation* 73: 1059-1062.

79. Lambert, C.P., and M.G. Flynn. 2002. Fatigue during high-intensity intermittent exercise. Applications to bodybuilding. *Sports Medicine* 32 (8): 511-522.

80. Langberg, H., L. Rosendal, and M. Kjaer. Training-induced changes in peritendinous type I collagen turnover determined by microdialysis in humans. *Journal of Physiology*, 534.1: 297-302, 2001.

81. Larsson, L. 1978. Morphological and functional characteristics of the ageing skeletal muscle in man. *Acta Physiologica Scandinavica* (Suppl) 457: 1-36.

82. Leveritt, M., and P.J. Abernethy. 1999. Effect of carbohydrate restriction on strength performance. *Journal of Strength and Conditioning Research* 13: 52-57.

83. MacDougall, J.D., G.R. Ward, D.G. Sale, and J.R. Sutton. 1977. Biochemical adaptation of human skeletal muscle to heavy resistance training and immobilization. *Journal of Applied Physiology* 43: 700-703.

84. MacDougall, J.D., M.J. Gibala, M.A. Tarnopolsky, J.R. MacDonald, S.A. Interisano, and K.E. Yarasheski. 1995. The time course for elevated muscle protein synthesis following heavy resistance exercise. *Canadian Journal of Applied Physiology* 20 (4): 480-486.

85. MacDougall, J.D., S. Ray, D.G. Sale, N. McCartney, P. Lee, and S. Garner. 1999. Muscle substrate utilization and lactate production during weightlifting. *Canadian Journal of Applied Physiology* 24: 209-215.

86. MacLaren, D.P., H. Gibson, M. Parry-Billings, and R.H.T. Edwards. 1989. A review of metabolic and physiological factors in fatigue. *Exercise and Sport Sciences Reviews* 17: 29-66.

87. Maddalozzo, G.F., and C.M. Snow. 2000. High intensity resistance training: Effects on bone in older men and women. *Calcified Tissue International* 66: 399-404.

88. Marcinik, E.J., J. Potts, G. Schlabach, S. Will, P. Dawson, and B.F. Hurley. 1991. Effects of strength training on lactate threshold and endurance performance. *Medicine and Science in Sports and Exercise* 23: 739-743.

89. Martyn-St James, M., and S. Carroll. 2006. Progressive high-intensity resistance training and bone mineral density changes among premenopausal women. Evidence of discordant site-specific skeletal effects. *Sports Medicine* 36: 683-704.

90. Masuda, K., T. Masuda, T. Sadoyama, M. Inaki, and S. Katsuta. 1999. Changes in surface EMG parameters during static and dynamic fatiguing contractions. *Journal of Electromyography and Kinesiology* 9 (1): 39-46.

91. McBride, J.M., T. Triplett-McBride, A.J. Davie, P.J. Abernethy, and R.U. Newton. 2003. Characteristics of titin in strength and power athletes. *European Journal of Applied Physiology* 88: 553-557.

92. Merton, P.A. 1954. Voluntary strength and fatigue. *Journal of Physiology (London)* 123: 553-564.

93. Miller, A.E.J., J.D. MacDougall, M.A. Tarnopolsky, and D.G. Sale. 1993. Gender differences in strength and muscle fiber characteristics. *European Journal of Applied Physiology* 66: 254-262.

94. Miller, B.F., J.L. Olesen, M. Hansen, S. Dossing, R.M. Crameri, R.J. Welling, H. Lanberg, A. Flyvbjerg, M. Kjaer, J.A. Babraj, K. Smith, and M.J. Rennie. Coordinated collagen and muscle protein synthesis in human patella tendon and quadriceps muscle after exercise. *Journal of Physiology*, 567.3: 1021-1033, 2005.

95. Milner-Brown, H.S., R.B. Stein, and R.G. Lee. 1975. Synchronization of human motor units: Possible roles of exercise and supraspinal reflexes. *Electroencephalography and Clinical Neurophysiology* 38: 245-254.

96. Moritani, T., and H.A. deVries. 1979. Neural factors vs. hypertrophy in the time course of muscle strength gain. *American Journal of Physical Medicine* 58: 115-130.

97. Moritani, T., and Y. Yoshitake. 1998. 1998 ISEK Congress Keynote Lecture. The use of surface electromyography in applied physiology. *Journal of Electromyography and Kinesiology* 8: 363-381.

98. Nelson, M.E., M.A. Fiatarone, C.M. Morganti, I. Trice, R.A. Greenberg, and W.J. Evans. 1994. Effects of high-intensity strength training on multiple risk factors for osteoporotic fractures. *Journal of the American Medical Association* 272: 1909-1914.

99. Osternig, L.R., J. Hamill, J.E. Lander, and R. Robertson. 1986. Co-activation of sprinter and distance runner muscles in isokinetic exercise. *Medicine and Science in Sports and Exercise* 18: 431-435.

100. Paavolainen, L., K. Häkkinen, I. Hamalainen, A. Nummela, and H. Rusko. 1999. Explosive-strength training improves 5-km running time by improving running economy and muscle power. *Journal of Applied Physiology* 86: 1527-1533.

101. Parcell, A.C., M.T. Wolstenhulme, and R.D. Sawyer. 2009. Structural protein alterations to resistance and endurance cycling exercise training. *Journal of Strength and Conditioning Research* 23: 359-365.

102. Patten, C., G. Kamen, and D.M. Rowland. 2001. Adaptations in maximal motor unit discharge rate to strength training in young and older adults. *Muscle and Nerve* 24 (4): 542-550.

103. Poehlman, E.T., W.F. Denino, T. Beckett, K.A. Kinaman, I.J. Dionne, R. Dvorak, and P.A. Ades. 2002. Effects of endurance and resistance training on total daily energy expenditure in young women: A controlled randomized trial. *Journal of Clinical Endocrinology and Metabolism* 87 (3): 1004-1009.

104. Pruitt, L.A., D.R. Taaffe, and R. Marcus. 1995. Effects of a one-year high-intensity versus low-intensity resistance training program on bone mineral density in older women. *Journal of Bone Mineral Research* 10: 1788-1795.

105. Psek, J.A., and E. Cafarelli. 1993. Behavior of coactive muscles during fatigue. *Journal of Applied Physiology* 74: 170-175.

106. Robergs, R.A., D.R. Pearson, D.L. Costill, W.J. Fink, D.D. Pascoe, M.A. Benedict, C.P. Lambert, and J.J. Zachweija. 1991. Muscle glycogenolysis during different intensities of weight-resistance exercise. *Journal of Applied Physiology* 70 (4): 1700-1706.

107. Rutherford, O.M., D.A. Jones, and D.J. Newham. 1986. Clinical and experimental application of percutaneous twitch superimposition technique for the study of human muscle activation. *Journal of Neurology, Neurosurgery, and Psychiatry* 49: 1288-1291.

108. Sale, D.G. 1992. Neural adaptation to strength training. In: *Strength and Power in Sport: The Encyclopedia of Sports Medicine,* P.V. Komi, ed. Oxford, England: Blackwell Scientific. pp. 249-265.

109. Sale, D.G., J.D. MacDougall, A.R.M. Upton, and A.J. McComas. 1983. Effects of strength training upon motoneuron excitability in man. *Medicine and Science in Sports and Exercise* 15: 57-62.

110. Schuenke, M.D., R.P. Mikat, and J.M. McBride. 2002. Effect of an acute period of resistance exercise on excess post-exercise oxygen consumption: Implications for body mass management. *European Journal of Applied Physiology* 86: 411-417.

111. Schwab, R., G.O. Johnson, T.J. Housh, J.E. Kinder, and J.P. Weir. 1993. Acute effects of different intensities of weightlifting on serum testosterone. *Medicine and Science in Sports and Exercise* 25: 1381-1385.

112. Staron, R.S., D.L. Karapondo, W.J. Kraemer, A.C. Fry, S.E. Gordon, J.E. Falkel, F.C. Hagerman, and R.S. Hikida. 1994. Skeletal muscle adaptations during early phase of heavy-resistance training in men and women. *Journal of Applied Physiology* 76: 1247-1255.

113. Staron, R.S., E.S. Malicky, M.J. Leonardi, J.E. Falkel, F.C. Hagerman, and G.A. Dudley. 1990. Muscle hypertrophy and fast fiber type conversions in heavy resistance-trained women. *European Journal of Applied Physiology* 60: 71-79.

114. Staron, R.S., M.J. Leonardi, D.L. Karapondo, E.S. Malicky, J.E. Falkel, F.G. Hagerman, and R.S. Hikida. 1991. Strength and skeletal muscle adaptations in heavy-resistance trained women after detraining and retraining. *Journal of Applied Physiology* 70 (2): 631-640.

115. Stone, M.H., R.E. Keith, J.T. Kearny, S.J. Fleck, G.D. Wilson, and N.T. Triplett. 1991. Overtraining: A review of the signs, symptoms, and possible causes. *Journal of Applied Sport Science Research* 5 (1): 35-50.

116. Stone, W.J., and S.P. Coulter. 1994. Strength/endurance effects from three resistance training protocols with women. *Journal of Strength and Conditioning Research* 8 (4): 231-234.

117. Tesch, P.A. 1992. Short- and long-term histochemical and biochemical adaptations in muscle. In: *Strength and Power in Sport: The Encyclopedia of Sports Medicine,* P. Komi, ed. Oxford, England: Blackwell Scientific. pp. 239-248.

118. Tesch, P.A., A. Thorsson, and E.B. Colliander. 1990. Effects of eccentric and concentric resistance training on skeletal muscle substrates, enzyme activities and capillary supply. *Acta Physiologica Scandinavica* 140: 575-580.

119. Thepaut-Mathieu, C., J. Van Hoecke, and B. Maton. 1988. Myoelectrical and mechanical changes linked to length specificity during isometric training. *Journal of Applied Physiology* 64: 1500-1505.

120. Tipton, K.D., and R.R. Wolfe. 2001. Exercise protein metabolism and muscle growth. *International Journal of Sport Nutrition and Exercise Metabolism* 11 (1): 109-132.

121. Vincent, K.R., and R.W. Braith. 2002. Resistance exercise and bone turnover in elderly men and women. *Medicine and Science in Sports and Exercise* 34: 17-23.

122. Vissing, K., M. Brink, S. Lonbro, H. Sorensen, K. Overgaard, K. Danborg, J. Mortensen, O. Elstrom, N. Rosenhoj, S. Ringgaard, J.L. Andersen, and P. Aagaard. 2008. Muscle adaptations to plyometric vs. resistance training in untrained young men. *Journal of Strength and Conditioning Research* 22: 1799-1809.

123. Weir, J.P., D.A. Keefe, J.F. Eaton, R.T. Augustine, and D.M. Tobin. 1998. Effect of fatigue on hamstring coactivation during isokinetic knee extensions. *European Journal of Applied Physiology* 78: 555-559.

124. Weir, J.P., D.J. Housh, T.J. Housh, and L.L. Weir. 1995. The effect of unilateral eccentric weight training detraining on joint angle specificity, cross-training, and the bilateral deficit. *Journal of Orthopaedic and Sports Physical Therapy* 22 (5): 207-215.

125. Weir, J.P., D.J. Housh, T.J. Housh, and L.L. Weir. 1997. The effect of unilateral concentric weight training and detraining on joint angle specificity, cross-training, and the bilateral deficit. *Journal of Orthopaedic and Sports Physical Therapy* 25: 264-270.

126. Weir, J.P., T.J. Housh, and L.L. Weir. 1994. Electromyographic evaluation of joint angle specificity and cross-training after isometric training. *Journal of Applied Physiology* 77: 197-201.

127. Weir, J.P., T.J. Housh, L.L. Weir, and G.O. Johnson. 1995. Effects of unilateral isometric strength training on joint angle specificity and cross-training. *European Journal of Applied Physiology* 70: 337-343.

128. Weir, J.P., T.J. Housh, S.A. Evans, and G.O. Johnson. 1993. The effect of dynamic constant external resistance training on the isokinetic torque-velocity curve. *International Journal of Sports Medicine* 14 (3): 124-128.

129. Westh, E., M. Kongsgaard, J. Bojsen-Moller, P. Aagaard, M. Hansen, M. Kjaer, and S.P. Magnusson. Effect of habitual exercise on the structural and mechanical properties of human tendon, in vivo, in men and women. *Scandinavian Journal of Medicine and Science in Sports,* 18: 23-30, 2008.

130. Winter, E.M., and R.J. Maughan. 1991. Strength and cross-sectional area of the quadriceps in men and women. *Journal of Physiology (London)* 438: 175.

131. Woolstenhulme, M.T., R.K. Conlee, M.J. Drummond, A.W. Stites, and A.C. Parcell. 2006. Temporal response of desmin and dystrophin proteins to progressive resistance exercise in human skeletal muscle. *Journal of Applied Physiology* 100: 1876-1882.

Physiological Responses and Adaptations to Aerobic Endurance Training

John P. McCarthy, PhD, and Jane L.P. Roy, PhD

After completing this chapter, you will be able to

- identify acute physiological responses to aerobic exercise,
- identify chronic physiological adaptations to aerobic endurance training,
- understand the factors that influence adaptations to aerobic endurance training,
- understand and identify the physiological factors associated with overtraining, and
- identify the physiological consequences of detraining.

The primary purpose of this chapter is to discuss the effects of aerobic exercise on the body's physiological systems and to explain the adaptations that occur. Acute responses occur immediately during a single exercise bout, whereas chronic training adaptations occur due to a series of repeated exercise bouts. The effects of aerobic exercise are regulated by the intensity, duration, and frequency of the activity. Paramount among these is intensity (e.g., %HRmax [% maximal heart rate]). In other words, the body adapts to an acute exercise stressor in proportion to that stressor. Generally speaking, then, if one exercises at a greater heart rate during aerobic exercise, the training adaptations will be greater than if one exercises at a lower heart rate. Of course, this assumes that frequency and duration are constant across training sessions.

It is the interplay of these components that results in aerobic physiological adaptations. With aerobic endurance training the body responds through alterations in many physiological processes and systems. The sections that follow explain in further detail exactly how these changes occur. The overall adaptation to recurring aerobic exercise is one that represents a more efficient body, resulting in less effort by all organs at the same exercise work rate.

Acute Responses to Aerobic Endurance Exercise

This section describes the acute effects of aerobic exercise on the cardiovascular, respiratory, and endocrine systems as well as the effects on metabolism.

The acute responses to aerobic exercise are summarized in table 6.1, and responses for most physiological variables (e.g., oxygen consumption [$\dot{V}O_2$], heart rate [HR]) are strongly related to exercise intensity.

Cardiovascular Responses

The cardiovascular system consists of two components, the heart and the vasculature (i.e., blood and blood vessels). For specific information with regard to the cardiovascular system's structure and function, refer to chapter 2. During aerobic exercise,

TABLE 6.1 Summary of Acute Responses to Aerobic Endurance Training

Variable	Response
CARDIOVASCULAR	
Heart rate	Increase
Stroke volume	Increase
Cardiac output	Increase
Total peripheral resistance	Decrease
Blood flow to coronary vasculature	Increase
Skeletal muscle blood flow	Increase
Splanchnic blood flow	Decrease
Mean arterial pressure	Increase
Systolic blood pressure	Increase
Diastolic blood pressure	No change or slight decrease
Rate–pressure product	Increase
Plasma volume	Decrease
Hematocrit	Increase
RESPIRATORY	
Pulmonary minute ventilation	Increase
Breathing rate	Increase
Tidal volume	Increase
RER or RQ	Increase
METABOLIC	
Oxygen consumption	Increase
Arteriovenous oxygen (a–$\bar{v}O_2$) difference	Increase
Blood lactate	Increase
Blood pH	Decrease
ENDOCRINE	
Catecholamines	Increase
Glucagon	Increase
Insulin	Decrease
Cortisol	Decrease—low to moderate intensity
	Increase—moderate to high intensity (>60% $\dot{V}O_2$max)
Growth hormone	Increase

RER = respiratory exchange ratio; RQ = respiratory quotient.

an increased stimulation or excitation of the heart occurs in order to supply blood to the exercising skeletal muscle. Although not the only reason for an increase in blood flow, a simple explanation is an increase in stimulation of the heart by the sympathetic nervous system and at the same time a reduction in parasympathetic nervous system stimulation. Because of the effect of the nervous system, the HR and stroke volume (SV, amount of blood ejected per beat from left ventricle) increase during exercise. The increase in HR and SV ultimately increases the cardiac output ($\dot{Q}$). The following formula helps to identify the relationship between HR and SV in determining $\dot{Q}$:

$$\dot{Q} \text{ (L/min)} = \text{HR (beats/min)} \times \text{SV (L/beat)} \qquad (6.1)$$

Stroke volume has been shown to increase to maximal levels at 40% to 60% of maximal oxygen consumption ($\dot{V}O_2$max) and plateau long before exhaustion (29). This finding is not conclusive, as other studies have indicated that SV continues to rise more linearly until exhaustion (65). During exercise, an increase in venous filling of the heart contributes to an increased pressure and stretching of the walls of the heart, resulting in an increase in elastic contractile force that is independent of neural and humoral factors. This is one explanation of why more blood is ejected from the left ventricle (increasing SV), and it is known as the **Frank-Starling mechanism** (59); that is, the stroke volume of the heart increases proportionally to the volume of blood filling the heart.

As aerobic exercise intensity increases from a resting state to maximal exercise, there is a 50% to 60% reduction in total peripheral resistance (TPR, resistance to blood flow in the systemic vascular system). This reduction in TPR is due to vasodilation that occurs in an effort to supply the working skeletal muscle with blood (36). During exercise, a greater proportion of blood is shunted to the exercising skeletal musculature where it is needed (24). At the same time, blood flow to other areas of the body, such as the splanchnic region, is decreased. Several mechanisms account for the changes in peripheral vasculature in response to aerobic exercise, but explaining them is beyond the scope of this chapter.

Blood pressure (BP, mmHg) is the force that is exerted by the blood on the vessels and drives blood through the circulatory system. Systolic blood pressure (SBP) and diastolic blood pressure (DBP) measures represent the pressure exerted on the vessels during ventricular systole (contraction) and diastole (relaxation), respectively. During aerobic endurance exercise involving large muscle groups, such as walking, jogging, cycling, and swimming, there is a linear increase in SBP in direct proportion to the exercise intensity and cardiac output and a negligible change in DBP (see figure 6.1). TPR also decreases (but $\dot{Q}$ increases to a greater extent) as the exercise intensity increases and has a major effect on blood pressure. As a result, mean arterial blood pressure (MAP) increases during exercise and can be expressed quantitatively by the following two formulas:

$$MAP = DBP + [.333 \times (SBP - DBP)] \quad \textbf{(6.2)}$$

$$MAP = \dot{Q} \times TPR \quad \textbf{(6.3)}$$

During exercise, the increase in BP helps facilitate the increase in blood flow through the vasculature and also increases the amount of plasma forced from the blood and into the intercellular space (and becoming part of the interstitial fluid). Thus, during exercise, a decrease in plasma volume and an increase in hematocrit (proportion of blood that consists of red blood cells) occur, even though the total number of red blood cells does not change (64, 71).

Coronary vasculature, composed of the right and left coronary arteries, vasodilates during exercise as a result of the increased oxygen demand placed on the heart muscle. The rate–pressure product (RPP) indicates how much oxygen the heart needs. It is a fairly easy measure to take and provides a good noninvasive index of how hard the heart is working (46). It is expressed quantitatively by the following formula:

$$RPP = HR \times SBP \quad \textbf{(6.4)}$$

> Cardiac output, heart rate, stroke volume, mean arterial blood pressure, coronary artery diameter, and rate pressure product increase during exercise.

Respiratory Responses

Pulmonary minute ventilation ($\dot{V}_E$) is the product of breathing rate (BR) and tidal volume (TV) and represents the amount of air moved into or out of the lungs in 1 minute. During exercise, $\dot{V}_E$ increases due to the body's increased oxygen requirement and consumption.

$$\dot{V}_E \text{ (L/min)} = BR \times TV \quad \textbf{(6.5)}$$

The respiratory quotient (RQ) is the ratio of the volume of carbon dioxide production ($\dot{V}CO_2$) to oxygen consumption ($\dot{V}O_2$) at the cellular level. This measure is commonly taken at the mouth rather than

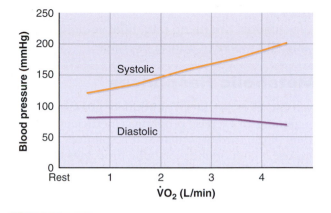

FIGURE 6.1 Blood pressure response to progressive aerobic endurance exercise.

Reprinted by permission from Hoffman 2002.

at the cell and is termed the **respiratory exchange ratio (RER)**. The RQ and RER are calculated by the same formula:

$$RQ \text{ or } RER = \dot{V}CO_2 / \dot{V}O_2 \quad \textbf{(6.6)}$$

The RQ can be used by exercise physiologists to estimate the proportion of fat and carbohydrate utilization during rest and steady-state exercise. The RQ is around 0.82 at rest (approximately 60% of energy derived from fat and 40% derived from carbohydrate) (46). As exercise intensity increases, both RQ and RER approach 1.0, and the proportion of energy derived from carbohydrates increases (see table 6.2). During very intense and maximal exercise, RER can increase to greater than 1.0 due to hyperventilation, which increases the amount of carbon dioxide expired in comparison to the amount of oxygen consumed. The RER is sometimes used as an indicator of exercise intensity, and RER values greater than 1.0 are sometimes used as a criterion measure as evidence of an individual's attaining $\dot{V}O_2$max during a progressive exercise test (46, 59, 71).

TABLE 6.2 Caloric Equivalence of the Respiratory Exchange Ratio (RER) and % kcal From Carbohydrates and Fats

	ENERGY	% KCAL	
RER	**kcal/L O_2**	**Carbohydrate**	**Fat**
0.71	4.69	0	100
0.75	4.74	16	84
0.80	4.80	33	67
0.85	4.86	51	49
0.90	4.92	68	32
0.95	4.99	84	16
1.00	5.05	100	0

Adapted by permission from Wilmore, Costill, and Kenney 2008.

Metabolic Responses

Aerobic exercise in an untrained person who is beginning an exercise program is inefficient. Limitations in the cardiovascular and respiratory systems impose a limit on the metabolic processes that take place in order to allow aerobic exercise to occur. Poor performance for a short time period is the ultimate result. During exercise the demand for adenosine triphosphate (ATP) is higher, so the body consumes more oxygen. The difference between the amount of oxygen in the arterial and mixed venous blood is the **arteriovenous oxygen difference (a–$\bar{v}$O$_2$ difference)**, and represents the extent to which oxygen is removed from the blood as it passes through the body. Normal values for resting arterial and venous oxygen per 100 ml of blood are 20 and 14 ml, respectively, and the normal resting a–$\bar{v}$O$_2$ difference is approximately 6 ml of oxygen per 100 ml of blood. This value increases almost linearly with exercise intensity and can reach approximately 18 ml of oxygen per 100 ml of blood at $\dot{V}$O$_2$max (71) (see figure 6.2). The volume of oxygen consumed ($\dot{V}$O$_2$) is determined as the product of $\dot{Q}$ and the a–$\bar{v}$O$_2$ difference, which is known as the **Fick equation:**

$$\dot{V}O_2 \text{ (L/min)} = \dot{Q} \times \text{a–}\bar{v}O_2 \text{ difference} \qquad \textbf{(6.7)}$$

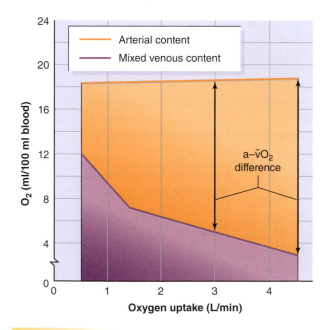

FIGURE 6.2 Changes in a–$\bar{v}$O$_2$ difference (arterial–mixed venous oxygen difference) from low levels to maximal levels of exercise.

Adapted by permission from Wilmore, Costill, and Kenney 2008.

During aerobic exercise the body's metabolism is increased, producing more CO_2 and lactate (which results in higher concentrations of H$^+$ ions). At high exercise intensities (and increased reliance on anaerobic pathways for energy production), lactate accumulates in the active muscles and produces a marked increase in blood acidity (decrease in pH) (19). See chapter 3 for a review of the energy systems as they pertain to aerobic exercise.

Endocrine Responses

In response to a bout of aerobic exercise, a major purpose of the endocrine system is to facilitate metabolism by maintaining the availability of carbohydrates (glucose) and fats (free fatty acids) that are needed to meet increased energy demands. Catecholamines also facilitate cardiovascular responses to enhance the delivery of oxygen and nutrients and the removal of waste products. Glands of major concern with regard to aerobic exercise include the pancreas, adrenal cortex, and adrenal medulla. The endocrine system is complex, and this section contains only basic information related to acute responses.

The pancreas is an endocrine gland that plays a major role in acute exercise metabolism because of the production and release of glucagon and insulin. These hormones release or uptake glucose from the tissues, which is vital to the survival of the body. Plasma glucagon stimulates an increase in plasma glucose concentration, whereas insulin facilitates glucose transport into the cells of the body. Due to the increased metabolic demands of acute exercise, glucagon secretion is increased whereas insulin secretion is decreased. An increase in plasma glucagon stimulates the conversion of glycogen to glucose, thus increasing the plasma glucose concentration so that more glucose is available to be transported into cells. During exercise, insulin plasma concentration decreases while there is improved insulin sensitivity and increased activation of non-insulin-mediated glucose transport into cells (9, 52). The increased glucagon release (and reduced insulin release) during acute exercise also enhances fat breakdown in tissue (lipolysis) and an increase in plasma fatty acids that make more fat available as a fuel for exercise.

Cortisol is the only substance released from the adrenal cortex that plays a direct role in metabolism. It is responsible for stimulating the conversion of proteins to be used by aerobic systems and in glycolysis, as well as for the maintenance of normal blood sugar levels; it also promotes the use of fats. Exercise intensity is a factor that affects the level of cortisol secretion, as plasma levels have been shown to decrease with low-intensity exercise and increase with moderate- to high-intensity exercise (13, 35). During exercise, growth hormone is secreted from the anterior pituitary, which assists cortisol and glucagon in making more fat and carbohydrate available in the plasma for the increased metabolism of exercise (46, 70).

The catecholamines (epinephrine and norepinephrine) are the "fight or flight hormones" that are released from the adrenal medulla when it is acted upon by the sympathetic nervous system during stressful situations. The adrenal medulla perceives exercise as a stressor and releases additional catecholamines during exercise. Catecholamine plasma concentration increases during exercise as these hormones help the body deliver blood and oxygen to the working muscles (e.g., by increasing heart rate and blood pressure) (71).

It is also important to note that, in general, during exercise of increasing intensity, progressive elevations in plasma hormone concentrations in glucagon, cortisol, growth hormone, epinephrine, and norepinephrine occur (46, 59) (see figure 6.3a). These changes are accompanied by a progressive decrease in insulin. Similar progressive changes in these hormones also occur as exercise of moderate intensity continues for a long duration (see figure 6.3b) (59).

Chronic Adaptations to Aerobic Exercise

In addition to understanding how the body's systems respond during bouts of aerobic exercise, personal trainers need to understand how the different body systems adapt to chronic aerobic exercise training.

This section describes the chronic effects of aerobic training on the cardiovascular, respiratory, and endocrine systems as well as the effects on skeletal muscle, bone and connective tissue, metabolism, body composition, and performance. To facilitate understanding of these training adaptations three summary tables are provided. Table 6.3 provides an overview of chronic adaptations at rest and during submaximal and maximal exercise for key cardiorespiratory and metabolic variables. Table 6.4 provides typical baseline and posttraining values for an initially inactive male, as well as comparison values for a male world-class endurance runner. Table 6.5 summarizes other chronic physiological and performance adaptations.

Cardiovascular Adaptations

Several terms are used to refer to maximal aerobic power, a key component for improving aerobic exercise performance. It is also known as $\dot{V}O_2max$, **maximal oxygen uptake,** *maximal oxygen consumption*, and **aerobic capacity.** Increasing maximal aerobic power relies greatly on the effective function and integration of the cardiovascular and respiratory systems. Oxygen uptake can be expressed by the Fick equation (6.7), presented earlier. The equation indicates that maximal aerobic power is dependent on the body's ability to deliver (i.e., cardiac output) and use (i.e., a–$\bar{v}O_2$ difference) oxygen. One of the hallmark adaptations to chronic aerobic training is an increase in maximal cardiac output that results primarily from an increase in stroke volume (46) (see figures 6.4 and 6.5). Aerobic endurance training does not affect maximal heart rate or decreases

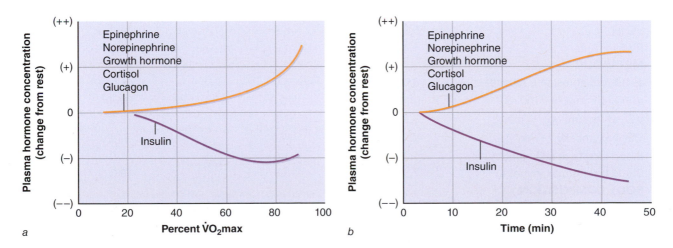

FIGURE 6.3 (a) Summary of the hormonal responses to exercise of increasing intensity. (b) Summary of the hormonal responses to moderate exercise of long duration.

TABLE 6.3 Chronic Cardiorespiratory and Metabolic Adaptations to Aerobic Endurance Training at Rest and During Exercise

Variable	Rest	Fixed submaximal exercise*	Maximal exercise
Heart rate	Decrease	Decrease	No change or slight decrease
Stroke volume	Increase	Increase	Increase
Cardiac output	No change	No change or slight decrease	Increase
Systolic blood pressure	Decrease	Decrease	Little or no change
Diastolic blood pressure	Decrease	Decrease	Little or no change
Pulmonary ventilation	No change	Decrease	Increase
Oxygen consumption	No change	No change or slight decrease	Increase
Arteriovenous oxygen difference	No change	No change or slight increase	Increase

*Responses in the fixed submaximal exercise column indicate adaptations comparing post- to pretraining responses at the same absolute (fixed) work rate.

TABLE 6.4 Effects of Aerobic Endurance Training in a Previously Inactive Man Along With Values for a Male World-Class Endurance Athlete

	SEDENTARY MALE SUBJECT		
Variables	Pretraining	Posttraining	World-class endurance runner
CARDIOVASCULAR			
HRrest (beats/min)	75	65	45
HRmax (beats/min)	185	183	174
SVrest (ml/beat)	60	70	100
SVmax (ml/beat)	120	140	200
$\dot{Q}$ at rest (L/min)	4.5	4.5	4.5
$\dot{Q}$max (L/min)	22.2	25.6	34.8
Heart volume (ml)	750	820	1,200
Blood volume (L)	4.7	5.1	6.0
Systolic BP at rest (mmHg)	135	130	120
Systolic BPmax (mmHg)	200	210	220
Diastolic BP at rest (mmHg)	78	76	65
Diastolic BPmax (mmHg)	82	80	65
RESPIRATORY			
$\dot{V}_E$ at rest (L/min)	7	6	6
$\dot{V}_E$max (L/min)	110	135	195
TV at rest (L)	0.5	0.5	0.5
TVmax (L)	2.75	3.0	3.9
VC (L)	5.8	6.0	6.2
RV (L)	1.4	1.2	1.2
METABOLIC			
a–$\bar{v}O_2$ diff at rest (ml/100 ml)	6.0	6.0	6.0
a–$\bar{v}O_2$ diff max (ml/100 ml)	14.5	15.0	16.0
$\dot{V}O_2$ at rest (ml · kg^{-1} · min^{-1})	3.5	3.5	3.5
$\dot{V}O_2$max (ml · kg^{-1} · min^{-1})	40.7	49.9	81.9
Blood lactate at rest (mmol/L)	1.0	1.0	1.0
Blood lactate max (mmol/L)	7.5	8.5	9.0
BODY COMPOSITION			
Weight (kg)	79	77	68
Fat weight (kg)	12.6	9.6	5.1
Fat-free weight (kg)	66.4	67.4	62.9
Fat (%)	16.0	12.5	7.5

HR = heart rate; SV = stroke volume; $\dot{Q}$ = cardiac output; BP = blood pressure; $\dot{V}_E$ = ventilation; TV = tidal volume; VC = vital capacity; RV = residual volume; a–$\bar{v}O_2$ diff = arterial–mixed venous oxygen difference; $\dot{V}O_2$ = oxygen consumption.

Adapted by permission from Wilmore, Costill, and Kenney 2008.

TABLE 6.5 Selected Chronic Adaptations to Aerobic Endurance Training

Variable	Chronic adaptation
HEART	
Left ventricular end-diastolic chamber diameter	Increase
Left ventricular muscle thickness	Increase
Coronary arteriole densities, diameters, or both	Increase
Myocardial capillary density	No change or increase
BLOOD	
Blood volume	Increase
Plasma volume	Increase
Red blood cell volume	Increase
RESPIRATORY SYSTEM	
Ventilatory muscle endurance	Increase
Respiratory muscle aerobic enzymes	Increase
SKELETAL MUSCLE	
Whole muscle cross-sectional areas	No change
Type I fiber cross-sectional areas	No change or small increase
Type IIa fiber cross-sectional areas	No change
Type IIx fiber cross-sectional areas	No change
Capillary density	Increase
Mitochondria density	Increase
Myoglobin	Increase
Glycogen stores	Increase
Triglyceride stores	Increase
Oxidative enzymes	Increase
METABOLIC	
Lactate threshold	Increase
SKELETAL SYSTEM	
Bone mineral density	No change or increase
BODY COMPOSITION	
Body mass	Decreases
Fat mass	Decreases
Fat-free mass	No change
% Body fat	Decreases
PERFORMANCE	
Cardiorespiratory endurance performance	Increase
Muscular strength	No change
Vertical jump	No change
Anaerobic power	No change
Sprint speed	No change

it slightly (see figure 6.6). Maximal cardiac output correlates closely with maximal aerobic power; so the higher the cardiac output, the higher the aerobic power. In response to aerobic endurance training, cardiac output remains essentially unchanged at rest and is either unchanged or slightly decreased at any fixed submaximal exercise intensity (46). At rest and at any fixed submaximal exercise intensity, adaptations include a decrease in heart rate and an increase in stroke volume (table 6.3). A training-induced reduction in heart rate has been shown to occur in two weeks (12), but depending on the intensity, duration, and frequency of training, may take up to 10 weeks (62). This response is believed to come from an increased parasympathetic influence, decreased sympathetic influence, and lower intrinsic heart rate (71).

Aerobic endurance training increases $\dot{V}O_2$max, which is generally regarded as the single best measure of aerobic fitness.

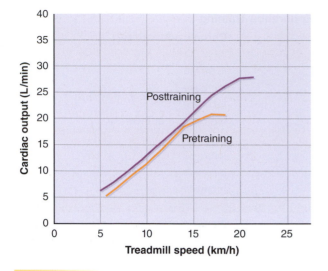

FIGURE 6.4 Changes in cardiac output with aerobic endurance training during walking, then jogging, and finally running on a treadmill as velocity increases.

Adapted by permission from Wilmore, Costill, and Kenney 2008.

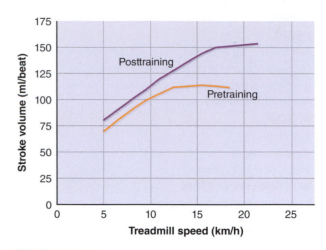

FIGURE 6.5 Changes in stroke volume with aerobic endurance training during walking, jogging, and running on a treadmill at increasing velocities.

Adapted by permission from Wilmore, Costill, and Kenney 2008.

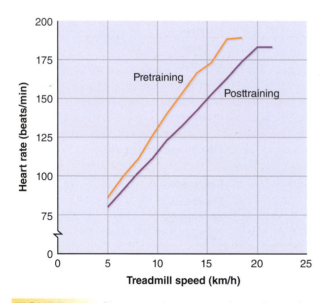

FIGURE 6.6 Changes in heart rate with aerobic endurance training during walking, jogging, and running on a treadmill at increasing velocities.

Adapted by permission from Wilmore, Costill, and Kenney 2008.

Long-term aerobic exercise training leads to moderate cardiac hypertrophy characterized by left ventricular cavity enlargement (i.e., increased volume) and increased myocardial wall thickness (4, 46). The increased left ventricular volume, along with increased ventricular filling time resulting from training-induced bradycardia (slower heart rate), and improved cardiac contractile function are major factors accounting for chronic stroke volume increases (46, 51). An increase in blood volume occurs very

quickly as an adaptation to aerobic endurance training and contributes to ventricular cavity enlargement and improvements in $\dot{V}O_2$max (64). Blood volume can be broken down into the two components of plasma volume and red blood cell volume. Aerobic exercise training induces a very rapid increase in plasma volume (a measurable change occurs within 24 hours), but the increase in red blood cell volume takes a few weeks (64) (see figure 6.7).

Many studies have investigated the effects of chronic aerobic endurance training on resting blood pressure. For individuals with normal BP, SBP/DBP values average only 3/2 mmHg lower with chronic aerobic endurance training; in people with hypertension (SBP >140 or DBP >90 mmHg), greater reductions are noted, with an average of 7/6 mmHg (57). It is also important to note that immediate reductions in resting blood pressure occur after a bout of aerobic exercise in both normotensive and hypertensive individuals, which may persist for up to 22 hours (38, 57). The term "postexercise hypotension" is used to describe these changes. At the same submaximal exercise work rate, chronic aerobic training also results in a decrease in SBP (39, 46). Since both SBP and HR are reduced at a given level of submaximal exercise with aerobic endurance training, it should be obvious that the RPP is also decreased, indicating a reduction in myocardial oxygen consumption and reduced workload on the heart (39, 46).

In trained peripheral skeletal muscle, prolonged aerobic training leads to an increase in the density of capillaries per unit of muscle (40). This allows for improved oxygen and substrate delivery and a

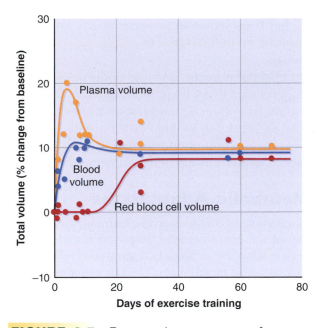

FIGURE 6.7 Estimated time course of percent changes in total blood volume, plasma volume, and red blood cell volume.

Adapted by permission from Wilmore, Costill, and Kenney 2008.

decrease in diffusion distance between blood and exercising muscle. Based on animal studies, it is also apparent that aerobic exercise training is linked with adaptations in the cardiac muscle vasculature, including increases in arteriole densities, arteriole diameters, or both (17). Myocardial capillary density has been shown to increase with swim training in young male rats; in larger animals (i.e., dogs and pigs) undergoing treadmill training, the number of capillaries increases in proportion to the added ventricular mass, and thus no change in capillary density occurs (17).

Aerobic endurance training reduces resting blood pressure in hypertensive individuals.

Respiratory Adaptations

With the respiratory system's large capacity to increase ventilation in response to exercise, as well as the relatively low oxygen (or energy expenditure) cost of breathing in terms of percentage of total body oxygen cost, the demands of aerobic endurance training on the human respiratory system are not as great as they are for other systems. Consequently, chronic aerobic training produces considerably less adaptation than occurs in the cardiovascular system and skeletal muscle (39, 46). For the great majority of healthy adults, the respiratory system is also not a limiting factor for performing maximal exercise

(14, 46, 71). There are, however, several important adaptations in the respiratory system that relate to aerobic performance enhancement.

Adaptations in pulmonary minute ventilation ($\dot{V}_E$) in response to chronic aerobic training occur during submaximal and maximal exercise, with no changes at rest. With aerobic endurance training, V_E values during a standardized submaximal work rate test may decrease by as much as 20% to 30% (71); in contrast, during maximal exercise, $\dot{V}_E$ may increase 15% to 25% or more (39). With aerobic endurance training, adaptations during submaximal exercise generally include an increase in tidal volume and a decrease in breathing frequency, while during maximal exercise both tidal volume and breathing frequency increase.

During moderate-intensity aerobic exercise, the oxygen cost of breathing averages 3% to 5% of total body oxygen cost and increases to 8% to 10% of total body cost at $\dot{V}O_2$max (15). With standardized submaximal exercise, after aerobic endurance training the percentage of the total body oxygen cost for breathing is reduced and the ventilatory equivalent for oxygen ($\dot{V}_E/\dot{V}O_2$) is lowered, indicating improvements in ventilatory efficiency (39, 46). This reduced oxygen cost for breathing enhances aerobic endurance performance by freeing more oxygen for use by exercising skeletal muscle (21) and by reducing the fatiguing effects of exercise on the diaphragm muscle (69). Specificity in respiratory training adaptations also occurs as can be illustrated through comparison of arm and leg aerobic training. Individuals performing arm training show an improvement in $\dot{V}_E/\dot{V}O_2$ with arm exercise, but not with leg exercise; and the opposite occurs in individuals training with leg cycling (60). It thus appears that local adaptations in trained muscle are responsible for adaptations in $\dot{V}_E/\dot{V}O_2$.

Ventilatory efficiency improves with aerobic endurance training; pulmonary minute ventilation decreases during submaximal exercise and increases during maximal exercise.

Skeletal Muscle Adaptations

Aerobic endurance training consists of a large number of rather continuous low-level muscle actions and thus elicits specific marked adaptations within trained skeletal muscle. Chronic aerobic training does not affect muscle size at the macroscopic level (whole muscle) and has little, if any, effect at the microscopic level (specific fiber type cross-sectional areas) (31, 48, 61). Aerobic exercise recruits predominantly type I (slow-twitch) muscle fibers, and the low-level muscle actions elicit either no change or small increases in cross-sectional areas of these fibers. Cross-sectional areas of both type IIa and IIx (fast-twitch) fibers do not change with aerobic endurance training. Small changes in fiber type distribution may occur in response to chronic aerobic training that shifts the distribution toward a larger percentage of more oxidative fibers, and this may translate into improved endurance performance (59, 71). One study, with a rather large sample size, showed that after 20 weeks of three day per week aerobic training, percent distribution of type IIx fibers decreased by 5%; there was no change in type IIa fibers, while percentage of type I fibers increased by 4% (61).

Major changes with aerobic endurance training in skeletal muscle that directly relate to enhanced endurance performance include an increase in capillary supply, an increase in mitochondrial density, and an enhancement in the activity of oxidative enzymes. With chronic aerobic exercise, capillary supply to the trained muscle increases, expressed as either the number of capillaries per muscle fiber or the number of capillaries per unit of cross-sectional area of muscle (capillary density) (61). More capillaries enable an improved exchange of oxygen, nutrients, and waste products between the blood and working muscle (71). Mitochondria, the energy powerhouses within cells, produce over 90% of the body's ATP (46). With chronic endurance training, both the number and size of mitochondria increase, as well as the activity of important oxidative enzymes (e.g., citrate synthase and succinate dehydrogenase) within the mitochondria that speed up the breakdown of nutrients to form ATP (46, 61, 71). Oxidative enzyme activity increases rapidly in response to aerobic endurance training; and with intense regular training, enzyme activity levels may double or triple (30 46, 71).

Intramuscular stores of glycogen are increased with chronic aerobic training (18, 46, 58). Fatigue in prolonged lower body aerobic exercise is associated with glycogen depletion in leg muscle type I and type IIa fibers (30, 46). The enhanced glycogen stores, together with the mitochondrial adaptations just mentioned, result in slower depletion of muscle glycogen stores, which generally translates into improved endurance performance. Myoglobin is an iron-containing protein that provides intramuscular oxygen stores, with higher concentrations in type I fibers than in type II fibers. Myoglobin oxygen stores are released to the mitochondria during the transition from rest to exercise and during intense exercise, when oxygen needs of the mitochondria greatly increase (46, 71). Aerobic endurance train-ing has been shown to increase muscle myoglobin stores by up to 80% (28, 71).

> In skeletal muscle, aerobic endurance train-ing induces three major changes that directly relate to enhanced endurance performance: (1) an increase in capillary density; (2) an increase in mitochondrial density; and (3) an enhancement in oxidative enzyme activity.

Metabolic Adaptations

In response to chronic aerobic training, the integra-tion of the cardiovascular, respiratory, and skeletal muscle adaptations already discussed is reflected in adaptations in metabolism (71). The major metabolic adaptations are an increased reliance on fat as energy and a coupled reduction in use of carbohydrates during submaximal exercise, an increase in lactate threshold, and an increase in maximal oxygen con-sumption. These changes translate into a greater capacity to perform at higher exercise intensities for prolonged periods.

Enhancement in blood supply (oxygen delivery) and increases in mitochondrial content (and mito-chondrial density) and aerobic enzymes in trained muscle greatly enhance the ability to produce ATP aerobically. These changes facilitate increased fatty acid use for energy during submaximal exercise (32, 34). They also serve to conserve glycogen stores (less use of carbohydrates), which are very important for maintaining high-intensity prolonged aerobic exercise (46, 71). The training adaptations in fat and carbohydrate metabolism are also reflected in decreases in the respiratory quotient at both fixed and relative submaximal exercise intensities (71).

Similar patterns for lactate production and accu-mulation are present in people who are untrained and those who have undergone aerobic endurance training, except that the threshold for lactate accu-mulation (blood lactate threshold) occurs at a higher percentage of a trained person's aerobic capacity (see figure 6.8). Untrained individuals with a lac-tate threshold occurring at 50% to 60% of maximal aerobic capacity can increase their threshold to 70% to 80%; while an endurance athlete who undertakes fairly intense training, and maybe with favorable genetic factors, may have a lactate threshold in the range of 80% to 90% of aerobic capacity (46). The enhancement in lactate threshold most likely is due to a combination of local adaptations that reduce lactate production and increase the rate of lactate removal (46, 71). Since a trained person's $\dot{V}O_2$max also increases with chronic aerobic training, the

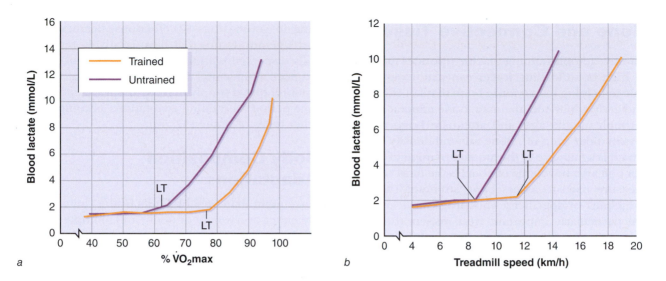

FIGURE 6.8   Changes in lactate threshold (LT) with training expressed as (a) a percentage of maximal oxygen uptake (%V̇O₂max) and (b) an increase in speed on the treadmill. Lactate threshold (LT) occurs at a speed of 5.2 miles per hour (8.4 km/h) in the untrained state and at 7.2 miles per hour (11.6 km/h) in the trained state.

Adapted by permission from Wilmore, Costill, and Kenney 2008.

enhancement in percentage of capacity where lactate threshold occurs effectively translates into a substantially higher work rate for sustained endurance performance.

Adaptations in resting, submaximal exercise, and maximal oxygen consumption are somewhat different in response to chronic aerobic training. Resting oxygen consumption (also known as *resting metabolic rate*) generally does not change (71, 72). After training, there is either no change or a slight decrease in submaximal exercise oxygen consumption at a fixed work rate. An improvement in exercise economy (i.e., performing the same amount of work at a lower energy cost) can account for a decrease in oxygen consumption at the same fixed work rate posttraining (46, 71). In response to 6 to 12 months of aerobic training, a wide range of percent improvements have been reported in maximal oxygen consumption (related to differences in training intensity, duration, or frequency and initial fitness levels or some combination of these); but the great majority of improvements fall in the range of 10% to 30% (2, 39).

Arteriovenous oxygen difference is a variable that could fall under cardiovascular, respiratory, or metabolic adaptation categories. As expressed by the Fick equation (6.7), $a-\bar{v}O_2$ difference can be a major contributor to improvement in V̇O₂max. With chronic aerobic training, $a-\bar{v}O_2$ difference increases particularly at maximal exercise. This increase is accomplished by both adaptations in skeletal muscle, which enhance extraction of oxygen during exercise, and a more effective distribution of blood flow to active tissue and away from inactive tissue (46).

Endocrine Adaptations

Aerobic endurance training generally leads to a blunted response in hormone release at the same absolute level of submaximal exercise. Comparisons between pre- and posttraining at the same absolute level of submaximal exercise represent a comparison of responses to aerobic exercise performed at any specific fixed (or absolute) submaximal work rate (such as a specific speed of running on a level treadmill). Training causes a reduction in the rise of plasma epinephrine, norepinephrine, glucagon, cortisol, and growth hormone in a person who performs the same absolute level of submaximal exercise posttraining as compared to pretraining (22, 46, 59, 73). Plasma insulin levels also decrease less in a trained person during submaximal exercise. At the tissue level, effects of exercise on insulin sensitivity are particularly important considering the high and increasing prevalence of diabetes in our society. An acute bout of moderate or intense exercise improves insulin sensitivity and decreases plasma glucose levels in persons with type 2 diabetes (1, 25, 27, 41, 46). These favorable changes usually deteriorate within 72 hours of the last exercise session. With regular exercise, the acute effects of enhanced insulin sensitivity can improve long-term glucose control. However, it appears that this enhanced long-term glucose control is not a consequence of chronic adaptation in muscle tissue function (1, 25, 46).

Bone and Connective Tissue

Chronic aerobic training that incorporates moderate to high bone loading forces can play a significant role in helping to maximize bone mass in childhood and early adulthood, maintain bone mineral content through middle age, and attenuate bone mineral loss in older age (42). Bone mineral density (BMD), which is a measure of the amount of mineral content per unit area or volume of bone, is the most common measure used to assess bone strength. The basic principles of specificity and progressive overload are particularly important with respect to adaptations in bone with exercise training. Only bone that is subject to chronic loading will undergo changes, and changes will occur only when the stimulus is greater than what the bone is accustomed to. Continued improvement also requires a progression in overload. Considering these basic principles, aerobic endurance training that incorporates moderate to high bone loading forces likely induces the most beneficial effects (42, 54, 58). Indeed, while walking training programs of up to one year in duration are not effective in preventing bone loss with aging (8), jogging with its higher-intensity bone loading forces has been shown to attenuate bone loss with aging (42, 50). Keep in mind that since BMD decreases in middle-aged and older adults, exercise that attenuates this loss should be viewed as beneficial (42, 53). Results are equivocal in a number of studies that have assessed the effect of aerobic and other types of training on BMD (42, 54, 58). Studies that report an increase in BMD favor relatively high-intensity weight-bearing aerobic exercise, plyometric or jump training, resistance training, or some combination of these (42, 53, 58). A combination of weight-bearing aerobic exercise (including jogging at least intermittently if walking is the main mode of exercise) and activities that involve jumping and resistance training (incorporating exercises that load all major muscle groups) is the recommended standard for maintaining bone health in adulthood (42).

There has been less research on the effects of aerobic endurance training on tendon, ligament, and cartilage than there has on the skeletal or cardiovascular systems and the research that has been done has focused primarily on animals (37). Tendon, ligament, and articular cartilage appear, like bone, to remodel in response to the mechanical stress placed on them (7, 55). Tendons and ligaments become stronger and stiffer when stressed with increased overload and weaker and less stiff with decreased overload (7, 37). Articular cartilage has been shown to become thicker with moderate volumes of run-

ning in young dogs (7). Tendons, ligaments, and cartilage are tissues that have relatively few living cells dispersed within an abundance of non-living extracellular material. This characteristic, along with a poorer blood supply to these tissues, prolongs the time period for training adaptations as compared to other types of tissue (37, 45).

Body Composition Adaptations

Since more than 66% of adults in the United States are either overweight or obese and multiple chronic diseases are associated with excess fatness, the effect of exercise on body composition is an important public health issue (56). Results from a number of studies with a wide range in months of physical activity intervention indicate that moderate-intensity aerobic activity of less than 150 minutes per week induces minimal weight loss; greater than 150 minutes per week of moderate activity induces a modest weight loss of about 4.4 to 6.6 pounds (2-3 kg); and moderate aerobic activity for 225 to 420 minutes per week induces an 11- to 16.5-pound (5-7.5 kg) weight loss (16). Thus, evidence supports a dose–response relationship between the amount of the aerobic activity performed and the amount of weight loss. A benefit of aerobic endurance training regarding body composition is that it induces reductions in fat mass while having a minimal effect on (or preserving) fat-free mass (6, 47, 67). Aerobic endurance training alone or in combination with an energy-restricted diet induces a greater loss in fat mass than an energy-restricted diet alone since the exercise promotes conservation of fat-free mass (46, 67).

> Health-related benefits of aerobic endurance exercise include enhanced insulin sensitivity, reduced body fat, and favorable effects on bone mineral density.

Performance Adaptations

Considering the physiologic adaptations just discussed, and keeping in mind that aerobic endurance training consists of fairly continuous low-level muscle actions, the effects of this type of training on specific types of performance should be evident. Aerobic endurance training is particularly effective in enhancing cardiovascular endurance performance, although it generally has no effect on types of performance that involve high levels of muscle activation or anaerobic metabolism. Thus, chronic aerobic endurance training generally does not improve muscular strength (26, 43, 47), vertical jump performance (26, 33, 47), anaerobic power (43), or sprint speed (26) in young adults. Although not discussed in this chapter, it should be kept in mind that chronic aerobic training also has many health-related benefits for a number of chronic visceral diseases and physical disabilities (23).

Factors That Influence Adaptations to Aerobic Endurance Training

The physiological adaptations to aerobic endurance training that have been addressed in this chapter are influenced by a number of individual factors. These include the types of activity that the person engages in (i.e., specificity), genetics, sex, and age. All these factors play a role in determining the success one may see with aerobic endurance training.

Specificity

The effects of exercise are all subject to the rule of specificity. This means that adaptations occur as a consequence of the training and in a fashion specifically related to the training. In short, if the exercise involves cycling, then the training adaptations will be most closely related to cycling performance. This is true also for running, swimming, or training on an ergometer or treadmill. The body seeks to adapt to the stress it encounters in as specific a manner as possible, a principle that has obvious implications for the design of training programs. While programming is beyond the scope of this chapter, it is important for the personal trainer to bear in mind that any exercise program will produce adaptations very closely related to the specific activities the client engages in.

Genetics

It is safe to say that each of us is born with a theoretical ceiling of human performance that we may attain. This ceiling is not absolute but rather falls within a range of values that is dependent on the training stimulus and motivation levels. However, there appears to be an absolute level that each of us is unable to exceed based on genetic factors we inherited from our ancestors. There is a saying that the best training begins with choosing the right parents. While we obviously do not have control over this factor, it does play a major role in our development. However, research has also shown that the body is not completely unchangeable. For example, people who undertake aerobic-type exercise for an extended period of time change fast-twitch muscle fibers so they take on more characteristics similar to those of slow-twitch fibers, which leads to improved aerobic performance. It has been estimated that genetic factors account for 20% to 30% of differences between individuals in maximal aerobic capacity and for about 50% of differences in maximal heart rate (5, 46).

Sex

The physiological changes due to aerobic exercise are similar for males and females. However, some basic differences affect the absolute amounts of the changes. Women on average have less muscle mass and more body fat than their male counterparts. They also have smaller hearts and lungs and an overall smaller blood volume. Research has shown that when males and females are matched for age, females typically have a lower cardiac output, stroke volume, and oxygen consumption than males when exercising at 50% of $\dot{V}O_2$max. Considering that females generally start an aerobic training program with smaller physiologic values, they generally show smaller absolute adaptations than males but very similar relative (percent) adaptations.

Age

As children mature, levels of absolute maximal aerobic power (L/min) increase. Females tend to reach their highest values for $\dot{V}O_2$max (L/min) between 12 and 15 years of age, while males do not reach their highest $\dot{V}O_2$max until 17 to 21 years of age (71). This period is followed by a plateau and then a gradual decrease as we age. Much of the decline can be negated through continued training regimens. Aerobic endurance–trained athletes who are older exhibit only slight declines during the fifth and sixth decades when they maintain training, whereas those who stop training show declines similar to those in untrained individuals. In five middle-aged men, 100% of the age-related decline in aerobic power that had occurred over 30 years was reversed by six months of aerobic endurance training (49). Figure 6.9 depicts changes in $\dot{V}O_2$max with age in both trained and untrained men.

Overtraining

When intensity, duration, frequency of training, or any combination of these factors exceeds an individual's capacity for adaptation, overreaching and overtraining may occur. Exceeding adaptation capacity without sufficient recovery normally leads to decrements in physical performance that are based

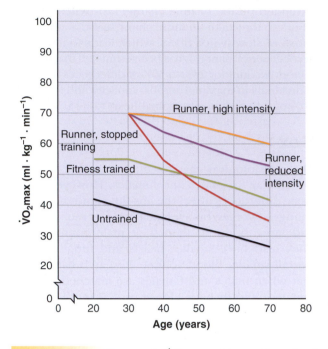

FIGURE 6.9 Changes in $\dot{V}O_2$max with age for trained and untrained men.

Adapted by permission from Wilmore, Costill, and Kenney 2008.

on complex interactions among several biological systems and psychological influences (3, 20, 44, 46, 68). **Overreaching** refers to short-term training, without sufficient recuperation, that exceeds an individual's capacity. Successful recovery from overreaching can occur within a few days or up to two weeks with an adequate recovery intervention (3, 46). While some authorities view overreaching as an unplanned and undesirable consequence of strenuous training, others view it as a training technique to enhance performance (3, 71). Although short-term overreaching results in a decrement in performance, when it is followed with appropriate recovery periods the result may be an enhanced performance as compared to baseline. Overtraining syndrome is more serious and results from untreated overreaching that produces long-term impairments in performance and other conditions that may require medical intervention.

Two types of overtraining have been theorized to exist; the difference is in the predominance of either the sympathetic or the parasympathetic nervous system (3, 44, 71). Apparently, aerobic endurance overtraining results predominantly from an excessive volume overload (parasympathetic dominant), whereas anaerobic or resistance overtraining (sympathetic dominant) primarily results from excessive high-intensity overload. These different types of overtraining have been reported to have different signs and symptoms, although performance decrements are a key common aspect of both. Discussion of the many complicated and not fully understood aspects of overtraining is beyond the scope of this chapter, and the reader is referred to other sources for more complete information on these concepts (3, 20, 44, 68).

A large number of markers for overreaching or overtraining have been identified by researchers. See the following sidebar for a list of some of the most common markers (i.e., signs and symptoms) of aerobic endurance overreaching, overtraining, or both (3, 20, 44, 46, 68).

There is a high degree of variability between individuals with regard to developing overtraining. Training practices that cause some individuals to thrive lead to overtraining in others. Unfortunately, there are also highly individualized responses and symptoms for overreaching and overtraining that make it difficult for clients and personal trainers to recognize (3, 46, 71). Besides a decrement in performance, people generally exhibit only a few, if any, other signs and symptoms of overreaching

Common Markers of Aerobic Endurance Overreaching or Overtraining

- Decreased performance
- Decreased maximal oxygen uptake
- Earlier onset of fatigue
- General malaise
- Loss of interest or enthusiasm for training
- Disturbed psychological mood states (increased depression, anxiety, fatigue or decreased vigor or a combination of these changes)

- Increased muscle soreness
- Decreased resting and maximal heart rate
- Increased submaximal exercise heart rate
- Decreased submaximal exercise plasma lactate concentration
- Increased sympathetic stress response
- Decreased catecholamine levels

or overtraining. Being familiar with each client's progression through training is essential for preventing overtraining. A decline in performance coupled with one or more of the easily recognizable markers (i.e., fatigue, malaise, loss of enthusiasm for training, increased soreness) should lead to suspicion of overtraining. Checking the heart rate response to a standardized submaximal exercise load would be another appropriate method to monitor clients undergoing strenuous aerobic endurance training. For prevention of overtraining, an important component would be a properly planned periodization program. It is critical for the client to have sufficient rest between training days to facilitate the recovery process. The amount of rest, however, depends on the duration and intensity of the training program and should be individualized for each client. Periods of high-volume or high-intensity training especially require sufficient recovery. Keep in mind that individuals undergoing strenuous and frequent endurance training also need sufficient carbohydrate intake to maintain muscle glycogen stores. Successive days of training can gradually reduce glycogen levels and impair performance (46, 71).

Detraining

The ways in which the body responds to detraining are analogous to the ways in which it responds to training. Once training is stopped, muscular endurance decreases after only two weeks. After four weeks, one study showed reductions in the trained muscles' respiratory ability, decreases in glycogen levels, and increases in lactate production that demonstrate obvious changes in the muscle metabolism (10). Another study showed a 7% decline in both $\dot{V}O_2max$ and maximal cardiac output, as well as 17% to 19% decreases in aerobic enzyme levels, after training was stopped for only 12 days (11). Another investigation demonstrated that when aerobically trained rats stopped training, there was a site-specific decrease in the BMD of the tibia (66).

Conclusion

Our interest in and understanding of the physiology of aerobic endurance training has greatly expanded in the last few decades. Aerobic endurance training is a potent stimulus to physiological changes in the cardiovascular, respiratory, skeletal muscle, metabolic, endocrine, and skeletal systems and has substantial effects on body composition and performance. To be a highly effective personal trainer, it is crucial to have a clear understanding of both the acute responses and chronic adaptations of the many physiological systems of the human body. Understanding how the body adapts to the overload of aerobic exercise is critical to designing effective exercise training programs, monitoring exercise responses and progress, and assessing training outcomes. The personal trainer must also recognize the effects that genetics, sex, age, specificity, overtraining, and detraining have on physiologic responses and adaptations.

Study Questions

1. A 35-year-old female began an exercise program four months ago in which she has been running on the treadmill four days per week. Which of the following describes the adaptations that are most likely to occur with this program?

   A. an increase in maximal exercise HR and a decrease in capillary density

   B. an increase in resting SBP and decrease in maximal a–$\bar{v}O_2$ difference

   C. an increase in mitochondrial density and a decrease in submaximal HR

   D. an increase in blood volume and a decrease in insulin sensitivity

2. Which of the following changes in trained skeletal muscle is an adaptation to chronic aerobic exercise?

   A. decreased mitochondria density

   B. increased concentration of aerobic enzymes

   C. increased cross-sectional area of type IIa fibers

   D. decreased capillary density

3. Which of the following is most likely to occur as a result of aerobic endurance overtraining?

   A. decreased $\dot{V}O_2max$

   B. increased muscle glycogen stores

   C. increased body fat percentage

   D. decreased blood volume

4. Which of the following measures decrease during an acute exercise bout?

    A. rate–pressure product, stroke volume, mean arterial pressure, hematocrit

    B. oxygen consumption, a–$\bar{v}O_2$ difference, systolic blood pressure, RER

    C. blood pH, blood flow to splanchnic region, plasma volume, insulin

    D. catecholamines, glucagon, stroke volume, tidal volume

Applied Knowledge Question

Complete the following chart to describe two ways the body adapts to chronic participation in an aerobic training program.

System	Two adaptations
Respiratory	
Metabolic	
Skeletal muscle	
Cardiovascular	
Endocrine	

References

1. Albright, A., M. Franz, G. Hornsby, A. Kriska, D. Marrero, I. Ullrich, and L.S. Verity. 2000. American College of Sports Medicine position stand. Exercise and type 2 diabetes. *Medicine and Science in Sports and Exercise* 32 (7): 1345-1360.

2. American College of Sports Medicine. 1998. Position stand on the recommended quantity and quality of exercise for developing and maintaining cardiorespiratory and muscular fitness, and flexibility in healthy adults. *Medicine and Science in Sports and Exercise* 30 (6): 975-991.

3. Armstrong, L.E., and J.L. VanHeest. 2002. The unknown mechanism of the overtraining syndrome: Clues from depression and psychoneuroimmunology. *Sports Medicine* 32 (3): 185-209.

4. Barbier, J., N. Ville, G. Kervio, G. Walther, and F. Carre. 2006. Sports-specific features of athlete's heart and their relation to echocardiographic parameters. *Herz* 31 (6): 531-543.

5. Bouchard, C., F.T. Dionne, J.A. Simoneau, and M.R. Boulay. 1992. Genetics of aerobic and anaerobic performances. *Exercise and Sport Sciences Reviews* 20: 27-58.

6. Broeder, C.E., K.A. Burrhus, L.S. Svanevik, J. Volpe, and J.H. Wilmore. 1997. Assessing body composition before and after resistance or endurance training. *Medicine and Science in Sports and Exercise* 29 (5): 705-712.

7. Buckwalter, J. A., and S.L.-Y. Woo. 1994. Effects of repetitive motion on the musculoskeletal tissues. In: *Orthopaedic Sports Medicine: Principles and Practice*, Vol. 1, J.C. DeLee and D. Drez, eds. Philadelphia: Saunders. pp. 60-72.

8. Cavanaugh, D.J., and C.E. Cann. 1988. Brisk walking does not stop bone loss in postmenopausal women. *Bone* 9 (4): 201-204.

9. Coggan, A.R. 1991. Plasma glucose metabolism during exercise in humans. *Sports Medicine* 11 (2): 102-124.

10. Costill, D.L., W.J. Fink, M. Hargreaves, D.S. King, R. Thomas, and R. Fielding. 1985. Metabolic characteristics of skeletal muscle during detraining from competitive swimming. *Medicine and Science in Sports and Exercise* 17 (3): 339-343.

11. Coyle, E.F., W.H. Martin III, D.R. Sinacore, M.J. Joyner, J.M. Hagberg, and J.O. Holloszy. 1984. Time course of loss of adaptations after stopping prolonged intense endurance training. *Journal of Applied Physiology* 57 (6): 1857-1864.

12. Dart, A.M., I.T. Meredith, and G.L. Jennings. 1992. Effects of 4 weeks endurance training on cardiac left ventricular structure and function. *Clinical and Experimental Pharmacology and Physiology* 19 (11): 777-783.

13. Davies, C.T., and J.D. Few. 1973. Effects of exercise on adrenocortical function. *Journal of Applied Physiology* 35 (6): 887-891.

14. Dempsey, J.A. 1986. J.B. Wolffe memorial lecture. Is the lung built for exercise? *Medicine and Science in Sports and Exercise* 18 (2): 143-155.

15. Dempsey, J.A., C.A. Harms, and D.M. Ainsworth. 1996. Respiratory muscle perfusion and energetics during exercise. *Medicine and Science in Sports and Exercise* 28 (9): 1123-1128.

16. Donnelly, J.E., S.N. Blair, J.M. Jakicic, M.M. Manore, J.W. Rankin, and B.K. Smith. 2009. American College of Sports Medicine position stand. Appropriate physical activity intervention strategies for weight loss and prevention of weight regain for adults. *Medicine and Science in Sports and Exercise* 41 (2): 459-471.

17. Duncker, D.J., and R.J. Bache. 2008. Regulation of coronary blood flow during exercise. *Physiology Reviews* 88 (3): 1009-1086.

18. Ebeling, P., R. Bourey, L. Koranyi, J.A. Tuominen, L.C. Groop, J. Henriksson, M. Mueckler, A. Sovijarvi, and V.A. Koivisto. 1993. Mechanism of enhanced insulin sensitivity in athletes. Increased blood flow, muscle glucose transport protein (GLUT-4) concentration, and glycogen synthase activity. *Journal of Clinical Investigation* 92 (4): 1623-1631.

19. Faude, O., W. Kindermann, and T. Meyer. 2009. Lactate threshold concepts: How valid are they? *Sports Medicine* 39 (6): 469-490.

20. Halson, S.L., and A.E. Jeukendrup. 2004. Does overtraining exist? An analysis of overreaching and overtraining research. *Sports Medicine* 34 (14): 967-981.

21. Harms, C.A., M.A. Babcock, S.R. McClaran, D.F. Pegelow, G.A. Nickele, W.B. Nelson, and J.A. Dempsey. 1997. Respi-

ratory muscle work compromises leg blood flow during maximal exercise. *Journal of Applied Physiology* 82 (5): 1573-1583.

22. Hartley, L.H., J.W. Mason, R.P. Hogan, L.G. Jones, T.A. Kotchen, E.H. Mougey, F.E. Wherry, L.L. Pennington, and P.T. Ricketts. 1972. Multiple hormonal responses to graded exercise in relation to physical training. *Journal of Applied Physiology* 33 (5): 602-606.

23. Haskell, W.L., I.M. Lee, R.R. Pate, K.E. Powell, S.N. Blair, B.A. Franklin, C.A. Macera, G.W. Heath, P.D. Thompson, and A. Bauman. 2007. Physical activity and public health: Updated recommendation for adults from the American College of Sports Medicine and the American Heart Association. *Medicine and Science in Sports and Exercise* 39 (8): 1423-1434.

24. Haughlin, M.H., R.J. Korthuis, D.J. Duncker, and R.J. Bache. 1996. Control of blood flow to cardiac and skeletal muscle during exercise. In: *Section 12: Exercise: Regulation and Integration of Multiple Systems,* L.B. Rowell and J.T. Shepherd, eds. New York: Oxford University Press. pp. 705-769.

25. Hawley, J.A., and S.J. Lessard. 2008. Exercise training-induced improvements in insulin action. *Acta Physiologica* 192 (1): 127-135.

26. Hennessy, L.C., and A.W.S. Watson. 1994. The interference effects of training for strength and endurance simultaneously. *Journal of Strength and Conditioning Research* 8 (1): 12-19.

27. Henriksen, E.J. 2002. Invited review: Effects of acute exercise and exercise training on insulin resistance. *Journal of Applied Physiology* 93 (2): 788-796.

28. Hickson, R.C. 1981. Skeletal muscle cytochrome c and myoglobin, endurance, and frequency of training. *Journal of Applied Physiology* 51 (3): 746-749.

29. Higginbotham, M.B., K.G. Morris, R.S. Williams, P.A. McHale, R.E. Coleman, and F.R. Cobb. 1986. Regulation of stroke volume during submaximal and maximal upright exercise in normal man. *Circulation Research* 58 (2): 281-291.

30. Holloszy, J.O., and E.F. Coyle. 1984. Adaptations of skeletal muscle to endurance exercise and their metabolic consequences. *Journal of Applied Physiology* 56 (4): 831-838.

31. Hoppeler, H. 1986. Exercise-induced ultrastructural changes in skeletal muscle. *International Journal of Sports Medicine* 7 (4): 187-204.

32. Horowitz, J.F. 2001. Regulation of lipid mobilization and oxidation during exercise in obesity. *Exercise and Sport Sciences Reviews* 29 (1): 42-46.

33. Hunter, G.R., R. Demment, and D Miller. 1987. Development of strength and maximum oxygen uptake during simultaneous training for strength and endurance. *Journal of Sports Medicine and Physical Fitness* 27 (3): 269-275.

34. Hurley, B.F., P.M. Nemeth, W.H. Martin III, J.M. Hagberg, G.P. Dalsky, and J.O. Holloszy. 1986. Muscle triglyceride utilization during exercise: Effect of training. *Journal of Applied Physiology* 60 (2): 562-567.

35. Jacks, D.E., J. Sowash, J. Anning, T. McGloughlin, and F. Andres. 2002. Effect of exercise at three exercise intensities on salivary cortisol. *Journal of Strength and Conditioning Research* 16 (2): 286-289.

36. Janicki, J.S., D.D. Sheriff, J.L. Robotham, and R.A. Wise. 1996. Cardiac output during exercise: Contributions of the cardiac, circulatory, and respiratory systems. In: *Section 12: Exercise: Regulation and Integration of Multiple Systems,* L.B. Rowell and J.T. Shepherd, eds. New York: Oxford University Press. pp. 651-704.

37. Jozsa, L., and P. Kannus. 1997. *Human Tendons: Anatomy, Physiology, and Pathology.* Champaign, IL: Human Kinetics.

38. Kenney, M.J., and D.R. Seals. 1993. Postexercise hypotension. Key features, mechanisms, and clinical significance. *Hypertension* 22 (5): 653-664.

39. Keteyian, S.J., and C.A. Brawner. 2006. Cardiopulmonary adaptations to exercise. In: *ACSM's Resource Manual for Guidelines for Exercise Testing and Prescription,* 5th ed., L.A. Kaminsky, ed. Philadelphia: Lippincott Williams & Wilkins. pp. 313-324.

40. Kiens, B., B. Essen-Gustavsson, N.J. Christensen, and B. Saltin. 1993. Skeletal muscle substrate utilization during submaximal exercise in man: Effect of endurance training. *Journal of Physiology* 469: 459-478.

41. King, D.S., P.J. Baldus, R.L. Sharp, L.D. Kesl, T.L. Feltmeyer, and M.S. Riddle. 1995. Time course for exercise-induced alterations in insulin action and glucose tolerance in middle-aged people. *Journal of Applied Physiology* 78 (1): 17-22.

42. Kohrt, W.M., S.A. Bloomfield, K.D. Little, M.E. Nelson, and V.R. Yingling. 2004. American College of Sports Medicine position stand: Physical activity and bone health. *Medicine and Science in Sports and Exercise* 36 (11): 1985-1996.

43. Kraemer, W.J., J.F. Patton, S.E. Gordon, E.A. Harman, M.R. Deschenes, K. Reynolds, R.U. Newton, N.T. Triplett, and J.E. Dziados. 1995. Compatibility of high-intensity strength and endurance training on hormonal and skeletal muscle adaptations. *Journal of Applied Physiology* 78 (3): 976-989.

44. Lehmann, M., C. Foster, and J. Keul. 1993. Overtraining in endurance athletes: A brief review. *Medicine and Science in Sports and Exercise* 25 (7): 854-862.

45. Mangine, B., G. Nuzzo, and G.L. Harrelson. 2004. Physiologic factors of rehabilitation. In: *Physical Rehabilitation of the Injured Athlete,* 3rd ed., J.R. Andrews, G.L. Harrelson, and K.E. Wilk, eds. Philadelphia: Saunders. pp. 13-33.

46. McArdle, W.D., F.I. Katch, and V.L. Katch. 2010. *Exercise Physiology: Nutrition, Energy, and Human Performance,* 7th ed. Philadelphia: Lippincott Williams & Wilkins.

47. McCarthy, J.P., J.C. Agre, B.K. Graf, M.A. Pozniak, and A.C. Vailas. 1995. Compatibility of adaptive responses with combining strength and endurance training. *Medicine and Science in Sports and Exercise* 27 (3): 429-436.

48. McCarthy, J.P., M.A. Pozniak, and J.C. Agre. 2002. Neuromuscular adaptations to concurrent strength and endurance training. *Medicine and Science in Sports and Exercise* 34 (3): 511-519.

49. McGuire, D.K., B.D. Levine, J.W. Williamson, P.G. Snell, C.G. Blomqvist, B. Saltin, and J.H. Mitchell. 2001. A 30-year follow-up of the Dallas Bedrest and Training Study: II. Effect of age on cardiovascular adaptation to exercise training. *Circulation* 104 (12): 1358-1366.

50. Michel, B.A., N.E. Lane, A. Bjorkengren, D.A. Bloch, and J.F. Fries. 1992. Impact of running on lumbar bone density: A 5-year longitudinal study. *Journal of Rheumatology* 19 (11): 1759-1763.

51. Mier, C.M., M.J. Turner, A.A. Ehsani, and R.J. Spina. 1997. Cardiovascular adaptations to 10 days of cycle exercise. *Journal of Applied Physiology* 83 (6): 1900-1906.

52. Mikines, K.J., B. Sonne, P.A. Farrell, B. Tronier, and H. Galbo. 1988. Effect of physical exercise on sensitivity and responsiveness to insulin in humans. *American Journal of Physiology: Endocrinology and Metabolism* 254 (3): E248-E259.

53. Nichols, D.L., and E.V. Essery. 2006. Osteoporosis and exercise. In: *ACSM's Resource Manual for Guidelines for Exercise Testing and Prescription,* 5th ed., L.A. Kaminsky, ed. Philadelphia: Lippincott Williams & Wilkins. pp. 489-499.

54. Nichols, D.L., C.F. Sanborn, and E.V. Essery. 2007. Bone density and young athletic women. An update. *Sports Medicine* 37 (11): 1001-1014.

55. Nordin, M., T. Lorenz, and M. Campello. 2001. Biomechanics of tendons and ligaments. In: *Basic Biomechanics of the Musculoskeletal System.* M. Nordin and V.H. Frankel, eds. Baltimore: Lippincott, Williams & Wilkins. pp. 102-125.

56. Ogden, C.L., M.D. Carroll, L R. Curtin, M.A. McDowell, C.J. Tabak, and K.M. Flegal. 2006. Prevalence of overweight and obesity in the United States, 1999-2004. *Journal of the American Medical Association* 295 (13): 1549-1555.

57. Pescatello, L.S., B.A. Franklin, R. Fagard, W.B. Farquhar, G.A. Kelley, and C.A. Ray. 2004. American College of Sports Medicine position stand. Exercise and hypertension. *Medicine and Science in Sports and Exercise* 36 (3): 533-553.

58. Plowman, S.A., and D.L. Smith. 2008. *Exercise Physiology for Health, Fitness, and Performance,* 2nd reprint ed. Philadelphia: Lippincott Williams & Wilkins.

59. Powers, S.K., and E.T. Howley. 2004. *Exercise Physiology: Theory and Application to Fitness and Performance,* 5th ed. New York, NY: McGraw Hill.

60. Rasmussen, B., K. Klausen, J.P. Clausen, and J. Trap-Jensen. 1975. Pulmonary ventilation, blood gases, and blood pH after training of the arms or the legs. *Journal of Applied Physiology* 38 (2): 250-256.

61. Rico-Sanz, J., T. Rankinen, D.R. Joanisse, A.S. Leon, J.S. Skinner, J.H. Wilmore, D.C. Rao, and C. Bouchard. 2003. Familial resemblance for muscle phenotypes in the HERI-TAGE Family Study. *Medicine and Science in Sports and Exercise* 35 (8): 1360-1366.

62. Rubal, B.J., A.R. Al-Muhailani, and J. Rosentswieg. 1987. Effects of physical conditioning on the heart size and wall thickness of college women. *Medicine and Science in Sports and Exercise* 19 (5): 423-429.

63. Saks, V., P. Dzeja, U. Schlattner, M. Vendelin, A. Terzic, and T. Wallimann. 2006. Cardiac system bioenergetics: Metabolic basis of the Frank-Starling law. *Journal of Physiology* 571 (2): 253-273.

64. Sawka, M.N., V.A. Convertino, E.R. Eichner, S.M. Schnieder, and A.J. Young. 2000. Blood volume: Importance and adaptations to exercise training, environmental stresses, and trauma/sickness. *Medicine and Science in Sports and Exercise* 32 (2): 332-348.

65. Scruggs, K.D., N.B. Martin, C.E. Broeder, Z. Hofman, E.L. Thomas, K.C. Wambsgans, and J.H. Wilmore. 1991. Stroke volume during submaximal exercise in endurance-trained normotensive subjects and in untrained hypertensive subjects with beta blockade (propranolol and pindolol). *American Journal of Cardiology* 67 (5): 416-421.

66. Shimamura, C., J. Iwamoto, T. Takeda, S. Ichimura, H. Abe, and Y. Toyama. 2002. Effect of decreased physical activity on bone mass in exercise-trained young rats. *Journal of Orthopaedic Science* 7 (3): 358-363.

67. Stiegler, P., and A. Cunliffe. 2006. The role of diet and exercise for the maintenance of fat-free mass and resting metabolic rate during weight loss. *Sports Medicine* 36 (3): 239-262.

68. Urhausen, A., and W. Kindermann. 2002. Diagnosis of overtraining: What tools do we have? *Sports Medicine* 32 (2): 95-102.

69. Vogiatzis, I., D. Athanasopoulos, R. Boushel, J.A. Guenette, M. Koskolou, M. Vasilopoulou, H. Wagner, C. Roussos, P.D. Wagner, and S. Zakynthinos. 2008. Contribution of respiratory muscle blood flow to exercise-induced diaphragmatic fatigue in trained cyclists. *Journal of Physiology* 586 (22): 5575-5587.

70. Widdowson, W.M., M.L. Healy, P.H. Sönksen, and J Gibney. 2009. The physiology of growth hormone and sport. *Growth Hormone & IGF Research* 19 (4): 308-319.

71. Wilmore, J.H., D.L. Costill, and W.L. Kenney. 2008. *Physiology of Sport and Exercise,* 4th ed. Champaign, IL: Human Kinetics.

72. Wilmore, J.H., P.R. Stanforth, L.A. Hudspeth, J. Gagnon, E.W. Daw, A.S. Leon, D.C. Rao, J.S. Skinner, and C. Bouchard. 1998. Alterations in resting metabolic rate as a consequence of 20 wk of endurance training: The HERITAGE Family Study. *American Journal of Clinical Nutrition* 68 (1): 66-71.

73. Zouhal, H., C. Jacob, P. Delamarche, and A. Gratas-Delamarche. 2008. Catecholamines and the effects of exercise, training and gender. *Sports Medicine* 38 (5): 401-423.

Nutrition in the Personal Training Setting

Marie Spano, MS

After completing this chapter, you will be able to

- identify a personal trainer's scope of practice and know when to refer clients to a nutrition professional,

- review a client's diet and estimate the client's energy expenditure and requirement,

- understand the changes in a client's nutritional and fluid requirements due to exercise,

- advise clients on guidelines for weight gain and weight loss, and

- recognize the role and appropriateness of dietary supplementation.

Nutrition and physical activity should be addressed in conjunction with one another. Focusing on one at the exclusion of the other will yield less than optimal results for clients. Personal trainers can enhance their overall effectiveness by maintaining a core knowledge of nutrition and by individualizing their nutrition advice. Nutrition assessment and recommendations should match the needs and goals of the client and will vary accordingly. Lastly, personal trainers should know when they need to refer their clients to a dietitian because the client's needs are outside of the trainer's scope of expertise or practice (38).

The author would like to acknowledge the contributions of Kristin J. Reimers, who wrote this chapter for the first edition of *NSCA's Essentials of Personal Training.*

Role of the Personal Trainer Regarding Nutrition

Television, newspapers, magazines, and websites are the major sources of nutrition information for most people. Nutrition information communicated as sound bites and advertisements can lead to consumer confusion. Personal trainers have the opportunity to help clear the confusion by serving as a source of credible nutrition information.

It is well within the personal trainer's scope of practice to address misinformation and to give general advice related to nutrition for physical performance, disease prevention, weight loss, and weight gain. A personal trainer would be conveying general nutrition knowledge if he or she said, for example, "According to the American Heart Association, omega-3 fatty acids from fatty fish like salmon or mackerel may benefit those who are at risk of developing cardiovascular disease." An important part of the core knowledge, from the standpoint of both ethics and safety, is the ability to recognize more complicated nutrition issues and know who to refer clients to.

Referral to a nutrition professional is indicated when the client has a disease state (i.e., diabetes, heart disease, gastrointestinal disease, eating disorder, osteoporosis, elevated cholesterol, etc.) that is affected by nutrition. This type of nutrition information is called *medical nutrition therapy* and falls under the scope of practice of a licensed nutritionist, dietitian, or registered dietitian (RD) (depending on the country and in the United States, on the state's licensure laws) (3). Referral is also indicated when the complexity of the nutrition issue is beyond the competence of the personal trainer, which will vary. Personal trainers should find a nutrition professional they feel comfortable referring their clients to and with whom they can communicate about clients. In the United States and Canada, registered dietitians can be located through state dietetic organizations; the American Dietetic Association (ADA) website, www.eatright.org; the Sports, Cardiovascular and Wellness Nutritionists website (SCAN, a dietetic practice group of the ADA), www.scandpg.org; and Dietitians of Canada, www.dietitians.ca. The European Federation of the Association of Dietitians, www.efad.org/everyone, provides links to each country's dietitian organization. Sports Dietitians Australia has a website where people can locate a sports dietitian: www.sportsdietitians.com.au/findasportsdietitian. In other countries, personal trainers will want to consult local dietetic organizations or national Web sites. To facilitate communication, the client should sign a release of information form so that the personal trainer and the nutrition professional can communicate about the client's training program and general nutrition needs.

> Personal trainers should refer clients to a dietitian when the client has a disease state, such as cardiovascular disease, that has a dietary component or when the complexity of the nutrition issue is beyond the competence of the personal trainer.

Who Can Provide Nutrition Counseling and Education?

Before assessing a client's diet, personal trainers should turn to their state dietetic licensing board or to their country's organization for dietetic regulations to find out the laws within their particular state that govern the provision of nutrition advice. In the United States, each state regulates the provision of nutrition information through licensure, statutory certification, or registration. According to the American Dietetic Association, definitions for these terms are as follows:

- **Licensing:** Statutes include an explicitly defined scope of practice, and performance of the profession is illegal unless a license has been obtained from the state.
- **Statutory certification:** Limits use of particular titles to persons meeting predetermined requirements, while persons not certified can still practice the occupation or profession.
- **Registration:** This is the least restrictive form of state regulation. As with certification, unregistered persons are permitted to practice the profession. Typically, exams are not given and enforcement of the registration requirement is minimal (3).

As an example, at the time of this writing, the scope of nutrition practice in Louisiana is clearly defined, and specific guidance on a person's diet is allowed only by a registered dietitian or nutritionist (25). But in Arizona, no licensure law exists, and any professional can offer nutrition advice (23). Various states and countries have different regulations governing whether or not personal trainers can provide dietary advice, and personal trainers should follow these guidelines.

Dietary Assessment

Should a client seek nutrition information that is within the scope of the personal trainer's practice, the personal trainer may want to assess the client's diet. If this is out of the scope of his or her practice, the personal trainer can work alongside a dietitian who assesses the client's diet.

A complete nutrition assessment includes dietary data, anthropometric data, biochemical data (lab tests), and a clinical examination (condition of skin, teeth, etc.). Although personal trainers are usually not involved in the comprehensive assessment, they may want to be familiar with the individual components of a comprehensive dietary assessment so they can work with the dietitian to provide their client the best service possible. (*Note:* The term *diet* as used throughout this chapter refers to the usual eating pattern of the individual, not a restrictive weight loss plan.)

Dietary Intake Data

Before the personal trainer can give valid nutrition advice, gleaning some information about the client's current diet is imperative. How balanced is the client's current diet? Is the client allergic to certain foods? Is the client vegetarian? Restricting food groups? Dieting to lose weight? Is he or she a sporadic eater? Has the individual just adopted a new way of eating? The answers to all of these questions and others may influence the personal trainer's advice to the client.

Gathering dietary intake data is a simple concept, but it is extremely complex to do. Most people have difficulty recalling fully and accurately what they ate in a given day. Research shows that there is a tendency to underestimate or underreport actual intake, especially in persons who are overweight. Keeping in mind these general shortcomings, personal trainers, again if under the scope of practice as allowed in their state, have three methods for gathering dietary intake data to choose from:

- Dietary recall
- Diet history
- Diet records

In a diet recall, clients report what they have eaten in the past 24 hours. With a diet history, clients answer questions about usual eating habits, likes and dislikes, eating schedule, medical history, weight history, and so forth. The diet record is typically a log, filled out for three days, in which the client records everything consumed (foods, beverages, and supplements).

The three-day diet record is considered the most valid of the three methods for assessing the diet of an individual. However, a valid record requires scrupulous recording as well as scrupulous analysis. The pitfall of this method is that recording food intake usually inhibits regular eating patterns, and recorded intake thus underestimates true intake. To get useful data, the personal trainer should ask only the most motivated clients to complete this process. The diet recall or diet history is more appropriate for many clients.

The personal trainer should never make assumptions about a client's eating habits. Assessing the client's diet is essential before one makes dietary recommendations.

Evaluating the Diet

When the personal trainer has successfully gathered dietary intake data, several options exist for evaluating the information. One way to evaluate the client's diet is to compare a client's diet to the recommendations given in the country's general dietary guidelines. In the United States, the U.S. Department of Agriculture (USDA) created **MyPlate** (46). For clients who are keenly interested in nutrition, a more detailed analysis of the diet using diet analysis software may be indicated. Both methods are reviewed here.

MyPlate

The USDA MyPlate (figure 7.1) is a reminder for healthy eating. The "my" in "MyPlate" signifies the importance of personalizing the recommendations to one's lifestyle, while the familiar plate symbol provides a visual representation of how much of one's diet should be made up of the following food groups:

1. Grains
2. Vegetables
3. Fruits
4. Protein
5. Dairy

USDA's website for MyPlate identifies three main dietary goals for Americans (46):

Balancing Calories
- Enjoy your food, but eat less.
- Avoid oversized portions.

Foods to Increase
- Make half your plate fruits and vegetables.
- Make at least half your grains whole grains.
- Switch to fat-free or low-fat (1%) milk.

Foods to Reduce
- Compare the sodium in foods like soup, bread, and frozen meals and choose the foods with lower numbers.
- Drink water instead of sugary drinks.

The USDA has also identified specific goals that relate to each of the main food groups. For instance, consumers are told to eat at least half their grains as whole grains, vary their vegetable intake, focus on fruits, eat more calcium-rich foods, and go lean with protein.

Though the older MyPyramid contained guidelines for "discretionary calories," MyPlate has replaced this with an "empty calories" category. Empty calories are calories from solid fats or added sugars that have no nutrients. Solid fats (i.e., fats solid at room temperature) include butter, beef fat, and shortening. Added sugars are sugars or syrups that are added during food processing or preparation. The USDA provides the following examples of

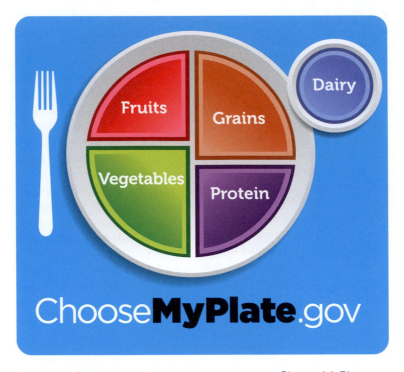

FIGURE 7.1   MyPlate. For more information and resources, go to www.ChooseMyPlate.gov.
U.S. Department of Agriculture/U.S. Department of Health and Human Services.

foods and beverages that provide the largest number of empty calories for Americans:

- Cakes, cookies, pastries, and donuts (contain both solid fat and added sugars)
- Sodas, energy drinks, sports drinks, and fruit drinks (contain added sugars)
- Cheese (contains solid fat)
- Pizza (contains solid fat)
- Ice cream (contains both solid fat and added sugars)
- Sausages, hot dogs, bacon, and ribs (contain solid fat)

Along with proving useful educational material, the MyPlate website (www.ChooseMyPlate.gov) contains tools that allow visitors to create customized meal plans, analyze their diets, and track their physical activity. This website is an excellent starting point for a personal trainer to use to help educate clients. Each food group in MyPlate provides key nutrients that are more difficult to acquire in the diet if that group is omitted.

The MyPlate website is an interactive tool that clients can use on their own or with a personal trainer's assistance. The Plan a Healthy Diet function allows users to enter data concerning their age, weight, height, gender, and physical activity level and in turn provides them with individualized directions for meeting their daily nutrition goals (see table 7.1 for an example). If consumers click on a food category, they'll be given more specific information on how to include that food group into their diet (46).

Computerized Diet Analysis

Computerized analysis can provide a snapshot of a client's diet, including vitamin and mineral intake. However, it is very important that the client accurately and completely record usual intake for at least three days. The client should input the amount of each food and beverage, specify how it was cooked, and give the brand name versus the generic term (e.g., "Wheaties" vs. just "bran flakes").

Even if the diet is recorded perfectly, the analysis will not be completely accurate because all software

TABLE 7.1   Example Menu Plan

Food group	Daily serving
Grains	10 oz
Vegetables	3.5 cups
Fruits	2.5 cups
Dairy	3 cups
Protein	7 oz

Menu plan is for a 22-year-old, 5'6", 140 lb male who exercises more than 60 minutes on most days of the week.

programs have shortcomings. For some foods in the database, values for certain vitamins and minerals are missing, meaning that analysis for those nutrients is also missing, which will result in an erroneously low intake value. Additionally, without fail, some foods that the client eats are not in the database, so it is necessary to make substitutions or type in the actual food data (and for processed foods, the results may not include values for all vitamins and minerals since this is not a requirement for food labels).

Before asking clients to assess their diet, it is helpful for personal trainers to complete a computerized diet analysis on themselves to recognize the bias that recording can impose on true habits. Additionally, analyzing one's own diet makes one aware of the level of detail needed to accurately assess a diet.

In many cases, the personal trainer does not have the training, time, knowledge, or resources to complete a computerized dietary analysis. This is an area in which many personal trainers turn to dietitians for assistance. Another option for motivated clients is to refer them to websites where they can enter their own diet and receive feedback (see the following list). These websites are excellent resources because they put the responsibility on the client. Additionally, some clients feel more comfortable asking questions and reporting intake in private situations. One drawback is that most of these websites do not have the extensive database that comes with food analysis programs, and they typically do not analyze food intake for all vitamins, minerals, types of fat, and so on. Instead, most tell the user only how many calories he or she has consumed, along with grams of fat, carbohydrates, and protein. A second drawback is that these sites cannot calculate calorie needs with the precision that a professional dietitian can.

Analysis of a client's diet is a detailed, time-consuming process that requires expertise. The personal trainer should consider referring the analysis to a dietitian or referring the client to self-directed diet analysis.

Energy

Energy is commonly measured in kilocalories (kcal). A kilocalorie is a measure of energy that equates to the heat required to raise the temperature of 1 kilogram of water 1 degree Celsius (or 2.2 pounds of water 1.8 degrees Fahrenheit). The general public refers to this as a *calorie*. (The terms *calorie* and *energy* are used interchangeably in this chapter.)

Factors Influencing Energy Requirements

Three factors make up the energy requirement of adults: resting metabolic rate, physical activity, and the thermic effect of food. Each of these factors can be affected directly or indirectly by age, genetics, body size, body composition, environmental temperature, training conditions, nontraining physical activity, and calorie intake. For infants, children, and teens, growth is another variable that increases the energy requirement.

Resting metabolic rate (RMR) is the largest contributor to total energy requirement, accounting for approximately 60% to 75% of daily energy expenditure. It is a measure of the calories required for maintaining normal body functions such as respiration, cardiac function, and thermoregulation (i.e., the energy a person would expend lying in bed all day and doing nothing). Factors that increase RMR include gaining lean body tissue, young age, growth, abnormal body temperature, menstrual cycle, and hyperthyroidism. Factors that decrease RMR include low caloric intake, loss of lean tissue, and hypothyroidism. All things equal, RMR can vary up to 20% between individuals due to normal genetic variations in metabolism.

The second largest component of energy requirement is physical activity. Of all the components, this one is the most variable. The amount of energy needed for physical activity depends on the intensity, duration, and frequency of training. It also depends on the environmental conditions; that is, extreme heat or cold increases calorie expenditure. When estimating how physically active a client is, the personal trainer needs to remember to ascertain how physically active the client is aside from structured exercise. Even if people have an exercise routine, those with the sedentary lifestyle of a desk job and sedentary leisure activities may be considered only lightly active.

Diet Analysis Websites

- www.sparkpeople.com: This website offers a food tracker, personalized meal plans, customized fitness plan, recipes, articles, and message boards.
- www.fitday.com: This website tracks food, exercise, and weight loss goals.
- www.ChooseMyPlate.gov: The MyPlate website allows users to track diet and physical activity and energy balance; in addition, it provides an analysis of food intake and physical fitness.

The **thermic effect of food** is the increase in energy expenditure above the RMR that can be measured for several hours following a meal. The thermic effect of food is the energy needed to digest and assimilate foods, approximately 7% to 10% of a person's total energy requirement.

Estimating Energy Requirements

A true estimation of energy requirement (i.e., energy expended in a day) is difficult to obtain directly. Therefore surrogate methods are often used. One such method is to measure calorie intake. This method is valid if the client is maintaining a stable body weight, because a stable body weight indicates that energy intake generally equals energy expenditure. For the motivated client who accurately records intake, the best way to determine energy requirement using this method is to assess the calorie intake from the three-day food log. If that is not possible, one can use mathematical equations that roughly estimate caloric expenditure. However, it is difficult to calculate energy needs because of the many variables affecting caloric requirements and the significant inter- and intraindividual variation. It is essential to stress that these equations are only estimates and are meant to serve as a frame of reference. Actual energy expenditure of individuals will vary widely. Table 7.2 lists factors that can be used for energy requirement estimation. For example, for a male who weighs 170 pounds (77 kg) and is highly physically active, the requirement would be 3,910 kcal (23 × 170).

Another method for calculating energy expenditure is to first calculate resting energy expenditure (REE), then multiply it by a factor based on activity level. Several equations for estimating REE exist. One set of REE equations , developed by the World Health Organization (14), is shown in table 7.3.

The result is the number of calories that are likely expended by the person in an average day. Clients wishing to maintain current body weight would need to consume the same number of calories that they expend.

It is difficult, if not impossible, to obtain an accurate estimate of a client's energy expenditure. The personal trainer can help the client base the estimation on intake or use an equation such as those provided in this chapter. Regardless of the method, these are rough estimates of the actual expenditure.

Nutrients

Once the personal trainer knows a client's dietary intake and energy requirements, he or she can assess general nutritional needs. To understand the relationship between the body and food, as well as to provide nutrition guidance, it is important to have an understanding of the six nutrients: protein, carbohydrate, fat, vitamins, minerals, and water.

Protein

For centuries, protein was considered the staple of the diet and the source of speed and strength for athletic endeavors. Although we now know that carbohydrates are the main energy source for humans, protein remains a main nutrient of interest, especially among bodybuilders, weightlifters, and others who engage in resistance training.

When answering the question "How much protein does my client need?" the personal trainer must consider two key factors, energy intake and source of protein. Protein may be used for energy when fewer calories are consumed than are expended. If this is the case, protein intake will not be used solely for the intended purpose of building and replacing lean tissue. Thus, when caloric intake goes down, the protein requirement goes up. Dietary protein requirements were derived from research on subjects who were consuming adequate calories. Requirements for clients who are dieting for weight loss are higher than standard requirements.

Additionally, protein requirements are based on "reference proteins" such as meat, fish, poultry,

TABLE 7.2 Estimated Daily Calorie Needs of Males and Females by Activity Level

Activity level	Male (kcal/pound)	Male (kcal/kg)	Female (kcal/pound)	Female (kcal/kg)
Light*	17	38	16	35
Moderate**	19	41	17	37
Heavy***	23	50	20	44

*Light activity level: Walking on a level surface at 2.5 to 3.0 miles per hour, garage work, electrical trades, carpentry, restaurant trades, housecleaning, child care, golf, sailing, table tennis.

**Moderate activity level: Walking 3.5 to 4.0 miles per hour, weeding and hoeing, carrying a load, cycling, skiing, tennis, dancing.

***Heavy activity level: Walking with load uphill, tree felling, heavy manual digging, basketball, climbing, football, soccer.

TABLE 7.3 Estimated Daily Calorie Needs Based on Resting Energy Expenditure (REE) and Activity Level

1. To calculate the REE, choose one of these six formulas [15]:

Age and sex	Kcal per day
Males 10 to 18 years	(17.686 × weight in kg) + 658.2
Males 19 to 30 years	(15.057 × weight in kg) + 692.2
Males 31 to 60 years	(11.472 × weight in kg) + 873.1
Males >60 years	(11.711 × weight in kg) + 587.7
Females 10 to 18 years	(13.384 × weight in kg) + 692.6
Females 19 to 30 years	(14.818 × weight in kg) + 486.6
Females 31 to 60 years	(8.126 × weight in kg) + 845.6
Females >60 years	(9.082 × weight in kg) + 658.5

2. then, multiply the REE by a factor to account for physical activity level (PAL) to estimate daily calorie needs:

Level of activity	PAL Value (×REE)
Sedentary or light activity lifestyle	1.40 to 1.69
Active or moderately active lifestyle	1.70 to 1.99
Vigorous or vigorously active lifestyle	2.00 to 2.40*

*PAL values greater than 2.40 are difficult to maintain over a long period of time.

Adapted from FAO 2004 (14).

dairy products, and eggs, which are considered high-quality proteins. If protein in the diet comes mostly from plants, the requirement is higher. The U.S. Recommended Dietary Allowance (RDA) for protein for healthy, sedentary adults is 0.8 g/kg of body weight for both men and women (31). The World Health Organization identifies the safe intake level, a level that is sufficient for 97.5% of the population, at 0.83 g protein/kg per day. The safe level ensures a low risk that needs will not be met but also includes the concept that there is no risk to individuals from excess protein intake up to levels considerably higher than 0.83 g/kg (51). Though the intake set by both of these organizations may be sufficient for nonactive healthy, young adults, it is not appropriate for clients who have greater protein needs to help offset protein–amino acid oxidation during exercise, repair muscle damage, and build lean tissue. A general recommendation for athletes is 1.2 to 2.0 g/kg per day depending on the sport, training intensity, total calorie intake, and overall health (10).

The personal trainer should be aware that excessively high protein intakes (e.g., greater than 4 g/kg body weight per day) are not indicated for clients with impaired renal function, those with low calcium intake, or those who are restricting fluid intake. These situations could be exacerbated by a high protein intake. For the most part, however, concerns about potential negative effects of high protein intakes are unfounded, especially in healthy individuals. Proteins consumed in excess of amounts needed for the synthesis of tissue are used for energy or are stored.

Carbohydrate

Carbohydrate is required for the complete metabolism of fatty acids. Roughly 50 to 100 g of carbohydrate (the equivalent of three to five pieces of bread) per day prevents **ketosis** (high levels of ketones in the bloodstream), which results from incomplete breakdown of fatty acids (50). Beyond that basal requirement, the role of carbohydrate is to provide fuel for energy, and thus the amount of carbohydrate needed by clients depends on their total energy requirement. Carbohydrate recommendations are also based on clients' mode of training.

Because dietary carbohydrate replaces muscle and liver glycogen used during high-intensity physical activity, a high-carbohydrate diet (up to 60-70% of total calories) is commonly recommended for physically active individuals (40). However, it is important to note that a variety of diets, with various carbohydrate, protein, and fat mixtures, have been shown to be equally effective in supporting training and performance. Which diet is appropriate depends upon a client's goals, training regimen, and fitness level (7, 8, 33, 34). Some physically active individuals may benefit from a high-carbohydrate diet, but others do not benefit; and they may experience negative effects such as an increase in serum triglycerides or weight gain. Individualizing carbohydrate intake based on the training program and diet history is imperative. In addition, incorporating the strategies of nutrient timing may be more important than overall carbohydrate intake. Nutrient timing involves the strategic timing of food and supplement intake to maximize muscle mass gains, alter body composition, and restore glycogen levels.

One important factor to consider in determining recommendations for carbohydrate intake is the training program. If a client is an aerobic endurance athlete, for example a distance runner, road cyclist, triathlete, or cross-country skier who trains aerobically for long durations (90 minutes or more daily), he or she should replenish glycogen levels by consuming approximately 7 to 10 g/kg body weight per day (19, 41, 42). This is equivalent to 600 to 750 g of carbohydrate (2,400-3,000 kcal from carbohydrate) per day for an individual weighing 165 pounds (75 kg). This level has been shown to adequately restore skeletal glycogen within 24 hours (1, 11, 20, 25, 26, 35).

However, the majority of physically active individuals do not train *aerobically* for more than an hour each day. Research on the carbohydrate needs of these individuals is sparse. Moderately low carbohydrate intake and muscle glycogen levels seem to have a minor impact, if any, on resistance training performance (30, 45, 47, 52). Intake of approximately half of that recommended for aerobic endurance exercise appears adequate to support training and performance of strength, sprint, and skill exercise; thus an intake of 5 to 6 g/kg body weight per day is reasonable (9, 41).

Dietary Fat

The human body has a low requirement of dietary fat. It is estimated that individuals should consume at least 3% of energy from omega-6 (linoleic) fatty acids and 0.5% to 1% from omega-3 (alpha linolenic acid) fatty acids to prevent true deficiency (12). Even though the requirement is low, inadequate fat intake is a potential problem for otherwise healthy individuals who overly restrict dietary fat. Very low-fat diets, such as those sometimes prescribed for patients with severe heart disease, are not recommended for healthy, active individuals. Diets with less than 15% fat may decrease testosterone production, thus possibly affecting metabolism and muscle development (48). And very low-fat diets may impair the absorption of fat-soluble vitamins.

Personal trainers need to be aware of their clients' perceptions about dietary fat and provide education on the importance of essential fatty acids (omega-3 and omega-6 fats). It is, of course, the overconsumption rather than the under consumption of fat that has held the attention of scientists, health care providers, and the general public for the past several decades, specifically with respect to the relationship between dietary fat and cardiovascular disease.

Approximately 34% of calories in the typical American diet are from fat (13). Dietary intake in most European countries is similar, with 34% of calories from fat in women and 36% in men (24). The recommendation for the general public from most health organizations is that fat should contribute 30% or less of the total calories consumed. It is recommended that 20% of the total calories (or two-thirds of the total fat intake) come from monounsaturated or polyunsaturated sources, that less than 10% come from saturated fats (one-third of total fat intake), and that minimal man-made trans fats from partially hydrogenated oils be consumed.

It is advisable for a personal trainer to consider the factors listed in the highlight box on the next page before making recommendations about decreasing dietary fat.

> Protein, carbohydrates, and fats are all essential nutrients. Excess or deficiency of any one will be problematic. The personal trainer should help clients stay focused on the total diet, not an individual nutrient.

Vitamins and Minerals

Dietary Reference Intakes (DRIs), which are used in the United States and Canada, are recommendations of the Food and Nutrition Board, Institute of Medicine, part of the U.S. National Academies, for the intake of vitamins and minerals, to be used for planning and assessing diets for healthy people (table 7.4). The DRIs are based on life stage groups, which take into account age, sex, pregnancy, and lactation. A personal trainer who has the computerized analysis of a client's diet can assess actual vitamin and mineral intake compared to the DRIs. Starting in 1997 the DRIs replaced the *Recommended Dietary Allowances* that had been published since 1941. Dietary Reference Intakes represent a different approach, with the emphasis on long-term health instead of deficiency diseases. The DRIs are split into four categories:

1. *Recommended Dietary Allowance (RDA)* is the intake that meets the nutrient needs of almost all (97% to 98%) healthy individuals in a specific age and sex group.

2. *Adequate Intake* is a goal intake when sufficient scientific information is unavailable to estimate the RDA.

3. *Estimated Average Requirement* is the intake that meets the estimated nutrient need of half the individuals in a specific group.

4. *Tolerable Upper Intake Level* is the maximum intake that is unlikely to pose risks of adverse health effects in almost all healthy individuals in a group.

When Should the Client Decrease Dietary Fat?

In general, there are three reasons for individuals to reduce dietary fat:

1. *Need to increase carbohydrate intake to support training* (see the earlier section on carbohydrate). In this case, to ensure adequate protein provision, fat is the nutrient to decrease so that caloric intake can remain similar while the person is increasing carbohydrate.

2. *Need to reduce total caloric intake to achieve weight loss.* Achieving a negative calorie balance is the only way to reduce body fat. Fat can be a source of excess calories because it is dense in calories (fat has 9 kcal/g vs. 4 kcal/g in carbohydrate and protein). Studies also suggest that the good flavor of high-fat foods increases the likelihood of over eating these foods. Thus, decreasing excess dietary fat can help reduce caloric intake. (The recommendation to reduce dietary fat should not be made before assessment of dietary intake. The individual may already have a low-fat diet.)

3. *Need to decrease elevated blood cholesterol.* Manipulation of fat and carbohydrate may be necessary if medically indicated for clients who have high blood cholesterol levels or a family history of heart disease. This diet therapy should be provided only by a registered dietitian.

TABLE 7.4 Dietary Reference Intakes for Individuals in Life Stage Group 19 to 30 Years (35)

Specific vitamin or mineral	Males	Females	Tolerable upper limit
Vitamin A (µg/day)	900	700	3,000
Vitamin C (mg/day)	75	75	2,000
Vitamin D (µg/day)	5*	5*	50
Vitamin E (mg/day)	15	15	1,000
Vitamin K (µg/day)	120*	75*	ND
Thiamin (mg/day)	1.2	1.0	ND
Riboflavin (mg/day)	1.3	1.0	ND
Niacin (mg/day)	16	14	35
Vitamin B_6 (mg/day)	1.3	1.2	100
Folate (µg/day)	400	400	1,000
Vitamin B_{12} (µg/day)	2.4	2.4	ND
Pantothenic acid (mg/day)	5*	5*	ND
Biotin (µg/day)	30*	25*	ND
Calcium (mg/day)	1,000*	1,000*	2,500
Chromium (µg/day)	35*	25*	ND
Copper (µg/day)	900	900	10,000
Iron (mg/day)	8	18	45
Magnesium (mg/day)	400	310	350
Phosphorus (mg/day)	700	700	4,000
Selenium (µg/day)	55	55	400
Zinc (mg/day)	11	8	40

Note: This table (taken from the Dietary Reference Intake reports, see www.nap.edu) presents Recommended Dietary Allowances (RDAs) in **bold type** and adequate intakes (AIs) in ordinary type followed by an asterisk. RDAs are set to meet the needs of almost all (97-98%) individuals in a group. The AI for adults and gender groups is believed to cover needs of all individuals in the group, but lack of data does not allow specifying the percentage of individuals covered by this intake. ND = not determined.

Adapted from The National Academy of Sciences and The National Academies (32).

Instead of being published in one volume as were the RDAs, the DRIs have been published as separate nutrient groups, each group having its own volume. The first book was published in 1997; several more have followed. The reader is referred to the Institute of Medicine's website at http://iom.edu, where DRI tables and links to the full texts of the reports are freely available. It is important to remember that the recommendations for nutrient intakes represent the state of the science at the time, and as such, continue to evolve.

Historically, focus has been on inadequate nutrient intake. However, both inadequate intakes and excessive intakes are problematic. Accordingly the DRIs include an upper limit, or the amount of a nutrient that may cause negative side effects. Excessively high vitamin and mineral intakes are not only unnecessary but can be harmful in some instances.

The European Food Safety Authority (EFSA) developed the Dietary Reference Values for nutrients. The micronutrient section was being worked on in 2010. At the time of this writing, the EFSA had set tolerable upper levels of intake (UL) for vitamins and minerals. Personal trainers can find up-to-date information concerning Dietary Reference Values at www.efsa.europa.eu.

Water

Fluid intake is a nonissue for some and an obsession for others. A variety of issues have set the stage for confusion about how much and what to drink. Surprisingly little research exists on the water requirements of humans. Research that does exist is primarily limited to hospitalized patients, soldiers, or serious athletes in hot environments. Assumptions that thirst will drive adequate water intake, and taking comfort in the fact that kidneys will do their job, have largely led scientists to overlook the issue of hydration in healthy individuals.

General Fluid Intake Guidelines

Unlike the situation with many other nutrients, it is impossible to set a general requirement for water. Common knowledge and folklore have put the requirement at anywhere from 64 ounces (1.9 L) per day to 2 gallons (7.5 L). Both could be right, depending on the situation. The reality is that water requirements change based on a variety of factors including environment, sweating, body surface area, calorie intake, body size, and lean muscle tissue, leading to tremendous inter- and intraindividual variation. Instead of looking at prescriptive amounts to be consumed each day, it is important for personal trainers to assess each client's situation and attempt to individualize recommendations.

The basic goal of fluid intake is to avoid dehydration, that is, maintain fluid balance. The state of fluid balance exists when the water that is lost from the body through urine, through insensible loss from skin and lungs, and through feces is replaced. The kidneys dilute or concentrate urine to keep the body's internal milieu unchanged regardless of significant changes in intake. Thirst is triggered at about 1% dehydration. Thus, encouraging fluid intake

based on thirst works quite well to maintain fluid balance for healthy adult individuals in temperature-controlled environments who are sedentary and who have plenty of fluid readily available.

The average fluid intake needed to offset fluid losses in sedentary adults may range from 1.5 to 2.7 quarts (1.4-2.6 L) per day. People often ask whether higher fluid intakes are healthful. The answer is unclear, but an emerging area of study on the relationship between disease prevention and fluid intake indicates that higher fluid intakes may be preventive against bladder cancer, kidney stones, gallstones, and colon cancer (6, 21, 29, 39).

It is impossible to set a generic water recommendation, such as eight glasses of water a day. Each individual's water requirement varies over time, as do requirements among various people.

Fluid Intake and Exercise

Although the answers regarding general fluid intake in sedentary conditions are unclear, more is known about fluid intake and exercise. Guidelines have been developed for individuals before, during, and after exercise.

Before Exercise   Approximately 5 to 7 ml of fluid per kilogram body weight should be consumed at least 4 hours prior to exercise. Additional fluid should be consumed 2 hours prior to exercise, approximately 3 to 5 ml/kg body weight if urine is dark and scant (39).

During Exercise   Preventing dehydration can be difficult for physically active people exercising in a warm environment. Continuous sweating during prolonged exercise can exceed 1.9 quarts (1.8 L) per hour, increasing water requirements significantly. Unless sweat losses are replaced, body temperature rises, leading to heat exhaustion, heatstroke, and even death. Paradoxically, during exercise, humans do not adequately replace sweat losses when fluids are consumed at will. In fact, most individuals replace only about two-thirds of the water they sweat off during exercise. Personal trainers must be aware of this tendency and make their clients aware of it as well. During times of high sweat loss under physical stress, a systematic approach to water replacement is necessary because thirst is not a reliable indicator of fluid needs in these situations.

After Exercise   Slight dehydration is common in almost all physical endeavors, and therefore rehydration is necessary. However, "preventive maintenance" is also important. Starting hydrated, as well as consuming fluids during activity, is a very important part of the systematic approach to hydration. After exercise, the main goal is to replace any fluid and electrolyte losses.

Clients should monitor sweat loss by checking body weight before and after physical activity. (For accuracy, clients should remove sweaty clothes before weighing.) Clients should drink 20 to 24 ounces (about 600 to 700 ml) of fluids for every pound lost (39). Sodium-rich foods or a sport drink should be used to stimulate thirst, replace lost electrolytes, and enhance rehydration. During the rehydration process, urine is produced before full rehydration occurs (43). Ideally, the amount of fluid clients need to replace should be measured into water bottles, pitchers, and so forth so that rehydration is not left to chance.

Clients who have a goal of weight loss may misperceive acute weight loss during a workout as loss of fat and therefore see it as positive. It is important for personal trainers to clarify with clients that the acute weight loss during a workout is water, not fat, and must be replaced by hydrating (preferably with the inclusion of sodium-rich foods or an electrolyte-enhanced sport beverage).

Monitoring Hydration Status

Although not as sensitive as weight change, other indicators of hydration status can be useful monitoring tools. Signs of dehydration include dark yellow, strong-smelling urine; decreased frequency of urination; rapid resting heart rate; and prolonged muscle soreness (4). Normal urine production for adults is about 1.2 quarts (1.1 L) per day, or 8 to 10 fluid ounces (237-296 ml) per urination four times per day. Normal urine is the color of light lemon juice, except in clients who are taking supplemental vitamins, which tend to make the urine bright yellow.

What to Drink Before and After Activity

All fluids, from beverages and from food, contribute to the body's fluid requirement. Juice and soft drinks are 89% water; milk is 90% water, and even pizza is 50% water. Before and after physical activity, water or other beverages such as milk, juice, carbonated or uncarbonated soft drinks, and sport drinks are suitable choices for fluid replacement. For clients who eat many fruits, vegetables, and soups, much of their water requirement may be coming from foods.

Whether consuming caffeine-containing beverages causes dehydration is a frequently asked question. Data show that tolerance to caffeine occurs in one to four days and that people who are tolerant do not experience increased urine output. Thus, caffeine-containing beverages contribute to hydration (16).

When significant sweating has occurred, consumption of sodium chloride (salt) in the form of beverages or food minimizes urine output and hastens recovery of water and electrolyte balance (27, 28). In practical terms, this means that consuming a wide variety of beverages and foods after training is important. In fact, most fluid consumption occurs during and around mealtimes.

> **All foods and fluids contribute to hydration, including foods like pizza and beverages like coffee.**

What to Drink During Activity

The goal of fluid replacement during exercise is to move the fluid from the mouth, through the gut, and into circulation rapidly and to provide a volume that matches sweat losses. The way to achieve this is to provide fluids that are absorbed rapidly and that the client finds palatable. A variety of fluids can serve as effective fluid replacement during exercise (18). Cool water is an ideal fluid replacement except during long-duration activity (endurance exercise, multiple games in a day, etc.)—when replacing sodium becomes very important to prevent a dangerous drop in blood sodium levels, called hyponatremia. Other options include commercial sport drinks or homemade sport drinks, such as diluted juice or diluted soft drinks. Although plain water can meet fluid requirements in most cases, some people find flavored drinks more palatable than water and consequently drink more (51). During aerobic endurance training, carbohydrate along with water intake can be helpful if activities last more than 60 to 90 minutes (5).

Commercial sport drinks contain water, sugars, and electrolytes (usually sodium, chloride, and potassium). The sugar content of sport drinks is slightly less than the amount in most soft drinks and juices. The carbohydrate concentration of commercial sport drinks ranges from 6% to 8%, a solution that tends to be absorbed rapidly.

Clients who are monitoring calorie intake in an effort to maintain or lose weight may be averse to consuming the extra calories in sport drinks. In this case, the cost to benefit of consuming carbohydrate must be examined. It is worth remembering that the benefits of carbohydrate during aerobic endurance training are important for competitive clients wanting to increase speed and aerobic endurance, but might be less so for a client who is training primarily for health and fitness and interested in weight loss.

Weight Gain

There are two basic reasons clients may attempt to gain weight: to improve physical appearance or enhance athletic performance. For weight gain in the form of muscle mass, a combination of diet and progressive resistance training is essential. However, genetic predisposition, body type, and compliance determine the client's progress. Muscle tissue is approximately 70% water, 22% protein, and 8% fatty acids and glycogen. If all the extra calories consumed are used for muscle growth during resistance training, then about 2,500 extra kilocalories are required for each 1-pound (0.45 kg) increase in lean tissue. This includes the energy needed for tissue assimilation as well as the energy expended during resistance training. Thus, 350 to 700 kcal above daily requirements would supply the calories needed to support a 1- to 2-pound (0.45 to 0.9 kg) weekly gain in lean tissue as well as the energy requirements of the resistance training program.

To accomplish increased caloric intake, it is recommended that clients eat larger portions of foods at mealtime, eat more total calories at each meal, eat frequently, and choose higher-calorie foods. To accommodate frequent eating, meal replacement drinks can come in handy, especially when a person is not hungry.

Gaining muscle increases protein requirements. Protein needs are estimated to be 1.2 to 2.0 g/kg body weight per day and may be higher if the client's primary source of protein is plant based. Plant proteins have a lower biological value than animal proteins.

> The two primary nutrition principles for weight gain are to increase calorie intake and to increase protein intake (or maintain at an adequate level).

Weight Loss

People who have weight loss as a goal, specifically fat loss, can be split into two general groups: those who are normal weight but want to lose body fat for aesthetic reasons and those who are overweight or obese, that is, have a body mass index (BMI) greater than 25 or 30, respectively. Chapter 11 includes procedures and norms related to BMI, while chapter 19 provides detailed information on weight loss. The following are general principles to be considered when a client embarks on a weight loss regimen:

- The ability to achieve and maintain minimal body fat is to some extent genetic.
- Whether clients can gain muscle and lose body fat simultaneously depends on their training program and nutrition intake. Previously untrained clients can lose body fat and gain lean body mass as a result of caloric restriction and training; however, it is more difficult for trained persons who already possess a low percentage of body fat to achieve body fat reduction without losing some lean body mass.

- An average loss of 1 to 2 pounds (about 0.5-1.0 kg) per week represents a daily caloric deficit of approximately 500 to 1,000 kcal, which can be achieved through a combination of dietary restriction and exercise. Faster rates of weight loss can lead to dehydration and decrease vitamin and mineral status as a result of the decreased food intake (17). Substantial weight loss by caloric restriction will result in loss of marked amounts of lean body mass (53). Fat loss rates vary depending on body composition, food intake, and training program. The rate of loss of 1% total body weight per week is a common guideline. For example, losing at a rate of 1%, a 110-pound (50 kg) client would strive for about a 1-pound (0.45 kg) weight loss per week, while a 331-pound (150 kg) client would aim to lose about 3 pounds (1.5 kg) per week.

- The diet should be composed of food low in energy density. Energy density refers to the calories per weight or volume of food. Examples of foods with low energy density are broth-based soup, salad greens, vegetables, and fruits. In general, foods with low energy density contain a high proportion of water and fiber. These are foods that people can eat in large portions without consuming excess calories. This can help control hunger and lower caloric intake (37).

- The diet should be nutritionally balanced and should provide a variety of foods.

> The guiding principle for weight loss is to help clients achieve a negative energy balance. Many clients think the issue is more complex than that, so the personal trainer should keep them focused on this principle.

Evaluating Weight Loss Diets

Weight loss diet plans are endless—high protein, low fat, low carbohydrate, this shake, that bar, fat burners, don't eat at night, eat six times a day, eat one time a day—and the list goes on and on. What makes things confusing is that every client can name at least one person for whom at least one of these methods has worked. In addition, each client can think of many people for whom nothing seems to work. The truth is, *any* method will lead to weight loss if, and only if, the person achieves a negative calorie balance. As personal trainers answer their clients' questions about diets they read about or see on TV, it is essential to keep in mind that people need to burn more calories than they consume for fat loss to occur.

Clearly, it is impossible to keep up with every new diet, and a personal trainer does not need to. Instead, one evaluates a diet not on the claims it makes, but by the foods (and therefore nutrients) that are included and excluded. Personal trainers can help clients spot fad diets by checking for signs like the following:

- The diet excludes one or more groups of foods, which means that it may be deficient in certain nutrients or that it is too restrictive for clients to stay on for the long term.

- It overemphasizes one particular food or type of food. The Cabbage Soup Diet is an example.

- It is very low in calories. Very low-calorie diets can lead to higher loss of lean tissue, are limited in nutrients, and may decrease compliance.

- The advocates discourage physical activity or indicate that it isn't necessary.

- The diet promises quick weight loss.

Last but not least, personal trainers need to talk to clients about what they are really doing, not what the diet plan says. Often, the two are different. Trainers can decipher nutrition misinformation by taking a close look at the source of the information and cross-referencing the information with trusted websites or sport nutrition experts.

In addition to foods, the personal trainer should examine whether a diet plan includes dietary supplements. Stimulants are commonly added to weight loss supplements. These types of supplements are generally contraindicated in individuals with high blood pressure or other medical conditions. Stimulants for weight loss should be used only under the supervision of a physician. In many cases, clients are not aware of all the ingredients in the supplement they ingest. The personal trainer can ask the client to bring in the container so they can review the contents together. At this time the personal trainer can gather information on any questionable ingredients.

Dietary Supplements

Dietary supplements cover the spectrum from traditional vitamin–mineral tablets to prohormones such as androstenedione. Because of the diversity of dietary supplements, it is difficult to give blanket recommendations or guidelines about them. The following is a brief overview of the science and regulation of dietary supplements.

Dietary Supplement Regulation

In the United States, dietary supplements are regulated under the Dietary Supplement Health and Education Act of 1994 (DSHEA). This act was a landmark law for supplements, affirming the status of dietary supplements as a category of food, not drugs, and defining dietary supplements as products "intended to supplement the diet." The ingredients of a supplement include vitamins, minerals, herbs or botanicals, amino acids, a substance that increases the total dietary intake, or variations and combinations thereof.

In January of 2000, the U.S. Food and Drug Administration ruled that supplement manufacturers can make claims on the label about the body's structure or function affected by the supplement but cannot claim to diagnose, prevent, cure, or treat disease. In other words, it is permissible to say that a calcium supplement will "help maintain bone health" but not permissible to say that calcium will "help prevent osteoporosis."

Although the Food and Drug Administration does not have the resources to monitor and test individual supplements, a few independent organizations offer quality testing and approval. One independent company, ConsumerLab.com, tests supplements for quality and purity and provides the results on its website. Supplements that pass the test can carry the ConsumerLab approved quality product seal on the label. An independent, voluntary organization called United States Pharmacopoeia (USP) is developing a pilot Dietary Supplement Certification Program. The acronym USP on the label is meant to assure the consumer that the label information is accurate and that the company follows good manufacturing practices. The World Anti-Doping Agency, the National Science Foundation, and Informed Choice also test supplements for banned substances.

Evaluating Supplement Regimens

It is estimated that 48% of U.S. adults take some kind of dietary supplement. Vitamin and mineral supplements remain the most commonly used. Although vitamin–mineral supplements are perceived to be without risk, excess intake of vitamins and minerals is not beneficial and, depending on the circumstance, potentially harmful. For example, excess iron can be dangerous for those with the genetic disorder called hemochomotasis, in which the body absorbs and stores excess iron in tissues, leading to multisystem failure.

When evaluating a client's supplement regimen, it is important to evaluate all sources of the nutrient. Because vitamins and minerals are often added to a variety of supplements (shakes, powders, etc.) as well as breakfast cereal, sport bars, and energy drinks, the likelihood of excessive intakes is increasing. Excessive intakes, especially of iron, calcium, zinc, magnesium, niacin, B_6, and vitamin A, should be corrected through changes in the supplement regimen.

A common finding is that the individual's supplementation choices do not match the inadequacies of the diet, causing excess intakes of some nutrients and not correcting the low intake of others. Helping a client adjust food and supplement choices to optimize the vitamin and mineral intake is a useful function of diet analysis.

Besides questions about vitamins and minerals, clients may have questions about other types of supplements such as creatine or amino acids. One way to make sense of the wide array of supplements is to categorize them. Most supplements fit into the categories shown in table 7.5. Evaluation of the particular supplement for a client depends on the individual's goals and situation. For example, meal replacement drinks and bars can be an excellent snack for busy people. Protein supplements can round out protein needs in those who don't eat enough dietary protein, and so on. If a client participates in National Collegiate Athletic Association, United States Olympic Committee, or other competitions where drug testing occurs, it is important to know that some supplements contain banned substances that could lead to a positive drug test. These individuals need to check with their sponsoring organizations for guidelines. For a comprehensive analysis on the efficacy and safety of various ergogenic aids, the reader is referred to the ISSN Exercise & Sports Nutrition Review: Research and Recommendations (www.jissn.com/content/7/1/7).

The Art of Making Dietary Recommendations

When a personal trainer is evaluating a client's eating habits and giving advice, it is important to keep a few concepts in mind. First, nutritional status is influenced by intake over a relatively long period. Short-term dietary inadequacies or excesses will typically have a minimal impact on long-term status. Additionally, the body can obtain the nutrients it needs through countless combinations of foods consumed over time. There is no "right way to eat" that applies to everyone. Generally speaking, an adequate diet provides nutrients the body needs, other components from food that promote health or prevent disease, and calories at the level needed to achieve desired body weight; and it does so in a way that matches the individual's preferences, lifestyle, training goals, and budget.

Conclusion

The most important thing for personal trainers is to operate under their scope of practice. Before assessing a client's diet, personal trainers should first

TABLE 7.5 Selected Dietary Supplement Categories

Category	Examples
Meal replacements	Drinks and bars
Protein sources	Drinks, powders
Amino acids	Glutamine, tyrosine, BCAAs, EAAs
Carbohydrate sources	Sport drinks, energy drinks, bars, gels
Pre- and prohormones*	Androstenedione, DHEA
Biochemicals/energy metabolites	Creatine, HMB, pyruvate, CLA
Herbs	Ginseng, St. John's wort, guarana

*Pre- and prohormones are substances that are precursors to or enhancers of hormone production.
CLA = conjugated linoleic acid; DHEA = dehydroepiandrosterone; HMB = beta-hydroxy-beta-methylbutyrate; BCAA = Branched chain amino acid; EAA = essential amino acid.

turn to their state dietetic licensing board to find out the laws within their particular state, province, or country that govern the provision of nutrition advice. Because nutrition is a complex field, just like personal training, the personal trainer can benefit from collaborating with a dietitian who specializes in sport nutrition.

The personal trainer can benefit from three fundamental tools when discussing nutrition with clients. One is factual information, such as that provided in this book, on which to base assessments and recommendations. The second tool is the individualized approach. Personal trainers are likely to find themselves recommending something to one client and advising the next client against the same thing (if they can make individual recommendations under their state dietitian or nutritionist licensure laws). The ability to match the recommendations to the individual's situation enhances the personal trainer's effectiveness exponentially. The third tool is a network of knowledgeable persons to consult or refer to when clients have nutrition issues outside the scope of the personal trainer's expertise. With these three tools, the personal trainer can help nutrition work for, not against, clients' health and fitness goals.

Study Questions

1. Taking into consideration REE, which of the following is the approximate daily caloric need of a 25-year-old, 125-pound (57 kg) female client who is moderately active?

   A. 1,333 kilocalories

   B. 1,600 kilocalories

   C. 2,000 kilocalories

   D. 2,263 kilocalories

2. An active male client lost 3 pounds (1.4 kg) during practice. How much fluid should he consume to replace sweat losses?

   A. 8 ounces per pound loss

   B. 60 ounces

   C. 16 ounces per pound loss

   D. 40 ounces

3. Approximately how much carbohydrate should an elite male cross country runner who weighs 150 pounds (68 kg) consume per day?

   A. 136 g

   B. 340 g

   C. 680 g

   D. 1,360 g

4. Which of the following is the recommended minimum protein intake for an active client?

   A. 1.0 g/kg body weight

   B. 0.83 g/kg body weight

   C. 1.2 g/kg body weight

   D. 2.0 g/kg body weight

Applied Knowledge Question

Assuming no deficiencies, special requirements, or additional needs, describe the general daily nutrient requirements for a 20-year-old, 240-pound (109 kg) professional male rugby player.

Nutrient	General daily requirements
Kilocalories	
Protein (grams)	
Carbohydrate (grams)	
Fat (percent of total kilocalories)	
Monounsaturated fat (percent of total fat intake)	
Polyunsaturated fat (percent of total fat intake)	
Saturated fat (percent of total fat intake)	
Vitamin A	
Vitamin E	
Calcium	
Iron	

References

1. Ahlborg, B., J. Bergstrom, J. Brohult, L. Ekelund, E. Hultman, and G. Maschio. 1967. Human muscle glycogen content and capacity for prolonged exercise after different diets. *Foersvarsmedicine* 3: 85-99.

2. American College of Sports Medicine. 1996. Position stand. Exercise and fluid replacement. *Medicine and Science in Sports and Exercise* 28: i-vii.

3. American Dietetic Association. 2009. Dietetics practitioner state licensure provisions. www.eatright.org/ada/files/State_Licensure_Summary_without_dfns_011409.pdf. Accessed 30 April 2010

4. Balsom, P.D., K. Wood, P. Olsson, and B. Ekblom. 1999. Carbohydrate intake and multiple sprint sports: With special reference to football (soccer). *International Journal of Sports Medicine* 20: 48-52.

5. Below, P.R., R. Mora-Rodriguez, J. Gonzalez-Alonso, and E.F. Coyle. 1995. Fluid and carbohydrate ingestion independently improve performance during 1 h of intense exercise. *Medicine and Science in Sports and Exercise* 27: 200-210.

6. Borghi, L., T. Meschi, F. Amato, A. Briganti, A. Novarini, and A. Giannini. 1996. Urinary volume, water, and recurrences in idiopathic calcium nephrolithiasis: A 5-year randomized prospective study. *Journal of Urology* 155: 839-843.

7. Brown, R.C., and C.M. Cox. 1998. Effects of high fat versus high carbohydrate diets on plasma lipids and lipoproteins in endurance athletes. *Medicine and Science in Sports and Exercise* 30: 1677-1683.

8. Burke, L.M. 2001. Nutritional needs for exercise in the heat. *Comparative Biochemistry and Physiology* 128: 735-748.

9. Burke, L.M., G.R. Collier, S.K. Beasley, P.G. Davis, P.A. Fricker, P. Heeley, K. Walder, and M. Hargreaves. 1995. Effect of coingestion of fat and protein with carbohydrate feedings on muscle glycogen storage. *Journal of Applied Physiology* 78: 2187-2192.

10. Campbell, B., R.B. Kreider, T. Ziegenfuss, P. La Bounty, M. Roberts, D. Burke, J. Landis, H. Lopez, and J. Antonio. 2007. International Society of Sports Nutrition position stand: Protein and exercise. *Journal of the International Society of Sports Nutrition* 4: 8.

11. Costill, D.L., W.M. Sherman, W.J Fink, C. Maresh, M. Witten, and J.M. Miller. 1981. The role of dietary carbohydrates in muscle glycogen resynthesis after strenuous running. *American Journal of Clinical Nutrition* 34: 1831-1836.

12. Davis, B. 1998. Essential fatty acids in vegetarian nutrition. *Vegetarian Diet* 7: 5-7.

13. Ernst, N.D., C.T. Sempos, R.R. Briefel, and M.B. Clark. 1997. Consistency between US dietary fat intake and serum total cholesterol concentrations: The National Health and Nutrition Examination Surveys. *American Journal of Clinical Nutrition* 66 (Suppl): 965S-972S.

14. Food and Agriculture Organization (FAO). 2004. *Human Energy Requirements.* Report of a Joint FAO/WHO/UNU Expert Consultation. Food And Nutrition Technical Report Series 1.Rome: Author.

15. Fogelholm, G.M., R. Koskinen, J. Laakso, T. Rankinen, and I. Ruokonen. 1993. Gradual and rapid weight loss: Effects on nutrition and performance in male athletes. *Medicine and Science in Sports and Exercise* 25: 371-373.

16. Grandjean, A.C., K.J. Reimers, K.E. Bannick, and M.C. Haven. 2000. The effect of caffeinated, non-caffeinated, caloric and non-caloric beverages on hydration. *Journal of the American College of Nutrition* 19: 591-600.

17. Grandjean, A.C., K.J. Reimers, and J.S. Ruud. 1998. Dietary habits of Olympic athletes. In: *Nutrition in Exercise and Sport,* I. Wolinsky, ed. Boca Raton, FL: CRC Press. pp. 421-430.

18. Horswill, C.A. 1998. Effective fluid replacement. *International Journal of Sport Nutrition* 8: 175-195.

19. Jacobs, K.A., and W.M. Sherman. 1999. The efficacy of carbohydrate supplementation and chronic high-carbohydrate diets for improving endurance performance. *International Journal of Sport Nutrition* 9: 92-115.

20. Kochan, R.G., D.R. Lamb, S.A. Lutz, C.V. Perrill, E.M. Reimann, and K.K. Schlende. 1979. Glycogen synthase activation in human skeletal muscle: Effects of diet and exercise. *American Journal of Physiology* 236: E660-E666.

21. Leitzmann, M.F., W.C. Willett, E.B. Rimm, M.J. Stampfer, D. Spiegelman, G.A. Colditz, and E. Giovannucci. 1999. A prospective study of coffee consumption and the risk of symptomatic gallstone disease in men. *Journal of the American Medical Association* 281: 2106-2112.

22. Lemon, P.W.R. 1998. Effects of exercise on dietary protein requirements. *International Journal of Sport Nutrition* 8: 426-447.

23. Licensure for Arizona RDs. Arizona Dietetic Association. www.eatrightarizona.org/Licensurehandout.pdf. Accessed January 1, 2010.

24. Linseisen, J., A.A. Welch, M. Ock, P. Amiano, C. Agnoli, P. Ferrari, E. Sonestedt, V. Chaj, H.B. Bueno-de-Mesquita, R. Kaaks, C. Weikert, M. Dorronsoro, L. Rodr, I. Ermini, A. Mattieloo, Y.T. van der Schouw, J. Manjer, S. Nilsson, M. Jenab, E. Lund, M. Brustad, J. Halkj, M.U. Jakobsen, K.T. Khaw, F. Crowe, C. Georgila, G. Misirli, M. Niravong, M. Touvier, S. Bingham, E. Riboli, and N. Slimani. Dietary fat intake in the European Prospective Investigation into Cancer and Nutrition: Results from the 24-h dietary recalls. *European Journal of Clinical Nutrition* 63: S61-S80.

25. Louisiana Board of Examiners in Dietetics and Nutrition. Rules and Regulations Title 46: Professional and Occupational Standards Part LXX: Registered Dieticians. www.lbedn.org/rules.pdf. Accessed May 31, 2009.

26. MacDougall, G.R., D.G. Ward, D.G. Sale, and J.R. Sutton. 1977. Muscle glycogen repletion after high intensity intermittent exercise. *Journal of Applied Physiology* 42: 129-132.

27. Maughan, R.J., J.B. Leiper, and S.M. Shirreffs. 1996. Restoration of fluid balance after exercise-induced dehydration: Effects of food and fluid intake. *European Journal of Applied Physiology* 73: 317-325.

28. Maughan, R.J., J.H. Owen, S.M. Shirreffs, and J.B. Leiper. 1994. Post-exercise rehydration in man: Effects of electrolyte addition to ingested fluids. *European Journal of Applied Physiology* 69: 209-215.

29. Michaud, D.S., D. Spiegelman, S.K. Clinton, E.B. Rimm, G.C. Curhan, W.C. Willett, and E.L. Giovannucci. 1999. Fluid intake and the risk of bladder cancer in men. *New England Journal of Medicine* 340: 1390-1397.

30. Mitchell, J.B., P.C. DiLauro, F.X. Pizza, and D.L. Cavender. 1997. The effect of pre-exercise carbohydrate status on resistance exercise performance. *International Journal of Sport Nutrition* 7: 185-196.

31. Muoio, D.M., J.J. Leddy, P.J. Horvath, A.B. Awad, and D.R. Pendergast. 1994. Effect of dietary fat on metabolic adjustments to maximal VO2 and endurance in runners. *Medicine and Science in Sports and Exercise* 26: 81-88.

32. National Academy of Sciences Institute of Medicine, Food and Nutrition Board. 2005. *Dietary Reference Intakes for Energy, Carbohydrate, Fiber, Fat, Fatty Acids, Cholesterol, Protein, and Amino Acids (Macronutrients).* Washington, DC: National Academies Press.

33. Pendergast, D.R., P.J. Horvath, J.J. Leddy, and J.T. Venkatraman. 1996. The role of dietary fat on performance, metabo-

lism, and health. *American Journal of Sports Medicine* 24: S53-S58.

34. Phinney, S.D., B.R. Bistrian, W.J. Evans, E. Gervino, and G.L. Blackburn. 1983. The human metabolic response to chronic ketosis without caloric restriction: Preservation of submaximal exercise capability with reduced carbohydrate oxidation. *Metabolism* 32: 769-776.

35. Piehl, K.S., S. Adolfsson, and K. Nazar. 1974. Glycogen storage and glycogen synthase activity in trained and untrained muscle of man. *Acta Physiologica Scandinavica* 90: 779-788.

36. Reimers, K.J. 1994. Evaluating a healthy, high performance diet. *Strength and Conditioning* 16: 28-30.

37. Rolls, B.J., V.H. Castellanos, J.C. Halford, A. Kilara, D. Panyam, C.L. Pelkman, G.P. Smith, and M.L. Thorwart. 1998. Volume of food consumed affects satiety in men. *American Journal of Clinical Nutrition* 67: 1170-1177.

38. Santana, J.C., J. Dawes, J. Antonio, and D.S. Kalman. 2007. The role of the fitness professional in providing sports/ exercise nutrition advice. *Strength and Conditioning Journal* 29 (30): 69-71.

39. Sawka, M.N., L.M. Burke, E.R. Eichner, R.J. Maughan, S.J. Montain, and N.S. Stachenfeld. 2007. Exercise and fluid replacement position stand. *Medicine and Science in Sports and Exercise* 39 (2): 377-389.

40. Sherman, W.M. 1995. Metabolism of sugars and physical performance. *American Journal of Clinical Nutrition* 62 (Suppl): 228S-241S.

41. Sherman, W.M., J.A. Doyle, D.R. Lamb, and R.H. Strauss. 1993. Dietary carbohydrate, muscle glycogen, and exercise performance during 7 d of training. *American Journal of Clinical Nutrition* 57: 27-31.

42. Sherman, W.M., and G.S. Wimer. 1991. Insufficient carbohydrate during training: Does it impair performance? *Sports Nutrition* 1 (1): 28-44.

43. Shirreffs, S.M., A.J. Taylor, J.B. Leiper, and R.J. Maughan. 1996. Post-exercise rehydration in man: Effects of volume consumed and drink sodium content. *Medicine and Science in Sports and Exercise* 28: 1260-1271.

44. Sugiura, K., and K. Kobayashi. 1998. Effect of carbohydrate ingestion on sprint performance following continuous and intermittent exercise. *Medicine and Science in Sports and Exercise* 30: 1624-1630.

45. Symons, J.D., and I. Jacobs. 1989. High-intensity exercise performance is not impaired by low intramuscular glycogen. *Medicine and Science in Sports and Exercise* 21: 550-557.

46. USDA MyPlate. www.ChooseMyPlate.gov. Accessed 26 June 2011.

47. Vandenberghe, K., P. Hespel, B.V. Eynde, R. Lysens, and E.A. Richter. 1995. No effect of glycogen level on glycogen metabolism during high intensity exercise. *Medicine and Science in Sports and Exercise* 27: 1278-1283.

48. Volek, J.S., W.J. Kraemer, J.A. Bush, T. Incledon, and M. Boetes. 1997. Testosterone and cortisol in relationship to dietary nutrients and resistance exercise. *Journal of Applied Physiology* 82: 49-54.

49. Walberg, J.L., M.K. Leidy, D.J. Sturgill, D.E. Hinkle, S.J. Ritchey, and D.R. Sebolt. 1987. Macronutrient needs in weight lifters during caloric restriction. *Medicine and Science in Sports and Exercise* 19: S70.

50. Wardlaw, G.M., and P.M. Insel. 1996. *Perspectives in Nutrition*. St. Louis: Mosby Year Book. p. 76.

51. Wilmore, J.H., A.R. Morton, H.J. Gilbey, and R.J. Wood. 1998. Role of taste preference on fluid intake during and after 90 min of running at 60% of VO₂max in the heat. *Medicine and Science in Sports and Exercise* 30: 587-595.

52. World Health Organization. 2007. *Protein and Amino Acid Requirements in Human Nutrition*. WHO Technical Report Series. Geneva: WHO Press. http://whqlibdoc.who.int/trs/ WHO_TRS_935_eng.pdf. Accessed 20 April 2010.

Exercise Psychology for the Personal Trainer

Bradley D. Hatfield, PhD, and Phil Kaplan, MS

After completing this chapter, you will be able to

- understand the psychological benefits of exercise,
- work with a client to set effective exercise goals,
- recognize the value of motivation, and
- implement methods to motivate a client.

Participation in physical activity results in desirable health consequences in terms of both acute responses and chronic adaptations in the physiological and psychological domains (75). Despite the well-known benefits of exercise, current estimates from the National Center for Health Statistics indicate that approximately 40% of American men and women are sedentary during their leisure time (10). According to one study, fewer than 50% of those who begin a program of regular physical activity will continue their involvement after six months (11). In addition, for those who do adhere, the level of improvement in muscular strength, cardiovascular fitness, and other fitness-related goals may be compromised by a lack of intensity and effort.

Thus for many people, the benefits of exercise remain elusive, and lack of compliance with programs offered by personal trainers results in a less than satisfactory experience for both the client and the personal trainer. Although the promotion of exercise behavior presents a significant challenge, understanding and implementing fundamental motivational principles can improve participation and program adherence as well as the intensity of effort during training sessions. Although it might appear that some individuals are naturally more motivated toward achievement than others, in actuality those motivated individuals are likely employing their own motivational strategies. If personal trainers can elicit a client's specific mental strategy for summoning motivation and can learn to stimulate a client to employ that strategy, it is possible to turn on motivation in much the same way one flips a switch on the wall to illuminate a room. This approach may hold the key to the realization of exercise and nutrition goals.

The first section of this chapter considers the psychological benefits of physical activity, including the anxiolytic (i.e., anxiety reducing) and antidepressive effects of exercise as well as the cognitive benefits, especially for persons who are older. It also outlines some of the scientific evidence for the role of genetic factors, which contribute to individual differences in the relationship between exercise participation and mental health. That is, some men and women may derive greater psychological and physiological benefit from exercise than others, supporting the notion that exercise is essential "medicine" for some. Educating clients about these benefits could provide additional motivation or energy for exercise. The second section deals with goals, goal orientations, and effective goal setting. The final sections cover motivation, reinforcement, the development of self-efficacy or confidence, and practical instructions for motivational techniques. Here the personal trainer will find specific steps to use to help clients minimize procrastination, overcome false beliefs, identify and modify self-talk, and employ mental imagery.

Mental Health Aspects of Exercise

In addition to the desirable physiological consequences of physical activity, there is ample scientific evidence that participation in physical activity has significant mental health benefits. Further, people who are aware of such benefits may be encouraged to increase commitment to regular exercise. Notable among the mental health benefits are a reduction of anxiety and depression, decreased reactivity to psychological stress, and enhanced cognition. In this section we discuss the psychological impact of exercise in order to help the personal trainer communicate such benefits to the client for educational and motivational purposes.

Stress Reduction Effects of Exercise: Evidence and Mechanisms

It is estimated that approximately 7.3% of the American population have anxiety-related disorders to the extent that treatment is warranted (44, 45). In addition, most people experience episodic, and sometimes extended, stress-related symptoms during the course of their lives. Regular physical exercise relieves both state and trait anxiety–related symptoms (59); *state anxiety* refers to short-term stress-related processes while *trait anxiety* refers to long-term processes. For many people, the alleviation of anxiety through physical activity likely provides a strong rationale for maintaining participation.

State anxiety can be defined as the actual experience of anxiety that is characterized by feelings of apprehension or threat and accompanied by increased physiological arousal, particularly as mediated by the autonomic nervous system (37, 72). State anxiety can largely be characterized by the flight-or-fight response first described by Cannon in 1929 (13)—relatively uncontrolled elevations in heart rate, blood pressure, and activity in the hypothalamic-pituitary-adrenal cortical (HPA) axis with heightened stress hormones such as cortisol. On the other hand, **trait anxiety** is a dispositional factor relating to the probability that a given person is likely to perceive situations as threatening (37, 72). Typically both forms of anxiety are measured by self-report scales such as the State-Trait Anxiety Inventory (72) or in terms of physiological variables such as muscle tension, blood pressure, or brain electrical activity. Clearly, both acute (i.e., state) and chronic (i.e., trait) anxiety represent negative psychological variables that one would want to avoid, and participation in physical activity effectively alleviates the symptoms associated with anxiety (59).

According to a recent review of the literature (45), there have been well over 100 scientific studies on the anxiety-reducing effects of exercise. Such a volume of research can be overwhelming, especially when some of the client investigations provide contradictory conclusions. Consequently, personal trainers may feel uncertain about their knowledge of the anxiety reduction effects of exercise, but clarification has been provided by meta-analytic (i.e., broad and integrative) reviews of the literature based on quantitative summaries of the relevant literature. Meta-analytic reviews suggest general patterns of the collective findings in the research literature, as opposed to highlighting individual studies, such that the personal trainer can see the "forest" instead of the "trees."

Small to moderate reductions in anxiety with physical activity have been consistently reported in the exercise psychology literature over the last 30 years (12, 41, 46, 48, 51, 59, 79, 80). These effects are typically observed for aerobic forms of exercise across a wide range of intensities, although low-intensity and higher-volume resistance training appears to be efficacious as well (4). (As one would expect, higher-intensity exercise [i.e., above ventilatory threshold] does not seem to provide immediate stress reduction benefits, although some people who are extremely well conditioned may derive a cathartic release from this type of activity.) Such an effect may be explained by the opponent-process theory of emotion advanced by Solomon and Corbit (71), which posits a rebound expression of positive affect on termination of a high-intensity exercise bout following the uncomfortable feelings and strain during exertion. The rebound "feel-better" effect following intense exercise may be due to the unmasking of physiological coping responses such as the release of beta endorphin and mood-altering central neurotransmitters (e.g., serotonin), which attenuate the stress of exercise during exertion but are no longer opposed by the stress processes once the work and effort stop (5). In this regard, the release of beta endorphin serves to manage or economize the hormonal response to work, as well as the ventilatory or breathing activity involved during exercise, which is a primary input to perceived exertion or the effort sense (36). The maintenance of these counteractive physiological responses—which manage exercise-induced strain—beyond the period of exertion may explain why the trained exercise participant derives a sense of satisfaction and substantial positive affect once a challenging and demanding workout is completed.

There are a number of possible explanations for the anxiety-reducing effects of exercise (36). One possibility is the rhythmic nature of many forms of physical activity and many exercise routines. People find that walking, running, or cycling at a steady pace for some period of time helps to promote mental and physical relaxation. Stair stepping and aerobic dance routines are often performed to a cadence or in time to music. The calming psychological effects of rhythmic exercise may be due to biological processes. It is possible that cerebral cortical arousal is inhibited due to a volley of afferent rhythmic impulses from the skeletal muscles during the exercise that provide afferent impulses or feedback to an inhibitory or "relaxation" site in the brain stem—and that this causes a "quieting" of the cognitive activity associated with anxiety or stress states (9, 36, 53). Interestingly, many workout routines are rhythmic in nature.

In addition, a number of studies have revealed that exercise alters the activity of the frontal region of the brain such that left frontal activation of the cerebral cortex is elevated relative to right-sided activation after exertion (58). On the basis of a number of investigations, Davidson (24) has clearly described the phenomenon of frontal asymmetry and provided evidence that relative left frontal activation (i.e., greater than right-sided activation), which can be measured with such technologies as brain electrical activity or electroencephalography (EEG), underlies positive affect and approach motivation to engage one's environment while right frontal activation underlies negative affect and withdrawal-oriented motivation. Some investigators have argued that the physiological changes experienced systemically during exercise reflexively influence the central nervous system and the brain, resulting in desirable changes in frontal asymmetry and mood (79, 80).

> **One reason for the anxiety-reducing effects of exercise is the rhythmic nature of the exercise stimulus.**

Another possible reason for the stress reduction effect of exercise has been termed the *thermogenic effect* (36, 59). According to this model, based on work with animals (77), the metabolic inefficiency of the human body that results in heat production during exercise causes a cascade of events leading to relaxation. The part of the brain known as the hypothalamus detects the elevation in the body's temperature and consequently promotes a cortical relaxation effect in an attempt to maintain homeostasis. This results in decreased activation of alpha and gamma motor neurons to the skeletal muscle extrafusal and intrafusal fibers, respectively. In turn, the reduction in muscle efference results in reduced muscle tension and less sensitivity of the muscle spindles to stretch. This "calming down" effect results, in turn, in less afferent stimulation or feedback to the brain stem arousal center (i.e., the reticular activating formation, RAF) and subsequently promotes a relaxation state.

As described earlier in relation to the opponent-process theory, the effects from the natural release of beta endorphin during exercise stress are maintained for some time after the cessation of exercise because of the half-life of hormonal action. Collectively such an effect, in concert with the rhythmic muscle afference and thermic effects of exercise, may underlie the altered state of mental and physical tension people typically experience immediately after working out.

It is also important to remember that exercise may take place either in a social context or in relative independence from others. In both cases, the exercise session may provide a diversion or time-out from daily concerns that occupy the participant's mind and cause stress (2). Additionally, a social setting may involve meaningful social interaction that could alleviate stress.

Finally, accomplishing the exercise goal may promote a significant sense of mastery or self-efficacy that can also serve to alter how a person feels after exercise. Overall, the change in psychological state from exercise is referred to as the "feel-better" phenomenon (54) and may result from a complex interaction of social and psychobiological factors that come together to change the overall psychological state of the exercise participant.

Antidepressive Effects of Exercise

As with anxiety, research evidence clearly and consistently reveals that physical exercise yields statistically significant and moderate effect sizes (i.e., reductions) both for men and women who are clinically depressed and for those experiencing less severe forms of depression, with the effects being somewhat larger for people with clinical depression (23, 56). Although depression is commonly treated by physicians with psychiatric intervention, psychotherapy, or electroconvulsive shock, exercise would seem to be a desirable alternative given its relative cost-effectiveness and lack of unwanted side effects. In addition, physical exercise appears to be as effective as medication in men and women experiencing clinical depression (8). Such efficacy of exercise to alleviate depression relative to pharmacological treatment is highly desirable in light of the negative side effects of drug treatment including cost, potential weight gain, and suicidal thoughts, as well as several other physiological effects such as muscle spasm and heart arrhythmias. In contrast, the side effects of exercise are generally if not universally desirable; these include reductions in body fat, cardiovascular disease, high blood pressure, certain cancers, and arthritis, as well as reductions in dementia and Alzheimer's disease. Because many people have episodic bouts of depression over stressful events in their lives, exercise appears to offer an appropriate and effective means of coping and feeling better.

As in the case of anxiety, exercise alleviates depression through several mechanisms. Two related possibilities center on the release of biogenic amines in the brain. Central levels of serotonin, an important neurotransmitter with antidepressant effects, are elevated during and following physical activity (16) as also are dopamine and its receptor binding sensitivity, thus reducing the likelihood of both depression and Parkinson's disease (73). There is strong evidence that physical activity maintains dopamine (an essential neurotransmitter involved in motor control processes) in the central nervous system (73). In addition, research reveals that this neurotransmitter is essential to the learning of motor skills as well as mental health (i.e., protection against depression) (73). Levels of norepinephrine, another neurotransmitter that is lowered during bouts of depression, are also increased with exercise (28).

Beyond the biogenic amine hypothesis, it is also likely that some people benefit from the social interaction that occurs in many exercise settings or from the sense of accomplishment or enhanced self-efficacy that stems from greater strength and flexibility in performing daily activities. This effect may be particularly important for people in older age groups, who may gain a sense of independence and experience decreased feelings of helplessness as a result of being physically fit. Such a perception, along with attendant elevations in muscular strength and endurance, may contribute to increased life satisfaction and opportunity to sustain independent living in the elderly.

> Serotonin and norepinephrine levels are lowered during bouts of depression, but exercise has an antidepressive effect because it naturally elevates these biogenic amines.

Cognitive Benefits

In addition to the emotional or affective benefits, exercise confers cognitive benefits. Cognition consists of memory, analytical thinking, planning, focus, concentration, and decision making. People who are physically fit seem to function more effectively than less physically active people on tasks involving such intellectual demands. The outcomes are particularly impressive in men and women in older age groups (i.e., 55 and older), who typically show some degree of cognitive decline in specific functions due to the aging process. In an early study demonstrating the advantageous effects of physical activity on the aging brain, the typical age-related increase in reaction time (RT) was moderated in physically active men compared to those who were less physically active (67). This effect was even more pronounced for complex or choice RT. Sedentary men showed large age-related increases in these RTs whereas physically active men showed little change (figure 8.1). Importantly, RT has been described as a fundamental index of the overall integrity of the central nervous system (CNS) (73).

Beyond the basic index of reaction time, mental performance more generally has been shown to be superior in physically fit versus sedentary people. In one study, men in their 60s who were physically fit achieved better mental performance on a complex battery of cognitive challenges than did sedentary men (31). In fact, the older men who were physically fit performed similarly to a group of younger college-aged men while also outperforming the sedentary men (figure 8.2).

Biological Mechanisms Underlying Cognitive Benefits: Vascular Changes

There are a number of possible explanations for the observed cognitive benefits of exercise in elderly persons. One postulate is that physical fitness decreases the decline in cerebral blood flow that normally occurs with aging (31) or exerts an angiogenic effect (i.e., formation of new blood vessels). Direct evidence for this possibility came from a study of brain blood flow in older retirees who

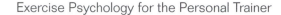

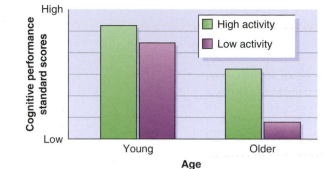

FIGURE 8.1 Choice reaction time: differences in reaction time at various ages, showing faster times with age in those who are physically active.

Adapted by permission from Sherwood and Selder 1979.

FIGURE 8.2 Cognitive performance of young and older men with low and high aerobic fitness levels.

Reprinted by permission from Dustman et al. 1990.

differed in their levels of physical activity (64). The retirees who were more active showed both superior cognitive functioning and increased perfusion of the cerebral cortex. Such an exercise-induced change would help to deliver oxygen and nutrients to the neural tissue and thereby support the neural processes underlying behavior.

Biological Mechanisms: Neurotrophic Factors

In addition to causing such vascular changes, exercise may lead to increases in the expression of genes that code for neurotrophic factors (agents that preserve and nourish brain tissue) (20). An animal study demonstrated that brain-derived neurotrophic factor (BDNF) increased in rats that engaged in voluntary wheel-running relative to those that were sedentary (74). Brain-derived neurotrophic factor effectively promotes the health of neurons or brain cells and the creation of new synapses or connections between neurons, thus increasing the thickness and integrity of brain tissue. More specifically, Tong and colleagues (74) reported an increase in BDNF expression in the rat hippocampus, a structure in the brain that is integrally involved in long-term or episodic memory–related processes. In light of such powerful neurobiological influences in animals, it seems likely that similar changes could occur in humans and contribute to the higher cognitive functioning seen in older physically fit participants. In support of this possibility, Colcombe and colleagues (18) reported a positive relationship between aerobic capacity, as measured by $\dot{V}O_2$max, and brain tissue density in several regions of the cerebral cortex (i.e., gray matter) as well as the white matter tracts, which allow for communication between various brain regions, in middle-aged men and women. That is, those who were characterized by higher

cardiovascular fitness exhibited denser tissue and reduced age-related decline in critical brain regions such as the prefrontal cortex that underlies executive functioning and reasoning. Importantly, the frontal brain region shows the greatest rate of decline in normal or nondemented aging, and fitness appears to be an effective antidote or prescription for this typical age-related decline. Thus there is tangible biological evidence that exercise and fitness slow the aging of the brain!

More specifically, the neurobiological benefits of exercise in the human brain may well contribute to the phenomenon of cognitive reserve, which is the resistance to age-related decline and pathology associated with forms of dementia like Alzheimer's disease (i.e., formation of plaques and tangles), particularly in the hippocampal region. This resilience to decline or ability to tolerate neurodegenerative processes is based on passive reserve or the biological integrity of the brain (i.e., thickness of brain tissue and preservation of vasculature), as well as active reserve or the strategic activation of neural processes to compensate for networks suffering from age-related decline and pathology. Importantly, it appears that exercise may maintain the youthfulness of the brain and the mind by contributing to passive reserve due to the neurotrophic and angiogenic effects. Figure 8.3 illustrates the relationship of cognitive reserve to cognitive function as it bestows relative resistance to cognitive decline (see top line in the figure relative to lower line), thus allowing for high-level functioning for a longer period of time. A high level of cognitive reserve also helps cope with the presence of preclinical pathology.

Neural Efficiency

One of the hallmarks of physically fit men and women is efficiency of musculoskeletal and cardiovascular

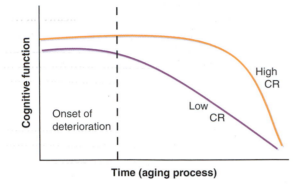

FIGURE 8.3 Cognitive performance of those characterized by high and low levels of cognitive reserve (CR) after the onset of cognitive decline.

function. For example, enhanced strength results in recruitment of fewer motor units to accomplish the lifting of a given (i.e., absolute) weight or resistance (27). Also, lowered heart rate is commonly observed in response to absolute work after exercise training. Such economy of physiological processes also seems to characterize the adaptations in the brain of those who are physically fit. For example, Dustman and colleagues (31) observed less activation in sensory regions of the brain in response to light stimulation in older fit men relative to their sedentary counterparts, while McDowell and colleagues (52) also observed a more adaptive cortical response during a basic decision-making challenge. Such a benefit to the CNS may enable resistance to fatigue over the course of sustained mental effort during daily activities. The efficiency of the brain may be due to the maintenance of neurotransmitter function as well as the neurotrophic effect; these likely work in concert with better oxygenation due to angiogenesis (38) to collectively preserve mental functioning.

Specificity and Cognitive Functioning

Just as with peripheral physiological adaptations to exercise training, the psychological benefits seem to be marked by the principle of specificity. The effects have been primarily observed for effortful cognitive tasks that involve fluid intelligence, while tasks characterized by crystallized intelligence appear to be relatively unaffected (17). *Fluid intelligence* refers to abstract reasoning and problem solving, whereas *crystallized intelligence* refers to accumulated factual knowledge and the ability to recognize words and recall facts (78). A classic study revealed that mental tasks involving the frontal lobe executive processes are most affected by physical activity involvement (40). Kramer and colleagues (40) postulated that this

exercise-induced benefit is most apparent for frontally mediated executive tasks because the frontal lobe is the fastest-aging area of the brain and therefore benefits most from the positive neurobiological effects we have described.

Interestingly, the frontal lobe in humans is the last region of the brain to mature and the first to show the effects of advanced age. The executive processes housed there are involved in working memory and in the coordination of complex attentional functions, as well as in the inhibition and control of behavior. Because this important area of the brain—serving some of the highest-order cognitive functions—is most susceptible to the deleterious effects of aging, it is reasonable to deduce that it would be most affected by the positive neurobiological changes we have discussed. In fact, older adults clearly manifest such specific effects of exercise; one study showed little difference in nonexecutive processes but significant improvement in executive processes in older men and women who engaged in aerobic training versus controls (40). Because nonexecutive processes, such as speed of word recognition, are less dependent on frontal lobe function and more dependent on other areas of the brain that age less rapidly, it is also reasonable to deduce that the biological benefits of exercise on the brain would be less apparent during the performance of such mental tasks. More recently, Bixby and colleagues (6) observed a significant and positive relationship between self-reported level of physical activity participation and executive performance as measured by the Stroop color-word test (i.e., the ability to quickly identify and name the ink color of words printed in conflicting text, such as naming "red" for the word "green" printed in red ink) but no such relationship for the nonexecutive elements of the test (i.e., speed of word and color naming). Importantly, this prominent effect of fitness on executive function was observed after controlling for differential levels of education and cognitive stimulation in the study participants. However, it is noteworthy that there are exercise-induced benefits across a variety of cognitive domains (i.e., speed, visual–spatial processing, and reasoning), but that the greatest magnitude of benefit seems to occur for executive tasks in older men and women (19).

Genetic Basis of Individual Differences in Response to Exercise and Physical Activity

Finally, a major recent development in exercise science has been work on the genetic basis of physiological adaptations to training. It seems that client differences in the response to exercise are highly dependent on genetic variation. An awareness of genetic factors has much to do with motivational concerns, as some clients respond favorably to aerobic endurance or resistance training while others may experience frustration in their attempts to improve their level of functioning or change their body composition. Such client variation also relates to the psychological benefits of exercise.

As an example of research on interactions between genes and exercise, one study revealed that cognitive decline in the elderly was particularly related to the presence of the apolipoprotein e4 allele (APOE e4) (66). That is, this particular gene is known to increase the risk for cognitive impairment and the likelihood of Alzheimer's disease in the elderly. Rovio et al. (2005) reported a reduction in the likelihood of dementia and Alzheimer's disease in older individuals who were physically active in midlife relative to those who were sedentary at midlife with the observed magnitude of effect (i.e., reduction) greater in APOE e4 carriers versus non-carriers (see figure 8.4). This kind of information suggests that the cost of inactivity is particularly high for some individuals and that scientific assessment and understanding of gene–exercise interactions may yield a major motivational impetus for those who are particularly at risk for dementia. Such individuals are ideally suited to achieving benefits from exercise in the form of protection from cognitive decline.

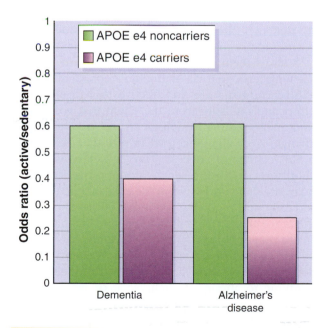

FIGURE 8.4 Risk of dementia and Alzheimer's disease as a function of physical activity level (i.e., high vs. low) in APOE e4 carriers and noncarriers showing the relative reduction in decline in active carriers.

Data from Rovio et al 2005. Leisure-time physical activity at midlife and the risk of dementia and Alzheimer's disease. *Lancet Neurol.* 4:705-711.

Insights into gene–exercise interactions may help people see the importance of a physically active lifestyle. These insights, along with the psychobiological changes discussed previously, substantiate the philosophical belief originating with the ancient Greeks, *mens sana in corpore sano* ("a healthy mind in a healthy body").

Importantly, the impact of exercise and physical fitness on the brain may be particularly important in those who are genetically at risk for dementia. Thus the promotion of a physically active lifestyle may move the threshold of symptoms to a later time or delay the onset of cognitive impairment.

Goal Setting

As described in the previous sections, physical activity and physical fitness confer substantial psychological and physiological benefits. However, the motivation and energy to engage in activity and exercise are critical elements in the achievement of such benefits. **Goal setting** is a powerful strategy for increasing the level of participation in exercise programs. This technique can be defined as a strategic approach to behavioral change by which progressive standards of success (i.e., goals) are set in an attempt to increasingly approximate a desired standard of achievement (i.e., the long-term goal). Importantly, systematic goal setting fosters a sense of mastery and success as people pursue the desired standard or target of achievement. Feelings of success and competency promote commitment and help maintain exercise behavior. Personal trainers can be instrumental in helping clients set goals that prove to be compelling and achievable.

Goal setting is not a one-size-fits-all endeavor. Rather than simply extracting information from an assessment and imposing goals on the client, it is important for the personal trainer to identify the client's true wants and needs and to act as a facilitator in uncovering the goals that the client is most compelled to achieve (34). Then, together, through directed conversation, the personal trainer and the client should identify goals that are measurable, achievable, and consistent with one another. In this manner, the goals or standards of successive achievement represent a series of attainable steps framed within a long-term goal that provides personal meaning to the participant (see figure 8.5).

Setting Goals for Feedback and Reinforcement

Feedback and reinforcement are critical to the success of a goal-setting program as each progressive

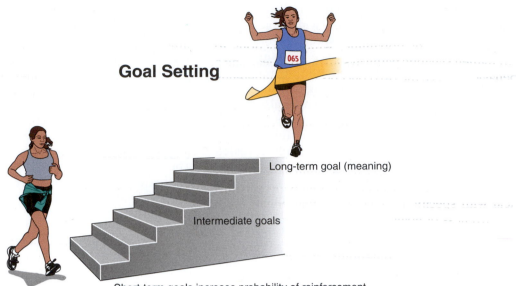

Goal Setting

Long-term goal (meaning)

Intermediate goals

Short-term goals increase probability of reinforcement

FIGURE 8.5   The progression of short-term and intermediate-term goals leads to a personally meaningful long-term goal.

goal is sought. For example, a client may want to change body composition by reducing the percentage of fat. The long-term goal could be to shed 60 pounds (27 kg) or achieve a target percentage of body fat. This could be accomplished by a series of short-term weight reduction goals to be achieved in specified time frames (22). **Feedback,** or knowledge of results, is inherent in the completion of or progress toward the short-term goal and leads to the cognitive evaluation of success or failure. Importantly, the realization of success or failure also invokes a corresponding emotional or affective state. Although the client may be far from the ultimate goal of losing 60 pounds, the positive mood or affective state that results from reaching the short-term goal will enhance commitment. Challenging goals that are difficult but within the present ability level of the client are superior to too-easy or very difficult goals in effecting behavior change (42).

> Goal setting is not a one-size-fits-all endeavor. Rather than simply extracting information from an assessment and imposing goals on the client, it is important to identify the client's true wants and needs.

The purpose of a **long-term goal** is to provide a meaningful pursuit for the client. Additionally, a personal trainer can assume that a goal selected by the client has a high level of meaning and purpose because it sets the direction of the short-term goals and provides a destination that the client values.

Thus it would seem prudent to conduct initial interviews with clients to assess not just their short-term needs but their core values. Clients are much more likely to pursue and maintain purposeful and meaningful physical activity over a lifetime than they are to maintain activity without purpose or meaning (55). For example, some people perceive themselves as runners and are so deeply committed to the activity that they are likely to maintain it indefinitely barring injury or chronic health problems.

A **short-term goal** provides a strategy to achieve the long-term goal via attainable steps. Challenging short-term goals are an effective tool to elicit the effort and intensity from the client that will result in a meaningful physiological and psychological change. A challenging goal is one that has about a 50% chance of success. Thus a well-constructed short-term goal represents a compromise between guaranteeing success, as in the case of a goal that is too easy, and requiring too much effort. Short-term goals are meaningless if they are not reasonably difficult; they will lead to going through the motions as opposed to investing real effort. If clients do not achieve a short-term goal initially, they will likely continue to attempt to achieve it or maintain the behavior (e.g., caloric restriction and walking activity in the case of weight reduction) in order to obtain the desired reinforcement. If a short-term goal is not attained in the specified time period, then it needs to be adjusted or replaced with another.

The power of behavioral reinforcement can be explained on both a psychological and a neurobiological level. Psychologically, the client may experience an increase in self-esteem or **self-efficacy** (3). Reinforcement on a neurobiological level consists of the release of dopamine, which functions to strengthen synaptic pathways involved in learning a behavior. In fact, the two concepts may be inherently linked. Accordingly, feedback and the associated reinforcement are critical to effective goal setting, but feedback cannot reliably occur when short-term goals are vague. Thus it is best to identify objective or highly quantifiable goals so that clients can target effort toward a clear standard resulting in unambiguous knowledge of results. The following sections deal with specific characteristics that enhance the effectiveness of goals.

> An effective yet challenging goal is one that has about a 50% chance of success.

Types of Goals

The specifics of the long-term and short-term goals vary according to the client. For example, a client's initial fitness level largely determines the number of short-term goals needed to achieve the desired long-term goal. Another general characteristic of goals concerns the amount of control that a client can exert over their attainment. Goals can be categorized as process, performance, and outcome goals depending on the level of personal control that the client has over them. **Process goals** are goals that clients have a high degree of personal control over, whereas **outcome goals** are goals that the client has little control over. **Performance goals** fall in between in relation to personal control.

Process Goals

The amount of effort applied during a workout is an example of a process goal. Other examples are exercise form and technique and positive attitude during an exercise routine. Regardless of the difficulty of the short-term goal, clients can experience success with a high degree of effort if they set a process goal. Such goals may be very important for maintenance of exercise behavior as success or goal accomplishment defined in other ways (i.e., outcome goals) becomes increasingly difficult, a situation that could result in the client's dropping out.

Outcome Goals

For some clients, process goals may not be fulfilling. Some need to see progress or accomplishments as gauged by social comparison. For example, they may want to be the fastest walker in the neighborhood walking group or the strongest lifter at the gym. Outcome goals are exemplified by social comparison

as in winning or in beating an opponent in a race. Such goals can be highly arousing and can induce great intensity of effort for individuals who like to compare themselves to others. However, outcome goals present less probability of success compared to process goals: Clients can guarantee the effort to achieve an advantage over the "opponent," but they cannot guarantee the outcome itself.

Performance Goals

Performance goals are more difficult to achieve than process goals and are typically stated in terms of a self-referenced personal performance standard for the client rather than in comparison to another client or an opponent. Performance goals are intermediate on the continuum of personal control ranging from low (outcome) to high (process). An example of personalized performance goals that challenge the client to focus on self-improvement in a personally meaningful way is based on the notion of a range or interval goal (57). For example, during a periodized resistance training program, a client may want to improve maximal strength in the squat or bench press exercise. Interval goals are calculated from the client's recent performance history in which a range of success is identified. The limits of the goal are established in the form of a lower (most attainable) and an upper (most challenging) boundary of success. The lower boundary is defined as the client's previous best 1-repetition maximum (1RM) performance. To determine the upper boundary, the client "computes" the average of recent performances (three to five) and determines the difference between the average and previous best performance. This difference yields an estimate of the client's performance variability. The difference is then added to the previous best to generate a highly challenging self-referenced level of success.

Overall, it seems appropriate to set a variety of goals or diversify one's goal-setting strategy so as to balance the client's underlying reasons for exercise while maintaining a reasonable probability of success and reinforcement.

Diversified Goal Setting

A successful goal-setting program should involve a diversity of goals, just as financial success entails a diversified financial portfolio (22). In addition, such diverse goals need to be formed within the context of a sound scientific strategy for long-term goal attainment. Thus the personal trainer needs to incorporate and integrate knowledge from the psychological, biomechanical, physiological, nutritional, and other relevant scientific domains.

As an example of a diversified goal-setting approach, think of a middle-aged client who wishes to run a 10K (6.2-mile) race in a time he or she can feel proud of. The long-term goal may be clearly stated in the form of a desired outcome that will be personally meaningful. Assume that this client has the talent and the ability to achieve the performance goal if he or she optimizes his effort and trains in a sound strategic manner. However, a number of motivational problems are bound to occur during the training of any client who is striving for a challenging standard of behavior. To overcome the disappointments that can occur if the client focuses on a single performance goal such as "finishing the race in less than an hour," the client should also set short-term goals using a goal diversification strategy in the context of a well-designed training program. On some training days, the client may set the goal of proper form during foot strike and mechanically sound arm swing and stride length. On other days, the client may stress resistance training goals to facilitate the efficiency of the lower extremities in an attempt to develop stamina. On still other days, he or she may concentrate on psychological goals such as positive focus and self-talk during a training run. Positive feedback from the attainment of such process goals can perpetuate the sense of desire and commitment to the long-term goal. Again, the basic principle is that a variety of goals associated with varying levels of personal control may well sustain commitment and adherence to the physical training program.

> A successful goal-setting program should include a diverse combination of short-term and long-term goals.

Goal Orientations

A concept that relates to goal diversification is individual differences—the differing personalities of clients. Consideration of individual differences in clients' perceptions of achievement situations helps to increase the effectiveness of goal setting (30, 61, 63). For example, clients who gauge their performance improvement on the basis of previous ability level are said to be *task involved*. On the other hand, ego-involved or other-referenced clients base their sense of improvement on comparison to the performance of one or more others (62). Such clients are highly aroused by social comparison and put forth greater effort in a situation that permits social comparison, especially if they perceive their own ability or fitness level to be high. A task involvement orientation, on the other hand, may relate to a higher need for personal control; task-involved clients may become

discouraged if inappropriate emphasis is placed on comparisons of their achievements to those of others. To be effective in goal setting, the personal trainer must consider these types of individual differences in goal orientation and perceived ability.

> The personal trainer should maintain focus on the client's desired goals and expected outcomes and should develop a sound plan of action with the client.

Tips for Effective Goal Setting

The following suggestions may help the personal trainer develop an effective goal-setting strategy. "Practical Principles of Effective Goal Setting" on page 135 summarizes the primary research-based elements of goal setting.

- Determine the client's perceived needs and desires, and agree on and plan out the long-term goals.

- Figure out the steps and the short-term goals that will lead to long-term achievement. If the goal is to run a marathon and the client has never run even 5 miles (8 km), the first goal might be to develop the habit of training four times per week; the second might be to run 2 miles (3.2 km); and the third might be to run in a 10K (6.2-mile) race. The short-term goals should progress from there, ultimately leading up to the point that the client can complete 26.2 miles (42.2 km).

- When starting out with a new client, clarify a preliminary goal based more on achievement than on a measured result. For example, one could set the goal of showing up at the gym three times per week for the first two weeks, or the goal of eating a healthy breakfast every morning. By beginning with goals that are simple to achieve and are free of the pressure of potential impending failure, the personal trainer creates a mind-set of achievement and helps to build a client's self-confidence. Once the client begins accumulating small achievements, the goals should become more challenging.

- Both the personal trainer and client should recognize that absence of required knowledge can often hinder the achievement of long-term goals. Evaluating the client's present level of knowledge will help to set a complementary knowledge-based goal, which might be to learn the names and functions of the major muscle groups or to read a series of recommended nutrition books.

- As time progresses and the client proves committed to the sessions and the result, it is appropriate to set more aggressive goals by identifying specific measures of achievement. These goals might typically include performance and achievement with direct measurement, such as "to bench press 200 pounds [90 kg]," "to walk 3 miles [4.8 km]," or "to lose 15 pounds [7 kg] of fat." These goals should be set in measurable terms so the personal trainer and client can easily discern the moment of achievement.

- Once measurable goals are clarified, attach a time frame to each goal. It is important to recognize that if a goal is not achieved by the assigned date, reevaluation and adjustment of action will move the client closer to the goal. Goals can and should be evaluated and adjusted at regular intervals, perhaps biweekly or monthly.

- Agree on a way to recognize whether or not the program is working. If a goal is to reduce waist girth, some clients may want to use a tape measure whereas others may find it psychologically more helpful to gauge progress by occasionally trying on a pair of pants that they have not worn in years.

- After setting goals, always check to make certain that the client believes they are attainable. If not, work on adjusting the client's belief

(i.e., by educating the client) or adjusting the goal.

- Examine the goals to make sure they are compatible with one another. If goals conflict, the client's chance for success may be compromised.

- Goals should be prioritized. If a client comes up with a long list of goals, it is best to first isolate three, for example, that are most important and then to put those three in order of importance.

Attach a time frame to each goal and note if a goal is not achieved by the assigned date. Goals can and should be evaluated and adjusted at regular intervals.

Motivation

According to its basic definition, **motivation** is a psychological construct that arouses and directs behavior (43). A **construct** is simply an internal drive or neural process that cannot be directly observed but must be indirectly inferred from observation of outward behavior. For example, a person who rises every day at dawn and works intensely at his or her job is considered to be highly motivated. There are many other examples of constructs in psychology, such as personality, ambition, and assertiveness. Although not directly observable, they yield powerful influence on behavior.

Practical Principles of Effective Goal Setting

1. Make goals specific, measurable, and observable.
2. Clearly identify time constraints.
3. Use moderately difficult goals (42).
4. Record goals and monitor progress.
5. Diversify process, performance, and outcomes.
6. Set short-range goals to achieve long-range goals.
7. Make sure goals are internalized (clients should participate or set their own).

The acronym "SMART" helps to capture these essential points (78):

Specific
Measurable
Action oriented
Realistic
Time bound

From Cox 2002 (22).

The basic definition suggests that motivation has two dimensions: (1) a directional aspect that influences the choices clients make about their time and commitment and (2) the intensity with which they pursue those choices. Such a definition helps clarify the concept of motivation but falls short of offering a strategy or clue regarding how to change behavior. Because regular exercise involvement is such a problem in our society, the following psychological principles are offered as a strategy to increase the level of participation.

Positive and Negative Reinforcement and Punishment

The use of goal setting is related to the concept of behaviorism, and to clarify the philosophy of motivational practices it is helpful to define the basic concepts used in behavioral or operant conditioning. Formalized by B.F. Skinner (69, 70), behaviorism as a view of learning holds that behavior is molded or shaped by its consequences. Accordingly, personal trainers can significantly influence exercise adherence by their reactions to a client's behaviors.

A **target behavior** (e.g., completing 45 minutes of a step aerobics class) is termed an *operant*, and the probability that an operant will be repeated in the future increases when the behavior is reinforced. On the other hand, the likelihood of the behavior's being repeated decreases when it is punished. **Reinforcement** is any act, object, or event that *increases* the likelihood of future operant behavior when the reinforcement follows the target behavior; and **punishment** is any act, object, or event that *decreases* the likelihood of future operant behavior when the punishment follows that behavior. Although personal trainers do not engage in purposeful punishment actions, understanding behaviorism can help trainers to clarify their own leadership philosophies and understand how they relate to enhancing client motivation.

> Reinforcement *increases* the likelihood that a behavior will be repeated, and punishment *decreases* the likelihood that a behavior will be repeated.

The terms *positive reinforcement* and *negative reinforcement* are often confused. Both terms refer to consequences that increase the probability of occurrence of a desired behavior or operant; but positive reinforcement "gives" something to the client in response to his behavior, and negative reinforcement "takes away" something (50). An example of positive

reinforcement is social approval or congratulations given to a client for completing a workout. An example of negative reinforcement is relieving the client of a disliked chore, such as mopping accumulated sweat from the floor around the exercise equipment, because of successful completion of the workout. In essence, something aversive is "removed" or taken away in order to reward behavior.

Conversely, a personal trainer who focuses on the shortcomings or deficiencies of the client subscribes to a punishing style of motivation since punishment following an event, by definition, decreases the probability of the event's occurring again. Positive punishment implies presentation of something aversive such as disapproval, while negative punishment implies removal of something in order to decrease the operant. Criticism of a client for poor exercise technique is an example of positive punishment. Removal of a privilege because of poor exercise technique or failure to complete an exercise goal is an example of negative punishment. Although it would seem appropriate for personal trainers to resort to reasonable forms of disapproval or punishment in the case of poor effort, a reinforcing style of leadership focuses on the progress of the client.

Self-Determination Theory

While new routines, new music, or a new piece of equipment can help a client continue to want to exercise, motivation runs deeper in the client's psyche. People are driven to act based on one of two possible stimuli. They either feel a compulsion to move toward a desire (pleasure) or feel a need to move away from pain. *Pain* does not mean only physical pain, although sometimes that may be an element to be considered; more commonly, it means emotional pain. When a situation becomes increasingly uncomfortable, a client's motivation to move away from the discomfort will increase.

Intrinsically motivated behavior is engaged in for the sense of enjoyment derived from it, while extrinsically motivated behavior is engaged to achieve another goal or outcome. In common terms, intrinsic motivation implies a true love for the experience of exercise and a sense of fun during its performance. Extrinsic motivation, on the other hand, implies a desire to be engaged in behavior to get an external reward. Although originally conceived as independent, the concepts of intrinsic and extrinsic motivation are tied together by the concept of **self-determination** or internalization (25, 26). In essence, self-determination implies that the individual is participating in the activity for his or her own fulfillment as opposed to trying to meet the expectations of others (which would be a "work" orientation). As such, intrinsic and extrinsic motivation represent important landmarks on a motivational continuum or range and are not essentially dichotomous unless one is referring to extremes.

> An intrinsically motivated client truly loves to exercise, whereas an extrinsically motivated client typically exercises only to achieve an external reward.

Clients who initially exhibit intrinsic motivation are more likely to maintain their exercise behavior than those who lack intrinsic motivation (65). Therefore, awareness of a client's location on the motivation continuum holds implications for the type of motivational approach that will be effective in enhancing enjoyment of an exercise program. Major points along the self-determination continuum have been identified (76) and can be summarized (22) as follows:

1. *Amotivation:* The client has a total lack of intrinsic or extrinsic motivation.

2. *External regulation:* The client engages in behavior to avoid punishment, not for personal satisfaction.

3. *Introjected regulation:* The client views exercise and training behavior as a means to a valued end (e.g., getting into correct starting position for resistance training exercise is partly internalized to please the personal trainer).

4. *Identified regulation:* The client accepts the personal trainer's instructions as beneficial but primarily follows the leadership of the personal trainer instead of initiating exercise behavior.

5. *Integrated regulation:* The client personally values exercise behavior, internalizes it, and freely engages in it; the client and the personal trainer agree on the goals for the client.

Clients develop greater commitment to their exercise goals if they are intrinsically motivated because they possess the desire to be competent and committed to achieving goals in which they have a personal stake (25). Although some people may be able to maintain their exercise behavior based solely on extrinsic reinforcement, those who are both intrinsically and extrinsically motivated probably enjoy physical activity and exercise training more, and this makes for a more positive experience for both the client and the personal trainer. Thus clients may have different preferences regarding involvement in goal setting, and the personal trainer can determine whether his or her participation is appropriate. That is, some individuals prefer to have goals formulated by the personal trainer, while others desire to actively participate in the goal-setting process. In general, consideration of client input in the goal-setting process seems well founded.

Effect of Rewards on Intrinsic Motivation

External rewards can play a role in increasing intrinsic motivation and exercise adherence. Although the personal trainer should not count solely on the value of ongoing extrinsic rewards, the promise of a T-shirt, a dinner gift certificate, or a 30-day complimentary health club membership can facilitate early compliance and follow-through. Given this, personal trainers might logically assume that they could enhance intrinsically motivated behavior by giving a client even more rewards. For example, if a client derives great satisfaction from running in 10K races, it might seem that a trophy or financial reward for each performance would result in even greater satisfaction. In actuality, external rewards or recognition can also reduce intrinsic motivation (25).

A well-known example (68) is the story of a retired psychology professor in need of peace and quiet who was disturbed by the sound of children playing on his lawn. Instead of punishing the playful (i.e., intrinsically motivated) behavior of the children, he gave each child 50 cents and heartily thanked them for the "entertainment" that they had afforded him. The children looked forward to returning the next day. At the end of their next romp on the man's lawn, he told them that he was short of money but that he was able to give them 25 cents. A little disappointed, the children returned on a third day and were even more disappointed when they learned that the man had no money to give. Alas, they never returned to play on the man's lawn again! What happened? Exactly what the professor had hoped! If a strong dependency is formed between behavior and reward, removal of the reward is likely to result in a lessening of the behavior. In this scenario, the reward is perceived as controlling (25). Rewards can be viewed as "controlling" if the recipient perceives a contingency or connection between the behavior and the reward.

When to Intervene With Motivational Efforts

To be the most effective at motivating a client, the personal trainer needs to be aware of the client's

stage of readiness for exercise participation. The transtheoretical model describes the process a client goes through as he or she "gets ready to start exercise" (7, 60):

1. *Precontemplation:* The person does not intend to increase physical activity and is not thinking about becoming physically active.

2. *Contemplation:* The person intends to increase physical activity and is giving it a thought now and then, but is not yet physically active.

3. *Preparation:* The person is engaging in some activity, accumulating at least 30 minutes of moderate-intensity physical activity at least one day per week, but not on most days of the week.

4. *Action:* The person is accumulating at least 30 minutes of moderate-intensity physical activity on five or more days of the week, but has done so for less than six months.

5. *Maintenance:* The person is accumulating at least 30 minutes of moderate-intensity physical activity on five or more days of the week, and has been doing so for six months or more.

Having identified the client's stage of readiness, the personal trainer can apply the appropriate processes for change or interventions in order to move the client to the next level with the ultimate goals of action and maintenance. The transtheoretical model may appear to be only common sense, but surveying prospective clients to individualize interventions may be helpful. The Stages of Exercise Scale (SES) (14) can be used to conveniently capture the stage of a prospective client. In general, the research has supported the efficacy of this approach (1, 15, 21, 49).

Self-Efficacy: Building Confidence

To have a truly successful experience with a client, it is important to consider the client's motivation in conjunction with his confidence about achieving the desired behaviors. For example, there are people who have a poor self-concept or social physique anxiety and therefore lack the confidence to engage in an exercise program (35). In his social cognitive theory, Bandura (3) described *self-efficacy* as a person's confidence in his or her own ability to perform specific actions leading to a successful behavioral outcome. Exercise self-efficacy is a powerful predictor of exercise behavior. Self-

efficacy is characterized by the degree to which the client is confident about performing the task and by the maintenance of that belief in the face of failure or obstacles. In other words, self-efficacy is related to persistence in striving for goal achievement. Four types of influences affect or build self-efficacy:

1. Performance accomplishments
2. Modeling effects
3. Verbal persuasion
4. Physiological arousal or anxiety

The successful performance of a behavior or of successive approximations of that behavior has the most powerful influence on enhancing self-efficacy for future behavior, and in that sense underscores the relationship of goal accomplishment to building confidence.

Observing others perform a target behavior can also increase self-efficacy by enhancing imitative behavior. For example, some clients may be more confident of effecting a significant behavioral change such as weight loss if they see others similar to themselves in age, gender, and body type reach the same goal.

Another positive influence on self-efficacy is verbal persuasion from a respected source. A person who is respected and who is known to possess expertise in a given area (e.g., strength development or bodybuilding) can significantly influence a client's self-efficacy by offering encouragement and stating, for example, that the client "has potential."

Finally, the client's own interpretation of his physiological state before or during exercise also exerts an influence on self-efficacy and can effectively decrease or increase confidence. For example, before performing a maximal repetition to determine 1RM strength in the bench press, the client may judge his level of arousal negatively ("I'm too nervous") or positively ("I'm ready").

> Achieving success has more impact than anything else on raising a client's self-efficacy.

Methods to Motivate a Client

Sometimes a particular psychological method is helpful in motivating a client. This section offers techniques for minimizing procrastination, overcoming false beliefs, identifying and modifying self-talk, and using mental imagery.

Minimizing Procrastination

The 14th-century philosopher Jean Buridan told the story of a mule that starved to death trying to decide between two equidistant bales of hay. The bales of hay were equally desirable, so the mule could not decide which way to go. The fable presents a valuable analogy for human indecision. Health and fitness are attributes desired by everyone, but only a disappointing margin of our population manages to commit to and maintain an exercise lifestyle. If people believe they have too many options that they must decide between—diets, devices, or personal trainers—the decision-making process itself often leads to stagnation. Personal trainers have to think beyond the personal training session and toward influencing clients to exercise not only today, or next week, but for the long haul. When a client procrastinates, he or she is weighing options, left in a frozen state of indecision, trying to decide if the perceived pain will outweigh the potential benefit.

Identifying False Beliefs

Because quick fixes are so often positioned as solutions, many clients have allowed flawed and misleading information into their belief systems. If, for example, a client believes that weight loss can be achieved only by severely restricting food intake, he or she is going to block out the personal trainer's suggestions of a more appropriate caloric intake. Further, many people have been conditioned to believe that exercise is not for them or that their bodies will not respond to exercise as the bodies of others do. "No pain, no gain" is another flawed belief. This belief increases a person's tendency to overtrain, which can sabotage the potential for results.

Practical Motivational Techniques

1. Have the client use an exercise log or journal to document baseline measurements and the details of each workout. Teach the client not only to use the journal as a report card for exercise sessions, but also to record emotions, meals, and perspectives on progress.

2. Begin clients with exercise sessions that involve familiar activities. Lack of familiarity with an exercise or exercise mode can frustrate clients and lead to a lack of desire to continue exercising.

3. Whenever possible, offer choices. Keep the client involved in decisions, but offer choices that are equally beneficial. Rather than having the client question whether he or she should exercise at all today, change the decision: "Would you rather do your warm-up on the elliptical climber or the exercise bike today?"

4. Provide feedback often. Look for small achievements. The personal trainer can notice and comment on increases in aerobic capacity, increases in strength, and decreases in body fat while providing exercise assistance. If, for example, the client moves up 5 pounds (2.5 kg) in a specific resistance training exercise, make it clear that progress is taking place.

5. Model the appropriate behavior for a fitness lifestyle. One of the best things a personal trainer can do for clients is to act as a role model and set an example of an exercise commitment.

6. Prepare the client for periods during which momentum may be disrupted. If the client understands that even the most dedicated individuals lower the intensity of their training occasionally, those unavoidable or undesired lapses are less likely to result in program abandonment.

7. Use social support resources. The personal trainer can check on a client's moods, responses, and adherence by tactful use of telephone contact, e-mail correspondence, and mailing of educational resources or motivational information. If possible, conversations with family members regarding the desired outcome and course of action can all contribute to motivation and adherence by providing a stronger support network at home.

8. Let the past go. If a client feels as if he or she failed to obtain the benefits of an exercise program in the past, focus instead on future goals.

9. Substitute a "do your best" outlook for a "be perfect" attitude. Clients who strive for perfection are guaranteed to hit a point of perceived failure. Teach clients to understand that giving total effort and commitment is the equivalent of excellence.

10. Agree on a motivational affirmation and have the client write it down.

Questions to Help Identify False Beliefs

To identify false beliefs, personal trainers can ask clients the following questions:

- What is your ideal approach to "getting in shape"?
- What have you tried in the past to achieve the fitness results you want?
- What exercise and nutrition strategies do you feel are important?
- What do you feel you need to do to reshape your body and improve your health and fitness?

Before a personal trainer can attempt to instill new empowering beliefs, he or she has to first identify, and then work to change, limiting false beliefs. The first step, therefore, in opening up a clear and effective line of communication between the personal trainer and client must involve a questioning process that includes discussion of the client's present beliefs about fitness and exercise. With education, reasoning, and reinforcement, the personal trainer can then help the client understand why the false beliefs are in fact deceptive and limiting. With that understanding, the false beliefs are weakened and ultimately dismissed, allowing the client to learn new, correct information.

"No pain, no gain" is a false belief that can encourage overtraining and diminish a client's potential for results.

Identifying and Modifying Self-Talk

Each client has his own "internal voice." Sometimes this is a source of motivation, but if this **self-talk** is negative, a person is less likely to accept even the most positively directed affirmations. Over time, strong and repetitive external encouragement can change a client's negative self-talk, but positive affirmations will have more effect if the client changes the negative self-talk first. The following are four simple exercises to identify and modify potentially negative self-talk:

1. Ask the client simply to notice self-talk throughout the day and realize that what he or she thinks creates mental pictures, words, and feelings.

2. Once the client has an awareness of the inner voice, direct him or her to identify it at the same point in time each day, ideally just before the scheduled personal training session. For example, if a client has a 5 p.m. personal training appointment each day, ask the client to write down what his or her self-

talk is saying at 4:45 p.m. during preparation for the workout.

3. Ask the client to draw a line down the middle of a sheet of paper and on the left-hand side write down precisely what his or her self-talk is saying. The client should then write down on the right-hand side what the self-talk *could* say that would be supportive or motivating instead. After the client has done this at a given time each day, encourage him or her to identify self-talk at several pertinent times each day (such as on waking or before going to bed), along with what the self-talk could say.

4. After identifying three common self-talk phrases (and three better phrases), the client should write the new phrases (affirmations) down and privately recite the better phrases, at first aloud five or six times each minute at the particular time of day the encouragement is desired, to instill the habit of vocalizing the "better" words. Once the personal trainer helps the client to create this habit, the client can shift to mentally "speaking" the words instead. With practice, clients' positive self-talk will motivate them toward success and achievement.

Mental Imagery

At the 1988 Olympic Games in Seoul, track and field athletes who had qualified for the Olympic trials participated in a survey (32). The survey showed that 83% of the athletes had practiced mental conditioning exercises. Since then, the popularity of mental imagery has grown immensely. The recognized value of mental conditioning for optimal performance is not limited to athletes. Mental conditioning is valuable in music (47), in military training (29), and in rehabilitation (33)—all arenas in which consistency of effort is required for excellence.

Relaxation Exercise for Mental Imagery

Mental imagery should be performed in a relaxed, tension-free state. Sport psychologists use several techniques to facilitate a state of relaxation. Progressive relaxation, developed by Jacobson (39), is one of the most commonly practiced techniques for mental imagery. In progressive relaxation the individual is asked to tighten each muscle group, one group at a time, and to follow each contraction with a full relaxation. The first step involves differentiating between the sensations of muscle tension and muscle relaxation. Although one might think the difference would be obvious, even when sitting in a relaxed position people are probably tensing many muscles. Before asking clients to perform a relaxation or mental imagery exercise, the personal trainer should become familiar with the relaxation process.

Visualization

Visualization involves using the ability of the brain to "draw" and "recall" mental images that can help a client learn how to create positive emotional responses and improve motivation. The following are three simple visualization exercises that can be performed in a relaxed state:

- Witnessing a past success: If a client has "seen" or experienced an achievement or witnessed her own excellence, the belief that such a performance is possible becomes concrete. Since the mind and nervous system are closely linked, perception of a remembered event might have the same "belief" power as an actual achievement.
- Witnessing a success yet to be: Even if a client has not yet achieved the desired goal or performance, with developed imagination skills he or she can create a mental movie of success as if it has already happened.
- Witnessing the value: Immediately before, during, or after a workout, the client mentally "sees" the result or valued outcome. This will greatly enhance the client's desire to achieve the outcome.

As a client's imagery becomes more powerful, the sensations the mental images bring about will become more powerful. Each time clients mentally see themselves achieving a goal, lifting the weight, transforming their body, or crossing the finish line, that vision will be accompanied by the feelings of winning and achievement.

Conclusion

The mental health aspects of exercise come from its anxiety-reducing and antidepressive benefits, both of which have special applications to new clients and individuals who are older. One method of encouraging regular participation in exercise is for the personal trainer and client to collectively set goals that are specific, measurable, action oriented, realistic, and time bound. Further, one of the roles of a personal trainer is to motivate clients expediently toward their established goals while minimizing delays, misconceptions, and negative self-talk via methods that include mental imagery and visualization.

Study Questions

1. All of the following describe how exercise provides cognitive benefits EXCEPT
    A. enhanced oxygen supply to the brain.
    B. greater genetic variation.
    C. improved neurotransmitter function.
    D. heightened neural efficiency.

2. Which of the following is an example of an outcome goal?
    A. "I want to do 60 sit-ups in 1 minute."
    B. "I want to do my best not to eat before going to bed tonight."
    C. "I want to be able to bench press more than my friend."
    D. "I want to lose 10 pounds of body fat."

3. Which of the following is an example of negative reinforcement used by a personal trainer with a client who just completed a month of consistently walking three times per week?
    A. "Good job! Next month, you do not have to take the time to fill out your own walking workout card—I'll do it for you!"
    B. "Good job! You won Walker of the Month"!
    C. "Walking? I thought we talked about you riding the bike instead of walking!"
    D. "Three times per week? It was supposed to be four times per week, so next month you won't be able to keep working out during your lunch hour."

4. On which of the following points along the self-determination continuum is a client who is highly intrinsically motivated?

   A. introjected

   B. integrated

   C. identified

   D. amotivated

Applied Knowledge Question

Using the seven "Practical Principles of Effective Goal Setting," develop an effective six-month goal-setting strategy for a client who says he wants to improve his 1RM leg press from 225 pounds (102 kg) to 315 pounds (143 kg).

References

1. Armstrong, C.A., J.F. Sallis, M.F. Howell, and C.R. Hofstetter. 1993. Stages of change, self-efficacy, and the adoption of vigorous exercise: A prospective analysis. *Journal of Sport and Exercise Psychology* 15: 390-402.

2. Bahrke, M.S., and W.P. Morgan. 1978. Anxiety reduction following exercise and meditation. *Cognitive Therapy and Research* 2: 323-333.

3. Bandura, A. 1997. *Self-Efficacy: The Exercise of Control.* San Francisco: Freeman.

4. Bartholomew, J.B., and D.E. Linder. 1998. State anxiety following resistance exercise: The role of gender and exercise intensity. *Journal of Behavioral Medicine* 21: 205-219.

5. Bixby, W.R., T.W. Spalding, and B.D. Hatfield. 2001. Temporal dynamics and dimensional specificity of the affective response to exercise of varying intensity: Differing pathways to a common outcome. *Journal of Sport and Exercise Psychology* 23: 171-190.

6. Bixby, W., T.W. Spalding, A.J. Haufler, S.P. Deeny, P.T. Mahlow, J. Zimmerman, and B.D. Hatfield. 2007. The unique relation of physical activity to executive function in older men and women. *Medicine and Science in Sports and Exercise* 39 (8): 1408-1416.

7. Blair, S.N., A.N. Dunn, B.H. Marcus, R.A. Carpenter, and P. Jaret. 2001. *Active Living Every Day.* Champaign, IL: Human Kinetics.

8. Blumenthal, J.A., M.A. Babyak, K.A. Moore, W.E. Craighead, S. Herman, P. Khatri, R. Waugh, M.A. Napolitano, L.M. Forman, M. Applebaum, M. Doraiswamy, and R. Krishman. 1999. Effects of exercise training on older patients with major depression. *Archives of Internal Medicine* 159: 2349-2356.

9. Bonvallet, M., and V. Bloch. 1961. Bulbar control of cortical arousal. *Science* 133: 1133-1134.

10. Brown, D. 2002. Study says 38 percent of adults are sedentary in leisure time. *Washington Post* (April 8): A2.

11. Buckworth, J., and R.K. Dishman. 2002. *Exercise Psychology.* Champaign, IL: Human Kinetics.

12. Calfas, K.J., and W.C. Taylor. 1994. Effects of physical activity on psychological variables in adolescents. *Pediatric Exercise Science* 6: 406-423.

13. Cannon, W.B. 1929. *Bodily Changes in Pain, Hunger, Fear, and Rage,* vol. 2. New York: Appleton.

14. Cardinal, B.J. 1995. The stages of exercise scale and stages of exercise behavior in female adults. *Journal of Sport Medicine and Physical Fitness* 35: 87-92.

15. Cardinal, B.J. 1997. Predicting exercise behavior using components of the transtheoretical model of behavior change. *Journal of Sport Behavior* 20: 272-283.

16. Chaouloff, F. 1997. The serotonin hypothesis. In: *Physical Activity and Mental Health,* W.P. Morgan, ed. Washington, DC: Taylor & Francis. pp. 179-198.

17. Chodzko-Zajko, W.J., and K.A. Moore. 1994. Physical fitness and cognitive functioning in aging. *Exercise and Sport Sciences Reviews* 22: 195-220.

18. Colcombe, S.J., K.I. Erickson, N. Raz, A.G. Webb, N.J. Cohen, E. McAuley, and A.F. Kramer. 2003. Aerobic fitness reduces brain tissue loss in aging humans. *Journal of Gerontology* 58A: 176-180.

19. Colcombe, S., and A.F. Kramer. 2003. Fitness effects on the cognitive function of older adults: A meta-analytic study. *Psychological Science* 14: 125-130.

20. Cotman, C.W., and C. Engesser-Cesar. 2002. Exercise enhances and protects brain function. *Exercise and Sport Sciences Reviews* 30: 75-79.

21. Courneya, K.S. 1995. Perceived severity of the consequences of physical inactivity across the stages of change in older adults. *Journal of Sport and Exercise Psychology* 17: 447-457.

22. Cox, R.H. 2002. *Sport Psychology: Concepts and Applications,* 5th ed. Boston: McGraw-Hill.

23. Craft, L.L., and D.M. Landers. 1998. The effect of exercise on clinical depression and depression resulting from mental illness: A meta-analysis. *Journal of Sport and Exercise Psychology* 20: 339-357.

24. Davidson, R.J. 1993. Cerebral asymmetry and emotion: Conceptual and methodological conundrums. *Cognition & Emotion* 7: 138.

25. Deci, E.L., and R.M. Ryan. 1985. *Intrinsic Motivation and Self-Determination in Human Behavior.* New York: Plenum Press.

26. Deci, E.L., and R.M. Ryan. 1991. A motivational approach to self: Integration in personality. In: *Nebraska Symposium on Motivation 1991: Vol. 38. Perspectives on Motivation: Current Theory and Research in Motivation,* R.A. Dienstbier, ed. Lincoln, NE: University of Nebraska Press. pp. 237-288.

27. deVries, H.A., and T.J. Housh. 1994. *Physiology of Exercise for Physical Education, Athletics, and Exercise Science.* Madison, WI: Brown and Benchmark.

28. Dishman, R.K. 1997. The norepinephrine hypothesis. In: *Physical Activity and Mental Health,* W.P. Morgan, ed. Washington, DC: Taylor & Francis. pp. 199-212.

29. Druckman, D., and J.A. Swets. 1988. *Enhancing Human Performance: Issues, Theories and Techniques.* Washington, DC: National Academy Press.

30. Duda, J.L. 1989. Relationships between task and ego orientation and the perceived purpose of sport among high school athletes. *Journal of Sport and Exercise Psychology* 11: 318-335.

31. Dustman, R.E., R.Y. Emmerson, R.O. Ruhling, D.E. Shearer, L.A. Steinhaus, S.C. Johnson, H.W. Bonekat, and J.W. Shigeoka. 1990. Age and fitness effects on EEG, ERPs, visual sensitivity, and cognition. *Neurobiology of Aging* 11: 193-200.

32. Golding, J., and S. Ungerleider. 1992. *Beyond Strength: Psychological Profiles of Olympic Athletes.* Madison, WI: Brown and Benchmark.

33. Groden, J., J.R. Cautela, P. LeVasseur, G. Groden, and M. Bausman. 1991. *Imagery Procedures for People With Special Needs: Video Guide.* Champaign, IL: Research Press.

34. Hall, H.K., and A.W. Kerr. 2001. Goal setting in sport and physical activity: Tracing empirical developments and establishing conceptual direction. In: *Advances in Motivation in Sport and Exercise,* G.C. Roberts, ed. Champaign, IL: Human Kinetics. pp. 183-234.

35. Hart, E.A., M.R. Leary, and W.J. Rejeski. 1989. The measurement of social physique anxiety. *Journal of Sport and Exercise Psychology* 11: 94-104.

36. Hatfield, B.D. 1991. Exercise and mental health: The mechanisms of exercise-induced psychological states. In: *Psychology of Sports, Exercise and Fitness,* L. Diamant, ed. Washington, DC: Hemisphere. pp. 17-50.

37. Iso-Ahola, S.E., and B.D. Hatfield. 1986. *Psychology of Sports: A Social Psychological Approach.* Dubuque, IA: Brown.

38. Issacs, K.R., B.J. Anderson, A.A. Alcantara, J.E. Black, and W.T. Greenough. 1992. Exercise and the brain: Angiogenesis in the adult rat cerebellum after vigorous physical activity and motor skill learning. *Journal of Cerebral Blood Flow and Metabolism* 12: 110-119.

39. Jacobson, E. 1974. *Progressive Relaxation.* Chicago: University of Chicago Press.

40. Kramer, A.F., S. Hahn, N.J. Cohen, M.T. Banich, E. McAuley, C.R. Harrison, J. Chason, E. Vakil, L. Bardell, R.A. Boileau, and A. Colcombe. 1999. Aging, fitness and neurocognitive function. *Nature* 400: 418-419.

41. Kugler, J., H. Seelback, and G.M. Kruskemper. 1994. Effects of rehabilitation exercise programmes on anxiety and depression in coronary patients: A meta-analysis. *British Journal of Clinical Psychology* 33: 401-410.

42. Kyllo, L.B., and D.M. Landers. 1995. Goal setting in sport and exercise: A research synthesis to resolve the controversy. *Journal of Sport and Exercise Psychology* 17: 117-137.

43. Landers, D.M. 1980. The arousal-performance relationship revisited. *Research Quarterly for Exercise and Sport* 51: 77-90.

44. Landers, D.M., and S.A. Arent. 2001. Physical activity and mental health. In: *Handbook of Sport Psychology,* 2nd ed., R.N. Singer, H.A. Hausenblas, and C.M. Janelle, eds. New York: Wiley. pp. 740-765.

45. Landers, D.M., and Arent, S.A. 2007. Physical activity and mental health. In: *Handbook of Sport Psychology,* 3rd ed., G. Tenenbaum and R.C. Eklund, eds. New York: Wiley. pp. 469-491.

46. Landers, D.M., and S.J. Petruzzello. 1994. Physical activity, fitness, and anxiety. In: *Physical Activity, Fitness, and Health,* C. Bouchard, R.J. Shepard, and T. Stevens, eds. Champaign, IL: Human Kinetics. pp. 868-882.

47. Lim, S., and L. Lipman. 1991. Mental practice and memorization of piano music. *Journal of General Psychology* 118: 21-30.

48. Long, B.C., and R. Van Stavel. 1995. Effects of exercise training on anxiety: A meta-analysis. *Journal of Applied Sport Psychology* 7: 167-189.

49. Marcus, B.H., C.A. Eaton, J.S. Rossi, and L.L. Harlow. 1994. Self-efficacy, decision making, and stages of change: An integrative model of physical exercise. *Journal of Applied Social Psychology* 24: 489-508.

50. Martens, R. 1975. *Social Psychology and Physical Activity.* New York: Harper & Row.

51. McDonald, D.G., and J.A. Hodgdon. 1991. *The Psychological Effects of Aerobic Fitness Training: Research and Theory.* New York: Springer-Verlag.

52. McDowell, K., S.E. Kerick, D.L. Santa Maria, and B.D. Hatfield. 2003. Aging, physical activity, and cognitive processing: An examination of P300. *Neurobiology of Aging* 24 (4): 597-606.

53. Meijer, E.H., F.T.Y. Smulders, and B.D. Hatfield. 2002. The effects of rhythmic physical activity and the EEG. Paper submitted for presentation at the annual meeting of the Society for Psychophysiological Research, Washington, DC.

54. Morgan, W.P. 1985. Affective beneficence of vigorous physical activity. *Medicine and Science in Sports and Exercise* 17: 94-100.

55. Morgan, W.P. 2001. Prescription of physical activity: A paradigm shift. *Quest* 53: 366-382.

56. North, T.C., P. McCullagh, and Z.V. Tran. 1990. Effects of exercise on depression. *Exercise and Sport Sciences Reviews* 18: 379-415.

57. O'Block, F.R., and F.H. Evans. 1984. Goal setting as a motivational technique: In: *Psychological Foundations of Sport,* J.M. Silva and R.S. Weinberg, eds. Champaign, IL: Human Kinetics. pp. 188-196.

58. Petruzzello, S.J., P. Ekkekakis, and E.E. Hall. 2006. Physical activity, affect and electroencephalogram studies. In: *Psychobiology of Physical Activity,* E.O Acevedo and P. Ekkekakis, eds. Champaign, IL: Human Kinetics. pp. 91-109.

59. Petruzzello, S.J., D.M. Landers, B.D. Hatfield, K.A. Kubitz, and W. Salazar. 1991. A meta-analysis an the anxiety-reducing effects of acute and chronic exercise. *Sports Medicine* 11: 143-182.

60. Prochaska, J.O., and B.H. Marcus. 1994. The transtheoretical model: The applications to exercise. In: *Advances in Exercise Adherence,* R.K. Dishman, ed. Champaign, IL: Human Kinetics. pp. 161-180.

61. Roberts, G.C. 1993. Motivation in sport: Understanding and enhancing the motivation and achievement of children. In: *Handbook of Research on Sport Psychology,* R.N. Singer, M. Murphy, and L.K. Tennant, eds. New York: Macmillan. pp. 405-420.

62. Roberts, G.C. 2001. Understanding the dynamics of motivation in physical activity: The influence of achievement goals on motivational processes. In: *Advances in Motivation in Sport and Exercise,* G.C. Roberts, ed. Champaign, IL: Human Kinetics. pp. 1-50.

63. Roberts, G.C., and D.C. Treasure. 1995. Achievement goals, motivation climate and achievement strategies and behaviors in sport. *International Journal of Sport Psychology* 26: 64-80.

64. Rogers, R.L., J.A. Meyer, and K.F. Mortel. 1990. After reaching retirement age physical activity sustains cerebral perfusion and cognition. *Journal of the American Geriatric Society* 38: 123-128.

65. Ryan, R.M., C.M. Frederick, D. Lepes, N. Rubio, and K.M. Sheldon. 1997. Intrinsic motivation and exercise adherence. *International Journal of Sport Psychology* 28: 335-354.

66. Schuit, A.J., E.J.M. Feskens, L.J. Launer, and D. Kromhout. 2001. Physical activity and cognitive decline, the role of apolipoprotein e4 allele. *Medicine and Science in Sports and Exercise* 33: 772-777.

67. Sherwood, D.E., and D.J. Selder. 1979. Cardiorespiratory health, reaction time and aging. *Medicine and Science in Sports* 11: 186-189.

68. Siedentop, D., and G. Ramey. 1977. Extrinsic rewards and intrinsic motivation. *Motor Skills: Theory Into Practice* 2: 49-62.

69. Skinner, B.F. 1938. *The Behavior of Organisms: An Experimental Analysis.* New York: Appleton Century Crofts.

70. Skinner, B.F. 1953. *Science and Human Behavior.* New York: Macmillan.

71. Solomon, R.L., and J.D. Corbit. 1973. An opponent-process theory of motivation: II. Cigarette addiction. *Journal of Abnormal Psychology* 81: 158-171.

72. Spielberger, C.D. 1983. *Manual for the State-Trait Anxiety Inventory (Form Y).* Palo Alto, CA: Consulting Psychologists Press.

73. Spirduso, W.W. 1983. Exercise and the aging brain. *Research Quarterly for Exercise and Sport* 54: 208-218.

74. Tong, L., H. Shen, V.M. Perreau, R. Balazas, and C.W. Cotman. 2001. Effects of exercise on gene-expression profile in the rat hippocampus. *Neurobiology of Disease* 8: 1046-1056.

75. U.S. Department of Health and Human Services. 1996. *Physical Activity and Health: A Report of the Surgeon General.* McLean, VA: International Medical.

76. Vallerand, R.J., and G.F. Losier. 1999. An integration analysis of intrinsic and extrinsic motivation in sport. *Journal of Applied Sport Psychology* 11: 142-169.

77. Von Euler, C., and V. Soderberg. 1957. The influence of hypothalamic thermoceptive structures on the electroencephalogram and gamma motor activity. *Electroencephalography and Clinical Neurophysiology* 9: 391-408.

78. Weinberg, R.S., and D. Gould. 1999. *Foundations of Sport and Exercise Psychology.* Champaign, IL: Human Kinetics.

79. Woo, M.., S. Kim, J. Kim, and B.D. Hatfield. (2010). The influence of exercise intensity on frontal electroencephalographic (EEG) asymmetry and self-reported affect. *Research Quarterly for Exercise and Sport 81: 349-359.*

80. Woo, M., S. Kim, J. Kim, S.J. Petruzzello, and B.D. Hatfield. 2009. Examining the exercise-affect dose-response relationship: Does duration influence frontal EEG asymmetry? *International Journal of Psychophysiology* 72 (2): 166-172.

PART II

Initial Consultation and Evaluation

Client Consultation and Health Appraisal

Tammy K. Evetovich, PhD, and Kristi R. Hinnerichs, PhD

After completing this chapter, you will be able to

- conduct an initial client interview to assess compatibility, develop goals, and establish a client–trainer agreement;
- understand the process of a preparticipation health appraisal screening;
- identify positive coronary risk factors associated with cardiovascular disease;
- evaluate and stratify the health status of potential clients; and
- recognize individuals requiring referral to health care professionals.

The scope of practice of the personal trainer involves the responsibility of interviewing potential clients to gather pertinent information regarding their personal health, lifestyle, and exercise readiness. The consultation process is a vital screening mechanism one can view as instrumental in appraising health status and developing comprehensive programs of exercise to safely and effectively meet the participant's individual objectives. This chapter covers the client consultation; preparticipation health screening; evaluation of coronary risk factors, disease, and lifestyle; interpretation of results; the referral process; and medical clearance.

The authors would like to acknowledge the contributions of John A.C. Kordich, who wrote this chapter for the first edition of *NSCA's Essentials of Personal Training*.

Purpose of Consultation and Health Appraisal

The NSCA-Certified Personal Trainer Job (Task) Analysis Committee has defined **scope of practice** for the personal training profession by characterizing personal trainers as follows:

Personal trainers are health/fitness professionals who use an individualized approach to assess, motivate, educate, and train clients regarding their health and fitness needs. They design safe and effective exercise programs and provide the guidance to help clients achieve their personal goals. In addition, they respond appropriately in emergency situations. Recognizing their area of expertise, personal trainers refer clients to other health care professionals when appropriate (33).

Chapter 9

Personal Trainers MATER

Personal trainers

- **Motivate** performance and compliance
- **Assess** health status
- **Train** clients safely and effectively to meet individual objectives
- **Educate** clients to be informed consumers
- **Refer** clients to health care professionals when necessary

The objective of the client consultation and health appraisal is directly in line with the scope of practice of the personal trainer. Perhaps the best way to describe the role and responsibilities of the personal trainer in the preparticipation screening process is through the acronym MATER.

The most important principle underlying the client consultation and **health appraisal** process is to screen participants for risk factors and symptoms of chronic cardiovascular, pulmonary, metabolic, and orthopedic diseases in order to optimize safety during exercise testing and participation. Thus this chapter focuses on assessing health status and stratifying risk as a basis for referral to health care professionals.

Delivery Process

Because the health and fitness industry is diverse, there is no specific standardized process for implementing the client consultation and health appraisal mechanism. However, typically, delivery of the process is predicated on four factors that dictate implementation:

1. Credentials of the personal trainer
2. Site of delivery
3. Specific population served
4. Legal statutes

Because of the differences in credentials, delivery sites, populations served, and legal issues, "Steps of the Client Consultation and Health Appraisal" provides an example of the steps that may be involved in the delivery of the consultation and preparticipation health appraisal screening process.

Client Consultation

Even though no recognized uniform process of administration appears to exist, there is agreement about the value of an initial interview as the first step in the client consultation to obtain and share essential information associated with the program delivery process (16, 28). The initial interview is a scheduled appointment intended as a mutual sharing of information with the expected outcomes of assessing client–trainer compatibility, discussing goals, and developing a client–trainer agreement.

> During the initial interview, the personal trainer and client assess compatibility, develop goals, and establish a client–trainer agreement.

Assessing Client–Trainer Compatibility

As the first step in determining trainer–client compatibility, the personal trainer provides a detailed description of the services available. Important information to convey to the potential client includes an explanation of the personal trainer's formal education, professional experience, certifications, and expertise or specializations, as well as the mission statement, success rate, and unique features of the program delivery system. Other important compo-

Steps of the Client Consultation and Health Appraisal

1. Schedule interview appointment.
2. Conduct interview.
3. Implement and complete health appraisal forms.
4. Evaluate for coronary risk factors, diagnosed disease, and lifestyle.
5. Assess and interpret results.
6. Refer to an allied health professional when necessary.
7. Obtain medical clearance and program recommendations.

nents that may affect suitability include logistical aspects regarding where and when services are available.

The personal trainer may also need to evaluate the level of exercise readiness by assessing the motivation and commitment of the individual. An attempt to predict compliance may begin with a discussion of past experiences, appreciation for exercise, availability of support, time management and organizational skills, and potential obstacles that may affect exercise adherence. Paper tests are available that are sensitive to predicting levels of exercise readiness and compliance. An attitudinal assessment form is shown on page 166.

The last step in determining compatibility is to assess suitability and appropriateness. It is important that the personal trainer and potential client agree to boundaries, roles, resources, and expectations and address concerns related to any of the issues or information discussed in the initial interview.

If facts are discovered during the initial interview that would establish incompatibility, it is important for the personal trainer to provide the person with an option to receive services through a referral process.

Discussion of Goals

If compatibility and suitability are established, the next step may be a discussion of goals. The main function of identifying objectives is to provide and define direction as it relates to purpose and motivation. Developing goals that are specific, measurable, action oriented, realistic, and time sensitive is a science and art and a vital element of the training process. Goal setting is discussed in chapter 8.

Establishing the Client–Trainer Agreement

After the personal trainer and client have identified and clarified goals, the next step may be to finalize the trainer–client agreement. Entering into an agreement under the elements of contract law requires a formal process that in most cases is legally driven. Components of a contract include written documentation describing the services, parties involved, expectations of those parties, time line of delivery, cost structure, and a payment process. Language of the contract should also cover the cancellation policy, termination of contract, and circumstances that would render the document void. An opportunity for discussion regarding the content of the contract should be provided during the consultation. The personal trainer should document and clarify questions and issues concerning the agreement before receipt

of acknowledgment of acceptance. The contract becomes valid when signed by both parties, assuming appropriate legal age and competency (23). An example of a personal training contract/agreement is provided on page 169. Personal training professionals should consult with an attorney to make sure that their contract/agreement is in accordance with their local city and state laws.

Preparticipation Health Appraisal Screening

The purpose of the preparticipation health appraisal screening process is to identify known diseases and positive risk factors associated with coronary artery disease, assess lifestyle factors that may require special considerations, and identify individuals who may require medical referral before starting an exercise program.

The first step in the preparticipation health appraisal screening process is to ask the client to complete relevant forms. The personal trainer should review the completed forms before services are provided and any activity occurs. It is essential that the process be cost-effective and time efficient in order to avoid unnecessary barriers to exercise for individuals who do not need a medical clearance to participate (30).

Health appraisal instruments are tools by which information is collected and evaluated to assess appropriateness for various levels of exercise and referral. Two instruments are commonly used: (1) **PAR-Q (Physical Activity Readiness Questionnaire)** and (2) Health/Medical Questionnaire.

Physical Activity Readiness Questionnaire

The PAR-Q, a tool developed in Canada, consists of a questionnaire that requires self-recall of observations and signs and symptoms experienced by the client, in addition to confirmation of diagnosis by a physician. The PAR-Q form appears on page 170.

The advantages of the PAR-Q are that it is cost-effective, easy to administer, and sensitive in that it identifies individuals who require additional medical screening while not excluding those who would benefit from participation in low-intensity activity (45). The PAR-Q appears to have limitations in that it was designed essentially to determine the safety of exercise and not necessarily the risk for coronary artery disease. Because of the limitations of the PAR-Q with respect to identifying positive **coronary risk factors,** medications, and contraindications to exercise, it is advisable for personal trainers to use an additional health appraisal instrument for more effective identification of these critical elements.

The Health/Medical Questionnaire is an effective tool for assessing the appropriateness of moderate and vigorous levels of exercise in that it can identify positive coronary risk factors associated with coronary artery disease, sudden cardiac death risk factors, existing diagnosed pathologies, orthopedic concerns, recent operations, personal history of suggested signs and symptoms, medications, supplements, and lifestyle management. A sample health/medical questionnaire appears on page 171.

Information gathered from both health appraisal tools is instrumental in identifying risk factors, stratifying the level of risk, and determining the appropriateness of testing and exercise. Reasons for which clients must seek a physician's clearance before exercise testing or participation are discussed later in this chapter.

Additional Screening

Additional screening forms that provide an opportunity to gather and exchange valuable information include lifestyle inventories, informed consent forms, and assumption of risk agreements.

Lifestyle Inventories

Lifestyle inventories vary in their format, substance, and depth. However, they usually consist of questions to evaluate personal choices and patterns related to dietary intake, management of stress, level of physical activity, and other practices that may affect the person's health. Although the specific benefits of the inventory results may be unclear, there appears to be some value in qualitatively and quantitatively assessing behaviors that may have a positive or negative impact on facilitating change in an individual's health and fitness. A personal trainer may use a lifestyle inventory to augment previously gathered health- and fitness-related information in an attempt to clarify and confirm personal issues possibly perceived as assets or obstacles to the client's success. In addition, the results of the inventory may provide valuable information for use in developing goals.

The vast majority of the existing standard lifestyle inventory assessments were developed for the average apparently healthy population. Persons with existing health-related conditions who have been previously diagnosed by a physician may not obtain valid and reliable information from the results of the inventories and therefore should rely on diagnos-

tic information from their physician for guidance. The form "Health Risk Analysis" on page 173 is an example of a lifestyle inventory.

Informed Consent

The informed consent form gives clients information about the content and process of the program delivery system. The essential elements of an informed consent include a detailed description of the program, the risks and the benefits associated with participation, a confidentiality clause, responsibilities of the participant, and documentation of acknowledgment and acceptance of the terms described within the form. It has been commonly accepted that the information on this form should be conveyed both verbally and in writing to the client prior to any testing or participation to ensure that the participant knows and understands the risks and circumstances associated with the program. See chapter 25 for a discussion of legal issues regarding informed consent forms. An example of an informed consent form appears on page 637 in chapter 25.

Release/Assumption of Risk Agreement

An **assumption of risk** or waiver is an agreement by a client, before beginning participation, to give up, relinquish, or waive the participant's rights to legal remedy (damages) in the event of injury, even when such injury arises as a result of provider negligence (2). The legal implications associated with the implementation and execution of the Release/Assumption of Risk Agreement appear to be unclear at best due to the various legal interpretations associated with waiver documents (see chapter 25). A release/assumption of risk agreement needs to identify the potential risks associated with participation and establish that the potential client understands those risks and voluntarily chooses to assume the responsibility. A signed assumption of risk may limit liability. If a trainer needs to prove in court that a participant was aware of how to avoid risks and assumed the risk of an activity, this type of document may prove helpful. However, acknowledgment of the content and authorization of this form does not relieve the personal trainer of the duty to perform in a competent and professional manner. An example of a release/assumption of risk agreement form appears on page 639 in chapter 25.

Children and Preparticipation Documents

As the number of overweight and obese children continues to grow, parents are employing personal trainers to help their children lose weight, increase their fitness level, and increase their self-esteem. In addition, some parents are enlisting the help of personal trainers to improve their child's sport performance. Unfortunately, little has been written about the medical and legal considerations for the participation of children in a training program. It is clear that parents or legal guardians should fill out a health history questionnaire for their child before he or she begins participation. *Preparticipation Physical Examination* (36) includes a preparticipation physical evaluation form that has been approved by the American Academy of Pediatrics and American Academy of Family Physicians as well as other organizations. This form may be helpful in determining whether a child should visit and get the permission of a physician prior to participation in a physical activity program. It is not so clear, however, whether waivers, parental consent forms, or assumption of risk documents for this age group are helpful and thus should be administered. With regard to assumption of risk or waiver agreements, parents do not have the right to execute such waivers on behalf of their children (22). Thus, it is difficult to free the personal trainer from liability in the event of an injury or claim. In fact, according to laws in many states, "children of particular ages (generally 7-14 years) are incapable of self-negligence" (22). Thus, a child's self-negligence is not sufficient to bar or limit any award of damages.

Given these concerns, it goes without saying that personal trainers of children need to be knowledgeable about safe and effective training methods and be aware of the unique psychological and physiological characteristics of younger populations. But although personal training for children involves unique legal and medical considerations, the benefits of physical activity in this age group are numerous (19). If personal trainers follow established training guidelines and safety procedures, they can decrease the risk of injury and protect themselves from liability.

Record Keeping

The personal trainer needs to develop a strategy to collect, organize, and store the vital information and materials obtained through the initial interview process. A record-keeping system to verify the completion and receipt of forms, along with other documentation concerning the status of the client, is instrumental in allowing one to move on to the next step of the preparticipation health appraisal screening process.

> The scope of practice of the personal trainer involves the responsibility to interview potential clients to gather and assess pertinent information regarding their personal health, medical conditions, and lifestyle in order to safely and effectively meet their individual health and fitness objectives.

Evaluation of Coronary Risk Factors, Disease, and Lifestyle

Once the appropriate forms are completed and the documentation is reviewed, it is necessary to evaluate the content of the information to identify any potential risks associated with the client's present health status. This evaluation helps the personal trainer stratify risk and refer clients to physicians as necessary. The key areas to evaluate include positive risk factors associated with **coronary artery disease (CAD),** medical conditions and diagnosed disease, and current lifestyle.

Coronary Artery Disease Risk Factors

Coronary artery disease is the leading cause of mortality in Western society (6). **Atherosclerosis** is a progressive degenerative process associated with CAD through which the endothelial lining of the arterial walls becomes hardened and the walls consequently lose elasticity. Over time, deposition of fat and plaque buildup occur and the artery wall narrows, which in turn occludes blood flow through the vascular system to the heart, causing heart tissue to die or leading to a **myocardial infarction.**

Although it is well documented that exercise is a protective preventive mechanism to deter this process, some individuals possess existing factors that put them at greater potential risk for a coronary episode because of the increased demand that exercise imposes on an already compromised system (34).

Identifiable positive risk factors are associated with the potential to acquire CAD. A *positive risk factor* may be defined as "an aspect of personal behavior or lifestyle, an environmental exposure or inherited characteristic, which, on the basis of epidemiologic evidence, is known to be associated with health related conditions considered important to prevent" (29). It is necessary to evaluate positive risk factors associated with CAD in order to identify individuals who may be at higher risk during exercise.

Positive Coronary Risk Factors

Epidemiological research suggests that a person's potential risk for developing CAD is associated with the positive coronary risk factors the person possesses. The greater the number and severity of those risk factors, the greater probability of CAD (26). The seven identifiable positive coronary risk factors that have a significant correlation to CAD are family history, smoking, hypertension, dyslipidemia, impaired fasting glucose levels, obesity, and sedentary lifestyle (see table 9.1, "Coronary Artery Disease Risk Factor Thresholds").

Age   The probability of developing CAD increases with age. Males are at a greater risk of having CAD than females are and they tend to develop it at younger ages. Following the most recent guidelines, reaching the threshold of ≥45 years for men and ≥55

years for women does not, by itself, move the client into the stratification of moderate risk.

Family History   Coronary artery disease appears to have a predisposing genetic connection and a tendency to be familial. Although it is difficult to ascertain whether a genetic code or an environmental influence is involved, it may be safe to speculate that people with a documented family history are more susceptible to CAD (27). Thus people with a family history possess a risk factor if a myocardial infarction, coronary revascularization, or sudden death occurred before 55 years of age in their biological father or another male first-degree relative (sibling or child), or before 65 years of age in their biological mother or other female first-degree relatives (3).

Cigarette Smoking   Overwhelming empirical evidence identifies cigarette smoking as a major positive

TABLE 9.1   Coronary Artery Disease Risk Factor Thresholds

Positive risk factors	Defining criteria
Age	Men ≥45 years; women ≥55 years
Family history	Myocardial infarction, coronary revascularization, or sudden death before 55 years of age in biological father or other male first-degree relative, or before 65 years of age in biological mother or other female first-degree relative
Cigarette smoking	Current cigarette smoker or someone who quit within the previous six months, or exposure to environmental tobacco smoke
Sedentary lifestyle	Not participating in at least 30 min of moderate intensity (40-60% $\dot{V}O_2$Reserve) physical activity on at least three days of the week for at least three months (47)*
Obesity†	Body mass index of ≥30 kg/m² or waist girth of >102 cm (40 in.) for men and >88 cm (35 in.) for women (17)
Hypertension	Systolic blood pressure ≥140 mmHg and/or diastolic ≥90 mmHg, confirmed by measurements on at least two separate occasions, or on antihypertensive medication**
Dyslipidemia	Low-density lipoprotein cholesterol (LDL-C) ≥130 mg/dl (3.37 mmol/L) or high-density lipoprotein cholesterol (HDL-C) of <40 mg/dl (1.04 mmol/L), or on lipid-lowering medication. If total serum cholesterol is all that is available, use ≥200 mg/dl (5.18 mmol/L)***
Prediabetes	Impaired fasting glucose (IFG) = fasting plasma glucose ≥100 mg/dl (5.50 mmol/L) but <126 mg/dl (6.93 mmol/L) or impaired glucose tolerance (IGT) = 2-h values in oral glucose tolerance test (OGTT) ≥140 mg/dl (7.70 mmol/L) but <200 mg/dl (11.00 mmol/L), confirmed by measurements on at least two separate occasions****
Negative risk factor	**Defining criteria**
High serum high-density lipoprotein cholesterol§	≥60 mg/dl (1.55 mmol/L)

*Pate, R.R., M. Pratt, S.N. Blair, et al. 1995. Physical activity and public health. A recommendation from the Centers for Disease Control and Prevention and the American College of Sports Medicine. *Journal of the American Medical Association* 1:273 (February, 5): 402-407.

**Chobanian, A.V., G.L. Bakris, H.R. Black, et al. 2003. The seventh report of the Joint National Committee on Prevention, Detection, Evaluation, and Treatment of High Blood Pressure: The JNC 7 report. *Journal of the American Medical Association* 289: 2560-2572.

***NCEP Expert Panel. 2002. Third report of National Cholesterol Education Program (NCEP) Expert Panel on Detection, Evaluation, and Treatment of High Blood Cholesterol in Adults (Adult Treatment Panel III). Final report. *Circulation* 106: 3143-3421.

****American Diabetes Association. 2007. Diagnosis and classification of diabetes mellitus. Diabetes Care 30 (suppl 1): S42-47.

†Professional opinions vary regarding the most appropriate markers and thresholds for obesity; therefore, exercise professionals should use clinical judgment when evaluating this risk factor.

§It is common to sum risk factors in making clinical judgments. If high-density lipoprotein (HDL-C) cholesterol is high, subtract one risk factor from the sum of positive risk factors because high HDL-C decreases coronary artery disease risk.

Adapted by permission from ACSM 2010.

risk factor for CAD (21). A linear relationship also appears to exist between the risk for cardiovascular disease and the volume of cigarette smoking and number of years a person smoked (14). Data suggest that the chemical makeup of cigarettes accentuates risk by elevating myocardial oxygen demand and reducing oxygen transport, causing the cardiovascular system to work harder to obtain a sufficient oxygen supply (15). In addition, cigarette smoking lowers high-density lipoprotein cholesterol, which has an impact on the acceleration of the atherosclerotic process (35). Persons who currently smoke cigarettes, and those who previously smoked but who have quit within the last six months, have a greater potential risk for CAD and have this positive risk factor (3).

Hypertension Hypertension is chronic, persistent sustained elevation of blood pressures (see table 11.2). Most individuals who are clinically diagnosed have essential hypertension, which by definition cannot be attributed to any specific cause. Secondary hypertension refers to elevated blood pressures caused by specific factors such as kidney disease and obesity (31).

Regardless of the etiology, hypertension is believed to predispose individuals to CAD through the direct vascular injury caused by high blood pressure and its adverse effects on the myocardium. These include increased wall stress, which dramatically increases the workload of the heart in pumping the extra blood required to overcome peripheral vascular resistance (44). In general, the higher the blood pressure, the greater the risk for CAD.

Dyslipidemia Cholesterol is a fatlike substance found in the tissues of the body that performs specific metabolic functions in the human organism. Cholesterol is carried in the bloodstream by molecular proteins known as *high-density lipoproteins* (HDLs) and *low-density lipoproteins* (LDLs). Evidence suggests that the LDL molecules release cholesterol, which penetrates the endothelial lining of the arterial wall and in turn contributes to the atherosclerotic plaque buildup that eventually leads to vascular occlusion and heart attacks (46). Research has strongly suggested that HDLs act as a protective mechanism by transporting cholesterol through the bloodstream to the liver, where it is metabolized and eliminated.

Epidemiological research has identified a strong relationship between high levels of total cholesterol, high LDL-cholesterol, and low HDL-cholesterol and a higher rate of CAD in both men and women (18). Individuals who have a total serum cholesterol of >200 mg/dl or an HDL-cholesterol of <35 mg/dl or an LDL >130 mg/dl or who are on lipid-lowering medication have a greater risk for CAD. It is important to note that the LDL may provide a more predictive value for CAD than the total cholesterol. In any event, people who have these values have a positive risk factor for CAD (3).

Impaired Fasting Glucose Levels Fasting blood glucose levels are markers to assess the body's metabolic function. Elevated levels of circulating glucose in the bloodstream cause a chemical imbalance that impedes the use of fats and glucose. As a result, individuals with this metabolic imbalance are more susceptible to atherosclerosis and have an increased risk for CAD (5). Elevated fasting glucose levels may also be early predictive values for the potential onset of diabetes. Individuals who present with fasting glucose values equal to or greater than 100 mg/dl, or 2-hour values in an oral glucose tolerance test equal to or greater than 140 mg/dl confirmed by measurements on at least two separate occasions, are considered to be at increased risk for CAD (3).

Obesity Obesity by medical definition is the accumulation and storage of excess body fat. The prevalence of obesity in the United States has reached epidemic proportions. An analysis of the relationship between obesity and CAD is confounded because of the connection between obesity and other risk factors such as physical inactivity, hypertension, hypercholesterolemia, and diabetes. However, evidence has suggested that obesity in and of itself may be considered an independent risk factor for CAD (24). In addition to the risk associated with accumulation of excess body fat, there may be an increased risk related to the location and deposition of stored visceral fat. Persons who store or accumulate excess body fat in the central waist or abdominal area appear to be at greater risk for CAD (17). The assessments and values associated with obesity as a positive risk factor include a body mass index (BMI) equal to or greater than 30 kg body weight per height in meters squared (30 kg/m²) or a waist girth >40 inches (102 cm) for men and 35 inches (88 cm) for women (3). Refer to chapter 11 for instructions on how to calculate BMI and measure waist girth.

Sedentary Lifestyle Physical inactivity or a sedentary lifestyle is recognized as a leading contributing factor to morbidity and mortality (see table 9.1). Numerous studies have linked a sedentary lifestyle or low fitness to a greater risk of CAD (47). Substantial evidence suggests that CAD risk for sedentary individuals is significantly greater than for those who are more physically active. Physical activity also has many beneficial effects on other CAD risk factors, for example by decreasing resting systolic and diastolic blood pressures, reducing triglyceride levels, increasing serum HDL-cholesterol levels, and enhancing glucose tolerance and insulin sensitivity (20). People who do not participate in a regular exercise program or meet the minimal physical activity recommendations (30 minutes or more of accumulated moderate-intensity activity on most, or preferably all, days of the week to expend approximately 200 to 250 calories per day) in the U.S. Surgeon General's report have a positive risk factor for CAD (3).

Negative Coronary Risk Factors

A negative coronary risk factor suggests a favorable influence that may contribute to the development of a protective cardiac benefit (32). High-density lipoproteins appear to provide a protective mechanism against CAD by removing cholesterol from the body and preventing plaque from forming in the arteries. Research suggests that increases in HDLs are consistent with decreased risk for CAD (12). Thus, persons who have a serum HDL-cholesterol of ≥ 60 mg/dl improve their cholesterol profile and decrease the risk of CAD (3). If HDL-cholesterol is high (≥ 60 mg/dl), the personal trainer subtracts one risk factor from the sum of positive risk factors shown in table 9.1. The results of this evaluation of CAD risk factors will affect risk stratification and referral, discussed later in this chapter.

> The personal trainer must be able to identify and understand positive risk factors and their association with CAD, as well as the potential concerns as they relate to safety.

Identification of Medical Conditions and Diagnosed Disease

Identifying and understanding positive risk factors and their association with CAD, as well as the potential concerns that exist when these risk factors are present, is an important responsibility of the personal trainer in the screening process. However, equally critical is the ability to identify signs and symptoms of various chronic cardiovascular, pulmonary, metabolic, and orthopedic diseases that may contraindicate exercise and could potentially exacerbate an existing condition, thus leading to an adverse impact on the individual's health. Persons who have evidence of a known disease, have symptoms of cardiovascular disease, or are presently on medications to control disease require special attention because of the increased potential risk.

Coronary Artery and Pulmonary Disease

Personal history plays a fundamental role in the process of early detection of CAD. Signs and symptoms suggestive of CAD are important guides in identifying individuals who are at higher risk for the future development of disease. People who exhibit signs and symptoms of a personal history associated with CAD present special safety concerns as to the appropriateness of participating in an exercise program. The health appraisal screening mechanisms mentioned earlier are intended to initially identify signs and symptoms that have been previously diagnosed or personally detected. However, the personal trainer needs to use enhanced observation throughout the client consultation and health appraisal process to identify and assess signs and symptoms suggestive of cardiovascular and pulmonary disease that the client may exhibit. The major signs or symptoms suggestive of cardiovascular and pulmonary disease are as follows:

- Pain, discomfort (or other anginal equivalent) in the chest, neck, jaw, arms, or other areas that may be due to ischemia (lack of blood flow)
- Shortness of breath at rest or with mild exertion
- Dizziness or syncope (fainting)
- Orthopnea (the need to sit up to breathe comfortably) or paroxysmal (sudden, unexpected attack) nocturnal dyspnea (shortness of breath at night)
- Ankle edema (swelling, water retention)
- Palpitations or tachycardia (rapid heart rate)
- Intermittent claudication (calf cramping)
- Known heart murmur
- Unusual fatigue or shortness of breath with usual activities

Adapted from ACSM 2010 (3).

It is important for personal trainers to understand that these signs and symptoms must be interpreted in a clinical setting for diagnostic purposes and that they are not all specific to cardiovascular, pulmonary, and metabolic disease (9). However, if an individual exhibits these signs or symptoms, it is the role and responsibility of the personal trainer to take appropriate action by referring the client to a physician for a medical examination.

Various pulmonary diseases affect the respiratory system's ability to transport oxygen during exercise to the tissue level via the cardiovascular system. The systematic breakdown that occurs as a result of inadequate oxygen supply creates a greater than normal demand on the cardiorespiratory system, in some cases markedly reducing exercise tolerance. Chronic bronchitis, emphysema, and asthma are considered to be syndromes associated with **chronic obstructive pulmonary disease (COPD)** and are the most common diagnosed diseases related to respiratory dysfunction. Chronic bronchitis is an inflammatory condition caused by persistent production of sputum due to a thickened bronchial wall, which in turn creates a reduction of airflow. Emphysema is a disease of the lung that affects the small airways. An enlargement of air spaces accompanied by the progressive destruction of alveolar-capillary units leads to elevated pulmonary vascular resistance, which in most cases can contribute to heart failure. Asthma is mostly due to a spasmodic contraction of smooth muscle around the bronchi that produces swelling of the mucosal cells lining the bronchi and an excessive secretion of mucus. Constriction of airway paths associated with asthma results in attacks that may be caused by allergic reactions, exercise, air quality factors, and stress (8). (Chapter 20 provides detailed information.)

Risk of Sudden Cardiac Death

Sudden cardiac death related to exercise is caused by cardiac arrest that occurs instantaneously with an abrupt change in an individual's preexisting clinical state or within a few minutes of that change (48). Exercise does not typically provoke cardiovascular events in healthy individuals with normal cardiovascular systems (3). In fact, regular physical activity is strongly advocated by the medical community in part because substantial epidemiological, clinical, and basic science evidence suggests that physical activity and exercise training delay the development of atherosclerosis and reduce the incidence of coronary heart disease events (4). However, vigorous physical activity can acutely and transiently increase the risk of acute myocardial infarction and sudden cardiac death in susceptible individuals (4).

Both younger (<35 years) and older populations are at risk of sudden cardiac death. However the underlying causes vary. Among young individuals, the most frequent cardiovascular abnormalities leading to sudden cardiac death include **hypertrophic cardiomyopathy,** coronary artery anomalies, **aortic stenosis,** aortic dissection and rupture (typically related to **Marfan syndrome**), **mitral valve prolapse,** various heart arrhythmias, and **myocarditis.** In all these conditions except Marfan syndrome, where aortic rupture is often the cause, ventricular arrhythmias are the immediate cause of death (4).

Older, previously asymptomatic individuals who experience sudden cardiac death often show evidence of acute coronary artery plaque disruption with acute **thrombotic occlusion** (4).

A thorough history as part of the Health/Medical Questionnaire (p. 172) can help the personal trainer identify potential risks for sudden cardiac death. Identification of one or more of the following conditions should warrant a referral for a cardiovascular examination.

- Chest pain or discomfort with physical exertion
- Unexplained dizziness or fainting, particularly when associated with physical exertion
- Excessive and unexplained shortness of breath or fatigue associated with exercise
- Prior recognition of a heart murmur
- Elevated systemic blood pressure
- Family history of sudden and unexpected death before age 50 in more than one relative
- Family history of disability from heart disease before age 50 in a close relative
- Family history of hypertrophic cardiomyopathy, long-QT syndrome, Marfan syndrome, or heart arrhythmias

Adapted from American Heart Association Council on Nutrition, Physical Activity, and Metabolism 2007 (7).

These items are taken from the American Heart Association recommendations for screening competitive athletes. Sudden cardiac death associated with moderate to intense physical activity is more prevalent in the competitive athlete population compared with the general population, which is why current screening guidelines are in place for competitive athletes (7). However, the medical and family history questions used to screen competitive athletes also apply to the general population, although the chance of encountering a person in the general population with an increased risk of sudden cardiac death is much smaller.

It is important for the personal trainer to remember that signs and symptoms must be interpreted in a clinical setting for diagnostic purposes and that they are not all specific to sudden cardiac death. However, if an individual identifies one or more of these risk factors, it is the role and responsibility of the personal trainer to take appropriate action through the referral process by recommending a medical examination by a physician before initiating any type of activity (4).

Personal trainers must keep in mind that the causes of exercise-related sudden cardiac death events are not strictly separated by age. Younger individuals may exhibit signs of early onset of cardiovascular disease, while older individuals may present with structural congenital cardiac abnormalities (4). It is important to understand the potential risk factor(s) for each individual. For those with or at risk for coronary heart disease, the benefits of regular physical activity outweigh the risks of sudden cardiac death. However, for individuals with diagnosed or difficult-to-detect cardiac diseases, the health risks of vigorous physical activity almost always exceed the benefits (4).

> For most individuals, the benefits of regular physical activity outweigh the risks of sudden cardiac death. However, for those with diagnosed or difficult-to-detect cardiac diseases, the risks almost always outweigh the benefits.

Sudden cardiac death in any population is an uncommon yet catastrophic event. Just one death is still one too many if it could have been prevented. An absolute rate of exercise-related death among younger athletes has been estimated to be 1 per 133,000 men and 1 per 769,000 women (4). These estimates include all sport-related nontraumatic deaths and are not restricted to cardiovascular events. The rate of sudden cardiac death during vigorous physical activity for the older population has been estimated at 1 per year for every 15,000 to 18,000 people (3). Sudden cardiac death, especially in the younger population, has stirred quite a controversy regarding preparticipation screening guidelines. (42). As a personal trainer, it is important to include sudden cardiac death risk factors in the Health/Medical Questionnaire in order to identify individuals who may be at risk for sudden cardiac death. It is also important to advance all clients according to individual readiness. Sudden cardiac death at all ages is more prevalent in those who perform activity that they are not accustomed to (4).

Metabolic Disease

As mentioned earlier, an impaired fasting glucose level has been identified as a positive risk factor for CAD and a potential predictor for the development of diabetes. Diabetes mellitus, a metabolic disease, affects the body's ability to metabolize blood glucose properly. The disease is characterized by hyperglycemia resulting from defects in insulin secretion (type 1), insulin action (type 2), or both. Persons with type 1 diabetes are insulin dependent, meaning that they require insulin injections to metabolize glucose. Persons with type 2 diabetes in most cases are able to produce insulin, but the tissue resists it, and consequently glycemic control is inadequate. Diabetes is known to be an independent contributing factor in the development of cardiovascular disease, increasing the potential for CAD, peripheral vascular disease, and congestive heart failure (3). Although physical activity and exercise along with dietary modifications and prescribed medications appear to have an impact on the regulation of glucose levels, diabetes still requires ongoing medical attention and warrants precautions (39). Chapter 19 provides information on working with clients who have diabetes. In addition, diabetes in a client affects risk stratification and referral, which are discussed later in this chapter.

Orthopedic Conditions and Disease

Even though orthopedic limitations and disease do not appear to present the same relative risk as those associated with cardiovascular function, musculoskeletal concerns are an important factor for the personal trainer to consider in assessing an individual's functional capacity and may require a physician's referral before initiation of a program. Common musculoskeletal concerns related to acute trauma, overuse, osteoarthritis, and lower back pain present issues and challenges that may need to be assessed on a case-by-case basis. Although these conditions may limit performance and are important to the personal trainer, dealing with individuals who have rheumatoid arthritis, who have had recent surgery, or who have diagnosed degenerative bone disease may involve greater concerns because of the potential implications regarding advanced complications. Issues related to orthopedic replacements, recent surgical procedures, osteoporosis, and rheumatoid arthritis may require communication with a physician and in most cases medical clearance. (Chapter 21 provides detailed information.)

Medications

Individuals being treated by a physician on an ongoing basis may be taking prescribed medications as a therapeutic measure to manage a diagnosed condition or disease. The chemical reactions that occur in the body may influence physiological responses during activity. Various medications may alter heart rate, blood pressures, cardiac function, and exercise capacity. It is important for the personal trainer to understand the classes of commonly used drugs and their effects. For example, beta-blocking medications commonly prescribed for persons with high blood pressure may affect normal increases in heart rates during exercise; as a result, people will have difficulty obtaining, and should not strive to achieve, training heart rates. In addition, monitoring intensity of exercise by using heart rates may be inappropriate because of the masking effect of the medications on heart rates, and therefore ratings of perceived exertion would provide a more effective mechanism to regulate intensity levels of exercise (38).

Lifestyle Evaluation

Identifying an individual's behavioral patterns concerning choices about dietary intake, physical activity, and stress management provides additional information for assessing potential health risks associated with current lifestyle. Evidence clearly suggests a strong relationship between lifestyle choices regarding dietary intake, physical activity, and the management of stress on the one hand and the potential risk of CAD and other leading causes of morbidity and premature mortality on the other (41). The results of this evaluation may influence risk stratification and referral, discussed later in this chapter.

Dietary Intake and Eating Habits

Because of the significant contributory impact of nutritional habits on health and performance, the personal trainer should consider encouraging clients to evaluate their current daily intake. Identifying, quantifying, and assessing a person's daily dietary intake gives the personal trainer valuable information for assessing overconsumption, underconsumption, and caloric imbalances that may be contributing factors in the development of disease. There is a solid link between dietary intake and the development of disease. The most evident connection is between dietary saturated fat and cholesterol and the development of atherosclerosis (13). Excessive alcohol consumption has also been associated with an increased risk for cardiovascular disease; and diets high in sodium can lead to chronic elevation of systolic blood pressure or, more importantly, can result in worsening of heart failure (25). Overconsumption of caloric intake may contribute to obesity and diabetes, and underconsumption may lead to degenerative bone diseases and psychological health issues related to disordered eating. An analysis of a typical dietary intake through documentation of a three-day or seven-day dietary record may be a starting point for assessing the health-related value of the individual's eating habits. A dietary recall or diet history, as discussed in chapter 7, may also be used. The information obtained through these methods may be instrumental as one part of a collective process to identify potential concerns in relation to the risk for disease. See chapter 7 for detailed guidance about seeking information on and evaluating clients' nutrition habits. In addition, strategies and methods have been developed for recognizing and referring individuals who exhibit signs and symptoms related to disordered eating. (Chapter 19 provides details.)

Exercise and Activity Pattern

Identifying patterns of physical activity and exercise helps the personal trainer to recognize individuals with little or no history of physical activity or exercise. As discussed earlier, physical inactivity is a major contributing positive risk factor associated with the development of CAD and requires evaluation to assess potential concerns and level of risk. An evaluation of physical activity and exercise patterns should include identifying the specific activity and the frequency, volume, and level of intensity (moderate, vigorous) of that activity, as well as documenting signs or symptoms associated with the activity, particularly shortness of breath or chest pains. Any musculoskeletal concerns related to joint discomfort or chronic pain should also be identified.

Stress Management

Epidemiological studies provide evidence that stress is related to the risk for CAD (37). Several investigations have linked stress with an increase in heart disease. In addition, several prospective studies suggest that "type A" behavior patterns may contribute to the overall risk for developing CAD (10). "Type A" behavior pattern characteristics include hostility, depression, chronic stress produced by situations involving "high demand and low control," and social isolation (1, 40). These lifestyle stress-related characteristics can be measured psychosocially and physiologically through emotional stress inventories and standard exercise testing (11, 43). Because of the implications of stress and its impact on developing CAD, it is important for the personal trainer to be able to identify the common signs and symptoms of stress overload and to develop intervention strategies to reduce health risks. The "Health Risk Analysis" form on page 173 can be used to assess a client's potential for stress and response to stressors. This inventory is to be completed during the preparticipation health screening.

Once the preparticipation health appraisal screening is complete, the personal trainer should evaluate the client's positive risk factors associated with CAD, medical conditions and diagnosed disease, and current lifestyle. The results of this evaluation will be used for risk stratification.

Interpretation of Results

After the preparticipation health appraisal screening process has taken place and a review and evaluation of coronary risk factors, disease, and lifestyle are complete, the next step in the screening process is to identify individuals who may be at increased risk and to stratify that risk. Stratifying risk for potential health-related concerns is a preliminary step in determining the appropriateness of activity and identifying clients who require referral before beginning an exercise program. In order to meaningfully interpret the results obtained through the screening process, the personal trainer uses the PAR-Q results and the initial risk stratification method to identify people who have a greater potential for risk and may require referral and a clearance from a physician.

PAR-Q

As mentioned earlier, the PAR-Q is easy to administer and is a cost-effective mechanism for initially screening individuals who are apparently healthy and want to engage in regular low-intensity exercise. The PAR-Q has also been shown to be useful for referring individuals who require additional medical screening while not excluding those who may benefit from exercise. After eliciting objective *yes* or *no* answers to seven questions related to signs and symptoms associated with CAD, orthopedic concerns, and diagnosis by a physician, the self-administered questionnaire form provides direction based on interpretation of the results and specifies recommendations as to the appropriateness of activity and the referral process. Specific recommendations related to this form are discussed later in this chapter in the "Referral Process" section.

Initial Risk Stratification

The intent of the initial **risk stratification** method is to use age, health status, personal symptoms, and coronary risk factor information to initially classify individuals into one of three risk strata for preliminary decision-making purposes (3). Table 9.2 provides criteria for the risk stratification process. It is nearly impossible for any set of guidelines or method to address all the potential situations that may arise. However, using a decision-making process to evaluate the information obtained through the initial health appraisal screening process, the personal trainer should be able to classify an individual into one of the three risk categories. Case study 9.1 illustrates how the personal trainer might stratify risk using the initial risk stratification process. The personal trainer might obtain the relevant information during the preparticipation health appraisal screening interview.

> The ability to stratify risk gives the personal trainer the foundation to eventually identify whether it is appropriate to assess and train an individual or refer the individual to a physician for medical clearance.

TABLE 9.2 ACSM's Initial Risk Stratification Table

Low risk	Asymptomatic men and women who have ≤ one CVD risk factor from table 9.1
Moderate risk	Asymptomatic men and women who have ≥ two risk factors from table 9.1
High risk	Individuals with ■ known cardiac, peripheral vascular, or cerebrovascular disease; chronic obstructive pulmonary disease, asthma, interstitial lung disease, or cystic fibrosis; or diabetes mellitus (type 1 and 2), thyroid disorders, renal or liver disease, or ■ one or more of the following signs or symptoms: -Heart murmur -Unexplained fatigue -Dizziness or fainting -Swelling of the ankles -Fast or irregular heartbeat -Unexplained shortness of breath -Intermittent lameness or pain in calf muscles -Breathing discomfort when not in upright position, or interrupted breathing at night -Pain or discomfort in the jaw, neck, chest, arms, or elsewhere that could be caused by lack of circulation

Adapted from ACSM 2010 (3).

Case Study 9.1

Stratifying Risk

Presentation

Ralph D. is a sedentary 36-year-old male tool and die engineer. His father survived a heart attack at age 70. Ralph reports that his blood pressure has been recorded at 136/86 mmHg and that his total cholesterol is 250 mg/dl, with an HDL of 45 mg/dl. His BMI has recently been measured at 30, his hip circumference is 40 inches (102 cm), and his waist girth is 47 inches (119 cm). Ralph reports no signs or symptoms and indicates that he quit smoking seven months ago.

Analysis

An evaluation of this scenario leads to the conclusion that Ralph presently has three positive coronary risk factors: hypercholesterolemia (total cholesterol >200 mg/dl), sedentary lifestyle, and obesity (waist girth >39 inches or 100 cm; BMI of 30). Consequently, Ralph would be classified according to the stratification as being at moderate risk.

Referral Process

The processes described so far (preparticipation health appraisal screening; evaluation of coronary risk factors, disease, and lifestyle; and interpretation of the information obtained through the initial interview and client consultation process) are intended to help identify individuals who will need a referral to a health care professional for **medical clearance** prior to participating in activity. The following referral processes may be implemented to assess readiness and appropriateness for exercise.

Medical Examinations

Regular medical examinations to evaluate health status are normally encouraged for preventive purposes for everyone. It is also reasonable to recommend that persons beginning a new program of activity or exercise consult with a physician prior to participation (3).

PAR-Q Recommendations

After a client has completed the PAR-Q, the personal trainer can derive recommendations from the seven-question form through the following analysis. If the client gave a *yes* answer *to one or more questions* (which are related to signs and symptoms associated with CAD, orthopedic concerns, and diagnosis by a physician), it is recommended that the individual contact his or her physician and tell the physician which questions elicited *yes* answers before increasing physical activity and taking part in a fitness appraisal or assessment. The client should seek recommendations from the physician regarding the level and progression of activity and restrictions associated with his or her specific needs. If the client gave *no* answers *to all questions,* there is reasonable assurance that it is suitable for him or her to engage in a graduated exercise program and a fitness appraisal or assessment. Note also the PAR-Q recommendation that a client who is or may be pregnant talk with her doctor before she starts becoming more active. Chapter 18 provides guidance about conditions in which pregnant women should cease exercising or seek physician advice.

> A client must seek physician clearance for exercise testing and participation if he or she answers *yes* to any PAR-Q questions, exhibits any signs or symptoms of cardiovascular or pulmonary disease, is stratified as moderate risk and wants to participate in vigorous exercise, or is stratified as high risk and wants to participate in moderate or vigorous exercise.

Recommendations for Current Medical Examinations and Exercise Testing

Suggested guidelines have been developed for determining when a diagnostic medical examination and submaximal or maximal exercise tests are appropriate before participation in moderate and vigorous exercise, and when a physician's supervision is required to monitor these tests. Figure 9.1 provides the American College of Sports Medicine recommendations for current medical examinations and exercise testing prior to participation and physician

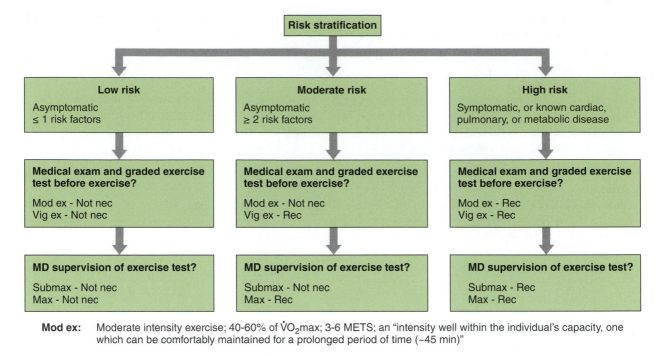

Mod ex: Moderate intensity exercise; 40-60% of $\dot{V}O_2$max; 3-6 METS; an "intensity well within the individual's capacity, one
           which can be comfortably maintained for a prolonged period of time (~45 min)"

Vig ex: Vigorous intensity exercise; >60% of $\dot{V}O_2$max; >6 METS; "exercise intense enough to represent a substantial
           cardiorespiratory challenge"

Not nec: Not necessary; a medical examination, exercise test, and physician supervision of exercise testing
           are not essential; however, they should not be viewed as inappropriate

Rec: Recommended; the MD should be in close proximity and readily available should there be an emergent need

FIGURE 9.1   Exercise testing and testing supervision recommendations based on risk stratification.
Reprinted by permission from ACSM 2010.

supervision of exercise tests (3). Guidelines and recommendations for medical examinations and exercise testing are interfaced with the initial risk stratification classifications for low, moderate, and high risk. The guidelines are consistent with the notion that as the intensity of the activity increases from moderate (40%-60% maximal oxygen uptake) to vigorous (>60% maximal oxygen uptake), there is a significant increase in potential risk for the participant. To help users better understand and interpret the recommended guidelines, figure 9.1 presents and defines the essential elements associated with medical examinations and exercise testing. The guidelines and recommendations for exercise testing clearly distinguish which exercise tests and stratification classifications require a physician's supervision. The personal trainer should note the difference between submaximal and maximal exercise tests in order to identify the appropriate recommendation regarding supervision. Submaximal and maximal exercise tests may be defined as follows:

A submaximal test is a nondiagnostic practical assessment, typically referred to as a *field test*, that is inexpensive, is easy to administer, and does not

normally require maximal effort. These tests are typically administered by certified personal trainers. It may also be necessary for a physician to be present at the testing if a patient is considered "high risk" (see table 9.2) in order to ensure the safety of the client. A maximal test is commonly performed in a clinical setting with use of specialized diagnostic equipment to assess an individual's functional capacity through maximal effort. Testing is relatively complex, and direct measurements are used to assess physiological responses. Because of the diagnostic capabilities and the high risk of cardiac complications, physicians often supervise the administration of these tests. The following recommendations apply to the levels of stratified risk (3):

Low risk: It is not necessary to have a current medical examination and an exercise test prior to participation in moderate and vigorous exercise. It is also not necessary for a physician to supervise a submaximal or maximal exercise test.

Moderate risk: It is not necessary to have a current medical examination and exercise test for moderate exercise; however, these are recommended for vigorous exercise. It is not necessary for a physician to supervise a submaximal exercise test, but physician supervision is recommended for a maximal test.

High risk: It is recommended that a current medical examination and exercise test be performed prior to moderate or vigorous exercise, and it is recommended that a physician supervise either a submaximal or a maximal exercise test.

The following case studies of information gained during the preparticipation health appraisal screening interview (case studies 9.2 through 9.4) provide examples of stratifying risk and making referrals based on recommendations for current medical examinations and exercise testing.

Medical Clearance

In the cases in which referral is considered necessary, it is the personal trainer's responsibility to encourage medical clearance as a reasonable and safe course of action. A recommendation to consult

---

Case Study 9.2

Moderate Risk Client

Presentation

Martha G. is a 56-year-old secretary. Her father died of an MI (myocardial infarction) at the age of 45. Martha reports that her LDL-cholesterol has been recorded at 125 mg/dl. Her BMI is 25. She reports that she has an active lifestyle that includes golf, tennis, and a daily walking routine.

Analysis

Martha has two positive coronary risk factors: age (over 55) and family history (her father died of an MI before the age of 55). She is thus classified as being at moderate risk. According to the guidelines and recommendations for medical examinations and exercise testing, it would not be necessary for Martha to have a current diagnostic medical examination and exercise test for moderate exercise; but these assessments would be recommended for vigorous exercise. In addition, it would not be necessary for a physician to supervise a submaximal test, but physician supervision would be recommended for a maximal test.

Case Study 9.3

High Risk Client

Presentation

Kathleen K. is a 47-year-old sedentary female. Kathleen reports a total cholesterol of 210 mg/dl with an HDL-cholesterol reading of 68 mg/dl. She stands five feet two inches (157 cm) tall, and her body weight is 110 pounds (50 kg) with a BMI of 20. Her blood pressure taken on two separate occasions is recorded as 120/80 mmHg. She reports that she was diagnosed with type 1 diabetes in early childhood.

Analysis

A review of the scenario shows that Kathleen has two positive coronary risk factors: a sedentary lifestyle and hypercholesterolemia (total cholesterol level >200 mg/dl). However, she presents an HDL-cholesterol level of 68 mg/dl, which gives her a negative risk factor (HDL-cholesterol >60 mg/dl) that cancels one of the positive risk factors—leaving her with one total positive risk factor. It would initially appear that her age (younger than 55) and one risk factor would classify her at low risk. However, the fact that she has been diagnosed with a metabolic disease (type 1 diabetes) places her in the stratification classification of high risk. Consequently, according to the guidelines and recommendations for medical examination and exercise testing, it would be necessary for Kathleen to have a diagnostic test and medical examination for both moderate and vigorous exercise. In addition, it would be recommended that a physician supervise both submaximal and maximal exercise tests.

Case Study 9.4

Effects of Family History

Presentation

Alex M. is a 20-year-old active male. He enjoys cycling, snow skiing, hiking, and running. On two separate occasions, Alex's blood pressure has been recorded as 145/85 mmHg. He stands six feet one inch (185 cm) tall, and his body weight is 176 pounds (80 kg) with a BMI of 23. He reports that his uncle died suddenly of unknown causes at the age of 34. Physicians determined that the cause of death was related to an unidentified heart condition. Alex's grandfather also died suddenly of unknown causes at the age of 47. No cause was ever determined.

Analysis

A review of the scenario shows that Alex has two risk factors for sudden cardiac death: blood pressure of 145/85 mmHg and a family history of sudden and unexpected death in two close family members before age 50, resulting from either a heart condition or unknown causes. Initially, with a healthy BMI, active lifestyle, and only one positive risk factor (high blood pressure), Alex would be classified as low risk. However, with the addition of Alex's family history, he is at an increased risk for sudden cardiac death. Based on recommendations, Alex would need to undergo a cardiovascular examination prior to initiating any physical activity under the supervision of the personal trainer.

with a physician prior to participation in an exercise program should not be considered an abdication of responsibility by the personal trainer, but rather a concerted effort to obtain valuable information and professional guidance to ensure safety and protection of the individual's health.

Physician Referral

Once medical clearance is recommended, the personal trainer should give the client a physician's referral form in order to obtain the necessary information about health status, physical limitations, and restrictions that would be required to make future fitness program recommendations. An example of a physician's referral form appears on page 178. The physician's referral form includes an assessment of the individual's functional capacity, a classification of ability to participate based on the evaluation, identification of preexisting conditions that may be worsened by exercise, prescribed medications, and fitness program recommendations. Chapter 25 includes discussion of the personal trainer's scope of practice as related to referral.

Program Recommendations

The physician recommendations provide the personal trainer with guidance and directions regarding what specific concerns and needs the individual has and which programs are appropriate. On the basis of the results obtained during the diagnostic medical examination and exercise tests, a physician may

recommend an unsupervised, supervised, or medically supervised exercise program.

- An unsupervised program is commonly recommended for people who are apparently healthy or presumably healthy with no apparent risks. This type of program recognizes the positive health-associated benefits that regular activity provides in relation to the relatively low risk involved in participation. These programs may be designed and initiated with the support of a personal trainer, the intended long-term eventual outcome being a combination of consistent weekly training sessions conducted by the personal trainer and other sessions that are self-directed and unsupervised.

- A supervised program may be recommended for people who have limitations or preexisting conditions that would restrict involvement but not limit participation. These programs are usually directed by a certified fitness professional, such as a certified personal trainer, who monitors intensity and modifies activity to meet the special concerns of the participant.

- A medically supervised program may be recommended for individuals who present a higher potential risk due to a predisposed condition, multiple risk factors, or an uncontrolled disease. These programs are directed and monitored by allied health professionals in clinical settings with immediately accessible emergency response capabilities.

Since there is no guarantee that the initial program recommendation resulting from a physician referral will meet the client's specific goals, it is important for those involved in the referral and recommendation process to monitor and readjust the program to ensure that it will be both safe and effective for the client.

> In cases in which referral is considered necessary, it is the personal trainer's responsibility to encourage medical clearance as a reasonable and safe course of action.

Conclusion

The client consultation and health appraisal process is directly in line with the scope of practice of the personal trainer to motivate, assess, train, educate, and refer when necessary. In order to develop programs of exercise that will safely and effectively meet the individual's objectives, the personal trainer needs to gather pertinent information and documentation that will be used to assess health status, evaluate potential for risk, and refer for medical clearance when necessary.

Study Questions

1. Which of the following should a personal trainer do during the initial meeting with a new client?

   I. Perform a submaximal bike test to estimate the client's $\dot{V}O_2$max.

   II. Have the client complete a medical history form.

   III. Evaluate the client's level of exercise readiness.

   IV. Discuss the client's goals for his or her exercise program.

   A. I and II only

   B. III and IV only

   C. I, II, and III only

   D. II, III, and IV only

2. Which of the following should be included in an informed consent?

   I. a summary of the client's testing results

   II. benefits associated with participation

   III. the client's exercise goals

   IV. responsibilities of the client

   A. I and III only

   B. II and IV only

   C. I, II, and III only

   D. II, III, and IV only

3. Which of the following factors discovered at a preparticipation health appraisal screening reveal a client's risk of coronary artery disease?

   I. HDL: 33 mg/dl

   II. family history: uncle died of stroke at age 42

   III. blood pressure: 128/88 mmHg; measured twice

   IV. quit smoking 60 days ago

   A. I and III only

   B. II and IV only

   C. I and IV only

   D. II and III only

4. Which of the following clients is in the highest risk stratification for coronary artery disease?

   A. 44-year-old male whose father died of a heart attack at 60 years of age

   B. 46-year-old male with a serum cholesterol reading of 205 mg/dl

   C. 48-year-old female with a BMI of 30

   D. 50-year-old female who has COPD

5. Which of the following conditions would indicate an increased risk for sudden cardiac death?

   I. disability from heart disease in a close relative >50 years of age

   II. prior recognition of a heart murmur

   III. sedentary lifestyle

   IV. unexplained shortness of breath and fatigue associated with exercise

   A. I and III only

   B. II and IV only

   C. I and IV only

   D. II and III only

Applied Knowledge Question

A 45-year-old sedentary male accountant wants to begin working with a personal trainer. After completing the initial interview and preparticipation health appraisal screening, the personal trainer learns the following information about the client:

Family history: both his father and grandmother had heart attacks at age 60

Cigarette smoking: nonsmoker

Resting blood pressure: 122/86 mmHg

Blood lipids: serum cholesterol 240 mg/dl; HDL 35 mg/dl

Fasting glucose: 100 mg/dl

BMI: 25

Evaluate and stratify his health status.

References

1. Almada, S.L., A.B. Zonderman, R.B. Shekelle, A.R. Dyer, M.L. Daviglus, P.T. Costa Jr., and J. Stamler. 1991. Neuroticism and cynicism and risk of death in middle-aged men: The Western Electric Study. *Psychosomatic Medicine* 53 (2): 165-175.

2. American College of Sports Medicine. 2006. *ACSM's Resource Manual for Guidelines for Exercise Testing and Prescription,* 5th ed. Baltimore: Williams & Wilkins.

3. American College of Sports Medicine. 2010. *ACSM's Guidelines for Exercise Testing and Prescription,* 8th ed. Philadelphia: Lippincott Williams & Williams.

4. American College of Sports Medicine, American Heart Association. 2007. Exercise and acute cardiovascular events: Placing the risks into perspective. *Medicine and Science in Sports and Exercise* 39 (5): 886-897.

5. American Diabetes Association. 1998. Report of the Expert Committee on the Diagnosis and Classification of Diabetes Mellitus. *Diabetes Care* 21: S5-S19.

6. American Heart Association. 2001. *2001 Heart and Stroke Statistical Update.* Dallas: American Heart Association.

7. American Heart Association Council on Nutrition, Physical Activity, and Metabolism. 2007. Recommendations and considerations related to preparticipation screening for cardiovascular abnormalities in competitive athletes: 2007 update: A scientific statement from the American Heart Association Council on Nutrition, Physical Activity, and Metabolism: Endorsed by the American College of Cardiology Foundation. *Circulation* 115 (12): 1643-1644.

8. American Thoracic Society. 1995. Standards for diagnosis and care of patients with chronic obstructive pulmonary disease. *American Journal of Respiratory and Critical Care Medicine* 152: S77-S120.

9. Brownson, R., P. Remington, and J. Davis, eds. 1998. *Chronic Disease Epidemiology and Control.* Washington, DC: American Public Health Association. pp. 379-382.

10. Burns, J., and E. Katkin. 1993. Psychological, situational, and gender predictors of cardiovascular reactivity to stress: A multi-variate approach. *Journal of Behavioral Medicine* 16: 445-466.

11. Carrol, D., J.R. Turner, and S. Rogers. 1987. Heart rate and oxygen consumption during mental arithmetic, video game, and graded static exercise. *Psychophysiology* 24 (1): 112-121.

12. Cholesterol: Up with the good. 1995. *Harvard Heart Letter* 5 (11): 3-4.

13. Committee on Diet and Health Food and Nutrition Board Co. 1989. *Diet and Health* 7.

14. Doll, R., and R. Peto. 1976. Mortality in relation to smoking: 20 years' observations on male British doctors. *British Medical Journal* 2: 1525-1536.

15. Donatelle, R.J. 2001. *Health: The Basics,* 5th ed. San Francisco: Benjamin Cummings.

16. Drought, H.J. 1990. Personal training: The initial consultation. *Conditioning Instructor* 1 (2): 2-3.

17. Expert Panel. 1998. Executive summary of the clinical guidelines on the identification, valuation, and treatment of overweight and obesity in adults. *Archives of Internal Medicine* 158: 1855-1867.

18. Expert Panel on Detection, Evaluation and Treatment of High Blood Cholesterol in Adults. 1993. Summary of the second report of the National Cholesterol Education Program (NCEP) Expert Panel on Detection, Evaluation and Treatment of High Blood Cholesterol in Adults (Adult Treatment Panel II). *Journal of the American Medical Association* 269: 3015-3023.

19. Faigenbaum, A.D., and W.L. Westcott. 2005. *Youth Strength Training,* 1st ed. Monterrey, CA: Healthy Learning Books and Videos.

20. Fletcher, G.F., G. Balady, S.N. Blair, J. Blumenthal, C. Caspersen, B. Chaitman, S. Epstein, E.S. Sivarajan Froelicher, V.F. Froelicher, I.L. Pina, and M.L. Pollock. 1996. Statement on exercise: Benefits and recommendations for physical activity programs for all Americans. A statement for health professionals by the Committee on Exercise and Cardiac Rehabilitation of the Council on Clinical Cardiology, American Heart Association. *Circulation* 94 (4): 857-862.

21. Glantz, S.A., and W.W. Parmley. 1996. Passive and active smoking. A problem for adults. *Circulation* 94 (4): 596-598.

22. Herbert, D.L. 1993. Medical, legal considerations for strength training for children. *National Strength and Conditioning Association Journal* 15 (6): 77.

23. Herbert, D.L., and W.G. Herbert. 1993. *Legal Aspects of Preventative and Rehabilitative Exercise Programs,* 3rd ed. Canton, OH: Professional Reports Corporation.

24. Hubert, H.B., M. Feinleib, P.M. McNamara, and W.P. Castelli. 1983. Obesity as an independent risk factor for cardiovascular disease: A 26-year follow-up of participants in the Framingham Heart Study. *Circulation* 67 (5): 968-977.

25. Joint National Committee on Detection, Evaluation, and Treatment of High Blood Pressure. 1993. The fifth report

of the Joint National Committee on Detection, Evaluation, and Treatment of High Blood Pressure (JNCV). *Archives of Internal Medicine* 153: 154-183.

26. Kannel, W.B., and T. Gordon. 1974. *The Framingham Study: An Epidemiological Investigation of Cardiovascular Disease.* Section 30. Public Health Service, NIH, DHEW Pub. No. 74-599. Washington, DC: U.S. Government Printing Office.

27. Klieman, C., and K. Osborne. 1991. *If It Runs in Your Family: Heart Disease: Reducing Your Risk.* New York: Bantam Books.

28. Kordich, J.A. 2000. Evaluating your client: Fitness assessment protocols and norms. In: *Essentials of Personal Training Symposium Study Guide.* Lincoln, NE: NSCA Certification Commission.

29. Last, J.M. 1988. *A Dictionary of Epidemiology,* 2nd ed. New York: Oxford University Press.

30. McInnis, K.J., and G.J. Balady. 1999. Higher cardiovascular risk clients in health clubs. *ACSM's Health and Fitness Journal* 3 (1): 19-24.

31. National Heart, Lung, and Blood Institute. 1993. National High Blood Pressure Education Program Working Group report on primary prevention of hypertension. *Archives of Internal Medicine* 153 (2): 186-208.

32. NIH Consensus Development Panel on Triglyceride, High Density Lipoprotein, and Coronary Heart Disease. 1993. Triglyceride, high-density lipoprotein, and coronary heart disease. *Journal of the American Medical Association* 269: 505-510.

33. NSCA-CPT Job Analysis Committee. 2001. *NSCA-CPT Content Description Manual.* Lincoln, NE: NSCA Certification Commission.

34. Olds, T., and K. Norton. 1999. *Pre-Exercise Health Screening Guide.* Champaign, IL: Human Kinetics.

35. Pasternak, R.C., S.M. Grundy, D. Levy, and P.D. Thompson. 1996. 27th Bethesda Conference: Matching the intensity of risk factor management with the hazard for coronary disease events. Task Force 3. Spectrum of risk factors for coronary heart disease. *Journal of the American College of Cardiology* 27 (5): 957-1047.

36. Physician and Sports Medicine. 2005. *Preparticipation Physical Evaluation,* 3rd ed. Minneapolis: McGraw-Hill.

37. Pieper, C., A. LaCroix, and R. Karasek. 1989. The relation of psychosocial dimensions on work with coronary heart disease risk factors: A meta-analysis of five United States databases. *American Journal of Epidemiology* 129: 483-494.

38. Pollock, M.L., D.T. Lowenthal, C. Foster, et al. 1991. Acute and chronic responses to exercise in patients treated with beta blockers. *Journal of Cardiopulmonary Rehabilitation* 11 (2): 132-144.

39. Report of the Expert Committee on the Diagnosis and Classification of Diabetes Mellitus. 1997. *Diabetes Care* 20 (7): 1183-1197.

40. Russek, L.G., S.H. King, S.J. Russek, and H.I. Russek. 1990. The Harvard Mastery of Stress Study 35-year follow-up: Prognostic significance of patterns of psychophysiological arousal and adaptation. *Psychological Medicine* 52: 271-285.

41. Schuler, G., R. Hambrecht, G. Schlierf, J. Niebauer, K. Hauer, J. Neumann, E. Hoberg, A. Drinkmann, F. Bacher, M. Grunze, et al. 1992. Regular physical exercise and low-fat diet: Effects on progression of coronary artery disease. *Circulation* 86 (1): 1-11.

42. Seto, G.K., and M.E. Pendleton. 2009. Preparticipation cardiovascular screening in young athletes: Current guidelines and dilemmas. *Current Sports Medicine Reports* 8 (2): 59-64.

43. Sims, J., and D. Carrol. 1990. Cardiovascular and metabolic activity at rest and during physical challenge in normotensives and subjects with mildly elevated blood pressure. *Psychophysiology* 27: 149-160.

44. The sixth report of the Joint National Committee on Prevention, Detection, Evaluation, and Treatment of High Blood Pressure (JNC VI). 1997. *Archives of Internal Medicine* 157: 2413-2446.

45. Thomas, S., J. Reading, and R.J. Shepard. 1992. Revision of the physical activity readiness questionnaire (PAR-Q). *Canadian Journal of Sport Sciences* 17: 338-345.

46. U.S. Department of Health and Human Services. 1989. *Report of the Expert Panel on Detection, Evaluation, and Treatment of High Blood Cholesterol in Adults.* Department of Health and Human Services, Public Health Services, NIH Pub. No. 89-2925. Washington, DC: U.S. Government Printing Office.

47. U.S. Department of Health and Human Services. 1996. *Physical Activity and Health: A Report of the Surgeon General.* Atlanta: U.S. Department of Health and Human Services, Centers for Disease Control and Prevention and Health Promotion.

48. Van Camp, S.P. 1992. Sudden death. *Clinics in Sports Medicine* 11 (2): 273-289.

The Attitudinal Assessment

The assessment should be viewed not only as an assessment of physical condition, but also as a gauge of attitude, outlook, and perspective. For each question, ask the client to rate him- or herself on a scale of 1 to 4. The first time you go through this exercise, your client might want to answer only the first section for each question (denoted with an asterisk [*]). You might come back whenever you feel the client is ready and complete the rest of each question. In the first part of each question, the assessment of where the client stands right now, the most motivated and driven athletes would likely have at least seven ratings of a 4 and not a single rating below a 3. Clients with three or more questions for which the answer was a 1 will need extra assistance to develop proper goals and may require frequent rewards, discussion, and education.

1. What would you consider your present attitude toward exercise?
1 - I can't stand the thought of it.
2 - I'll do it because I know I should, but I don't enjoy it.
3 - I don't mind exercise, and I know it is beneficial.
4 - I am motivated to exercise.

*Your answer: _____

How would you like to feel about exercise, if you could change your feelings?

Your answer: _____

Describe why and any specifics of how you would like to change your feelings about exercise and how those feelings might bring about positive change in your life:

2. What would you consider your present attitude toward goal achievement?
1 - I feel that whatever happens, happens, and I'll roll with the punches.
2 - I set goals and believe it adds clarity and gives me some control over my outcome.
3 - I write down my goals and believe it is a very valuable exercise in determining my future performance and achievement.
4 - I have written goals and I review them often. I believe I have the power to achieve anything I desire and know that setting goals is a vital part of achievement.

*Your answer: _____

How would you like to feel about goal achievement, if you could change your feelings?

Your answer: _____

Describe why and any specifics of how you would like to change your feelings about goal achievement and how those feelings might bring about positive change in your life:

3. How important to you are the concepts of health and well-being?
1 - I don't need to put any effort into bettering my health.
2 - I make certain I devote some time and effort into bettering my physical body.
3 - I am committed to maintaining and working to improve my health and physical well-being.
4 - My health and well-being are the foundation of all that I achieve, and they must remain my top priorities.

*Your answer: _____

How would you like to feel about the concepts of health and well-being, if you could change your feelings?

Your answer: _____

Describe why and any specifics of how you would like to change your feelings about the concepts of health and well-being and how those feelings might bring about positive change in your life:

4. How strong and driving is your desire for improvement?

1 - I'm really pretty satisfied with the way things are. Striving for improvement might leave me frustrated and disappointed.

2 - I'd like to improve but don't know that it's worth all the work involved.

3 - I love feeling as if I've bettered myself and am open to any suggestions for improvement.

4 - I'm driven to excel and am committed to striving for consistent and ongoing improvement.

*Your answer: _____

How strong and driven would you like to feel about improvement?

Your answer: _____

Describe why and any specifics of how you would like to change your feelings about improvement and how those feelings might bring about positive change in your life:

5. How do you feel about yourself and your abilities (self-esteem)?

1 - I am not comfortable with the way I look, feel, or perform in most situations.

2 - I would love to change many things about myself although I am proud of who I am.

3 - I'm very good at the things I must do, take pride in many of my achievements, and am quite able to handle myself in most situations.

4 - I have great strength, ability, and pride.

*Your answer: _____

How would you like to feel about yourself and your abilities, if you could change your feelings?

Your answer: _____

Describe why and any specifics of how you would like to change your feelings about yourself and your abilities and how those feelings might bring about positive change in your life:

6. How do you feel about your present physical condition in terms of the way you look?

1 - I would like to completely change my body.

2 - There are many things about my reflection in the mirror that I'm not comfortable with.

3 - For the most part I look OK, and I can look really good in the right clothing, but I do feel uncomfortable with a few things about my physical appearance.

4 - I am proud of my body and am comfortable in any manner of dress in appropriate situations.

*Your answer: _____

How would you like to feel about the way you look, if you could change your feelings?

Your answer: _____

Describe why and any specifics of how you would like to change your feelings about the way you look and how those feelings might bring about positive change in your life:

7. How do you feel about your present physical condition in terms of overall health?

1 - I wish I felt healthy.

2 - I feel healthy for my age compared to most people I meet.

3 - I maintain a high level of health.

4 - I am extremely healthy.

*Your answer: _____

How would you like to feel about yourself and your abilities, if you could change your feelings?

Your answer: _____

Describe why and any specifics of how you would like to change your feelings about yourself and your abilities and how those feelings might bring about positive change in your life:

(continued)

8. How do you feel about your physical condition in terms of your performance in any chosen physical fields of endeavor (sports, training, etc.)?

1 - I feel as if I'm in very poor condition and am uncomfortable when faced with a physical challenge.
2 - I am not comfortable with my performance abilities; however, I am comfortable training to improve.
3 - I feel pretty good about my ability to perform physically although I would like to improve.
4 - I have exceptional physical abilities and enjoy being called upon to display them.

*Your answer: _____

How would you like to feel about your performance, if you could change your feelings?

Your answer: _____

Describe why and any specifics of how you would like to change your feelings about your performance and how those feelings might bring about positive change in your life:

9. How strongly do you believe that you can improve your body?

1 - I believe most of my physical shortcomings are genetic, and most efforts to change would be a waste of time.
2 - I've seen many people change their bodies for the better and am sure with enough effort I can see some improvement.
3 - I strongly believe the proper combination of exercise and nutrition can bring about some improvement.
4 - I know without question that with the proper combination of exercise and nutrition I can bring about dramatic changes in my body.

*Your answer: _____

How would you like to feel about your ability to improve your body, if you could change your feelings?

Your answer: _____

Describe why and any specifics of how you would like to change your feelings about your ability to improve your body and how those feelings might bring about positive change in your life:

10. When you begin a program or set a goal, how likely are you to follow through to its fruition?

1 - I've never been real good at following things through to the end.
2 - With the right motivation and some evidence of results I think I might stick to a program.
3 - I have the patience and ability to commit to a program and will give it a chance in order to assess it value.
4 - Once I set a goal, there's no stopping me.

*Your answer: _____

How would you like to feel about following through on goals, if you could change your feelings?

Your answer: _____

Describe why and any specifics of how you would like to change your feelings about following through on goals and how those feelings might bring about positive change in your life:

From NSCA, 2012, *NSCA's essentials of personal training*, 2nd ed., J. Coburn and M. Malek (eds.), (Champaign, IL: Human Kinetics).

Personal Training Contract/Agreement

Congratulations on your decision to participate in an exercise program! With the help of your personal trainer, you greatly improve your ability to accomplish your training goals faster, safer, and with maximum benefits. The details of these training sessions can be used for a lifetime.

In order to maximize progress, it will be necessary for you to follow program guidelines during supervised and (if applicable) unsupervised training days. Remember, exercise and healthy eating are EQUALLY important!

During your exercise program, every effort will be made to assure your safety. However, as with any exercise program, there are risks, including increased heart stress and the chance of musculoskeletal injuries. In volunteering for this program, you agree to assume responsibility for these risks and waive any possibility for personal damage. You also agree that, to your knowledge, you have no limiting physical conditions or disability that would preclude an exercise program.

By signing below, you accept full responsibility for your own health and well-being AND you acknowledge an understanding that no responsibility is assumed by the leaders of the program.

It is recommended that all program participants work with their personal trainer three (3) times per week. However, due to scheduling conflicts and financial considerations, a combination of supervised and unsupervised workouts is possible.

Personal Training Terms and Conditions

1. Personal training sessions that are not rescheduled or canceled 24 hours in advance will result in forfeiture of the session and a loss of the financial investment at the rate of one session.

2. Clients arriving late will receive the remaining scheduled session time, unless other arrangements have been previously made with the trainer.

3. The expiration policy requires completion of all personal training sessions within 120 days from the date of the contract. Personal training sessions are void after this time period.

4. No personal training refunds will be issued for any reason, including but not limited to relocation, illness, and unused sessions.

Description of program:

Total investment: _____

Method of payment: _____

WE WISH YOU THE BEST OF LUCK ON YOUR NEW PERSONAL TRAINING PROGRAM!

_____
Participant's name (please print clearly)

_____   Date: _____
Participant's signature

_____   Date: _____
Parent/guardian's signature (if needed)

_____   Date: _____
Witness' signature

From NSCA, 2012, *NSCA's essentials of personal training*, 2nd ed., J. Coburn and M. Malek (eds.), (Champaign, IL: Human Kinetics).

Physical Activity Readiness
Questionnaire - PAR-Q
(revised 2002)

PAR-Q & YOU

(A Questionnaire for People Aged 15 to 69)

Regular physical activity is fun and healthy, and increasingly more people are starting to become more active every day. Being more active is very safe for most people. However, some people should check with their doctor before they start becoming much more physically active.

If you are planning to become much more physically active than you are now, start by answering the seven questions in the box below. If you are between the ages of 15 and 69, the PAR-Q will tell you if you should check with your doctor before you start. If you are over 69 years of age, and you are not used to being very active, check with your doctor.

Common sense is your best guide when you answer these questions. Please read the questions carefully and answer each one honestly: check YES or NO.

YES	NO	
❑	❑	1. Has your doctor ever said that you have a heart condition <u>and</u> that you should only do physical activity recommended by a doctor?
❑	❑	2. Do you feel pain in your chest when you do physical activity?
❑	❑	3. In the past month, have you had chest pain when you were not doing physical activity?
❑	❑	4. Do you lose your balance because of dizziness or do you ever lose consciousness?
❑	❑	5. Do you have a bone or joint problem (for example, back, knee or hip) that could be made worse by a change in your physical activity?
❑	❑	6. Is your doctor currently prescribing drugs (for example, water pills) for your blood pressure or heart condition?
❑	❑	7. Do you know of <u>any other reason</u> why you should not do physical activity?

If **you** **answered**

YES to one or more questions

Talk with your doctor by phone or in person BEFORE you start becoming much more physically active or BEFORE you have a fitness appraisal. Tell your doctor about the PAR-Q and which questions you answered YES.

- You may be able to do any activity you want — as long as you start slowly and build up gradually. Or, you may need to restrict your activities to those which are safe for you. Talk with your doctor about the kinds of activities you wish to participate in and follow his/her advice.
- Find out which community programs are safe and helpful for you.

NO to all questions

If you answered NO honestly to <u>all</u> PAR-Q questions, you can be reasonably sure that you can:

- start becoming much more physically active – begin slowly and build up gradually. This is the safest and easiest way to go.
- take part in a fitness appraisal – this is an excellent way to determine your basic fitness so that you can plan the best way for you to live actively. It is also highly recommended that you have your blood pressure evaluated. If your reading is over 144/94, talk with your doctor before you start becoming much more physically active.

DELAY BECOMING MUCH MORE ACTIVE:

- if you are not feeling well because of a temporary illness such as a cold or a fever – wait until you feel better; or
- if you are or may be pregnant – talk to your doctor before you start becoming more active.

PLEASE NOTE: If your health changes so that you then answer YES to any of the above questions, tell your fitness or health professional. Ask whether you should change your physical activity plan.

<u>Informed Use of the PAR-Q:</u> The Canadian Society for Exercise Physiology, Health Canada, and their agents assume no liability for persons who undertake physical activity, and if in doubt after completing this questionnaire, consult your doctor prior to physical activity.

No changes permitted. You are encouraged to photocopy the PAR-Q but only if you use the entire form.

NOTE: If the PAR-Q is being given to a person before he or she participates in a physical activity program or a fitness appraisal, this section may be used for legal or administrative purposes.

"I have read, understood and completed this questionnaire. Any questions I had were answered to my full satisfaction."

NAME _____

SIGNATURE _____ DATE _____

SIGNATURE OF PARENT _____ WITNESS _____
____or GUARDIAN (for participants under the age of majority)

Note: This physical activity clearance is valid for a maximum of 12 months from the date it is completed and becomes invalid if your condition changes so that you would answer YES to any of the seven questions.

© Canadian Society for Exercise Physiology   Supported by: [Canada flag] Health   Santé
                                                                    Canada   Canada

Health/Medical Questionnaire

Date: _____

Name: _____ Date of birth: _____ Soc. Sec. #: _____

Address: _____

                         Street   City   State   Zip

Phone (H): _____ (W): _____ E-mail address: _____

In case of emergency, whom may we contact?

Name: _____ Relationship: _____

Phone (H): _____ (W): _____

Personal physician

Name: _____ Phone: _____ Fax: _____

Present/Past History

Have you had OR do you presently have any of the following conditions? (Check if *yes*.)

- ___ Rheumatic fever
- ___ Recent operation
- ___ Edema (swelling of ankles)
- ___ High blood pressure
- ___ Injury to back or knees
- ___ Low blood pressure
- ___ Seizures
- ___ Lung disease
- ___ Heart attack
- ___ Fainting or dizziness with or without physical exertion
- ___ Diabetes
- ___ High cholesterol
- ___ Orthopnea (the need to sit up to breathe comfortably) or paroxysmal (sudden, unexpected attack) nocturnal dyspnea (shortness of breath at night)
- ___ Shortness of breath at rest or with mild exertion
- ___ Chest pains
- ___ Palpitations or tachycardia (unusually strong or rapid heartbeat)
- ___ Intermittent claudication (calf cramping)
- ___ Pain, discomfort in the chest, neck, jaw, arms, or other areas with or without physical exertion
- ___ Known heart murmur
- ___ Unusual fatigue or shortness of breath with usual activities
- ___ Temporary loss of visual acuity or speech, or short-term numbness or weakness in one side, arm, or leg of your body
- ___ Other

Family History

Have any of your first-degree relatives (parent, sibling, or child) experienced the following conditions? (Check if *yes*.) In addition, please identify at what age the condition occurred.

- ___ Heart arrhythmia
- ___ Heart attack
- ___ Heart operation
- ___ Congenital heart disease
- ___ Premature death before age 50
- ___ Significant disability secondary to a heart condition
- ___ Marfan syndrome
- ___ High blood pressure
- ___ High cholesterol
- ___ Diabetes
- ___ Other major illness _____

(continued)

Explain checked items: _____

_____

_____

Activity History

1. How were you referred to this program? (Please be specific.) _____

_____

2. Why are you enrolling in this program? (Please be specific.) _____

_____

3. Are you presently employed? Yes ___ No ___

4. What is your present occupational position? _____

5. Name of company: _____

6. Have you ever worked with a personal trainer before? Yes ___ No ___

7. Date of your last physical examination performed by a physician:

8. Do you participate in a regular exercise program at this time? Yes ___ No ___ If yes, briefly describe:

_____

9. Can you currently walk 4 miles briskly without fatigue? Yes ___ No ___

10. Have you ever performed resistance training exercises in the past? Yes ___ No ___

11. Do you have injuries (bone or muscle disabilities) that may interfere with exercising? Yes ___ No ___ If yes, briefly describe: _____

_____

12. Do you smoke? Yes ___ No ___ If yes, how much per day and what was your age when you started?

    Amount per day _____ Age _____

13. What is your body weight now? ____ What was it one year ago? ____ At age 21? ____

14. Do you follow or have you recently followed any specific dietary intake plan, and in general how do you feel about your nutritional habits? _____

_____

15. List the medications you are presently taking. _____

_____

16. List in order your personal health and fitness objectives.

    a. _____

    _____

    b. _____

    _____

    c. _____

    _____

From NSCA, 2012, *NSCA's essentials of personal training*, 2nd ed., J. Coburn and M. Malek (eds.), (Champaign, IL: Human Kinetics).

Health Risk Analysis Form

This health risk analysis form helps to identify positive and negative aspects of health behavior. Although many of the effects are based on real findings from large epidemiological investigations, the estimates are generalized and should not be taken too literally. Accurately predicting how long you will live or when you will die is impossible.

Plus one (+1) represents a positive effect that could add a year to your life or life to your years, and minus one (–1) indicates a loss in the quantity or quality of life. A zero (0) indicates no shortening or lengthening of your longevity. If none of the categories listed for a factor apply to you, enter 0. Complete each section and record the totals in section VIII.

Section I: Coronary Heart Disease (CHD) Risk Factors

Cholesterol or total cholesterol to HDL ratio					Score
<160	160–200	200–240	240–280	>280	
<3	3–4	4–5	5–6	>6	
+2	+1	–1	–2	–4	

Blood pressure (choose your highest number for either value)					Score
<110	110–120	120–150	150–170	170	
60–80	60–80	80–90	90–100	>100	
+1	0	–1	–2	–4	

Smoking					Score
Never	Quit	Smoke cigar or pipe or close family member smokes	One pack of cigarettes daily	Two or more packs daily	
+1	0	–1	–3	–5	

Heredity					Score
No family history of CHD	One close relative over 60 with CHD	Two close relatives over 60 with CHD	One close relative under 60 with CHD	Two or more close relatives under 60 with CHD	
+2	0	–1	–2	–4	

Body mass index (BMI, use table 11.8 on page 236)					Score
19–25	<19	26–30	31–40*	>40*	
+2	0	–1	–3	–5	

*If waist is under 40 in. (102 cm) subtract one less (e.g., –2 or –4).

Gender					Score
Female under 55 years	Female over 55 years	Male	Stocky male	Bald, stocky male	
0	–1	–1	–2	–4	

Stress					Score
Phlegmatic, unhurried, generally happy	Ambitious but generally relaxed	Sometimes hard-driving, time-conscious, competitive	Hard-driving, time-conscious, competitive (type A)	Type A with repressed hostility	
+1	0	0	–1	–3	

Physical activity					Score
High intensity, 60 min most days	Moderate, 30 min most days	Moderate, 20–30 min, 3–5 times per week	Light, 10–20 min, 1–2 times per week	Little or none	
+3	+2	+1	–1	–3	

TOTAL: I. CHD risk factors					

(continued)

Section II: Health Habits (Related to Good Health and Longevity)

Breakfast					Score
Daily	Sometimes	None	Coffee	Coffee and doughnut	
+1	0	−1	−2	−3	
Regular meals					**Score**
Three or more	Two daily	Not regular	Fad diets	Starve and stuff	
+1	0	−1	−2	−3	
Sleep					**Score**
7–8 hr	8–9 hr	6–7 hr	>9 hr	<6 hr	
+1	0	0	−1	−2	
Alcohol					**Score**
None	Women 3/wk	Men 1–2 daily	3–6 daily	>6 daily	
+1	+1	+1	−2	−4	
TOTAL: II. Health habits					

Section III: Medical Factors

Medical exam and screening tests (blood pressure, diabetes, glaucoma)					Score
Regular tests, see doctor when necessary	Periodic medical exam and selected tests	Periodic medical exam	Sometimes get tests	No tests or medical exams	
+1	+1	0	0	−1	
Heart					**Score**
No history of problems, self or family	Some history	Rheumatic fever as child, no murmur now	Rheumatic fever as a child, have murmur	Have ECG abnormality or angina pectoris	
+2	0	−1	−2	−3	
Lung (including pneumonia and tuberculosis)					**Score**
No problem	Some past problem	Mild asthma or bronchitis	Emphysema, severe asthma, or bronchitis	Severe lung problems	
+1	0	−1	−1	−3	
Digestive tract					**Score**
No problem	Occasional diarrhea, loss of appetite	Frequent diarrhea or stomach upset	Ulcers, colitis, gall bladder, or liver problems	Severe gastrointestinal disorders	
+1	0	−1	−2	−3	
Diabetes					**Score**
No problem or family history	Controlled hypoglycemia (low blood sugar)	Hypoglycemia and family history	Mild diabetes (diet and exercise)	Diabetes (insulin)	
+1	0	−1	−2	−4	
Drugs					**Score**
Seldom take	Minimal but regular use of aspirin or other drugs	Heavy use of aspirin or other drugs	Regular use of mood-altering or psychogenic drugs	Heavy use of mood-altering or psychogenic drugs	
+1	0	−1	−2	−3	
TOTAL: III. Medical factors					

Section IV: Safety Factors

Driving in car					Score
<7,000 mi (11,000 km) per year, mostly local	7,000–10,000 mi (11,000–16,000 km) per year, local and some highway	10,000–15,000 mi (16,000–24,000 km) per year, local and high-way	>15,000 mi (24,000 km) per year, highway and some local	>15,000 mi (24,000 km) per year, mostly highway	
+1	0	0	–1	–2	

Using seat belts					Score
Always	Most of time (>75%)	On highway only	Seldom (<25%)	Never	
+1	0	–1	–2	–4	

Risk-taking behavior (Motorcycle, skydive, mountain climb, fly small plane, etc.)					Score
Some with careful preparation	Never	Occasional	Often	Try anything for thrills	
+1	0	–1	–1	–2	
TOTAL: IV. Safety factors					

Section V: Personal Factors

Diet					Score
Low fat, low calories	Balanced complex carbohydrate	High protein, limited fat	Extra calories, low carbohydrate	Fad diets and fat	
+2	+1	Unknown.	–1	–2	

Longevity					Score
Grandparents lived past 90, parents past 80	Grandparents lived past 80, parents past 70	Grandparents lived past 70, parents past 60	Few relatives lived past 60	Few relatives lived past 50	
+2	+1	0	–1	–3	

Love and marriage					Score
Happily married	Married	Unmarried	Divorced	Extramarital relationship(s)	
+2	+1	0	–1	–3	

Education					Score
Postgraduate or master craftsman	College graduate or skilled craftsman	Some college or trade school	High school graduate	Grade school graduate	
+1	+1	0	–1	–2	

Job satisfaction					Score
Enjoy job, see results, room for advancement	Enjoy job, see some results, able to advance	Job OK, no results, nowhere to go	Dislike job	Hate job	
+1	+1	0	–1	–2	

Social					Score
Have some close friends	Have some friends	Have no good friends	Stuck with people I don't enjoy	Have no friends at all	
+1	0	–1	–2	–3	

Race					Score
White or Asian	Black or Hispanic	American Indian			
0	–1	–2			
TOTAL: V. Personal factors					

(continued)

Section VI: Psychological Factors

Outlook					Score
Feel good about present and future	Satisfied	Unsure about present or future	Unhappy in present, don't look forward to future	Miserable, rather not get out of bed	
+1	0	−1	−2	−3	
Depression					**Score**
No family history of depression	Some family history, feel OK	Family history and mildly depressed	Sometimes feel life isn't worth living	Thoughts of suicide	
+1	0	−1	−2	−3	
Anxiety					**Score**
Seldom anxious	Occasionally anxious	Often anxious	Always anxious	Panic attacks	
+1	0	−1	−2	−3	
Relaxation					**Score**
Relax or meditate daily	Relax often	Seldom relax	Usually tense	Always tense	
+1	0	−1	−2	−3	
TOTAL: VI. Psychological factors					

Section VII: For Women Only

Health care					Score
Regular breast and Pap tests	Occasional breast and Pap tests	Never have exams	Treated disorder	Untreated cancer	
+1	0	−1	−2	−4	
Birth control pill					**Score**
Never used	Quit 5 years ago	Still use, under 30 years	Use pill and smoke	Use pill, smoke, over 35	
+1	0	0	−2	−3	
TOTAL: VII. For women only					

Section VIII: Scoring Summary

You can now estimate your longevity. Add your total score from the previous sections to your normal life expectancy (from the chart below) to find your longevity estimate. If you would like to improve your longevity estimate, go back and decide on some lifestyle areas you would like to improve.

Category		Score (+ or − from previous sections)
I.	CHD risk factors	_____
II.	Health habits	_____
III.	Medical factors	_____
IV.	Safety factors	_____
V.	Personal factors	_____
VI.	Psychological factors	_____
VII.	For women only	_____
Total		_____ + _____ = _____
		Total from sections I-VII Life expectancy (from the following table)

Life Expectancy

Nearest age	EXPECTANCY (ALL RACES)	
	Male	Female
20	76.1	81.0
25	76.5	81.1
30	76.9	81.3
35	77.2	81.4
40	77.6	81.7
45	78.1	82.0
50	78.8	82.5
55	79.7	83.0
60	80.7	83.8
65	82.0	84.7
70	83.6	85.9

From NSCA, 2012, *NSCA's essentials of personal training*, 2nd ed., J. Coburn and M. Malek (eds.), (Champaign, IL: Human Kinetics). Adapted, by permission, from B. Sharkey and S. Gaskill, 2007, *Fitness and health*, 6th ed. (Champaign, IL: Human Kinetics), 64-68; Data from Life Expectancy from CDC, National Vital Statistics Reports, June 2010.

Physician's Referral Form Pertaining to a Fitness Evaluation and Preventive Program of Exercise

Dear Doctor:

Your patient _____ has contacted us regarding the fitness evaluation conducted by _____. The program is designed to evaluate the individual's fitness status prior to embarking on an exercise program. From this evaluation, an exercise prescription is formulated. In addition, other parameters related to a health improvement program are discussed with the participant. It is important to understand that this program is preventive and is not intended to be rehabilitative in nature.

The fitness testing includes: _____
_____
_____

A comprehensive consultation will be provided to the participant that serves to review the test results and explain recommendations for an individualized fitness program.

A summary of test results and our recommendations will be kept on file and may be made available to you upon request.

In the interest of your patient and for our information, please complete the following:

A. Has this patient undergone a physical examination within the last year to assess functional capacity to perform exercise? Yes ___ No ___

B. I consider this patient (please check one):

___ Class I: presumably healthy without apparent heart disease eligible to participate in an unsupervised program

___ Class II: presumably healthy with one or more risk factors for heart disease eligible to participate in a supervised program

___ Class III: patient not eligible for this program, and a medically supervised program is recommended

C. Does this patient have any preexisting medical/orthopedic condition(s) requiring continued or long-term medical treatment or follow-up? Yes ___ No ___

Please explain: _____
_____

D. Are you aware of any medical condition(s) that this patient may have or may have had that could be worsened by exercise? Yes ___ No ___

E. Please list any currently prescribed medication(s): _____
_____
_____

F. Please provide specific recommendations and/or list any restrictions concerning this patient's present health status as it relates to active participation in a fitness program. _____
_____
_____
_____

Comments: _____
_____
_____

Referring physician's signature: _____

Date: _____ Client's name: _____

Phone (H): _____ Phone (W): _____

Address: _____ _____

From NSCA, 2012, *NSCA's essentials of personal training,* 2nd ed., J. Coburn and M. Malek (eds.), (Champaign, IL: Human Kinetics).

Fitness Assessment Selection and Administration

Sharon Rana, PhD, and Jason B. White, PhD

After completing this chapter, you will be able to

- explain the purposes of performing physical assessments on a client,

- evaluate a test's validity and reliability,

- apply risk stratification criteria to an individual client to determine suitability for specific tests, and

- select appropriate tests for individual clients.

After conducting the client consultation and health appraisal, the personal trainer needs to gather more information about the client's current level of fitness and skills before developing a program. There is no "one size fits all" test or battery of assessments that will suit each client and circumstance. Selecting appropriate physical assessments requires thoughtful consideration of the client's health and exercise history, personal goals, and the personal trainer's own experience and training in conducting various assessments. Choosing valid and reliable tests suitable for individual clients and conducting them accurately requires practice on the part of the personal trainer. The availability and appropriateness of equipment and facilities, environmental factors, and the client's pre-assessment preparation influence test selection and implementation. Having determined the assessment protocols, the personal trainer must conduct them accurately, record and manage the data, and interpret the results. Communicating the results to the client in an individualized program that incorporates his or her goals and interests is the "personal" in personal training. Implementation of the program requires formative and summative evaluation of the program, reassessment of the client's fitness levels and goals, and subsequent adjustments to the program in an ongoing cycle.

The authors would like to acknowledge the contributions of John A.C. Kordich and Susan L. Heinrich, who wrote this chapter for the first edition of NSCA's Essentials of Personal Training.

Chapter 10

Purposes of Assessment

The purposes of assessment are to gather baseline data and to provide a basis for developing goals and effective exercise programs. Gathering and evaluating the various pieces of information give the personal trainer a broader perspective of the client. The process and the data collected assist the trainer in identifying potential areas of injury and reasonable starting points for recommended intensities and volumes of exercise based on the goals and fitness outcomes.

Gathering Baseline Data

There are many valid reasons for administering assessments to clients. The data collected provide

- a baseline for future comparisons of improvement or rate of progress;
- identification of current strengths and weaknesses that may affect program emphasis on specific components;
- assistance in establishing appropriate intensities and volumes of exercise;
- assistance in clarification of short-, intermediate-, and long-term goals;
- identification of areas of potential injury or contraindications prior to program initiation, which may lead to referral to a physician or other health care professionals; and
- a record demonstrating prudent judgment and appropriate scope of practice in program design should client injuries develop after a program has begun (22, 37).

The assessment process may fall within the services typically provided to all clients, may constitute an additional revenue stream for the personal trainer, or may do both. However, subjecting clients to a seemingly endless barrage of assessments that have little or no relevance to their program goals is a violation of the trust the client places in the personal trainer to gather necessary information to design a program.

Goal and Program Development

The personal trainer can use physical assessment information in conjunction with personal information gathered about the client to plan a time-efficient, specific program that will help the client achieve his or her goals. Understanding personal characteristics and current lifestyle factors about the client helps the personal trainer plan sessions that are reasonable in length, frequency, intensity, and complexity so that the client is more likely to continue adhering to the program. Developing goals with a client is critical for both program design and motivation. (Refer to chapter 8 for more details on motivating clients.)

When possible and appropriate, choosing specific tests that are congruent with clients' goals or preferred mode of exercise may give them a clearer picture of their progress and may be more motivating. For highly trained clients, choosing an exercise ergometer that most closely matches their mode of exercise (treadmill, cycle, swim flume) leads to a more accurate assessment of their performance (6, 18, 56). For average or deconditioned clients, the type of test is not as much of a factor in assessing aerobic function; however, a treadmill test will usually produce the highest maximal $\dot{V}O_2$ scores (34, 35). Clients who seldom if ever ride a bike may experience local muscular fatigue and as a result achieve a lower estimated $\dot{V}O_2$max value on a bike test compared to a treadmill test (20, 34). In addition, if clients are tested on a cycle ergometer but will not be riding a bike in their program, they may overlook some of the indicators of their improved performance during the training period.

A timed mile can be easily repeated on occasion during a walking program; if the client can cover the distance more quickly or easily with a lower exercise heart rate or rating of perceived exertion (RPE), the client knows immediately that he or she is making progress. In this instance an appropriate test may match the type of activity the client enjoys doing. However, for clients who are overweight or who have lower body joint issues that make weight-bearing activities painful, the advantages of a non-weight-bearing cycle test may override any concerns about slightly lower estimates of maximal oxygen consumption. Additionally, since cycling tests give results independent of body weight, they are more accurate indicators of progress for a person on a weight loss program than is a treadmill test, whose results are directly related to an individual's body weight (31, 56). Assessment of health- or skill-related fitness components, or both, provides the personal trainer and client with baseline information that will be used to develop safe, effective, and appropriately challenging goals.

Choosing Appropriate Assessments

A primary duty of the personal trainer is to facilitate improvements in the client's physical well-being without causing harm. With the exception of assessing cardiovascular disease risk factors, there is no standardized battery of tests one can give each client before designing an appropriate program (25, 43, 51). The first step in individualizing the personal trainer's approach to each client is determining the specific tests to give to measure various parameters of health- and skill-related fitness. Those decisions are made based on the client's apparent health and level of cardiovascular disease risk, as well as the desired program outcomes expressed by the client. In order for the personal trainer to conduct meaningful assessments, appropriate tests must be chosen. Given the wide range of fitness tests available, it is wise for the personal trainer to become educated about which assessments provide the best information for a given client. Assessment is the act of measuring a specific component using a well-constructed, valid, and reliable test and then evaluating and interpreting the results (34). If the evaluation is done in accordance with the client's goals, the results will be more meaningful to the client. Assessment can be formal, following specific test protocols, or informal, through observation of the client performing specific activities and exercises.

Formative and Summative Evaluation

There are two ways of looking at assessments—as formative or summative evaluations. Formative evaluations include formal assessment with a specified **test protocol,** as well as the subjective observations the personal trainer makes during each interaction with the client. The formative assessments take place before a program begins and periodically throughout the training period. They offer the personal trainer opportunities to *formulate* or plan a program, give the client feedback, and make modifications to the program while it is still in progress.

Although this chapter concerns selecting the specific assessment instruments, it is important to keep in mind that *every* observation of a client provides important data about the client that the personal trainer must consider in designing, implementing, and modifying that client's program. Subjective observations are variable between evaluators and might include noticing posture, gait, exercise technique, response to cardiovascular exercise, comments or body language relating to specific exercises or suggestions, and daily energy levels in each exercise session. These provide immediate opportunities for the personal trainer to focus on educating, motivating, and modifying activities for the client. Data from specific test protocols provide

objective evidence that the personal trainer can compare to relevant standards to interpret the client's performance.

Summative evaluations are final evaluations made when a client completes a specified training period, class, or season. They represent the *sum total* of what has been accomplished in a given period. The same assessments used at the beginning and midpoint of an exercise program can and generally should be used to provide the final evaluation, but how the results are used will differ. For example, if a client has a flexibility goal for a specific joint, the formative evaluation would have included an initial measurement of the range of motion in the joint and a realistic goal for improved flexibility of that joint. The program might include a variety of stretching techniques for that joint with periodic repetitions of the test so the client knows the amount of progress he or she is making toward the goal. At the end of the specified period, the same test is repeated under similar conditions, and the client and personal trainer can determine whether the stated goals were achieved in that time: This evaluation is a *summary* of what was achieved during the specified training period.

Assessment Terminology

Before selecting tests to use with a specific client, the personal trainer must have an understanding of the terminology specific to tests, measurements, and evaluation, and to some extent of the process by which tests are developed. The purpose of this chapter is not to list or explain all of the possible choices of assessment instruments available for each health- and skill-related component and each type of client—sedentary, athletic, healthy, or medically compromised. As new research and tests are reported, personal trainers need to evaluate new information and decide whether it has a place in the battery of tests used for their particular clientele. A test may be excellent in terms of validity and reliability but still not be appropriate for a specific client—for example, a near-maximal exertion running test would not be appropriate for a deconditioned adult (25, 40). Additionally, although some tests may be excellent for measuring a specific component or trait, they may require equipment, facilities, or expertise that the personal trainer does not have (e.g., hydrostatic weighing). Conversely, the fact that a particular piece of equipment or computer-generated test battery is available does not make it appropriate for all clients. For example, if a client is visibly obese, it might not be necessary or accurate to assess body composition via the skinfold method, but it would be fine to simply use body mass index until weight loss occurs. The personal trainer must sort through the information and select tests appropriate to each client while recognizing that some clients will be more interested in personal progress than in multiple formal assessments. The objective of the personal trainer in selecting assessments for the client is to reduce error and increase the accuracy of the assessment. Questions to answer in attempting to improve the accuracy of a test include the following:

- How reliable and objective was the assessment?
- Was it valid?
- Was the equipment calibrated and did it produce accurate results?
- Was the subject physically or emotionally influenced by anything before or during the test that may have affected the results?
- Was the test protocol followed carefully and were data collected accurately?

When these factors receive adequate attention, the personal trainer may confidently and accurately interpret data and apply the results.

Reliability and Objectivity

Reliability is a measure of repeatability or consistency of a test or an observation (34). To determine if a measurement is reliable, one must measure the same trait under the same conditions, with no intervention (e.g., physical conditioning, diet) before a subsequent measurement is performed. If the results of the test are the same from one trial to another, the test is reliable. A common method of determining reliability of a test is the **test–retest method.** This is when a test is repeated with the same individual or group within one to three days, and sometimes up to one week later if the test is particularly strenuous (50). In order for a test to be reliable, the person conducting the test must be consistent in his or her administration of it. This is called *intrarater reliability* and can be determined as just described. However, a personal trainer could be consistent but not accurate. Therefore, scores collected by different personal trainers on the same client without intervention should be compared in order to determine interrater reliability or objectivity (5, 34, 50). If more than one personal trainer can consistently get the same result from a client, the test is objective rather than subjective. It is not practical to test a client multiple times per day or week on the same assessment, so the personal trainer must look for assessments that were proven to have good reliability when they were developed. However, the

fact that an assessment had good reliability when developed is meaningless if the personal trainer does not take the time to practice giving the assessment under very strict and standardized conditions (13). Factors affecting reliability will be discussed in a following section; those that have to do with the personal trainer can include competence, confidence, concentration on the task, familiarity with the instrument, and motivation (6).

Validity

Validity indicates that a test measures what it is supposed to measure (50). In other words, is the test score a "truthful" score (34)? Does the assessment instrument really test what it claims to be testing? For example, when selecting a test for aerobic capacity, one must choose a test that is long enough and is sufficiently intense to require provision of energy primarily from the aerobic system. Therefore, the 50 m dash sprint test would not give a valid or truthful measure of aerobic capacity ($\dot{V}O_2max$). For a test to be valid, it must also be relevant (34). The relevance indicates how well the test matches the objectives of testing. In the example just mentioned, a test of speed is not relevant for assessing aerobic capacity. A body mass index (BMI) measurement is a relevant indicator of overweight status in a fairly sedentary population, but it is not relevant to a group of athletes with increased lean muscle mass and a low percentage of body fat (23, 26, 41). *Face validity*, then, means that the test appears to test what it is supposed to test (21, 50). In this sense, a 1RM (1-repetition maximum) test is a valid measure of muscular strength, but not muscular flexibility. A related term is *content validity*, which indicates that an expert has determined that a test covers all topics or abilities that it should (21, 50). For example, a volleyball athlete should be tested on more than just jumping ability in order to cover all skills performed in that particular sport.

Construct validity is a theoretical concept meaning that a test is able to differentiate between performance abilities. In other words, if a test is a sport skill-related test, those with the given sport skills should score better on the test than those who take the test without having previously acquired the skills (21, 34, 50).

Criterion-related validity allows personal trainers to use tests in the field or in the fitness center, instead of tests that can be performed only in a laboratory setting or with expensive equipment, because the laboratory test results and field test results have been statistically compared with each other (34). A maximal-exertion stress test should be given only in a tightly controlled environment, with medical personnel and equipment on hand (40, 42,

51). Since that is not practical in a fitness center setting, personal trainers can select a submaximal cardiovascular endurance test, such as a treadmill test, a step test, or a cycle ergometer test that has been statistically correlated to the maximal exertion tests on the basis of certain assumptions. The assumptions are that the more fit the individual is, the more work she or he should be able to do at a given heart rate and the more total work he or she should be able to perform before reaching maximal heart rate (51). The results on the submaximal tests are not precisely the same as those on the maximal test, nor will the estimated $\dot{V}O_2max$ score on different types of submaximal tests identically match each other. However, if the margin of error between the submaximal and maximal tests is small and the test is reliable and valid, then it is a good test. The following should serve as an example of these points.

Hydrostatic weighing is an **indirect measure** or estimate of body fatness, based on the assumption that the body is made up of fat mass and fat-free mass (23, 55). An autopsy is a **direct measure,** but because it cannot be used on living individuals it is not a useful measure. Other common methods (field methods) of assessing body composition such as skinfold assessments, bioelectrical impedance (BIA), near-infrared interactance (NIR), or anthropometric measures, are doubly indirect (12). This means that the statistical relationship is with hydrostatic weighing and that the standard error of estimating body composition is established against hydrostatic weighing, not against the direct method. The error involved in assessing body composition with a doubly indirect test may be higher than with an indirect test. Also, when a specific test is selected to assess a client, the same test should be used for any further testing of the given fitness component. A skinfold estimate of body fatness cannot be reliably compared to an estimate made by means of BIA or NIR, for example (23). (See chapter 11 for further discussion.)

> A valid test is one that measures what it purports to measure. A reliable test is one that can be repeated with accuracy, by the same tester or another. A good assessment instrument is both valid and reliable.

Factors That Affect Reliability and Validity

All tests have a **standard error of measurement.** This is the difference between a person's observed score—what the result was—and that person's true score, a theoretically errorless score. For example,

when choosing to assess body composition using the skinfold technique, a personal trainer will never know the client's actual percent fat (true score), but instead will only be able to estimate the percent fat (observed score) knowing that this estimation will involve some error. Empirically any test result consists of a true score and error. All test results contain the true value of the factor being measured as well as the errors associated with the test itself. Measurement error can arise from several sources, including the client, the personal trainer, the equipment, or the environment (34).

Client Factors

In the process of identifying and selecting appropriate tests, it is important to consider factors that may influence client performance and subsequently have an impact on the validity and the reliability of the assessment results. The key client factors to consider in selecting tests include health status and functional capacity, age, sex, and pretraining status.

Health Status and Functional Capacity The health status and functional capacity of a client dictate which assessments are appropriate. Information gathered during the preparticipation screening process (see chapter 9) should be used to identify potential physical limitations. Understanding those limits provides a context for selecting assessments that will reasonably match the capabilities of the individual. As an example, if an individual is sedentary, over the age of 60, and has a functional aerobic capacity of 5 METs (MET = metabolic equivalent; 1 MET is equal to an oxygen consumption of $3.5 \ ml \cdot kg^{-1} \cdot min^{-1}$ and is an estimate of a person's oxygen consumption at rest), it may be unreasonable for that person to perform the YMCA step test or 1.5-mile (2.4 km) run. Both of these assessments may require a greater metabolic level of performance than 5 METs and in some instances may be considered near-maximal tests for deconditioned individuals (2, 25, 51). Also, client fatigue (and motivation), whether a function of recent activities, food and fluid intake, or sleeping patterns or due to the number and physical demands of the assessments being administered in one session, will influence the assessment outcomes (6).

Age Chronological age and maturity may influence testing performance. For example, the 1.5-mile (2.4 km) run is considered a standard field test to measure aerobic capacity for apparently healthy college-age men and women. However, this same assessment will not appropriately measure aerobic ability of preadolescents, primarily because of the immature physical development of the cardiovascular system and the experiential maturity needed to cover the distance by pacing (11). A better choice for children may be the timed 1-mile run, the 9-minute run for distance, or the PACER (7, 32, 52); and for older clients who are lower-risk individuals, a 1-mile walk test has been recommended as a safer field test (39).

Sex Sex-specific biological factors may influence performances in a variety of activities or assessments such as the chin-up, push-up, and bench press to assess muscular endurance of the upper extremities. Several differences between men and women appear to influence performance: Women tend to have more body fat and less muscle, a smaller shoulder mass that supports less muscle tissue, and as a result less of a mechanical advantage for muscles working at the shoulder (14, 53). For example, the chin-up test appears to provide reliable results for males; however, it may in some cases fail to differentiate between strength and muscular endurance for females. As a result, the flexed arm hang is sometimes used as an alternative method to assess muscular endurance, through a static rather than a dynamic muscular action, by measuring the length of time the flexed elbow hang position can be sustained. Also, push-up tests to measure dynamic muscular fitness of the upper extremities include a variation to accommodate for the differences in upper body strength; this modification uses the same standard military push-up position as for men with the exceptions that the knees are flexed, the lower legs are in contact with the testing surface, and the ankles are plantarflexed (29, 51). In addition, the YMCA fixed-load bench press test provides different fixed loads for men and women (35 pounds [15.8 kg] for women and 80 pounds [36 kg] for men), illustrating the sex-specific differences related to client factors that one needs to consider when selecting appropriate tests (19). (See chapter 11 for the complete procedures for these tests.)

Pretraining Status The pretraining status of the client may affect test selection when the skills required for the test and the relative level of exertion are considered. Caution should be emphasized in assessment of untrained, deconditioned individuals, even when they express a desire to achieve high performance levels. For example, the 1.5-mile (2.4 km) run test and the 12-minute run test are considered near-maximal-exertion tests, as they require the individual to cover distance as quickly as possible (2, 25, 38, 51). A deconditioned client should have a period of at least four to six weeks of aerobic conditioning before participating in either of these assessments (40). Clients who are unaccustomed to pacing themselves may do better on subsequent trials of a 1-mile (1.6 km) walk test as they learn to adjust their initial pace with a

practice trial (34, 38). Similarly, clients who do not have an opportunity to practice a footwork pattern for an agility test may not get an accurate score. Allowing the client time to practice the movement pattern will yield a better indication of the person's agility (34); however, some argue that practicing a movement pattern decreases the likelihood that a test actually measures agility because it will then require no cognitive or reactive component (45).

Likewise, a 1-repetition maximum (1RM) test in the squat movement may be appropriate for a conditioned individual who has previous experience with that free weight movement pattern. However, for someone with no pretraining experience, the lack of motor skill and the intensity required for the exercise may create an unacceptably high risk for injury (3, 15, 27, 30). The greater the load, the more stress the joints, muscles, bones, and connective tissues experience (3, 4, 47). In order to improve safety and reliability, it may be necessary to modify the test to one that estimates maximal strength with a submaximal load, such as a 10RM (30). One or more practice sessions of the specific exercise with a lighter load to learn the proper technique may be necessary. For the untrained person, adaptations in the coordination of the neuromuscular system may account for most of the initial strength gains in a resistance training program (3, 15, 33). Even so, a familiarization period may be prudent to acquaint the untrained individual with the new skill involved in the movement and to protect the person from injury. The length of the familiarization period varies by client and the relative intensity required by the strength test chosen. Also, some muscular endurance tests may involve resistances heavy enough to permit only a limited number of repetitions to be performed by untrained clients. For example, clients with weak or smaller upper body muscles (e.g., younger and older clients, some women, sedentary clients) will not be able to complete very many repetitions (e.g., <6) in the push-up test because their body weight—even using the modified body position—is simply too heavy. For these clients, the push-up test becomes one that can be used to assess muscular *strength*. If this is the case, another test of upper body muscle endurance could be utilized, such as the YMCA bench press test, which will be more accurate if the client has experience with lifting.

Personal Trainer Factors

The level of experience and training of the personal trainer has an impact on the selection of assessments. To maintain objectivity and reduce intrarater error, testing protocols that require adept technical skills need to match the abilities of the personal trainer. As an example, theoretical prediction errors of ±3.5% or less body fat are considered acceptable on various equations and combinations of skinfold measurements to assess body composition (23), but tester error may account for 3% to 9% variability between raters (interrater reliability) (23). Errors can be further compounded by failure to follow a protocol, inaccurate identification of measurement sites, improperly calibrated equipment, and the choice of prediction equations (23). Taking accurate skinfold measurements is a complicated skill that requires about 100 practice opportunities on different clients in order for the personal trainer to gain adequate proficiency (23). To develop intrarater consistency, the personal trainer should do the measurements on different sites and body types (23). The relative test difficulty and the type of measurement required can affect outcomes. It is not reasonable to expect a personal trainer to read through a protocol, administer an assessment to a client, and get good results without practice. Some tests require quite a bit more skill and practice than others. For example, relatively little skill on the part of the personal trainer is required to manage a stopwatch and monitor heart rate for a timed 1-mile (1.6 km) walk or run test. On the other hand, the skills required to get reliable results on a noncomputerized cycle ergometer test are much more complex and involved (e.g., monitoring and adjusting the workload and pedal cadence on the ergometer; obtaining heart rates every minute of the test) (24, 43).

A personal trainer who is unfamiliar with administration of an assessment should not select it but should continue his or her professional development by taking time to practice administration of the assessment for use with future clients.

Equipment Factors

Any mechanism or device used to measure work, performance, or physiological response requires calibration, or the adjusting of the device to ensure precision, in order to accurately measure the specific trait being assessed. Through calibration one checks the accuracy of a measuring device to provide an accurate reading. Reliability, validity, and objectivity of the assessment are directly affected by the accuracy of the measurement tool. Common mechanisms and devices used in the assessment process that require calibration are cycle, stepping, and treadmill ergometers; blood pressure sphygmomanometers; skinfold calipers and body composition mechanisms; metronomes; and other electronic devices used to measure time, distance, and power. To ensure the accuracy of equipment, it is important to institute a scheduled plan for checking and calibrating mechanisms and devices according to manufacturer specification and based on warranty recommendations (25, 37, 51).

Environmental Factors

Climatic elements and the physical setting of the environment present potential concerns that may influence client performance and safety. Consequently when one is selecting and administering tests, it is necessary to consider environmental planning and quality control assurance related to weather, altitude, air pollution, and the physical setting of a facility.

Temperature and Humidity The environment poses challenges and issues related to physiological responses that may have an impact on test administration and performance. High heat and humidity and cold weather exposure need to be considered in the selection of assessments. High ambient temperatures in combination with high humidity inhibit the body's thermoregulatory system from dissipating heat, which impedes physical endurance performance, poses health risks, and affects test results. The personal trainer should be aware of the thresholds of a combined temperature and humidity above which participation in continuous activity may increase the risk of heat injury and also affect performance (1, 10). For example, between 65° and 72° Fahrenheit (18.4-22.2° Celsius) and 65.1% and 72.0% humidity, the risk of exertional heatstroke begins to rise (1, 10). Geographic areas that experience high temperatures along with high humidity may not be suitable for outdoor tests to assess aerobic endurance since performance may be affected. Furthermore, a period of acclimatization to higher temperatures (and humidity) may be necessary for testing in an area with seasonal fluctuations in temperatures (49).

Exposure to cold temperatures, less than 25° Fahrenheit (−4° Celsius), may not have a significant impact on the performance and health of younger apparently healthy individuals; however, older people and those who have cardiovascular and circulatory disorders and respiratory problems may need to use caution. Cold exposure may stimulate the sympathetic nervous system, which can affect total peripheral resistance, arterial pressure, myocardial contraction, and cardiac work (40, 54). Of particular concern are outdoor performances that require significant effort of the upper extremities. Clients with respiratory conditions, particularly asthma, may also be more prone to problems in cold temperatures, as cold air may trigger a bronchial spasm (48, 51).

Altitude Altitude can also impair aerobic endurance performance. Tests to measure aerobic endurance may not correlate with normative performance data when assessment takes place at altitudes higher than 1,900 feet (580 m) (17). In addition, individuals not acclimated to altitude changes may require an adaptation period of 9 to 12 days before engaging in aerobic endurance assessments (51).

Air Pollution Another environmental consideration is the **air quality index (AQI)**. This is a measure of air quality as it relates to pollutants. Pollution can have a negative effect on performance and health by decreasing the ability of the blood to transport oxygen, by increasing the resistance in the airways, and by altering the perception of effort for a given task (16, 40). The AQI is usually reported in local weather forecasts, and the personal trainer should become knowledgeable about which groups of individuals are sensitive to given levels of the AQI (40). See figure 10.1 for more information regarding AQI and health concerns.

Test Setting Issues associated with health and environmental control are important factors related to assessment validity and reliability. To minimize external distractions and the potential anxiety related to the assessment process, the testing area should be quiet and private. The personal trainer should project a positive, relaxed, confident demeanor; and the process should be clearly explained and not rushed. The testing room should be well equipped with comfortable furnishings and standardized and calibrated testing devices. The room temperature should be set at 68° to 72° Fahrenheit (20-22° Celsius), 60% or less humidity, and air circulation should be six to eight exchanges per hour (51). Physical facilities must be inspected for deficiencies, and safety procedures need to be clearly documented and posted. Appropriate emergency equipment must be operable and immediately available in the event that an incident requires an emergency response (8, 43, 51). (See chapter 24 for more details about recommended facility characteristics.)

> The integrity of the assessment process depends on the validity and reliability of the assessments selected and proper administration by a trained fitness professional. Personal trainers should take care to enhance reliability by consistently attending to controllable factors related to the client, personal trainer, equipment, and environment.

Air quality index levels of health concern	Numerical value	Meaning
Good	0-50	Air quality is considered satisfactory, and air pollution poses little or no risk.
Moderate	51-100	Air quality is acceptable; however, for some pollutants there may be a moderate health concern for a very small number of people wo are unusually sensitive to air pollution.
Unhealthy for sensitive groups	101-150	Members of sensitive groups may experience health effects. The general public is not likely to be affected.
Unhealthy	151-200	Everyone may begin to experience health effects. Members of sensitive groups may experience more serious health effects.
Very unhealthy	201-300	Health alert: everyone may experience more serious health effects.
Hazardous	>300	Health warnings of emergency conditions. The entire population is more likely to be affected.

FIGURE 10.1 Air quality index levels.

Reprinted from http://airnow.gov/index.cfm?action=aqibasics.aqi.

Assessment Case Studies

The most important required assessments for initiating and designing an exercise program are of the client's cardiovascular disease risk and potential contraindications for specific activities due to known musculoskeletal limitations or diseases. The outcome of the health screening process and risk stratification dictates the selection and administration of all other assessments. Before selecting the assessment instruments for each client, the personal trainer must also consider other factors, including the client's exercise goals, exercise history, and attitudes about assessments; his or her own experience and skill in performing the assessments; and the equipment and facilities available. In most cases, more than one assessment instrument may be used to collect the information needed to design a program. The next section further explores these concepts using two case studies. (Refer to table 9.2 on p. 158 for details on risk stratification.)

> Selecting valid, reliable, and safe assessments that will provide meaningful results requires an understanding of the health status, risk stratification, and goals of the client; level of experience of the personal trainer; availability of equipment; and the specific test characteristics associated with the assessment.

Case Study 10.1

Maria G.

Maria G. is a 57-year-old grandmother of four who has been active most of her life. She is 65 inches (165 cm) tall and weighs 145 pounds (66 kg). She participated in step aerobics and spinning classes three or four times per week at her old club before she moved to be closer to her daughters' families. She is planning on resuming those activities at her new club. She also enjoys occasional games of recreational tennis and golf with her friends. She would like to increase her strength, as she is helping more with the toddlers and finds carrying them and their gear tiring. She has never been a smoker, although her husband still smokes a pack a day. Her father died at age 73 in a car accident, and her 82-year-old mother is still alive.

Last month, a local hospital sponsored a health fair, and Maria took full advantage of the screening opportunities. Her average blood pressure was 129/79 mmHg (millimeters of mercury). Her total cholesterol was 231 mg/dl (milligrams per deciliter) with a low-density lipoprotein (LDL) count of 150 mg/dl and a high-density lipoprotein (HDL) score of 65 mg/dl. Her fasting glucose was 93 mg/dl. She also had her body fat tested with a handheld BIA device and was told she was 28% fat. She has no other health problems. See the "Individual Assessment Recording Form for Maria" on the following page for a summary of the assessment findings.

Individual Assessment Recording Form for Maria

(Pretest)　　Posttest　　(circle one)

Client's name: __Maria G.__　　　　　　　　　　　　　　Age: __57__

Goals: __Increase muscular strength; maintain aerobic capacity and body composition; improve balance and blood lipid profile.__

Preparticipation screening notes: __In "moderate" risk category; need to receive physician's release prior to prescribing "vigorous" activity exercise program.__

Assessment dates: __8/9/11; 8/11/11__

Comments: __Will reevaluate % body fat using skinfold calipers; she previously was active but has not exercised recently; wants to begin aerobic classes again; recently completed lipid screening (cholesterol: 231 mg/dl; LDL: 150 mg/dl; HDL: 65 mg/dl; fasting glucose: 93 mg/dl); husband is smoker.__

Vital signs	Score or result	Classification*	Examples and norm- and criterion-referenced standards (chapter 11)
Resting blood pressure	129/79	Prehypertensive	Table 11.2
Resting heart rate	72 beats/min	Average	Table 11.1
Body composition measures	**Score or result**	**Classification**	
Height	65 in. (165 cm)	Percentile: ~75th	Table 11.7
Weight	145 lb (66 kg)		
Body mass index (BMI)	24.1	Normal	Table 11.8
Waist circumference	29 in. (74 cm)	Under the 88 cm cutoff	Table 11.5
Hip circumference	36 in. (91 cm)	–	–
Waist-to-hip ratio	0.81	Moderate risk	Table 11.12
Percent body fat Method: BIA	28%	Percentile: ~60th Criterion: leaner than average	Percentile: table 11.11 Criterion: table 11.11
Cardiovascular endurance	**Score or result**	**Classification**	
Åstrand-Rhyming cycle test initial work rate: 450 kg · m^{-1} · min^{-1}	28.64 ml · kg^{-1} · min^{-1}	Percentile: ~55th Criterion: good	Percentile: table 11.16 Criterion: table 11.18
Muscular endurance	**Score or result**	**Classification**	
YMCA bench press test weight: 35 lb	9 reps at 35 lb (16 kg)	Percentile: 50th	Table 11.24
Muscular strength	**Score or result**	**Classification**	
Estimate a 1 RM bench press with a submaximal load	1 RM estimated as 60 lb, which is ~41% of body weight	Percentile: ~90th	
Flexibility	**Score or result**	**Classification**	
YMCA sit-and-reach test	13 in. (33 cm)	Percentile: 30th	Table 11.27
Other tests	**Score or result**	**Classification**	
Thomas hip range of motion test**	Both tested legs remained on floor	Adequate hip flexor flexibility	
One-foot stand test, eyes open***	Right: 6 s Left: 9 s	Below average	

*Classification refers to either the norm- or criterion-referenced standard, depending on the test and protocol. Refer to the examples and the norm- and criterion-referenced standards provided in chapter 11 for a further explanation of how the classification labels were assigned to Maria.'s results.

**Protocol and normative data in Howley and Franks (25).

***Protocol and normative data in Springer et al. (46).

Risk Factor Analysis

What is Maria's risk stratification (see tables 9.1 and 9.2)? Maria has three positive risk factors from the screening: age, smoking, and dyslipidemia. First, Maria is over 55, which counts as one risk factor. Second, while Maria is not herself a smoker, her husband is, and this means that she has significant exposure to environmental tobacco smoke. Finally, both her total and LDL-cholesterol are above the threshold levels for risk (200 mg/dl for total cholesterol and 130 mg/dl for LDL-cholesterol). However, Maria's HDL level of 65 mg/dl is above the 60 mg/dl level, which is a positive high number that cancels one of the risk factors. Maria's blood pressure and blood glucose are normal, and her BMI score of 24.1 does not indicate an overweight condition. Her percentage of body fat at 28% is in the "leaner than average" category for a woman her age. Maria does not have a significant family history of cardiovascular disease. Since Maria's net total of two risk factors places classifies her as moderate risk she should not participate in *maximal* exercise testing or in a *vigorous* exercise program until she obtains a physician's release (see figure 9.1).

Assessment Recommendations

What assessment recommendations would be appropriate for this client? For assessment of cardiovascular endurance, the personal trainer has several choices of activities. Since Maria has been consistently active in aerobic exercise, she would be a candidate for one of the tests that require some preconditioning (e.g., 1.5-mile [2.4 km] run test, 12-minute run test, and the multistage YMCA cycle ergometer test) (25, 51). However, because of her moderate-risk status due to her age, these near-maximal tests must be deemed inappropriate for her at this time without a physician's release. Single-stage or graded treadmill tests, walking tests, cycling tests, and step tests (12-inch [30 cm] step or lower) would be acceptable choices since she has no joint complaints and used to participate in two of the three activities.

Since Maria has not been performing a resistance training program, all maximal (1RM) strength tests are not recommended. Performing a muscular endurance test such as the YMCA fixed-weight bench press test may pose no problem since she has been active; but the activity has not been in a resistance program, and the exercises are unfamiliar. It would be best to wait until Maria is comfortable with the mechanics of performing the exercises and becomes better trained to perform standardized strength assessment. However, because of her weak upper body, the personal trainer could choose to use a submaximal load on the bench press to estimate Maria's 1RM and thus her relative strength in order to assess baseline upper body strength. The personal trainer could allow the client to practice the bench press movement prior to performing the submaximal test so the results would be more valid, as long as full rest is given between the practice and the actual assessment.

If Maria had expressed concerns related to body weight or body size, it would be prudent to repeat a test for body composition under the prescribed conditions to get the baseline data for future comparisons, since the testing conditions at the health fair are unknown. For measures of body fat, it is recommended that the same test be administered under the same conditions by the same tester (23). Therefore, the personal trainer can retest Maria with, for example, skinfold calipers if he or she is skilled in using this tool. Circumference measures would also provide baseline data for health risks related to excess abdominal fat and allow Maria to track changes in her body after participating in an exercise program. (See chapter 11 for further discussion of how to perform these anthropometric measurements.)

Maria has not expressed a desire to improve athletic performance, and therefore tests for agility, speed, and power are not necessary at this time. Balance, reaction time, and coordination issues related to her activities of daily living may become more apparent and require further investigation or programming in the future. If the client continues to participate in tennis and golf, she may welcome some activities related to improved performance after the personal trainer has designed a program to meet her current goal of increased functional strength.

Paul C.

Paul C. is a 28-year-old accountant in a very busy office. He is 6 feet (183 cm) tall and weighs 260 pounds (118 kg) and has never smoked or used tobacco products. Paul's father had two heart attacks prior to his death at age 47, and Paul's 34-year-old brother recently underwent triple-bypass surgery after experiencing chest pains. His mother has type 2 diabetes, which is under control. Paul has not had his fasting blood glucose measured. During the initial interview, his blood pressure measured 150/96 mmHg; his percentage of body fat was 30, and his waist measurement was 41 inches (104 cm) compared to a hip measurement of 44 inches (112 cm). His last cholesterol test was over six months ago, and he does not recall the numbers but states "The doctor didn't say anything, so I guess it was okay." Paul has developed asthma, induced by seasonal allergies and exercise. He has an inhaler of albuterol and finds that activity easily winds him, sometimes precipitating an asthma attack. He also reports some intermittent pain in his left knee, probably related to a fall several months ago. He has not had the knee examined by the doctor. Paul has come in at his wife's insistence because she is concerned that he is as much a candidate for a heart attack as his brother was. He has never been active or enjoyed exercise and is concerned about how to fit activity into his busy work schedule.

Risk Factor Analysis

What is Paul's risk stratification (see figure 9.1)? Paul has a number of risk factors at this time. He has a significant family history with both his father and brother having experienced heart attacks or cardiovascular disease prior to age 55. His BMI is 35.3, which places him in very high-risk obesity class II (see table 11.5) (23, 51). The other anthropometric measures support the fact that his excess visceral fat, stored in the abdominal area, puts Paul at high risk of cardiovascular disease, stroke, and diabetes type 2; body fat is ≥30% (see table 11.10); waist circumference is >40 inches (102 cm) (23, 51); waist-to-hip ratio is above .94 (see table 11.12) (23, 51). By his own admission, he is not an active person. His blood pressure is high; two consecutive high blood pressure readings on either systolic (>140 mmHg) or diastolic (>90 mmHg) indicate a referral to a physician for evaluation (see table 11.2). His fasting glucose is unknown at this time. Paul reports no other signs or symptoms of cardiovascular disease, but his blood cholesterol is also presently unknown. In addition to the four risk factors he presents (family history, obesity, inactivity, high blood pressure), he has a known disease, asthma, and an undiagnosed orthopedic problem (left knee). Paul should be advised not to do any activities until his physician releases him.

Assessment Recommendations

Given Paul's situation, his physician may designate him as a high-risk client and may choose to perform a diagnostic stress test on this client. If that is the case and Paul is released for a limited activity program, the personal trainer can use the maximal heart rate and maximal oxygen consumption data from the stress test in designing the exercise program. If Paul is not stress tested and is released for moderate exercise, the assessment of cardiovascular function will be submaximal, with a bike test as possibly the most appropriate since it is non-weight bearing and may put the least stress on his left knee. Additional consideration needs to be given to some of the other information provided by this client. He is not an active person, does not particularly enjoy exercise, and is already erecting roadblocks in terms of finding time to exercise. He appears to be in the contemplation, or possibly preparation, stage of readiness for lifestyle change (36). (See chapter 8, p. 135, for more information about psychological readiness for exercise.) Also, the personal trainer could have Paul complete "The Attitudinal Assessment" form (p. 135), which gauges attitudes toward exercise. While awaiting the physician's release, Paul may benefit from sessions to discuss his readiness to change lifestyle behaviors, goal setting, strategies to enhance his adherence to a program, and consultation with a nutrition specialist.

Administration and Organization of Fitness Assessments

Administration of the fitness assessment requires advanced preparation and organization to ensure psychometrically sound results and safe outcomes. When organizing and administering the fitness assessment process, one must pay close attention to the details of preparation and the implementation of factors that will have an impact on obtaining safe, accurate, and meaningful results.

Test Preparation

Appropriate and valuable test outcomes are predicated on the ability of the personal trainer to prepare clients by educating them as to the content of the test, pretest requirements, and expectations of the assessment process. Preparation to evaluate someone's level of fitness requires the personal trainer to execute preassessment screening procedures, review safety considerations, select appropriate assessments, select facilities and verify accuracy of equipment, and perform record-keeping responsibilities. See page 199 for the "Test Preparation and Implementation Checklist."

Conduct Preassessment Screening Procedures and Review Safety Considerations

The implementation of a fitness assessment procedure should occur only after a thorough preactivity screening that includes an initial interview, execution of a health appraisal tool, completion of appropriate forms, and, when required, recommendations from a physician regarding the management of medical contraindications (see chapter 9). Documented risks are associated with exercise testing; however, evidence suggests that complications are relatively low (.06% or 6 per 10,000) (51).

Verify Appropriateness of Selected Assessments

Selecting valid, reliable, and safe assessments that will provide meaningful results requires an understanding of the goals and health status of the client, level of experience of the personal trainer, and the specific test characteristics associated with the assessment.

Select Facilities and Verify Accuracy of Equipment

Ease of administration, cost-effectiveness, availability of equipment, and the facility setting influence the selection and implementation of the assessment process. Two types of assessments, laboratory tests and field tests, may be administered to yield valuable results; but in most situations they are administered under different conditions. Laboratory tests, in most cases, are performed in clinical facilities using specialized diagnostic equipment to assess an individual's maximal functional capacity. Examples of laboratory tests include the use of a metabolic cart to measure oxygen consumption and hydrostatic weighing to measure body composition. Testing is relatively complex, and direct-measurement tools are used to reduce data error and quantify results based on physiological responses. Because of the diagnostic capabilities of the tests and the high risk of cardiac complications, allied health professionals are responsible for administering the assessment and evaluation process of laboratory tests. For these tests, it is helpful to have equipment such as the following:

- Bicycle ergometer or treadmill
- Equipment for measuring body composition (e.g., skinfold calipers)
- Equipment for measuring flexibility (e.g., goniometer or sit-and-reach box)
- Equipment for measuring the force of muscular contraction (e.g., dynamometer)
- Perceived exertion chart
- Stopwatch
- Metronome
- Sphygmomanometer
- Stethoscope
- Tape measure
- Body weight scale
- First aid kit
- Automated external defibrillator (AED) (9)

Field tests are practical assessments that are inexpensive, are easy to administer, require less equipment, are less time-consuming, can be performed at various venues, and may be more efficient for evaluating large groups. Examples of field tests include walk/run tests, agility tests, and 1RM tests. The assessments may be submaximal or maximal and are usually administered by a certified fitness professional. These assessments, which are not diagnostic, use indirect measurements to quantify and extrapolate performance results. The major concerns with the maximal assessments are the potential risks that exist as a result of an individual's putting forth a maximal effort without being monitored with diagnostic devices. Because of the cost of laboratory equipment and the consideration of ease of administration, it may not be practical or appropriate for the personal trainer to implement laboratory testing. In any case, one can use field tests effectively and efficiently to obtain the information needed to assess performance and compare to norm- or criterion-referenced standards.

Instruct Client on Preassessment Protocols

An appointment for the assessment should be scheduled in advance in order for the client to adequately prepare mentally and physically for the event. The client should receive pretest instructions in preparation for the assessment. These include

- adequate rest (e.g., 6 to 8 hours the night before and no vigorous exercise 24 hours preceding the test);
- moderate food intake (e.g., a light meal or snack 2 to 4 hours prior to the test);
- adequate hydration (e.g., six to eight glasses of water the day before the test and at least two cups [0.5 L] of water in the 2 hours prior to the test);
- abstinence from chemicals that accelerate heart rate (with the exception of prescribed medications);
- proper attire (e.g., loose-fitting clothing, sturdy, tied athletic shoes);
- specific testing procedures and expectations before, during, and after the test; and
- conditions for terminating a test.

It is important for clients to be told that they may terminate a test for any reason at any time. Also, occasionally it may be necessary, for safety reasons, for the personal trainer to terminate a test before its completion. Reasons for stopping a test when performed without direct involvement of a physi-

cian or electrocardiographic monitoring are listed in table 10.1. If a test must be terminated abruptly, it should be followed by a 5 to 15 minute cool down period when possible.

Prepare Record-Keeping System

An organized method to collect, record, and store data is critical in reducing the incidence of error and is instrumental to the evaluation and interpretation of testing results. Creating a systematic method for collecting and storing data is one of the professional responsibilities associated with the role of the personal trainer. In addition, documentation may provide evidence of reasonable and prudent care in the event that the standard of care is questioned and litigation is pursued (37, 44).

A systematic approach to data collection would include manual recording forms or software programs that allow documentation of raw scores expressed in specific units of measurement. Recording devices should also contain vital client information related to the assessment process and provide space for comments pertaining to the collection of data during the process. In addition, the data collection system should be organized so that testing results can be retrieved from it in a time-efficient manner. This feature is especially important when one is making pretest-to-posttest comparisons during the reassessment process. The system should also have a protective mechanism to ensure confidentiality. See the blank copy of the "Individual Assessment Recording Form" (used in case study 10.1) as an example of an assessment recording form that you may use.

Test Implementation

Organizing and implementing an assessment procedure requires the personal trainer's detailed attention to a number of tasks: identifying the sequence of the

TABLE 10.1   Indications for Terminating Exercise Testing

Onset of angina or angina-like symptoms
Drop in systolic BP of >10 mmHg from baseline BP despite an increase in workload
Excessive rise in BP: systolic pressure >250 mmHg or diastolic pressure >115 mmHg
Shortness of breath, wheezing, leg cramps, or claudication
Signs of poor perfusion (e.g., ataxia, dizziness, pallor, cyanosis, cold or clammy skin, or nausea)
Failure of HR to rise with increased exercise intensity
Noticeable change in heart rhythm
Client's request to stop
Physical or verbal manifestations of severe fatigue
Failure of the testing equipment

Reprinted from ACSM 2010 (51).

assessments, defining and following testing protocols, collecting and interpreting data, and scheduling a review of the results. Refer to the "Test Preparation and Implementation Checklist" on page 199.

Determine Sequence of Assessments

Organization of a testing procedure demands that the personal trainer identify and determine the proper order of the testing to ensure optimal performance and adequate rest and recovery to yield accurate results. Test order is influenced by many factors: number of clients to be tested, components to be evaluated, skill involved, energy system demand, time available, and the specific goal of the client. Many clients do not require a battery of tests as inclusive as the lists that follow. One can use various strategies related to test order; however, the following are examples of logical sequences for clients with general fitness or athletic performance-related goals (21):

General Fitness

1. Resting tests (e.g., resting heart rate, blood pressure, height, weight, body composition)
2. Nonfatiguing tests (e.g., flexibility, balance)
3. Muscular strength tests
4. Local muscular endurance tests (e.g., YMCA bench press test, partial curl-up test)
5. Submaximal aerobic capacity tests (e.g., step test, Rockport walking test, Åstrand-Ryhming cycle ergometer test, 1.5-mile [2.4 km] run, 12-minute run/walk)

Athletic Performance

1. Resting tests (e.g., resting heart rate, blood pressure, height, weight, body composition)
2. Nonfatiguing tests (e.g., flexibility, vertical jump)
3. Agility tests (e.g., T-test)
4. Maximum power and strength tests (e.g., 3RM power clean, 1RM bench press)
5. Sprint tests (e.g., 40-yard [37 m] sprint)
6. Local muscular endurance tests (e.g., 1-minute sit-up test, push-up test)
7. Anaerobic capacity tests (e.g., 300-yard [275 m] shuttle run)
8. Maximal or submaximal aerobic capacity tests (e.g., maximum treadmill test, 1.5-mile [2.4 km] run, YMCA cycle ergometer test)

If possible, it is most appropriate to schedule assessments to measure maximum aerobic capacity on a separate day. However, if all assessments are performed on the same day, maximum aerobic tests should be performed last, after a minimum of an hour-long rest recovery period (21). Note that some organizations recommend assessing aerobic capacity prior to muscular fitness or flexibility due to elevated heart rate from previously performed assessments (51). However, the recommended minimum recovery of an hour prior to an aerobic capacity assessment should avoid the problem.

Define and Follow Test Protocols

Individuals to be assessed should receive precise instructions regarding the test prior to the scheduled assessment appointment. The clarity and simplicity of instructions have a direct impact on the reliability and objectivity of a test (5). Test instructions should define the protocols, including the purpose of the test, directions on implementation, performance guidelines regarding technique and disqualification, test scoring, and recommendations for maximizing performance. The personal trainer should also provide a demonstration of appropriate test performance and should give the client an opportunity to practice and ask questions concerning the protocol.

It is the responsibility of the personal trainer to ensure that testing protocols are followed safely and efficiently. To enhance reliability, strict standardized procedures should be followed with each client each time the test is administered. Also, the test selected for the pretest should be repeated as the posttest so that a reliable comparison of scores can be made. The personal trainer should institute an adequate warm-up and cool-down procedure when warranted and implement spotting practices when required by the testing protocol.

> Administration of the assessments should follow a standardized procedure including mental and physical preparation of the client, verification of the accuracy of the equipment, application of the specific test protocol, ensuring safety throughout the process, and performance of record-keeping responsibilities.

Interpretation and Review of Results

The data collected through the assessment process provide baseline information for the client. The interpretation of the baseline data is dependent on the specific purpose of the assessment and the goals of the client. Common ways to explain data to a client are through norm-referenced and criterion-referenced standards (see chapter 11).

Norm-Referenced Standards

The two reference perspectives for comparison of data involve **norm-referenced standards** and **criterion-referenced standards.** Norm-referenced standards are used to compare the performance of an individual against the performance of others in a like category. Chapter 11 provides several tables demonstrating **percentile** values for various fitness measures. The results show how the men and women in the study *performed*. In other words, the percentile scores compare the actual "best, worst, and in-between" performance scores of each participant. Table 11.14, for example, compares a client's scores from a modified Balke treadmill test against scores of all the other participants of the same gender. The first and last finishers were off the respective ends of this chart, and the rest were statistically divided into percentile rankings. Some clients may confuse percentile scores with "percent scores" such as those they may have received in school, with 70% generally being a "passing grade." Therefore, a personal trainer should be able to interpret the test results for clients and educate them on the relative value of their scores. As table 11.14 shows, a score at the 50th percentile (meaning that the person performed better than roughly half of the performers and was outperformed by half) is an average performance.

Many clients are content to know their raw (performance) score and whether they get stronger, faster, or more flexible after training. Clients who are very unfit or who have had negative experiences with fitness testing in the past may have no interest in knowing how poorly they performed compared to others. Other clients feel more motivated with use of the normative data to articulate performance goals and feel a sense of achievement as they "climb the chart." Although using the normative approach may provide positive feedback related to performance, it does not address the health-related status of the individual based on desirable health standards.

Criterion-Referenced Standards

What norm-referenced standards do not do is let the client know whether the performance met a health standard. A health standard could be defined as the lowest performance that would allow an individual to maintain good health and lessen the risk of chronic diseases (40). Another way of stating

this is to say that a criterion is a specific, minimal standard—one that theoretically each person can strive for, as it is not compared to how other individuals perform. Criterion-referenced standards are set against a combination of normative data and the best judgment of the experts in a given field to identify a specific level of achievement (34). Criterion-referenced standards that have been matched to healthy levels of fitness provide reasonable goals for most people to achieve for improved health. For example, table 11.5 demonstrates standards of health by showing a client's disease risk based on waist circumference and BMI. If a female client had a waist circumference greater than 35 inches and also was in the overweight category according to BMI, she would have a high risk of diseases such as diabetes or coronary heart disease. As another example, table 11.2 demonstrates the criterion-referenced standards for blood pressure, or whether a client would be considered hypertensive or not.

Unfortunately, there is disagreement on the exact level of performance that accurately reflects a health standard (34). At least four criterion-referenced health-related fitness batteries of tests are given to school-age children in the United States, but each has a different criterion denoting acceptable performance levels for health (28, 34). There is no consensus on what determines minimal health standards for adults in all areas, either (34). For example, despite the normative values for maximal aerobic power presented in table 11.14, some data suggest that, for males between 20 and 29 years of age, a score below the 20th percentile or $38.1 \text{ ml} \cdot \text{kg}^{-1} \cdot \text{min}^{-1}$ would represent a health-related criterion standard (about $31.6 \text{ ml} \cdot \text{kg}^{-1} \cdot \text{min}^{-1}$ for women in the same age group) (51). Does this mean that a client achieving a score higher than the 20th or 30th percentile on any fitness test is healthy? Not necessarily. The problem is that exact cutoffs for health for each component of fitness for all segments of the adult population have not been identified and universally accepted. For a deconditioned client who scores at or near the bottom of a column on a norm-referenced table, the results may be demoralizing if the client thinks, mistakenly, that he or she must score at or near the top to be *healthy*.

Where they exist, criterion-referenced data provide a reasonable estimate of the level of fitness required for health. In the absence of criterion-referenced data for a test chosen for a particular client, the best way to use the normative tables is to encourage clients with goals related to health to strive for fitness improvements until they reach the "average" or higher levels for a given component, and then to maintain their level of performance (25).

Applying Norm- and Criterion-Referenced Standards

If a 39-year-old woman had a $\dot{V}O_2$max of 32 ml · kg^{-1} · min^{-1}, she scored at the 40th percentile (33.8 is the closest score and she's just barely above that), meaning that 60% of the women her age have a higher $\dot{V}O_2$max and 40% have a lower $\dot{V}O_2$max (see table 11.17). This $\dot{V}O_2$max is slightly below average for her age. What the score does not tell her is whether this represents a healthy level of cardiovascular fitness. On the other hand, 29.9 ml · kg^{-1} · min^{-1} is the minimal criterion for health in aerobic power (not noted in this norm-referenced table), and she has achieved a score that exceeds the health standard. The personal trainer and client would need to discuss her interests, performance goals, current program, and time available to determine together how she will maintain (minimal goal) or improve her current level of fitness.

Clients with average or higher levels of performance initially or after training may have already achieved a healthy level of fitness, but may be motivated to improve both health and performance by setting higher performance goals using the norm-referenced tables (25).

The personal trainer should schedule a review of results immediately or shortly following the assessment process. The client should receive an illustrated summary of the test results, along with an explanation of personal strengths and areas identified that may have room for improvement. It is important to note that testing data are neither good nor bad—they are baseline data to provide a foundation for positive change.

Reassessment

Once the assessments are complete and the personal trainer has reviewed the results with the client, the program is designed and implemented based on the client's goals. The initial assessments, intermediate assessments (repetitions of some or all of the initial assessments), anecdotal records, and exercise logs documenting client progress are all part of the formative evaluation of the client, providing frequent opportunities for feedback and guidance. A time frame for accomplishing goals is set, and posttests are scheduled for that time. This date may be eight or more weeks from program initiation. Some goals may require more or less time for completion. In any case, the summative evaluation should be scheduled just after the posttesting is complete to discuss the client's degree of achievement, review the strengths and weaknesses of the initial program, set new goals, and modify the program where appropriate. It is important to keep in mind that formative evaluations are a measure of *progress toward a goal,* and the summative evaluation is a measure of the *degree of attainment of a stated goal.* For most clients, regardless of whether norm- or criterion-referenced standards are used, it is more appropriate to have them compare their own performances over time than to the skills or fitness levels of others.

Conclusion

If the personal trainer is truly providing individualized programming for his or her clients, the process begins with a thoughtful evaluation of the client's total circumstances—age, health, past experiences with exercise, current training status, exercise readiness, personal interests, and goals. Once these are identified, the personal trainer must consider the appropriateness of various valid and reliable tests that will yield meaningful baseline data from which a program can be developed. The personal trainer must further consider his or her own skills, equipment availability and appropriateness, and environmental factors in selecting the assessment(s) to gather these data. A system of record keeping and storage must be developed to facilitate communication with the client after the initial testing and subsequent follow-up assessments. The entire process is part art and part science. It takes energy and initiative to continually search for assessment protocols relevant to one's clientele and to practice administering and interpreting them correctly. The personal trainer who does so will increase his or her knowledge, skills, and confidence; and both the personal trainer and the clients will benefit from the effort.

Study Questions

1. Which one of the following tests used to estimate $\dot{V}O_2$max would likely be inappropriate for a 43-year-old sedentary male client who has not yet been cleared by his family physician for participation in a supervised exercise program?

   A. Åstrand-Ryhming cycle ergometer test

   B. YMCA cycle ergometer test

   C. Rockport walking test

   D. 1.5-mile (2.4 km) run

2. A personal trainer performs hydrostatic weighing for a client. The client then proceeds to have the same hydrostatic weighing test performed under the same conditions a day later, but the body fat percentage is 10 points higher. In this case, the hydrostatic weighing performed by the personal trainer is

   A. reliable.

   B. valid.

   C. valid and reliable.

   D. neither valid nor reliable.

3. A new client has completed a YMCA cycle ergometer test, but upon completion of the test her personal trainer notices the machine was not properly calibrated prior to testing. Which of the following was affected by a lack of calibration?

   A. objectivity

   B. intrarater reliability

   C. the standard error of measurement

   D. interrater objectivity

4. Which of the following is a recommended sequence of tests that promotes the most accurate results when assessing general fitness?

   I. Rockport walking test

   II. sit-and-reach test

   III. push-up test

   IV. skinfold measurements

   A. I, II, III, IV

   B. IV, III, II, I

   C. I, III, II, IV

   D. IV, II, III, I

Applied Knowledge Question

The following are four client examples with a fitness component to be tested. Identify two appropriate fitness assessment tests for each client based on that client's background.

Client	Description	Fitness component to be tested	Test 1	Test 2
27-year-old male	Has been participating in 5 km runs for three years	Cardiorespiratory endurance		
33-year-old female	Has been resistance training consistently for 10 years	Muscular strength		
41-year-old female	Has been diagnosed as obese by her physician	Body composition		
11-year-old male	Has no exercise experience or training	Muscular endurance		

References

1. Armstrong, L.E., D.J. Casa, M. Millard-Stafford, D.S. Moran, S.W. Pyne, and W.O. Roberts. 2007. Exertional heat illness during training and competition. *Medicine and Science in Sports and Exercise*, 39 (3): 556-572.

2. Åstrand, I. 1960. Aerobic work capacity in men and women with special reference to age. *Acta Physiologica Scandinavica* 49 (169): 45-60.

3. Baechle, T.R., and R.W. Earle. 2006. *Weight Training: Steps to Success*. Champaign, IL: Human Kinetics.

4. Baechle, T.R., R.W. Earle, and D. Wathen. 2008. Resistance training. In: *Essentials of Strength Training and Conditioning*, 3rd ed., T.R. Baechle and R.W. Earle, eds. Champaign, IL: Human Kinetics. pp. 382-412.

5. Baumgartner, T.A., and A.S. Jackson. 1995. *Measurement for Evaluation*, 5th ed. Dubuque, IA: Brown.

6. Bilodeau, B., B. Roy, and M. Boulay. 1995. Upper-body testing of cross-country skiers. *Medicine and Science in Sports and Exercise* 27 (11): 1557-1562.

7. Buono, M.J., J.J. Roby, F.G. Micale, J.F. Sallis, and W.E. Shepard. 1991. Validity and reliability of predicting maximum oxygen uptake via field tests in children and adolescents. *Pediatric Exercise Science* 3 (3): 250-255.

8. Carver, S. 2003. Injury prevention and treatment. In: *Health Fitness Instructor's Handbook*, 4th ed., E.T. Howley and B.D. Franks, eds. Champaign, IL: Human Kinetics. pp. 393-420.

9. Caton, M. 1998. Equipment selection, purchase, and maintenance. In: *ACSM's Resource Manual for Guidelines for Exercise Testing and Prescription*, 3rd ed., J.L. Roitman, ed. Baltimore: Lippincott Williams & Wilkins. pp. 625-631.

10. Coris, E., A. Ramirez, and D. Van Durme. 2004. Heat illness in athletes: The dangerous combination of heat, humidity and exercise. *Sports Medicine* 34 (1): 9-16.

11. Daniels, J., N. Oldridge, F. Nagel, and B. White. 1978. Differences and changes in VO_2 among young runners 10-18 years of age. *Medicine and Science in Sports* 17: 200-203.

12. Deurenberg, P., and M. Durenberg-Yap. 2003. Validity of body composition methods across ethic population groups. *Acta Diabetologica* 40: S246-S249.

13. Earle, R.W., and T.R. Baechle, eds. 2004. *NSCA's Essentials of Personal Training*. Champaign, IL: Human Kinetics.

14. Faigenbaum, A. 2008. Age and sex-related differences and their implications for resistance exercise. In: *Essentials of Strength Training and Conditioning*, 3rd ed., T.R. Baechle and R.W. Earle, eds. Champaign, IL: Human Kinetics. pp. 142-158.

15. Fleck, S.J., and W.J. Kraemer. 2004. *Designing Resistance Training Programs*, 3rd ed. Champaign, IL: Human Kinetics.

16. Frampton, M. 2007. Does inhalation of ultrafine particles cause pulmonary vascular effects in humans? *Inhalation Toxicology* 19: 75-79.

17. Fulco, C.S., P.B. Rock, and A. Cymerman. Maximal and submaximal exercise performance at altitude. *Aviation, Space, and Environmental Medicine* 69 (8): 793-801.

18. Gergley, T., W. McArdle, P. DeJesus, M. Toner, S. Jacobowitz, and R. Spina. 1984. Specificity of arm training on aerobic power during swimming and running. *Medicine and Science in Sports and Exercise* 16 (4): 349-354.

19. Golding, L.A., ed. 2000. *YMCA Fitness Testing and Assessment Manual*. Champaign, IL: Human Kinetics.

20. Hambrecht, R., G. Schuler, T. Muth, M. Grunze, C. Marburger, J. Niebauer, et al. 1992. Greater diagnostic sensitivity of treadmill versus cycle exercise testing of asymptomatic men with coronary artery disease. *American Journal of Cardiology* 70 (2): 141-146.

21. Harman, E. 2008. Principles of test selection and administration. In: *Essentials of Strength Training and Conditioning*, 3rd ed., T.R. Baechle and R.W. Earle, eds. Champaign, IL: Human Kinetics. pp. 238-247.

22. Herbert, D.L. 1996. Legal and professional responsibilities of personal training. In: *The Business of Personal Training*, S.O. Roberts, ed. Champaign, IL: Human Kinetics. pp. 53-63.

23. Heyward, V.H., and D.R. Wagner. 2004. *Applied Body Composition Assessment*, 2nd ed. Champaign, IL: Human Kinetics.

24. Housh, T.J., J.T. Cramer, J.P. Weir, T.W. Beck, and G.O. Johnson. 2009. *Physical Fitness Laboratories on a Budget*. Scottsdale, AZ: Holcomb Hathaway.

25. Howley, E.T., and B.D. Franks. 2003. *Health Fitness Instructor's Handbook*, 4th ed. Champaign, IL: Human Kinetics.

26. Katch, F., and V. Katch. 1984. The body composition profile. Techniques of measurement and applications. *Clinics in Sports Medicine* 3 (1): 31-63.

27. Kraemer, W.J., and S.J. Fleck. 2007. *Optimizing Strength Training*. Champaign, IL: Human Kinetics.

28. Lacy, A.C., and D.N. Hastad. 2007. *Measurement and Evaluation in Physical Education and Exercise Science*, 5th ed. San Francisco: Pearson Education.

29. Laughlin, N., and P. Busk. 2007. Relationships between selected muscle endurance tasks and gender. *Journal of Strength and Conditioning Research* 21 (2): 400-404.

30. Mayhew, J.L., B.D. Johnson, M.J. LaMonte, D. Lauber, and W. Kemmler. 2008. Accuracy of prediction equations for determining one repetition maximum bench press in women before and after resistance training. *Journal of Strength and Conditioning Research* 22 (5): 1570-1577.

31. McArdle, W.D., F.I. Katch, and V.L. Katch. 2001. *Exercise Physiology: Energy, Nutrition, and Human Performance*, 5th ed. Philadelphia: Lippincott Williams & Wilkins.

32. McClain, J.J., G.J. Welk, M. Ihmels, and J. Schaben. 2006. Comparison of two versions of the PACER aerobic fitness test. *Journal of Physical Activity and Health* 3 (Suppl 2): S47-S57.

33. Moritani, T., and H. deVries. 1979. Neutral factors versus hypertrophy in the time course of muscle strength gain. *American Journal of Physical Medicine* 58 (3): 115-130.

34. Morrow Jr., J.R., A.W. Jackson, J.G. Disch, and D.P. Mood. 2005. *Measurement and Evaluation in Human Performance*, 3rd ed. Champaign, IL: Human Kinetics.

35. Myers, J., N. Buchanan, D. Walsh, M. Kraemer, P. McAuley, M. Hamilton-Wessler, et al. 1991. Comparison of the ramp versus standard exercise protocols. *Journal of the American College of Cardiology* 17 (6): 1334-1342.

36. Napolitano, M.A., B. Lewis, J.A. Whiteley, and B.H. Marcus. 2006. Principles of health behavior change. In: *ACSM's Resource Manual for Guidelines for Exercise Testing and Prescription*, L.A. Kaminsky, ed. Philadelphia: Lippincott Williams & Wilkins. pp. 545-557.

37. National Strength and Conditioning Association. 2001. NSCA's strength & conditioning professional standards and guidelines. http://www.nsca-lift.org/Publications/posstatements.shtml. Accessed October 20, 2010.

38. Noonan, V., and E. Dean. 2000. Submaximal exercise testing: Clinical application and interpretation. *Physical Therapy* 80 (8): 782-807.

39. O'Brien, C.P. 1999. Are current exercise test protocols appropriate for older patients? *Coronary Artery Disease* 10: 43-46.

40. Powers, S.K., and E.T. Howley. 2009. *Exercise Physiology: Theory and Application to Fitness and Performance,* 7th ed. Boston: McGraw-Hill.

41. Prentice, A.M., and S.A. Jebb. 2001. Beyond body mass index. *Obesity Reviews* 2: 141-147.

42. Rodgers, G., J. Ayanian, G. Balady, J. Beasley, K. Brown, E. Gervino, et al. 2000. American College of Cardiology/ American Heart Association Clinical Competence statement on stress testing: A report of the American College of Cardiology/American Heart Association/American College of Physicians—American Society of Internal Medicine Task Force on Clinical Competence. *Journal of the American College of Cardiology* 36 (4): 1441-1453.

43. Rozenek, R., and T.W. Storer. 1997. Client assessment tools for the personal fitness trainer. *Strength and Conditioning* (June): 52-63.

44. Rusk, D.B. 1996. Creating your own personal training business. In: *The Business of Personal Training,* S.O. Roberts, ed. Champaign, IL: Human Kinetics. pp. 23-30.

45. Sheppard, J.M., and W.B. Young. 2006. Agility literature review: Classifications, training and testing. *Journal of Sports Sciences* 24 (9): 919-932.

46. Springer, B.A., R. Marin, T. Chan, H. Roberts, and N.W. Gill. 2007. Normative values for the unimpeded stance test with eyes open and closed. *Journal of Geriatric Physical Therapy* 30 (1): 8-15.

47. Soutine, H. 2007. Physical activity and health: Musculoskeletal issues. *Advances in Physiotherapy* 9 (2): 65-75.

48. Tan, R., and S. Spector. 1998. Exercise-induced asthma. *Sports Medicine* 25 (1): 1-6.

49. Terrados, N., and R.J. Maughan. 1995. Exercise in the heat: Strategies to minimize the adverse effects on performance. *Journal of Sports Sciences* 13: S55-S62.

50. Thomas, J.R., J.K. Nelson, and S.J. Silverman. 2005. *Research Methods in Physical Activity,* 5th ed. Champaign, IL: Human Kinetics.

51. Thompson, W.R., N.F. Gordon, and L.S. Pescatello, eds. 2010. *ACSM's Guidelines for Exercise Testing and Prescription,* 8th ed. Philadelphia: Lippincott Williams & Wilkins.

52. Turley, K.R., J.H. Wilmore, B. Simons-Morton, J.M. Williston, J.R. Epping, and G. Dahlstrom. 1994. The reliability and validity of the 9-minute run in third-grade children. *Pediatric Exercise Science* 6: 178-187.

53. van den Tillaar, R., and G. Ettema. 2004. Effect of body size and gender in overarm throwing performance. *European Journal of Applied Physiology* 91 (4): 413-418.

54. Victor, R., W. Leimbach, D. Seals, B. Wallin, and A. Mark. 1987. Effects of the cold pressor test on muscle sympathetic nerve activity in humans. *Hypertension* 9 (5): 429-436.

55. Wang, Z., S. Heshka, R. Pierson, and S. Heymsfield. 1995. Systematic organization of body-composition methodology: An overview with emphasis on component-based methods. *American Journal of Clinical Nutrition* 61 (3): 457-465.

56. Wilmore, J.H., D.L. Costill, and W.L. Kenney. 2008. *Physiology of Sport and Exercise,* 4th ed. Champaign, IL: Human Kinetics.

Test Preparation and Implementation Checklist

Client's name: _____

Personal trainer's name: _____

Test preparation	√	Date/comments
1. Verify appropriateness of selected assessments:		
a. Identify and evaluate client's specific goals.		
b. Assess professional expertise associated with the tests to determine appropriateness of current skill level to obtain accurate results.		
c. Evaluate the characteristics of tests to determine congruency with client's goals and to assess the risk-to-benefit relationship.		
2. Review safety considerations:		
a. Conduct a preparticipation health appraisal screening.		
b. Obtain a physician referral, medical clearance, or both.		
c. Distribute and collect completed informed consent and screening forms.		
d. Review emergency procedures.		
3. Select facilities and verify accuracy of equipment:		
a. Identify tests that are easy to administer and are cost-effective.		
b. Select appropriate equipment and confirm availability.		
c. Calibrate equipment.		
d. Provide a testing atmosphere that is calm, private, and relaxed.		
e. Make sure that the assessment area is safe, clean, set up, and ready for testing.		
f. Evaluate room temperature and humidity (68-72° F [20-22° C]; 60% humidity).		
4. Instruct client on preassessment protocols:		
a. Provide clients with pretest instructions. • Adequate rest (6-8 h the night before testing) • Moderate dietary intake (including adequate hydration) • Abstinence from chemicals that accelerate heart rates (except for presently prescribed medications) • Appropriate attire (loose-fitting clothing and sturdy shoes)		
b. Explain conditions for starting and stopping procedures of the protocol.		
5. Prepare record-keeping system:		
a. Create and supply a recording form or system.		
b. Develop a storage and retrieval system for data that is secure and confidential.		
Test implementation	**√**	**Date/comments**
1. Determine sequence of assessments:		
a. Establish an organized and appropriate testing order.		
b. Develop an appointment schedule for testing.		
2. Define and follow test protocols:		
a. Provide written test directions and guidelines to client.		
b. Explain technique, reasons for disqualification, and test scoring.		
c. Demonstrate test performance and allow time to practice.		
d. Provide an opportunity for client to ask questions regarding the tests.		
e. Implement an adequate warm-up and cool-down procedure.		
f. Spot the client when appropriate.		

From NSCA, 2012, *NSCA's essentials of personal training*, 2nd ed., J. Coburn and M. Malek (eds.), (Champaign, IL: Human Kinetics).

Individual Assessment Recording Form

Pretest   Posttest   (circle one)

Client's name: _____   Age: _____

Goals: _____

_____

Preparticipation screening notes: _____

_____

Assessment dates: _____

Comments: _____

_____

Vital signs	Score or result	Classification
Resting blood pressure		
Resting heart rate		
Body composition measures	**Score or result**	**Classification**
Height		
Weight		
Body mass index (BMI)		
Waist circumference		
Hip circumference		
Waist-to-hip ratio		
%body fat (method: _____)		
Cardiorespiratory endurance	**Score or result**	**Classification**
$\dot{V}O_2$max		
Other: _____		
Muscular endurance	**Score or result**	**Classification**
YMCA bench press		
Partial curl-up		
Prone double straight-leg raise		
Other: _____		
Muscular strength	**Score or result**	**Classification**
1RM bench press		
1RM leg press		
Other: _____		
Flexibility	**Score or result**	**Classification**
Sit-and-reach		
Other: _____		
Other tests	**Score or result**	**Classification**
Other: _____		
Other: _____		
Other: _____		

From NSCA, 2012, *NSCA's essentials of personal training*, 2nd ed., J. Coburn and M. Malek (eds.), (Champaign, IL: Human Kinetics).

Fitness Testing Protocols and Norms

Eric D. Ryan, PhD, and Joel T. Cramer, PhD

After completing this chapter, you will be able to

- understand the protocols for selected fitness tests,

- correctly administer the selected fitness tests,

- attain valid and reliable measurements of your clients' fitness levels and select appropriate tests for individual clients, and

- compare your clients' results with normative data.

As discussed in chapter 10, personal trainers must choose valid and reliable tests that are suitable for an individual client. To do this effectively, the personal trainer must administer tests accurately and record and interpret the results. This chapter describes the most frequently used and widely applicable fitness testing protocols for assessing a client's vital signs, body composition, cardiovascular endurance, muscular strength, muscular endurance, and flexibility. Specific descriptive or normative data are also provided for each protocol. More fitness testing protocols are available, but many do not have associated descriptive and normative data and thus are not included here.

Exercise Testing Protocols

Vital Signs

Body Composition

Cardiovascular Endurance

Muscular Strength

Muscular Endurance

Flexibility

Vital Signs

Many of the assessments that a personal trainer performs during a fitness evaluation involve two basic tasks: taking the client's pulse and blood pressure. Sometimes these assessments are performed with the client in a resting state (e.g., measuring resting heart rate); but monitoring heart rate and blood pressure changes with exercise—especially aerobic exercise—is an effective method to determine appropriate exercise intensity (i.e., keeping the client's exercise heart rate in the prescribed target zone).

Heart Rate

Most adults have a resting heart rate (HR), or *pulse*, between 60 and 80 beats per minute (beats/min), with the average HR for females 7 to 10 beats/min greater than that for males (19). A normal resting heart rate can be anywhere between 60 and 100 beats/min. Those slower than 60 beats/min are classified as bradycardia and those higher than 100 beats/min as tachycardia (15). Table 11.1 (p. 203) provides resting HR norm values. Three commonly used field techniques for assessing resting HR may be particularly useful for personal trainers: (a) palpation, (b) auscultation, and (c) the use of heart rate monitors.

Equipment

Depending on the specific procedure used to assess HR, any one or a combination of the following devices may be necessary.

- Stopwatch
- Stethoscope
- Heart rate monitor

Palpation Procedure

Palpation is probably the most common and certainly the most cost-effective method for assessing both resting and exercise HR.

1. Use the tips of the index and middle fingers to palpate the pulse. Avoid using the thumb, because its inherent pulse may be confusing and potentially confounding. Any one of the following anatomical landmarks can be used to palpate the pulse:
   - Brachial artery: the anterior-medial aspect of the arm just distal to the belly of the biceps brachii muscle, 1 inch (2 to 3 cm) superior to the antecubital fossa (15).
   - Carotid artery: on the anterior surface of the neck just lateral to the larynx (19). This position is illustrated in figure 11.1a. *Note:* Avoid applying too much pressure to this location when palpating for HR. Baroreceptors located in the arch of the aorta and the carotid sinuses can sense increases in applied pressure and will feed back to the medulla to decrease HR. Thus, use of the carotid site for measuring HR, if done incorrectly, can result in artificially low HR values.
   - Radial artery: on the anterior-lateral surface of the wrist, in line with the base of the thumb (19). This position is illustrated in figure 11.1b.
   - Temporal artery: the lateral side of the cranium on the anterior portion of the temporal fossa, usually along the hairline at the level of the eyes.
2. If you are using a stopwatch to keep the time while counting beats, and if you start the stopwatch simultaneously with the first beat, count the first beat as zero. If the stopwatch has been running, count the first beat as one (19). The HR should be counted for 6, 10, 15, 30, or 60 seconds.
3. If the HR is counted for less than a full minute, use the following multipliers to convert your measurement to beats per minute: ×10 for 6 seconds; ×6 for 10 seconds; ×4 for 15 seconds; and ×2 for 30 seconds.

Typically, the shorter-duration HR counts (6, 10, and 15 seconds) are used during exercise and postexercise conditions (19). Not only are short-duration HR counts more time efficient;

Locating the Pulse

Radial Pulse

- Bend the elbow with the arm at the side. The palm of the hand should be up.
- The radial artery is located on the inside of the wrist near the base of the thumb.
- Using the middle (long) and index (pointer) fingers, gently feel for the radial artery.

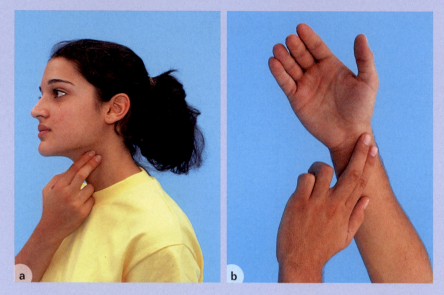

FIGURE 11.1 *(a)* Carotid pulse determination and *(b)* radial pulse determination.

Carotid Pulse

- Using the middle (long) and index (pointer) fingers, gently feel the carotid artery on either side of the neck, in the space between the windpipe (trachea) and muscle (right or left sternocleidomastoid), beneath the lower jawbone.
- Caution: Some pressure needs to be applied to allow one to feel the pulse, but too much pressure may cause reduced blood flow to the head. Therefore it is important to be careful not to press too hard on the artery and not to press on both arteries at the same time.

Example 11.1

Converting Pulse Measurements

12 heartbeats counted during a 6-second period:

12 beats per 6 s × 10 = 120 beats/min

18 heartbeats counted during a 10-second period:

18 beats per 10 s × 6 = 108 beats/min

24 heartbeats counted during a 15-second period:

24 beats per 15 s × 4 = 96 beats/min

41 heartbeats counted during a 30-second period:

41 beats per 30 s × 2 = 82 beats/min

Factors Affecting Heart Rate Assessment

- Smoking and tobacco products ($\uparrow$ resting HR; $\uparrow$ or $\leftarrow$ exercise HR)
- Caffeine ($\uparrow$ or $\leftarrow$ resting and exercise HR—responses to caffeine consumption are quite variable and depend on previous exposure or consumption; therefore, caffeine consumption should be avoided prior to HR measurements)
- Environmental temperature extremes ($\uparrow$ resting and exercise HR in hot environmental temperatures; HR responses can be quite variable in cold environmental temperatures and largely dependent on a client's body composition, acclimatization, and metabolism)
- Altitude ($\uparrow$ HR at altitudes greater than approximately 4,000 feet [1,200 m])
- Stress ($\uparrow$ resting and exercise HR)
- Food digestion ($\uparrow$ resting and exercise HR)
- Body position ($\downarrow$ HR when supine, $\uparrow$ HR from supine to seated position or standing position)
- Time of day ($\downarrow$ HR first thing in the morning, $\uparrow$ or $\leftarrow$ during afternoon or evening hours)
- Medications ($\uparrow$, $\leftarrow$, or $\downarrow$ resting and exercise HR—responses to medications are quite variable and contingent on the specific medication)

Note: $\uparrow$ = increase; $\downarrow$ = decrease; $\leftarrow$ = no significant change.

From Kordich 2002 (18).

they may also provide a more accurate representation of momentary HR due to the immediate fluctuations that often occur with changes in exercise intensity. Resting HR, however, is generally assessed with the longer-duration HR counts (30 and 60 seconds) to reduce the risk of miscounts and measurement error.

Auscultation Procedure

Auscultation requires the use of a stethoscope. The bell of the stethoscope should be placed directly on the skin over the third intercostal space just left of the sternum (19). The sounds heard from the heart beating should be counted for either 30 or 60 seconds (19). Refer to previously given instructions for the correct conversion factor for the 30-second HR count.

Heart Rate Monitor Procedure

Digital display HR monitors are becoming increasingly popular because of their validity, stability, and functionality (23). One drawback, however, is the cost of HR monitoring equipment. Nevertheless, personal trainers may find that these monitors are a very efficient and convenient way to assess HR at rest and during exercise.

Blood Pressure

Blood pressure (BP) can be defined as the forces of blood acting against vessel walls (8). The sounds that are emitted as a result of these vibratory forces are called **Korotkoff sounds.** The detection and disappearance of Korotkoff sounds under controlled pressure environments are the basis of most BP measurement methods. Although there are various invasive and noninvasive techniques for determining BP (8), **sphygmomanometry** is the most commonly used field technique and as such gives personal trainers a convenient tool for evaluating their clients' BP. One can also use a mercury or an **aneroid sphygmomanometer.** However, both of these require the use of an inflatable air bladder–containing cuff and a stethoscope to **auscultate** the Korotkoff sounds; thus this procedure is also commonly referred to as the *cuff* or *auscultatory method* (8).

Repeated BP measurements are important for detecting hypertension (table 11.2, p. 233; [27]) and for monitoring the antihypertensive effects of an exercise program or dietary changes (8). When assessing BP, it is imperative to use calibrated equipment that meets certification standards (37) and to follow standardized protocol (34). It is recommended that BP readings be taken with a mercury sphygmomanometer. However, recently calibrated aneroid sphygmomanometers or validated electronic devices are being used more frequently, although their accuracy has been questioned compared to that of traditional mercury sphygmomanometers (35).

Equipment

- Mercury or aneroid sphygmomanometer
- Air bladder–containing cuff
- Stethoscope

Procedure

1. Instruct the client to refrain from smoking or ingesting caffeine at least 30 minutes prior to BP measurements (34).

2. Have the client sit upright in a chair that supports the back with either the right or the left arm and forearm exposed, supinated, and supported at the level of the heart (differences between right and left arm BP measurements are marginal). *Note:* If exposing the arm by rolling or bunching up the sleeves of clothing causes any occlusion of circulation above the cuff site, ask the client to remove the constricting clothing articles (19).

3. Select the appropriate cuff size for the client. See table 11.3 (p. 233) for the correct cuff size based on the client's arm circumference. To determine the arm circumference, have the client stand with arms hanging freely at the sides, and take the arm circumference measurements midway between the acromion process of the scapula and the olecranon process of the ulna (19), roughly midway between the shoulder and elbow.

4. Begin BP measurements only after the client has rested for a minimum of 5 minutes in the position described in step 2 (35).

5. Place the cuff on the arm so that the air bladder is directly over the brachial artery (some cuffs have a line indicating the specific placement over the brachial artery). The bottom edge of the cuff should be 1 inch (2.5 cm) above the antecubital space (8).

6. With the client's palm facing up, place the stethoscope firmly, but not hard enough to indent the skin, over the antecubital space (8). *Note:* Most personal trainers find it easier to use their dominant hand to control the bladder airflow by placing the air bulb in the palm and using the thumb and forefinger to control the pressure release. The nondominant hand is then used to hold the stethoscope (8).

7. Position the sphygmomanometer so that the center of the mercury column or aneroid dial is at eye level and the air bladder tubing is not overlapping, obstructing, or being allowed to freely contact the stethoscope head or tubing (19). See figure 11.2 for common errors in performing a BP assessment.

8. Once the cuff, stethoscope, and sphygmomanometer are in place, quickly inflate the air bladder either (a) to 160 mmHg or (b) to 20 mmHg above the anticipated systolic BP. Upon maximum inflation, turn the air release screw counterclockwise to release the pressure slowly at a rate of 2 or 3 mmHg per second (8).

9. Record both systolic blood pressure (SBP) and diastolic blood pressure (DBP) measurements in even numbers using units of millimeters of mercury (mmHg) to the nearest 2 mmHg on the sphygmomanometer. To do this it is necessary during cuff deflation to make a mental note of the pressure corresponding with the first audible detection of Korotkoff sounds via auscultation, or SBP. The pressure at which the Korotkoff sounds disappear is the DBP (8). *Note:* Traditionally, Korotkoff sounds occur as sharp "thud" noises that can be similar to the sounds of gentle finger tapping on the stethoscope head (bell). Consequently, Korotkoff sounds are also similar to the extraneous noises often made when the air bladder tubing is allowed to bump against the stethoscope bell, so it is important to take great care to avoid these erroneous and potentially confusing noises (19).

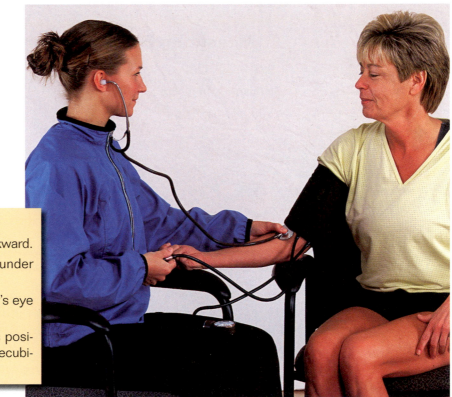

COMMON ERRORS

- The stethoscope is on backward.
- The stethoscope bell is under the cuff.
- The dial is not at the tester's eye level.
- The blood pressure cuff is positioned too close to the antecubital space.

FIGURE 11.2   Common errors in performing a blood pressure assessment.

10. Upon the disappearance of the Korotkoff sounds, carefully observe the manometer for an additional 10 to 20 mmHg of deflation to confirm the absence of sounds. Once the absence of sounds is confirmed, release the remaining pressure rapidly and remove the cuff (8).

11. After a minimum of 2 minutes' rest, measure BP again using the same technique. If the two consecutive measurements of either the SBP or the DBP differ by more than 5 mmHg, take a third BP measurement and record the average of the three SBP and the average of the three DBP measurements as the final scores (i.e., the SBP and the DBP; see example 11.2, Client A). If the consecutive measurements of neither the SBP nor the DBP differ by more than 5 mmHg, average the two SBP scores and average the two DBP scores to determine the final BP (see example 11.2, Client B) (8).

12. Once a client's BP has been determined, it can be classified from table 11.4.

Tips for Blood Pressure Measurement

1. The client should be seated comfortably with the back supported and the legs not crossed.
2. The upper arm should be bare and have no restrictive clothing.
3. The client's arm should be completely relaxed and supported at approximately heart level.
4. The bladder of the cuff should cover at least 80% of the client's upper arm.
5. The cuff should be deflated at 2 or 3 mm/s, with the first and last audible sounds taken as the SBP and DBP, respectively.
6. Both the client and tester should remain quiet during testing.

Based on Pickering et al. (35)

Example 11.2

Measuring Blood Pressure

Client A	SBP (mmHg)	DBP (mmHg)	Client B	SBP (mmHg)	DBP (mmHg)
Trial 1	132	78	Trial 1	110	68
Trial 2	126	80	Trial 2	114	66
Difference	6	2	Difference	4	2
Trial 3 (required)	130	78	Trial 3 (not required)	–	–
Averaged final score	**129**	**79**	**Averaged final score**	**112**	**67**

Factors Affecting Blood Pressure Assessment

- Smoking and tobacco products (↑ resting and exercise)
- Caffeine (BP responses to caffeine consumption are quite variable and depend on previous exposure and consumption; therefore, caffeine consumption should be avoided prior to BP measurements)
- Stress (↑ resting and exercise)
- Body position (↓ when supine, ↑ from supine to seated position or standing position)
- Time of day (↓ first thing in the morning, ↑ or ← during afternoon or evening hours)
- Medications (↑, ←, or ↓ resting and exercise BP—responses to medications are quite variable and contingent on the specific medication)

↑ = increase; ↓ = decrease; ← = no significant change.

From Kordich 2002 (21).

Body Composition

The measurement of body composition is of great interest to personal trainers and their clients. A variety of methods are available, each with its own advantages and disadvantages. Regardless of the method chosen, the personal trainer must be meticulous in following the appropriate protocol and must take great care in measuring and evaluating clients.

Anthropometry

Anthropometry, which is the science of measurement applied to the human body, generally includes measurements of height, weight, and selected body girths. Measurement of height requires a flat wall against which the client stands, a measuring tape attached or unattached to the wall, and a rectangular object placed concurrently against both the client's head and the wall. More detailed instructions for measuring height are given later in this section.

The most accurate body mass or body weight measurement is performed with a certified balance beam scale (of the type normally found in physicians' offices), which is generally more reliable than a spring scale and should be calibrated on a regular basis. A calibrated electronic scale is an acceptable alternative. Clients should be weighed while wearing minimal dry clothing (e.g., gym shorts and T-shirt, no shoes). For comparison measurements at a later date, they should dress similarly and be weighed at the same time of day. The most reliable body mass (weight) measurements are made in the morning upon rising, after elimination and before ingestion of food or fluids. Level of hydration can result in variability of body mass (weight). Thus, clients should be encouraged to avoid eating salty food (which increases water retention) the day before weighing and to go to bed normally hydrated.

The most reliable girth measurements are usually obtained with the aid of a flexible measuring tape equipped with a spring-loaded attachment at the end that, when pulled out to a specified mark, exerts a fixed amount of tension on the tape—for example, a Gulick tape (2). Girth measurements can be made at the beginning of a training or incentive period for comparison with subsequent measurements.

Body Mass Index

Personal trainers often use the body mass index (BMI) to examine **body mass** related to **stature.** Body mass index is a somewhat more accurate indicator of body fat than are estimates based simply on height and weight (e.g., height–weight tables).

$$\text{BMI (kg/m}^2\text{)} = \text{Body weight (kg)} \div \text{Height}^2 \text{ (m}^2\text{)} \qquad \textbf{(11.1)}$$

Once a client's BMI has been determined, this value can be compared to those in table 11.5 (p. 234). To calculate BMI, it is necessary to have the client's height and weight. The following instructions describe how to accurately measure height and weight.

Height

Height is a basic anthropometric measurement for which "stature" is a more accurate term (8). Although stature can be measured in several different ways, the two most common techniques involve (a) using an anthropometer typically located on the upright of a standard platform scale and (b) simply having a client stand with the back against a flat wall. The anthropometer method is convenient but requires access to a standard platform scale. The use of a wall is cost-effective but requires a right-angled device to simultaneously slide against the wall and contact the top of the client's head (crown). Regardless of the specific technique used, the following standard protocol is recommended for assessing a client's stature (8).

Equipment

Depending on the procedure used to assess a client's stature, one of the following devices is necessary.

- Standard platform scale with anthropometer arm
- Flat, ridged, right-angled device (to simultaneously slide against a wall and rest on top of client's crown)

Procedure

1. Ask the client remove all footwear.
2. Instruct the client to stand as erect as possible with feet flat on the floor and heels together facing away from wall or stadiometer.
3. Instruct the client to horizontally align the lowest point of the orbit of the eye with the opening of the ear.
4. Immediately before taking the measurement, instruct the client to take a deep breath and hold until the measurement has been taken.
5. Rest the anthropometer arm or measurement angle gently on the crown of the client's head.
6. Mark the wall or stabilize the anthropometer, and record the measurement to the nearest centimeter. If only inches are available as a unit of measure, then record the value to the nearest 1/4 to 1/2 inch and convert the measurement in inches to centimeters.
7. Once a client's height has been measured, the value can be compared to those in tables 11.6 and 11.7 (p. 234).

Weight

The term *weight* is defined as the mass of an object under the normal acceleration due to gravity; therefore, a more accurate term to characterize body weight is *body mass* (8). An accurate measurement of body mass can be taken only with a calibrated and certified scale. One of the types of scales most commonly used is the platform-beam scale. The personal trainer should adhere to the following standard protocol when assessing a client's body mass (8).

Equipment

- Calibrated and certified scale

Procedure

1. Ask the client to remove as much clothing and jewelry as feasible.
2. Instruct the client to step gently onto the scale and remain as still as possible throughout the measurement.
3. Record the weight to the nearest 1/4 pound or, when a sensitive metric scale is available, to the nearest 0.02 kg (8).
4. Convert the measurement in pounds to kilograms using the following equation:

$$\text{pounds (lb)} \div 2.2046 = \text{kilograms (kg)} \tag{11.2}$$

5. Body weight measurements can be compared to the values in table 11.8 on page 236. For example, for a 36-year-old female client who is 60 inches (152.4 cm) tall and weighs 135 pounds (61.2 kg), table 11.8 indicates that she is classified as overweight based on her BMI.

Example 11.3

Calculating BMI

Client A

A female client is measured with a height of 65 inches and a weight of 145 pounds.

Stature	= 65 inches × 0.0254 = 1.651 meters
Mass	= 145 pounds ÷ 2.2046 = 65.8 kilograms
BMI	= 65.8 ÷ (1.651 × 1.651) = 65.8 ÷ 2.726
	= 24.1

From table 11.5, a BMI of 24.1 is normal.

Client B

A male client is measured with a height of 69 inches and a weight of 214 pounds.

Stature	= 69 inches × 0.0254 = 1.753 meters
Mass	= 214 pounds ÷ 2.2046 = 97.1 kilograms
BMI	= 97.1 ÷ (1.753 × 1.753) = 97.1 ÷ 3.073
	= 31.6

From table 11.5, a BMI of 31.6 is consistent with Class I obesity.

Factors Affecting Body Mass Assessment

- Previous meals (↑ after meal consumption)
- Time of day (↓ first thing in the morning, ↑ during afternoon or evening hours)
- Hydration status (↓ when dehydrated; body mass will ↓ postexercise due to sweat loss)

↑ = increase; ↓ = decrease; ←→ = no significant change.

Skinfolds

A skinfold (SKF) indirectly measures the thickness of subcutaneous fat tissue. Skinfold measurements are highly correlated with body density measurements from underwater weighing. Percent body fat estimated from skinfolds is valid and can be reliably measured by properly trained personal trainers.

Equipment

- Skinfold caliper
- Nonelastic (i.e., plastic or metal) tape measure
- Pen or other marking device

General Considerations for Skinfold Testing

- Take all skinfold measurements on the right side of the body.
- Take the skinfold measurements when the client's skin is dry and free of lotion. In addition, skinfold measurements should always be taken before exercise. Exercise-induced changes in the hydration status of different body tissues can significantly affect the thickness of a skinfold.
- Carefully identify, measure, and mark the skinfold site.
- Grasp the skinfold firmly between the thumb and fingers. The placement of the thumb and fingers should be at least 1 cm (0.4 inches) away from the site to be measured.
- Lift the fold by placing the thumb and index finger approximately 8 cm (3 inches) apart on a line that is perpendicular to the long axis of the skinfold. The long axis is parallel to the natural cleavage lines of the skin. The thicker the fat tissue layer, the greater the separation between the thumb and finger as the fold is lifted.
- Keep the fold elevated while taking the measurement.
- Place the jaws of the caliper perpendicular to the fold, 1 cm (0.4 inches) away from the thumb and index finger, and release the jaw pressure slowly.
- Record the skinfold measurement after 1 to 2 seconds (but within 4 seconds) after the jaw pressure has been released.
- If the caliper is not equipped with a digital display (Skyndex II), read the dial of the caliper to the nearest 0.2 mm (Harpenden), 0.5 mm (Lange or Lafayette), or 1 mm (Slim Guide, The Body Caliper, or Accu-Measure). Studies have been conducted to compare skinfold measurements and body composition estimates from different types of calipers (13, 30). The practical implications, however, regarding any potential variations among skinfold calipers are marginal.
- Take a minimum of two measurements at each site. If the values vary by more than 2 mm or 10%, take an additional measurement.

Harrison et al. 1988 (16).

Procedure for Specific Skinfold Sites

1. Select an appropriate combination of skinfold sites for the client from the following list.

   - Chest
   - Triceps
   - Abdomen
   - Thigh
   - Midaxilla
   - Subscapula
   - Suprailium
   - Medial calf

2. Carefully identify and mark the appropriate skinfold sites:

   - *Chest:* Take a diagonal fold half the distance between the anterior axillary line (imaginary line extending from the front of the armpit downward) and the nipple for men (figure 11.3*a*), and one-third of the distance from the anterior axillary line to the nipple for women.
   - *Midaxilla:* Take a vertical fold on the midaxillary line (imaginary line extending from the middle of the armpit downward; it divides the body into front and back halves) at the level of the xiphoid process (bottom of the sternum) (figure 11.3*b*).

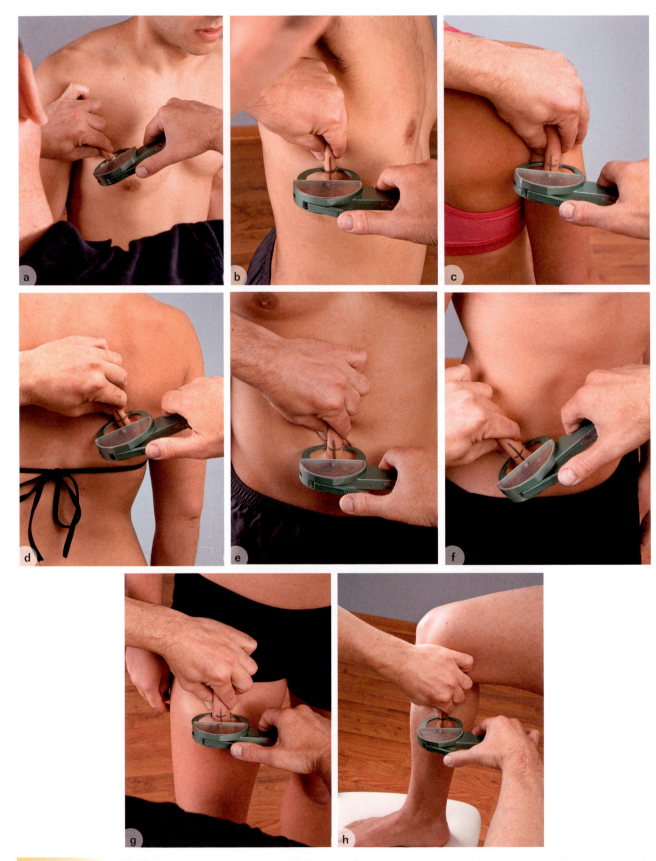

FIGURE 11.3   Skinfold measurements: (*a*) chest skinfold, (*b*) midaxilla skinfold, (*c*) triceps skinfold, (*d*) subscapula skinfold, (*e*) abdomen skinfold, (*f*) suprailium skinfold, (*g*) thigh skinfold, and (*h*) medial calf skinfold.

- *Triceps:* Take a vertical fold on the posterior midline of the upper arm (over the triceps muscle), halfway between the acromion (top of shoulder) and olecranon processes (elbow); the elbow should be extended and relaxed (figure 11.3c).

- *Subscapula:* Take a fold on a diagonal line coming from the vertebral (medial) border to 1 to 2 cm (0.4 to 0.8 inches) from the inferior angle (bottommost point) of the scapula (figure 11.3d).

- *Abdomen:* Take a vertical fold at a lateral distance of approximately 2 cm (1 inch) from the umbilicus (figure 11.3e).

- *Suprailium:* Take a diagonal fold above the crest of the ilium (top of the pelvis) at the spot where an imaginary line would come down from the anterior axillary line (figure 11.3f).

- *Thigh:* Take a vertical fold on the anterior aspect of the thigh midway between hip and knee joints (figure 11.3g).

- *Medial calf:* Have the client place the right leg on a bench with the knee flexed at 90°. On the medial border, mark the level of the greatest calf girth. Raise a vertical skinfold on the medial side of the right calf 1 cm (0.4 inches) above the mark, and measure the fold at the maximal girth (figure 11.3h).

3. Using the appropriate population-specific equation from table 11.9 (p. 236), calculate the estimated body density from the skinfold measurements.

4. Enter the body density into the appropriate population-specific equation from table 11.10 (p. 237) to calculate the percent body fat.

5. Compare the percent body fat to the normative values in table 11.11 (p. 238).

From ACSM 2010 (2)

BIA and NIR Techniques for Measuring Body Composition

Bioelectrical impedance analysis (BIA) has been developed as a method for measuring body composition. Bioelectrical impedance analysis works via measurement of the amount of impedance or resistance to a small, painless electrical current passed through the body between two electrodes, which are often placed on the wrist and ankle (12). The underlying concept is that leaner clients conduct this electrical current with less resistance than those who are carrying more adipose tissue. Some authors have suggested that BIA methods for determining body composition are roughly as accurate as skinfold techniques except for clients who are either very lean or obese, in which cases BIA is not as accurate (10). Others, however, have questioned the validity and sensitivity of BIA body composition assessments (12, 27) and have stated that BIA measurements can be easily and significantly affected by factors such as hydration status, skin temperature, and racial characteristics (27). However, recent research has reported that BIA analyses are acceptable field techniques to measure body composition in Caucasian men and women (30, 31). Future studies are needed to determine if BIA analyses are acceptable in other races.

The **near-infrared interactance (NIR)** method of measuring body composition is derived from its use in agriculture to assess body composition in animals, quality of meats, and lipid concentrations in grains (27). This method works on the principles of the wavelength changes of light that is absorbed and reflected by different tissues in the body at various anatomical sites, such as the biceps, triceps, subscapula, suprailium, and thigh (12). Equipment for NIR consists of a fiber-optic probe or "light wand" that emits low-level electromagnetic radiation light waves (12). Most authors (12, 27) agree, however, that NIR body composition measurements (a) are not as accurate as skinfolds, (b) are not sensitive to changes in body composition, and (c) can produce large measurement errors. However, recently NIR (Futrex 6100XL) has been shown to produce acceptable estimates of percent fat in Caucasian women (30). Future studies are needed to determine if the Futrex 6100XL is acceptable in males and in other races.

Waist-to-Hip Girth Ratio

Although not truly a measure of body composition per se, measurement of the waist-to-hip ratio is a valuable tool for assessing relative fat distribution and risk of disease. People with more fat in the trunk, particularly abdominal fat, are at increased risk for a variety of cardiovascular and metabolic diseases (2).

Equipment

- Nonelastic (i.e., plastic or metal) tape measure

Procedure

1. Place tape measure around girth of waist (smallest girth around the abdomen) and hip (largest girth measured around the buttocks). See figures 11.4 and 11.5.
2. Hold zero end of tape in one hand, positioned below the other part of the tape, which is held in the other hand.
3. Apply tension to the tape so that it fits snugly around the body part but does not indent the skin or compress the subcutaneous tissue.
4. Align the tape in a horizontal plane, parallel to the floor.
5. To determine the waist-to-hip ratio, divide the waist circumference by the hip circumference.
6. Use table 11.12 (p. 239) to assess risk.

From Heyward 1998 (18).

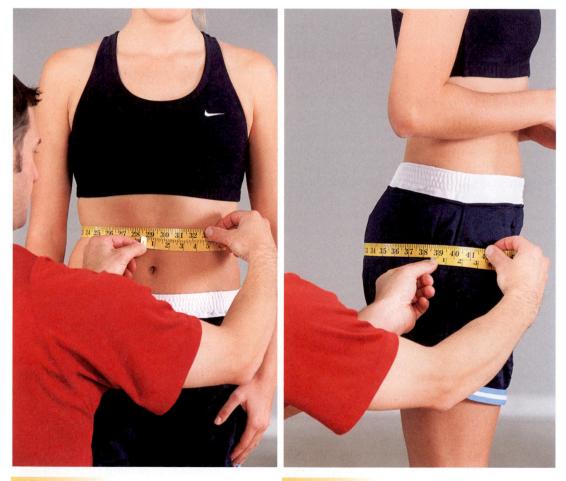

FIGURE 11.4 Waist circumference measurement.

FIGURE 11.5 Hip circumference measurement.

Assumptions and Solutions for Submaximal Exercise Tests

Assumption 1: Heart rate measurements must be **steady state.**

Solution: Heart rate can fluctuate dramatically with sudden changes in work rate. To ensure that HR has achieved steady state, personal trainers should record HR values at the end of a constant work rate stage or after 2 or 3 minutes of exercise at a constant work rate (1). Steady-state HR is defined as two consecutive HR measurements that are within five beats/min of each other (2).

Assumption 2: True maximal HR for a given age must be the same for all clients.

Solution: For any given age, maximal HR can vary as much as ±10 to 12 beats/min across individuals (2); therefore, the typical equation to calculate age-predicted maximal HR can introduce an unknown error into the model for submaximal estimation of $\dot{V}O_2$max.

$$\text{Age-predicted maximal HR (beats/min)} = 220 - \text{Age (years)} \qquad \textbf{(11.3)}$$

Assumption 3: The relationship between HR and work rate must be strong, positive, and linear.

Solution: The positive relationship between HR and workload is most linear between 50% and 90% of maximal HR (8). One should consider this when extrapolating HR versus work rate data points. In example 11.4, only the HR values at stages 2, 3, and 4 should be used to estimate $\dot{V}O_2$max since those HR values are between 50% and 90% of the age-predicted maximal HR.

Assumption 4: Mechanical efficiency ($\dot{V}O_2$ at a given work rate) is the same for all clients.

Solution: Personal trainers should choose a test that is specific to the client's existing cardiovascular exercise mode(s), daily activities, or both. For example, if a client typically goes for long walks three or four times per week, the Rockport walking test or a submaximal treadmill walking test might be the best indicator of that client's $\dot{V}O_2$max.

Cardiovascular Endurance

The personal trainer can use submaximal cardiovascular endurance tests to attain a reasonably accurate estimation of a client's $\dot{V}O_2$max (2). Submaximal exercise tests are used most often because of high equipment expenses, the personnel needed, and the increased risks associated with maximal tests. See table 10.1 for a list of indicators a personal trainer should look for that would require immediate termination of an exercise test. The concept behind a submaximal test is to monitor HR, BP, or rating of perceived exertion (RPE)—or some combination of these—during exercise until a predetermined percentage of the client's predicted maximal HR is achieved, at which point the test is terminated. To get a true measure of a client's cardiovascular endurance, one would need to conduct a maximal test, taking the client to his or her extreme limits of HR and oxygen consumption rate ($\dot{V}O_2$max). Maximal tests, however, are not safe or necessary for many clients and sometimes cannot be conducted without physician supervision; thus submaximal tests are used instead. By their very nature, submaximal tests provide *estimations* of a client's $\dot{V}O_2$max. However, most submaximal exercise testing protocols, such as those presented in this chapter, provide a valid, reliable, specific, and sensitive estimation of $\dot{V}O_2$max. And, as with many estimation techniques, there are certain assumptions that must be considered. Refer to the outline on this page to understand the basic assumptions underlying a submaximal exercise test as well as some potential solutions that the personal trainer should consider.

General Procedures for Cycle Ergometer Testing

1. Ensure that the cycle ergometer has been recently and correctly calibrated.
2. Adjust the seat height so that there is a slight flexion at the knee joint (about 5°) at maximal leg extension (lowest pedal position) with the ball of the foot on the pedal (19).

3. The client should be seated on the cycle ergometer in an upright position with the hands properly positioned on the handlebars (19). Ask the client to maintain the same grip and posture throughout the duration of the test.

4. Establish the pedaling cadence before setting the resistance (19). If a metronome is necessary to set the pedaling cadence, set it at twice the desired cadence so that one full pedal revolution occurs for every two metronome beats (e.g., set the metronome at 100 for a test requiring a pedaling cadence of 50 revolutions per minute [rpm]) (19).

5. Set the workload. The workload on a cycle ergometer usually refers to the work rate. Work rate is defined as a power output and is measured in units of kilogram-meters per minute (kg · m · min^{-1}) or watts (W) that can be calculated with the following equation:

$$\text{Work rate (kg} \cdot \text{m} \cdot \text{min}^{-1}) = \text{Resistance (kg)} \times \text{Distance (m)} \times \text{Cadence (rpm)} \quad \textbf{(11.4)}$$

where resistance = the amount of friction placed on the flywheel (usually in kilograms or kiloponds),

distance = the distance the flywheel travels as a result of one pedal revolution (meters), and

cadence = the pedaling cadence (revolutions per minute). The work rate in watts can now be calculated by the following equation:

$$\text{Work rate (W)} = \text{Work rate (kg} \cdot \text{m} \cdot \text{min}^{-1}) \div 6.12. \quad \textbf{(11.5)}$$

■ Setting the work rate on an electronically braked cycle ergometer is usually simple, because these expensive ergometers often have computer- or digitally interfaced work rate settings that automatically adjust the resistance based on the pedaling cadence to maintain a predetermined work rate.

■ On a mechanically braked ergometer, maintaining a work rate is more difficult. Mechanically braked cycle ergometers have a flywheel "braked" by a belt that adds resistance by friction as it is tightened. Since the work rate is controlled by the resistance and the pedaling cadence, both must remain constant to maintain the work rate.

6. Check the resistance setting frequently during the test to avoid the unexpected increases or decreases that are common with use of mechanically braked cycle ergometers (19).

7. Continuously monitor the appearance and symptoms of the client (see table 10.1) for a list of general indications for stopping an exercise test in low-risk adults (1).

8. During multistage tests (i.e., the YMCA cycle ergometer test):

■ Assess HR during the end of each stage or until steady-state HR is achieved. For example, if the client is working through a 3-minute stage, measure his or her HR during the final 15 to 30 seconds of the second and third minutes. If the consecutive HR measurements are not within five beats/min of each other, continue the stage for one more minute and measure HR again (see HR testing protocol [3]).

■ Assess BP near the end of each stage and repeatedly in the case of a hypo- or hypertensive response (see BP testing protocol [3]).

■ Assess RPE near the end of each stage using either the 6 to 20 or the 0 to 10 RPE scale (1).

9. Once you have terminated the test, initiate an appropriate cool-down. The cool-down can be an active recovery period consisting of light pedaling at a resistance equal to or less than the starting resistance. Or, if the client is uncomfortable or is experiencing signs and symptoms (table 10.1), a passive recovery may be necessary (2).

10. During the cool-down, monitor HR, BP, and signs and symptoms regularly for at least 4 minutes. If unusual or abnormal responses occur, further monitoring of the recovery period will be necessary (2).

YMCA Cycle Ergometer Test

The YMCA cycle ergometer test is a submaximal, multistage exercise test for cardiovascular endurance. This popular test is designed to progress the client to 85% of his or her predicted maximal HR using 3-minute stages of increasing work rate.

Equipment

- Mechanically or electrically braked cycle ergometer
- Metronome (if the cycle ergometer does not have an rpm gauge)
- Stopwatch
- Heart rate and BP measurement equipment (see "Heart Rate" and "Blood Pressure" sections earlier in this chapter)
- Rating of perceived exertion scale

Procedure

1. Instruct the client to begin pedaling at 50 rpm and maintain this cadence throughout the duration of the test.
2. Set the work rate for the 1st three-minute stage at 150 kg $\cdot$ m $\cdot$ min^{-1} (0.5 kg at 50 rpm).
3. Measure the client's HR during the final 15-30 seconds of the second and third minute of the 1st stage; if they are not within six beats/min of each other, continue the stage for one more minute.
4. See table 11.13 (p. 239) for directions on how to set the work rate for the remaining stages. If the client's HR at the end of the 1st stage is:
   - <80 beats/min, set the work rate for the 2nd stage at 750 kg $\cdot$ m $\cdot$ min^{-1} (2.5 kg at 50 rpm)
   - 80-89 beats/min, set the work rate for the 2nd stage at 600 kg $\cdot$ m $\cdot$ min^{-1} (2.0 kg at 50 rpm)
   - 90-100 beats/min, set the work rate for the 2nd stage at 450 kg $\cdot$ m $\cdot$ min^{-1} (1.5 kg at 50 rpm)
   - >100 beats/min, set the work rate for the 2nd stage at 300 kg $\cdot$ m $\cdot$ min^{-1} (1.0 kg at 50 rpm)
5. Measure the client's HR during the final 15-30 seconds of the second and third minute of the 2nd stage; if they are not within six beats/min of each other, continue the stage for one more minute.
6. Set the 3rd and 4th three-minute stages (if required) according to table 11.13 (work rates for the 3rd and 4th stages are located in the rows below the 2nd stage). Be sure to measure the client's HR in the final 15-30 seconds of the second and third minute of each stage; if they are not within six beats/min of each other, continue each stage for one more minute.
7. Terminate the test when the client reaches 85% of his or her age-predicted maximal HR or if the client meets one of the criteria listed in table 10.1.

Reprinted by permission from ACSM 2010.

Estimating $\dot{V}O_2$max From the YMCA Cycle Ergometer Test

When the test is complete, the personal trainer should have the following data:

- Body weight (kg)
- Age-predicted maximal HR
- At least two HR measurements at each work rate up to 85% of the age-predicted maximal HR
- A BP measurement at each work rate
- An RPE assessment at each work rate

To attain an estimation of the client's $\dot{V}O_2$max:

1. Plot the HR (Y-axis in beats/min) versus work rate (X-axis in kg $\cdot$ m $\cdot$ min^{-1} or W) on a graph (example 11.4).

2. Construct a horizontal line at the age-predicted maximal HR value (A in 11.6).

3. Extrapolate the data by drawing a line of best fit for the HR values between 50% and 90% of the age-predicted maximal HR (B in figure 11.6).

Example 11.4

YMCA Cycle Ergometer Test

Client A, a 23-year-old male client who weighs 181 pounds (82 kg), has just completed a YMCA cycle ergometer test with the following data:

Resting HR = 62 beats/min

Resting BP = 124/78 mmHg

Age-predicted maximal HR = 197 beats/min = 220 − 23 = 197 beats/min (from equation 11.3).

85% age-predicted maximal HR = 0.85 × 197 beats/min = 167 beats/min

Stage	Work rate	Elapsed time	HR	Average HR*	BP	RPE
1	150 kg · m · min⁻¹	2:00	88 beats/min			
1	150 kg · m · min⁻¹	3:00	88 beats/min	88 beats/min*	134/82 mmHg	9
2	600 kg · m · min⁻¹	5:00	132 beats/min			
2	600 kg · m · min⁻¹	6:00	136 beats/min	134 beats/min*	148/76 mmHg	13
3	750 kg · m · min⁻¹	8:00	154 beats/min			
3	750 kg · m · min⁻¹	9:00	158 beats/min	156 beats/min*	152/80 mmHg	15
4	900 kg · m · min⁻¹	11:00	164 beats/min			
4	900 kg · m · min⁻¹	12:00	168 beats/min	166 beats/min*	160/82 mmHg	17

*Average HR was calculated by averaging the two consecutive HR values at each work rate.

Step 1: Plot all of the average HR measurements (Y-axis) versus the corresponding work rates (X-axis) on a graph.

Step 2: Construct a horizontal line (A in figure 11.6) at 197 beats/min (the age-predicted maximum HR).

Step 3: Construct a line of best fit (B in figure 11.6) for the plotted data points (from step 1) and extend the line beyond the horizontal line at 197 beats/min (A in figure 11.6).

Step 4: Construct a vertical line (D in figure 11.6) from the intersection (C in figure 11.6) of lines A and B that extends to the X-axis.

Step 5: Identify the X-axis value that corresponds with the vertical line D. This value is the predicted maximal work rate that will be used to calculate the estimated $\dot{V}O_2$max (E in figure 11.6). In this example, it is 1,172 kg · m · min⁻¹.

Step 6: Use equation 11.5 to convert the kg · m · min⁻¹ value to watts.

$$\text{Work rate (W)} = \text{Work rate (kg · m · min}^{-1}) \div 6.12 \qquad \textbf{(11.5)}$$

From step 5, predicted maximal work rate (kg · m · min⁻¹) = 1,175 kg · m · min⁻¹

Predicted maximal work rate (W) = 1,175 kg · m · min⁻¹ ÷ 6.12 = 192 W

Step 7: Use equation 11.2 to convert the client's body weight in pounds to kilograms.

$$\text{pounds (lb)} \div 2.2046 = \text{kilograms (kg)} \qquad \textbf{(11.2)}$$

Body weight (lb) = 181 lb

181 lb ÷ 2.2046 = 82 kg

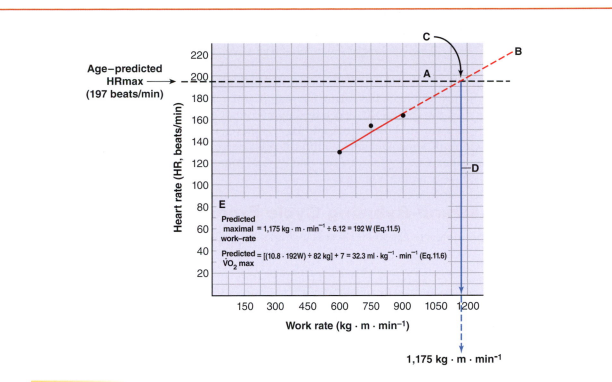

FIGURE 11.6   Using data from example 11.4, this figure illustrates how to graph a client's submaximal YMCA test data and how to construct the horizontal line for predicted maximal HR (A), extrapolate the line of best fit (B), identify the intersection (C), construct a vertical line for predicted maximal work rate (D), and use equations 11.5 and 11.6 to determine the predicted $\dot{V}O_2$max (E).

Step 8: Use equation 11.6 (from [2]) to determine the predicted $\dot{V}O_2$max score in ml · kg^{-1} · min^{-1}.

$$\dot{V}O_2\text{max (ml} \cdot \text{kg}^{-1} \cdot \text{min}^{-1}) = [(10.8 \times W) \div BW] + 7 \qquad \textbf{(11.6)}$$

From step 6, predicted maximal work rate (W) = 192 W

Body weight (kg) = 82 kg

$$\dot{V}O_2\text{max (ml} \cdot \text{kg}^{-1} \cdot \text{min}^{-1}) = [(10.8 \times 192) \div 82] + 7 = 32.3 \text{ ml} \cdot \text{kg}^{-1} \cdot \text{min}^{-1}$$

Step 9: Use table 11.14 (1) to compare this client's predicted $\dot{V}O_2$max of 32.3 ml · kg^{-1} · min^{-1} to normative values; 32.3 ml · kg^{-1} · min^{-1} for a 23-year-old male ranks at less than the 10th percentile. Therefore, more than 90% of the population have higher $\dot{V}O_2$max scores, while less than 10% have a lower $\dot{V}O_2$max.

From Golding 2000 (14).

4. Continue the line of best fit (B) beyond the final data point until it crosses the horizontal line (A) representing the age-predicted maximal HR. Construct a vertical line from the intersection (C in figure 11.6) of the line of best fit and the horizontal age-predicted maximal HR line. Extend the vertical line to the X-axis and record the corresponding work rate value (D in figure 11.6). This X value is the predicted maximal work rate that will be used to calculate the estimated $\dot{V}O_2$max (E in figure 11.6).

5. If the predicted maximal work rate is in kg · m · min^{-1}, it will need to be converted to watts (W). Use equation 11.5 to convert the kg · m · min^{-1} value to W.

6. Use the following equation (from [2]) to calculate the predicted $\dot{V}O_2$max value in milliliters per kilogram per minute (ml · kg^{-1} · min^{-1}):

$$\dot{V}O_2\text{max (ml · kg}^{-1}\text{ · min}^{-1}) = [(10.8 \times W) \div BW] + 7 \tag{11.6}$$

where W = the predicted maximal work rate (in watts) and BW = body weight (kg).

7. Once a client's $\dot{V}O_2$max has been estimated (ml · kg^{-1} · min^{-1}), use table 11.14 (p. 239) to rank the client's $\dot{V}O_2$max based on his or her age. For example, if the $\dot{V}O_2$max has just been estimated to be 36.7 ml · kg^{-1} · min^{-1} for a 46-year-old male client, that client would rank approximately within the 30th percentile when compared to others his age. In other words, one can say that 30% of men his age have a lower $\dot{V}O_2$max, while 70% have a higher $\dot{V}O_2$max.

Åstrand-Ryhming Cycle Ergometer Test

The Åstrand-Ryhming cycle ergometer test is a single-stage test (5). Total duration of the test is 6 minutes.

Equipment
- Mechanically or electrically braked cycle ergometer
- Metronome (if the cycle ergometer does not have an rpm gauge)
- Stopwatch

Procedure
1. Set the pedaling cadence at 50 rpm.
2. Set the work rate. Work rates used for the Åstrand-Ryhming test are chosen based on gender and fitness level (8). Note that for estimating a client's fitness level (unconditioned vs. conditioned) prior to the Åstrand-Ryhming test to determine the starting work rate, the recommendation is to always choose the more conservative work rate (unconditioned) if there is any question about the client's current status.

Males, unconditioned	300 or 600 kg · m · min^{-1}
Males, conditioned	600 or 900 kg · m · min^{-1}
Females, unconditioned	300 or 450 kg · m · min^{-1}
Females, conditioned	450 or 600 kg · m · min^{-1}

3. Instruct the client to begin pedaling. Once the proper cadence is achieved, start the stopwatch. After 2 minutes, take a HR measurement.
   - If the HR is ≥120 beats/min, have the client continue the selected work rate throughout the 6-minute test duration.
   - If the HR after 2 minutes is <120, increase the resistance to the next highest increment or until the HR measurement is ≥120 beats/min after 2 minutes of riding at a constant work rate.
4. Take HR measurements at the end of the fifth and sixth minutes of the test, average them, and use this average value to estimate $\dot{V}O_2$max in liters per minute (L/min) from table 11.15 (p. 240) for males and table 11.16 (p. 240) for females.
5. Once the $\dot{V}O_2$max is estimated, it must be corrected for the age of the client. To obtain the age-corrected $\dot{V}O_2$max estimation, multiply the unaltered $\dot{V}O_2$max value (L/min) from table 11.15 or table 11.16 by the appropriate age correction factor in table 11.17 (p. 241).
6. After age correction of the $\dot{V}O_2$max estimation (L/min), it can be converted to ml · kg^{-1} · min^{-1} by the following equation:

$$\dot{V}O_2\text{max (ml · kg}^{-1}\text{ · min}^{-1}) = \dot{V}O_2\text{max in L/min} \times 1{,}000 \div BW \tag{11.7}$$

where BW = body weight in kilograms (kg).

7. Compare the age-corrected $\dot{V}O_2$max estimations (ml · kg^{-1} · min^{-1}) from the Åstrand-Ryhming test to the normative values listed in table 11.18 (p. 241) (8).

Example 11.5

Åstrand-Ryhming Cycle Ergometer Test

A 57-year-old female client who weighs 145 pounds (66 kg) has just completed the Åstrand-Ryhming cycle ergometer test. The following data were recorded:

Work rate = 450 kg · m · min^{-1}

Heart rate after second minute = 122 beats/min

Heart rate after fifth minute = 129 beats/min

Heart rate after sixth minute = 135 beats/min

Step 1. (129 beats/min + 135 beats/min) ÷ 2 = 132 beats/min average.

Step 2. Estimated $\dot{V}O_2$max value from table 11.16 for an average HR of 132 beats/min and a work rate of 450 kg · m · min^{-1} = 2.7 L/min.

Step 3. Age correction factor from table 11.17 for a 57-year-old client = 0.70.

Step 4. 2.7 L/min × 0.70 age correction factor = 1.89 L/min.

Step 5. (1.89 L/min × 1,000) ÷ 66 kg = 28.64 ml · kg^{-1} · min^{-1}.

Step 6. Aerobic fitness category from table 11.18 for 28.64 ml · kg^{-1} · min^{-1} for a 57-year-old female = Good.

Step 7. Percentile rank from table 11.14 for 28.64 ml · kg^{-1} · min^{-1} for a 57-year-old female: ~55%.

YMCA Step Test

The YMCA step test is a basic, inexpensive cardiovascular endurance test that can be easily administered individually or to large groups. This test classifies fitness levels based on the postexercise HR response but does not provide an estimation of $\dot{V}O_2$max. The objective of the YMCA step test is to have the client step up and down to a set cadence for 3 minutes and to measure the HR recovery response immediately after the test.

Equipment

- 12-inch (30 cm) step bench or box
- Metronome set at 96 beats/min
- Stopwatch

Procedure

1. For familiarization, the client should listen to the cadence prior to stepping.
2. Instruct the client to step "up, up, down, down" to a cadence of 96 beats/min, which allows 24 steps per minute. It does not matter which foot leads or if the foot lead changes during the test.
3. Have the client continue stepping for 3 minutes.
4. Immediately after the final step, help the client sit down and, within 5 seconds, measure the HR for 1 minute.
5. Compare the 1-minute recovery HR value to the normative values in table 11.19 (p. 242).

Distance Run and Walk Test Considerations

Distance run tests are based on the assumption that a more "fit" client will be able to run a given distance in less time or run a greater distance in a given period of time. These tests are practical, inexpensive, less time-consuming than other tests, and easy to administer to large groups. They also can be used to classify the cardiovascular endurance level of healthy men under 40 years of age and healthy women under 50 years of age. The personal trainer cannot, however, use field tests to detect or control for cardiac episodes because HR and BP are typically not monitored during the performance of these tests.

It is important to note that these field tests are effort-based assessments and are suited for clients who can run (or walk briskly) for either 12 minutes, 1.5 miles (2.4 km), or 1 mile (1.6 km). Examples of clients for whom these tests are appropriate are those who have been training for several weeks and those who regularly use running or fast walking as a mode of cardiovascular exercise. Other tests for $\dot{V}O_2$max such as the Åstrand-Ryhming cycle ergometer test or the YMCA step test are recommended for clients who do not meet these criteria.

From Golding 2000 (14).

12-Minute Run/Walk

The 12-minute run/walk test is a field test designed to measure the distance traveled over 12 minutes of running/walking. After distance is recorded as the test score, it is used in a regression equation (equation 11.8) to estimate $\dot{V}O_2$max.

Equipment

- 400 m (437-yard) track or flat course with measured distances so that the number of laps completed can be easily counted and multiplied by the course distance
- Visible place markers—may be necessary to divide the course into predetermined section lengths (e.g., every one-fourth or one-half of a lap) so that the exact distance covered in 12 minutes can be determined quickly
- Stopwatch

Procedure

1. Instruct the client to run as far as possible during the 12-minute duration. Walking is allowed; however, the objective of this test is to cover as much distance as possible in 12 minutes.

2. Record the total distance completed in meters. For example, a client has just completed five full laps and one-fourth of the last lap (5.25 laps). Since there are 400 m per lap, the client completed 2,100 m (5.25 laps × 400 m = 2,100 m).

3. Use the following equation (from [14]) to estimate the client's $\dot{V}O_2$max (ml · kg^{-1} · min^{-1}):

$$\dot{V}O_2\text{max (ml} \cdot \text{kg}^{-1} \cdot \text{min}^{-1}) = (0.0268 \times D) - 11.3 \qquad \textbf{(11.8)}$$

where D = distance completed in meters.

4. You can then compare estimated $\dot{V}O_2$max scores to the normative values listed in table 11.14 (2).

Example 11.6

12-Minute Run/Walk

A 31-year-old female client who weighs 128 pounds (58 kg) has just completed the 12-minute run. The following data were recorded:

12-min run distance = 1.16 miles (6,109 feet; 1,862 m)

1. [0.0268 × (1,862 m)] − 11.3 = 38.60 ml · kg^{-1} · min^{-1}.

2. Percentile rank from table 11.14 for 38.60 ml · kg^{-1} · min^{-1} for a 31-year-old female = 80th percentile.

1.5-Mile Run

The 1.5-mile run is a field test designed to measure the time it takes for a client to run 1.5 miles. Once the time is recorded as the test score, it is used in a regression equation (equation 11.9) to estimate $\dot{V}O_2$max.

Equipment

- 400 m (437-yard) track or flat course with the 1.5-mile (2.4 km) distance measured (to measure the course, use an odometer or measuring wheel [14])
- Stopwatch

Procedure

1. Instruct clients to cover the 1.5-mile (2.4 km) distance in the fastest possible time. Walking is allowed, but the objective is to complete the distance in as short a time as possible.

2. Call out or record the elapsed time (in minutes and seconds, 00:00) as the client crosses the finish line.

3. Convert the seconds to minutes by dividing the seconds by 60. For example, if a client's time for the test is 12:30, the run time is converted to 12.5 minutes (30 ÷ 60 seconds = 0.5 minutes).

4. Use the following equation (from [14]) to estimate the client's $\dot{V}O_2$max (ml · kg^{-1} · min^{-1}):

$$\dot{V}O_2\text{max (ml · kg}^{-1}\text{ · min}^{-1}\text{)} = 88.02 - (0.1656 \times BW) \hspace{1cm} \text{(11.9)}$$
$$- (2.76 \times time + (3.716 \times gender^*)$$

where BW = body weight in kilograms (kg) and time = 1.5-mile run time to completion (to the nearest hundredth of a minute, 0.00 min).

*For gender, substitute 1 for males and 0 for females.

5. Estimated $\dot{V}O_2$max scores can be compared to the normative values listed in table 11.14 (2).

Example 11.7

1.5-Mile Run

A 28-year-old male client who weighs 171 pounds (77.6 kg) has just completed the 1.5-mile (2.4 km) run. The following data were recorded:

1.5-mile run time = 8:52 min:s

1. 52 s ÷ 60 s = 0.87 min, so 8:52 min:s = 8.87 min.
2. 88.02 − [0.1656 × (77.6)] − [2.763 (8.87)] + [3.716 × (1 *for males*)] = 54.40 ml · kg^{-1} · min^{-1}.
3. Percentile rank from table 11.14 for 54.40 ml · kg^{-1} · min^{-1} for a 28-year-old male = over 90th percentile.

Rockport Walking Test

The Rockport walking test has been developed to estimate $\dot{V}O_2$max for men and women ages 18 to 69 years (20). Because this test requires only walking at a fast pace, it is useful for testing older or sedentary clients.

Equipment

- Stopwatch
- Measured 1.0-mile (1.6 km) walking course that is flat and uninterrupted (preferably an outdoor track)

Procedure

1. Instruct the client to walk 1.0 mile (1.6 km) as briskly as possible.

2. Immediately after the test, calculate the client's HR (in beats per minute) using a 15-second HR count duration (see "Heart Rate" section earlier in this chapter).

3. Convert the seconds to minutes by dividing the seconds by 60 (see step 3 for the 1.5-mile run procedure).

4. Estimate the client's $\dot{V}O_2$max (ml · kg^{-1} · min^{-1}) using the following equation (from [22]):

$$\dot{V}O_2\text{max (ml · kg}^{-1} \cdot \text{min}^{-1}) = 132.853 - (0.0769 \times BW) \hspace{1cm} \textbf{(11.10)}$$
$$- (0.3877 \times age) + (6.315 \times gender^*)$$
$$- (3.2649 \times time) - (0.1565 \times HR)$$

where BW = body weight in pounds, age = age in years, time = 1.0-mile walk time to completion (to the nearest hundredth of a minute, 0.00 minutes), and HR = heart rate in beats per minute.

*For gender, substitute 1 for males and 0 for females.

5. Estimated $\dot{V}O_2$max scores can be compared to the normative values listed in table 11.14 (2).

6. 1.0-mile walk times can also be compared to the normative values listed in table 11.20 (p. 242) (32).

1-Mile Run

The 1-mile run has been developed to estimate cardiovascular endurance for children ages 6 to 17 years (32).

Equipment

- Stopwatch
- A flat and uninterrupted 1.0-mile (1.6 km) course (e.g., an outdoor track)

Procedure

1. Instruct clients to cover the 1-mile (1.6 km) distance in the fastest possible time. Walking may be interspersed with running, but the client should try to complete the distance in the fastest time possible.

2. Record the elapsed time (in minutes and seconds, 00:00) as the client crosses the finish line.

3. Convert the seconds to minutes by dividing the seconds by 60 (see step 3 for the 1.5-mile run procedure).

4. Compare the recorded time to the normative values listed in table 11.21 (p. 242) (32).

Example 11.8

Rockport Walking Test

A 52-year-old male client who weighs 228 pounds (103.4 kg) has just completed the Rockport walking test. The following data were recorded:

Posttest HR = 159 beats/min

1.0-mile walk time = 10:35 min:s

1. 35 s ÷ 60 s = 0.58 min; 10:35 min:s = 10.58 min.

2. 132.853 − [0.0769 × (228 pounds)] − [0.3877 × (52)] + [6.315 × (1 *for males*)] − [3.2649 × (10.58 min)] − [0.1565 × (159)] = 42.05 ml · kg^{-1} · min^{-1}.

3. Percentile rank from table 11.14 for 42.05 ml · kg^{-1} · min^{-1} for a 52-year-old male = 80th to 90th percentile.

4. Rating from table 11.20 for 10:35 min:s = Good.

5. Percentile rank from table 11.20 for 10:35 min:s = over 90th percentile.

Non-Exercise-Based Estimation of $\dot{V}O_2$max

Non-exercise-based equations have been developed by Malek and colleagues (21, 22) to estimate a client's $\dot{V}O_2$max from various demographic and descriptive variables. These equations have been used to provide reasonable estimates of $\dot{V}O_2$max for both trained and untrained men and women. In addition, the errors associated with these equations range between ±10% to 15% of $\dot{V}O_2$max, which are similar to the errors often encountered with exercise-based estimates of $\dot{V}O_2$max (21, 22). Overall, non-exercise-based equations for the prediction of $\dot{V}O_2$max can be very useful, especially when the risk of conducting an exercise-based $\dot{V}O_2$max assessment is too high or unknown for clients who may be susceptible to exercise-induced stress.

Equipment

- Standard platform scale with anthropometer arm or flat, ridged, right-angled device (to simultaneously slide against a wall and rest on top of client's crown)
- Calibrated and certified scale
- Rating of perceived exertion scale

Procedure

1. Record the client's height in centimeters, body weight in kilograms, and age in years.
2. Estimate the typical intensity of training using the Borg RPE scale (e.g., 6-20).
3. Indicate the number of hours per week your client exercises.
4. Indicate the number of years your client has been training consistently with no more than one month without exercise.
5. Determine the natural log of the years of training. That is, enter the client's years of training and then hit "LN," or the natural log, on a handheld calculator.
6. Determine $\dot{V}O_2$max in L/min using the following equations.
7. Calculate $\dot{V}O_2$max in $ml \cdot kg^{-1} \cdot min^{-1}$ using equation 11.7.
8. Compare your client's scores to table 11.14.

Equations

Population	Equation for predicting $\dot{V}O_2$max (L/min)
Untrained males	$(0.046 \times H) - (0.021 \times A) - 4.31$
Untrained females	$(0.046 \times H) - (0.021 \times A) - 4.93$
Aerobically trained males*	$(27.387 \times BW) + (26.634 \times H) - (27.572 \times A) + (26.161 \times D) + (114.904 \times I) + (506.752 \times Y) - 4609.791$
Aerobically trained females*	$(18.528 \times BW) + (11.993 \times H) - (17.197 \times A) + (23.522 \times D) + (62.118 \times I) + (278.262 \times Y) - 1375.878$

H = height in cm; A = age in years; BW = body weight in kg; D = duration of training in hours per week; I = intensity of training using the Borg scale; Y = natural log of years training.
*Aerobically trained is defined as having participated in continuous aerobic exercise for a minimum of 1 hour per workout session, three or more sessions per week, for at least the last 18 months (21, 22)

Muscular Strength

Muscular strength is an important component of physical fitness. A minimal level of muscular strength is needed to perform daily activities, especially as one ages, and to participate in recreational or occupational activities without undue risk of injury. Strength may be expressed either as absolute strength or as relative strength. Absolute strength is simply the raw strength score a person achieves. Relative strength is usually expressed relative to body weight.

1-Repetition Maximum Bench Press

A 1-repetition maximum (1RM) bench press test may be used to measure upper body strength. Because free weights are used, this test requires skill on the part of the client being tested.

Equipment

- Adjustable barbell and weight plates that allow resistance increments of 5 to 90 pounds (approximately 2.5-40 kg).

Procedure

Provide a spotter and closely observe technique. See page 308 for proper bench press technique. Then, follow these steps for determining a 1RM:

1. Instruct the client to warm up with a light resistance that easily allows 5 to 10 reps at 40% to 60% of his or her estimated 1RM.

2. Provide a 1-minute rest period.

3. Estimate a warm-up load that will allow the client to complete three to five reps by adding as follows:

Body area	Absolute increase or percent increase
Upper body exercise	10-20 pounds (4-9 kg) or 5-10%
Lower body exercise	30-40 pounds (14-18 kg) or 10-20%

4. Provide a 2-minute rest period.

5. Estimate a conservative, near-maximum load that will allow the client to complete two or three reps by adding as follows:

Body area	Absolute increase or percent increase
Upper body exercise	10-20 pounds (4-9 kg) or 5-10%
Lower body exercise	30-40 pounds (14-18 kg) or 10-20%

6. Provide a 2- to 4-minute rest period.

7. Make a load increase:

Body area	Absolute increase or percent increase
Upper body exercise	10-20 pounds (4-9 kg) or 5-10%
Lower body exercise	30-40 pounds (14-18 kg) or 10-20%

8. Instruct the client to attempt a 1RM.

9. If the client was successful, provide a 2- to 4-minute rest period and go to back to step 7. If the client failed, provide a 2- to 4-minute rest period and decrease the load as follows:

Body area	Absolute decrease or percent decrease
Upper body exercise	5-10 pounds (2-4 kg) or 2.5-5%
Lower body exercise	15-20 pounds (7-9 kg) or 5-10%

   And then go back to step 8.

10. Continue increasing or decreasing the load until the client can complete one repetition with proper exercise technique. Ideally, the client's 1RM will be measured within three testing sets.

11. Record the 1RM value as the maximum weight lifted (i.e., the client's absolute strength) for the last successful attempt.

Once you have completed these steps, divide the 1RM value by the client's body weight to determine relative strength. Then, compare the relative strength value to values in table 11.22 (p. 242). (*Note:* The norms in table 11.22 were established using a Universal bench press machine.)

From Baechle, Earle 2008 (6) and Kraemer, Ratamess, Fry, and French 2006 (22).

1-Repetition Maximum Leg Press

The 1RM leg press may be used to measure lower body strength. Chapter 13 provides a detailed account of client and spotter responsibilities during most lower body exercises. Personal trainers should be familiar with the guidelines in chapter 13 before attempting 1RM trials.

Equipment

- Universal leg press machine. This resistance training device is less common than many others and therefore may be difficult to find. The personal trainer can instead opt to use a different exercise such as an angled hip sled or horizontal leg press to assess a client's lower body muscular strength. Note, however, that the normative data shown in table 11.23 (p. 243) will apply only if a Universal leg press machine is used.

Procedure

1. Have the client sit in the seat of the leg press machine and place the feet on the upper pair of foot plates.
2. Adjust the seat to standardize the knee angle at approximately 120°.
3. Follow the steps for determining a 1RM described in the "1-Repetition Maximum Bench Press" section to assess the client's leg press 1RM (5).
4. Divide the 1RM value by the client's body weight to determine relative strength.
5. If the Universal leg press machine was used, compare the relative strength value to values in table 11.23.

From Baumgartner, Jackson, Mahar, and Rowe 2007 (7).

Estimating a 1-Repetition Maximum

For safety or technique reasons, or both, many personal trainers prefer not to have their clients perform 1RM testing. Fortunately, it is possible to estimate a client's 1RM from a submaximal resistance. This involves having the client perform as many repetitions as possible with a submaximal resistance. More detailed instructions can be found elsewhere (6), and the process for estimating starting loads for a resistance training program is described in chapter 15.

Muscular Endurance

Muscular endurance is the ability of a muscle or muscle group to exert submaximal force for extended periods. Along with muscular strength, muscular endurance is important for performing the activities of daily living, as well as in recreational and occupational pursuits. Muscular endurance may be assessed during static and dynamic muscle actions.

YMCA Bench Press Test

The YMCA bench press test is used to measure upper body muscular endurance. This is a test of absolute muscular endurance; that is, the resistance is the same for all members of a given gender.

Equipment

- Adjustable barbell and weight plates
- Metronome

Procedure

1. Spot the client and closely observe the technique.
2. Set the resistance at 80 pounds (36.3 kg) for male clients, 35 pounds (15.9 kg) for female clients.
3. See page 308 for proper bench press technique.
4. Set the metronome cadence at 60 beats/min to establish a rate of 30 repetitions per minute.
5. Have the client, beginning with the arms extended and a shoulder-width grip, lower the weight to the chest. Then, without pausing, the client should raise the bar to full arm's length. The movement should be smooth and controlled, with the bar reaching its highest and lowest positions with each beat of the metronome.

6. Terminate the test when the client can no longer lift the barbell in cadence with the metronome.

7. Compare the client's score to values in table 11.24 (p. 244).

Partial Curl-Up Test

The partial curl-up test measures the endurance of the abdominal muscles. It is often favored over the sit-up test because it eliminates the use of the hip flexor muscles.

Equipment

- Metronome
- Ruler
- Masking tape
- Mat

Procedure

1. Direct the client to assume a supine position on a mat with the knees at 90° (figure 11.7a). The arms are at the side (on the floor), with the fingers touching a 4-inch (10 cm) piece of masking tape (placed on the floor perpendicular to the fingers). A second piece of masking tape is placed 10 cm beyond (but parallel to) the first.

2. Set a metronome to 50 beats/min and have the individual do slow, controlled curl-ups to lift the shoulder blades off the mat (trunk makes a 30° angle with the mat; figure 11.7b) in time with the metronome (25 curl-ups per minute). The low back should be flattened before curling up.

3. Direct the client to perform as many curl-ups as possible without pausing, up to a maximum of 25.

4. Compare the client's score to table 11.25 (p. 244).

Adapted from American College of Sports Medicine 2010 (2).

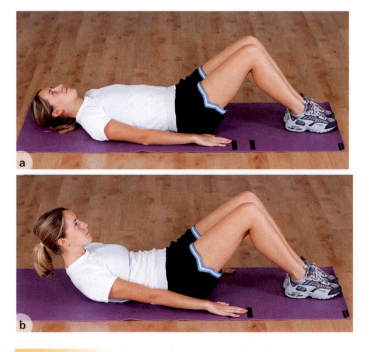

FIGURE 11.7 Curl-up: *(a)* beginning position and *(b)* end position.

Prone Double Straight-Leg Raise Test

The prone double straight-leg raise test has been shown to be a useful test for examining low back muscular endurance and predicting potential low back pain (3, 24).

Equipment

- A training or massage table

Procedure

1. Have the client begin the test in the prone position, legs extended, hands underneath the forehead, and forearms perpendicular to the body (figure 11.8*a*).
2. Instruct the client to raise both legs to the point of knee clearance from the table (figure 11.8*b*).
3. You can monitor the test by sliding one hand under the thighs.
4. Record the test duration in seconds.
5. Terminate the test when client can no longer maintain knee clearance from the table.
6. Compare your client's score to the values in table 11.26 (p. 244).

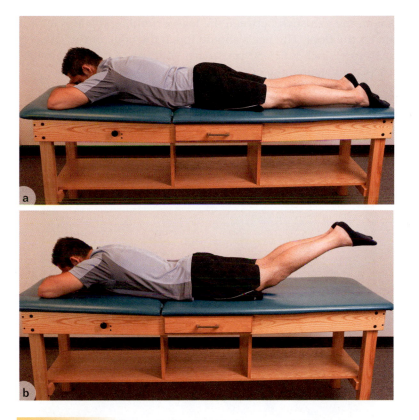

FIGURE 11.8 Prone double straight-leg raise: *(a)* beginning position and *(b)* legs raised position.

Flexibility

Flexibility refers to the range of motion (ROM) around a joint (e.g., shoulder) or a series of joints (e.g., vertebral column). It is believed to be related to the development of a number of musculoskeletal disorders, for example low back pain. There is no single test that can measure whole-body flexibility. Separate tests need to be administered for each area of interest. Traditionally, personal trainers have focused on tests that measure the flexibility of joints believed to be associated with risk of developing low back pain.

Sit and Reach

The sit-and-reach test is often used to measure hip and low back flexibility. Although the sit-and-reach test is commonly seen as an indicator of previous back discomfort, its ability to predict the incidence of low back pain is limited (19). Nonetheless, a lack of hip and low back flexibility, along with poor muscular strength and endurance of the abdominal muscles, is believed to be predictive of low back pain.

Equipment

- Yardstick or sit-and-reach box
- Adhesive tape
- Measuring tape

Procedure

1. Have the client warm up and perform some moderate stretching prior to the test. All testing should be done without shoes. The test should be performed with slow, controlled stretches.

2. For the YMCA sit-and-reach test, place a yardstick on the floor and place tape across the yardstick at a right angle to the 15-inch (38 cm) mark (see figure 11.9a). The client then sits with the yardstick between the legs, extending the legs at right angles to the taped line on the floor. The heels should touch the edge of the taped line and should be about 10 to 12 inches (25-30 cm) apart. With use of a sit-and-reach box, the heels should be placed against the edge of the box (see figure 11.10a).

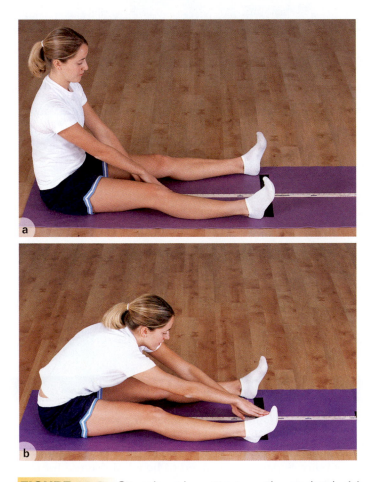

FIGURE 11.9   Sit-and-reach positioning with a yardstick: (a) beginning position and (b) end position.

3. Have the client reach forward slowly with both hands, moving as far as possible and holding the terminal position. The fingers should overlap and should be in contact with the yardstick (figure 11.9b) or sit-and-reach box (figure 11.10b).

4. The score is the most distant point reached. Use the best of two trials as the score. The knees must stay extended throughout the test, but the tester should not press the client's legs down.

5. Compare the test results using either table 11.27 (YMCA sit-and-reach test) or 11.28 (sit-and-reach box). Note that the norms for the YMCA sit-and-reach test use a "zero point" (the zero point is the point at which the client reaches the toes) of 15 inches (38 cm), while the sit-and-reach box typically uses a zero point set at 26 cm. When using a different zero point, be sure to adjust the client's score before using the norm tables. For example, if the box has a zero point of 23, add 3 cm to the client's score before consulting table 11.28 (or subtract 3 cm from the norms in the table before comparing the client's score to table 11.28).

From ACSM 2010 (2).

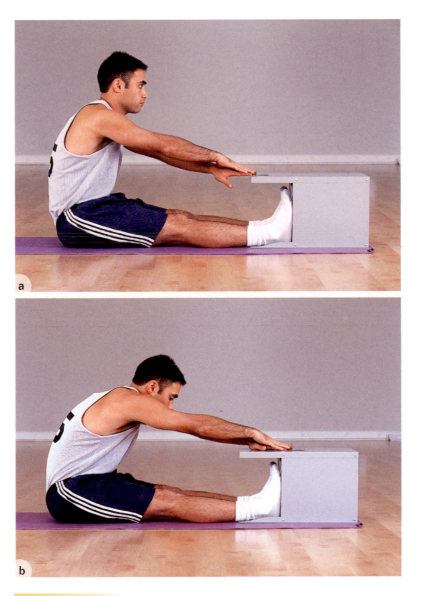

FIGURE 11.10 Sit-and-reach positioning with a sit-and-reach box: (a) beginning position and (b) end position.

Conclusion

Typically the personal trainer has the challenge of working with clients who have a broad spectrum of fitness or exercise capabilities. To gather baseline assessments, the personal trainer may test for a variety of fitness parameters such as HR, BP, body composition, cardiovascular endurance, muscular strength, muscular endurance, and flexibility and then make comparisons to established sets of descriptive or normative data. The resulting conclusions can then form the basis for the client's exercise prescription.

Study Questions

1. A 40-year-old female client's resting blood pressure was 115/72 during the initial assessment. When measuring her blood pressure one month later, to what level of mercury (Hg) should the bladder be inflated?

    A. 115 mm

    B. 125 mm

    C. 135 mm

    D. 150 mm

2. All of the following skinfold sites are appropriate for performing a three-site skinfold for a 45-year-old male client EXCEPT

    A. chest.

    B. suprailium.

    C. abdomen.

    D. thigh.

3. Calculate the estimated $\dot{V}O_2max$ value for a 38-year-old male client who weighs 88 kg and ran 1.5 miles in 13:30.

    A. $34.5 \: ml \cdot kg^{-1} \cdot min^{-1}$

    B. $36.2 \: ml \cdot kg^{-1} \cdot min^{-1}$

    C. $39.9 \: ml \cdot kg^{-1} \cdot min^{-1}$

    D. $41.5 \: ml \cdot kg^{-1} \cdot min^{-1}$

4. Which of the following is an assessment of local muscular endurance for a 38-year-old female client?

    A. bench press 35 pounds at 60 beats/min until failure

    B. 12-minute run/walk

    C. Åstrand-Ryhming cycle ergometer test

    D. YMCA step test

Applied Knowledge Question

A 28-year-old female recently hired a personal trainer. Her fitness evaluation indicated the following information:

Height: 66 inches

Weight: 150 pounds

Resting heart rate: 75 beats/min

Resting BP: 128/82

Body fat: 20%

$\dot{V}O_2max$: $26 \: ml \cdot kg^{-1} \cdot min^{-1}$

1RM bench press: 140 pounds

1RM leg press: 310 pounds

Partial curl-up test (1 minute): 25

Which of the fitness evaluation results is below average for this client and should be given attention when setting goals? How do you know this to be true?

TABLE 11.1 Norms for Resting Heart Rate (beats/min)

Rating	18-25 M	18-25 F	26-35 M	26-35 F	36-45 M	36-45 F	46-55 M	46-55 F	56-65 M	56-65 F	>65 M	>65 F
Excellent	40-54	42-57	36-53	39-57	37-55	40-58	35-56	43-58	42-56	42-59	40-55	49-59
Good	57-59	59-63	55-59	60-62	58-60	61-63	58-61	61-64	59-61	61-64	57-61	60-64
Above average	61-65	64-67	61-63	64-66	62-64	65-67	63-65	65-69	63-65	65-68	62-65	66-68
Average	66-69	68-71	65-67	68-70	66-69	69-71	66-70	70-72	68-71	69-72	66-69	70-72
Below average	70-72	72-76	69-71	72-74	70-72	72-75	72-74	73-76	72-75	73-77	70-73	73-76
Poor	74-78	77-81	74-78	77-81	75-80	77-81	77-81	77-82	76-80	79-81	74-79	79-83
Very poor	82-103	84-103	81-102	84-102	83-101	83-102	84-103	85-104	84-103	84-103	83-103	86-97

Adapted from Golding 2000 (14).

TABLE 11.2 Classification of Blood Pressure for Adults 18 Years or Older[a]

Systolic BP (mmHg)[b]	Category	Diastolic BP (mmHg)
<120	Normal	<80
120-139	Prehypertension	80-89
140-159	Stage 1 hypertension	90-99
≥160	Stage 2 hypertension	≥100

[a]For individuals not taking antihypertensive medication and not acutely ill. Based on average of two or more readings on two or more occasions.
[b]When systolic and diastolic pressures fall into different categories, use the higher category for classification.

Adapted from The Seventh Report of the Joint National Committee on Detection, Evaluation, and Treatment of High Blood Pressure, 2003 (33).

TABLE 11.3 Guidelines for Type of Blood Pressure Cuff

Cuff type	Arm circumference (cm)	Bladder width × length (cm)
Smaller child	≤17	4 × 13
Larger child	18-25	10 × 18
Standard adult	26-33	12 × 26
Larger adult	34-42	16 × 33
Obese adult (thigh cuff)	43-50	20 × 42

Reprinted by permission from Heyward 2010.

TABLE 11.4 Percentile Norms for Blood Pressure in Active Men and Women

%	Systolic (mmHg) 20-29 years	30-39 years	40-49 years	50-59 years	60+ years	Diastolic (mmHg) 20-29 years	30-39 years	40-49 years	50-59 years	60+ years
MEN										
90	110	108	110	110	112	70	70	70	72	70
80	112	110	111	116	120	72	74	76	78	76
70	118	116	118	120	124	78	78	80	80	80
60	120	120	120	122	130	80	80	80	80	80
50	121	120	121	128	131	80	80	80	82	81
40	128	124	126	130	140	80	81	84	86	84
30	130	130	130	138	140	84	85	88	90	88
20	136	132	138	140	150	88	90	90	90	90
10	140	140	142	150	160	90	92	98	100	98

(continued)

TABLE 11.4 *(continued)*

%	Systolic (mmHg)					Diastolic (mmHg)				
	20-29 years	30-39 years	40-49 years	50-59 years	60+ years	20-29 years	30-39 years	40-49 years	50-59 years	60+ years
WOMEN										
90	100	100	100	108	120	63	65	65	69	70
80	101	104	105	110	120	68	70	70	70	75
70	106	110	110	118	125	70	70	70	75	76
60	110	110	112	120	128	72	74	75	79	80
50	112	114	118	122	130	75	76	80	80	80
40	118	118	120	130	136	78	80	80	82	80
30	120	120	120	134	140	80	80	80	85	84
20	120	122	130	140	142	80	82	82	90	88
10	130	130	138	148	160	82	90	90	92	98

Adapted from Pollock, Wilmore, and Fox, III 1978 (36).

TABLE 11.5 Classification of Overweight and Obesity by Body Mass Index (BMI), Waist Circumference, and Associated Disease Risks

	BMI (kg/m²)	Obesity class	Disease* risk relative to normal weight and waist circumference	
			Men ≤102 cm (≤40 in.) Women ≤88 cm (≤35 in.)	Men >102 cm (>40 in.) Women >88 cm (>35 in.)
Underweight	<18.5		–	–
Normal	18.5-24.9		–	–
Overweight	25.0-29.9		Increased	High
Obesity	30.0-34.9	I	High	Very high
	35.0-39.9	II	Very high	Very high
Extreme obesity	≥40.0	III	Extremely high	Extremely high

*Disease risk for type 2 diabetes, hypertension, and coronary heart disease.

Reprinted from NIH; NHLBI 1998 (34).

TABLE 11.6 Average Stature and Percentiles for American Men (cm)

Race, ethnicity, and age	Mean	Percentile								
		5th	10th	15th	25th	50th	75th	85th	90th	95th
ALL RACES AND ETHNICITIES										
20 years and over	176.3	163.6	166.6	168.4	171.3	176.3	181.5	184.4	186.0	188.7
20-29 years	177.6	164.2	167.1	169.3	172.3	177.8	183.0	185.3	186.8	190.1
30-39 years	176.4	162.7	165.9	167.9	171.4	176.4	181.5	184.6	186.4	189.6
40-49 years	177.1	165.6	168.2	169.8	172.3	177.0	181.8	184.6	186.2	188.0
50-59 years	176.6	165.1	167.2	168.8	171.4	176.6	181.5	184.6	186.5	189.1
60-69 years	175.4	163.1	166.2	167.8	170.5	175.3	180.7	182.7	184.8	187.2
70-79 years	173.8	162.1	164.1	166.3	168.6	174.0	178.5	180.4	182.9	185.7
80 years and over	170.7	159.2	161.7	163.4	166.4	170.7	175.0	177.8	179.0	181.2
NON-HISPANIC WHITE										
20 years and over	177.5	166.0	168.5	170.2	172.6	177.4	182.4	184.9	186.5	189.1
20-39 years	178.9	167.4	170.1	171.9	174.4	178.9	183.4	185.7	187.7	190.3
40-59 years	178.0	167.3	169.2	170.8	173.1	177.9	182.8	185.2	186.6	188.8
60 years and over	174.6	162.6	165.2	167.1	169.8	174.6	179.7	182.2	183.7	186.4

Race, ethnicity, and age	Mean	Percentile								
		5th	10th	15th	25th	50th	75th	85th	90th	95th
NON-HISPANIC BLACK										
20 years and over	177.2	165.4	167.8	169.8	172.3	177.0	181.9	184.7	186.4	189.6
20-39 years	178.0	166.3	167.9	170.1	173.1	177.7	183.0	185.2	187.1	190.6
40-59 years	177.4	166.0	168.6	170.3	172.7	177.2	181.6	184.5	186.6	189.0
60 years and over	174.3	163.0	164.7	166.8	169.4	174.0	179.1	181.8	183.5	185.7
MEXICAN AMERICAN										
20 years and over	170.3	158.7	161.1	163.0	165.2	170.4	174.9	177.0	178.9	182.0
20-39 years	170.6	158.3	161.2	163.3	165.3	170.6	175.2	177.6	180.5	183.7
40-59 years	170.2	159.4	161.4	163.3	165.6	170.8	174.9	176.3	178.1	180.1
60 years and over	167.8	157.7	159.4	160.8	163.4	167.8	172.4	173.7	175.1	176.9

Reprinted from McDowell et al. 2008 (28).

TABLE 11.7 Average Stature and Percentiles for American Women (cm)

Race, ethnicity, and age	Mean	Percentile								
		5th	10th	15th	25th	50th	75th	85th	90th	95th
ALL RACE AND ETHNICITY GROUPS										
20 years and over	162.2	150.7	153.3	154.9	157.7	162.2	166.7	169.1	170.8	173.1
20-29 years	163.2	152.2	154.8	156.5	158.7	163	167.9	169.8	171.4	172.8
30-39 years	163.2	152.4	154.4	156.2	158.9	163	167.6	170.4	172	174.2
40-49 years	163.1	152.1	153.9	155.8	158.5	163.1	167.6	169.8	171.9	174
50-59 years	162.2	150.7	153.3	155.4	158.1	162.1	166.8	168.7	170.3	172.4
60-69 years	161.8	151.9	153.8	155.1	157.6	161.9	165.9	168	170	171.5
70-79 years	159.2	149	150.9	152.6	155	159	163.7	165.5	167.4	169.4
80 years and over	156	146.2	148	149.4	151.7	155.8	159.7	162.3	164.3	166.1
NON-HISPANIC WHITE										
20 years and over	163	152.1	154.4	156.3	158.7	163	167.5	169.7	171.3	173.6
20-39 years	164.8	154.7	157.2	158.6	160.7	164.7	168.9	171.1	172.4	174.4
40-59 years	163.6	152.6	155.5	157.5	159.4	163.4	167.7	169.9	171.8	174
60 years and over	160.2	149.7	152	153.6	155.9	159.8	164.5	166.7	168.6	170.5
NON-HISPANIC BLACK										
20 years and over	162.7	151.5	153.9	155.5	158.2	162.7	167	169.6	171	173.8
20-39 years	163.2	151.6	154.7	156.3	158.5	163	167.3	170.1	171.8	174.5
40-59 years	163.2	152.2	154.1	155.9	158.7	163.5	167.5	169.7	171.2	173.7
60 years and over	160.6	150	152.6	153.6	156.2	160.5	165.2	166.8	169	170.5
MEXICAN AMERICAN										
20 years and over	157.8	147.3	149.8	151.1	153.6	157.8	161.9	164.3	166.2	168.1
20-39 years	158.7	148.2	150.7	152.5	154.6	159	162.6	165	166.6	168.9
40-59 years	157.7	*	149.9	151.1	153.5	157.6	161.7	164	165.8	*
60 years and over	153.9	144.9	145.9	147.4	150.1	154	158.1	159.7	161.6	164.3

*Figure does not meet standards of reliability.

Reprinted from McDowell et al. 2008 (28).

TABLE 11.8 Body Mass Index Chart

BMI	NORMAL (HEALTHY) WEIGHT						OVERWEIGHT					OBESE					
	19	20	21	22	23	24	25	26	27	28	29	30	31	32	33	34	35
HEIGHT (IN.)	BODY WEIGHT (LB)																
58	91	96	100	105	110	115	119	124	129	134	138	143	148	153	158	162	167
59	94	99	104	109	114	119	124	128	133	138	143	148	153	158	163	168	173
60	97	102	107	112	118	123	128	133	138	143	148	153	158	163	168	174	179
61	100	106	111	116	122	127	132	137	143	148	153	158	164	169	174	180	185
62	104	109	115	120	126	131	136	142	147	153	158	164	169	175	180	186	191
63	107	113	118	124	130	135	141	146	152	158	163	169	175	180	186	191	197
64	110	116	122	128	134	140	145	151	157	163	169	174	180	186	192	197	204
65	114	120	126	132	138	144	150	156	162	168	174	180	186	192	198	204	210
66	118	124	130	136	142	148	155	161	167	173	179	186	192	198	204	210	216
67	121	127	134	140	146	153	159	166	172	178	185	191	198	204	211	217	223
68	125	131	138	144	151	158	164	171	177	184	190	197	203	210	216	223	230
69	128	135	142	149	155	162	169	176	182	189	196	203	209	216	223	230	236
70	132	139	146	153	160	167	174	181	188	195	202	209	216	222	229	236	243
71	136	143	150	157	165	172	179	186	193	200	208	215	222	229	236	243	250
72	140	147	154	162	169	177	184	191	199	206	213	221	228	235	242	250	258
73	144	151	159	166	174	182	189	197	204	212	219	227	235	242	250	257	265
74	148	155	164	171	179	186	194	202	210	218	225	233	241	249	256	264	272
75	152	160	168	176	184	192	200	208	216	224	232	240	248	256	264	272	279
76	156	164	172	180	189	197	205	213	221	230	238	246	254	263	271	279	287

Reprinted from Heyward 2010 (19).

TABLE 11.9 Skinfold Prediction Equations

SKF sites	Population	Equation	Ref
Σ7SKF (chest + abdomen + thigh + triceps + subscapular + suprailiac + midaxilla)	Black or Hispanic women, 18-55 yr	$Db (g \cdot cc^{-1}) = 1.0970 - 0.00046971 (\Sigma7SKF) + 0.00000056 (\Sigma7SKF)^2 - 0.00012828 (age)$	[1]
	Black men or male athletes, 18-61 yr	$Db (g \cdot cc^{-1}) = 1.1120 - 0.00043499 (\Sigma7SKF) + 0.00000055 (\Sigma7SKF)^2 - 0.00028826 (age)$	[2]
Σ4SKF (triceps + anterior suprailiac + abdomen + thigh)	Female athletes, 18-29 yr	$Db (g \cdot cc^{-1}) = 1.096095 - 0.0006952 (\Sigma4SKF) + 0.0000011 (\Sigma4SKF)^2 - 0.0000714 (age)$	[1]
Σ3SKF (triceps + suprailiac + thigh)	White or anorexic women, 18-55 yr	$Db (g \cdot cc^{-1}) = 1.0994921 - 0.0009929 (\Sigma3SKF) + 0.0000023 (\Sigma3SKF)^2 - 0.0001392 (age)$	[1]
Σ3SKF (chest + abdomen + thigh)	White men, 18-61 yr	$Db (g \cdot cc^{-1}) = 1.109380 - 0.0008267 (\Sigma3SKF) + 0.0000016 (\Sigma3SKF)^2 - 0.0002574 (age)$	[2]
Σ3SKF (abdomen + thigh + triceps)	Black or white collegiate athletes, 18-34 yr	$\%BF = 8.997 + 0.2468 (\Sigma3SKF) - 6.343 (gender^a) - 1.998 (race^b)$	[3]
Σ2SKF (triceps + calf)	Black or white boys, 6-17 yr Black or white girls, 6-17 yr	$\%BF = 0.735 (\Sigma2SKF) + 1.2$ $\%BF = 0.610 (\Sigma2SKF) + 5.1$	[4]

ΣSKF = sum of skinfolds (mm). Use population-specific conversion formulas to calculate %BF (percent body fat) from Db (body density). [a]Male athletes = 1; female athletes = 0. [b]Black athletes = 1; white athletes = 0.

[1] Jackson et al., 1980. Generalized equations for predicting body density of women. *MSSE* 12: 175–182. [2] Jackson and Pollock. 1978. Generalized equations for predicting body density of men. *Brit J Nutr* 40: 497–504. [3] Evans et al. 2005. Skinfold prediction equation for athletes developed using a four-component model. *MSSE* 37: 2006-2011. [4] Slaughter et al.1988. Skinfold equations for estimation of body fatness in children and youth. *Hum Biol* 60: 709–723.

Reprinted by permission from Heyward 2010.

TABLE 11.10 Population-Specific Equations for Calculating the Estimated Percent Body Fat From Body Density (Db)

Population	Age (years)	Gender	%BF[a]	FFB$_d$ (g · cc^{-1})*
RACE AND ETHNICITY				
African American	9-17	Female	(5.24/Db) − 4.82	1.088
	19-45	Male	(4.86/Db) − 4.39	1.106
	24-79	Female	(4.85/Db) − 4.39	1.106
American Indian	18-62	Male	(4.97/Db) − 4.52	1.099
	18-60	Female	(4.81/Db) − 4.34	1.108
Asian: Japanese Native	18-48	Male	(4.97/Db) − 4.52	1.099
	18-48	Female	(4.76/Db) − 4.28	1.111
	61-78	Male	(4.87/Db) − 4.41	1.105
	61-78	Female	(4.95/Db) − 4.50	1.100
Asian: Singaporean (Chinese, Indian, Malay)		Male	(4.94/Db) − 4.48	1.102
		Female	(4.84/Db) − 4.37	1.107
White	8-12	Male	(5.27/Db) − 4.85	1.086
	8-12	Female	(5.27/Db) − 4.85	1.086
	13-17	Male	(5.12/Db) − 4.69	1.092
	13-17	Female	(5.19/Db) − 4.76	1.090
	18-59	Male	(4.95/Db) − 4.50	1.100
	18-59	Female	(4.96/Db) − 4.51	1.101
	60-90	Male	(4.97/Db) − 4.52	1.099
	60-90	Female	(5.02/Db) − 4.57	1.098
Hispanic		Male	NA	NA
	20-40	Female	(4.87/Db) − 4.41	1.105
ATHLETES				
Resistance trained	24 ± 4	Male	(5.21/Db) − 4.78	1.089
	35 ± 6	Female	(4.97/Db) − 4.52	1.099
Endurance trained	21 ± 2	Male	(5.03/Db) − 4.59	1.097
	21 ± 4	Female	(4.95/Db) − 4.50	1.100
All sports	18-22	Male	(5.12/Db) − 4.68	1.093
	18-22	Female	(4.97/Db) − 4.52	1.099
CLINICAL POPULATIONS				
Anorexia nervosa	15-44	Female	(4.96/Db) − 4.51	1.101
Obesity	17-62	Female	(4.95/Db) − 4.50	1.100
Spinal cord injury (paraplegic or quadriplegic)	18-73	Male	(4.67/Db) − 4.18	1.116
		Female	(4.70/Db) − 4.22	1.114

FFB$_d$ = fat-free body density; Db = body density; %BF = percent body fat; NA = no data available for this population subgroup.
[a]Multiply value by 100 to calculate %BF.
*FFB$_d$ based on average values reported in selected research articles.

Reprinted by permission from Heyward and Wagner 2004.

TABLE 11.11 Criterion Scores and Normative Values for Percent Body Fat for Males and Females

Score or value	Age (years)						
MALE RATING (CRITERION SCORES)							
	6-17**	18-25	26-35	36-45	46-55	56-65	66+
Very lean	<5 (not recommended)	3-7	4-10	5-13	8-16	11-17	12-18
Lean (low)	5-10	8-10	11-13	15-17	17-19	19-21	19-20
Leaner than average	–	11-12	14-16	18-20	20-22	22-23	21-22
Average (mid)	11-25	13-15	17-19	21-22	23-24	24-25	23-24
Fatter than average	–	16-18	20-22	23-25	25-27	26-27	25-26
Fat (upper)	26-31	19-21	23-26	26-28	28-30	28-29	27-29
Overfat (obesity)	>31	23-35	27-38	29-39	31-40	31-40	30-39
MALE PERCENTILES (NORMATIVE REFERENCES)*							
		20-29	30-39	40-49	50-59	60-69	70-79
90		7.9	11.9	14.9	16.7	17.6	17.8
80		10.5	14.5	17.4	19.1	19.7	20.4
70		12.7	16.5	19.1	20.7	21.3	21.6
60		14.8	18.2	20.6	22.1	22.6	23.1
50		16.6	19.7	21.9	23.2	23.7	24.1
40		18.6	21.3	23.4	24.6	25.2	24.8
30		20.6	23.0	24.8	26.0	25.4	26.0
20		23.1	24.9	26.6	27.8	28.4	27.6
10		26.3	27.8	29.2	30.3	30.9	30.4
FEMALE RATING (CRITERION SCORES)*							
	6-17**	18-25	26-35	36-45	46-55	56-65	66+
Very lean	<12 (not recommended)	9-17	7-16	9-18	12-21	12-22	11-20
Lean (low)	12-15	18-19	18-20	19-22	23-25	24-26	22-25
Leaner than average	–	20-21	21-22	23-25	26-28	27-29	26-28
Average (mid)	16-30	22-23	23-25	26-28	29-30	30-32	29-31
Fatter than average	–	24-26	26-28	29-31	31-33	33-35	32-34
Fat (upper)	31-36	27-30	29-32	32-35	34-37	36-38	35-37
Overfat (obesity)	>36	32-43	34-46	37-47	39-50	39-49	38-45
FEMALE PERCENTILES (NORMATIVE REFERENCES)*							
		20-29	30-39	40-49	50-59	60-69	70-79
90		14.8	15.6	17.2	19.4	19.8	20.3
80		16.5	17.4	19.8	22.5	23.2	24.0
70		18.0	19.1	21.9	25.1	25.9	26.2
60		19.4	20.8	23.8	27.0	27.9	28.6
50		21.0	22.6	25.6	28.8	29.8	30.4
40		22.7	24.6	27.6	30.4	31.3	31.8
30		24.5	26.7	29.6	32.5	33.3	33.9
20		27.1	29.1	31.9	34.5	35.4	36.0
10		31.4	33.0	35.4	36.7	37.3	38.2

When personal trainers assess a client's body composition, they must account for a standard error of the estimate (SEE) and report a range of percentages that the client falls into. Note that the minimum SEE for population-specific skinfold equations is ±3% to 5%. Therefore, if a 25-year-old male client's body fat is measured at 24%, there is a minimum of a 6% range (21%-27%) that suggests a criterion-reference score of "fat." Note that reporting a client's body fat percentage with an SEE range can also cover any gaps and overlaps in the criterion-referenced norms shown. For example, what is the criterion score for a 30-year-old male with 29% body fat? The minimum SEE of ±3% places this client between 26% and 32% and therefore would suggest a criterion-reference score of "fat-overfat" or "borderline overfat."

*Data for male and female rating (criterion scores), ages 18-66+, are adapted from Morrow et al. 2011 (27).

**Data for male and female rating (criterion scores), ages 6-17, are from Lohman, Houtkooper, and Going 1997 (24).

***Data for male and female percentiles (normative references) are reprinted from ACSM 2010 (2).

Adapted from Golding 2000 (14).

TABLE 11.12 Waist-to-Hip Circumference Ratio Norms for Men and Women

Age	Risk			
	Low	Moderate	High	Very high
MEN				
20-29	<0.83	0.83-0.88	0.89-0.94	>0.94
30-39	<0.84	0.84-0.91	0.92-0.96	>0.96
40-49	<0.88	0.88-0.95	0.96-1.00	>1.00
50-59	<0.90	0.90-0.96	0.97-1.02	>1.02
60-69	<0.91	0.91-0.98	0.99-1.03	>1.03
WOMEN				
20-29	<0.71	0.71-0.77	0.78-0.82	>0.82
30-39	<0.72	0.72-0.78	0.79-0.84	>0.84
40-49	<0.73	0.73-0.79	0.80-0.87	>0.87
50-59	<0.74	0.74-0.81	0.82-0.88	>0.88
60-69	<0.76	0.76-0.83	0.84-0.90	>0.90

Adapted from Bray and Gray 1988 (9).

TABLE 11.13 YMCA Cycle Ergometry Protocol

1st stage	150 kg · m · min^{-1} (0.5 kg)			
	HR <80 beats/min	HR 80-89 beats/min	HR 90-100 beats/min	HR >100 beats/min
2nd stage	750 kg · m · min^{-1} (2.5 kg)*	600 kg · m · min^{-1} (2.0 kg)	450 kg · m · min^{-1} (1.5 kg)	300 kg · m · min^{-1} (1.0 kg)
3rd stage	900 kg · m · min^{-1} (3.0 kg)	750 kg · m · min^{-1} (2.5 kg)	600 kg · m · min^{-1} (2.0 kg)	450 kg · m · min^{-1} (1.5 kg)
4th stage	1,050 kg · m · min^{-1} (3.5 kg)	900 kg · m · min^{-1} (3.0 kg)	750 kg · m · min^{-1} (2.5 kg)	600 kg · m · min^{-1} (2.0 kg)

*Resistance settings shown here are appropriate for an ergometer with a flywheel that is geared to travel 6 meters per pedal revolution.

Reprinted by permission from ACSM 2010.

TABLE 11.14 Percentile Values for Maximal Aerobic Power ($\dot{V}O_2$max; ml · kg^{-1} · min^{-1})

	Age (years)						Age (years)				
Percentile	20-29	30-39	40-49	50-59	60-69	Percentile	20-29	30-39	40-49	50-59	60-69
MALES						**FEMALES**					
90	54.0	52.5	51.1	46.8	43.2	90	47.5	44.7	42.4	38.1	34.6
80	51.1	47.5	46.8	43.3	39.5	80	44.0	41.0	38.9	35.2	32.3
70	48.2	46.8	44.2	41.0	36.7	70	41.1	38.8	36.7	32.9	30.2
60	45.7	44.4	42.4	38.3	35.0	60	39.5	36.7	35.1	31.4	29.1
50	43.9	42.4	40.4	36.7	33.1	50	37.4	35.2	33.3	30.2	27.5
40	42.2	42.2	38.4	35.2	31.4	40	35.5	33.8	31.6	28.7	26.6
30	40.3	38.5	36.7	33.2	29.4	30	33.8	32.3	29.7	27.3	24.9
20	38.1	36.7	34.6	31.1	27.4	20	31.6	29.9	28.0	25.5	23.7
10	35.2	33.8	31.8	28.4	24.1	10	29.4	27.4	25.6	23.7	21.7

Adapted from ACSM 2010 (2).

TABLE 11.15 Prediction of Maximal Oxygen Consumption (L/min) From Heart Rate and Cycling Power in Men

HR (beats/min)	Power (kg · m · min⁻¹; watts) 300; 50	600; 100	900; 150	1,200; 200	1,500; 250	HR (beats/min)	Power (kg · m · min⁻¹; watts) 600; 100	900; 150	1,200; 200	1,500; 250
120	2.2	3.5	4.8			146	2.4	3.3	4.4	5.5
121	2.2	3.4	4.7			147	2.4	3.3	4.4	5.5
122	2.2	3.4	4.6			148	2.4	3.2	4.3	5.4
123	2.1	3.4	4.6			149	2.3	3.2	4.3	5.4
124	2.1	3.3	4.5	6.0		150	2.3	3.2	4.2	5.3
125	2.0	3.2	4.4	5.9		151	2.3	3.1	4.2	5.2
126	2.0	3.2	4.4	5.8		152	2.3	3.1	4.1	5.2
127	2.0	3.1	4.3	5.7		153	2.2	3.0	4.1	5.1
128	2.0	3.1	4.2	5.6		154	2.2	3.0	4.0	5.1
129	1.9	3.0	4.2	5.6		155	2.2	3.0	4.0	5.0
130	1.9	3.0	4.1	5.5		156	2.2	2.9	4.0	5.0
131	1.9	2.9	4.0	5.4		157	2.1	2.9	3.9	4.9
132	1.8	2.9	4.0	5.3		158	2.1	2.9	3.9	4.9
133	1.8	2.8	3.9	5.3		159	2.1	2.8	3.8	4.8
134	1.8	2.8	3.9	5.2		160	2.1	2.8	3.8	4.8
135	1.7	2.8	3.8	5.1		161	2.0	2.8	3.7	4.7
136	1.7	2.7	3.8	5.0		162	2.0	2.8	3.7	4.6
137	1.7	2.7	3.7	5.0		163	2.0	2.8	3.7	4.6
138	1.6	2.7	3.7	4.9		164	2.0	2.7	3.6	4.5
139	1.6	2.6	3.6	4.8		165	2.0	2.7	3.6	4.5
140	1.6	2.6	3.6	4.8	6.0	166	1.9	2.7	3.6	4.4
141		2.6	3.5	4.7	5.9	167	1.9	2.6	3.5	4.4
142		2.5	5.5	4.6	5.8	168	1.9	2.6	3.5	4.3
143		2.5	3.4	4.6	5.7	169	1.9	2.6	3.5	4.3
144		2.5	3.4	4.5	5.7	170	1.8	2.6	3.4	4.3
145		2.4	3.4	4.5	5.6					

Adapted by permission from Åstrand 1960.

TABLE 11.16 Prediction of Maximal Oxygen Consumption (L/min) From Heart Rate and Cycling Power in Women

HR (beats/min)	Power (kg · m · min⁻¹; watts) 300; 50	600; 100	900; 150	1,200; 200	1,500; 250	HR (beats/min)	Power (kg · m · min⁻¹; watts) 600; 100	900; 150	1,200; 200	1,500; 250
120	2.6	3.4	4.1	4.8		146	1.6	2.2	2.6	3.2
121	2.5	3.3	4.0	4.8		147	1.6	2.1	2.6	3.1
122	2.5	3.2	3.9	4.7		148	1.6	2.1	2.6	3.1
123	2.4	3.1	3.9	4.6		149		2.1	2.6	3.0
124	2.4	3.1	3.8	4.5		150		2.0	2.5	3.0
125	2.3	3.0	3.7	4.4		151		2.0	2.5	3.0
126	2.3	3.0	3.7	4.4		152		2.0	2.5	2.9
127	2.2	2.9	3.5	4.2		153		2.0	2.4	2.9
128	2.2	2.8	3.5	4.2		154		2.0	2.4	2.8
129	2.2	2.8	3.4	4.1		155		1.9	2.4	2.8
130	2.1	2.7	3.4	4.0	4.7	156		1.9	2.3	2.8
131	2.1	2.7	3.4	4.0	4.6	157		1.9	2.3	2.7

HR (beats/min)	Power (kg · m · min⁻¹; watts) 300; 50	600; 100	900; 150	1,200; 200	1,500; 250	HR (beats/min)	Power (kg · m · min⁻¹; watts) 600; 100	900; 150	1,200; 200	1,500; 250
132	2.0	2.7	3.3	4.0	4.5	158		1.8	2.3	2.7
133	2.0	2.6	3.2	3.8	4.4	159		1.8	2.2	2.7
134	2.0	2.6	3.2	3.8	4.4	160		1.8	2.2	2.6
135	2.0	2.6	3.1	3.7	4.3	161		1.8	2.2	2.6
136	1.9	2.5	3.1	3.6	4.2	162		1.8	2.2	2.6
137	1.9	2.5	3.0	3.6	4.2	163		1.7	2.2	2.6
138	1.8	2.4	2.9	3.5	4.1	164		1.7	2.1	2.5
139	1.8	2.4	2.8	3.5	4.0	165		1.7	2.1	2.5
140	1.8	2.4	2.8	3.4	4.0	166		1.7	2.1	2.5
141	1.8	2.3	2.8	3.4	3.9	167		1.6	2.1	2.4
142	1.7	2.3	2.8	3.3	3.9	168		1.6	2.0	2.4
143	1.7	2.2	2.7	3.3	3.8	169		1.6	2.0	2.4
144	1.7	2.2	2.7	3.2	3.8	170		1.6	2.0	2.4
145	1.6	2.2	2.7	3.2	3.7					

Adapted by permission from Åstrand 1960.

TABLE 11.17 Age Correction Factors (CF) for Age-Adjusted Maximal Oxygen Consumption

Age	CF	Age	CF	Age	CF	Age	CF	Age	CF
15	1.10	25	1.00	35	0.87	45	0.78	55	0.71
16	1.10	26	0.99	36	0.86	46	0.77	56	0.70
17	1.09	27	0.98	37	0.85	47	0.77	57	0.70
18	1.07	28	0.96	38	0.85	48	0.76	58	0.69
19	1.06	29	0.95	39	0.84	49	0.76	59	0.69
20	1.05	30	0.93	40	0.83	50	0.75	60	0.68
21	1.04	31	0.93	41	0.82	51	0.74	61	0.67
22	1.03	32	0.91	42	0.81	52	0.73	62	0.67
23	1.02	33	0.90	43	0.80	53	0.73	63	0.66
24	1.01	34	0.88	44	0.79	54	0.72	64	0.66

Adapted by permission from Åstrand 1960.

TABLE 11.18 Norms for Evaluating Åstrand-Ryhming Cycle Test Performance

Age	Aerobic fitness categories Very high	High	Good	Average	Fair	Low
	Maximal oxygen consumption (ml · kg⁻¹ · min⁻¹)					
MEN						
20-29	>61	53-61	43-52	34-42	25-33	<25
30-39	>57	49-57	39-48	31-38	23-30	<23
40-49	>53	45-53	36-44	27-35	20-26	<20
50-59	>49	43-49	34-42	25-33	18-24	<18
60-69	>45	41-45	31-40	23-30	16-22	<16
WOMEN						
20-29	>57	49-57	38-48	31-37	24-30	<24
30-39	>53	45-53	34-44	28-33	20-27	<20
40-49	>50	42-50	31-41	24-30	17-23	<17
50-59	>42	38-42	28-37	21-27	15-20	<15
60-69	>39	35-39	24-34	18-23	13-17	<13

Reprinted from Adams 2002 (1).

TABLE 11.19 Male and Female Norms for Recovery Heart Rate Following the 3-Minute Step Test (beats/min)

Rating	Age (years)					
	18-25	26-35	36-45	46-55	56-65	66+
MALE						
Excellent	70-78	73-79	72-81	78-84	72-82	72-86
Good	82-88	83-88	86-94	89-96	89-97	89-95
Above average	91-97	91-97	98-102	99-103	98-101	97-102
Average	101-104	101-106	105-111	109-115	105-111	104-113
Below average	107-114	109-116	113-118	118-121	113-118	114-119
Poor	118-126	119-126	120-128	124-130	122-128	122-128
Very poor	131-164	130-164	132-168	135-158	131-150	133-152
FEMALE						
Excellent	72-83	72-86	74-87	76-93	74-92	73-86
Good	88-97	91-97	93-101	96-102	97-103	93-100
Above average	100-106	103-110	104-109	106-113	106-111	104-114
Average	110-116	112-118	111-117	117-120	113-117	117-121
Below average	118-124	121-127	120-127	121-126	119-127	123-127
Poor	128-137	129-135	130-138	127-133	129-136	129-134
Very poor	142-155	141-154	143-152	138-152	142-151	135-151

Reprinted from Morrow et al. 2011 (32).

TABLE 11.20 Norms for the Rockport Walk Test

Clients aged 30-69 years (min:s)		
Rating	Males	Females
Excellent	<10:12	<11:40
Good	10:13-11:42	11:41-13:08
High average	11:43-13:13	13:09-14:36
Low average	13:14-14:44	14:37-16:04
Fair	14:45-16:23	16:05-17:31
Poor	>16:24	>17:32
Clients aged 18-30 years (min:s)		
Percentile	Males	Females
90	11:08	11:45
75	11:42	12:49
50	12:38	13:15
25	13:38	14:12
10	14:37	15:03

Reprinted from Morrow et al. 2011 (32).

TABLE 11.21 Norms for 1-Mile Run (min:s)

	Percentile					
	Boys			Girls		
Age	85	50	15	85	50	15
6	10:15	12:36	16:30	11:20	13:12	16:45
7	9:22	11:40	15:00	10:36	12:56	16:00
8	8:48	11:05	14:10	10:02	12:30	15:19
9	8:31	10:30	12:59	9:30	11:52	14:57
10	7:57	9:48	13:07	9:19	11:22	14:00
11	7:32	9:20	12:29	9:02	11:17	14:16
12	7:11	8:40	11:30	8:23	11:05	14:12
13	6:50	8:06	10:39	8:13	10:23	14:10
14	6:26	7:44	10:18	7:59	10:06	12:56
15	6:20	7:30	9:34	8:08	9:58	13:33
16	6:08	7:10	9:22	8:23	10:31	14:16
17	6:06	7:04	8:56	8:15	10:22	13:03

Data from The President's Council on Fitness, Sports & Nutrition 2010 (38).

TABLE 11.22 Relative Strength Norms for 1RM Bench Press

Percentile rankings* for men	Age				
	20-29	30-39	40-49	50-59	60+
90	1.48	1.24	1.10	0.97	0.89
80	1.32	1.12	1.00	0.90	0.82
70	1.22	1.04	0.93	0.84	0.77
60	1.14	0.98	0.88	0.79	0.72
50	1.06	0.93	0.84	0.75	0.68
40	0.99	0.88	0.80	0.71	0.66
30	0.93	0.83	0.76	0.68	0.63
20	0.88	0.78	0.72	0.63	0.57
10	0.80	0.71	0.65	0.57	0.53

Percentile rankings* for women	Age					
	20-29	30-39	40-49	50-59	60-69	70+
90	0.54	0.49	0.46	0.40	0.41	0.44
80	0.49	0.45	0.40	0.37	0.38	0.39
70	0.42	0.42	0.38	0.35	0.36	0.33
60	0.41	0.41	0.37	0.33	0.32	0.31
50	0.40	0.38	0.34	0.31	0.30	0.27
40	0.37	0.37	0.32	0.28	0.29	0.25
30	0.35	0.34	0.30	0.26	0.28	0.24
20	0.33	0.32	0.27	0.23	0.26	0.21
10	0.30	0.27	0.23	0.19	0.25	0.20

Norms were established using a Universal bench press machine.

*Descriptors for percentile rankings: 90 = well above average; 70 = above average; 50 = average; 30 = below average; 10 = well below average.
Data for women provided by the Women's Exercise Research Center, The George Washington University Medical Center, Washington, D.C., 1998.
Data for men provided by The Cooper Institute for Aerobics Research, *The Physical Fitness Specialist Manual*, The Cooper Institute, Dallas, TX, 2005.

Reprinted from Heyward 2010 (19).

TABLE 11.23 Relative Strength Norms for 1RM Leg Press

Percentile rankings* for men	Age				
	20-29	30-39	40-49	50-59	60+
90	2.27	2.07	1.92	1.80	1.73
80	2.13	1.93	1.82	1.71	1.62
70	2.05	1.85	1.74	1.64	1.56
60	1.97	1.77	1.68	1.58	1.49
50	1.91	1.71	1.62	1.52	1.43
40	1.83	1.65	1.57	1.46	1.38
30	1.74	1.59	1.51	1.39	1.30
20	1.63	1.52	1.44	1.32	1.25
10	1.51	1.43	1.35	1.22	1.16

Percentile rankings* for women	Age					
	20-29	30-39	40-49	50-59	60-69	70+
90	2.05	1.73	1.63	1.51	1.40	1.27
80	1.66	1.50	1.46	1.30	1.25	1.12
70	1.42	1.47	1.35	1.24	1.18	1.10
60	1.36	1.32	1.26	1.18	1.15	0.95
50	1.32	1.26	1.19	1.09	1.08	0.89
40	1.25	1.21	1.12	1.03	1.04	0.83
30	1.23	1.16	1.03	0.95	0.98	0.82
20	1.13	1.09	0.94	0.86	0.94	0.79
10	1.02	0.94	0.76	0.75	0.84	0.75

Norms were established using a Universal leg press machine.

*Descriptors for percentile rankings: 70 = above average; 50 = average; 30 = below average; 10 = well below average.
Data for women provided by the Women's Exercise Research Center, The George Washington University Medical Center, Washington, D.C., 1998.
Data for men provided by The Cooper Institute for Aerobics Research, *The Physical Fitness Specialist Manual*, The Cooper Institute, Dallas, TX, 2005.

Reprinted from Heyward 2010 (19).

TABLE 11.24 YMCA Bench Press Norms

Percentile	Age											
	18-25		26-35		36-45		46-55		56-65		>65	
	M	F	M	F	M	F	M	F	M	F	M	F
90	44	42	41	40	36	33	28	29	24	24	20	18
80	37	34	33	32	29	28	22	22	20	20	14	14
70	33	28	29	28	25	24	20	18	14	14	10	10
60	29	25	26	24	22	21	16	14	12	12	10	8
50	26	21	22	21	20	17	13	12	10	9	8	6
40	22	18	20	17	17	14	11	9	8	6	6	4
30	20	16	17	14	14	12	9	7	5	5	4	3
20	16	12	13	12	10	8	6	5	3	3	2	1
10	10	6	9	6	6	4	2	1	1	1	1	0

Note: Score is number of repetitions completed in 1 minute using 80-pound barbell for men and 35-pound barbell for women.

Adapted from Golding 2000 (14).

TABLE 11.25 Percentiles by Age Groups and Gender for Partial Curl-Up

Rating	Age (years)					
	15-19	20-29	30-39	40-49	50-59	60-69
MEN						
Excellent	25	25	25	25	25	25
Very good	23-24	21-24	18-24	18-24	17-24	16-24
Good	21-22	16-20	15-17	13-17	11-16	11-15
Fair	16-20	11-15	11-14	6-12	8-10	6-10
Needs improvement	≤15	≤10	≤10	≤5	≤7	≤5
WOMEN						
Excellent	25	25	25	25	25	25
Very good	22-24	18-24	19-24	19-24	19-24	17-24
Good	17-21	14-17	10-18	11-18	10-18	8-16
Fair	12-16	5-13	6-9	4-10	6-9	3-7
Needs improvement	≤11	≤4	≤5	≤3	≤5	≤2

Reprinted from CSEP 2003 (11).

TABLE 11.26 Normative Percentile Data in Seconds for Prone Double Straight-Leg Raise

Percentile	Age group									
	19-29		30-39		40-49		50-59		60+	
	M	F	M	F	M	F	M	F	M	F
75	130	126	123	111	95	87	80	83	60	40
50	88	74	73	73	55	45	48	37	22	23
25	55	49	45	45	35	29	22	18	11	7

Reprinted from McIntosh et al. 1998 (29).

TABLE 11.27 Percentiles by Age Groups and Gender for YMCA Sit-and-Reach Test (inches)

Percentile	Age 18-25 M	F	26-35 M	F	36-45 M	F	46-55 M	F	56-65 M	F	>65 M	F
90	22	24	21	23	21	22	19	21	17	20	17	20
80	20	22	19	21	19	21	17	20	15	19	15	18
70	19	21	17	20	17	19	15	18	13	17	13	17
60	18	20	17	20	16	18	14	17	13	16	12	17
50	17	19	15	19	15	17	13	16	11	15	10	15
40	15	18	14	17	13	16	11	14	9	14	9	14
30	14	17	13	16	13	15	10	14	9	13	8	13
20	13	16	11	15	11	14	9	12	7	11	7	11
10	11	14	9	13	7	12	6	10	5	9	4	9

These norms are based on a yardstick placed so that the "zero" point is set at 15 inches (38 cm).

Adapted from Golding 2000 (14).

TABLE 11.28 Fitness Categories by Age Groups for Trunk Forward Flexion Using a Sit-and-Reach Box (cm)

Category*	Age 20-29 M	F	30-39 M	F	40-49 M	F	50-59 M	F	60-69 M	F
Excellent	40	41	38	41	35	38	35	39	33	35
Very good	39	40	37	40	34	37	34	38	32	34
	34	37	33	36	29	34	28	33	25	31
Good	33	36	32	35	28	33	27	32	24	30
	30	33	28	32	24	30	24	30	20	27
Fair	29	32	27	31	23	29	23	29	19	26
	25	28	23	27	18	25	16	25	15	23
Needs improvement	24	27	22	26	17	24	15	24	14	22

These norms are based on a sit-and-reach box in which the "zero" point is set at 26 cm. When using a box in which the "zero" point is set at 23 cm, subtract 3 cm from each value in this table.

Reprinted from CSEP 2003 (11).

Age	Percentile Boys 85	50	15	Girls 85	50	15
5	30	25	21	31	27	22
6	31	26	20	32	27	22
7	30	25	19	32	27	22
8	31	25	20	33	28	21
9	31	25	20	33	28	21
10	30	25	18	33	28	21
11	31	25	18	34	29	22
12	31	26	18	36	30	22
13	33	26	18	38	31	22
14	36	28	21	40	33	24
15	37	30	22	43	36	28
16	38	30	21	42	34	26
17+	41	34	25	42	35	28

Adapted from The President's Council on Fitness, Sports & Nutrition 2010 (38).

References

1. Adams, G. 2002. *Exercise Physiology Laboratory Manual.* 4th ed. New York: McGraw-Hill Companies.

2. American College of Sports Medicine. 2010. *ACSM's Guidelines for Exercise Testing and Prescription,* 8th ed., W.R. Thompson, N.F. Gordon, and L.S. Pescatello, eds. Philadelphia: Lippincott Williams & Wilkins.

3. American College of Sports Medicine. 2010. *ACSM's Resource Manual for Guidelines for Exercise Testing and Prescription,* 6th ed. Philadelphia: Lippincott Williams & Wilkins.

4. Arab, A.M., M. Salavati, I. Ebrahimi, and M.E. Mousavi. 2007. Sensitivity, specificity and predictive value of the clinical trunk muscle endurance tests in low back pain. *Clinical Rehabilitation* 21 (7): 640-647.

5. Åstrand, P.-O., and I. Ryhming. 1954. A nomogram for calculation of aerobic capacity (physical fitness) from pulse rate during submaximal work. *Journal of Applied Physiology* 7: 218-221.

6. Baechle, T.R., and R. Earle. 2008. Resistance training and spotting techniques. In: *Essentials of Strength Training and Conditioning,* 3rd ed., T.R. Baechle and R.W. Earle, eds. Champaign, IL: Human Kinetics. pp. 325-375.

7. Baumgartner, T.A., A.S. Jackson, M.T. Mahar, and D.A. Rowe. 2007. *Measurement for Evaluation in Physical Education and Exercise Science,* 8th ed. Boston: McGraw-Hill.

8. Beam, W., and G. Adams. 2011. *Exercise Physiology Laboratory Manual,* 6th ed. New York: McGraw-Hill.

9. Bray, G. and D. Gray. 1988. Obesity Part I—Pathogenesis. *Western Journal of Medicine* 149: 432.

10. Brooks, G.A., T.D. Fahey, and K.M. Baldwin. 2005. *Exercise Physiology: Human Bioenergetics and Its Applications,* 4th ed. New York: McGraw-Hill.

11. Canadian Society for Exercise Physiology (CSEP). 2003. *The Canadian Physical Activity, Fitness & Lifestyle Approach: CSEP-Health & Fitness Program's Health-Related Appraisal and Counselling Strategy.* 3rd ed. Ontario, Canada: Author.

12. Devries, H.A., and T.J. Housh. 1994. *Physiology of Exercise for Physical Education, Athletics, and Exercise Science,* 5th ed. Madison, WI: Brown and Benchmark.

13. Eckerson, J.M., J.R. Stout, T.K. Evetovich, T.J. Housh, G.O. Johnson, and N. Worrell. 1998. Validity of self-assessment techniques for estimating percent fat in men and women. *Journal of Strength and Conditioning Research* 12: 243-247.

14. Golding, L.A. 2000. *YMCA Fitness Testing and Assessment Manual,* 4th ed. Champaign, IL: Human Kinetics.

15. Grenier, S.G., C. Russell, and S.M. McGill. 2003. Relationships between lumbar flexibility, sit-and-reach test, and a previous history of low back discomfort in industrial workers. *Applied Physiology, Nutrition, and Metabolism* 28 (2): 165-177.

16. Harrison, G.G., E.R. Buskirk, J.E. Carter Lindsay, F.E. Johnston, T.G. Lohman, M.L. Pollock, A.F. Roche, and J.H. Wilmore. 1988. Skinfold thicknesses and measurement technique. In: *Anthropometric Standardization Reference Manual,* T.G. Lohman, A.F. Roche, and R. Martorell, eds. Champaign, IL: Human Kinetics. pp. 55-70.

17. Heyward, V. and D. Wagner, 2004, Applied body composition assessment, 2nd ed. Champaign, IL: Human Kinetics.

18. Heyward, V.H. 1998. *Advanced Fitness Assessment and Exercise Prescription.* Champaign, IL: Human Kinetics.

19. Heyward, V.H. 2010. *Advanced Fitness Assessment and Exercise Prescription,* 6th ed. Champaign, IL: Human Kinetics.

20. Kline, G.M., J.P. Porcari, R. Hintermeister, P.S. Freedson, A. Ward, R.F. McCarron, J. Ross, and J.M. Rippe. 1987. Estimation of $\dot{V}O_2$max from a one-mile track walk, gender, age, and body weight. *Medicine and Science in Sports and Exercise* 19: 253-259.

21. Kordich, J.A. 2002. *Evaluating Your Client: Fitness Assessment and Protocol Norms.* Lincoln, NE: NSCA Certification Commission.

22. Kraemer W.J., N.A. Ratamess, A.C. Fry, and D.N. French. 2006. Strength training: Development and evaluation of methodology. In: *Physiological Assessment of Human Fitness,* P.J. Maud and C. Foster, eds. Champaign, IL: Human Kinetics. pp. 119-150.

23. Leger, L., and M. Thivierge. 1988. Heart rate monitors: Validity, stability, and functionality. *Physician and Sports-Medicine* 16: 143-151.

24. Lohman, T., L. Houtkooper, and S. Going. Body fat measurement goes high-tech: not all are created equal. *ACSM's Health Fit J* 1997;7:30-35.

25. Malek, M.H., T.J. Housh, D.E. Berger, J.W. Coburn, and T.W. Beck. 2004. A new non-exercise based VO$_2$max equation for aerobically trained females. *Medicine and Science in Sports and Exercise* 36: 1804-1810.

26. Malek, M.H., T.J. Housh, D.E. Berger, J.W. Coburn, and T.W. Beck. 2004. A new non-exercise based VO$_2$max equation for aerobically trained men. *Journal of Strength and Conditioning Research* 19: 559-565.

27. McArdle, W.D., F.I. Katch, and V.L. Katch. 2009. *Exercise Physiology: Nutrition, Energy, and Human Performance,* 7th ed. Philadelphia: Lippincott Williams & Wilkins.

28. McDowell, M., Fryar, C., Ogden, C., & Flegal, K. (2008). Anthropometric Reference Data for Children and Adults: United States, 2003-2006. *National Health Statistics Reports* (10).

29. McIntosh, G., L. Wilson, M. Affleck, and H. Hall. 1998. Trunk and lower extremity muscle endurance: Normative data for adults. *Journal of Rehabilitation Outcome Measures* 2: 20-39.

30. Moon, J.R., H.R. Hull, S.E. Tobkin, M. Teramoto, M. Karabulut, M.D. Roberts, E.D. Ryan, S.J. Kim, V.J. Dalbo, A.A. Walter, A.E. Smith, J.T. Cramer, and J.R. Stout. 2007. Percent body fat estimations in college women using field and laboratory methods: A three-compartment model approach. *Journal of the International Society of Sports Nutrition* 4: 16.

31. Moon, J.R., S.E. Tobkin, A.E. Smith, M.D. Roberts, E.D. Ryan, S.J. Kim, V.J. Dalbo, C.M. Lockwood, A.A. Walter, J.T. Cramer, T.W. Beck, and J.R. Stout. 2009. Percent body fat estimations in college men using field and laboratory methods: A three-compartment model approach. *Dynamic Medicine* 7: 7.

32. Morrow, J., A. Jackson, J. Disch, and D. Mood. 2011. *Measurement and Evaluation in Human Performance,* 4th ed. Champaign, IL: Human Kinetics.

33. National Heart, Lung, and Blood Institute Joint National Committee on Prevention, Detection, Evaluation, and Treatment of High Blood Pressure and National High Blood Pressure Education Program Coordinating Committee. 2003. The seventh report of the Joint National Committee on Prevention, Detection, Evaluation, and Treatment of High Blood Pressure: The JNC 7 report. *Journal of the American Medical Association* 289: 2560-2572.

34. National Institutes of Health, National Heart, Lung, and Blood Institute, 1998, Clinical Guidelines on the Identification, Evaluation and Treatment of Overweight and Obesity in Adults (Executive Summary). NIH Publication 98-4083.

Available online at www.nhlbi.nih.gov. Accessed January 27, 2011.

35. Pickering, T.G., Hall, J.E., Appel, L.J., Falkner, B.E., Graves, J., Hill, M.N., Jones, D.W., Kurtz, T., Sheps, S.G., and E.J. Roccella. 2005. Recommendations for blood pressure measurement in humans and experimental animals. Part 1: Blood pressure measurement in humans. A statement for professionals from the Subcommittee of Professional and Public Education of the American Heart Association Council on High Blood Pressure Research. *Hypertension* 45: 142-161.

36. Pollock, M., J. Wilmore and S. Fox III. 1978. *Health and Fitness Through Physical Activity*. New York: Wiley.

37. Prisant, L.M., B.S. Alpert, C.B. Robbins, A.S. Berson, M. Hayes, M.L. Cohen, and S.G. Sheps. 1995. American National Standard for nonautomated sphygmomanometers. Summary report. *American Journal of Hypertension* 8: 210-213.

38. The President's Council on Fitness, Sports & Nutrition. Normative Data. 2010. *The President's Challenge 2010*. www.presidentschallenge.org/tools-resources/docs/normative_data_spreadsheet.xls. Accessed November 18, 2010.

PART III

Exercise Technique

Flexibility, Body Weight, and Stability Ball Exercises

Allen Hedrick, MA

After completing this chapter, you will be able to

- describe the benefits of participating in a flexibility training program,

- understand the factors that affect flexibility,

- explain the value of warming up prior to participating in flexibility training,

- list and explain the various types of flexibility training,

- supervise a flexibility training program emphasizing a combination of dynamic and static stretching, and

- supervise exercises using body weight only and stability balls.

This chapter covers four major topics. The first is flexibility training, which forms an important part of an overall conditioning program. The second topic is warm-up, with discussion of both its importance and the techniques used for warming up prior to physical activity. This is followed by a discussion of body weight exercises and stability ball training, which highlights the potential benefits of these training methods. Finally, the chapter presents detailed instructions for recommended static and dynamic flexibility movements, and for suggested body weight and stability ball exercises.

Defining Flexibility

Those involved in supervising conditioning or rehabilitation programs typically use some form of stretching. Despite this, there is still a lot of confusion about flexibility training in terms of its scientific basis (9, 10). Much of the confusion results from the notion that people must achieve extreme levels of flexibility in order to reduce the chance of injury and to improve movement capabilities (14). This does not accurately represent the role that flexibility plays in training. Flexibility is an important piece of the training puzzle; but, like other aspects of training, it must be based on the needs of the individual.

A logical starting point for alleviating some of the confusion is to consider definitions of *flexibility*. According to the most common definition, **flexibility** is the range of motion of a joint or a series of joints (4, 7, 8). For personal trainers, who are concerned with improving clients' movement performance and reducing their chances of injury, a more relevant definition might be the ability of a joint to move freely through the full normal range of motion (ROM) (30).

Flexibility Training as Part of the Total Exercise Program

Although a later section of the chapter discusses warm-up in more detail, it is important to note here that each training session should begin with a warm-up designed to elevate core temperature. After completing the warm-up session, the client may or may not need to immediately participate in flexibility training, depending on the nature of the activity to follow. For example, if the clients are going to participate in a dynamic activity (e.g., basketball, racquetball) following the warm-up, they will need to engage in flexibility training first. If they are going to participate in a less dynamic activity (e.g., stationary bike, stair climber), they can work on flexibility after the training session is complete.

> Every workout, no matter the time constraints of the client, should be preceded by a warm-up session. However, when the flexibility training should occur depends on the nature of the activity that is to take place during the workout.

Benefits of Flexibility Training

Developing flexibility is an important goal of any training program. Achieving optimum flexibility helps eliminate awkward and inefficient movement by allowing joints to move freely through a full normal ROM, and it may also provide increased resistance to muscle injury (3, 22, 23, 24, 32, 36). Improving flexibility is a fundamental element of any training program because ROM may enhance the ability to perform various movement skills,

especially those that require a high level of flexibility (i.e., serving a tennis ball, picking up a bag of groceries off the floor) (4, 8, 9, 30, 37, 42, 47). It is important to note that while great athletes may have above-average flexibility, this may not be why they are successful. The ability to move effectively depends on strength with coordination, and being flexible can enhance this ability in certain situations (14). The goal of flexibility training is not to get to a point at which the client has no joint stability, but rather to achieve strength combined with flexibility that can allow the client to better control his or her movements (14).

Flexibility training is also important in injury prevention (4, 8, 9, 10, 20, 25, 30, 32, 37, 42, 47). Among the more common problems seen in individuals with poor flexibility is lower back pain potentially resulting from tight quadriceps, iliopsoas, and back muscles (and possibly a corresponding weakness in the abdominal muscles and hamstrings). A lack of flexibility may also increase the incidence of muscle tears resulting from tight muscles on one or both sides of a joint (9). The accepted rule regarding the role of flexibility in injury prevention is that a normal ROM (i.e., the ROM common to most individuals) in each joint will reduce the chance for injury (10). If a client is involved in a sport or activity that requires greater than normal ROM, then more emphasis should be placed on increasing flexibility to help protect against injury.

Because of these important benefits, it is recommended that trainers supervise stretching just as they would any other part of the training session. Doing this communicates the importance of the warm-up and stretching period and may encourage clients to keep their attention focused on the task at hand (25).

> Flexibility training is important because of the role that flexibility plays in improving movement performance and reducing the opportunity for injury.

Factors Affecting Flexibility

A number of physiological, lifestyle, and environmental factors influence flexibility. While some of these are out of the client's control, such as joint structure, age, and sex, factors like muscle and connective tissue elasticity, core temperature, activity level, and the client's training program can have a profound influence on ROM, and these can be influenced by training (4, 19).

Joint Structure

One of the primary limiting factors in static ROM is the structure of the joint itself (10). Because of joint structure, there is a limit to how much movement is available. Joint structures vary between individuals, and the personal trainer must consider this variation when evaluating flexibility.

Joint structure also varies between joints. Some joints offer a reduced range of movement compared to others by virtue of their construction. The hinge-type joints of the knee and elbow allow only backward and forward movements (flexion and extension), so knee and elbow ROM is significantly less than that of the shoulder or hip (4). The ball and socket joints of the hip and shoulder allow movements in all anatomical planes and have the greatest ROM of all joints (4, 9, 19, 30).

Flexibility is joint specific. That is, it is common to have above-average flexibility in one joint and below-average ROM in another (7, 12). Thus flexibility needs to be thought of not as a general characteristic but instead as a characteristic specific to a particular joint and joint action (30). For this reason, it is a fallacy to think that a single flexibility test can provide an accurate measure of overall flexibility (12, 25).

Muscle and Connective Tissue

Connective tissue (muscles, ligaments, and tendons) is the area of emphasis during ROM exercise. This is because, under normal circumstances, connective tissues are the major structures limiting joint ROM. These connective tissue structures include ligamentous joint capsules, tendons, and muscles (24, 25). While muscle is not usually thought of as a connective tissue structure, evidence indicates that when a relaxed muscle is stretched during ROM exercise, the majority of the resistance to the stretch comes from the extensive connective tissue framework and sheathing within and around the muscle (24). Thus, improvements in ROM as a result of stretching are primarily due to the connective tissue adaptations (4).

Most of the difference between individuals in static ROM is due to the elastic properties of the muscle and tendons attached across the joints (10). "Stiff" muscles and tendons reduce the ROM, while "compliant" muscles and tendons increase ROM.

It is these elastic properties that are altered as a result of stretching exercises. When a muscle is held for a period of time under tension in a static stretch, the passive tension in the muscle declines; that is, the muscle "gives" a little, or relaxes. This is called a *viscoelastic stretch relaxation response* (10). *Passive tension* is defined as the amount of external force required to lengthen the relaxed muscle (10).

Obviously the more pliable the muscle, the less external force required. This increased pliability can be sustained for up to 90 minutes after the stretch.

The muscles crossing over or adjacent to a joint will also affect flexibility (7). In any movement, the active contraction of a muscle (agonistic) occurs simultaneously with the relaxation or stretching of the antagonistic muscle. The more easily the antagonistic muscles yield, the less energy is spent overcoming their resistance. The capacity of a muscle fiber to lengthen improves as a result of flexibility training. However, flexibility is often limited, regardless of the amount of training, if the antagonistic muscles are not relaxed or if there is a lack of coordination between contraction (agonists) and relaxation (antagonists).

Hyperlaxity

While it is fairly uncommon, some individuals are born with a tissue structure that predisposes them to **hyperlaxity.** Hyperlaxity allows the joints of the body to achieve a ROM that exceeds what is considered normal (37). If it has been determined that a client has joint hyperlaxity, the personal trainer should use caution when implementing the stretching program and should ensure that the client has been assessed by a health care professional. It is important to avoid overstretching the client and creating even greater levels of laxity in the surrounding supportive tissues. Poor selection of stretching exercises can also cause problems because excessive ROM in the joint can increase the opportunity for injury.

Age

Age also plays a role in flexibility. Investigators have found that elementary school children become less flexible with age, reaching a low point between ages 10 and 12 (4, 8, 12, 25, 30). Flexibility normally improves at this point but never reaches the level seen during early childhood (24). This decrease in flexibility is due to a gradual loss of elasticity in the muscle (7). There are few significant changes in flexibility between early and late puberty.

From the anatomical point of view, childhood, and more specifically the period before puberty, is the ideal time to start a flexibility program (7, 8) because young clients still have a high level of flexibility. During this stage, training programs should be aimed at developing flexibility in all joints.

Sex

Sex also plays a role in flexibility; with females typically having greater flexibility than males (4, 9,

12, 22, 25). Research shows that elementary school girls are superior to boys in flexibility, and it is likely that this difference exists throughout adult life (24). The higher flexibility in females is generally due to anatomical variations in joint structures (22). The biggest differences are seen in the trunk (flexion and extension), hips, and ankles (7). The decrease in flexibility seen in boys at puberty is thought to be related to increases in muscle size, stature, and muscle strength.

Temperature

Temperature is another factor that influences flexibility, as ROM is positively affected by an increase in either core temperature (4, 9, 12, 30) or external temperature (30). The positive effect of increased core temperature on ROM points to the importance of warming up prior to participating in flexibility training. Warm-up is discussed later in the chapter.

Activity Level

As would be expected, evidence indicates that people who are physically active tend to be more flexible than inactive individuals. The decrease in flexibility in inactive individuals primarily occurs because connective tissues tend to become less pliable when exposed only to limited ROMs (4, 24, 30). A decrease in activity level will typically result in an increase in percent body fat and a decrease in the pliability of connective tissue. Further, an increase in fat deposits around the joints creates obstructions to ROM (24).

Resistance Training

A well-designed and properly executed resistance training program, using exercises that are performed through a full range of motion, can also increase flexibility. However, a resistance training program emphasizing high loads performed through less than full ROM can decrease flexibility (4). Therefore resistance training programs should be designed to develop both agonist and antagonist muscles, and all exercises must be performed through the full available ROM of the involved joints (4). While improper strength training can impair flexibility, the reason is not usually that the person has become too muscular or "muscle bound." Instead, the decrease occurs because of the improper development of a muscle or a group of muscles around a joint, resulting in a restriction of motion at that joint (9, 14). For example, a person with large biceps and deltoids may have difficulty stretching the triceps, racking a power clean, or holding a bar while performing the front squat (4). This is another reason resistance

training programs should be designed to develop both agonist and antagonistic muscles and to take all the involved joints through the full available ROM.

> Flexibility is influenced by a variety of factors. Some of these factors (joint structure, age, and sex) cannot be influenced by training. However, core temperature during flexibility training, overall activity level, participation in a well-designed resistance training program, and stretching on a regular basis can all affect flexibility and can be positively influenced by the personal trainer.

Elasticity and Plasticity

Flexibility training targets two different tissue adaptations, elastic and plastic. **Elasticity** refers to the ability to return to original resting length after a passive stretch (4). Thus elasticity provides a temporary change in length. In contrast, **plasticity** refers to the tendency to assume a new and greater length after a passive stretch, even after the load is removed (4, 24).

Muscle has elastic properties only. However, ligaments and tendons have both plastic and elastic properties. When connective tissue is stretched, some of the elongation occurs in the elastic tissue elements and some occurs in the plastic elements. When the stretch is removed, the elastic deformation recovers, but the plastic deformation remains (24).

Stretching techniques should be designed primarily to produce a plastic elongation if a permanent increase in ROM is the goal. During stretching, the proportion of elastic and plastic deformation can vary, depending on how and under what conditions the flexibility training occurs. Stretching to the point of mild discomfort, holding the stretched position for a period of time, and stretching only when the core temperature has been elevated will help emphasize plastic stretching (24).

Types of Flexibility Training

A number of stretching techniques can be used to maintain or increase flexibility. The most common of these methods are ballistic, dynamic, static, and various proprioceptive neuromuscular facilitation (PNF) techniques (8, 24, 25, 30).

Flexibility training can be further categorized into active and passive stretching exercises. Active stretching occurs when the person who is stretching supplies the force of the stretch. For example, during the sitting toe touch, the client supplies the force for the forward lean that stretches the hamstrings and low back (4). In contrast, passive stretching occurs when a partner or stretching device provides the force for the stretch (4).

The most important aspect of designing an effective flexibility training program is to ensure correct performance of exercises, regardless of the flexibility training method (10). For example, one technique commonly used to stretch the hamstrings is the toe touch stretch. However, this position requires lower back flexion, which posteriorly rotates the pelvis, decreasing the effectiveness of the stretch for the hamstrings. A better method to stretch the hamstrings is to place one foot slightly in front of the other, leaning forward from the hips and keeping the back arched. Supporting upper body weight with the hands on the rear leg, the client should feel the stretch in the front leg. This position ensures that the back does not flex and that the pelvis remains tilted forward, keeping the hamstrings optimally lengthened (10). Good technique is necessary to bring about optimal increases in flexibility.

Ballistic Stretching

Ballistic stretching (bouncing) is a rapid, jerky, uncontrolled movement. During ballistic stretching the body part is put into motion, and its momentum takes it through the ROM until the muscles are stretched to the limit (4, 7, 8, 24, 30, 47).

Ballistic stretching, though widely used in the past, is no longer considered an acceptable method for increasing ROM in any joint. One reason for this is that, because the movements are performed at high speeds, the rate and degree of stretch and the force applied to induce the stretch are difficult to control (24). A second reason is that this type of stretching may increase the risk of injury to the muscles and connective tissues, especially when there has been a previous injury (4, 30). This increased opportunity for injury occurs because there is a danger of exceeding the extensibility limits of the tissue being stretched (47).

In comparison to static stretching, ballistic stretching has four distinct disadvantages (3):

1. Increased danger of exceeding the extensibility limits of tissues involved
2. Higher energy requirements
3. Greater likelihood of causing muscular soreness
4. Activation of the stretch reflex

Two of the sensory organs within skeletal muscle that function as protective mechanisms against injury during passive and active stretching are the muscle spindles, which are located within the center of the muscle (30), and the Golgi tendon organ, which is located at the musculotendon junction. Muscle spindles initiate the stretch reflex, while the Golgi tendon organ initiates the Golgi tendon reflex.

The stretch reflex occurs in response to the extent and rapidity of a muscle stretch. When the muscle spindles are not stimulated, the muscle relaxes, allowing a greater stretch. During a rapid stretching movement, however, a sensory neuron from the muscle spindle innervates a motor neuron in the spine. The motor neuron then causes a muscle action of the previously stretched extrafusal muscle fibers; this is the stretch reflex (4). When the client bounces, for instance, the muscles respond by contracting to protect themselves from overstretching. Thus, internal tension develops in the muscle and prevents it from being fully stretched (24). A familiar example of this reflex is the knee jerk response. When the patellar tendon is struck, the tendon, and consequently the quadriceps muscle, experiences a slight but rapid stretch. The induced stretch results in activation of muscle spindle receptors within the quadriceps, causing the lower leg to jerk (24). Since motion is limited by this reflexive muscle action, stimulation of the muscle spindle and the subsequent activation of the stretch reflex should be avoided during stretching.

In addition to the stretch reflex, when excessive force is generated in the muscle, the Golgi tendon organ causes a reflex opposite that of the muscle spindle by inhibiting muscle contraction and causing the muscle to relax. This reflex helps to avoid injury by preventing the muscle from developing too much force or tension during active stretching (30).

Static Stretching

The most commonly used method of increasing flexibility is **static stretching.** A slow, constant speed is used, with the stretched position held for 30 seconds (4). Static stretching involves relaxing and simultaneous lengthening of the stretched muscle. Because of the slow speed of the stretches, static stretching does not activate the stretch reflex of the muscle. Thus, the risk for injury is lower than during ballistic stretching (4). Although injury to muscles or connective tissue may result if the static stretch is too intense, there are no real disadvantages to static stretching in terms of injury potential as long as proper technique is used. However, recent research suggests that static stretching prior to taking part in a dynamic activity (running, jumping, throwing) may have a negative effect on performance (15, 24).

Those just starting a flexibility training program may find it difficult to hold a stretch for 30 seconds. In these cases the personal trainer may wish to start the client with 15 or 20 seconds of holding and gradually progress to 30 seconds as the client gains experience and focus. Increasing the length of time the stretched position is held from 30 seconds to 60 seconds does not result in improved flexibility (30).

Movement into the final static stretch position should occur slowly and only to a point of minor discomfort. As the stretched position is held, the feeling of tension should diminish. If it does not, the stretched position should be slightly reduced. Using this procedure should assist in eliminating activation of the stretch reflex (24).

> To avoid activation of the stretch reflex, the client should move into the final static stretch position slowly and only to a point of minor discomfort. As the stretched position is held, the feeling of tension should diminish; if it does not, the stretched position should be slightly reduced.

Proprioceptive Neuromuscular Facilitation

Proprioceptive neuromuscular facilitation (PNF) stretching was originally developed as a technique to relax muscles that demonstrated increased tone or activity. It has since expanded to the conditioning of both athletes and the general population as a method of increasing ROM (4).

Proprioceptive neuromuscular facilitation is widely accepted as an effective method of increasing ROM (14, 18, 28, 43, 52). These techniques are normally performed with a partner and make use of both passive movement and active (concentric and isometric) muscle actions (10, 25, 30). While there are a variety of PNF techniques, perhaps the most common method (the hold-relax method) involves taking the muscle or joint into a static stretch position while keeping the muscle relaxed. After this static stretch position is held for about 10 seconds, the muscle is contracted for 6 seconds with a strong isometric contraction against an external fixed object (i.e., a force acting in the direction of the stretch). The partner should not allow the client to have any movement in the joint. Following a very brief (1-2 second) rest, another passive stretch is performed for 30 seconds, potentially resulting in a greater stretch. The isometric contraction will result in stimulation of the Golgi tendon organs; this may help to maintain low muscle tension during the second stretching maneuver, allowing connective tissue length to further increase and resulting in increased ROM (24).

Recommendations for Static Stretching

The following recommendations can be made to clients who are implementing a static flexibility training program (47):

- Stretching should be preceded by a warm up of 5 to 15 minutes, until a light sweat appears.

- Emphasize slow, smooth movements and coordinate deep breathing. Have clients inhale deeply and then exhale as they stretch to the point of mild discomfort. Then, have them ease back slightly and hold the stretch for 30 seconds as they breathe normally. Finally, have clients exhale as they slowly stretch further, again to the point of mild discomfort. Repeat three times and emphasize the importance of staying relaxed.

- Properly performed stretches should cause no more than mild discomfort. If clients feel pain, they are stretching too far.

- Ensure that clients do not lock their joints.

- To reduce the chance of activating the stretch reflex, discourage bouncing.

- Large muscle groups should be stretched first and the same routine should be repeated every training day. As areas that are less flexible become apparent, a greater emphasis can be placed on performing additional stretches for those muscle groups and joints.

- Stretches should be done at least three times per week and, in order to track performance improvements, should be done at the same time of day. Clients are least flexible in the morning because core temperature is the lowest at that time, so stretching early in the morning without first elevating core temperature is not advantageous in enhancing flexibility.

- The ideal time to stretch is after aerobic activity or resistance training, when the core temperature is maximally elevated.

Proprioceptive neuromuscular facilitation stretching may be superior to other stretching methods because it assists muscular relaxation, potentially assisting in increased ROM (14, 26, 28, 37, 43, 52). A study evaluating increases in ROM resulting from static and PNF stretching procedures showed that while both resulted in increased flexibility, subjects using the PNF method gained the most ROM. Despite this, not everyone agrees that PNF is the best method. Even though some studies suggest that PNF produces better results, PNF techniques can be impractical to use. One of the limitations of using PNF methods in a group setting is that a partner is typically required. The partner has to take great care not to overstretch the muscle. In addition, PNF can be dangerous unless each person is familiar with the appropriate techniques, because too much emphasis can be placed on flexibility and not enough on correct technique (13). The injury potential from PNF may be a concern especially with children or with groups of youngsters because of a lack of attention to detail (13). For this reason and also because the research pointing to the effectiveness of PNF has been disputed in some studies, great caution needs to be used in the implementation of a PNF program with this age group (9).

Because of the issues just mentioned, PNF methods have limited application in personal training settings. A significant level of training is needed to safely implement PNF methods. Because a partner is needed, PNF can be more time-consuming than other methods. Further, because static and dynamic flexibility methods are effective at increasing flexibility and because most clients will not need to achieve superior flexibility levels, PNF methods are not generally required in this setting. If the personal trainer has been trained in PNF methods and if the client has a drastic lack of ROM in one or more joints, PNF methods might be used.

Dynamic Stretching

Dynamic and ballistic stretching are similar in that both allow for faster movements to occur during training. However, **dynamic stretching** avoids bouncing and includes movements specific to a sport or movement pattern (4). An example of a dynamic stretch is a lunge walk in which the client exaggerates the length of the stride and bends the back leg so that he or she ends up in a position in which the front knee is over the toe (but not in front of it) and the back knee is just off the floor with the torso held in an upright position.

Often flexibility is measured using tests that measure static flexibility such as the sit and reach.

However, research has shown that there is no relationship between static flexibility and dynamic performance. There are few instances in which the ability to achieve a high degree of static flexibility is advantageous (23). With reference to the principle of specificity, **dynamic flexibility** may be more appropriate because it more closely simulates movements that occur in daily activities. An example is the everyday movement of reaching for an item on the top shelf at the grocery store, at home, or in the workplace. Dynamic arm circles, which are done with fluidity of movement, may more closely resemble reaching overhead in everyday life than would a position in which the arms are held statically over the head.

Much about stretching methods needs to be investigated before all the definitive answers can be given. However, the fitness professional should closely examine certain stretching techniques and determine the best time to use them. In particular, static stretching as part of a warm-up is very common, yet neither research nor logic suggests that static stretches will do much to help prevent injuries or improve muscle function before an activity. Instead, performed after warm-up, active mobility exercises—those that take the muscles dynamically through the full ROM, starting slowly and building up to movement-specific speeds—are more appropriate for developing active ROM for daily activities (10).

Dynamic stretching emphasizes functionally based movements. As training progresses, advancing from a standing position to a walk or a skip can enhance the specificity of dynamic stretching exercises. Adjusting from static stretching to dynamic exercises is not difficult. Often the stretching exercise is the same but is preceded and followed by some form of movement.

Personal trainers who wish to implement dynamic flexibility training in a client's program should begin dynamic stretches with low volume and low intensity because dynamic flexibility exercises require balance and coordination. Furthermore, dynamic flexibility training when introduced may lead to soreness for a short period of time because it represents a new stress to the body.

Many of the guidelines established for static flexibility training programs are also applicable to dynamic flexibility training. As already discussed, a warm-up period should occur prior to any flexibility training. Frequency should be two to five times per week, depending on the flexibility requirements of the activities the client is preparing for and his or her flexibility. Because dynamic flexibility training uses movement, each stretch should be repeated over a distance of 20 to 25 yards (about 18 to 23 m).

As the client becomes better able to perform each drill, the exercises can be performed in combinations. For example, a knee tuck and a lunge walk can be combined, alternating legs after performance of each movement. The possible combinations of exercises are nearly limitless. There are two primary advantages of combining movements. First, the variety is greater so the program is less likely to become monotonous. Second, combining stretches is more time efficient because the client is stretching a larger number of muscle groups rather than duplicating the same stretch repeatedly. This is important because many clients have limited time to devote to their training programs.

A later section of this chapter describes and illustrates a number of dynamic flexibility exercises. Since dynamic flexibility exercises are based on movements that occur both in sport and in everyday life, this selection of exercises does not represent an all-inclusive list of dynamic stretches. The number and types of dynamic stretches that can be used is limited only by the creativity of those designing the programs.

> **Dynamic stretching may be the most appropriate type of flexibility training for improving movement capability before a workout. If additional flexibility work is needed, performance of static flexibility exercises postworkout is effective.**

Recommended Flexibility Routine and Guidelines

A combination of dynamic and static flexibility training is recommended when the goal of training is increased ROM. Dynamic flexibility training is often associated with training athletes. However, dynamic flexibility training can also be successfully used in a nonathletic population. Increasing flexibility is

Recommendations for Dynamic Stretching

The following are recommendations for implementing a dynamic flexibility training program (19):

- Moderation and common sense are important. Flexibility is just one component of fitness and should not be overemphasized.
- The stretch should never be forced. If the stretch hurts, it should be discontinued.
- Flexibility training should be combined with strength training.
- Flexibility should be joint specific based on the needs of the client and the requirements of the activity.
- Ballistic stretching should be avoided.
- Stretching movements that position the body in the most functional stance possible, relative to the involved joints and musculature to be stretched and the activity requirements of the client, should be emphasized.
- It is important to make use of gravity, body weight, and ground reaction forces when stretching. Further, changes in planes and proprioceptive demand should be considered to further enhance improvements in flexibility.
- The dynamic flexibility training program should be specific to the demands of the sport or activities the client takes part in. The individual flexibility requirements of the client are also an important consideration.
- Improvements in flexibility can occur from day to day. Additionally, once increases in ROM have occurred, it is easy to maintain that ROM. Maintaining flexibility requires less work than improving it does.
- Clients should stretch the large muscle groups first and repeat the same routine every training day. As areas that are less flexible become apparent, a greater emphasis can be placed on performing additional stretches for those muscle groups and joints.
- Train for dynamic flexibility at least three times per week or along with each exercise session. In order to track performance improvements, clients should be consistent with the time of day they perform dynamic flexibility training, remembering that they are least flexible in the morning.
- Stretching should take place after the core temperature has been elevated.

of value during any type of movement regardless of whether that movement is occurring during an athletic competition or during performance of the multitude of movements that occur during daily life. The more functional the training, the more benefit it provides to those taking part in the training program.

Using dynamic flexibility alone can have limitations, however. Some of the dynamic stretches require a significant level of strength and mobility. This may preclude clients from performing some of the more demanding dynamic flexibility exercises. Further, some joints and muscle groups (i.e., neck, shoulders) may be more effectively stretched using static stretching techniques as compared to dynamic flexibility techniques.

Warm-Up

Clients should regularly perform preparatory exercises before undertaking vigorous activities. These preparatory exercises or movements are generally referred to as a *warm-up*.

Warm-up and stretching are not the same thing. Warm-up is an activity that raises the total body temperature, as well as temperature of the muscles, to prepare the body for vigorous exercise (4). Warming up is a part of the foundation of a successful practice session. Getting fully warmed up, mentally and physically, is a key aspect of attaining the training intensity required to achieve optimal results. A warm-up period is also important for increasing core temperature, thus improving the pliability of the muscles (15, 24, 40, 47, 57). A warm-up increases flexibility because muscle elasticity is dependent on blood flow to the target muscle (51). Cold muscles with low blood flow are more susceptible to injury or damage than muscles with a greater amount of blood flow (51).

Unfortunately, many clients attempt to take shortcuts in the warm-up procedure, which may translate into poor performance and increased injury risks (26). While the psychological aspects of warm-up have not yet been adequately investigated, research indicates that individuals who perform a warm-up prior to their main activity tend to be more mentally tuned or prepared (51).

Most research indicates that the major benefits of warm-up are related to temperature-dependent physiological processes. An increase in body temperature following a warm-up helps to produce the following effects (40):

- Increase in blood flow to the muscles
- Increase in the sensitivity of nerve receptors

- Increase in the disassociation of oxygen from hemoglobin and myoglobin
- Increase in the speed of nerve impulse transmissions
- Reduction in muscle viscosity
- Lowering of the energy rates of metabolic chemical reactions

The increase in tissue temperature that occurs during warm-up is the result of three physiological processes: the friction of the sliding filaments during muscular action, the metabolism of fuels, and the dilation of intramuscular blood vessels (19).

The following physiological changes take place during warm-up and theoretically should enhance performance (25).

1. Temperature increases within the muscles that are recruited during the warm-up session. A warmed muscle contracts more forcefully and relaxes more quickly. As a result, both speed and strength should be enhanced during exercise.

2. Temperature of the blood increases as it travels through the working muscle. As blood temperature rises, the amount of oxygen it can hold decreases, and more oxygen is unloaded to the working muscles.

3. Range of motion around joints is increased.

Range of motion is increased following a warm-up period because elevated core temperatures lower muscle, tendon, and ligament viscosity (51). This decrease in viscosity enables achievement of the best possible results and reduces the potential risk of stretching-induced injuries. It also reduces muscle and joint stiffness and provides protection against sudden, unexpected movements (19). It has been reported that excessive stretching when the tissue temperatures are relatively low increases the risk of connective tissue damage (51).

For the reasons just outlined, stretching should occur only after a warm-up (8, 13, 30, 51) or after the workout (19). Postworkout flexibility training also has a regenerative effect, restoring the muscles to their resting length, stimulating blood flow, and reducing muscle spasm (19). The physiological responses that occur due to a warm-up warrant the use of warm-up as a method to prepare the body for flexibility training (17). Body temperature should be elevated to a point that the client has broken into a light sweat before beginning flexibility work (25).

Unfortunately, many clients' preactivity warm-up program consists primarily of static stretching.

There are three distinct disadvantages to using static stretching to increase core temperature (1):

1. Because static stretching is a passive activity, minimal friction of the sliding filaments occurs.
2. There is little, if any, increase in the rate of fuels being metabolized.
3. There is no need for the intramuscular blood vessels to dilate in response to static stretching.

For these reasons, clients who begin exercise sessions with static stretching experience only a minimal increase in core body temperature (23) and are thus missing out on the benefits of an increased core temperature and decreased muscle viscosity. Warming up, mentally and physically, is a key aspect of achieving a training intensity required to achieve optimal results.

> Flexibility training should never be used as a method of warming up. Instead, flexibility training should occur only after core temperature has been elevated to a point that the client is beginning to perspire.

Types of Warm-Up

Regardless of the warm-up method chosen, the general purpose of warming up prior to physical activity is to increase muscle temperature (23). There are three types of warm-up methods—passive, general, and specific (23, 31, 51).

Passive Warm-Up

Passive warm-up involves such methods as hot showers, heating pads, or massage. Much of the research (18, 46, 50), but not all (25), has shown that passive warm-up methods can have a positive effect. One obvious advantage of a passive warm-up is that it does not prefatigue a client before an exercise session; once elevated temperatures are achieved, this increase in temperature can be preserved prior to physical activity with minimal energy expenditure (51). Unfortunately, passive warm-up procedures (e.g., moist heat pack) may not be practical in many settings.

General Warm-Up

General warm-up involves basic activities that require movement of the major muscle groups, such as jogging, cycling, or jumping rope (51). General warm-up increases heart rate, blood flow, deep muscle temperature, respiration rate, viscosity of joint fluids, and perspiration (4). The increase in muscle temperature allows greater flexibility (4), which prepares the body for movements (4). Thus, general warm-up seems more appropriate than passive when the goal is preparing the body for demanding physical activity.

Specific Warm-Up

Unlike general warm-up, **specific warm-up** includes movements that are an actual part of the activity, such as slow jogging before going out on a run or performing light repetitions of bench presses before progressing to the workout weight (4, 25, 51). Specific warm-up appears to be the most desirable method because it increases the temperature of the particular muscles that will be used in subsequent, more strenuous activity and also serves as a mental rehearsal of the event, allowing complex skills to be performed more effectively (23, 31).

Warm-Up Guidelines

The amount, intensity, and duration of warm-up should ideally be adjusted to every individual depending on his or her current level of fitness. The length of the warm-up period depends on climate and physical conditioning level. In general, the warm-up activity should last approximately 5 to 15 minutes, long enough for the individual to break into a light sweat (47).

As conditioning improves, the intensity and duration of the warm-up need to increase to bring about the desired increase in core temperature, again demonstrated by the client's breaking into a slight sweat. As a client becomes better conditioned, the thermoregulatory system is better able to respond to the heat produced during exercise, meaning the client is likely to exercise at a higher body temperature than would a less-conditioned client. Consequently, compared to a less conditioned person, a well-conditioned individual probably requires a longer or more intense warm-up, or one that is both longer and more intense, to achieve an optimal level of body temperature (51).

Body Weight and Stability Ball Exercises

Personal trainers may work with a client who does not have access to traditional weight training equipment or simply prefers not to train in a health club setting. This does not mean that the client cannot perform resistance training activities, but it does mean that the personal trainer will have to be creative in his or her approach.

One possible solution is to have the client perform a series of **body weight exercises** or stability ball exercises. As long as the stress of the exercise is of an appropriate intensity, the body will adapt by increasing muscle size or strength. Further, caloric expenditure will occur during activity; and as the intensity of the activity increases, so will the rate of caloric expenditure.

It is important to remember that the mode of exercise is not the most important variable in this setting. For example, clients can train the pectoralis and triceps muscle groups by performing a free weight bench press, a bench press on a selectorized machine, or push-ups on the floor or off of a stability ball. As long as the intensity is at the necessary threshold, adaptation will occur in the working muscle groups, regardless of the mode of training.

Body Weight Training

Body weight training is simply a mode of resistance training in which the resistance is provided by the body rather than by an external weight such as a barbell or the weight stack of a selectorized machine. In cases in which no equipment is available or if the client prefers this type of training, body weight training is a viable option. The personal trainer needs to be aware that the ability to develop maximal strength or power (or both) with body weight training will be eliminated because it cannot provide the intensity necessary to develop these physiological adaptations. However, if the goal of training is to develop basic strength levels or muscular endurance or both, body weight training is acceptable. To gain maximal benefits from this type of training, the emphasis must be on performing each exercise in a slow, controlled manner with perfect technique.

Stability Ball Training

The use of stability balls has increased significantly (29, 48). Initially, stability balls were used primarily by individuals with low back problems in physical therapy clinics (35, 52). However, stability balls are now more commonly used in orthopedic rehabilitation programs, with the physically active in fitness centers, in physical education classes, and with special needs populations and the elderly. Many fitness and rehabilitation facilities incorporate stability balls into their training programs, and the use of stability balls has expanded into sport conditioning programs (56).

The primary motivation for the use of stability balls in these applications is the belief that an unstable surface will provide a greater challenge to the trunk muscles, increase dynamic balance, and possibly help to stabilize the spine in order to prevent injuries (2). Additionally, while a primary emphasis with stability balls has been and continues to be trunk training, it is now common to see stability balls used in conjunction with strength training for multiple muscle groups, not just the trunk (35).

Research Findings

The use of unstable training has been purported in the popular literature to enhance sport-specific training through increased activation of stabilizers and trunk muscles (2). Further, several practitioners have suggested that stability ball exercises are most effective for training core stability. Research on the use of unstable platforms and their effects on force and muscle activation of the upper body musculature is scant (48) and has produced mixed results.

- *Stability balls and core activation.* Some studies show that stability training increases abdominal muscle activity, activating more motor units of the stabilizing muscles than traditional exercises and thus improving overall balance and core stability (16, 29). In addition, stability balls stimulate parts of the cerebellum, vestibular system, and brainstem, which are responsible for posture, balance, and body control (29). Initial scientific support for stability ball training came from observations of greater activation of the rectus abdominis and external obliques during abdominal curl-ups on the stability ball compared with a stable surface (54). Research since has shown that use of a stability ball versus a stable surface leads to greater activation of the external obliques, transverse abdominis, internal obliques, erector spinae, and rectus abdominis, as well as the abdominal stabilizers (6, 34, 41), suggesting that exercises intended to strengthen or increase the endurance of the core stabilizers should involve a destabilizing component (6). However, other studies do not show significant differences in abdominal muscle electromyography with the ball versus a stable surface (2, 35, 49).

- *Stability balls and core training.* Training the core has become an area of emphasis in athletic strength and conditioning programs, health and fitness centers, and rehabilitation facilities (21). Prevailing beliefs hold that training the core is important for improving performance and reducing the risk of injuries and that core strengthening is vital to improving athletic performance (44). Use of stability balls is most commonly associated with core training. Research has also shown that the stability ball provides a wider range of movement than most training modes (2).

Stability ball training has been used for many years in physical therapy settings to strengthen the musculature responsible for spinal stability (11), though little research has been performed to show that it improves spine stabilization or helps decrease the risk of back pain (11). However, stability ball exercises that require a neutral spine position may be appropriate for targeting the specific muscles that stabilize the spine during the early phase of training; they also may improve trunk endurance because of the high percentage of slow-twitch fibers recruited to maintain a neutral position.

Increasing back strength may provide some protection from low back pain when greater forces are required to perform a task (6, 21). Further, the spine may become unstable because of weak trunk stabilizer muscles, and a lack of back muscle endurance is strongly associated with low back pain.

- *Other potential benefits.* Stability ball training may offer a number of additional potential benefits:

  □ Improved balance, joint stability, proprioception, and neuromuscular control decrease the incidence of injury (29).

  □ Heart rate response and oxygen consumption rates increase (29).

  □ Strength, stability, balance, posture, proprioception, and flexibility in pregnant women increase. These adaptations result in stronger abdominal muscles, which help to support the baby, decrease the incidence of back pain, and reduce the chances of accidental falls (29).

- *Stability balls in sport performance training programs.* Few investigations have examined the effect of stability ball training on physical performance. Stability ball training enhanced core stability in swimmers, but this did not transfer to improved swim times (45). Thus stability ball training might not be specific to the core stability requirements of swimming (57). In runners, stability ball training significantly improved core stability but did not improve running performance (5, 16, 48) or running posture (5, 16). Thus the anecdotal evidence supporting the use of stability ball training to enhance physical performance has not been scientifically substantiated (48), and there is no guarantee that improvements in core strength and power will transfer to improvements in sport performance (56).

- *Importance of training specificity.* As with all training endeavors, the principle of specificity must be emphasized for optimal results (48, 56). With regard to the trunk, training in a supine or prone position on the stability ball may not transfer effectively to sports or activities performed predominantly in upright positions (56). However, specificity also dictates that training activities should simulate the demands of a sport as closely as possible (56), and in some situations the use of a stability ball can increase the degree of specificity. Mogul skiing, shooting a puck in hockey, and surfing, for example, all involve generating forces under unstable conditions. Additionally, most sports involve a combination of stabilizing and force-producing functions (e.g., forehand in tennis, baseball pitcher windup), and resistance training under unstable conditions provides similar challenges to the neuromuscular system (2).

Another important aspect of specificity is core stability requirements. Free weight exercises performed on a stable surface might be more transferable to sport performance than exercises performed on a stability ball (56). Resistance training exercises can be altered to place greater emphasis on core stability (e.g., squats and deadlifts performed with dumbbells while standing on one leg; power cleans and push presses performed unilaterally with dumbbells, trunk rotation exercises performed with cables or medicine balls) (57).

- *Effect of unstable base on force output.* The value of unstable training for the limb musculature remains a matter of debate (33). A recognized limiting factor with strength training under unstable conditions is reduced force-generating capabilities (2, 33, 38, 48, 55), as limb muscles must assist in joint stability (2).

Isometric force output during unstable resistance exercise is significantly lower than during stable conditions. Thus some have recommended that resistance training be performed under stable conditions when the goal is to improve muscle strength and athletic performance. An intensity level of at least 80% of maximum is required to yield strength gains, and this level of intensity is not possible under unstable conditions (33). Similarly in healthy subjects, the stimulus provided by stability ball training is insufficiently intense to increase muscular strength and thus does not appear to provide a training advantage (38). Squats and deadlifts performed under stable conditions at intensities as low as 50% of 1RM were shown to be more challenging to the neuromuscular system than stability ball exercises (38), suggesting their superiority for increasing muscular strength and hypertrophy of the back extensors.

The reduced force-generation capabilities elicited by unstable training have led to the suggestion that instability training devices should be used to "augment" traditional training methods (55). Nuzzo and colleagues (38), however, suggested that such training be "excluded" or "limited" because of the apparent lack of evidence that it improves strength or hypertrophy or measures related to athletic performance.

■ Stability ball training provides some unique advantages that warrant its continued use by personal trainers. However, there are also disadvantages. As with all types of training, the personal trainer must emphasize the concept of specificity and the client's primary goals when deciding whether to include the stability ball in a training program. The following is a review of the advantages and disadvantages.

Advantages

- Injuries are decreased as a result of improved balance, joint stability, proprioception, and neuromuscular control (29).
- Heart rate response and oxygen consumption rates are increased (29).
- Abdominal strength, stability, balance, posture, proprioception, and flexibility are increased in pregnant women (see chapter 18) (29).
- For some sports that involve a degree of instability, using a stability ball can increase the degree of training specificity (2).

Disadvantages

- Some studies have confirmed increased core stability with the use of stability balls, but this did not result in improved sport performance (45).
- Under unstable conditions, training at an intensity necessary to bring about increases in strength in trained individuals is not possible (2, 33, 38, 48, 55).
- Sport performance might be better enhanced by free weight exercises performed on a stable surface than exercises performed on a stability ball (56).

In light of some of the disadvantages described previously, personal trainers might choose to incorporate instability into training programs via methods other than stability ball training. Two such methods are described here.

■ *Emphasis on structural multijoint exercises.* Instead of emphasizing stability ball training, personal trainers should focus on structural multijoint exercises like squats and deadlifts because the intensity can be continually increased through changes in external loading (38). Additionally, because these are multijoint exercises that recruit multiple major muscle groups, they may be more time efficient than numerous stability ball exercises (38). However, because of its advantages, stability ball training should be viewed as an important supplement to more traditional methods of resistance training so that clients obtain the benefits of each training mode.

■ *Instability with free weight training.* Instability can be influenced not only by the base of support, but also by the implements used. Free weight training has been promoted as more beneficial than machines for training athletes partially due to the instability it offers (2). Free weight training can provide a moderate degree of instability (56). The use of water-filled implements can further increase the instability because of the active fluid resistance of the water (27). Another way to augment instability in free weight training is to emphasize unilateral over bilateral dumbbell training (6). Many activities in daily life and in sport are unilateral. Unilateral exercises allow a higher degree of movement specificity than bilateral training and stimulate the trunk stabilizers more (6).

Safety and Correct Sizing

Because of their inherent instability, safety is a major concern with stability balls (29). Proper exercise technique must be emphasized to protect people from falling. It is important that people start off with basic, less complex exercises and increase the complexity over time (29). Jakubek (29) suggests using sandbags as stabilizing wedges. Further, people with long hair should tie it back so it does not get caught during movements. Finally, during stability ball training people need to use common sense; if an exercise causes pain, the movement should be discontinued (29).

Another aspect of safety with the use of stability balls is making sure the ball is correctly sized (29). The individual should sit on the ball; the size is correct if the thighs are slightly above parallel to the ground.

Correct Positioning of the Stability Ball

An important but often overlooked aspect of maximizing the effectiveness of stability ball training is the positioning of the ball relative to the body. One investigation showed a significant increase in abdominal muscle activity when a crunch was performed on a stability ball in comparison to the same movement performed on the floor, but only when the ball was correctly placed (49). When the ball was placed high on the back, at the level of the inferior border of the scapula, abdominal muscle activity was significantly decreased as compared to that with either a lower ball position or a crunch performed on a stable surface. Placing the ball lower on the back requires elevation of a greater portion

Guidelines for Stability Ball Training

As with any training method, it is important for the personal trainer to adhere to training guidelines to ensure that clients are maximizing their time and effort with the stability ball. Guidelines include the following:

1. *The stability ball should be fully inflated so that it is firm.*

2. *The stability ball should be the correct size for the client.* To determine the correct size, have the client sit on the ball with feet on the floor. In this position the thighs should be parallel or slightly above parallel to the floor. If the client has low back pain, the thighs should be slightly above parallel, with the knees lower than the hips.

3. *As with other modes of training, a warm-up session of 5 to 15 minutes should precede the actual workout.* Activities such as brisk walking or jogging, walking up stairs, or calisthenics types of activities (i.e., jumping jacks, mountain climbers) can be used during the warm-up period. Warm-up activities performed on the stability ball have the advantage of training the stabilizing muscle groups, improving balance and coordination (53).

4. *Allow time for the client to become familiar with the ball.* A client may be able to demonstrate superior strength in traditional types of exercises but still find stability ball exercises extremely challenging. This is especially true for clients who perform a majority of their training on machines. When an exercise is performed on a machine, the stabilizing muscles are not activated. Thus when clients begin to use a stability ball, they may fatigue very rapidly, which leads to poorly performed repetitions.

5. *Emphasize correct technique.* Attention to detail is critical when clients perform exercises on a stability ball. Many stability ball exercises look easy, but the slightest deviation from correct technique or position can have a negative effect on performance of the exercise. This is especially important to remember as the client becomes fatigued and it becomes more and more difficult to perform the exercise correctly.

6. *The number of sets and repetitions performed will depend on the fitness level of the client.* Clients can perform the exercises in circuit training fashion, or can perform the full number of sets on each exercise before advancing to the next exercise, depending on their fitness goals. As with beginning any exercise routine, clients should start with low volume and low intensity (e.g., 1 × 8) and gradually adjust the training variables as their fitness level improves (e.g., 3 × 15).

of the trunk during the crunch motion and requires greater trunk stabilization in the horizontal position because there is no support for the upper trunk from either the floor or the ball. Thus performing the crunch using the lower ball placement requires more abdominal muscle activity than either performing using the higher ball placement or performing a traditional crunch (49).

Individuals with abdominal muscle weakness can use a high ball placement, allowing them to perform the crunch motion with less effort than would be needed on a stable bench or the floor. As their condition and fitness improves, the ball can gradually be positioned lower on the back to increase the training load and thus increase abdominal muscle activity (49).

Conclusion

Personal trainers typically incorporate some form of stretching into their clients' programs, and it is important that they and their clients have a clear understanding of what flexibility is and how it relates to conditioning in general. Defined as the ROM of a joint or a series of joints, flexibility helps a joint to move freely through a full normal ROM and helps to improve performance and prevent injury. Many factors affect a client's flexibility, including joint structure, muscle and connective tissue, sex, temperature, and resistance training. Warm-up—which is not to be confused with stretching—is part of the foundation of an effective workout, increasing the client's body temperature and ROM.

Ballistic, static, and various PNF techniques are the stretching techniques most commonly used to maintain or increase flexibility, although dynamic stretching—while still somewhat controversial—is also gaining acceptance. In designing flexibility programs, the personal trainer is well advised to incorporate a combination of dynamic and static flexibility training. For some clients, it is appropriate to use a series of body weight or stability ball exercises or to use a combination of the two.

Flexibility, Body Weight, and Stability Ball Exercises

Static Flexibility Exercises

Look Right and Left

1. Stand or sit with the head and neck upright.
2. Turn the head to the right using a submaximal concentric muscle action.
3. Turn the head to the left using a submaximal concentric muscle action.

Primary Muscles Stretched
Sternocleidomastoid

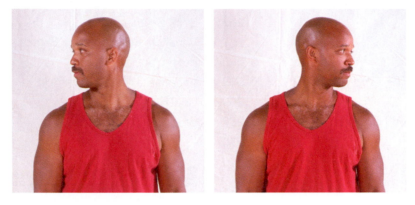

Common Errors

- Turning the torso as the head turns
- Not turning the head through the full comfortable range of motion

Neck Flexion and Extension

1. Standing or sitting with head and neck upright, flex the neck by tucking the chin toward the chest.
2. If the chin touches the chest, try to touch the chin lower on the chest.
3. Extend the neck by trying to come as close as possible to touching the head to the back.

Primary Muscles Stretched
Sternocleidomastoid, suboccipitals, splenae

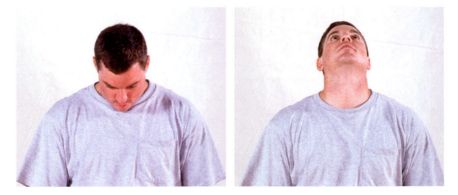

Common Errors

- Failing to go through a complete range of motion, either during flexion or extension
- Using a jerky, explosive type of action rather than pushing against, or resisting against, the force being applied to the head; all movements should be slow, continuous, and steady
- Using movements in the trunk, arms, or other parts of the body to assist in the movement at the neck; there should be no movement other than what is occurring at the neck

Hands Behind Back

1. Stand erect and reach behind the back with both arms.
2. Clasp the hands together and fully extend the elbows.
3. Slightly flex the knees and look straight ahead.
4. Raise the arms until a stretch is felt.

Common Errors

- Allowing the elbows to flex
- Flexing the torso forward or looking down at the floor

Primary Muscles Stretched
Anterior deltoids, pectoralis major

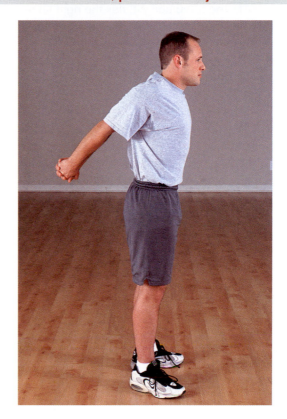

Behind-Neck Stretch

1. Stand erect and raise the right arm to position it next to the right side of the head.
2. Flex the right elbow to allow the right hand to touch the back of the neck or upper back.
3. Raise the left arm to grasp the right elbow with the left hand.
4. Pull the right elbow toward (and behind) the head with the left hand (i.e., increase shoulder abduction) until a stretch is felt.
5. Repeat the stretch with the right hand grasping and pulling the left elbow.

Common Errors

- Flexing the torso forward or rounding the shoulders

Primary Muscles Stretched
Triceps brachii, latissimus dorsi

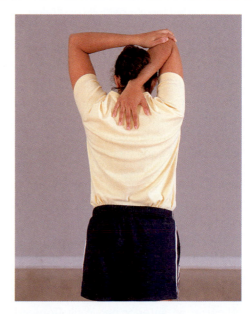

Pretzel

1. Sit on the floor with the legs next to each other and extended away from the body.
2. With the torso upright, flex the right knee, cross it over the left leg, and place the right foot on the floor to the outside of the left knee.
3. Twist the torso to the right to position the back of the left elbow against the outside of the right knee.
4. Place the right palm on the floor 12 to 16 inches (30-40 cm) behind the hips.
5. Keeping the buttocks on the floor, use the right knee to hold the left elbow stationary while twisting the head and shoulders to the right until a stretch is felt.
6. Repeat the stretch with the left foot placed to the outside of the right knee and the right elbow against the outside of the left knee.

Primary Muscles Stretched
Internal oblique, external oblique, piriformis, erector spinae

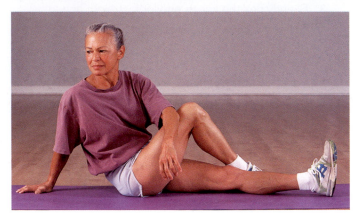

Common Errors

- Placing the elbow on the front of the thigh (rather than to the outside of the knee)
- Allowing the buttocks to rise off of the floor

Forward Lunge

1. From a standing position, take an exaggerated step forward with the right leg.
2. Flex the right knee until it is positioned over the right foot.
3. Keep the right foot on the floor with both feet pointed straight ahead.
4. Keep the left leg almost fully extended; the heel can be off the floor, if needed.
5. Place the hands on the top of the right thigh or on the hips and look straight ahead.
6. With the torso fully upright, move the hips forward and slightly downward until a stretch is felt.
7. Repeat the stretch with the left leg positioned ahead of the body (i.e., lunge with the left leg).

Primary Muscles Stretched
Iliopsoas, rectus femoris, gluteus maximus, hamstrings

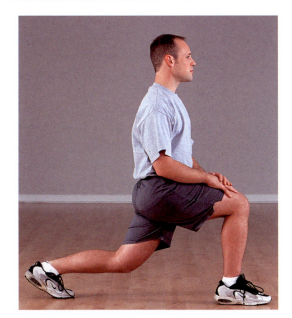

Common Errors

- Allowing the lead knee to flex beyond the toes of the lead foot
- Allowing the heel of the lead foot to lift off of the floor
- Flexing the torso forward or looking down at the floor
- Allowing an anterior pelvic tilt (forward pelvis tilt and increased low-back arch)

Lying Knee to Chest

1. Lie supine with the legs next to each other and extended away from the body.
2. Flex the right knee and hip to elevate the right thigh toward the chest.
3. Grasp the back of the right thigh (underneath the right knee).
4. Keep the left leg in the same starting position.
5. Use the arms to pull the right thigh further toward the chest until a stretch is felt.
6. Repeat the stretch with the left knee pulled to the chest and the right leg extended away from the body.

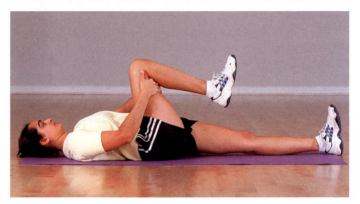

Primary Muscles Stretched
Gluteus maximus, hamstrings, erector spinae

Common Errors

- Grasping the front of the flexed knee (rather than the back of the thigh)
- Flexing the neck or arching the back
- Lifting the opposite leg off of the floor

Semistraddle (Modified Hurdler's Stretch)

1. Sit on the floor with the right leg extended away from the body and the sole of the left foot pressed against (or near to) the inside of the right knee.
2. The outside of the left leg will be touching or nearly touching the floor.
3. Keeping the back flat, lean forward at the hips and grasp the toes of the right foot with the right hand.
4. Pull the toes of the right foot toward the upper body as the torso is flexed toward the right leg until a stretch is felt.
5. Repeat the stretch with the left leg extended away from the body and the sole of the right foot pressed against (or near to) the inside of the left knee.

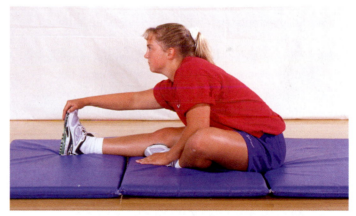

Primary Muscles Stretched
Hamstrings, erector spinae, gastrocnemius

Common Errors

- Allowing the extended thigh to externally rotate
- Rounding the shoulders or curling the torso toward the extended leg (rather than flexing the torso at the hips)
- Allowing the knee of the extended leg to flex

Butterfly

1. Sit on the floor with the torso upright.
2. Flex the hips and knees and externally rotate the thighs to bring the soles of the feet together.
3. Lean forward at the hips and grasp the feet and move them toward the body.
4. Place the elbows on the inside of the legs.
5. Keeping the back flat, slightly push the elbows down, pull the feet toward the upper body, and flex the torso forward until a stretch is felt.

Common Errors

- Rounding the shoulders or curling the torso toward the feet (rather than flexing the torso at the hips)

Primary Muscles Stretched
Hip adductors, gracilis

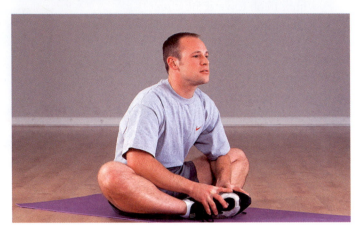

Wall Stretch

1. Stand facing a wall with the feet shoulder-width apart and the toes about 12 inches (30 cm) from the wall.
2. Lean forward and place the hands on the wall.
3. Step back about 2 feet (61 cm) with the left leg and slightly flex the right knee.
4. Fully extend the left knee and keep the left heel on the floor.
5. Allow the elbows to flex to move the hips and torso closer to the wall until a stretch is felt.
6. Repeat the stretch with the right leg positioned behind the body (i.e., step back with the right leg).

Common Errors

- Moving the torso closer to the wall without also moving the hips forward
- Allowing the heel of the stepped-back foot to lift off of the floor

Primary Muscles Stretched
Gastrocnemius, soleus (and Achilles tendon)

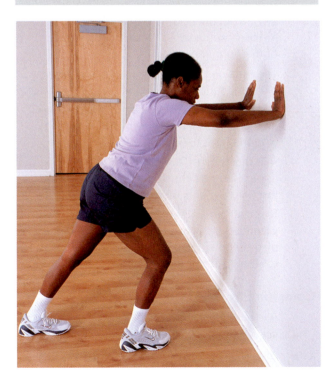

Dynamic Flexibility Exercises

Arm Circle

1. While slowly walking over the prescribed distance, move the arms in wide circles, progressing from a position in which the arms are directly at the sides to a position in which the arms are directly overhead.
2. Allow movement to occur only at the shoulder joints (i.e., keep the elbows fully extended).
3. Perform the arm circles both forward and backward through a full comfortable ROM.

Common Errors

- Allowing the torso to flex and extend as the arms move in circles

Primary Muscles Stretched
Deltoids, latissimus dorsi, pectoralis major

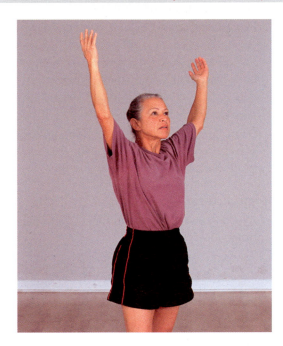

Arm Swing

1. Flex the arms at the shoulders to position the arms parallel to the floor in front of the body.
2. While slowly walking over the prescribed distance, swing the arms in unison to the right so the left arm is in front of the chest, the fingers of the left hand are pointing directly lateral to the right shoulder, and the right arm is behind the body.
3. Immediately reverse the movement direction to swing the arms in unison to the left.
4. Allow movement to occur only at the shoulder joints (i.e., keep the torso and head facing forward).
5. Alternate the arm swings to the right and left through a full comfortable ROM.

Common Errors

- Allowing the torso or neck to rotate in the direction of the arm swing

Primary Muscles Stretched
Latissimus dorsi, teres major, anterior and posterior deltoids, pectoralis major

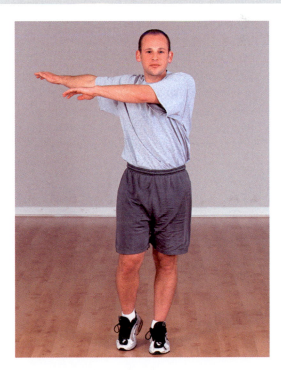

Lunge Walk

1. Clasp the hands behind the head.
2. From a standing position, take an exaggerated step forward with the left leg.
3. Flex the left knee until it is positioned over the left foot.
4. Slightly flex the right knee to be just off the floor; both feet should be pointed straight ahead.
5. Keep the torso erect (or leaning back slightly) and look straight ahead.
6. Pause for a count in the bottom lunged position, stand up, and then repeat with the right leg, progressing forward with each step.

Common Errors

- Allowing the lead knee to flex beyond the toes of the lead foot
- Touching the knee of the trailing leg to the floor
- Flexing the torso forward or looking down at the floor

Primary Muscles Stretched
Iliopsoas, rectus femoris, gluteus maximus, hamstrings

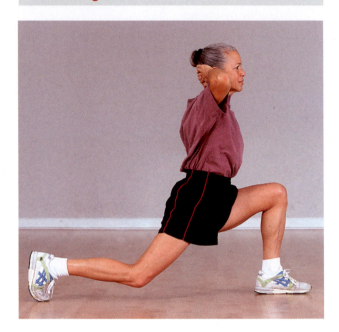

Variation: Reverse Lunge Walk

1. Clasp the hands behind the head.
2. From a standing position, take an exaggerated step backward with the right leg.
3. Flex the left knee until it is positioned over the left foot.
4. Slightly flex the right knee to be just off the floor; both feet should be pointed straight ahead.
5. Keep the torso erect (or leaning back slightly) and look straight ahead.
6. Pause for a count in the bottom lunged position, stand up, and then repeat with the left leg, progressing backward with each step.

Primary Muscles Stretched
Iliopsoas, rectus femoris, gluteus maximus, hamstrings

Common Errors

- Allowing the lead knee to flex beyond the toes of the lead foot
- Touching the knee of the trailing leg to the floor
- Flexing the torso forward or looking down at the floor

Hockey Lunge Walk

1. Clasp the hands behind the head.
2. From a standing position, take an exaggerated step forward and diagonally to the right with the right leg.
3. Place the right foot on the floor 10 to 12 inches (25-30 cm) wider than the placement of the lead foot during the lunge walk exercise (p. 272).
4. Keep the toes of both feet pointing straight ahead.
5. Flex the right knee until it is positioned over the right foot.
6. Slightly flex the left knee to be just off the floor.
7. Keep the torso erect (or leaning back slightly) and look straight ahead.
8. Pause for a count in the bottom lunged position, stand up, and then repeat with the left leg, progressing forward with each step.

Common Errors

- Allowing the lead knee to flex beyond the toes of the lead foot
- Touching the knee of the trailing leg to the floor
- Flexing the torso forward or looking down at the floor
- Stepping too laterally or pointing the feet medially or laterally

Variation: Walking Side Lunge

1. Clasp the hands behind the head.
2. Turn sideways, with the right shoulder pointing in the desired movement direction.
3. From a standing position, take an exaggerated lateral step to the right with the right foot.
4. Keeping the left knee straight, flex the right knee until it is positioned over the right foot and allow the hips to sink back and to the right.
5. Keep the torso erect and look straight ahead.
6. Pause for a count in the bottom lunged position, then stand back up, pivot on the right foot, and repeat with the left leg.

Primary Muscles Stretched
Iliopsoas, rectus femoris, gluteus maximus, hamstrings, hip adductors

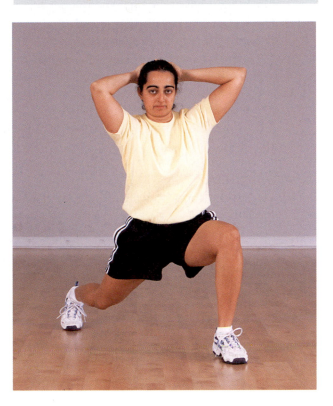

Primary Muscles Stretched
Iliopsoas, rectus femoris, gluteus maximus, hamstrings, hip adductors

Common Errors

- Allowing the lead knee to flex beyond the toes of the lead foot
- Flexing the knee of the trailing leg
- Flexing the torso forward or looking down at the floor

Walking Knee Tuck

1. From a standing position, step forward with the left leg and flex the right hip and knee to move the right thigh toward the chest.

2. Grasp the front of the right knee/upper shin.

3. Use the arms to pull the right knee farther up and squeeze the right thigh against the chest.

4. Pause for a count in the knee tuck position, then step back down with the right leg, shift the body weight to the right leg, and repeat with the left leg, progressing forward with each step.

5. Try to pull the knee slightly higher with each repetition.

Common Errors

- Flexing the torso forward or looking down at the floor

Primary Muscles Stretched
Gluteus maximus, hamstrings

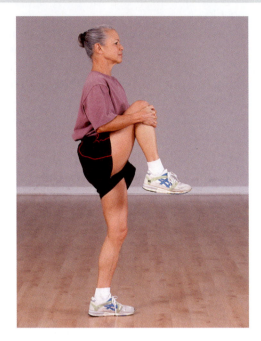

Walking Knee Over Hurdle

1. Imagine facing a line of hurdles approximately 3 feet (91 cm) tall, where the hurdles are on alternating sides of the body. The first hurdle is to the right side; the second hurdle, which is a short distance beyond the first, is to the left side, and so on.

2. From a standing position, flex the right hip and knee then abduct the right thigh to be parallel with the floor.

3. Lead the right knee over the first imaginary hurdle that is on the right.

4. Pause for a count in the highest thigh position, then step back down with the right leg, shift the body weight to the right leg, and repeat with the left leg, progressing forward with each step.

5. Try to lift the thigh slightly higher over the hurdle with each repetition.

Common Errors

- Leaning the torso too far away from the hurdle (rather than emphasizing hip abduction)
- Leading with the torso or the head over the hurdle (rather than with the lead knee)

Primary Muscles Stretched
Hip adductors

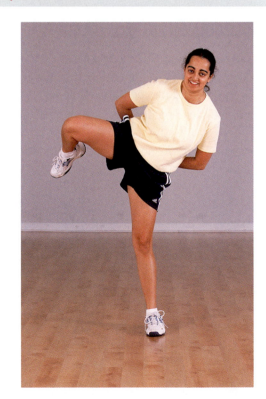

Body Weight Exercises

Abdominal Crunch

1. Assume a supine position on the floor.
2. Flex the hips and knees and place the heels on a box.
3. Place the hands behind or at the sides of the head (to hold its weight only) or fold the arms across the chest or abdomen.
4. Curl the torso until the upper back is off of the floor. Client should maintain a tucked or neutral head and neck position.
5. Keep the feet, buttocks, and lower back stationary at all times.
6. After completing the crunch, allow the torso to uncurl back down to the starting position.

Common Errors

- Raising the hips or feet
- Pulling the head with the hands
- Flexing the torso to a fully seated position

Primary Muscles Trained
Rectus abdominis

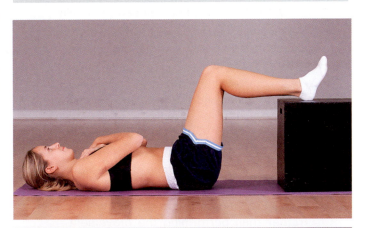

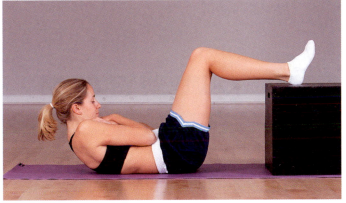

Variation: Twisting Crunch

1. Assume a supine position on the floor.
2. Flex the hips and knees and place the heels on a box or bench.
3. Place the hands behind or at the sides of the head (to hold its weight only) or fold the arms across the chest or abdomen.
4. Twist (rotate) the torso to move the right shoulder toward the left thigh.
5. Continue flexing and twisting the torso until the upper back is off of the floor.
6. Keep the feet, buttocks, and lower back stationary at all times.
7. After completing the crunch, allow the torso to uncurl and untwist back down to the starting position.
8. Alternate the direction of the twist with each repetition.

Primary Muscles Trained
Rectus abdominis, internal and external oblique

Common Errors

- Raising the hips or feet
- Pulling the head with the hands

Back Extension

1. Assume a prone position on the floor with the knees fully extended and the toes pointed down to the floor.

2. Clasp the hands behind the head.

3. Keeping the toes in contact with the floor, extend the torso (i.e., arch the back) to lift the chest off the floor.

4. After completing the extension, allow the chest to lower and return to the starting position.

Common Errors

- Flexing the knees or lifting the toes off the floor

- Rapidly rocking up and down on the hips (rather than performing the movement under control)

Primary Muscles Trained
Erector spinae

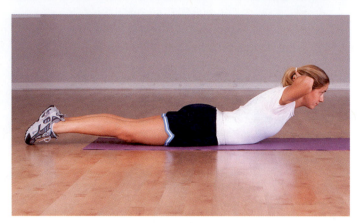

Variation: Twisting Back Extension

1. Assume a prone position on the floor with the knees fully extended and the toes pointed down to the floor.

2. Clasp the hands behind the head.

3. Keep the toes in contact with the floor.

4. Extend and twist (rotate) the torso to move the right shoulder up and to the left.

5. Continue extending and twisting the torso until the chest is off of the floor.

6. Keep the feet, buttocks, and lower back on the floor at all times.

7. After completing the extension, allow the chest to lower and untwist back down to the starting position.

8. Alternate the direction of the twist with each repetition.

Primary Muscles Trained
Erector spinae

Common Errors

- Flexing the knees or lifting the toes off the floor

- Rapidly rocking back and forth on the hips (rather than performing the movement under control)

Push-Up

1. Assume a prone position on the floor with the knees fully extended and the toes pointed down to the floor.
2. Place the hands on the floor, palms down, about 2 to 3 inches (5-8 cm) wider than shoulder-width apart with the elbows pointed outward.
3. Keeping the body in a straight line and the toes in contact with the floor, push against the floor with the hands to fully extend the elbows.
4. After completing the push-up, lower the body by allowing the elbows to flex to a 90° angle. Alternatively, the personal trainer can place a soft object about the size of rolled-up socks or a foam half-roller on the floor beneath the client's chest and count the repetitions only when the client's chest touches the socks or roller.

Common Errors

- Allowing the hips to sag or rise up (rather than keeping the body in a straight line)
- Performing the exercise through a reduced ROM

Primary Muscles Trained
Pectoralis major, anterior deltoid, triceps brachii

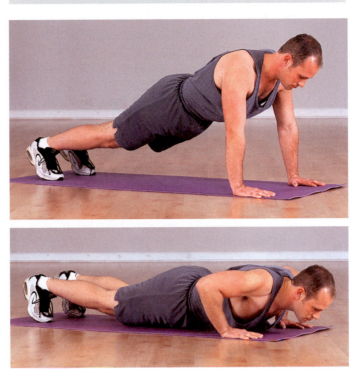

Variation: Modified Push-Up

1. Modify the standard push-up technique by having the client assume a kneeling position, with the knees flexed to 90° and the ankles crossed.

Common Errors

- Allowing the hips to sag or rise up (rather than keeping the body in a straight line)
- Performing the exercise through a reduced ROM

Primary Muscles Trained
Pectoralis major, anterior deltoid, triceps brachii

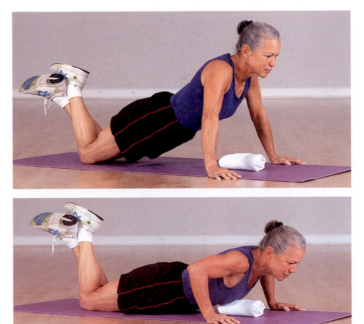

Heel Raise

1. Stand on the floor or on the edge of a stair step, with one hand at the side or on the hip.

2. Place one hand on the wall or stair railing to assist in balance.

3. The feet should be close together and flat on the floor. If on a stair step, place the balls of the feet on the edge of the step, with the rear portion of the feet extending off the step.

4. Elevate up onto the toes, then lower the heels through the full comfortable ROM.

Common Errors

- Using a ballistic movement to achieve a brief full range of motion contraction instead of slowing lifting and holding a full range of motion position

- Failing to achieve a true comfortable full range of motion position

Primary Muscles Trained
Gastrocnemius, soleus

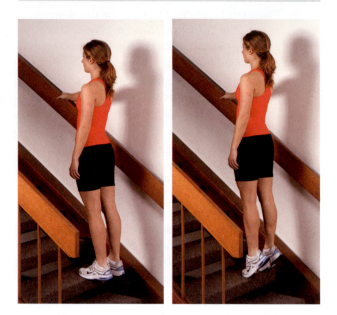

Step-Up

1. Stand facing a chair, bench, or other sturdy object. The height of the object should be such that when you place your foot on the object your knee is at about hip height.

2. Place your right foot on the object. Make sure your entire foot is on the object.

3. Using your right leg to lift you, step up on the object, so that you are standing on both legs on top of the object.

4. Leaving your left foot on the object, step down with your right foot.

5. Step back up with your right foot.

Common Errors

- Not placing the entire foot on the step, increasing the opportunity for the foot to slip off the step

- Pushing off with the foot on the floor to assist in the movement; rising to the step should occur as a result of muscular action originating from the leg placed on the step and not both legs

Primary Muscles Trained
Gluteus maximus, semimembranosus, semitendinosus, biceps femoris, vastus lateralis, vastus intermedius, vastus medialis, rectus femoris

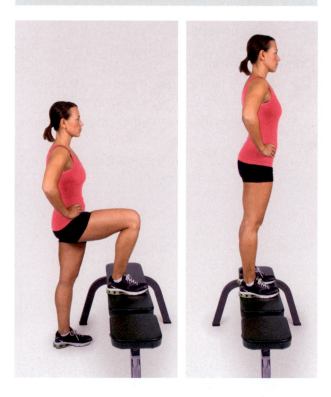

Stability Ball Exercises

Extended Abdominal Crunch

1. Lie supine on the stability ball with the lower-to-middle section of the back on the apex of the ball.
2. Place the feet flat on the floor about hip-width apart with the thighs, hips, and lower abdomen approximately parallel to the floor.
3. Place the hands behind or at the sides of the head (to hold its weight only) or fold the arms across the chest or abdomen.
4. Curl the torso to raise it 30° to 40° from the starting position.
5. Keep the feet on the floor and the thighs and hips stationary.
6. After completing the crunch, allow the torso to uncurl back down to the starting position.

Common Errors

- Raising the feet off the floor
- Allowing the hips to drop down off the side of the ball
- Pulling the head with the hands

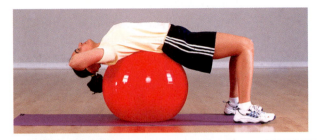

Primary Muscles Trained
Rectus abdominis

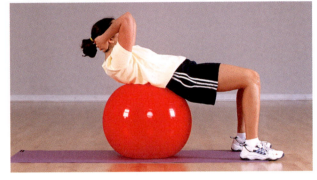

Supine Leg Curl

1. Lie supine on the floor with the legs next to each other and extended away from the body.
2. Abduct the arms 90° away from the torso with the palms facing the floor.
3. Lift the hips off the floor to position the lower calves and back of the heels on the apex of the stability ball.
4. Begin the exercise with the feet, knees, hips, and shoulders in a straight line.
5. Keeping the upper body in the same position, flex the knees (which will cause the ball to roll backward) to bring the heels toward the buttocks.
6. Continue flexing the knees to a 90° angle; the soles of the feet will finish near the apex of the ball.
7. Keep the knees, hips, and shoulders in a straight line.
8. After completing the leg curl, allow the knees to extend and the ball to roll forward to the starting position.

Common Errors

- Allowing the hips to flex or sag (rather than keeping them in line with the knees and shoulders)

Primary Muscles Trained
Hamstrings, gluteus maximus, erector spinae

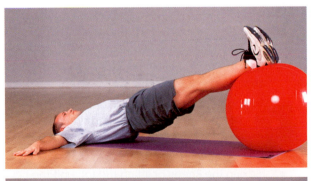

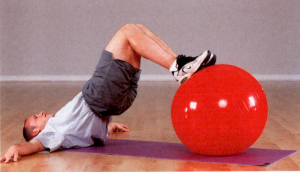

Supine Hip Lift

1. Lie supine on the floor with the legs next to each other and extended away from the body.
2. Abduct the arms 90° away from the torso with the palms facing the floor.
3. Keeping the hips on the floor, position the back of the heels on the apex of the stability ball.
4. Begin the exercise with the feet, knees, and hips in a straight line.
5. Keeping the upper body in the same position, lift (extend) the hips until the feet, knees, hips, and shoulders are in a straight line.
6. After completing the hip lift, allow the hips to lower and return to the starting position.

Common Errors

- Allowing the knees to flex (rather than keeping them in line with the feet and hips)

Primary Muscles Trained
Erector spinae, gluteus maximus, hamstrings

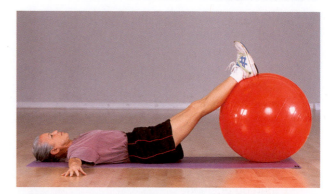

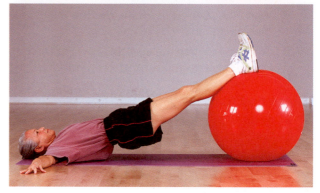

Back Hyperextension

1. Lie prone on the stability ball with the navel positioned on the apex of the ball.
2. Place the feet (toes) on the floor at least 12 inches (30 cm) apart with the knees fully extended.
3. Clasp the hands behind the head.
4. Keeping the toes in contact with the floor, elevate the torso until it is fully extended (arched) and the chest is off the ball.
5. After completing the extension, allow the torso to lower and return to the starting position.

Common Errors

- Flexing the knees or lifting the toes off the floor
- Allowing the navel to move off the apex of the ball as the torso extends

Primary Muscles Trained
Erector spinae

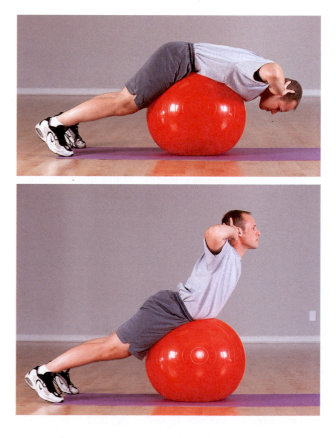

Reverse Back Hyperextension

1. Lie prone on the stability ball with the navel positioned on the apex of the ball.
2. Place the hands (palms) on the floor at least 12 inches (30 cm) apart with the elbows fully extended.
3. Begin the exercise with the knees extended and the toes in contact with the floor.
4. Keeping the hands in contact with the floor, elevate legs with the knees held in extension until the hips are fully extended.
5. After completing the reverse extension, allow the legs to lower and return to the starting position.

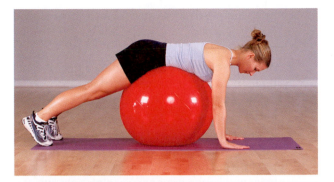

Common Errors

- Flexing the knees or lifting the hands off the floor
- Allowing the navel to move off the apex of the ball as the legs are raised

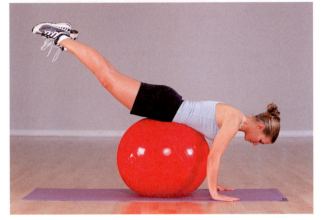

Primary Muscles Trained
Gluteus maximus, erector spinae, hamstrings

Elbow Bridge

1. Kneel next to the stability ball and place the elbows and the back of the upper forearms on the ball.
2. While keeping the elbows/forearms on the ball, roll the ball forward or reposition the kneeling location to create about a 90° angle at the elbows, shoulders, and knees.
3. Keeping the knees and toes on the floor and the elbows on the ball, begin the exercise by extending the knees to roll the ball forward until the elbows, shoulders, hips, and knees are nearly in a straight line and the back of the upper arms are on the ball.
4. After completing the elbow bridge, flex the knees to roll the ball backward to return to the starting position.

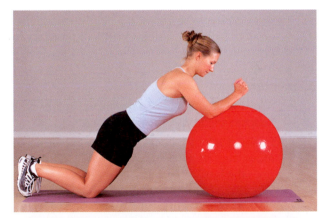

Common Errors

- Arching the back as the knees extend
- Raising the feet off the floor

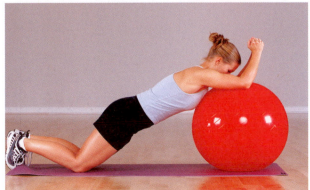

Primary Muscles Trained
Rectus abdominis, internal and external obliques, quadratus lumborum, latissimus dorsi, teres major, erector spinae

Variation: Straight Arm Roll-Out

1. Kneeling next to the stability ball, fully extend the elbows and place the hands on the stability ball.
2. While keeping the hands on the ball, roll the ball forward or reposition the kneeling location to create about a 90° angle at the shoulders and knees.
3. Keeping the knees and toes on the floor, begin the exercise by extending the knees to roll the ball forward until the hands, elbows, shoulders, hips, and knees are nearly in a straight line and the arms are across the ball.
4. After completing the roll-out, flex the knees to roll the ball backward to return to the starting position.

Primary Muscles Trained
Rectus abdominis, internal and external obliques, quadratus lumborum, latissimus dorsi, teres major, erector spinae

Common Errors

- Arching the back as the knees extend
- Raising the feet off the floor

Stability Ball Push-Up

1. Assume a push-up position (see p. 277) with the shins and the instep of the feet on the stability ball and the elbows fully extended.
2. Position the feet, knees, hips, and shoulders in a straight line.
3. Allow the elbows to flex to lower the face to a position 1 to 2 inches (2.5-5 cm) from the floor while keeping the body in a straight line.
4. After reaching the lowest position, push with the arms to extend the elbows back to the starting position.

Common Errors

- Allowing the hips to sag or rise up (rather than keeping the body in a straight line)
- Pushing slightly backward with the arms to move the body backward or roll the knees onto the ball

Primary Muscles Trained
Pectoralis major, anterior deltoid, triceps brachii

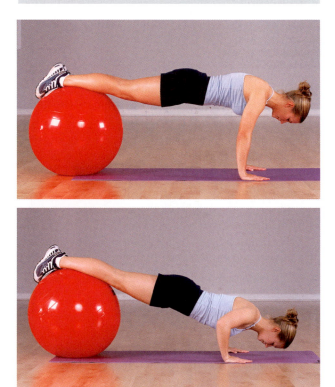

Pike Roll Out and In

1. Assume a push-up position (see p. 277) with the instep of the feet on the stability ball and the elbows fully extended.
2. Position the feet, knees, hips, and shoulders in a straight line.
3. Keeping the knees and elbows fully extended, begin the exercise by flexing the hips to roll the ball forward until the toes are on top of the ball and the hips are directly over the shoulders.
4. After reaching the pike position, allow the hips to extend back to the starting position.

Common Errors

- Arching the back in the push-up position
- Hyperextending the neck in the pike position

Primary Muscles Trained
Rectus abdominis, internal and external obliques, quadratus lumborum, hip flexors

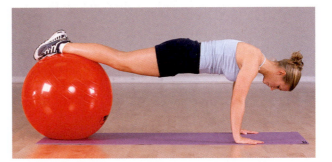

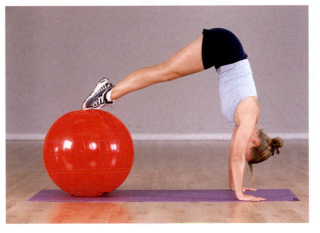

Variation: Knee to Chest (Jack knife)

1. Assume a push-up position (see p. 277) with the instep of the feet on the stability ball and the elbows fully extended.
2. Position the feet, knees, hips, and shoulders in a straight line.
3. Keeping the elbows fully extended, begin the exercise by raising the hips slightly and flexing the hips and knees to roll the ball forward until the hips and knees are fully flexed and the knees are near the torso.
4. After reaching the knee-to-chest position, allow the hips and knees to extend back to the starting position.

Primary Muscles Trained
Rectus abdominis, internal and external obliques, quadratus lumborum, hip flexors

Common Errors

- Arching the back in the push-up position
- Allowing the elbows to flex in the knee-to-chest position

Study Questions

1. All of the following are appropriate activities to use as a warm-up EXCEPT

    A. stationary cycling.

    B. jumping rope.

    C. dynamic flexibility.

    D. jogging.

2. Which of the following pre-exercise activities has the HIGHEST transference to athletic performance?

    A. PNF stretching

    B. specific warm-up

    C. static stretching

    D. general warm-up

3. Incorporating stability ball training into the strength and conditioning programs of athletes has resulted in which of the following findings?

    I. improved transference to athletic performance

    II. negligible transference to athletic performance

    III. enhanced core stability

    IV. reduced core stability

    A. I and III only

    B. II and III only

    C. II and IV only

    D. I and IV only

4. All of the following have been shown to be an advantage of stability ball training EXCEPT

    A. reduced injury risk.

    B. increased heart rate response.

    C. enhanced maximal strength.

    D. improved performance on unstable surfaces.

Applied Knowledge Question

The personal trainer evaluates the fitness level of a 46-year-old female who participates in a competitive tennis league and determines that the client needs to increase the flexibility and muscular strength of the hip extensors to improve performance levels.

a. What static flexibility exercises focus on the hip extensors?

b. What dynamic flexibility exercises involve the hip extensors?

c. What body-weight exercises strengthen the hip extensors?

d. What stability ball exercises actively (concentrically not isometrically) train the hip extensors?

References

1. Anderson, B. and E. Burke. 1991. Scientific, medical, and practical aspects of stretching. *Clinics in Sports Medicine,* 10 (1):63-86.

2. Anderson, K.G., and D.G. Behm. 2004. Maintenance of EMG activity and loss of force output with instability. *Journal of Strength and Conditioning Research* 18 (3): 637-640.

3. Bandy, W.D., J.M. Irion, and M. Briggler. 1998. The effect of static and dynamic range of motion training on the flexibility of the hamstring muscles. *Journal of Sports Physical Therapy* 27 (4): 295-300.

4. Baechle, T.R., and R.W. Earle, eds. 2000. *Essentials of Strength Training and Conditioning,* 2nd ed. Champaign, IL: Human Kinetics.

5. Barnes, D. 2002. What type of strength training do distance runners need? *Modern Athlete and Coach* 40(2): 35-37.

6. Behm, D.G., A.M. Leonard, W.B. Young, A.C. Bonney, and S.N. MacKinnon. 2005. Trunk muscle electromyographic activity with unstable and unilateral exercises. *Journal of Strength and Conditioning Research* 19 (1): 193-201.

7. Bompa, T.O. 1995. *From Childhood to Champion Athlete.* Toronto: Veritas.

8. Bompa, T.O. 2000. *Total Training for Young Champions.* Champaign, IL: Human Kinetics.

9. Bourne, G. 1995. The basic facts about flexibility in a nutshell. *Modern Athlete and Coach* 33 (2): 3-4, 35.

10. Brandon, R. 1998. What science has to say about the performance benefits of flexibility training. *Peak Performance* (September), 6-9.

11. Carter, J.M., W.C. Beam, S.G. McMahan, M.K. Barr, and L.E. Brown. 2006. The effects of stability ball training on spinal stability in sedentary individuals. *Journal of Strength and Conditioning Research* 20 (2): 429-435.

12. Chek, P. 1998. Swiss ball exercise. *Sports Coach* 21 (3): 27-29.

13. Collins, P. 2001. How to make use of Swiss ball training. *Modern Athlete and Coach* 39 (4): 34-36.

14. Cornelius, W.J., and M.M. Hinson. 1980. The relationship between isometric contractions of hip extensions and sub-

sequent flexibility in males. *Sports Medicine and Physical Fitness* 20: 75-80.

15. Cornwell, A., A.G. Nelson, and B. Sideaway. 2002. Acute effects of stretching on the neuromuscular properties of the triceps surae muscle complex. *European Journal of Applied Physiology* 86 (5): 428-434.

16. Cosio-Lima, L.M., K.L. Reynolds, C. Winter, V. Paolone, and M.T. Jones. 2003. Effects of physical ball and conventional floor exercises. *Journal of Strength and Conditioning Research* 17: 475-483.

17. Franklin, A.J., C.F. Finch, and C.A. Sherman. 2001. Warm-up practices of golfers: Are they adequate? *British Journal of Sports Medicine* 35 (2): 125-127.

18. Funk, D., A.M. Swank, K.J. Adams, and D. Treolo. 2001. Efficacy of moist heat pack application over static stretching on hamstring flexibility. *Journal of Strength and Conditioning Research* 15 (1): 123-126.

19. Gambetta, V. 1997. Stretching the truth; the fallacies of flexibility. *Sports Coach* 20 (3): 7-9.

20. Gesztesi, B. 1999. Stretching during exercise. *Strength and Conditioning Journal* 21 (6): 44.

21. Hamlyn, N., D.G. Behm, and W.B. Young. 2007. Trunk muscle activation during dynamic weight-training exercises and isometric instability activities. *Journal of Strength and Conditioning Research* 21 (4): 1108-1112.

22. Hardy, L., and D. Jones. 1986. Dynamic flexibility and proprioceptive neuromuscular facilitation. *Research Quarterly for Exercise and Sport* 57 (2): 150-153.

23. Hedrick, A. 1992. Physiological responses to warm-up. *National Strength and Conditioning Association Journal* 14 (5): 25-27.

24. Hedrick, A. 1993. Flexibility and the conditioning program. *National Strength and Conditioning Association Journal* 15 (4): 62-66.

25. Hedrick, A. 2000. Dynamic flexibility training. *Strength and Conditioning Journal* 22 (5): 33-38.

26. Hedrick, A. 2000. Volleyball coaches guide to warm-up and flexibility training. *Performance Conditioning Volleyball* 8 (3): 1-4.

27. Hedrick, A. 2003. Using uncommon implements in the training programs of athletes. *Strength and Conditioning Journal* 25 (4): 18-22.

28. Holt, L.E., T.M. Travis, and T. Okia. 1970. Comparative study of three stretching techniques. *Perceptual and Motor Skills* 31: 611-616.

29. Jakubek, M.D. 2007. Stability balls: Reviewing the literature regarding their use and effectiveness. *Strength and Conditioning Journal* 29 (5): 58-63.

30. Karp, J.R. 2000. Flexibility for fitness. *Fitness Management* (April), 52-54.

31. Kato, Y., T. Ikata, H. Takia, S. Takata, K. Sairyo, and K. Iwanaga. 2000. Effects of specific warm-ups at various intensities on energy metabolism during subsequent exercise. Journal of Sports Medicine and Physical Fitness 40 (2): 126-130.

32. Kokkonen, J., A.G. Nelson, and A. Cornwell. 1998. Acute muscle stretching inhibits maximal strength performance. *Research Quarterly for Exercise and Sport* 69 (4): 411-415.

33. Koshida, S., Y. Urabe, K. Miyashita, K. Iwai, and A. Kagimori. 2008. Muscular outputs during dynamic bench press under stable versus unstable conditions. *Journal of Strength and Conditioning Research* 22 (5): 1584-1588.

34. Marshall, P.W.M., and B.A. Murphy. 2005. Core stability on and off a Swiss ball. *Archives of Physical Medicine and Rehabilitation* 86: 242-249.

35. Marshall, P.W.M., and B.A. Murphy. 2006. Increased deltoid and abdominal muscle activity during Swiss ball bench press. *Journal of Strength and Conditioning Research* 20 (4): 745-750.

36. McBride, J. 1995. Dynamic warm-up and flexibility: A key to basketball success. *Coaching Women's Basketball* (Summer): 15-17.

37. Ninos, J. 1999. When could stretching be harmful? *Strength and Conditioning Journal* 21 (5): 57-58.

38. Nuzzo, J.L., G.O. McCaulley, P. Cormie, M.J. Cavill, and J.M. McBride. 2008. Trunk muscle activity during stability ball and free weight exercises. *Journal of Strength and Conditioning Research* 22 (1): 95-102.

39. O'Brien, B., W. Payne, P. Gastin, and C. Burge. 1997. A comparison of active and passive warm-ups in energy system contribution and performance in moderate heat. *Australian Journal of Science and Medicine in Sport* 29 (4): 106-109.

40. Poe, C.M. 1995. Principles of off-ice strength, power, and flexibility training for figure skaters. *Skating* 72 (9): 22-30.

41. Purton, J., B. Humphries, and G. Warman. 2001. Comparison of peak muscular activation between Ab-roller and exercise ball. Honors thesis, Central Queensland University, Rockhampton, Queensland.

42. Ross, M. 1999. Stretching the hip flexors. *Strength and Conditioning Journal* 21 (3): 71-72.

43. Sady, S.P., M. Wortman, and D. Blanke. 1982. Flexibility training: Ballistic, static, or proprioceptive neuromuscular facilitation? *Archives of Physical Medicine and Rehabilitation* 63: 261-263.

44. Sato, K., and M. Mokha. 2008. Does core strength training influence running kinetics, lower extremity stability, and 5000-m performance in runners? *Journal of Strength and Conditioning Research* 23 (1): 133-140.

45. Schibek, J.S., K.M. Guskiewicz, W.E. Prentice, S. Mays, and J.M. Davis. 2001. The effect of core stabilization training on functional performance in swimming. Master's thesis, University of North Carolina, Chapel Hill.

46. Shellock, F.G., and W.E. Prentice. 1985. Warming-up and stretching for improved physical performance and prevention of sports-related injuries. *Sports Medicine* 2 (4): 267-278.

47. Sobel, T., T.S. Ellenbecker, and E.P. Roetert. 1995. Flexibility training for tennis. *Strength and Conditioning Journal* 17 (6): 43-51.

48. Stanton, R., P.R. Reaburn, and B. Humphries. 2004. The effect of short-term Swiss ball training on core stability and running economy. *Journal of Strength and Conditioning Research* 18 (3): 522-528.

49. Sternlight, E., S. Rugg, L.L. Fujii, K.G. Tomomitsu, and M.M. Seki. 2007. Electromyographic comparison of a stability ball crunch with a traditional crunch. *Journal of Strength and Conditioning Research* 21 (2): 506-509.

50. Stricker, T., T. Malone, and W.E. Garrett. 1990. The effects of passive warming on muscle injury. *American Journal of Sports Medicine* 18 (2): 141-145.

51. Tancred, T., and B. Tancred. 1995. An examination of the benefits of warm-up: A review. *New Studies in Athletics* 10 (4): 35-41.

52. Tanigawa, M.C. 1972. Comparison of the hold relax procedure and passive mobilization on increasing muscle length. *Physical Therapy* 52: 725-735.

53. Thomas, M. 2000. The functional warm-up. *Strength and Conditioning Journal* 22 (2): 51-53.

54. Vera-Garcia, F.J., S.G. Grenier, and S. McGill. 2000. Abdominal muscle response during curl-ups on both stable and unstable surfaces. *Physical Therapy* 80: 564-569.

55. Wahl, J.M., and D.G. Behm. 2008. Not all instability training devices enhance muscle activation in highly resistance-trained individuals. *Journal of Strength and Conditioning Research* 22 (4): 1360-1370.

56. Willardson, J. 2007. Core stability training: Applications to sports conditioning programs. *Journal of Strength and Conditioning Research* 21 (3): 979-985.

57. Wirth, V.J., B.L. Van Luten, D. Mistry, E. Saliba, and F.C. McCue. 1998. Temperature changes in deep muscles during upper and lower extremity exercise. *Journal of Athletic Training* 33 (3): 211-215.

Resistance Training Exercise Techniques

John F. Graham, MS

> **After completing this chapter, you will be able to**
>
> - comprehend the fundamental techniques for performing and instructing proper form for resistance training exercises,
>
> - describe proper spotting techniques as well as situations in which they are needed,
>
> - define appropriate training equipment and apparel, and
>
> - recognize common resistance exercise technique errors.

One of the personal trainer's most important responsibilities to clients is to instruct and manage their exercise technique to ensure maximum benefit from resistance training in the safest possible environment. This chapter explains the benefits and physiological aspects of resistance training, safety, and resistance training technique. The chapter concludes with a detailed description of resistance training exercise techniques and spotting techniques.

Fundamental Exercise Technique Guidelines

Several basic guidelines apply to performing nearly all resistance (weight) training exercises. The client

The author would like to acknowledge the contributions of Thomas R. Baechle and Roger W. Earle to this chapter. Much of the content is directly attributed to their work in the first edition of *NSCA's Essentials of Personal Training.*

has to grasp some type of barbell, dumbbell, or handle; place his or her body in an optimal position; and follow a recommended movement and breathing pattern to promote safe and effective exercise technique.

Handgrip Types and Widths

The most frequently used handgrip positions in resistance training exercises are the **pronated grip,** with the palms down and the knuckles up (also called the **overhand grip**), and the **supinated grip**, with the palms up and the knuckles down (also called the **underhand grip**) (figure 13.1, *a* and *b*). Examples of exercises that use these handgrips are the shoulder press, which uses a pronated grip, and the wrist curl, which uses a supinated grip. Some exercises, such as the dumbbell hammer curl and a version of the machine seated shoulder press, use a **neutral grip.** With this grip, the palms face in and the knuckles point out to the side, as in a handshake.

A grip that is often recommended for spotting the barbell (e.g., for the free weight bench press exercise) is the **alternated grip,** in which one hand is pronated and the other is supinated (figure 13.1*c*). In the pronated, supinated, and alternated grips, the thumb is wrapped around the barbell so that the barbell is fully held by the hand. This thumb position creates a **closed grip.** When the thumb does not wrap around the barbell but instead is placed next to the index finger, the position is called an **open** or **false grip** (figure 13.1*d*). When a client is preparing to perform a free weight resistance training exercise using a barbell, it is also important for the personal trainer to instruct the client to place the hands a certain distance from each other. This placement is called the **grip width.** The four standard grip widths, shown in figure 13.2, are close, hip-width, shoulder-width, and wide. For most exercises, the hands are placed shoulder-width apart on the barbell. A client's body dimensions influence the decisions regarding

actual hand placement, however. For all of the grip widths, the hand position should result in an evenly balanced barbell.

Starting Position

For all resistance training exercises, it is critical that the personal trainer instruct the client to "assume" or get into a correct initial body position. Demonstration of a new exercise given to a client should begin with how to establish a starting position. From this position, the client is able to maintain correct body alignment throughout the exercise, thereby placing the stress only on the targeted muscles. Standing exercises (e.g., back squat, barbell bent-over row, barbell upright row) typically require the client's feet to be at or between hip-width or shoulder-width apart with the feet flat on the floor. Establishing a secure position in or on a machine typically requires the personal trainer to change the seat height, the position of all adjustable body and limb pads, or both the seat height and pad positions, to align the joint(s) involved in the exercise with the axis of the machine. For example, preparing a client to perform the leg (knee) extension exercise requires the personal trainer to adjust the position of the back pad forward or backward, the cam on the range limiter, and the ankle pad up or down to place the client's knee joints in line with the machine axis.

> Every demonstration of a new exercise given to a client should begin with establishing a stable starting position.

Five-Point Body Contact Position

Some free weight and machine exercises are performed while the client is seated (e.g., leg press, shoulder press) or lying down on the back facing up (**supine;** e.g., dumbbell bench press, supine triceps extension, dumbbell fly). The exercises performed on a chair-like seat or a torso-length bench require the personal trainer to instruct the client to position his or her body in a **five-point body contact position** so that these body parts or segments contact the seat or bench and the floor or foot platform:

- Back of the head
- Upper back and rear shoulders
- Lower back and buttocks
- Right foot
- Left foot

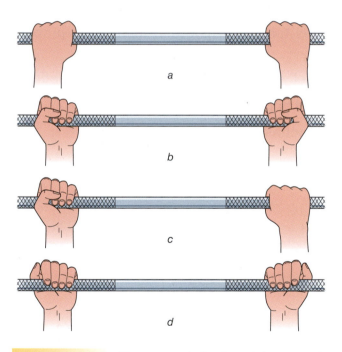

FIGURE 13.1 Recommended grips: (*a*) pronated, closed; (*b*) supinated, closed; (*c*) alternated, closed; (*d*) supinated, open.

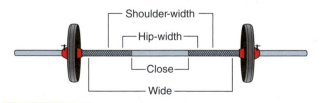

FIGURE 13.2 Choices for grip widths: close, hip-width, shoulder-width, wide.

For **prone** exercises, the client lies facedown (e.g., leg [knee] curl, back hyperextension); and most of the front surface of the client's body is in contact with the floor or machine pads and handles. For example, the proper position for the leg (knee) curl exercise involves these five contact points:

- Chin (or one cheek if the head is turned to the side)
- Chest and stomach
- Hips and front of the thighs
- Right hand
- Left hand

Breathing Considerations

The best general recommendation personal trainers can give to their clients about when and how to breathe during a resistance exercise is to exhale through the **sticking point** (the most difficult part of the exercise) during the concentric or exertion phase and inhale during the easier part of the exercise (the eccentric phase). Typically, the sticking point occurs soon after the transition from the eccentric to the concentric phase. For example, since the sticking point of the barbell incline press exercise is reached when the barbell is about halfway up, the client should exhale through this portion of the movement. As the barbell is lowered back down to the starting position, the client should inhale. This breathing strategy applies to nearly all resistance training exercises. A personal trainer can tell a client to "breathe out during the hardest part of the exercise and breathe in during the easier part of the exercise."

Valsalva Maneuver

Some exercises might require a variation to the typical breathing method for optimal performance. For these particular exercises it may be helpful for the personal trainer to explain to certain clients a different breathing pattern. For example, clients who are resistance trained and will perform **structural exercises** (those that load the vertebral column; e.g., back squat, push press) or exercises that stress the lower back (e.g., bent-over row, deadlift, shoulder press) may benefit from temporarily holding their breath during the exercise.

This course of action produces what is referred to as the **Valsalva maneuver.** In this breathing practice, the glottis (the narrowest part of the larynx) is closed to keep air from escaping the lungs while the muscles of the abdomen and rib cage contract. This results in the person's trying to exhale against a closed "throat." The outcome is that the diaphragm

and the deep muscles of the torso contract and generate intra-abdominal pressure against the **fluid ball,** which aids in supporting the vertebral column internally, from the inside out, and significantly reduces the effort required of other muscles (e.g., the low back muscles during the back squat exercise) to perform the exercise (5). Thus, the client is better able to maintain correct posture and body alignment. The following are two breathing options, with sample verbal directions, that a personal trainer can give to advanced clients who are performing exercises that involve the Valsalva maneuver.

- *Option 1:* Inhale during the eccentric phase until just before starting the concentric phase; hold the breath through the sticking point; then exhale. Verbal directions: "Take a breath in during the easiest part of the exercise; hold your breath until the hardest part of the exercise is completed, and then exhale."
- *Option 2:* Inhale prior to beginning a **repetition;** hold the breath through the sticking point of the concentric phase; then exhale. Verbal directions: "Take a breath in before starting a repetition; hold your breath until the hardest part of the exercise is completed, and then exhale."

For an example of option 1, advanced clients attempting to lift heavy loads for the back squat exercise can take a breath in as they descend to the bottom or low position, perform the Valsalva maneuver and continue to hold the breath until right after the sticking point of the upward movement, and then exhale through the rest of the concentric phase back up to the starting or standing body position.

Despite its advantages, the Valsalva maneuver causes an increase in the pressure in the chest that can have the undesirable side effect of exerting compressive forces on the heart, making venous return more difficult. Also, the Valsalva maneuver can momentarily raise blood pressure to high levels that may cause dizziness, rapid-onset fatigue, blood vessel rupture, disorientation, and blackouts. Therefore, a personal trainer should not permit clients with any known or suspected cardiovascular, metabolic, or respiratory condition to hold their breath during resistance exercise. Personal trainers who conduct maximum or near-maximum muscular strength tests need to be aware of the advantages and disadvantages of encouraging or allowing their clients to use the Valsalva maneuver. While it is important that the vertebral column be internally supported during these testing situations for safety and technique reasons, it is recommended that a client not overextend the time that the breath is held.

Even resistance-trained and technique-experienced clients should be advised to hold their breath only momentarily (e.g., 1 to 2 seconds).

> A personal trainer should not permit clients with any known or suspected cardiovascular, metabolic, or respiratory condition to breath-hold during resistance exercise.

Weightlifting Belt Recommendations

Weight belts have been shown to increase intra-abdominal pressure during performance of a resistance training exercise (19, 21, 22). Therefore, the use of a weight belt can contribute to injury-free training by decreasing the compressive forces on the vertebral column. Despite this benefit, if a client uses a weight belt for all resistance training exercises, the muscles of the lower back and abdomen may become unaccustomed to supporting the torso (19). Then, if the client performs an exercise without a weight belt, the weaker torso muscles may not be capable of generating enough intra-abdominal pressure to decrease the chance of injury. When determining whether or not a client should wear a weight belt during a resistance training exercise, the personal trainer should base the decision on the following guidelines:

- A weight belt is recommended for ground-based, structural exercises that load the trunk and place stress on the lower back (e.g., back and front squat, standing shoulder press, deadlift) *and* involve lifting maximal or near-maximal loads. (Both conditions should exist; it is not necessary, for example, for the client to wear a weight belt when lifting lighter loads even when performing a structural exercise.)
- A weight belt is not needed for an exercise that does not directly load the trunk even if it places stress on the lower back (e.g., lat pulldown, bench press, biceps curl, leg extension).

> A weight belt is recommended for ground-based, structural exercises that involve lifting maximal or near-maximal loads.

Spotting Resistance Training Exercises

When a client is performing a resistance training exercise, the personal trainer's primary responsibil-ity is the client's safety. In addition to teaching and reinforcing proper exercise technique, the personal trainer may also serve as a spotter by physically assisting clients in completing the exercise to help protect them from injury. This need for a spotter is typically associated with free weight exercises. Bars, dumbbells, and weight plates that are not restricted to a fixed movement path increase the possibility that a client will lose control and become injured. A spot can be given for a machine exercise, but it is not as necessary because clients are not exposed to the possibility that a bar, dumbbell, or weight plate could fall on them. This advantage does not imply that machine exercises do not require supervision or assistance, however (e.g., a client may need help with maintaining proper speed and range of motion).

A personal trainer may assist a client with **forced repetitions** (repetitions that are successfully performed with help from another person), but this type of assistance should not be confused with or substituted for spotting for safety.

Four free weight exercise conditions require a spotter. These include exercises that are performed

- overhead (e.g., standing shoulder press),
- over the face (e.g., bench press, lying triceps extension),
- with a bar on the upper back and shoulders (e.g., back squat), or
- with a bar positioned on the front of the shoulders or clavicles (e.g., front squat).

Spotting Overhead or Over-the-Face Exercises

Many overhead and over-the-face resistance training exercises place the client in a sitting or standing position (e.g., shoulder press, overhead dumbbell triceps extension) or a supine position (e.g., bench press, dumbbell chest fly, lying triceps extension, dumbbell pullover). Because of the location of the barbell or dumbbell above the client's head or face, the potential for serious injury is greater during the performance of these exercises compared to most others. Also, to be effective at providing enough assistance to spot an overhead exercise, the personal trainer must be at least as tall as the client. If this is not the case, then the personal trainer should modify the exercise so that the client is in a seated position. Some types of bench press and shoulder press benches have a small platform that places the spotter in a better position for spotting overhead or over-the-face exercises.

Barbell Exercises

When spotting over-the-face barbell exercises, the personal trainer should grasp the bar between the client's hands using an alternated grip. This helps to keep the bar from rolling out of the personal trainer's hands and onto the client's head, face, or neck. Also the personal trainer should take a position as close to the client as possible—without creating a distraction—in order to be able to grab the bar quickly if necessary. Finally, to create a stable base of support, the personal trainer, if possible, should be in a flat-back rather than rounded-back position, with the feet flat on the floor in a staggered stance. With some bench frames there may not be enough room for the staggered stance, however.

Dumbbell Exercises

It is common to see people receiving spotting assistance at their upper arms or elbows while performing an overhead or over-the-face dumbbell exercise. This spotting technique may lead to injury if the individual's elbows quickly collapse while the spotter is lifting the upper arms or elbows. If that happens, the spotter probably will not be able to prevent the dumbbells from landing on the client's head, face, neck, or chest. The personal trainer should instead spot the client's wrists (figure 13.3) very near to the dumbbell. For exercises that require the client to use two hands to hold one dumbbell (e.g., dumbbell pullover) or only one hand at a time to perform an exercise (e.g., overhead dumbbell triceps extension), the personal trainer should spot the lowest half of the dumbbell itself, that is, the end closest to the floor.

> When a client is performing an overhead or over-the-face dumbbell exercise, the personal trainer should spot the client's wrists close to the dumbbell, not the upper arms or elbows.

Spotting Exercises With the Bar on the Back or Front Shoulders

Exercises that involve placing the bar across the shoulders at the base of the neck or the upper back (e.g., back squat, lunge, step-up) or on the front of the shoulders and across the clavicles (e.g., front squat) should also be spotted. As with the overhead or over-the-face exercises, in order to be an effective spotter the personal trainer needs to be strong enough to handle the load lifted and needs to be at least as tall as the client. There are a variety of methods that can be used to spot these types of exercises. For example, the spotter can stand behind and very close to the client (without impeding the execution of the exercise) and be prepared to "hug and lift" the client if he or she is not able to complete the set. To further guard against injury or accident, these types of exercises should be performed, if possible,

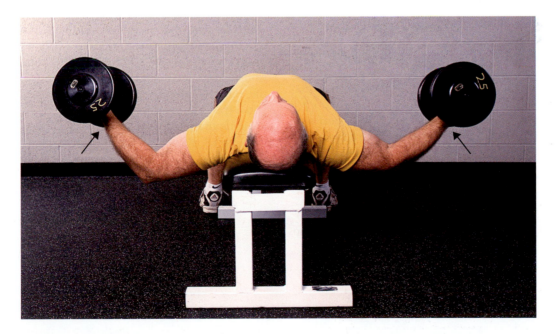

FIGURE 13.3 The arrows point to where the personal trainer should grasp the client's wrists when spotting a dumbbell exercise.

inside a squat rack with the crossbars placed just below the lowest position the bar will reach during the downward movement phase.

Spotting Power Exercises

As a rule, "explosive" or simply "power" exercises (e.g., power clean, hang clean, push jerk, high pull, snatch) should not be spotted. Fast-moving bars are difficult for a personal trainer to spot and catch; trying to do so may result in injury to one or both parties. Because of this dynamic situation, power exercises should be performed in a segregated area or on a lifting platform in case the client "misses" (fails to complete a repetition) or loses control of the bar. Instead of physically spotting the bar during a missed lift, the personal trainer should teach the client to push the bar away or simply drop it. Clients should be instructed that if the bar begins to fall behind their head, they should simultaneously let go of the bar and step or jump forward. It is also important to remove any equipment from the area in and around the space where power exercises are performed.

> Power exercises should be performed in a segregated area or on a lifting platform without the use of a spotter.

Number of Spotters

Once a personal trainer decides that a client requires a spot for an exercise, the next step is to determine how many spotters are necessary. If the load is beyond the personal trainer's ability to handle effectively, an additional spotter must be used. For example, it is common to use one spotter at each end of the bar during the front or back squat exercise. This technique requires spotters who are experienced, because the spotters have to perfectly synchronize when and how much they assist the client to keep the bar even and balanced. When excessively heavy loads are involved, three spotters may be appropriate.

Communication

Communication is the responsibility of both the client and the personal trainer. A client should be instructed to tell the personal trainer when he is ready to move the bar, dumbbells, or machine handles into the starting position (called a **liftoff**). If the client needs help during the **set**, he should quickly ask or signal the personal trainer; and after the last repetition the personal trainer should help the client move the bar back onto the supports (called *racking the bar*). Poor communication may cause the personal trainer to spot the client too soon, too late, or improperly. Therefore, the personal trainer should discuss all of these issues with the client before the beginning of a set.

Conclusion

Personal trainers are responsible for teaching clients proper resistance training exercise technique to maximize the training effect of the exercises and create the safest training environment. This includes not only instructions on how to perform an exercise, but also proper breathing guidelines and weight belt recommendations. The personal trainer must also know when and how to spot a client during a resistance training exercise and how to recognize and correct mistakes in a client's exercise technique. A personal trainer should be familiar with all of the exercises described in this chapter and should realize that there has been no attempt to explain or provide photos of all possible technique and spotting variations. The checklists on the following pages offer the most commonly accepted guidelines for resistance training exercise technique (7, 8, 24). Readers are encouraged to see references 1 through 4, 6, 9 through 18, 20, and 23 for supplementary guidelines.

Resistance Training Exercises

Abdominal Exercises

Bent Knee Sit-Up

Starting Position

Assume a supine position on a floor mat.

Flex the knees to bring the heels near the buttocks.

Fold the arms across the chest or abdomen.

Upward Movement Phase

Flex the neck to move the chin to the chest.

Keeping the feet, buttocks, and lower back flat and stationary on the mat, curl the torso toward the thighs until the upper back is off the mat.

Keep the arms folded across the chest or abdomen.

Downward Movement Phase

Allow the torso, then the neck, to uncurl and extend back to the starting position.

Keep the feet, buttocks, lower back, and arms in the same position.

Common Errors

- Raising the feet off the mat during the upward movement phase
- Raising the hips off the mat during the downward movement phase

Primary Muscle Trained
Rectus abdominis

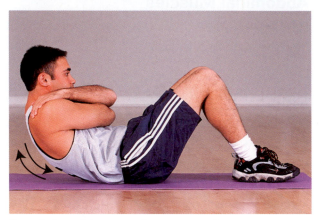

Completion of the upward movement phase.

Machine Abdominal Crunch

Starting Position

Sit in the machine with the upper chest pressed against the chest pad; if there are handles instead, grasp them with a closed, pronated or neutral grip.

Forward Movement Phase

Flex the neck to move the chin to the chest.

Keeping the feet, legs, and buttocks stationary, curl the torso toward the thighs.

Keep the upper chest pressed against the pad (or keep a grip on the handles).

Backward Movement Phase

Allow the torso, then the neck, to uncurl and extend back to the starting position.

Keep the feet, legs, buttocks, and arms in the same position.

Keep the upper chest pressed against the pad (or keep a grip on the handles).

Common Errors

- Raising the hips off the seat during the forward movement phase
- Pulling with the legs or hands to help curl the torso forward

Primary Muscle Trained
Rectus abdominis

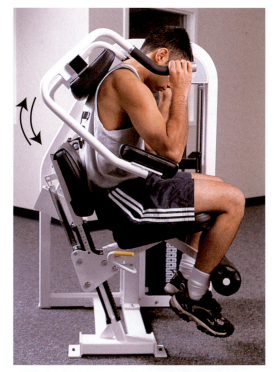

Completion of the forward movement phase.

Back

Bent-Over Row

Starting Position

Grasp the bar with a closed, pronated grip wider than shoulder-width.

Lift the bar from the floor to a position at the front of the thighs using the first pull phase of the power clean exercise.

Adjust the feet to assume a shoulder-width stance with the knees slightly to moderately flexed.

Flex the torso forward so that it is slightly above parallel to the floor.

Assume a flat-back torso position with the shoulders back and the chest out.

Focus the eyes a short distance ahead of the feet.

Allow the bar to hang with the elbows fully extended.

Adjust the position of the knees, hips, and torso to suspend the weight plates off the floor.

Upward Movement Phase

Pull the bar up toward the lower chest or upper abdomen.

Keep the elbows pointed away from the sides of the body with the wrists straight.

Keep the torso rigid, back flat, and knees in the same flexed position.

Touch the bar to the sternum or upper abdomen. At the highest bar position, the elbows should be higher than the torso.

Downward Movement Phase

Allow the elbows to slowly extend back to the starting position.

Keep the torso rigid, back flat, and knees in the same flexed position.

After the set is completed, squat down to return the bar to the floor.

Common Errors

- Jerking the upper body, shrugging the shoulders, extending the torso, extending the knees, curling the bar in the hands, or rising up on the toes to help raise the bar
- Allowing the upper back to round (losing the flat-back position) during the movement

Primary Muscles Trained
Latissimus dorsi, teres major, rhomboid, posterior deltoid

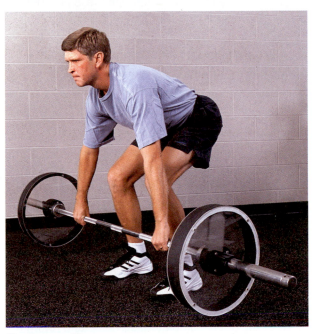

Starting position.

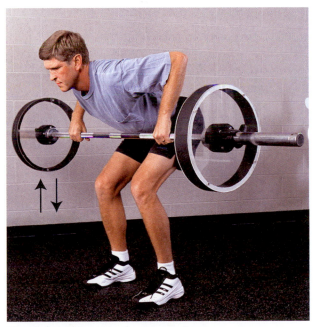

Upward and downward movements.

Lat Pulldown

Starting Position

Grasp the bar with a closed, pronated grip wider than shoulder-width.

Sit facing the machine stack with the legs under the thigh pads and the feet flat on the floor.

Slightly lean the torso backward to create a path for the bar to pass by the face.

Allow the elbows to fully extend.

In this position, the weight to be lifted will be suspended above the rest of the stack.

Downward Movement Phase

Pull the bar down and toward the upper chest; the elbows should move down and back and the chest up and out as the bar is lowered.

Keep the feet, legs, and torso in the same position.

Touch the bar to the clavicles or upper chest.

Upward Movement Phase

Allow the elbows to slowly extend back to the starting position.

Keep the feet, legs, and torso in the same position.

After the set is completed, stand up and return the weight to its resting position.

Common Errors

- Using an open grip on the bar
- Contracting the abdominal muscles and flexing the torso to assist in the downward movement phase
- Not fully extending the elbows during the upward movement phase
- Pulling the bar down behind the head to the back of the neck.

Primary Muscles Trained
Latissimus dorsi, teres major, rhomboid, posterior deltoid

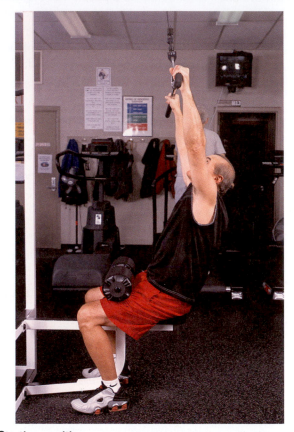

Starting position.

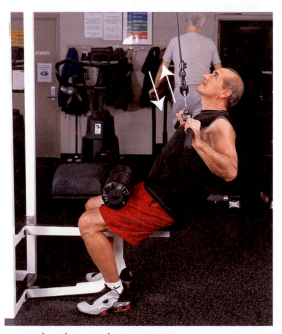

Downward and upward movements.

Low Pulley Seated Row

Starting Position

Facing the machine, sit on the floor (or on the long seat pad, if available).

Place the feet on the machine frame or foot supports.

Flex the knees and hips to reach forward and grasp the handle with a closed, neutral grip.

Pull the handle back and assume an erect seated position with the torso perpendicular to the floor, knees slightly flexed, and the feet and legs parallel to each other.

Allow the elbows to fully extend with the arms about parallel to the floor.

In this position, the weight to be lifted will be suspended above the rest of the stack.

Backward Movement Phase

Pull the handle toward the chest or upper abdomen.

Maintain an erect torso position with the knees in the same slightly flexed position.

Touch the handle to the sternum or abdomen.

Forward Movement Phase

Allow the elbows to slowly extend back to the starting position.

Maintain an erect torso position with the knees in the same slightly flexed position.

After the set is completed, flex the knees and hips to reach forward and return the weight to its resting position.

Common Errors

- Jerking the upper body or leaning back during the backward movement phase
- Curling the handle toward the torso during the backward movement phase
- Flexing the torso forward during the forward movement phase

Primary Muscles Trained
Latissimus dorsi, teres major, rhomboid, posterior deltoid

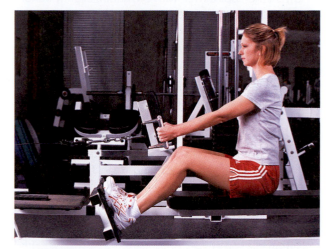

Starting position.

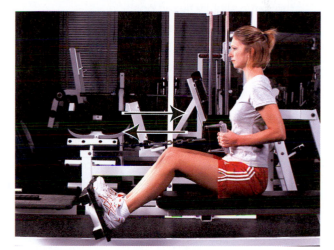

Backward and forward movements.

Seated Row (Resistance Band)

Starting Position

Grasp the handles of the resistance band with a closed, neutral grip.

Sit on the floor or mat with the knees slightly flexed, and evenly wrap the resistance band around the insteps of the feet.

Assume an erect position with the torso perpendicular to the floor.

Hold on to the handles with the elbows fully extended, the arms about parallel to the floor, and the palms facing each other.

In this position, the resistance band should be nearly taut (not stretched); if it is not, take up the slack by wrapping the resistance band further around the feet.

Backward Movement Phase

Pull the handles toward the chest or upper abdomen.

Maintain an erect torso position with the knees in the same slightly flexed position.

Touch the hands to the sides of the torso.

Forward Movement Phase

Allow the elbows to slowly extend back to the starting position.

Maintain an erect torso position with the knees in the same slightly flexed position.

Common Errors

- Jerking the upper body or leaning back during the backward movement phase
- Curling the handles toward the torso during the backward movement phase
- Flexing the torso forward during the forward movement phase

Primary Muscles Trained
Latissimus dorsi, teres major, rhomboid, posterior deltoid

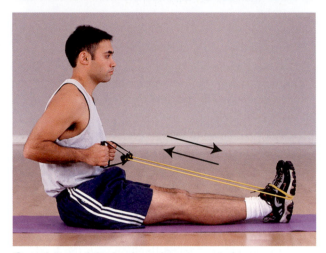

Completion of the backward movement phase.

Machine Back Extension

Starting Position

Sit in the machine with the upper back pressed against the back pad.

Flex the torso forward and move the body back to align the hips with the axis of the machine.

Place the feet on the machine frame or foot supports.

Grasp the handles or the sides of the seat.

Backward Movement Phase

Keeping the thighs and feet stationary, extend the torso (lean backward).

Keep the upper back firmly pressed against the back pad.

Maintain a tight grip on the handles or the sides of the seat.

Forward Movement Phase

Allow the torso to flex (lean forward) back to the starting position.

Keep the upper back firmly pressed against the back pad and the thighs and feet stationary.

Maintain a tight grip on the handles or the sides of the seat.

Common Errors

- Pushing with the legs or rising off the seat during the backward movement phase
- Arching the back at the end of the backward movement phase

Primary Muscle Trained
Erector spinae

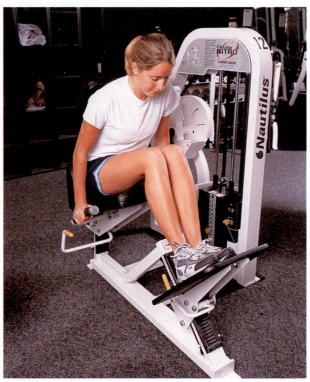

Starting position.

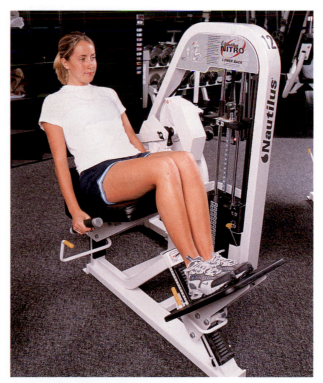

Backward and forward movements.

Arms (Biceps)

Biceps Curl (Bar)

Starting Position

Grasp the bar with a closed, supinated grip at or slightly wider than shoulder-width.

Stand erect with the feet shoulder-width apart and knees slightly flexed.

Position the bar in front of the thighs with the elbows fully extended.

Position the upper arms against the sides of the torso and perpendicular to the floor.

Upward Movement Phase

Flex the elbows to move the bar in an upward arc toward the shoulders.

Keep the torso erect, the upper arms stationary, and the knees in the same slightly flexed position.

Flex the elbows until the bar is within 4 to 6 inches (10-15 cm) of the shoulders.

Downward Movement Phase

Allow the elbows to slowly extend back to the starting position.

Keep the torso, upper arms, and knees in the same position.

Common Errors

■ Jerking the upper body, shrugging the shoulders, extending the torso, extending the knees, swinging the bar, or rising up on the toes to help raise the bar

■ Moving the elbows away from the sides of the torso (backward during the downward movement phase or forward during the upward movement phase)

■ Keeping the elbows partially flexed at the end of the downward movement phase (a shortened range of motion)

■ Bouncing the bar off the thighs to add momentum to help with the next repetition

Primary Muscles Trained
Brachialis, biceps brachii (especially), brachioradialis

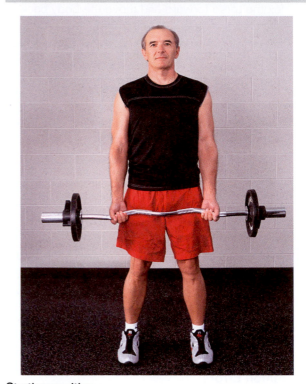

Starting position.

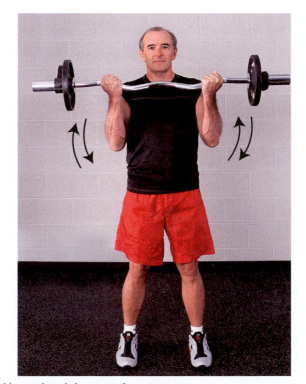

Upward and downward movements.

Biceps Curl (Resistance Band)

Starting Position

Grasp the handles of the resistance band with a closed, supinated grip.

Position the feet shoulder-width apart with the arches of both feet on top of a middle section of the resistance band.

Stand erect with the knees slightly flexed.

Position the handles outside of the thighs with the arms at the sides and the palms facing forward.

In this position, the resistance band should be nearly taut (not stretched); if not, take up the slack by widening the stance or selecting a shorter band.

Upward Movement Phase

Flex the elbows to move the handles in an upward arc toward the shoulders.

Keep the torso erect, the upper arms stationary, and the knees in the same slightly flexed position.

Flex the elbows until the hands are within 4 to 6 inches (10-15 cm) of the shoulders.

Downward Movement Phase

Allow the elbows to slowly extend back to the starting position.

Keep the torso, upper arms, and knees in the same position.

Common Errors

- Shrugging the shoulders to help raise the handles upward
- Moving the elbows away from the sides of the torso (backward during the downward movement phase or forward during the upward movement phase)
- Keeping the elbows partially flexed at the end of the downward movement phase (a shortened range of motion)

Primary Muscles Trained
Brachialis, biceps brachii (especially), brachioradialis

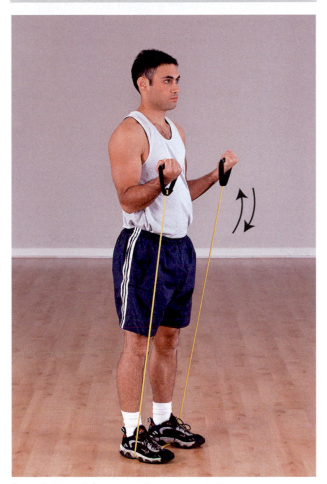

Completion of the upward movement phase.

Machine (Preacher) Biceps Curl

Starting Position

Assume a seated position facing the chest pad of the machine.

Grasp the handles with a closed, supinated grip with the elbows fully extended.

Position the upper arms on the angled upper arm pad(s), and align the elbows with the axis of the machine.

Place the feet on the machine frame, foot supports, or floor.

Sit erect and press the torso against the chest pad. If necessary, adjust the pad to position the torso perpendicular to the floor.

Upward Movement Phase

Keeping the torso, thighs, and feet stationary, flex the elbows to move the handles toward the face and shoulders.

Keep the torso and upper arms firmly pressed against their pads.

Flex the elbows until the handles are within 4 to 6 inches (10-15 cm) of the face and shoulders.

Downward Movement Phase

Allow the elbows to slowly extend back to the starting position.

Keep the torso and upper arms firmly pressed against their pads.

Common Errors

- Lifting the upper arms off the angled upper arm pad(s) during the upward movement phase
- Jerking the upper body or leaning back during the upward movement phase
- Rising off the seat during the downward movement phase
- Keeping the elbows partially flexed at the end of the downward movement phase (a shortened range of motion)

Primary Muscles Trained
Brachialis, biceps brachii (especially), brachioradialis

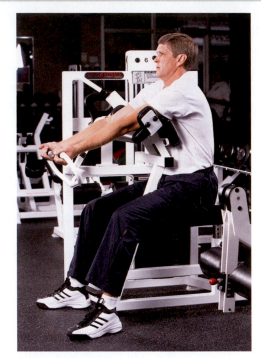

Starting position.

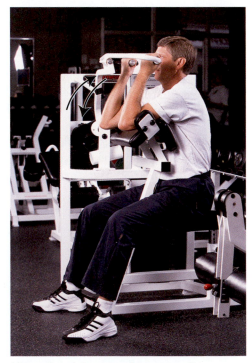

Upward and downward movements.

Arms (Triceps)

Triceps Extension (Resistance Band)

Starting Position

Grasp the handles of the resistance band with a closed, pronated grip.

Sit on the floor or mat with the buttocks on top of a middle section of the resistance band.

Assume an erect position with the torso perpendicular to the floor and the legs crossed in front of the body.

Position the arms and handles behind the head and upper back with the elbows flexed and the palms facing up.

In this position, the resistance band should be nearly taut (not stretched); if not, select a shorter band.

Upward Movement Phase

Keeping the wrist rigid, push one handle upward until the elbow is fully extended.

Maintain an erect torso position with the legs in the same position.

Downward Movement Phase

Allow the elbow to flex to slowly move the handle down to the starting position.

Maintain an erect torso position with the legs in the same position.

At the completion of the set, repeat the movement with the other arm.

Common Errors

- Excessively arching the back during the upward movement phase
- Flexing the torso or head forward during the downward movement phase

Primary Muscle Trained
Triceps brachii

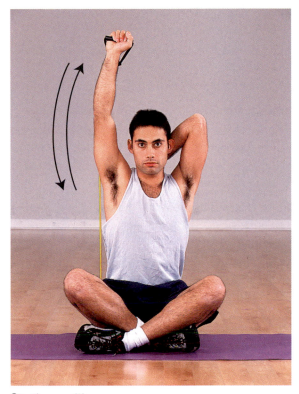

Starting position.

Lying Triceps Extension

A spotter is required for this exercise, but in order to show proper exercise technique the head-on photo does not include the spotter.

Client: Starting Position

Assume a supine position on a bench in the five-point body contact position.

On a signal, take the bar from the personal trainer.

Grasp the bar with a closed, pronated grip about 12 inches (30 cm) apart.

Position the bar over the chest with the elbows fully extended and the arms parallel.

Point the elbows away from the face.

Personal Trainer: Starting Position

At the client's signal, grasp the bar with a closed, alternated grip (not where the client will grasp the bar, however) and lift it from the floor.

Stand erect and very close to the head of the bench (but not so close as to distract the client).

Place the feet shoulder-width apart with the knees slightly flexed.

At the client's signal, place the bar in the client's hands.

Guide the bar to a position over the client's chest.

Release the bar smoothly.

Client: Downward Movement Phase

Allow the elbows to slowly flex to lower the bar toward the nose, eyes, forehead, or the top of the head depending on the length of the arms.

Keep the wrists rigid and the elbows pointing away from the face.

Keep the upper arms parallel to each other and perpendicular to the floor.

Lower the bar to touch the top of the head or forehead.

Maintain the five-point body contact position.

Personal Trainer: Downward Movement Phase

Keep the hands in the alternated grip position close to—but not touching—the bar as it descends.

Slightly flex the knees, hips, and torso and keep the back flat when following the bar.

Client: Upward Movement Phase

Push the bar upward until the elbows are fully extended.

Keep the wrists rigid and the elbows pointing away from the face.

Keep the upper arms parallel to each other and perpendicular to the floor.

Maintain the five-point body contact position.

At the completion of the set, signal the personal trainer to take the bar.

Personal Trainer: Upward Movement Phase

Keep the hands in the alternated grip position close to—but not touching—the bar as it ascends.

Slightly extend the knees, hips, and torso and keep the back flat when following the bar.

At the client's signal, grasp the bar with an alternated grip, take it from the client, and return it to the floor.

Common Errors

- Allowing the elbows to flare out to the sides during the movement
- Moving the upper arms away from their perpendicular position in relation to the floor
- Arching the back or raising the hips off the bench during the upward movement phase

Primary Muscle Trained
Triceps brachii

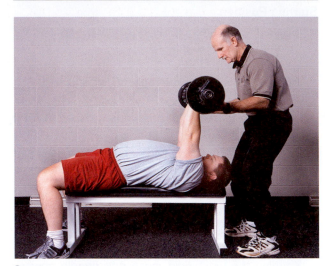

Starting position.

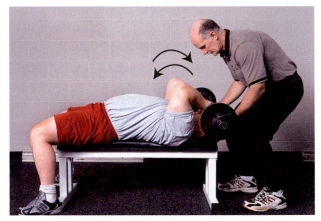

Downward and upward movements.

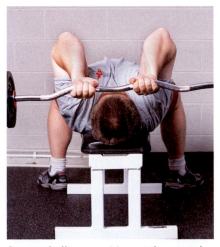

Arm and elbow position at the completion of the downward movement phase.

Triceps Pushdown

Starting Position

Grasp the bar with a closed, pronated grip 6 to 12 inches (15-30 cm) apart. A minimum recommended grip width is close enough for the tips of the thumbs to touch each other when they are extended along the bar. A maximum grip width is one in which the forearms are parallel to each other.

Stand erect with feet shoulder-width apart and knees slightly flexed.

Pull the bar down and position the upper arms against the sides of the torso with the arms flexed.

Adjust the degree of elbow flexion to position the forearms approximately parallel to the floor.

Stand close enough to the machine to allow the cable to hang straight down when it is held in the starting position.

Keep the head in a neutral position with the cable directly in front of the nose.

Keep the torso in position by holding the

- shoulders back,
- upper arms and elbows against the sides of the body, and
- abdominal muscles contracted throughout the exercise.

In this position, the weight to be lifted will be suspended above the rest of the stack.

Downward Movement Phase

Push the bar down until the elbows are fully extended.

Keep the torso and the upper arms stationary.

Upward Movement Phase

Allow the elbows to slowly flex back to the starting position.

Keep the torso, upper arms, and knees in the same position.

After the set is completed, guide the bar upward to move the weight back to its resting position.

Common Errors

- Moving the elbows away from the sides of the torso (backward during the downward movement phase or forward during the upward movement phase)
- Flexing the torso during the downward movement phase
- Forcefully locking out the elbows during the downward movement phase
- Turning the head to the side during the movement

Primary Muscle Trained
Triceps brachii

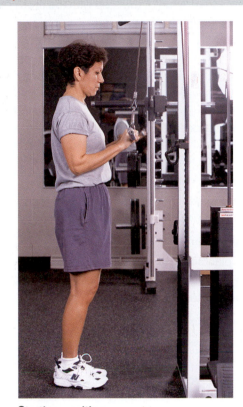

Starting position.

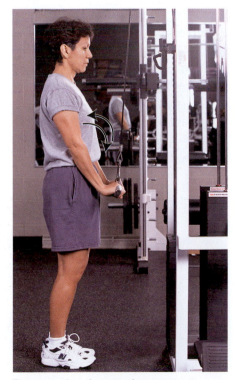

Downward and upward movements.

Calves

Machine Standing Calf (Heel) Raise

Starting Position

Facing the machine, place the balls of the feet on the nearest edge of the step with the toes pointing straight ahead.

Move under the shoulder pads and stand erect with the hips under the shoulders.

Position the feet and legs parallel to each other.

Slightly plantarflex the feet and ankles to lift the thigh pads to remove the supports. If there are none, then the position of the shoulder pads needs to be low enough that the exercise can be performed through a full range of motion.

Extend the knees fully, but not forcefully.

Allow the heels to drop down lower than the step in a comfortable, stretched position.

Upward Movement Phase

Fully plantarflex the feet and ankles.

Keep the torso erect, legs and feet parallel, and knees extended.

Downward Movement Phase

Allow the heels to slowly lower back to the starting position.

Maintain the same body position.

After the set is completed, slightly flex the knees, replace the supports, and move out from under the shoulder pads.

Common Errors

- Allowing the ankles to invert or evert (i.e., rising up on the big or little toes, respectively) during the upward movement phase

- Allowing the knees to flex during the downward movement phase or extend during the upward movement phase

- Bouncing the weight to add momentum to help with the next repetition

Primary Muscles Trained
Soleus, gastrocnemius (especially)

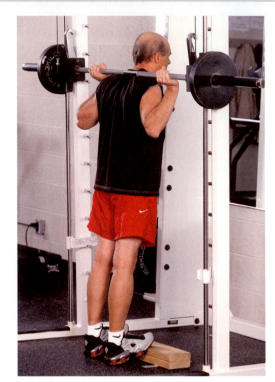

Starting position.

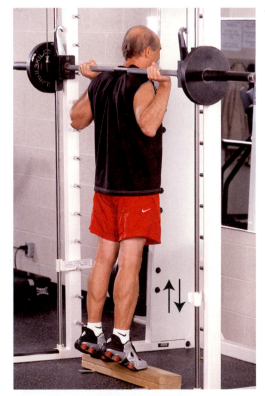

Upward and downward movements.

Machine Seated Calf (Heel) Raise

Starting Position

Sit erect on the seat and place the knees and lower thighs under the pads with the thighs parallel to the floor.

Place the balls of the feet on the nearest edge of the step with the toes pointing straight ahead.

Position the feet and legs parallel to each other.

Slightly plantarflex the feet and ankles to lift the thigh pads to remove the supports.

Allow the heels to drop down lower than the step in a comfortable, stretched position.

Upward Movement Phase

Keeping the torso erect and the legs and feet parallel, fully plantarflex the feet and ankles.

Downward Movement Phase

Allow the heels to slowly lower back to the starting position.

Maintain the same body position.

After the set is completed, replace the supports and remove the feet.

Common Errors

- Allowing the ankles to invert or evert (i.e., rising up on the big or little toes, respectively) during the upward movement phase

- Pulling with the hands or jerking the torso to help raise the weight

- Bouncing the weight to add momentum to help with the next repetition

Primary Muscles Trained
Soleus (especially), gastrocnemius

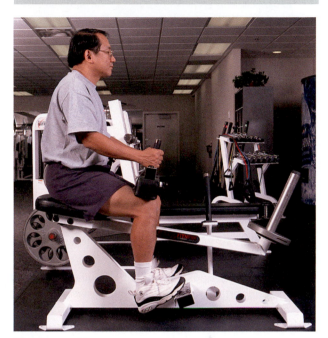

Starting position.

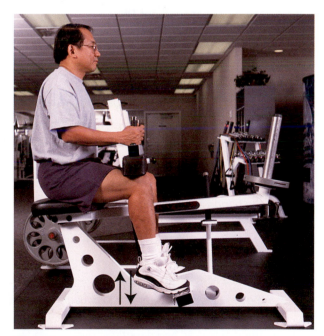

Upward and downward movements.

Chest

Flat Barbell Bench Press

Client: Starting Position

Assume a supine position on a bench in the five-point body contact position.

Place the body on the bench so that the eyes are below the bar.

Grasp the bar with a closed, pronated grip slightly wider than shoulder-width.

Signal the personal trainer for a liftoff.

Guide the bar to a position over the chest with the elbows fully extended.

Personal Trainer: Starting Position

Stand erect and very close to the head of the bench (but not so close as to distract the client).

Place the feet shoulder-width apart, in a staggered stance, with the knees slightly flexed.

Grasp the bar with a closed, alternated grip inside the client's hands.

At the client's signal, assist with moving the bar off the supports and to a height that allows the client's elbows to be fully extended.

Guide the bar to a position over the client's chest.

Release the bar smoothly.

Client: Downward Movement Phase

Allow the bar to lower to touch the chest at approximately nipple level.

Allow the elbows to move down past the torso and slightly away from the body.

Keep the wrists rigid and directly above the elbows.

Keep the forearms approximately perpendicular to the floor and parallel to each other.

Maintain the five-point body contact position.

Personal Trainer: Downward Movement Phase

Keep the hands in the alternated grip position close to—but not touching—the bar as it descends.

Slightly flex the knees, hips, and torso and keep the back flat when following the bar.

Client: Upward Movement Phase

Push the bar upward and very slightly backward until the elbows are fully extended.

Keep the wrists rigid and directly above the elbows.

Maintain the five-point body contact position.

After the set is completed, signal the personal trainer for assistance in racking the bar.

Keep a grip on the bar until it is racked.

Personal Trainer: Upward Movement Phase

Keep the hands in the alternated grip position close to—but not touching—the bar as it ascends.

Primary Muscles Trained
Pectoralis major, anterior deltoid, serratus anterior, pectoralis minor, triceps brachii

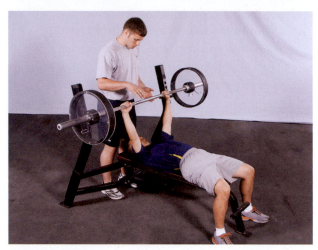

Starting position.

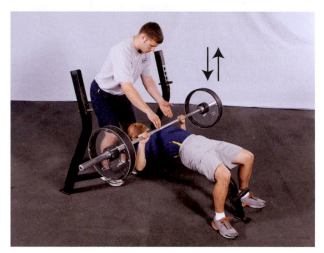

Downward and upward movements.

Slightly extend the knees, hips, and torso and keep the back flat when following the bar.

At the client's signal after the set is completed, grasp the bar with an alternated grip inside the client's hands and help to rack the bar.

Common Errors

- Bouncing the bar on the chest during the upward movement phase to help raise the bar past the sticking point
- Lifting the buttocks off the bench
- Raising the head off the bench during the movement

Flat Dumbbell Fly

A spotter is required for this exercise, but in order to show proper exercise technique the photos do not include the spotter.

Client: Starting Position

Assume a supine position on a bench in the five-point body contact position.

On a signal, take the dumbbells from the personal trainer (one at a time) and position them near to or on the chest.

Rotate the dumbbells to a neutral grip position.

Signal the personal trainer for assistance to move the dumbbells into an extended elbow position over the chest with the arms parallel to each other.

Slightly flex the elbows and point them out to the sides.

Personal Trainer: Starting Position

At the client's signal, lift the dumbbells from the floor into the client's hands (one at a time).

While the client adjusts the dumbbells, position one knee on the floor with the foot of the other leg forward and flat on the floor (or kneel on both knees) very close to the head of the bench (but not so close as to distract the client).

Grasp the client's wrists.

At the client's signal, assist with moving dumbbells to a position over the client's chest.

Release the client's wrists smoothly.

Client: Downward Movement Phase

Allow the dumbbells to lower at the same rate in a wide arc until they are level with the shoulders or chest.

Keep the dumbbell handles parallel to each other as the elbows move downward.

Keep the wrists rigid and the elbows held in a slightly flexed position.

Keep the dumbbells in line with the elbows and shoulders.

Maintain the five-point body contact position.

Personal Trainer: Downward Movement Phase

Keep the hands near—but not touching—the client's wrists as the dumbbells descend.

Client: Upward Movement Phase

Pull the dumbbells up toward each other in a wide arc back to the starting position; imagine the arc formed by the arms when hugging a very large tree trunk.

Keep the wrists rigid and the elbows held in a slightly flexed position.

Keep the dumbbells in line with the elbows and shoulders.

Maintain the five-point body contact position.

Primary Muscles Trained
Pectoralis major, anterior deltoid

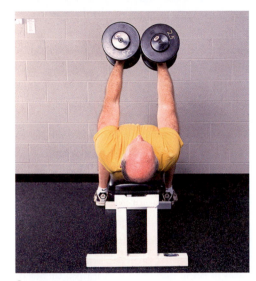

Starting position.

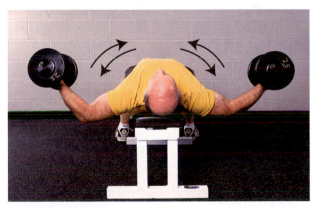

Downward and upward movements.

At the completion of the set, first slowly lower the dumbbells to the chest and armpit area then signal the personal trainer to return them to the floor.

Personal Trainer: Upward Movement Phase

Keep the hands near—but not touching—the client's wrists as the dumbbells ascend.

At the client's signal, take the dumbbells from the client and return them to the floor.

Common Errors

- Allowing the elbows to flex and extend during the movement
- Lifting the buttocks off the bench
- Raising the head off the bench during the movement
- Lowering the dumbbells below chest level.

Pec Deck (Butterfly)

Starting Position

Sit in the machine with the head, back, hips, and buttocks pressed against their pads.

If the seat is adjustable, move it up or down to

- position the thighs parallel to the floor with the feet flat in the starting seated position,
- position the shoulders slightly above the bottom of the forearm pads (or in line with the elbow pads, depending on the type of machine), and
- position the upper arms parallel to the floor (or slightly above parallel) when the elbows are flexed to 90° with the hands holding on to the handles.

Grasp the handles with

- a closed, neutral grip;
- the elbows flexed at right angles (90°); and
- the forearms pressed against the small vertical pads near the handgrips. (If the machine has elbow pads, press the inside of the elbows against them.)

If the handles are too far back to be grasped from the seated position, push down on the foot pedal (if available), or request the assistance of a spotter.

Begin the exercise with the handles together in front of the face.

Backward Movement Phase

Begin the exercise by allowing both handles to swing out and back slowly and under control.

Keep the wrists erect, the forearms and elbows next to the arm pads, and the upper arms approximately parallel to the floor.

Allow the handles to move back so they are level with the chest.

Forward Movement Phase

Move the handles out and then toward each other, under control, by squeezing the forearms and elbows together.

Use the entire arm to exert pressure against the pads to squeeze the handles together.

At the completion of the set, guide the handles backward to their resting position.

Common Errors

- Positioning the seat too low or too high
- Pushing the handles together with the hands or the palms of the hands
- Swinging the handles back to add momentum to help with the next repetition
- Flexing the torso forward to help move the handles together

Primary Muscle Trained
Pectoralis major

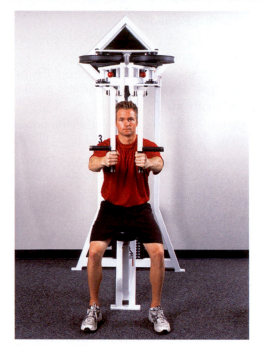
Starting position.

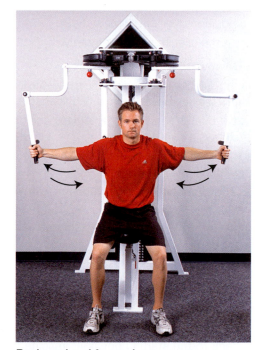
Backward and forward movements.

Chest Press (Resistance Band)

Starting Position

Grasp the handles of the resistance band with a closed, pronated grip, and evenly wrap the band around the upper back at nipple height.

Stand erect with the feet shoulder-width apart and the knees slightly flexed.

Position the handles to the outside of the chest at nipple height with the palms facing down.

In this position, the resistance band should be nearly taut (not stretched); if not, select a shorter band.

Forward Movement Phase

Push the handles away from the chest until the elbows are fully extended.

Keep the arms parallel to the floor.

Maintain the erect standing position with the heels on the floor and the knees slightly flexed.

Backward Movement Phase

Allow the handles to slowly move backward to the starting position.

Keep the arms parallel to the floor.

Maintain the erect standing position with the heels on the floor and the knees slightly flexed.

Common Errors

- Forcefully locking out the elbows at the end of the forward movement phase
- Shortening the range of motion during the backward movement phase

Primary Muscles Trained
Pectoralis major, anterior deltoid, triceps brachii

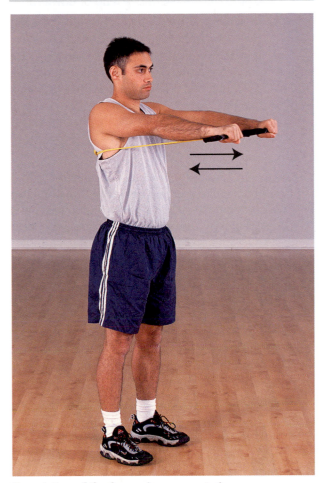

Completion of the forward movement phase.

Vertical Chest Press

Starting Position

Sit in the machine with the head, back, hips, and buttocks pressed against their pads.

If the seat is adjustable, move it up or down to

- position the thighs parallel to the floor with the feet flat in the starting seated position,
- put the body in line with the handgrips (an imaginary line connecting both handgrips should cross the front of the chest at nipple height), and
- position the arms parallel to the floor with the elbows extended and holding on to the handgrips.

Grasp the handles with a closed, pronated grip. If the handles are too far back to be grasped from the seated position, push down on the foot pedal (if available) or request the assistance of a spotter to move the handles slightly forward.

Forward Movement Phase

Push the handles away from the chest until the elbows are fully extended.

Maintain the five-point body contact position.

Backward Movement Phase

Allow the handles to slowly move backward so that they are level with the chest.

Maintain the five-point body contact position.

At the completion of the set, guide the handles backward to their resting position.

Common Errors

- Positioning the seat too low or too high
- Arching the back or pushing with the legs during the forward movement phase
- Flexing the torso forward to help move the handles forward
- Forcefully locking out the elbows at the end of the forward movement phase
- Shortening the range of motion during the backward movement phase

Primary Muscles Trained
Pectoralis major, anterior deltoid, triceps brachii

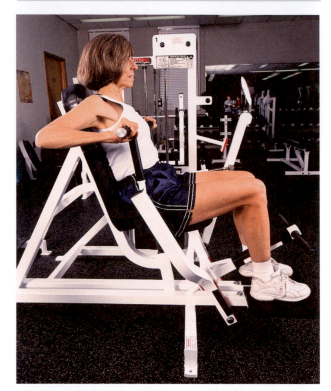

Starting position.

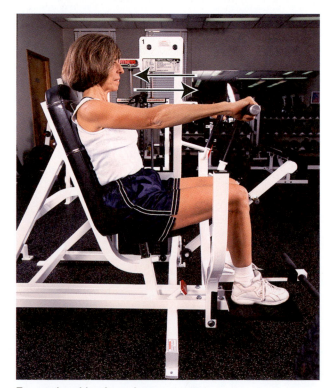

Forward and backward movements.

Hip and Thigh

Leg Press

Starting Position

Sit in the machine with the back, hips, and buttocks pressed against their pads. (If the horizontal position of the foot platform or the seat is adjustable, move it forward or backward to allow the thighs to be parallel to the foot platform when seated in the starting position.)

Place the feet flat in the middle of the platform in a hip-width position with the toes slightly pointed out.

Position the thighs and lower legs parallel to each other.

Grasp the handles or the sides of the seat.

Forward Movement Phase

Extend the hips and knees to push the foot platform forward (note that in some machines, the foot platform is fixed and the seat will move backward during this phase).

Push to a fully extended position while maintaining the same upper body position and the heels in contact with the platform.

Backward Movement Phase

Allow the hips and knees to slowly flex to lower the weight.

Keep the hips and buttocks on the seat and the back flat against the back pad.

Keep the legs parallel to each other.

Continue flexing the hips and knees until the thighs are parallel to the foot platform.

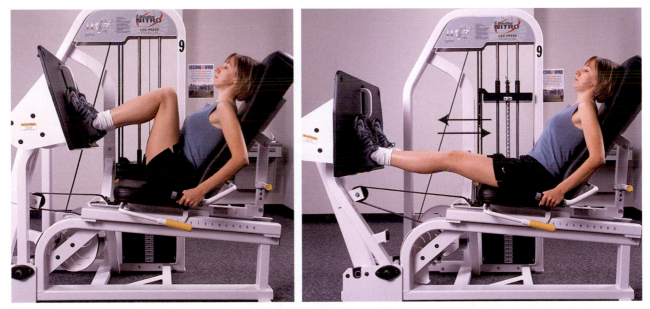

Starting position.

Forward and backward movements.

Common Errors

- Allowing the heels to lift off the platform, the buttocks to lose contact with the seat, or the hands to let go during the movement
- Allowing the knees to move in (via hip adduction) or out (hip abduction) during the movement
- Locking the knees out at the end of the forward movement phase

Back Squat

Client: Starting Position

Step under the bar and position the feet parallel to each other.

Place the hands on the bar using the "high bar position" technique:

- Grasp the bar with a closed, pronated grip slightly wider than shoulder-width.

- Dip the head under the bar and move the body to place the bar evenly above the posterior deltoids at the base of the neck.

Lift the elbows up to create a shelf for the bar to rest on.

Hold the chest up and out.

Pull the scapulae toward each other.

Tilt the head slightly up.

Once in position, signal the spotters for a liftoff.

Extend the hips and knees to lift the bar off the rack, and take one or two steps backward.

Position the feet shoulder-width or wider apart and even with each other, with the toes slightly pointed outward.

Keep the elbows lifted up and backward to keep the bar on the shoulders.

Two Spotters: Starting Position

Stand erect at opposite ends of the bar with the feet shoulder-width apart and the knees slightly flexed.

Grasp the end of the bar by cupping the hands together with the palms facing upward.

At the client's signal, assist with lifting and balancing the bar as it is moved out of the rack.

Release the bar smoothly in unison with the other spotter.

Hold the hands 2 to 3 inches (5 to 8 cm) below the ends of the bar.

Move sideways in unison with the client as the client moves backward.

Once the client is in position, assume a hip-width stance with the knees slightly flexed and the torso erect.

Client: Downward Movement Phase

Allow the hips and knees to slowly flex while keeping the torso-to-floor angle constant.

Maintain a position with the back flat, elbows high, and the chest up and out.

Keep the heels on the floor and the knees aligned over the feet.

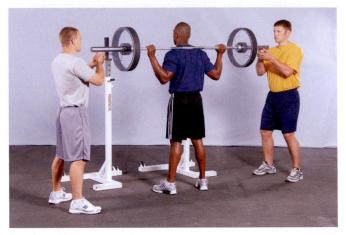

Primary Muscles Trained
Gluteus maximus, hamstrings, quadriceps

Starting position.

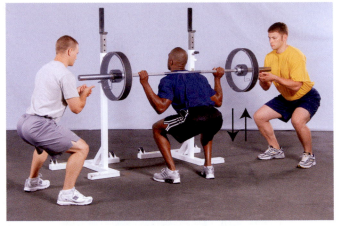

Downward and upward movements (high bar).

Continue allowing the hips and knees to flex until one of these three events first occurs (this determines client's maximum range of motion; the lowest or "bottom" position):

- The thighs are parallel to the floor.

- The trunk begins to round or flex forward.

- The heels rise off the floor.

Two Spotters: Downward Movement Phase

Keep the cupped hands close to—but not touching—the bar as it descends.

Slightly flex the knees, hips, and torso and keep the back flat when following the bar.

Client: Upward Movement Phase

Extend the hips and knees at the same rate to keep the torso-to-floor angle constant.

Maintain a position with the back flat, elbows high, and the chest up and out.

Keep the heels on the floor and the knees aligned over the feet.

Continue extending the hips and knees to reach the starting position.

After the set is completed, step forward and rack the bar.

Two Spotters: Upward Movement Phase

Keep the cupped hands close to—but not touching—the bar as it ascends.

Slightly extend the knees, hips, and torso and keep the back flat when following the bar.

After the set is completed, help the client rack the bar.

Common Errors

- Allowing the heels to lift off the floor, the torso to flex further forward, or the upper back to round during the upward movement phase
- Allowing the knees to move in (via hip adduction) or out (hip abduction) during the movement
- Allowing the arms to relax or the elbows to drop down and forward

Squat (Resistance Band)

Starting Position

Grasp the handles of the resistance band with a closed, pronated grip.

Position the feet shoulder-width apart with the toes slightly pointed outward and the arches of both feet on top of a middle section of the resistance band.

Position the handles to the outside and level with the top of the shoulders, palms facing forward.

Create a flat-back position with the chest held up and out and the shoulders back.

Flex the hips and knees to assume the lowest desired squat position.

In this position, the resistance band should be nearly taut (not stretched); if not, select a shorter band.

Upward Movement Phase

Extend the hips and knees at the same rate to keep the torso-to-floor angle constant.

Maintain the flat-back position with the chest held up and out.

Keep the heels on the floor and the knees aligned over the feet.

Continue extending the hips and knees to a fully standing position.

Downward Movement Phase

Allow the hips and knees to slowly flex while keeping the torso-to-floor angle relatively constant.

Maintain the flat-back position with the chest held up and out.

Keep the heels on the floor and the knees aligned over the feet.

Continue allowing the hips and knees to flex until reaching the lowest desired squat position.

Primary Muscles Trained
Gluteus maximus, hamstrings, quadriceps

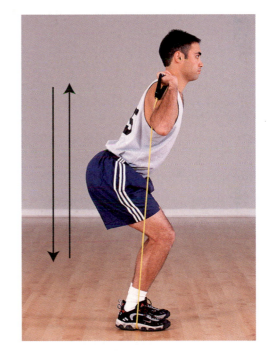

Completion of the upward movement phase.

Common Errors

- Allowing the heels to lift off the floor, the torso to flex further forward, or the upper back to round during the upward movement phase
- Allowing the knees to move in (via hip adduction) or out (hip abduction) during the movement

Front Squat

Client: Starting Position

Walk up to the bar and position the feet parallel to each other.

Place the hands on the bar using the "parallel arm position" technique:

- Grasp the bar with a closed, pronated grip slightly wider than shoulder-width.
- Move the body to place the bar evenly on top of the anterior deltoids and clavicles.
- Fully flex the elbows and hyperextend the wrists to position the upper arms parallel to the floor. The back of the hands should be either on top of or just to the outside of the shoulders, right next to where the bar is resting on the deltoids.
- Hold the chest up and out.
- Pull the scapulae toward each other.
- Tilt the head slightly up.
- Once in position, signal the spotters for a liftoff.
- Extend the hips and knees to lift the bar off the rack, and take one or two steps backward.
- Position the feet shoulder-width or wider apart, and even with each other, with the toes slightly pointed outward.
- Keep the elbows lifted up and forward to keep the bar on the shoulders.

Two Spotters: Starting Position

Stand erect at opposite ends of the bar with the feet shoulder-width apart and the knees slightly flexed.

Grasp the end of the bar by cupping the hands together with the palms facing upward.

At the client's signal, assist with lifting and balancing the bar as it is moved out of the rack.

Release the bar smoothly in unison with the other spotter.

Hold the hands 2 to 3 inches (5 to 8 cm) below the ends of the bar.

Move sideways in unison with the client as the client moves backward.

Once the client is in position, assume a hip-width stance with the knees slightly flexed and the torso erect.

Primary Muscles Trained
Gluteus maximus, quadriceps, hamstrings

Client: Downward Movement Phase

Allow the hips and knees to slowly flex while keeping the torso-to-floor angle relatively constant.

Maintain a position with the back flat, elbows high, and the chest up and out.

Keep the heels on the floor and the knees aligned over the feet.

Continue allowing the hips and knees to flex until one of these three events first occurs (this determines client's maximum range of motion; the lowest or "bottom" position):

- The thighs are parallel to the floor.
- The trunk begins to round or flex forward.
- The heels rise off the floor.

Two Spotters: Downward Movement Phase

Keep the cupped hands close to—but not touching—the bar as it descends.

Slightly flex the knees, hips, and torso and keep the back flat when following the bar.

Client: Upward Movement Phase

Extend the hips and knees at the same rate to keep the torso-to-floor angle constant.

Maintain a position with the back flat, elbows high, and the chest up and out.

Keep the heels on the floor and the knees aligned over the feet.

Continue extending the hips and knees to reach the starting position.

After the set is completed, step forward and rack the bar.

Two Spotters: Upward Movement Phase

Keep the cupped hands close to—but not touching—the bar as it ascends.

Slightly extend the knees, hips, and torso and keep the back flat when following the bar.

After the set is completed, help the client rack the bar.

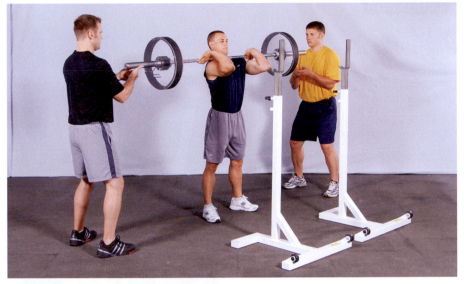

Starting position.

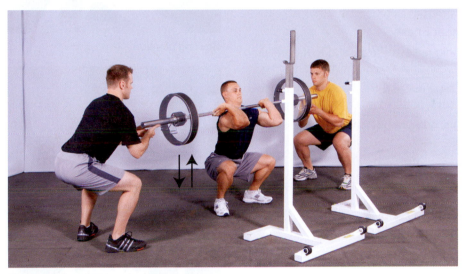

Downward and upward movements.

Common Errors

- Allowing the heels to lift off the floor, the torso to flex forward, or the upper back to round during the upward movement phase
- Allowing the knees to move in (via hip adduction) or out (hip abduction) during the movement
- Allowing the arms to relax or the elbows to drop down and backward

Leg (Knee) Extension

Starting Position

Sit in the machine with the thighs and back in the center of their pads (not to the left or right side) and the knees aligned with the axis of the machine. If the back pad is adjustable, move it forward or backward to

- align the knees with the axis of the machine and
- position the buttocks and thighs so that the backs of the knees are touching the front end of the seat.

Hook the feet under the ankle pad or pads; if the pad is adjustable, position it so it is in contact with the instep of the foot.

Position the thighs, lower legs, and feet parallel to each other.

Grasp the handles or the sides of the seat.

Upward Movement Phase

Keeping the thighs, lower legs, and feet parallel to each other, extend the knees until they are straight.

Keep the torso erect and the back firmly pressed against the back pad.

Maintain a tight grip on the handles or the sides of the seat.

Downward Movement Phase

Allow the knees to slowly flex back to the starting position.

Keep the thighs, lower legs, and feet parallel to each other.

Keep the torso erect and the back firmly pressed against the back pad.

Maintain a tight grip on the handles or the sides of the seat.

Common Errors

- Allowing the hips or buttocks to lift off the seat during the upward movement phase
- Swinging the legs or jerking the torso backward to help raise the weight
- Forcefully locking out the knees at the end of the upward movement phase

Primary Muscles Trained
Quadriceps

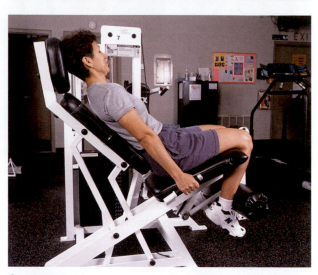

Starting position.

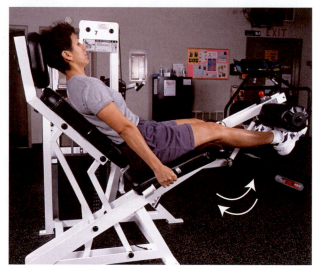

Upward and downward movements.

318

Forward Lunge

Client: Starting Position

Grasp the bar with a closed, pronated grip slightly wider than shoulder-width.

Step under the bar and position the feet parallel to each other.

Place the bar evenly on the upper back and shoulders above the posterior deltoids at the base of the neck.

Lift the elbows up to create a shelf for the bar to rest on.

Hold the chest up and out.

Pull the scapulae toward each other.

Tilt the head slightly up.

Once in position, signal the spotter for a liftoff.

Extend the hips and knees to lift the bar off the rack, and take two or three steps backward.

Place the feet hip-width apart with the toes pointed ahead.

Personal Trainer: Starting Position

Stand erect and very close to the client (but not close enough to be a distraction).

Place the feet shoulder-width apart with the knees slightly flexed.

At the client's signal, assist with lifting and balancing the bar as it is moved out of the rack.

Move in unison with the client as the client moves backward to the starting position.

Once the client is in position, assume a hip-width stance with the knees slightly flexed and the torso erect.

Position the hands near the client's hips, waist, or torso.

Client: Forward Movement Phase

Take one exaggerated step directly forward with one leg (the lead leg).

Keep the torso erect as the lead foot moves forward and contacts the floor.

Keep the trailing foot in the starting position, but allow the trailing knee to slightly flex.

Plant the lead foot flat on the floor pointing straight ahead or slightly inward. To help maintain balance, place this foot directly ahead from its initial position with the lead ankle, knee, and hip in one vertical plane.

Allow the lead hip and knee to slowly flex. Once balance has shifted to be even on both feet, flex the lead knee to lower the trailing knee toward the

Primary Muscles Trained
Gluteus maximus, hamstrings, quadriceps, iliopsoas (of the trailing leg), soleus and gastrocnemius (of the lead leg)

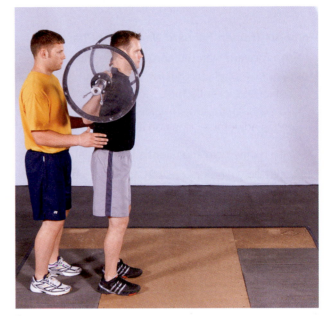

Starting position.

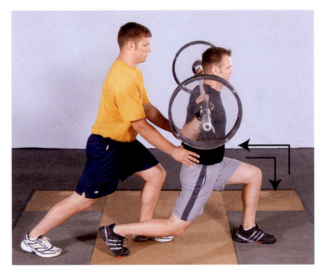

Forward and backward movements.

floor. The trailing knee will flex somewhat further, but not to the same degree as the lead knee.

Keep the lead knee directly over the lead foot (which remains flat on the floor).

Lower the trailing knee—still slightly flexed—until it is 1 to 2 inches (3 to 5 cm) above the floor. At this

(continued)

319

point, the lead knee will be flexed to about 90° with the lower leg perpendicular to the floor.

Balance the weight evenly between the ball of the trailing foot and the entire lead foot.

Keep the torso perpendicular to the floor by "sitting back" on the trailing leg. Actual lunge depth, however, depends primarily on individual hip joint flexibility.

Personal Trainer: Forward Movement Phase

Step forward with the same foot as the client.

Plant the lead foot 12 to 18 inches (30-45 cm) behind the client's foot.

Flex the lead knee as the client's lead knee flexes.

Keep the torso erect.

Keep hands near the client's hips, waist, or torso.

Assist only when necessary to keep the client balanced.

Client: Backward Movement Phase

Shift the balance forward to the lead foot, and forcefully push off the floor by extending the lead hip and knee. As the lead foot moves back toward the trailing foot, balance will shift back to the trailing foot. This will cause the heel of the trailing foot to regain contact with the floor.

Maintain the same torso position.

Bring the lead foot back to a position next to the trailing foot.

Stand erect in the starting position, pause, and then alternate lead legs.

After the set is completed, step forward and rack the bar.

Personal Trainer: Backward Movement Phase

Push backward with the lead leg in unison with the client.

Bring the lead foot back to a position next to the trailing foot.

Keep hands near the client's hips, waist, or torso.

Stand erect in the starting position, pause to wait for the client, and alternate lead legs.

Assist only when necessary to keep the client balanced.

After the set is completed, help the client rack the bar.

Common Errors

- Stepping out too shallowly, causing the lead knee to extend past the lead foot
- Allowing the torso to flex forward during the forward movement phase
- Quickly jerking the torso backward during the backward movement phase
- Stutter-stepping backward during the backward movement phase
- Not maintaining a neutral pelvis or spine

Leg (Knee) Curl

Starting Position

Assume a prone position on the machine with the hips and torso in the center of their pads (not to the left or right side) and the knees aligned with the axis of the machine.

Hook the feet under the ankle pad or pads; if the pad is adjustable, position it so it is in contact with the back of the heel just above the top of the shoe.

Once in proper position, the knees should be hanging slightly off the bottom edge of the thigh pad.

Position the thighs, lower legs, and feet parallel to each other.

Grasp the handles or the sides of the chest pad.

Upward Movement Phase

Keeping the thighs, lower legs, and feet parallel to each other, flex the knees until the ankle pad nearly touches the buttocks.

Keep the torso stationary.

Maintain a tight grip on the handles or the sides of the chest pad.

Downward Movement Phase

Allow the knees to slowly extend back to the starting position.

Keep the thighs, lower legs, and feet parallel to each other.

Keep the torso stationary.

Maintain a tight grip on the handles or the sides of the chest pad.

Primary Muscles Trained
Hamstrings

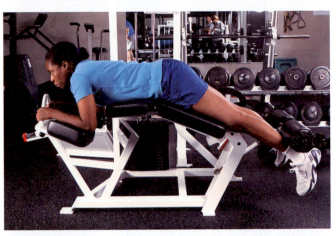
Starting position.

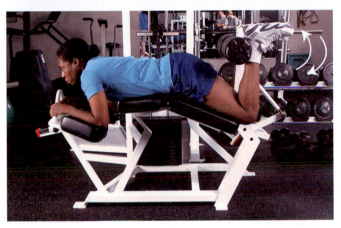
Upward and downward movements.

Common Errors

- Allowing the hips to rise (using hip flexion) during the upward movement phase
- Swinging the legs backward to help raise the weight
- Locking out the knees at the end of the downward movement phase

Shoulders

Shoulder Press (Bar)

Client: Starting Position

Sit on a shoulder press bench and lean back to assume the five-point body contact position. If the seat can be adjusted, modify its height to

- position the thighs parallel to the floor (with the feet flat) and
- allow the bar to move in and out of the rack without hitting the top of the head (the seat is too high) or having to half-stand up to reach the rack (the seat is too low).

Grasp the bar with a closed, pronated grip slightly wider than shoulder-width.

Signal the personal trainer for a liftoff.

Press the bar over the head until the elbows are fully extended.

Personal Trainer: Starting Position

Stand erect on the step at the back of the bench or on the spotter's platform (if present) with the feet shoulder-width apart, if there is enough room, and the knees slightly flexed.

Grasp the bar with a closed, alternated grip inside the client's hands.

At the client's signal, assist with moving the bar off the rack.

Guide the bar to a position over the client's head.

Release the bar (or wrists) smoothly.

Client: Downward Movement Phase

Allow the elbows to slowly flex to lower the bar toward the head.

Keep the wrists rigid and directly above the elbows. The width of the grip will determine how parallel the forearms are to each other.

Extend the neck slightly to allow the bar to pass by the face as the bar is lowered to touch the clavicles and anterior deltoids.

Maintain the five-point body contact position.

Personal Trainer: Downward Movement Phase

Keep the hands in the alternated grip position close to—but not touching—the bar as it descends.

Slightly flex the knees, hips, and torso and keep the back flat when following the bar.

Primary Muscles Trained
Anterior and medial deltoids, trapezius, triceps brachii

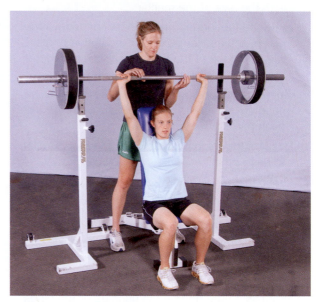

Starting position.

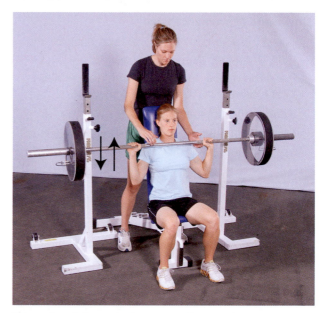

Upward and downward movements.

Client: Upward Movement Phase

Push the bar upward until the elbows are fully extended.

Extend the neck slightly to allow the bar to pass by the face as it is raised.

Keep the wrists rigid and directly above the elbows.

Maintain the five-point body contact position.

After the set is completed, signal the personal trainer for assistance in racking the bar.

Keep a grip on the bar until it is racked.

Upward Movement Phase: Personal Trainer

Keep the hands in the alternated grip position close to—but not touching—the bar as it ascends.

Slightly extend the knees, hips, and torso and keep the back flat when following the bar.

After the set is completed, help the client rack the bar.

Common Errors

- Pushing with the legs or rising off the seat to help raise the bar upward
- Excessively arching the back during the upward movement phase

Shoulder Press (Resistance Band)

Starting Position

Grasp the handles of the resistance band with a closed, pronated grip.

Sit on the floor or mat with the buttocks on top of a middle section of the resistance band.

Assume an erect position with the torso perpendicular to the floor and the legs together and extended away from the body.

Slightly flex the hips and knees for balance.

Position the handles to the outside and level with the top of the shoulders with the palms facing forward.

In this position, the resistance band should be nearly taut (not stretched); if not, select a shorter band.

Upward Movement Phase

Push the handles upward until the elbows are fully extended.

Keep the wrists rigid and directly above the elbows.

Maintain an erect torso position with the legs in the same position.

Downward Movement Phase

Allow the handles to slowly move backward to the starting position.

Maintain an erect torso position with the legs in the same position.

Common Errors

- Excessively arching the back during the upward movement phase
- Flexing the torso forward during the downward movement phase

Primary Muscles Trained
Anterior and medial deltoids, trapezius, triceps brachii

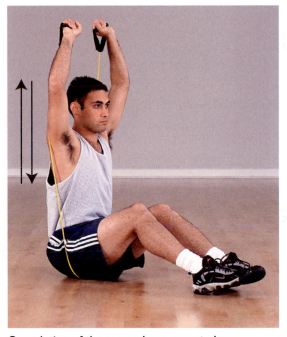

Completion of the upward movement phase.

Dumbbell Lateral Raise

Starting Position

Grasp two dumbbells with a closed, neutral grip.

Position the feet shoulder- or hip-width apart, knees slightly flexed, torso erect, shoulders back, and eyes focused ahead.

Move the dumbbells to the front of the thighs, positioning them with the palms facing each other.

Slightly flex the elbows and hold this flexed position throughout the exercise.

Upward Movement Phase

Raise the dumbbells up and out to the sides; the elbows and upper arms should rise together and ahead of (and slightly higher than) the forearms and hands/dumbbells. This movement is similar to pouring liquid out of a plastic jug.

Maintain an erect upper body position with the knees slightly flexed and feet flat.

Continue raising the dumbbells until the arms are approximately parallel to the floor or nearly level with the shoulders. At the highest position, the elbows and upper arms will be slightly higher than the forearms and hands/dumbbells.

Downward Movement Phase

Allow the dumbbells to lower slowly back to the starting position.

Keep the knees slightly flexed, feet flat on the floor, and eyes focused ahead.

Common Errors

- Extending or flexing the elbows during the movement
- Shrugging the shoulders, flexing the torso backward, extending the knees, or rising up on the toes to help raise the dumbbells upward
- Flexing the torso forward or allowing the body's weight to shift toward the toes during the downward movement phase

Primary Muscles Trained
Deltoids, trapezius

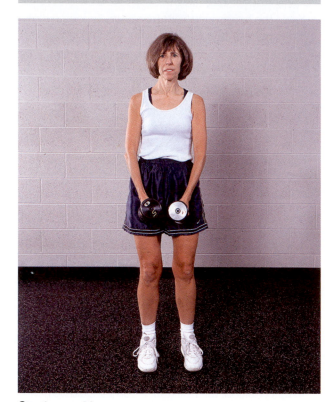

Starting position.

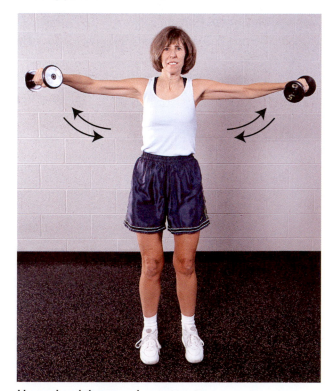

Upward and downward movements.

Lateral Raise (Resistance Band)

Starting Position

Grasp the handles of the resistance band with a closed, neutral grip.

Position the feet shoulder-width apart with the arches of both feet on top of a middle section of the resistance band.

Stand erect with the knees slightly flexed.

Position the handles outside of the thighs with the arms at the sides and the palms facing inward.

In this position, the resistance band should be nearly taut (not stretched); if not, take up the slack by widening the stance or selecting a shorter band.

Upward Movement Phase

Pull the handles up and out to the sides; the hands, forearms, elbows, and upper arms should rise together.

Maintain an erect body position with the knees slightly flexed and feet flat.

Continue raising the handles until the arms are approximately parallel to the floor or nearly level with the shoulders.

Downward Movement Phase

Allow the handles to slowly move back to the starting position.

Maintain an erect body position with the knees slightly flexed and feet flat.

Common Errors

- Extending or flexing the elbows during the movement
- Shrugging the shoulders to help raise the handles upward

Primary Muscles Trained
Deltoids, trapezius

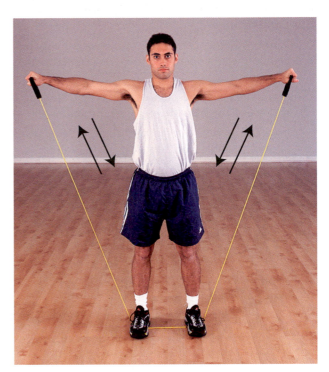

Completion of the upward movement phase.

Whole Body

Power Clean

This exercise consists of four phases (first pull, scoop, second pull, and catch), but there is no pause between them; the bar is lifted (pulled up) from the floor to the front of the shoulders in one continuous movement.

Starting Position

Stand with the feet placed between hip- and shoulder-width apart with the toes pointed slightly outward.

Squat down with the hips lower than the shoulders and grasp the bar with a closed, pronated grip.

Place the hands on the bar slightly wider than shoulder-width apart, outside of the knees, with the elbows fully extended.

Place the feet flat on the floor and position the bar approximately 1 inch (3 cm) in front of the shins and over the balls of the feet.

Position the body with the

- back flat or slightly arched,
- trapezius relaxed and slightly stretched,
- chest held up and out,
- scapulae retracted,
- head in line with the spine or slightly hyperextended,
- shoulders over or slightly in front of the bar, and
- eyes focused straight ahead or slightly upward.

Upward Movement Phase: First Pull

Lift the bar off the floor by forcefully extending the hips and knees.

Keep the torso-to-floor angle constant.

Do not let the hips rise before the shoulders.

Maintain a flat-back position.

Keep the elbows fully extended, the head neutral in relation to the spine, and the shoulders over or slightly ahead of the bar.

As the bar is raised, keep it as close to the shins as possible.

Upward Movement Phase: Scoop (Transition)

As the bar rises just above the knees, thrust the hips forward and slightly re-flex the knees to move the thighs against and the knees under the bar.

Keep the back flat or slightly arched, the elbows fully extended and pointing out to the sides, and the head in line with the spine.

Upward Movement Phase: Second Pull

Forcefully and quickly extend the hips and knees and plantarflex the ankles.

Keep the bar near to or in contact with the front of the thighs.

Keep the bar as close to the body as possible.

Keep the back flat, the elbows pointing out to the sides, and the head in line with the spine.

Keep the shoulders over the bar and the elbows extended as long as possible.

When the lower body joints reach full extension, rapidly shrug the shoulders upward, but do not allow the elbows to flex yet.

As the shoulders reach their highest elevation, flex the elbows to begin pulling the body under the bar.

Because of the explosive nature of this phase, the torso will be erect or slightly hyperextended, the head will be tilted slightly back, and the feet may lose contact with the floor.

Upward Movement Phase: Catch

After the lower body has fully extended and the bar reaches near-maximal height, pull the body under the bar and rotate the arms around and under the bar.

Simultaneously, the hips and knees flex into a quarter squat position.

Once the arms are under the bar, lift the elbows to position the upper arms parallel to the floor.

Rack the bar across the front of clavicles and anterior deltoids.

The bar should be caught at the anterior deltoids and clavicles with the

- head facing forward,
- neck neutral or slightly hyperextended,
- wrists hyperextended,
- elbows fully flexed,
- upper arms parallel to the floor,
- back flat or slightly arched,
- knees and hips slightly flexed to absorb the impact of the weight,
- feet flat on the floor, and
- the body's weight over the middle of the feet.

Stand up by extending the hips and knees to a fully erect position.

Downward Movement Phase

Lower the bar to the thighs by gradually reducing the muscular tension of the arms to allow a controlled descent.

Simultaneously flex the hips and knees to cushion the impact of the bar on the thighs.

Squat down with the elbows fully extended until the bar touches the floor.

Common Errors

- Allowing the hips to rise before the shoulders during the first pull
- Allowing the upper back to round (i.e., losing the flat-back position), especially during the first pull
- Extending the knees faster than the hips, before the hips, or both
- Allowing the bar to travel upward too far away from the body
- Using a "reverse curl" movement to move the bar into the catch position

Primary Muscles Trained
Gluteus maximus, hamstrings, quadriceps, soleus, gastrocnemius, deltoids, trapezius

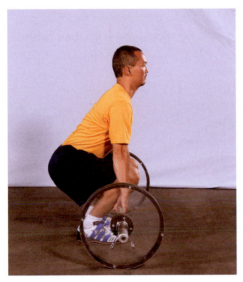

Starting position.

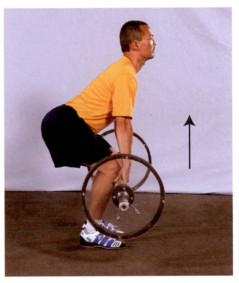

First pull.

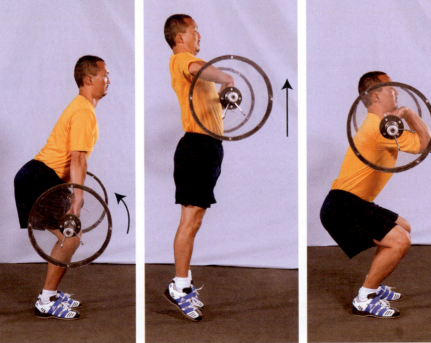

Scoop.

Second pull

Catch.

Study Questions

1. Which of the following lower-body exercises is a single-joint exercise?

   A. back squat

   B. front squat

   C. leg (knee) extension

   D. forward lunge

2. All of the following exercises require one or more spotters EXCEPT

   A. lying supine triceps extension.

   B. biceps curl (barbell).

   C. flat barbell bench press.

   D. back squat.

3. Which of the following is the PRIMARY reason for using proper footwear while resistance training?

   A. etiquette

   B. technique improvement

   C. safety

   D. equipment maintenance

4. Which of the following handgrips is used in performing a power snatch exercise?

   A. pronated with closed grip

   B. supinated with closed grip

   C. pronated with hook grip

   D. supinated with hook grip

Applied Knowledge Question

An experienced resistance training participant is performing a 1RM exercise in the back squat with two spotters. Where should each spotter be positioned and what are his or her responsibilities?

References

1. Barnes, M., and K.E. Cinea. 2007. Explosive movements. In: *Strength Training,* L.E. Brown, ed. Champaign, IL: Human Kinetics.

2. Barnes, M., and K.E. Cinea. 2007. Lower body exercises. In: *Strength Training,* L.E. Brown, ed. Champaign, IL: Human Kinetics.

3. Barnes, M., and K.E. Cinea. 2007. Torso exercises. In: *Strength Training,* L.E. Brown, ed. Champaign, IL: Human Kinetics.

4. Barnes, M., and K.E. Cinea. 2007. Upper body exercises. In: *Strength Training,* L.E. Brown, ed. Champaign, IL: Human Kinetics.

5. Cholewicki, J., K. Juluru, and S. McGill. 1999. Intra-abdominal pressure mechanism for stabilizing the lumbar spine. *Journal of Biomechanics* 32 (1): 13–17.

6. Delavier, F. 2006. *Strength Training Anatomy.* Champaign, IL: Human Kinetics.

7. Earle, R.W., and T.R. Baechle. 2008. Resistance training and spotting techniques. In: *Essentials of Strength Training and Conditioning,* 3rd ed., T.R. Baechle and R.W. Earle, eds. Champaign, IL: Human Kinetics.

8. Faigenbaum, A., and W. Westcott. 2009. *Youth Strength Training.* Champaign, IL: Human Kinetics.

9. Graham, J.F. 2000. Exercise technique: Power clean. *Strength and Conditioning Journal* 22 (6): 63-65.

10. Graham, J.F. 2001. Exercise technique: Back squat. *Strength and Conditioning Journal* 23 (5): 28-29.

11. Graham, J.F. 2002. Exercise technique: Barbell lunge. *Strength and Conditioning Journal* 24 (5): 30-32.

12. Graham, J.F. 2002. Exercise technique: Front squat. *Strength and Conditioning Journal* 24 (3): 75-76.

13. Graham, J.F. 2003. Exercise technique: Barbell bench press. *Strength and Conditioning Journal* 25 (3): 50-51.

14. Graham, J.F. 2003. Exercise technique: Front lat pulldown. *Strength and Conditioning Journal* 25 (5): 42-43.

15. Graham, J.F. 2004. Exercise technique: Barbell upright row. *Strength and Conditioning Journal* 26 (5): 60-61.

16. Graham, J.F. 2005. Exercise technique: Leg curl. *Strength and Conditioning Journal* 27 (1): 59-60.

17. Graham, J.F. 2008. Exercise technique: Barbell overhead press. *Strength and Conditioning Journal* 30 (3): 70-71.

18. Graham, J.F. 2008. Resistance exercise techniques and spotting. In: *Conditioning for Strength and Human Performance,* T.J. Chandler and L.E. Brown, eds. Philadelphia: Lippincott Williams & Wilkins.

19. Harman, E.A., R.M. Rosenstein, P.N. Frykman, and G.A. Nigro. 1989. Effects of a belt on intra-abdominal pressure during weightlifting. *Medicine and Science in Sports and Exercise* 21 (2): 186-190.

20. Hoffman, J.R., and N.A. Ratamess. 2006. *A Practical Guide to Developing Resistance Training Programs.* Monterey, CA: Coaches Choice.

21. Lander, J.E., J.R. Hundley, and R.L. Simonton. 1990. The effectiveness of weight-belts during multiple repetitions of the squat exercise. *Medicine and Science in Sports and Exercise* 24 (5): 603-609.

22. Lander, J.E., R.L. Simonton, and J.K.F. Giacobbe. 1990. The effectiveness of weight-belts during the squat exercise. *Medicine and Science in Sports and Exercise* 22 (1): 117-126.

23. Newton, H. 2002. *Explosive Lifting for Sports.* Champaign, IL: Human Kinetics.

24. NSCA Certification Commission. 2008. *Exercise Technique Manual for Resistance Training,* 2nd ed. Champaign, IL: Human Kinetics.

Cardiovascular Training Methods

Travis W. Beck, PhD

After completing this chapter, you will be able to

- provide recommendations relevant to cardiovascular activities, including hydration, clothing, footwear, and warm-up and cool-down activities;

- provide advice regarding proper exercise technique on treadmills, rowing machines, stair climbers, elliptical trainers, and stationary bicycles;

- teach clients safe participation in group exercise classes; and

- match clients with cardiovascular activities that are compatible with their preferences and physical capabilities.

The purpose of this chapter is to provide an overview of important considerations when one is prescribing cardiovascular exercise activities. These activities can be classified into machine (e.g., treadmill, stair climber, elliptical trainer) and non-machine (e.g., walking, running, swimming) exercises. A single chapter cannot provide a complete description of these activities; but the most important aspects of proper exercise technique, hydration status, and sound programming are covered. Since personal trainers often work with various types of clients, some of whom may have special needs, knowledge of techniques for incorporating variety

The author would like to acknowledge the contributions of J. Henry "Hank" Drought, who wrote this chapter for the first edition of *NCSA's Essentials of Personal Training*.

into the training program can help to achieve many different training goals.

Safe Participation

The six variables that should be considered to ensure safe participation in cardiovascular activities are (1) proper hydration; (2) appropriate clothing and footwear; (3) warm-up and cool-down; (4) prescription of exercise frequency, intensity, and duration; (5) proper breathing techniques; and (6) exercise program variation. The following sections address these variables.

Hydration

Water makes up roughly 60% of the body mass and functions in regulating body temperature, acting as a solvent for glucose, minerals, amino acids, and vitamins, and provides a cushion and lubricant for joints. Thus, water is particularly important during high-intensity exercise in hot environments, when the body can lose as much as 2 to 4 quarts (about 2 to 3.8 L) of water every hour (30). The digestive system can absorb only approximately 1 quart (about 1 L) per hour. Thus, fluid replacement is most critical when high-intensity exercise is performed for an extended time period in a hot, humid environment. Generally speaking, water is the best fluid replacement for exercise durations of less than 1 hour, but sport drinks with sodium and glucose are recommended for durations greater than 1 hour (27, 30). In addition, although perspiration rates can vary widely among individuals and in different environments, approximately 5 to 7 ml of fluid per kilogram body weight should be consumed at least 4 hours prior to exercise. Furthermore, clients should be encouraged to weigh themselves before and after exercise and to replace each pound that is lost with 20 to 24 ounces (about 0.6 to 0.7 L) of fluid (28).

Clothing and Footwear

Comfortable, loose-fitting clothing is important during aerobic activities because it allows for ease of movement. In very hot environments, the clothing should be as light as possible, while layered clothing should be used in the cold. A great deal of the body's heat is lost through the head and extremities in cold weather, so hats, gloves, and scarves are recommended to prevent excessive heat loss. Proper footwear is also very important for weight-bearing activities such as walking and running. Generally speaking, shoes should provide cushioning, stability, and comfort while maintaining flexibility. The

primary factor determining the quality of a running shoe is its compression capabilities, 50% of which are lost within 300 to 500 miles (483 to 805 km) of use (15). Of course, some running shoes are better than others; but in general, most running shoes should be replaced after 300 to 500 miles of use or every six months, whichever comes first. Runners with a high body weight or an unusual gait (e.g., over- or underpronation) may require more frequent shoe replacement. Tables 14.1 and 14.2 provide recommendations for shoe selection based on the type of activity and foot strike characteristics, and figure 14.1 provides an illustration of overpronation and underpronation.

Running shoes are generally made with three different types of forms: straight, semicurved, or curved (figure 14.2). Overpronators may benefit from a motion-control shoe with a straight last. Underpronators may favor a shoe with a curved last that allows greater foot range of motion. Neutral foot strikers may benefit from shoes with a semicurved last and moderate direction- and foot-control features (14). A consultation with a podiatrist to analyze running biomechanics may be helpful for proper shoe selection.

Warm-Up and Cool-Down

Warm-up and cool-down activities help the cardiovascular and musculoskeletal systems adjust to the workload used during the exercise. If the training program requires exercise at a target heart rate, a 5- to 15-minute warm-up should be used to gradually increase heart rate to the target level, and the exercise session should be followed by a 5- to 15-minute cool-down to reduce heart rate. If desired, 5 to 15 minutes of low-intensity stretching exercises can also be used to help loosen up stiff muscles and joints

TABLE 14.1 Shoe Selection Based on Activity

Activity	GENERAL SHOE CHARACTERISTICS	
	Cushion	Lateral stability
Walking	Moderate	Moderate
Running	High	Low
Aerobics	Moderate to high	Moderate to high
Racket sports	Moderate	High
Cross-training	Moderate to high	Moderate to high

TABLE 14.2 Shoe Selection Based on Foot Strike

Type of foot strike	Specific shoe characteristics
Neutral	Semicurved last; moderate motion control
Overpronators	Straight last; high motion control
Underpronators (supinators)	Curved last; high motion flexibility or straight (figure 14.2)

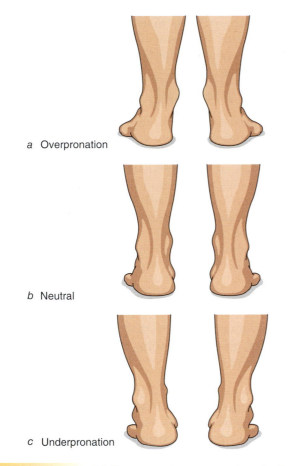

a Overpronation

b Neutral

c Underpronation

FIGURE 14.1 (a) Overpronation occurs when the foot collapses too far inward on the arch with each foot strike. (b) Neutral foot strike. (c) Underpronation (supination) occurs when foot strikes are too much on the outsides of the feet and have too little inward roll.

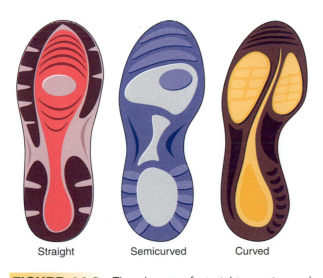

Straight   Semicurved   Curved

FIGURE 14.2 The shapes of straight, semicurved, and curved lasts. Overpronators may benefit from straight lasts, neutral foot strikers from semicurved lasts, and underpronators (supinators) from curved lasts.

after the warm-up or as part of the cool-down (see chapter 12).

Exercise Frequency, Intensity, and Duration

The following are general guidelines for frequency, intensity, and duration of cardiovascular exercise (2).

- Frequency: 2 to 5 sessions per week
- Intensity: 50% to 85% of heart rate reserve
- Duration: 20 to 60 minutes

Generally speaking, most clients are capable of performing a single exercise session continuously. Deconditioned clients, however, may benefit from intermittent bouts performed throughout the day. Chapter 16 provides information on designing aerobic endurance training programs.

Proper Breathing Techniques

It is important for clients to understand that it is not necessary to exercise in a state of breathlessness to achieve cardiovascular benefits. In general, breathing during cardiovascular exercise should be relaxed and regular. A general recommendation is that clients should be able to carry on a casual conversation while exercising and breathing through both the nose and mouth. However, competitive clients may require more advanced training techniques, such as sprint or interval training, that elicit high heart and breathing rates.

Exercise Program Variation

Exercise program variation is important for reducing the chances of overuse injuries. It is also important to remember, however, that introducing new exercises into a program will usually require decreases in intensity. For example, a client who has been riding a stationary bike for 30 minutes three times per week may not be able to immediately switch to treadmill running for 30 minutes three times per week. Instead, the client should be gradually acclimated to the new activity. In addition, each exercise presents a unique stress, thereby eliciting adaptations that are specific to that modality. General adaptations to the cardiovascular and pulmonary systems carry over well from one exercise to the next, but the client's musculoskeletal system and connective tissues will not be accustomed to the mechanical stresses of running if she is usually cycling. Thus, personal trainers should pay careful attention to their clients as they adapt from one exercise modality to the next.

In keeping with the principle of specificity, a client's ability to perform one exercise modality does not completely transfer to another. Personal trainers should pay attention to proper progression when adding activities to a program or substituting new activities.

Training on Cardiovascular Machines

Common cardiovascular machines include treadmills, stair climbers, elliptical trainers, stationary bicycles, and rowing machines. This section discusses the primary muscles used with each piece of equipment and the techniques that should be considered with use of the equipment.

Treadmill

Primary muscles used: quadriceps, hamstrings, gluteals, iliopsoas, tibialis anterior, gastrocnemius, and soleus

Both walking and running can be performed on a treadmill. Important advantages of the treadmill include the conveniences of indoor exercise, handrail support, controlled speed and elevation, and a soft landing surface to reduce the impact forces associated with foot strike.

Stepping on the Belt

Most clients will be familiar with a treadmill and how to step on the belt to begin exercising. However, elderly clients and those undergoing cardiac rehabilitation may need assistance to help them become acclimated to using a treadmill. Personal trainers can do the following to assist clients in need of help on a treadmill:

1. Instruct the client to hold on to the handrails while straddling the belt. Turn the treadmill on and set the speed to 1.0 miles per hour. When the belt begins moving, instruct the client to step on the belt with one foot and then the other to begin walking. Some clients may find it useful to "paw" the belt with one foot several times before stepping on to become acclimated to the speed.

2. Instruct clients to continue to hold the handrails if they feel unsure about their balance. Once they feel comfortable, however, they should let go of the handrails and swing their arms in a natural walking motion.

3. Instruct clients that they should try to stay toward the front of the treadmill and on the center of the belt to reduce the risk for falling.

Treadmill Running

Clients accustomed to running outdoors will find it easier to run indoors on a treadmill, assuming the running speed is the same. This difference is caused by the lack of air resistance on a treadmill, so the body has only to keep up with the belt speed rather than propel itself forward. Thus, treadmill running at a given speed has a lower energy cost than running at the same speed outdoors. One can offset this difference by increasing the treadmill grade to approximately 1% (18). See figure 14.3.

Stair Climber

Primary muscles used: quadriceps, hamstrings, gluteals, erector spinae, gastrocnemius, and soleus

The ground reaction forces at the knee during nonmachine stair climbing can be three to four times body weight (25). Escalator-type stair climber machines help to reduce these knee stresses because the downward stroke of the leg is assisted by the moving step. A disadvantage, however, is that these

Reducing Handrail Usage

When possible, personal trainers should strive to reduce handrail usage among their clients for both the treadmill and stair climber. General procedures for achieving this include instructing the client to hold the handrails in the following progression.

1. Two hands lightly
2. The fingers of two hands
3. One hand, with the other arm swinging at the side
4. The fingers of one hand
5. Only one finger of one hand

Clients should progress through steps 1 to 5 in order until they can release the handrails completely. For both the treadmill and stair climber, clients who use the handrails tend to support too much of their body weight, thereby reducing the workload demands. Excessive handrail usage can also compromise postural alignment, thereby increasing the risk for lower back injury.

machines do not allow for variations in step height, which can make their use difficult for very short clients. Pedal-based stair climbers allow for adjustment of stepping depth, and generally speaking, a greater stepping depth requires more muscle activation. An important drawback is that deconditioned clients may not be able to use a stair climber even at the lowest work levels (1).

Body Position

The manufacturers design stair climbers to be used with the client facing and stepping forward onto the pedals. Thus, reversing the body position and facing out is not recommended because it can place excessive stress on the lower back, thereby increasing the risk for injury.

Hip movement during stair climbing is beneficial. However, uncontrolled and exaggerated hip movement should be discouraged. Extreme side-to-side rocking at the hips indicates excessive stepping

depth and usually results in compromised postural alignment due to too much forward flexion at the spine (31). The personal trainer should reduce the stepping depth, speed, or both until the client can comfortably balance the torso over the hips and maintain good postural alignment.

Range of Movement

Height and fitness level are the primary determinants of stair stepping depth. An appropriate range of movement is usually from 4 to 8 inches (10 to 20 cm) (19). Excessive depth is usually indicated by side-to-side rocking of the hips, while a depth that is too shallow will not properly stress the target muscles, and, in turn, the cardiovascular system. Generally speaking, all clients should strive to achieve a stepping depth that promotes proper posture and works the muscles adequately.

Stepping Speed

Stepping speed generally ranges from 43 to 95 steps per minute (29). A stepping speed that is too fast usually results in (1) excessive hip movement to keep up with the stepping depth or (2) short, fast steps that result in a stepping depth that is too shallow. Both of these extremes should be discouraged; but it is important for the client to become comfortable with a stepping speed that elicits the appropriate metabolic demands yet encourages proper biomechanics.

> When clients are performing stair climbing, elliptical trainer, or stationary bicycling exercise, the knee should not come forward in front of the toe when the leg is in the flexed position. This produces added strain on the knee and can cause injury.

Elliptical Trainer

Primary muscles used: quadriceps, hamstrings, gluteals, iliopsoas, tibialis anterior, gastrocnemius, and soleus

Elliptical trainers are useful because they combine the motions involved in stair climbing with those in walking or running. The advantage of elliptical trainers is that they are very low impact, and most models allow the upper body to contribute at least partially to the movement. This is important from a practical standpoint because it increases the amount of muscle mass involved in the activity and therefore the total caloric expenditure. The following sections present important considerations with use of an elliptical trainer.

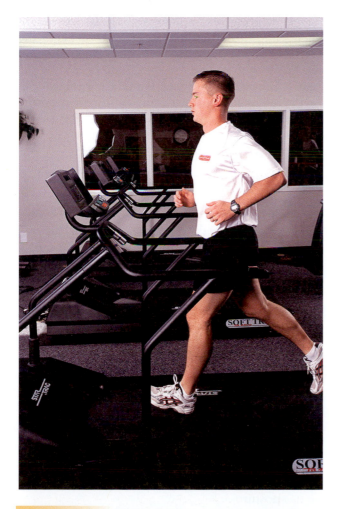

FIGURE 14.3 Treadmill running at a given speed uses less energy than running outdoors. Increasing the treadmill's incline to 1% will offset this difference.

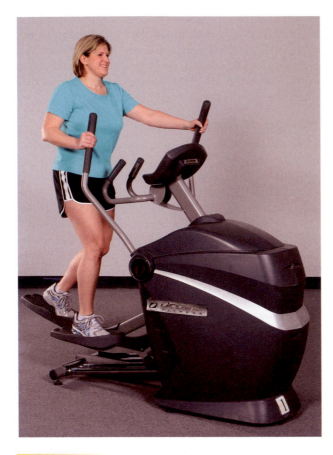

FIGURE 14.4 Proper elliptical trainer exercise technique: head up, looking straight ahead, torso balanced over hips with no excessive forward lean.

Foot Placement and Handrail Usage

The whole foot should be in contact with the pedal surface at all times unless the machine requires lifting of the heel (e.g., figure 14.4). In addition, although many elliptical trainers do not have side handrails, the handrails on those that do should be used only for balancing purposes.

Body Position and Knee Placement

All clients who use the elliptical trainer should remain upright with the torso balanced over the hips. In addition, the knees should not come in front of the toes, since this position places additional strain on the joint that can lead to injury.

Cadence, Elevation, Resistance, and Direction of Movement

Generally speaking, movements with slow cadences resemble the walking motion, while those with fast cadences are closer to a running movement. Motions on medium-level inclines resemble walking and running up hills, while those on high inclines are

similar to stair climbing. Another unique feature of elliptical trainers is that they allow pedaling in both the forward and reverse directions, which allows the muscles to work in slightly different ways. Thus, changing the direction of movement may be a useful method for introducing variation into the exercise program.

> Low-impact cardiovascular training machines (e.g., elliptical trainers, stationary bicycles), as well as swimming, can be used for clients who have orthopedic problems like arthritis and low back pain.

Stationary Bicycles

Primary muscles used: quadriceps, hamstrings, gluteals, tibialis anterior, gastrocnemius, and soleus

Stationary cycling has the advantage that it is non-weight bearing and nonimpact. Thus, overweight clients and those with orthopedic problems of the low back, knees, ankles, or feet may benefit from the fact that their body weight is supported by the seat. A drawback, however, is that the exercise can be limited by local muscle fatigue, thereby resulting in a suboptimal cardiovascular stimulus. The following sections discuss some important aspects of use of a stationary bicycle.

Seat Height

The seat height should allow for a slight bend in the knee joint at the bottom of the pedal stroke, which permits maximum extension of the leg without locking of the knee joint (figure 14.5). A general guideline is that the seat height should be at approximately midhip level when the client is standing next to the bicycle. Most clients can readjust the seat height if they feel that the range of motion is too short or too long.

Handlebars and Body Positioning

Handlebar positioning should allow the back to be tilted forward from the hips, but not excessively rounded. Some stationary bicycles use "bullhorn" handlebars that allow for a variety of hand positions, including the following:

1. A palms-facing-down grip on the front of the handlebar, which requires a more upright posture

2. A neutral palms-facing-in grip on the sides of the handlebar, which uses more forward lean

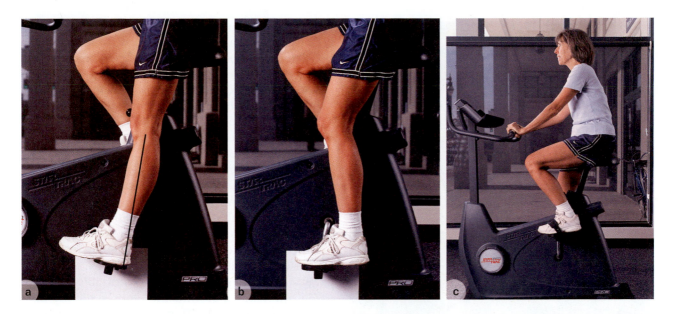

FIGURE 14.5 Proper seat height adjustment: (a) leg straight with knee locked and heel on pedal; (b) knee slightly bent with ball of foot on pedal; (c) with the pedal at 12 o'clock, the knee will be about even with the hips and approximately parallel with the floor.

3. A position in which the forearms rest on the sides of the handlebar, thereby supporting much of the upper body weight and encouraging forward lean

Many clients will find it useful to adjust their hand positioning during longer rides, although some stationary bicycles do not allow for handlebar adjustments.

Cadence and Pedaling Action

In general, the most economical pedaling cadence ranges from 60 to 100 revolutions per minute (rpm), with beginners preferring lower pedaling rates and trained cyclists preferring higher cadences. Pedaling at too high a cadence, however, results in wasted energy due to added muscular work needed to stabilize the trunk (16, 20, 21, 24, 32). Most clients are able to sense the pedaling cadence that allows for the greatest economy. In addition, most of the force production during cycling is applied in a forward and downward direction during the downstroke. For most clients, the upstroke contributes very little to the overall power output, and the quadriceps femoris and gluteal muscles generate nearly all of the power needed for the movement. In some cases, the calf muscles can aid in the downstroke, but they do not contribute significantly to the overall power output.

Semirecumbent Bikes

Many training facilities have semirecumbent bikes that provide back support and a wider seat that is particularly beneficial for overweight clients, those with low back pain, and pregnant women. Heart rate, oxygen consumption rate, and rating of perceived exertion on a semirecumbent bike are typically lower than on an upright bike (given the same workload). There are two primary reasons for this phenomenon: (1) The back support of a semirecumbent bike reduces the workload placed on postural muscles, and (2) the semirecumbent position prevents the heart from having to pump blood vertically against gravity (10). Figure 14.6 shows proper body positioning on a semirecumbent bike.

Group Indoor Cycling

Group indoor cycling generally provides a higher-intensity workout than is performed during individual cycling. This form of cycling is usually performed with music in a class atmosphere, with instructors guiding the class on a simulated ride that lasts anywhere from 30 to 45 minutes. It is important to point out that beginners should usually develop a good baseline level of conditioning before starting a cycling class. They should do this on their own time; and when they feel they are ready, they should start with a beginning-level class and progress to more advanced classes.

Group indoor cycling bikes typically additionally allow fore (forward) and aft (backward) seat adjustments. When set properly, fore and aft seat adjustments encourage optimal force production on the downstroke and better safety for the knee. To adjust the fore and aft seat position, the client

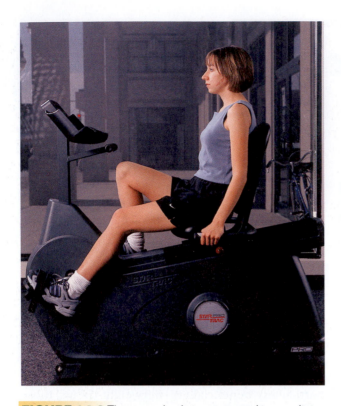

FIGURE 14.6 The upper body is supported in a reclining position on a semirecumbent bike; the seat is adjusted to allow a slight bend at the knee (similar to the situation with a standard stationary bike).

should set the pedals parallel to the floor at 3 and 9 o'clock, then adjust the seat forward or backward so that at 3 o'clock the knee does not come forward in front of the toe. A plumb line dropped from the tibial tuberosity (small bump just below the kneecap) should contact the ball of the foot at the center of the pedal. The knee should not come forward in front of the toe, since this reduces optimal force output and may lead to knee injuries (22).

Group indoor cycling bikes also allow handlebar height adjustments. Handlebar height is largely a function of individual preference, but normally the handlebar should be set level with the tip of the saddle. Novices and clients with poor back flexibility may prefer the handlebar higher to allow a more upright sitting posture (figure 14.7a). Either way, the arms should be a comfortable distance from the handlebar with the elbows slightly bent at a minimum of 15°. The angle between the torso and the upper arm typically measures approximately 90° (or slightly less) (12, 22). Some bikes also include handlebar fore and aft positioning, which allows further adjustment to maximize comfort. A more forward-leaning upper body "racing" posture (figure 14.7b) is used more often during group indoor cycling than for standard stationary bicycling on electronic and generator-driven bikes.

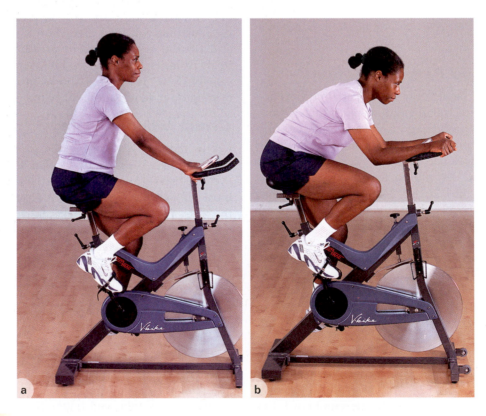

FIGURE 14.7 Proper body position on group cycling bike (a) when not racing and (b) when racing.

Rowing Machines

Primary muscles used: quadriceps, hamstrings, gluteals, tibialis anterior, gastrocnemius, soleus, biceps brachii, brachioradialis, brachialis, rectus abdominis, posterior and medial deltoids, trapezius, latissimus dorsi, teres major, erector spinae, and flexor and extensor carpi ulnaris

Rowing is a very good non-weight-bearing activity that stimulates both the upper and lower body. Since a very large portion of the entire muscle mass is used to perform the rowing motion, the risk for local muscle fatigue is low. The only disadvantage is that many clients are not familiar with the movement, and beginners tend to perform the row too much with their upper body. In addition, those with low back pain tend to round the back too much. Proper body positioning is very important in rowing (see figure 14.8).

Starting Position and the Drive

For the starting position, clients should have their head upright, looking straight ahead, with an upright back and slight forward lean. The arms are straight in front of the body, and the hips and knees are flexed. From this position, they should perform the drive by extending the hips and legs forcefully while leaning the torso back slightly. Only after the hips and legs have been extended should the arms be used to pull the handle to the abdomen.

The Finish, Recovery, and Catch

For the finish, the legs are fully extended, the torso leans backward slightly, the elbows are flexed, and the handle is pulled into the abdomen. The recovery, in turn, involves extension of the elbows followed by a forward lean of the torso at the hip joint. The catch resumes the starting position. Specifically, the torso leans forward slightly at the hips, the arms are straight, and the shins are vertical in preparation for the next stroke.

Resistance and Cadence

Although rowing machines use various designs, a very common design uses air as the resistance. Specifically, an air vent controls the amount of air that reaches the flywheel. As more air is allowed through the vent, the resistance on the flywheel increases. All beginners should start at a low resistance and increase the workload as their conditioning improves. Most recreational rowers row at a moderate cadence of approximately 20 to 25 strokes per minute, and elite rowers generally row at a faster rate (e.g., 25-35 strokes per minute).

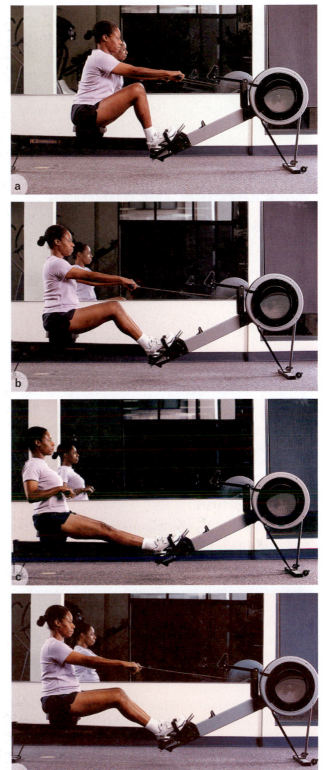

FIGURE 14.8 Proper body position on the rowing machine: (a) starting position (and the catch); (b) the drive; (c) the finish; (d) the recovery.

> The cardiovascular training modality chosen should conform to equipment availability; it should also be comfortable for the client and help the client achieve his or her fitness goals. It is important to start the client's program at a level that matches the client's fitness level and then progress slowly.

Nonmachine Cardiovascular Exercise Techniques

Nonmachine exercises like walking and running are generally less expensive than machine activities and are often easy to fit into a client's schedule. This section deals with walking, running, swimming, group exercise classes, and aqua exercise.

Walking

Primary muscles used: quadriceps, hamstrings, gluteals, iliopsoas, tibialis anterior, gastrocnemius, and soleus

Any walking, regardless of the biomechanics used, is good for beginners. However, as conditioning improves, clients should strive to achieve the proper body position, foot strike, hip action, and arm action as explained next.

Body Position

Proper posture is very important during walking because it improves efficiency and decreases strain on the lower back and entire vertebral column. Clients should be told that proper posture is characterized by "walking tall" and should imagine a string that pulls the head upward and straightens the vertebral column. The shoulders should be relaxed but not rounded, and the upper body should be positioned directly over the hips.

Foot Strike

Foot strike during walking occurs when the heel strikes the ground and the body weight is transferred through the foot in a gentle rolling action from the heel to the ball of the foot. Abnormal foot strike patterns are usually characterized by excessive weight transfer to either the inside or outside of the foot (see figure 14.1), neither of which is healthy, and the result is potential injury.

Hip Action

People can increase walking speed by increasing **stride frequency**, **stride length,** or both. Beginners

may find it useful to do some light stretching before walking to improve hip mobility. Improved hip movement ensures adequate stride length. Gradually increasing stride frequency, stride length, or both is an excellent way to increase training intensity during walking.

Arm Action

Arm and leg action should be coordinated during walking, with the left arm swinging forward with the right leg, the right arm with the left leg. At fast walking speeds, the elbows should be flexed such that the joint angle is 90° and the hands are brought upward to chest level. This swinging action from the hips to the chest and back helps to propel the body forward.

Race Walking

There are two primary differences between normal walking and race walking. First, the rules of competitive race walking require one foot to be in contact with the ground at all times. Second, the leg must be fully extended from the time the foot lands until the body passes over the supporting leg. Competitive race walkers improve performance by maximizing stride length. This is accomplished by increasing hip rotation (i.e., the "pelvic roll" commonly used in race walking) (see figure 14.9).

The success of competitive race walkers is dictated by their ability to consistently produce stride

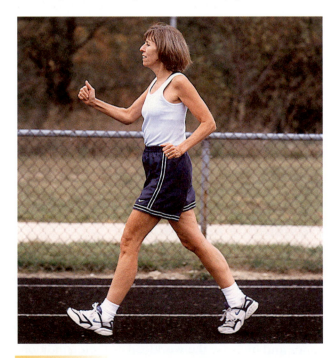

FIGURE 14.9 Proper race walking technique dictates that one foot must always be in contact with the ground, and the support leg must remain straight. Race walkers increase stride length with increased hip rotation.

lengths just a few inches longer than a normal stride length. Many clients are unsure, however, when it is appropriate to incorporate running into their program. Generally speaking, when a client can walk roughly 4 miles (6.4 km) without becoming fatigued, he should start a walk/run program. These programs alternate periods of walking and running (e.g., a 1- to 2-minute run followed by a 3- to 5-minute walk), with this sequence repeated for the necessary duration. Progression is accomplished as the amount of running time is increased until running is continuous. It is important to remember, however, that running is a high-impact activity. Overweight clients and those with orthopedic problems may require low-impact cardiovascular activities such as cycling or swimming.

Running

Primary muscles used: quadriceps, hamstrings, gluteals, iliopsoas, tibialis anterior, gastrocnemius, and soleus

Running produces outstanding cardiovascular benefits and, like walking, is a low-cost exercise. Running is time efficient for conditioned clients and is sport specific for recreational athletes whose sport involves running. The net energy cost of running is generally greater than for walking and therefore requires specific techniques to conserve energy and reduce the risk of impact injury. Bouncing with each step should be avoided because it wastes energy through vertical displacement and increases shock. The heel–ball method is the safest foot strike for running long distances because the impact is well absorbed by the entire foot. Foot strike abnormalities, like overpronation and underpronation, have greater consequences during running than during walking because of the foot strike impact.

Body Position and Foot Strike

Running is similar to walking in that clients should be told to "run tall" by keeping the head upright, the shoulders relaxed, and the torso balanced over the hips. Foot strike is achieved through a heel-to-ball rolling action. Specifically, the heel touches the ground first, and the body weight is spread through the foot with a gentle rolling action (figure 14.10). Thus, it is important for clients to concentrate on preventing the foot from slapping the ground as they run, since this can cause orthopedic problems. Instead, running should be thought of as a gliding motion with as little impact force as possible.

Arm Action

During long-distance running, the arms hang from relaxed shoulders and are bent at the elbows. Some arm action occurs from the shoulders, but too much shoulder movement wastes energy. Much of the arm movement comes from the lower arm (forearm, wrist, and hand) by means of hinging at the elbow. In this way, the elbow is unlocked, and the angle at the elbow opens during the arm downswing and closes during the upswing. The forearms are carried between the waist and chest. If the arms are carried too high, the shoulders and upper back become fatigued. If the arms are carried too low, excessive forward lean may occur. The hands are gently cupped, and the thumb softly touches the index finger. The hands should not be clenched into fists. On the forward swing, the hands reach chest height. On the backward swing, the hands reach the hips at the side of the body. The arms and hands also move slightly inward, but the hands do not cross the midline of the body. The wrists should be relaxed but not held too loosely.

Stride Length

Running speed, like walking speed, is determined by stride length and stride frequency. To improve

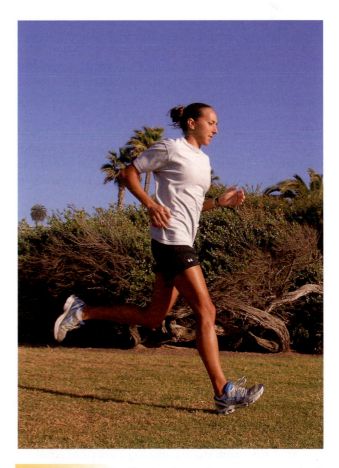

FIGURE 14.10 During long-distance or treadmill running, proper foot strike involves contact with the heel and then a gentle "rolling" action toward the ball of the foot for push-off.

running performance, it is necessary to increase stride length, stride frequency, or both. A client's exact stride length depends on leg length, flexibility, strength, coordination, and level of fatigue. With each running step, the feet should land approximately under the hips. If the foot hits too far in front of the body's center of gravity, greater shock and a slight braking effect will occur. This is **overstriding.** Braking, as well as too much time spent in the air, makes overstriding inefficient. Many runners overreach with the front leg and foot in an effort to improve stride length. This is counterproductive and will likely cause braking. **Understriding** (taking too short a stride) also wastes energy, since it prevents the body from advancing far enough with each stride. The best way to improve stride length is to increase rear leg drive by improving strength and to increase range of motion by improving flexibility. Plyometric exercises may also increase rear leg drive and may be added to the program when appropriate.

Stride Frequency

To increase stride frequency, the client should be instructed to simply take quicker, softer, relaxed steps and keep the feet low to the ground. Plyometric exercises, when appropriate, may also be used to increase stride frequency. People who are running for health benefits may not see the importance of improving stride frequency and stride length, since speed and racing are not the goal. One safety reason is worth mentioning, though. A slow overstride usually results in a raised center of gravity and more time spent in the air. This leads to a harder landing and greater impact. Therefore, a slow overstride may cause not only loss of speed, but also an increased risk of injury.

Swimming

Primary muscles used: dependent on the stroke being used, but can be nearly a full-body activity

The four competitive swimming strokes are the front stroke, backstroke, breaststroke, and butterfly. All strokes can provide an excellent stimulus to the cardiovascular system and are very low impact. It is recommended, however, that American Red Cross–certified Water Safety Instructors be used to teach clients with no swimming experience before they begin any exercise program. A discussion of proper technique for all strokes is beyond the scope of this chapter; the following is a brief discussion of instruction on the front stroke.

The front stroke (also known as **freestyle** or **front crawl**) is the most popular and fastest stroke. Since this stroke uses both the upper and lower body, it is highly dependent on proper coordination, and it also provides an excellent stimulus to the cardiovascular system (4).

Body Position

With freestyle swimming, the body is prone and straight, the head should be held in a natural position with the eyes looking at the bottom of the pool or slightly forward. Extraneous lateral or vertical movements should be avoided as much as possible, since they reduce horizontal velocity. This straight and streamlined position also incorporates a body roll that is initiated by the hips and then includes the shoulders, legs, and feet. The head should be turned only to take a breath, and this turning should just be an extension of the body roll, which involves four basic steps: (1) rotation of the hips, (2) lifting of the recovery arm, (3) forward propulsion by the pulling arm, and (4) leg kick that produces lateral force as the legs roll with the rest of the body. Body roll not only allows easier breathing and improves arm propulsion but also reduces drag forces and decreases shoulder stresses.

Arm Stroke

The arm stroke action in the front stroke is very important because it provides as much as 80% to 90% of the propulsion force needed to move the body through the water. The arm stroke consists of three phases: (1) the entry/catch phase, (2) the power phase, and (3) the recovery phase. Entry of the hand occurs in front of the shoulder and slightly lateral to the midline of the body. The elbow should be flexed slightly and held high, which allows the arm to enter the water cleanly and ensures an effective pulling position. The fingertips, hand, forearm, elbow, and shoulder all enter the water in the same location and in sequential order. The catch occurs just after entry and allows the hand and forearm to "catch" the water in front of the shoulder. The catch is important because it properly positions the hand and arm so that they can pull effectively during the stroke. This action should be thought of as "feeling" for the water, similar to the way a mountain climber grabs a piece of rock with an outstretched arm to pull the body upward.

The power phase is important because it is the primary propulsive phase of the arm stroke. The power phase involves pulling the body forward through the water by accelerating the hand and forearm backward with a pulling action. This action occurs in an "S"-shaped pattern in which the hand sweeps downward and slightly outward. The hand and arm then move slightly inward and backward toward the chest and middle of the body as the elbow is bent to roughly 90°. The hand is then rotated to a neutral position with the palm facing backward, and the arm is extended outward, upward, and backward past the thigh. The last portion of the backward pull past the thigh is the most forceful portion of the power phase and is when the arm has maximum pulling capacity. In addition, this last part of the stroke should be coupled with the body roll to maximize propulsion. However, the "S"-shaped movements are very subtle and span a width of only 4 to 8 inches (10 to 20 cm) (see figure 14.11). The fingers should not be held together tightly, but should be comfortable and relaxed.

The final phase involves recovery and prepares the arm for another pull. First, the elbow is lifted high out of the water and the hand is turned inward toward the legs. The high elbow position allows the forearm to hang downward. Once the hand has cleared the water, it is brought forward and in position for the next power phase.

Leg Kick

The primary functions of the leg kick are to balance the body and help maintain a horizontal position. In most swimmers, the leg kick does not contribute meaningfully to forward propulsion (13, 17). During the front stroke, the leg kick is best described as a flutter kick that ranges in amplitude from 12 to 15 inches (30 to 40 cm). The downward thrust of the kick is the power portion and the one that provides the most propulsion. The foot should remain plantarflexed, with the kick originating from the hips and continuing with very slight knee extension and

flexion. During the recovery portion of the kick (the upward thrust), the leg rises until the heel is just above the surface of the water.

Many swimmers use a two-beat kick, with the feet kicking two times for every arm cycle. It is important, however, to acknowledge that with long-distance swimming, emphasis should be placed on kicking just fast enough to stay afloat to conserve energy. Elite swimmers usually try to maximize kicking propulsion. For example, high-level sprint swimmers primarily use a six-beat kick because they are not concerned with conserving energy.

Breathing

Breathing should occur when the head turns to the side as a natural part of the body rotation. The head should stay level, with the forehead just higher than the chin. A breath can then be taken in the trough created by the head when it turns. Many beginners make the mistake of lifting the head, which causes the hips to sink. After the inhale, the head is turned back into the water with the body roll. At low intensities, it is possible to exhale through the nose only; but during maximal efforts, it is important to exhale forcefully through the mouth and nose to ensure exhalation of all the air.

Group Exercise Classes

Primary muscles used: dependent on the exercises involved, but can be nearly a full-body activity

The traditional aerobics classes of the past have evolved to include many group exercise classes, including kickboxing, step classes, group resistance

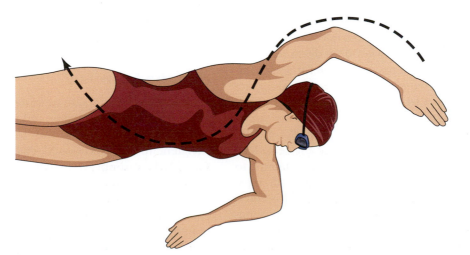

FIGURE 14.11 The subtle "S"-shaped hand pattern during the power phase of the freestyle (front crawl) arm stroke in swimming.

Adapted by permission from Maglisch 2003.

training, aqua exercises, tai chi, and fitness yoga (3). These classes typically provide various cardio-vascular activities that are choreographed with music. The purpose of this section is not to cover the various cardiovascular classes in depth. Instead, it presents a brief discussion of aerobics, step classes, kickboxing, and aqua exercise. Safety is very important during group exercise, particularly good posture and body position. As with most exercises, the shoulders should be relaxed but not rounded, and the torso should be kept upright. In addition, during all activities that require knee flexion, the knee joint should not come in front of the toes.

> Clients in group exercise classes should maintain good posture, aligning the ear, shoulder, and hip; slightly contract the abdominal and gluteal muscles to prevent excessive back arching; and ensure that when they flex the knee joint, the knee does not come in front of the toe.

Traditional Aerobics

Traditional aerobics classes range in duration from 45 to 75 minutes. Each class session usually begins with a warm-up and preworkout stretching, followed by the aerobic activity, cool-down, and postworkout stretching. Each section uses a different time requirement, based on the emphasis of the class session.

The aerobics portion of a class can be low impact, moderate impact, high impact, or a combination of these. In low-impact aerobics, one foot remains in contact with the floor at all times; and ways of altering intensity include changing the amount of muscle mass used, lifting and lowering the center of gravity, and changing the range of motion and tempo, as well as side-to-side and forward and backward traveling. Low-impact aerobics is very good for deconditioned, beginning, or obese clients as well as for senior clients and pregnant women, since the vertical impact forces range from 1 to 1.25 times body weight (11). In moderate-impact aerobics, one foot is in contact with the floor at all times, and the center of gravity is raised and lowered on the balls of the feet. This results in vertical impact forces that range from 2 to 2.5 times body weight (11). With high-impact aerobics, both feet leave the floor as the body is lifted into the air. This movement occurs through running, jumping, hopping, and leaping. Obviously, this type of workout is vigorous and is appropriate only for well-conditioned clients. The vertical impact forces of high-impact aerobics are greater than three times body weight (11).

Step Training

Step training uses a small platform ranging in height from 4 to 12 inches (10 to 30 cm). The participants step up and down to music while performing various movements and sequences using large muscle groups. Intensity can be increased simply by raising the step height, but this form of training should not be used for clients who have knee problems. Simply stepping up and down on a bench 6 to 8 inches (15 to 20 cm) high produces impact forces of approximately 1.4 to 1.5 times body weight, which is roughly the same as those for brisk walking. However, when the stepping speed is increased and propulsive moves are added, the impact forces may get as high as 2.5 times body weight (9, 23, 28). Thus, propulsive moves should always be directed up onto the platform, and never down onto the floor. In addition, it is recommended that the step height for beginners produce a maximum of 60° of knee flexion to reduce the risk for knee injury (9, 26).

Kickboxing

Kickboxing simulates martial arts training by using choreographed kicks and punching moves. These classes usually involve "shadow boxing" sessions rather than contact sparring against an opponent. They are usually 45 to 90 minutes in duration and should devote adequate time to warm-up, cool-down, and stretching.

Beginners should be encouraged to learn the kickboxing moves correctly, since injuries often occur when clients try to do too much too soon. Beginners may also require at least one day of rest between classes to recover from workouts. More advanced clients can use punching combinations, speed kicking, and kicks above the waist after they have properly warmed up. Some advanced clients even prefer to progress to heavy bags, speed bags, and other punching and kicking equipment.

Aquatic Exercise

Aquatic exercise is a safe training modality because the buoyancy of the water reduces the impact of landing on joints. Thus, this form of exercise is excellent for deconditioned clients or those who are elderly, are obese, or have low back pain (7). Aqua exercise has the advantage that swimming expertise is not necessary. In addition, some obese clients may appreciate the fact that their entire body is submerged in the water rather than exposed for others to see. Proper hydration is important during aquatic exercise. Clients often neglect this aspect of aquatic exercise because they may not be sweating at high rates. However, respiration causes fluid loss as well, so clients should be instructed to drink plenty of fluids after workouts.

Aquatic exercises can be performed in shallow or deep water with an upright body position. Generally speaking, a body submerged to the waist bears 50% of its weight, one submerged to the chest bears 25% to 35%, and one submerged to the neck bears only 10% (5, 6). The basic aquatic movements include walking, jogging, kicking, jumping, and scissors. Walking can be done with high knees, backward, sideways, and on toes to provide variation. Jogging can be performed either in place or with a traveling motion. Greater speed of movement results in higher intensity, and additional arm movements can be used to add variety. Kicking movements with one leg can be forward, sideways, and backward; other kicking movements are knee lifts and leg curls. During all movements, the client should avoid hyperextension of the legs. Clients can also perform swimming flutter kicks when seated at the side of the pool or lying prone and holding on to the side of the pool. Participants can perform jumping activities on one or both feet, and rebounding from the bottom of the pool increases intensity. Jumping variations include jumping jacks, traveling jumps, jumping with a twist, frog jumps, and leaps (8). All participants should learn proper landing technique before performing jumping movements. A proper landing is a toe–ball–heel landing with "soft" knees (extended but not locked) directly over the ankles

to absorb body weight impact and reduce the risk of injury. Scissors movements involve simultaneous arm and leg actions that are similar to those in cross-country skiing. Larger-amplitude movements and rebounding off the pool bottom can increase workout intensity.

Other aquatic exercises include squats, lunges, leg extension and flexion, and forearm flexion and extension, just to name a few. It is also important to point out that clients who are elite runners can use aquatic exercise or deep water running (or both) as a supplement to dryland running if they are injured. This allows them to maintain both a high level of cardiovascular conditioning and running specificity. The feet can touch the bottom of the pool, or flotation devices can help the client stay afloat.

Conclusion

All cardiovascular activities should be performed with proper technique, since poor technique can lead to injuries. The personal trainer is responsible for helping clients choose activities that are appropriate for their capabilities. However, when possible, variety should be added to the program to decrease the chance for overuse injuries. Long-term adherence to the proper exercise program is an important key to maintaining a high level of physical fitness throughout one's life.

Study Questions

1. Which of the following is correct regarding the amount of fluid that should be ingested for every pound of body weight lost during exercise?

   A. one cup

   B. one gallon

   C. 10 to 14 ounces

   D. 20 to 24 ounces

2. Which of the following is the first action to perform when using a treadmill?

   A. set the treadmill incline to 0°

   B. hold on to the handrails while straddling the belt

   C. walk/run toward the front part of the treadmill deck

   D. turn on the machine to a speed of no more than 1 mile per hour (0.6 km/h)

3. Which of the following instructions should be given to a client for using a stair climber?

   A. "Place your entire foot on the pedal to start, but allow the heels to lift off as each pedal rises."

   B. "Lean forward slightly, especially as the workout becomes harder."

   C. "Lock out the knees at the bottom of each step."

   D. "Hold the handrails for balance if necessary."

4. Which of the following describes correct body position on a stationary bicycle?

   A. With the ball of the foot on the upward pedal, the knee is above the height of the hips.

   B. With the heel of the foot on the downward pedal, the leg is straight.

   C. With the heel of the foot on the upward pedal, the knee is even with height of the hips.

   D. With the ball of the foot on the downward pedal, the leg is straight.

Applied Knowledge Question

Explain the similarities and differences in the exercise technique guidelines (e.g., body position, foot strike, arm action) that a personal trainer gives a client for *walking* and *running*.

References

1. American College of Sports Medicine. 2010. *ACSM's Resource Manual for Guidelines for Exercise Testing and Prescription,* 6th ed. Philadelphia: Lippincott Williams & Wilkins.

2. American College of Sports Medicine. 2009. *ACSM's Guidelines for Exercise Testing and Prescription,* 8th ed. Baltimore: Lippincott Williams & Wilkins.

3. American Council on Exercise. 2008. *Group Fitness Instructor Manual. 2nd ed.* San Diego: Author.

4. American Red Cross. 1992. *Swimming and Diving.* Boston: American Red Cross. pp. 112-119, 236.

5. Aquatic Exercise Association. 2010. *Aquatic Fitness Professional Manual,* 6th ed. Nokomis, FL: Author.

6. Aquatic Exercise Association. 2001. *The Water Well Newsletter 6.*

7. Ariyoshi, M., K. Sonoda, K. Nagata, T. Mashima, M. Zenmyo, C. Paku, Y. Takamiya, H. Yoshimatsu, Y. Hirai, H. Yasunaga, H. Akashi, H. Imayama, T. Shimokobe, A. Inoue, and Y. Mutoh. 1999. Efficacy of aquatic exercises for patients with low-back pain. *Kurume Medical Journal* 46 (2): 91-96.

8. Bonelli, S. 2001. *Aquatic Exercise.* San Diego: American Council on Exercise.

9. Bonelli, S. 2000. *Step Training.* San Diego: American Council on Exercise.

10. Bonzheim, S.C., B.A. Franklin, C. Dewitt, C. Marks, B. Goslin, R. Jarski, and S. Dann. 1992. Physiologic responses to recumbent versus upright cycle ergometry, and implications for exercise prescription in patients with coronary artery disease. *American Journal of Cardiology* 69 (1): 40-44.

11. Bricker, K. 2000. *Traditional Aerobics.* San Diego: American Council on Exercise.

12. Burke, E.R., ed. 1988. *The Science of Cycling.* Champaign, IL: Human Kinetics.

13. Deschodt, V.J., L.M. Arsac, and A.H. Rouard. 1999. Relative contribution of arms and legs in humans to propulsion in 25-m sprint front-crawl swimming. *European Journal of Applied Physiology and Occupational Physiology* 80 (3): 192-199.

14. Evans, M. 1997. *Endurance Athlete's Edge.* Champaign, IL: Human Kinetics. pp. 75-77, 93.

15. Glover, B., and S.L. Florence Glover. 1999. *The Competitive Runner's Handbook,* rev. ed. New York: Penguin Books. pp. 336-337.

16. Hagberg, J.M., J.P. Mullin, M.D. Giese, and E. Spitznagel. 1981. Effect of pedaling rate on submaximal exercise responses of competitive cyclists. *Journal of Applied Physiology* 51 (2): 447-451.

17. Hobson, W., C. Campbell, and M. Vickers. 2001. *Swim, Bike, Run.* Champaign, IL: Human Kinetics. pp. 45-54.

18. Jones, A.M., and J.H. Doust. 1996. A 1% treadmill grade most accurately reflects the energetic cost of outdoor running. *Journal of Sports Science* 14 (4): 321-327.

19. Kordich, J.A. 1994. *Stair Machine. Treadmill. Teaching Technique Series.* Colorado Springs, CO: National Strength and Conditioning Association.

20. Lepers, R., G.Y. Millet, N.A. Maffiuletti, C. Hausswirth, and J. Brisswalter. 2001. Effect of pedaling rates on physiological response during endurance cycling. *European Journal of Applied Physiology* 85 (3-4): 392-395.

21. Lucia, A., J. Hoyos, and J.L. Chicharro. 2001. Preferred pedaling cadence in professional cycling. *Medicine and Science in Sports and Exercise* 33 (8): 1361-1366.

22. Mad Dogg Athletics. 2010. The spinning program – keeping it safe. www.spinning.com/images/Keep_it_Safe.pdf. Accessed Feb. 2, 2011.

23. Michaud, T., J. Rodriguez-Zavas, C. Armstrong, et al. 1993. Ground reaction forces in high impact and low impact aerobic dance. *Journal of Sports Medicine and Physical Fitness* 33: 359-366.

24. Neptune, R.R., and W. Herzog. 1999. The association between negative muscle work and pedaling rate. *Journal of Biomechanics* 32 (10): 1021-1026.

25. Nordin, M., and V.H. Frankel. 2001. *Basic Biomechanics of the Musculoskeletal System.* 3rd ed. Philadelphia: Lea & Febiger.

26. Reilly, D., and M. Martens. 1972. Experimental analysis of quadriceps muscle force and patellofemoral joint reaction force for various activities. *Acta Orthopaedica Scandanavica* 43:16-37.

27. Sawka, M.N., L.M. Burke, E.R. Eichner, R.J. Maughan, S.J. Montain, and N.S. Stachenfeld. 2007. American College of Sports Medicine position stand. Exercise and fluid replacement. *Medicine and Science In Sports and Exercise* 39 (2): 377-390.

28. Scharff-Olson, M., and H. Williford. 1998. Step aerobics fulfills its promise. *ACSM's Health & Fitness Journal* 2: 32-37.

29. Shih, J., Y.T. Wang, and M.H. Moeinzadeh. 1996. Effect of speed and experience on kinetic and kinematic factors during exercise on a stair-climbing machine. *Journal of Sport Rehabilitation* 5 (3): 224-233.

30. Sizer, F., and E. Whitney. 2011. *Nutrition: Concepts and Controversies,* 12th ed. Pacific Cove, CA: Brooks Cole.

31. Stairmaster Health & Fitness Products. 2001. *Stair Climbing: From Head to Toe.* Kirkland, WA: Stairmaster Health & Fitness Products.

32. Takaishi, T., Y. Yasuda, T. Ono, and T. Moritani. 1996. Optimal pedaling rate estimated from neuromuscular fatigue for cyclists. *Medicine and Science in Sports and Exercise* 28 (12): 1492-1497.

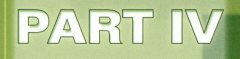

Program Design

Resistance Training Program Design

G. Gregory Haff, PhD, and Erin E. Haff, MA

After completing this chapter, you will be able to

- understand the application of specificity, overload, variation, progression, and sequencing;

- select exercises, determine training frequency, and arrange exercises in a specific sequence;

- determine loading through the appropriate use of 1-repetition maximum, body weight, or repetition maximum testing;

- assign training loads, volumes, and rest period lengths based on client needs and appropriate sequential training methods;

- add variation between training sessions, training days, and training weeks; and

- determine when training loads need to be increased or varied.

Designing a safe and effective resistance training program is a multifaceted process in which the personal trainer must consider and manipulate specific training variables to achieve specific goals. While many personal trainers consider the resistance training program separate from the aerobic exercise or sprint interval program, it is important to consider all elements of the training plan when constructing the resistance training program. Regardless of the client's goals, the best approach begins with an initial consultation to determine the client's goals, an evaluation of the client's health or medical history, and a fitness assessment (see chapters 9, 10, and 11). At this time the personal trainer can find out about the client's experience with resistance training and perform a cursory evaluation of his or her technical capabilities. The information gathered at this time will assist the personal trainer in the development of the overall training program, which will include factors such as how often the client will train, the types of exercises selected, the training loads, the repetition and set schemes, the order of exercises, and the rest intervals. To facilitate continued improvements, the personal trainer should consider a periodized training plan. Periodization can ensure that appropriate training variation and progression are used so as to minimize the potential for overtraining while maximizing improvements in the targeted training outcomes.

General Training Principles

Four basic principles should guide the development of effective resistance training programs: specificity, overload, variation, and progression. Any program that does not address all of these principles can result in a failure to meet client goals, poor adherence to the exercise plan, and potential litigation as a result of an increased risk of injury.

Specificity

The principle of **specificity** is a foundational aspect of every effective training program. *Specificity of training* refers to training a client in a specific way to produce a targeted change or result. The personal trainer can accomplish this by targeting specific muscle groups, energetic systems, movement velocities, movement patterns, or muscle action types (31, 107, 117). For example, if a client wants to strengthen his or her leg muscles, the personal trainer would select exercises such as the back squat because of its emphasis on lower body development. This type of specificity is often referred to as *muscle group specificity* (31).

Another method of applying specificity to a client's training program is to target specific movement patterns. Movement pattern specificity is generally used in work with athletes or clients who wish to develop strength that translates to a specific activity or sport. For example, if the client is a volleyball player, the personal trainer takes into account the fact that volleyball involves repeated jumping movements. The personal trainer could target these movements by incorporating exercises such as back squats (or front squats), power cleans, and power snatches into the program because they mimic the jumping movements in volleyball. The more similar the resistance training exercise is to the movement pattern, the greater the likelihood of translation to the targeted activity (104). Exercises such as the Olympic lifts (i.e., cleans, snatches, etc.) appear to offer the most translation to sports because their movement patterns are similar to those used in many sports and activities.

Overload

Overload refers to a training stress or intensity that is greater than what a client is used to. If a program fails to adhere to the principle of overload, it will produce limited results. The most common methods

of inducing overload include increasing the weight lifted, having the client perform more repetitions or sets of a given exercise, shortening the rest interval between sets, and increasing the number of training sessions in a week. While overload is an essential component of a resistance training program, the personal trainer should apply overload systematically and should adhere to the principles of progression and variation. Overload must be progressive to allow sufficient time for the client to adapt to the new training stimulus.

Variation

Variation refers to the manipulation of specific training variables (4, 117) such as volume, intensity, exercise selection, frequency of training, rest interval, and speed of movement (117). The application of appropriate training variation is essential when one is attempting to ensure long-term adaptation (65, 72, 113, 117). The best way to apply training variation is through use of the principles of periodization (117), which refers to the logical phasic manipulation of training factors to optimize specific training outcomes at specific time points (90). If appropriate training variation is not incorporated in the program, the rate of improvement will plateau (4, 117) or decrease, resulting in what is termed "monotonous program overtraining" (106). The variation in the resistance training plan should not be haphazard, and the sequencing of training factors should be appropriate (45, 89, 117). For example, clients who want to target power and strength development may undergo periods of training designed to target muscular strength followed by a period of power development. This type of sequencing has been shown to result in significantly greater improvements in performance compared to a program that lacks planned or sequenced variation (45).

Progression

Regardless of how effective a training program is, it should not continue indefinitely without modification. As the client adapts to the training plan, the training stress or intensity must be altered to continue to induce positive adaptations. The process of altering training stress as a client adapts is termed **progressive overload.** The stress is changed as the client becomes better trained (31), allowing him or her to continue advancing toward a specific training goal (4). Progression in resistance training must be applied systematically (4) and in proportion to the client's training status. Often the effective application of progression in a program requires appropriate variation strategies and the use of periodized training models.

Sequential Steps for Designing a Resistance Training Program

To design an effective resistance training program, the personal trainer must make specific decisions about the manipulation of the **program design variables,** such as the training frequency, exercises used and how they are arranged, the structure of the program, the rest periods between sets, and the overall progression of the program. To facilitate the decision-making process, the personal trainer should consider a sequential approach. The culmination of this process is the establishment of a periodized training plan that increases the likelihood of the clients' achieving their predetermined training goals. The first step is to conduct an initial fitness consultation and evaluation, which serves as the foundation for the subsequent steps that are generally associated with the sequential approach.

1. Initial consultation and fitness evaluation
2. Determination of training frequency
3. Exercise selection
4. Arrangement of exercises (exercise order)
5. Training load: resistance and repetitions
6. Training volume: repetitions and sets
7. Rest periods
8. Training variation
9. Sequencing the training plan
10. Progression

Successful resistance training programs must incorporate **specificity, overload, variation, and progression. Ignoring any of these factors** can limit the program's ability to stimulate the desired outcome, decrease adherence to the program, and increase the probability of injury and legal risk.

Initial Fitness Consultation and Evaluation

Before any exercise program begins, it is essential that the personal trainer conduct an initial client consultation to assess compatibility, establish a client–trainer agreement, discuss the client's exercise goals, and determine the client's level of commitment (see chapter 9). After this discussion, the personal trainer needs to evaluate the client's exercise history and current level of fitness, identify strengths and weaknesses, identify areas of potential risk for injury, determine if contraindications to exercise exist, and refine the goals for the program (see chapters 9 and 10).

The initial consultation is an essential component of the resistance training program design process in that it gives the personal trainer valuable information about the client's training status. More specific information will be collected as the personal trainer assesses the client's initial resistance training status and resistance exercise technique experience, conducts a fitness evaluation and analyzes the results, and determines the client's primary goals

Initial Resistance Training Status and Experience

The client's current training status and experience with resistance training will exert a significant impact on the training program to be developed. General information about the client's experience with resistance training can be gathered during the initial meeting (or soon afterward) when the client's exercise history is discussed.

The first step in determining the client's resistance training status is to have the client answer the general exercise history questions listed on the Health/Medical Questionnaire on page 171. The personal trainer then needs to obtain more specific information about the client's resistance training status and experience. A way to do this is to ask the client five basic questions (26):

1. Do you currently participate in a resistance training program?
2. How long have you been following a regular (one or more times per week) resistance training program?

3. How many times per week do you resistance train?

4. How intense (or difficult) are your resistance training workouts?

5. What types of resistance training exercises do you perform and how many of them can you perform with proper technique?

These questions can be used to establish a basic understanding of the client's resistance training experience and as a tool for establishing a general classification of the training status. Table 15.1 offers one approach for classifying resistance training status on a continuum from beginner to advanced. When the client's answers to the five questions match those shown in at least three of the five columns in one row, the estimated or predicted resistance training status is the one shown in the right-hand column. While this basic classification system is useful, it is important to realize that pigeonholing a client into a generalized training classification is difficult. Therefore the personal trainer must also make decisions about the client's responses based on professional knowledge and experience.

TABLE 15.1 A Method for Classifying Resistance Training Status

Question 1 Do you currently participate in a resistance training program?*	Question 2 How long have you been following a regular (one or more times per week) resistance training program?	Question 3 How many times per week do you resistance train?	Question 4 How intense (or difficult) are your resistance training workouts?	Question 5 What types of resistance training exercises do you perform and how many of them can you perform with proper technique?**	Estimated resistance training classification***
No	n/a	n/a	n/a	None	Beginner
Yes	≤2 months	1-2	Low intensity	3 to 5 machine exercises	
	4 to 6 months	2-3	Low to medium intensity	6 to 10 machine core and assistance exercises; 3 to 5 free weight assistance exercises	
Yes	8 to 10 months	3	Medium intensity	11 to 15 machine core and assistance exercises; 6 to 10 free weight assistance exercises; 3 to 5 free weight core exercises	Intermediate
Yes	1 year	4	Medium to high intensity	>15 free weight and machine core and assistance exercises	
Yes	1 to 1 1/2 years	4	High intensity	>15 free weight and machine core and assistance exercises; 3 to 5 power/explosive exercises	Advanced
Yes	≥2 years	≥5	Very high intensity	>15 free weight and machine core and assistance exercises; most power/explosive exercises	

*If a client is not currently following a resistance training program but was participating in a regular resistance training plan in the past four to six weeks, the personal trainer could consider the answer to question 1 a *yes* and the client could answer questions 2 through 5 based on that recent program. The decision to equate participation in a recent program with participation in a current resistance training program is based entirely on the personal trainer's professional judgment regarding the particular client.

**As determined or evaluated by a qualified personal trainer; refer to section "Types of Resistance Training Exercises" on page /bb/ for a description of the various types of resistance training exercises.

***Classification of resistance training status is determined when the client's answers match the answers shown in at least three of the five columns in one row pertaining to resistance training exercise history and technique experience.

The personal trainer should realize that this method of classifying resistance training status will not apply to every client; the unique characteristics of each client need to be considered.

Adapted from Baechle and Earle 2000 (8) and Earle and Baechle 2004 (26).

For example, if the client is not currently participating in a resistance training program but was following a regular training plan within the past four to six weeks, the answer to question 1 can be considered *yes*. In this case, the personal trainer would ask the client to answer questions 2 through 5 based on the recent training program. The decision to consider a recent resistance training program a "current" program is based solely on the personal trainer's professional judgment regarding the individual client's ability.

Fitness Evaluation

Typically the fitness evaluation involves an assessment of the client's resting heart rate and blood pressure, body composition, height, weight, girth, muscular strength and endurance, cardiorespiratory fitness or endurance, and flexibility. In the context of this chapter, the fitness evaluation focuses on assessing or estimating the client's muscular strength and endurance. Chapters 10 and 11 provide more information on fitness assessments.

After the fitness evaluation is completed, the personal trainer should compare the results with the normative or descriptive data presented in chapter 11. This comparison allows the personal trainer to determine the client's current level of fitness, establish a baseline for future comparisons as training status improves, and identify any strengths and weaknesses to base goals on. Additionally, the initial assessment may reveal contraindications to exercise that may require referring the client to a medical professional.

Primary Resistance Training Goal

Establishing the client's training goals is a very important part of the resistance training program design process. In keeping with the specificity principle, the client must train in specific ways in order to achieve desired results. Four primary resistance training goals include muscular endurance, hypertrophy (muscular size or tone), muscular strength, and muscular power.

Often the client's goals are not clearly identifiable. For example, it is uncommon for clients to say "I want to follow a resistance training program for hypertrophy"; they may say something more like "I want to have flatter abs." When the training goals are established during the initial consultation and fitness evaluation, the personal trainer will have to match the resistance training goals with the desires expressed by the client. Frequently during the consultation, the personal trainer needs to educate clients about the various goals that resistance training can address.

Muscular Endurance

A client may express a desire to improve muscular endurance with statements like "I want to have better endurance" or "I want to increase my stamina." Resistance training that targets muscular endurance, which is often termed *strength endurance training*, would address these goals by enhancing the ability of the targeted muscles to perform at a submaximal level for many repetitions or an extended period of time. The appropriate application of a resistance training program has great potential to improve muscular endurance (12, 50, 61, 116). Muscular endurance is commonly viewed as a part of aerobic exercise, as the muscle may contract thousands of times during a 20-minute activity such as running.

Hypertrophy

Statements like "I want my arms to be bigger," "I want more size," "I want to be more sculpted," or "I want to change my body shape" suggest that the client wants to follow a program that will result in muscular hypertrophy or increased tone. *Hypertrophy* refers to an increase in muscle size, and hypertrophy training typically leads to an increase in fat-free mass and a reduction in percent body fat.

Muscular Strength

Of the four resistance training goals, muscular strength is the easiest to establish. Clients often state this goal directly—"I want to get stronger." While this is a common goal for athletes interested in a resistance training program designed to enhance their athletic performance (114, 115, 116), it may also be a goal for other clients. For example, older clients may say things like "I want to be able to carry my golf bag" or "I want to be able to get up and down the stairs better." Current scientific literature suggests that older adults can improve their ability to engage in activities of daily living by increasing their muscular strength through performance of appropriate training programs (46, 57).

In comparison to resistance training programs that target muscular endurance or hypertrophy, a program that targets the development of muscular strength uses heavier training loads. Therefore it is prudent for people to develop muscular endurance and hypertrophy before engaging in a program that targets muscular strength improvements.

Muscular Power

Traditionally, resistance training programs that target **muscular power** have been used only with athletes or clients who want to improve their sport performance abilities. Typically, statements like "I want to jump higher" or "I need to improve my speed and agility" suggest that the client would like to improve muscular power. Training programs that target muscular power have great potential to improve sport performance (11, 55, 130). To maximize the benefits of these types of programs, it is prudent to sequence the client's training program. For example, it has been shown that improvements in speed and jumping ability are greater when a program targeting muscular strength is performed for a period of time prior to a program targeting muscular power (45).

While power training has generally been used with athletes, contemporary literature suggests that it also has a place in work with older adult and nonathletic populations. Recent evidence indicates that older adults who engage in power training experience improvements in their ability to engage in activities of daily living (46) and in functional performance (47, 48).

Determination of Training Frequency

Training **frequency** refers to the number of workouts a client will undertake during one week. Many factors contribute to the determination of the optimal frequency for an individual client. Factors such as the types of exercises used, the number of muscle groups trained per session, the structure of the program (volume and intensity), and the client's training status and overall fitness level dictate the training frequency (4). The client's work schedule, social schedule, and family obligations will also strongly influence how frequently the client can train.

Influential Factors

The primary factor that the personal trainer should consider when determining training frequency is the client's training status and overall level of fitness. Lesser-trained clients usually require more rest between workouts, which lowers the frequency, and highly trained clients will be able to tolerate more frequency. However, the personal trainer may need to reduce the frequency of resistance training if the client's overall amount of physical (24) or psychological stress (106) is high as a consequence of other demands (e.g., work, social, or academic schedule; other forms of exercise; or some combination of all demands). For example, if the client is a construction worker who performs repetitive lifting tasks in his or her job, he or she may not want or be able to

tolerate more than two or three days per week of resistance training.

An influential factor that many personal trainers overlook is how the different components of the training program interact (58, 59, 90). Many personal trainers plan resistance, endurance, agility, and plyometric training without considering how each factor affects the overall workload. It is essential to examine how the various training activities interact and to take the client's overall workload into account. For example, if the client is running 30 minutes a day, five days per week, he or she may be able to tolerate only two days per week of resistance training.

Guidelines for Determining Training Frequency

When determining the training frequency it is important to plan sufficient recovery into the program. A general rule that many personal trainers follow is to allow at least one day (but no more than three) between workouts that stress the same muscle group or groups (5, 14, 54, 85). More specific guidelines depend on a client's overall resistance training status (table 15.2). Most novice or beginner clients can experience the benefits of resistance training with as few as two or three days per week (4, 19, 51, 86, 95). However, individuals who are already accustomed to resistance training can only maintain their strength gains and cannot increase strength levels with one or two days per week (4, 35). In general, the more frequent the sessions, the greater the strength gains (4, 34).

Novice or Beginner Resistance Training Status

The recommendation for the novice or the beginner to resistance training is to use frequencies of two or three days per week when training the entire body (4, 19, 22, 25, 51, 95). With this frequency, resistance training days should be nonconsecutive (i.e., Monday and Thursday; Tuesday, Thursday, and Saturday;

TABLE 15.2 General Guidelines for Resistance Training Frequency

Resistance training status	Recommended number of sessions per week
Novice or beginner	2-3
Intermediate	3 if using total body training
	4 if using a split routine
Advanced	4-6*

*Advanced resistance trainers may perform multiple sessions in one day.

Adapted from Ratamess et al. 2007 (92).

or Monday, Wednesday, and Friday) to allow for appropriate recovery between sessions. As a general rule novice clients should have 1 to 3 days between resistance training session, but never more than 3, in order to facilitate recovery. If, for example, the client were to train on Monday and Wednesday, the amount of time between the Wednesday and the next Monday training session would be greater than three days and result in a less effective training program (35, 54). As the client progresses from the novice to the intermediate level, a change in frequency is not always necessary (4). However, increasing the frequency to three or four days per week allows for greater program flexibility.

Intermediate Resistance Training Status

A general recommendation for the client who has achieved an intermediate training status is to increase the training frequency to three or four days per week (4). However, this increase will mean that the client trains two or more days in a row. A common strategy is to use a split routine, which spreads four or more workouts evenly across the week. With this structure, the client can train only one part of the body (i.e., upper back or lower body) (70), certain muscle areas (e.g., chest, back, or legs) (70), or certain movement patterns (i.e., "push" or "pull") (117) during a session. This structure allows for an increase in frequency while still allowing sufficient time for recovery between sessions (85, 95).

A common example of a four time per week split routine for the intermediate client includes upper body exercises on Monday and Thursday and lower body exercises on Tuesday and Friday (70). Even though the client is training two days in row, changing the targeted muscle groups ensures adequate recovery. Additionally, there are two days of rest between sessions that target the same muscle groups, which allows for greater recovery between similar sessions (95). With this type of frequency split, the nonresistance training or rest days are consistently Wednesday, Saturday, and Sunday. More importantly, when training specific muscle groups or body parts, this split allows for maximization of results because the client can use higher volumes (95).

Advanced Resistance Training Status

Depending on their goals, intermediate clients may need to increase their training frequency as they become more experienced and are reclassified as advanced in status. The general recommendation is for advanced individuals to resistance train four to six days per week to allow for an increase in train-ing stimulus (4). It is common for these clients to use double split routines (44), performing two sessions on the same day, which increases the number of training sessions from 8 to 12 per week (4, 110). Strong evidence in the scientific literature supports the concept of performing multiple short training sessions in one day (4, 44, 110).

Another method for increasing the frequency from five to six days is to use a "three days on, one day off" **split routine.** With this structure, three distinct workouts target specific muscle groups, and the client completes one workout on three consecutive days and rests on the fourth day. A common strategy is to divide the program into upper body "push" exercises (i.e., chest, shoulders, triceps), lower body exercises, and upper body "pull" exercises (i.e., upper back, trapezius, and biceps). In this type of structure the workouts are on unspecified days; that is, the rest day is not the same each week.

Exercise Selection

The selection of exercises to be incorporated into the client's training program is influenced by the principle of specificity, the equipment available, the client's resistance training experience, and the amount of time the client has to dedicate to training. Once the personal trainer considers these issues, he or she can make exercise selections that maximize the training adaptations and increase the chances of achieving the client's specific training goals.

Influential Factors

When selecting exercises, the personal trainer should make decisions based on the specific needs of the client and the target goals established in the initial consultation with the client. Many factors will affect this decision-making process, including how much time a client has to dedicate to training. The time available can have a large impact on the number and complexity of exercises chosen for a given training session. For example, performing the back squat to target lower body development takes significantly less time than performing leg curls and leg extensions.

An additional factor is the equipment available to the client. Even if an exercise is effective, goal specific, and efficient it cannot be a major part of a client's training plan if the equipment is not available. To account for this before planning the program, the personal trainer needs to gather an equipment inventory for the facility in which the client intends to train. This important step can help avoid wasting time in constructing the training plan.

Another factor that will dictate the selection of exercises is whether or not the client can perform the exercise correctly. If the client is inexperienced in or unfamiliar with proper technique for an exercise, or if the extent of the client's experience is unknown, the personal trainer must provide a complete demonstration, explanation, and familiarization period in which to teach the client appropriate technique. This may require beginning the client with remedial exercises that can build a foundation for more complex exercises in future programs. Inexperienced clients are often taught machine exercises and free weight assistance exercises first because these require less skill than many of the core exercises (31, 107, 124). (In this context, *core exercises* does not refer to exercises targeting the abdominal core. See the next section on types of resistance training exercises.) Following these recommendations can be effective in reducing the potential for litigation, decreasing injury risk, promoting adherence, and improving the overall effectiveness of the program.

Types of Resistance Training Exercises

There are a plethora of exercises from which to construct a resistance training program. These exercises can be classified as either core or assistance exercises based on the size of the muscles recruited, the complexity of the movement pattern, and the degree of contribution toward the client's training goals.

Core Exercises

Core exercises should form the bulk of a program because they are more effective than assistance exercises in helping clients achieve their specific training goals. Generally, an exercise is classified as a core exercise if it

- involves two or more primary joints, which would make it a **multijoint exercise,** and
- engages large muscles while activating synergistic muscles.

One multijoint large-muscle exercise has the potential to activate as many muscles or muscle groups as four to eight small-muscle, single-joint assistance exercises (112). A program that uses core exercises appropriately is more efficient than one that uses many small-muscle exercises.

The personal trainer has many core exercises to choose from when constructing a program (see chapter 13). An example is the bench press, which involves movement at the shoulder and elbow joint while recruiting the chest muscles with synergistic help from the anterior deltoids and the triceps brachii.

If a core exercise loads the axial skeleton (places a load on the spine) (i.e., power clean, squat, front squat, shoulder press, etc.), it is further classified as a structural exercise. Structural exercises require the muscles of the torso to maintain an erect or near-erect position. For example, during the squat, the barbell loads the axial skeleton, and the musculature of the torso must maintain a near-erect position as the client descends and ascends. Structural exercises that are performed very quickly, such as the power clean or power snatch, are also classified as **power** or **explosive exercises** (e.g., push press, snatch or clean pull, high pull, push jerk). These types of exercises are extremely effective because they provide a multidimensional training stimulus through the engagement of a large amount of muscle mass and result in a large caloric expenditure (101).

> In the context of resistance training, *core exercises* refer to exercises that engage large muscles and multiple joints.

Assistance Exercises

Assistance exercises supplementary exercises that are performed to maintain muscular balance across a joint, help prevent injury, rehabilitate a previous injury, or isolate a specific muscle group or muscle. Exercises are classified as assistance exercises if they

- are **single-joint exercises,** engaging only one primary joint, and
- recruit a small amount of muscle mass (i.e., a small muscle group or area).

Assistance exercises should not be the major components of the program; they should be considered a secondary emphasis in relation to the more effective core exercises.

One of the most popular assistance exercises is the barbell biceps curl. This exercise engages a small amount of muscle mass (biceps brachii, brachialis, and brachioradialis) and involves movement of only a single joint (elbow joint). The "pec deck" and dumbbell fly are also classified as assistance exercises even though they engage the muscles of the chest. They involve movement only at the shoulder and place primary emphasis on the chest musculature.

Guidelines for Choosing Exercises

Selection of the exercises for a training program should meet the individual client's needs, whether the client is an elite athlete or a novice, is severely detrained, or has been recently injured.

For a novice or untrained individual, the personal trainer should pay more attention to developing a training base, probably with assistance exercises or basic core exercises. In this situation one may decide to target specific muscle groups or train each muscle group. This strategy involves choosing one exercise per muscle group: chest, shoulders, upper back, hips and thighs, biceps, triceps, abdominal muscles, and calves (6, 85). As the client becomes better trained, the number of exercises per muscle group can be increased (85). Typically, this type of program uses small-muscle or single-joint exercises but programs should progressively incorporate more multijoint large-muscle or core exercises.

Employing multijoint large-muscle exercises can magnify the adaptive response and increase the overall metabolic cost of the training program. An example is the squat and press. This complex exercise engages a large amount of muscle mass, substantially increases the metabolic cost of training, and produces a substantial training effect. Other examples are exercises such as power cleans, power snatches, and pulls. These all train the entire body and appear to be extremely effective training methods for athletes (104) and clinical populations (57). With athletes, the more closely the exercise relates to the sporting movement pattern, the more likely the strength gains developed will translate to the sport (15, 31, 107, 117, 120, 121, 131). For example, when working with a volleyball or basketball player, the personal trainer should consider using exercises such as the power clean or power snatch since they involve a jumping movement, which is important in these sports. (See chapter 23 for guidelines on selecting exercises for particular sports.)

In work with clients who have special needs, such as lower back problems or recent injuries, it is important to adapt the training program to address these issues. The exercises should be selected with guidance from the appropriate medical professional. It is essential that a training program for these clients avoid exercises that are contraindicated or not recommended. For example, if a client was recently released from the care of a physical therapist for a shoulder impingement, the physical therapist may prescribe the dumbbell lateral raise in place of the overhead shoulder press to work the deltoid muscle group

Exercise Order

The **exercise order** or arrangement refers to the order in which the exercises are performed during the workout. The exercise order is dependent on many factors but is most strongly influenced by the type and characteristics of the exercises selected.

Influential Factors

Factors that influence the order of exercises include the goals of the client, the fatigue-generating potential of the exercise, and the type of exercise (core or assistance).

One method for ordering exercises is to place them in a descending order of priority or application to the client's goals, activity, or, in the case of athletes, sport. With this type of structure, the client performs the exercises that target his or her individual goals earlier in the workout when fatigue is lowest, performing less goal-specific exercises toward the end of the session.

A second method for arranging exercises is based on their type (core or assistance). With this method, core exercises are performed first, and assistance exercises are performed later in the session. This arrangement allows the client to perform the more complex, multijoint core exercises under minimal levels of fatigue. In general, the personal trainer should attempt to maximize the client's ability to tolerate the training loads and complete all the exercises in one session by arranging the exercises to manage fatigue.

Guidelines for Arranging Exercises

There are many ways to arrange exercises in a training session (31). The ordering of exercises can be categorized into several primary methods, such as placing power and core exercises before assistance exercises, alternating "push" and "pull" exercises, and alternating upper and lower body exercises. There are also combination methods and secondary arrangement methods (tables 15.3 and 15.4).

Placing Power and Core Exercises Before Assistance Exercise

One of the most commonly used guidelines is to order the exercises as follows:

Power exercises → Core exercises → Assistance exercises

Conceptually, since power exercises and core exercises are often multijoint exercises and assistance exercises are typically single-joint exercises, the following is another possible order:

Multijoint exercises → Single-joint exercises

TABLE 15.3 Sample Exercise Order for Resistance Training Based on Exercise Type and Muscle Mass Activated

	SAMPLE EXERCISE ORDER: POWER → CORE → ASSISTANCE			
Exercise order	Exercise	Exercise classification		
1	Power clean	Power exercises	Multijoint exercises	Large-muscle exercises
2	Push press			
3	Front squat	Core exercises		
4	Bench press			
5	Triceps press-down	Assistance exercises	Single-joint exercises	Small-muscle exercises
6	Wrist curl			
7	Seated heel raise			

	SAMPLE EXERCISE ORDER: MULTIJOINT → SINGLE JOINT			
Exercise order	Exercise	Exercise classification		
1	Squat + press		Multijoint exercises	Large-muscle exercises
2	Back squat			
3	Incline bench press			
4	Leg curl		Single-joint exercises	Small-muscle exercises
5	Three-way shoulder			

	SAMPLE EXERCISE ORDER: LARGE MUSCLE → SMALL MUSCLE			
Exercise order	Exercise	Exercise classification		
1	Power snatch	Power exercises	Multijoint exercises	Large-muscle exercises
2	Overhead squat	Core exercises		
3	Snatch grip Romanian deadlift			
4	Bent-over row	Assistance exercises	Single-joint exercises	Small-muscle exercises
5	Lateral raise			
6	Abdominal crunch			

These are simply examples of how exercises may be sequenced and do not represent complete resistance training workouts.

TABLE 15.4 Examples of Alternate Exercise Ordering Systems

	SAMPLE EXERCISE ORDER: ALTERNATING "PUSH" AND "PULL" EXERCISES			
Exercise order	Exercise	Exercise classification		
1	Back squat	Push	Core	Multijoint
2	Leg curl	Pull	Assistance	Single joint
3	Standing heel raise	Push	Assistance	Single joint
4	Upright row	Pull	Assistance	Single joint
5	Incline bench press	Push	Core	Multijoint
6	Dumbbell biceps curl	Pull	Assistance	Single joint
7	Shoulder press	Push	Core	Multijoint
8	Lat pulldown	Pull	Assistance	Multijoint

	SAMPLE EXERCISE ORDER: ALTERNATING UPPER AND LOWER BODY EXERCISES			
Exercise order	Exercise	Exercise classification		
1	Leg press	Lower body	Core	Multijoint
2	Bench press	Upper body	Core	Multijoint
3	Lunge	Lower body	Core	Multijoint
4	Shoulder shrug	Upper body	Assistance	Single joint
5	Leg extension	Lower body	Assistance	Single joint
6	Dumbbell shoulder press	Upper body	Core	Multijoint
7	Leg curl	Lower body	Assistance	Single joint
8	Triceps extension	Upper body	Assistance	Single joint

These are simply examples of how exercises may be sequenced and do not represent complete resistance training workouts.

Another way to think about exercise order is to consider the amount of muscle mass activated with the exercise. Large-muscle exercises, which are generally core or multijoint exercises, should be performed prior to single-joint exercise:

Large-muscle exercises → Small-muscle exercises

Regardless of the way one conceptualizes these exercise sequences, the basic structures noted here should be considered to be the most effective exercise sequencing methods for the majority of clients.

These arrangements of exercises are effective because power or multijoint exercises require more effort, skill, and focus than single-joint assistance exercises (31) and should be performed when the client is fresh (31, 30). Historically it has been recommended that only athletes use power exercises, such as the Olympic lifts and their derivatives; but contemporary literature suggests that all populations can use power exercises to achieve their training goals (20, 57, 64). In fact, one study in adults showed that transfer of training effects to activities of daily living was greater with power training than with strength training (46). Therefore, the personal trainer should consider the use of these types of exercises not only with athletes, but with all clients.

Alternating "Push" and "Pull" Exercises

Another method of arranging exercises is to alternate "push" exercises (e.g., vertical chest press and triceps press-down) with "pull" exercises (e.g., seated row and dumbbell biceps curl) (8). It has been suggested that this system allows rest between exercises and guarantees that the same muscle group is not used for two exercises in a row (8). While the push–pull system is commonly used, it is important to remember that core exercises can activate a vast array of muscles and that many will use the same muscle groups. For example, if a client performs the back squat (a "pushing" exercise) followed by the leg curl (a "pulling" exercise), the hamstrings will be activated in both exercises.

Alternating Upper and Lower Body Exercises

A traditional approach to ordering exercises requires the client to alternate between upper and lower body exercises (31). This type of ordering is typically used with a circuit weight training program and short rest intervals. As with the push–pull system, this ordering may be best suited for machine-based training or

when the predominant exercises selected are those classified as small-muscle or assistance exercises.

Combination Arrangement Methods

It is possible to combine the most common methods of arranging exercises. Two or three of the previously mentioned methods can be combined: for example, core exercises and then assistance exercises that alternate push and pull. Often with a combination arrangement, a lower body exercise precedes an upper body exercise.

Secondary Arrangement Methods

Two popular secondary methods involve completing a set of two different exercises in succession without an intervening rest interval. If the two exercises coupled together train the same muscle group (e.g., incline bench press and incline dumbbell fly), the set is considered a **compound set** (8). Compound sets are often used by bodybuilders in an attempt to induce muscular hypertrophy (31).

Another secondary arrangement, which is termed a *super set*, uses the performance of two exercises that activate opposing or antagonistic muscle groups (e.g., biceps curl and triceps press) with no rest between each exercise (8, 31, 107). Super setting is popular among bodybuilders, individuals who are attempting to increase muscular endurance, and individuals with limited time for training (31).

Training Load: Resistance and Repetitions

The training **load** or the amount of weight to be used in a resistance training program is one of the most important factors to consider in the design of a training program. There are many ways to determine the training load. The assigned load will exert a large impact on the number of repetitions that can be performed and ultimately the types of physiological and performance adaptations stimulated. Ultimately the interplay between the load and **volume** of training (repetitions × sets × resistance) is dictated by the type of training program established and the intended goals of the program.

Before assigning the training load and the repetitions to be performed in each set, the personal trainer must test the client. The purpose of testing is to determine the client's abilities to handle specific loads in a series of selected exercises. Once the personal trainer establishes these abilities, he or she can assign training loads.

Influential Factors

The load, the number of repetitions, and the targeted outcomes of a resistance training program are strongly related. For example, higher loads (>80% of 1-repetition maximum [1RM]) performed for fewer repetitions (three to five) target the development of muscular strength. Lifting lighter loads (<70% of 1RM) for higher repetitions (>10 repetitions) results in improvements in muscular endurance. In its most basic form, a client's training program would address specific goals and target them with selected repetition and load relationships. This, however, is a gross simplification of the training process. Regardless of the client's goals, the training plan should include periods in which muscular endurance, strength, and potentially power are developed. Sequencing different repetition and loading schemes will magnify training adaptations and provide a greater chance of accomplishing the client's goals (45, 90, 117).

Percentage of 1-Repetition Maximum Relationship

The **repetition maximum (RM)** is the maximum load that the client can handle in a specific exercise for specific number of repetitions. As the load becomes heavier, the number of repetitions that the client can perform will decrease. Eventually the load will become so heavy that the client can perform only one repetition; this is the **1-repetition maximum (1RM)**. Conversely, the lighter the load, the more repetitions the client can perform. This association between 1RM and repetitions has been termed the percentage of 1RM (%1RM)–repetitions relationship.

Load assignments are best accomplished with the use of percentages of the 1RM (3, 9, 38, 62, 63, 101, 102, 107) or of a specified targeted maximum repetition range. For example, table 15.5 indicates that if a client's 1RM is 200 pounds (91 kg), he or she should be able to perform eight repetitions with around 160 pounds (73 kg). If his or her 10RM is 150 pounds (68 kg), we can estimate his or her 1RM as around 200 pounds (91 kg). By using these relationships, the personal trainer can estimate the training loads to prescribe for the client. It is important to note that the numbers in table 15.5 are only estimates and that these values can vary slightly depending on the training status of the client and the exercises used in the program (6, 8, 9, 15, 17, 18, 27, 28, 80, 123).

An alternative method is to use an intensity that allows for performance of a specific number of repetitions, or what is known as a **repetition maximum**

TABLE 15.5 Percentage of 1-Repetition Maximum to Repetitions Relationship

% 1-repetition maximum	Estimated number of repetitions
100	1
95	2
93	3
90	4
87	5
85	6
83	7
80	8
77	9
75	10
70	11
67	12
65	15
60	20

The percentage to repetition maximum will vary slightly (±0.5-2.0%) depending on the training status of the client.

Adapted from Baechle and Earle 1989, 2000 (7,9); Baechle, Earle, and Wathen 2008 (10); Bompa and Haff 2009 (15); Bryzychi 1993, 2000 (17,18); Epley 1985, 2004 (27, 28); Mayhew et al. 1995 (80); Wathen 1994 (123).

(RM) target. With use of this method, the client lifts the heaviest load he or she can for the selected repetition scheme (31, 38, 68, 71). For example, if the client were to perform three sets at a 12RM load, he or she would use the heaviest weight that would allow him to perform three sets with no less or more than 12 repetitions. A similar method, using what is called the RM target zone, is to assign a range such as 3- to 5RM (31). When a **repetition maximum zone (RM target zone)** is prescribed, the client uses the heaviest weight he or she can to perform the exercise for the number of repetitions within the range. The RM target and RM target zone methods for assigning load are problematic because in both instances the client is required to train to muscular failure. The scientific literature shows clearly that training to failure results in reduced training adaptations (87) and may increase the client's risk for overtraining and experiencing injuries (60). Therefore it is prudent for personal trainers to avoid both the RM target and the RM target zone methods when establishing the client's training load.

Limitations in the Percent 1-Repetition Maximum Relationship

While the %RM–repetitions relationship is an excellent tool for prescribing intensities in resistance training, it is important to realize a number of limitations that may affect its accuracy.

1. While there appears to be a relationship between the %1RM and the number of repetitions that can be performed, several studies suggest that the relationship is not as robust as was once thought (52, 76, 78, 79, 80, 82).

2. Training status appears to influence the relationship between repetitions and %1RM, with trained individuals being able to perform more repetitions at a given %1RM (52, 53, 79, 100, 118).

3. When working with the %1RM–repetitions relationship, it is important to remember that the number of repetitions performed at a specific %1RM is related only to a single set and not to multiple sets. With multiple sets, fatigue will cause a reduction in the number of repetitions that can be performed in later sets, thus altering the %1RM–repetitions relationship (123).

4. The %1RM–repetitions association is for the most part based on research on the bench press, back squat, and power clean (31, 118). The relationship between %1RM and repetitions does not likely apply to all exercises (52, 53, 100) and should be applied with care in work with clients.

5. The mode of resistance training appears to affect the number of repetitions that can be performed at a given %1RM. Generally, more repetitions can be performed at any given %1RM with machine-based exercises (e.g., vertical chest press) than with free weight exercises (e.g., bench press) (52, 53).

6. More repetitions can be performed at any given %1RM for core exercises compared to assistance exercises (91, 118).

7. The order of exercises may also affect the number of repetitions that can be performed at any given %1RM. Whether it is a core or assistance exercise, placing an exercise toward the end of the workout results in a decrease in the number of repetitions (103).

When using the %1RM–repetitions relationships presented in table 15.5, the personal trainer will probably have greater success estimating with loads of ≥75% of 1RM performed with ≤10 repetitions (17, 21, 81, 122), because the %1RM–repetitions relationship becomes increasingly inaccurate as the load decreases and the number of repetitions increases (8). Therefore the information presented in table 15.5 should be used only as a guide and not to derive hard and fast rules.

Guidelines for Assessing Load Capabilities

Before assigning training loads, the personal trainer must perform some form of assessment in order to estimate the client's capabilities. The following are methods for accomplishing this:

1. Directly assessing the 1RM
2. Estimating the 1RM
3. Using a percentage of the client's body weight for testing
4. Repetition maximum testing

One or more of these methods can be used depending on the client's training status, technical proficiency, and the type of exercise being tested (9).

Assessing the 1-Repetition Maximum

The personal trainer must determine the 1RM in order to use the %1RM–repetitions relationships presented in table 15.5. As a general rule, the 1RM test poses minimal risks to both clinical and athletic clients (98, 99); and it is considered the gold standard of muscular strength assessments (56). The biggest issue with the 1RM test is whether or not the client has the technique needed to perform the exercise correctly with increasing loads. If technique is lacking, it may be best to use other methods. While use of a test-established 1RM is the most accurate way to determine loading, it is also possible to use a submaximal load to estimate the 1RM (8, 53). It is important to note that using estimations from submaximal loads may result in overestimation of the 1RM (73, 80, 82, 93, 125) which could lead to a problem in prescribing training intensities.

As a rule, clients who have never lifted, who are classified as untrained, have been recently injured, or are under medical supervision should not perform a 1RM test. It may be prudent to reserve this type of testing for more advanced clients who have developed the appropriate technical base and can perform the test exercise using appropriate technique with various loads.

In selecting the exercises to be tested with a 1RM, the personal trainer should choose only those exercises that can be performed safely, accurately, and consistently (8). In general, the larger multijoint core exercises are best suited for 1RM testing because heavy loads are better tolerated with these exercises. As a rule, 1RM testing should not be used with assistance exercises because of the large physiological stress placed on the smaller muscle groups across a single joint (10). It is important to use sound judgment when selecting exercises for a 1RM test.

As one example, even though the lunge and step-up are large-muscle multijoint exercises, they are not typically used with 1RM testing because of the uneven loads they place on the lower body. The uneven loads can increase the potential for injury and accidents. The bent-over row is another exercise that would not be assessed with 1RM testing. While this exercise does activate the large muscle joints of the upper back and functions across several joints, it is likely that during a 1RM test the weaker muscles of the lower back may not be able to maintain appropriate body positions, which would increase the risk of injury and result in an inaccurate assessment of strength. Once an exercise has been deemed acceptable for testing and if the client is of appropriate training status, the personal trainer should select the appropriate 1RM testing protocol as explained in chapter 11.

Estimating the 1-Repetition Maximum

If the client is unable to perform an actual 1RM test, there are several ways in which the 1RM can be estimated. Such estimation procedures can be used to develop the loading structure and resistance training plan.

1. Use of repetition maximum tests
2. Use of prediction equations

One way to estimate a client's 1RM is to use a repetition maximum (RM) test, which then becomes an estimate of the 1RM. The best means of ensuring accuracy is to use lower numbers of repetitions (5-10) such as a 6RM or 10RM (i.e., the heaviest load the client can lift 6 or 10 times with proper technique). Once the 6- or 10RM is established, table 15.6 can be used to estimate the 1RM. As a basic rule, the RM should be determined within three testing sets.

TABLE 15.6   Estimating a 1-Repetition Maximum From a Training Load

	MAX REPETITIONS												
1	**2**	**3**	**4**	**5**	**6**	**7**	**8**	**9**	**10**	**12**	**15**	**20**
					% OF REPETITION MAX								
100	**95**	**93**	**90**	**87**	**85**	**83**	**80**	**77**	**75**	**67**	**65**	**60**
10	10	9	9	9	9	8	8	8	8	7	7	6
15	14	14	14	13	13	12	12	12	11	10	10	9
20	19	19	18	17	17	17	16	15	15	13	13	12
25	24	23	23	22	21	21	20	19	19	17	16	15
30	29	28	27	26	26	25	24	23	23	20	20	18
35	33	33	32	30	30	29	28	27	26	23	23	21
40	38	37	36	35	34	33	32	31	30	27	26	24
45	43	42	41	39	38	37	36	35	34	30	29	27
50	48	47	45	44	43	42	40	39	38	34	33	30
55	52	51	50	48	47	46	44	42	41	37	36	33
60	57	56	54	52	51	50	48	46	45	40	39	36
65	62	60	59	57	55	54	52	50	49	44	42	39
70	67	65	63	61	60	58	56	54	53	47	46	42
75	71	70	68	65	64	62	60	58	56	50	49	45
80	76	74	72	70	68	66	64	62	60	54	52	48
85	81	79	77	74	72	71	68	65	64	57	55	51
90	86	84	81	78	77	75	72	69	68	60	59	54
95	90	88	86	83	81	79	76	73	71	64	62	57
100	95	93	90	87	85	83	80	77	75	67	65	60
105	100	98	95	91	89	87	84	81	79	70	68	63
110	105	102	99	96	94	91	88	85	83	74	72	66
115	109	107	104	100	98	95	92	89	86	77	75	69
120	114	112	108	104	102	100	96	92	90	80	78	72
125	119	116	113	109	106	104	100	96	94	84	81	75
130	124	121	117	113	111	108	104	100	98	87	85	78
135	128	126	122	117	115	112	108	104	101	90	88	81

*LOAD IN POUNDS OR KILOGRAMS**

*Whenever possible, round down to the nearest 5 lb or 2.5 kg increment.

LOAD IN POUNDS OR KILOGRAMS*						MAX REPETITIONS							
	1	2	3	4	5	6	7	8	9	10	12	15	20
						% OF REPETITION MAX							
	100	95	93	90	87	85	83	80	77	75	67	65	60
	140	133	130	126	122	119	116	112	108	105	94	91	84
	145	138	135	131	126	123	120	116	112	109	97	94	87
	150	143	140	135	131	128	125	120	116	113	101	98	90
	155	147	144	140	135	132	129	124	119	116	104	101	93
	160	152	149	144	139	136	133	128	123	120	107	104	96
	165	157	153	149	144	140	137	132	127	124	111	107	99
	170	162	158	153	148	145	141	136	131	128	114	111	102
	175	166	163	158	152	149	145	140	135	131	117	114	105
	180	171	167	162	157	153	149	144	139	135	121	117	108
	185	176	172	167	161	157	154	148	142	139	124	120	111
	190	181	177	171	165	162	158	152	146	143	127	124	114
	195	185	181	176	170	166	162	156	150	146	131	127	117
	200	190	186	180	174	170	166	160	154	150	134	130	120
	205	195	191	185	178	174	170	164	158	154	137	133	123
	210	200	195	189	183	179	174	168	162	158	141	137	126
	215	204	200	194	187	183	178	172	166	161	144	140	129
	220	209	205	198	191	187	183	176	169	165	147	143	132
	225	214	209	203	196	191	187	180	173	169	151	146	135
	230	219	214	207	200	196	191	184	177	173	154	150	138
	235	223	219	212	204	200	195	188	181	176	157	153	141
	240	228	223	216	209	204	199	192	185	180	161	156	144
	245	233	228	221	213	208	203	196	189	184	164	159	147
	250	238	233	225	218	213	208	200	193	188	168	163	150
	255	242	237	230	222	217	212	204	196	191	171	166	153
	260	247	242	234	226	221	216	208	200	195	174	169	156
	265	252	246	239	231	225	220	212	204	199	178	172	159
	270	257	251	243	235	230	224	216	208	203	181	176	162
	275	261	256	248	239	234	228	220	212	206	184	179	165
	280	266	260	252	244	238	232	224	216	210	188	182	168
	285	271	265	257	248	242	237	228	219	214	191	185	171
	290	276	270	261	252	247	241	232	223	218	194	189	174
	295	280	274	266	257	251	245	236	227	221	198	192	177
	300	285	279	270	261	255	249	240	231	225	201	195	180
	305	290	284	275	265	259	253	244	235	229	204	198	183
	310	295	288	279	270	264	257	248	239	233	208	202	186
	315	299	293	284	274	268	261	252	243	236	211	205	189
	320	304	298	288	278	272	266	256	246	240	214	208	192
	325	309	302	293	283	276	270	260	250	244	218	211	195
	330	314	307	297	287	281	274	264	254	248	221	215	198
	335	318	312	302	291	285	278	268	258	251	224	218	201
	340	323	316	306	296	289	282	272	262	255	228	221	204
	345	328	321	311	300	293	286	276	266	259	231	224	207
	350	333	326	315	305	298	291	280	270	263	235	228	210
	355	337	330	320	309	302	295	284	273	266	238	231	213
	360	342	335	324	313	306	299	288	277	270	241	234	216
	365	347	339	329	318	310	303	292	281	274	245	237	219
	370	352	344	333	322	315	307	296	285	278	248	241	222

*Whenever possible, round down to the nearest 5 lb or 2.5 kg increment.

(continued)

361

TABLE 15.6 *(continued)*

						MAX REPETITIONS							
1	**2**	**3**	**4**	**5**	**6**	**7**	**8**	**9**	**10**	**12**	**15**	**20**	
						% OF REPETITION MAX							
100	**95**	**93**	**90**	**87**	**85**	**83**	**80**	**77**	**75**	**67**	**65**	**60**	
375	356	349	338	326	319	311	300	289	281	251	244	225	
380	361	353	342	331	323	315	304	293	285	255	247	228	
385	366	358	347	335	327	320	308	296	289	258	250	231	
390	371	363	351	339	332	324	312	300	293	261	254	234	
395	375	367	356	344	336	328	316	304	296	265	257	237	
400	380	372	360	348	340	332	320	308	300	268	260	240	
405	385	377	365	352	344	336	324	312	304	271	263	243	
410	390	381	369	357	349	340	328	316	308	275	267	246	
415	394	386	374	361	353	344	332	320	311	278	270	249	
420	399	391	378	365	357	349	336	323	315	281	273	252	
425	404	395	383	370	361	353	340	327	319	285	276	255	
430	409	400	387	374	366	357	344	331	323	288	280	258	
435	413	405	392	378	370	361	348	335	326	291	283	261	
440	418	409	396	383	374	365	352	339	330	295	286	264	
445	423	414	401	387	378	369	356	343	334	298	289	267	
450	428	419	405	392	383	374	360	347	338	302	293	270	
455	432	423	410	396	387	378	364	350	341	305	296	273	
460	437	428	414	400	391	382	368	354	345	308	299	276	
465	442	432	419	405	395	386	372	358	349	312	302	279	
470	447	437	423	409	400	390	376	362	353	315	306	282	
475	451	442	428	413	404	394	380	366	356	318	309	285	
480	456	446	432	418	408	398	384	370	360	322	312	288	
485	461	451	437	422	412	403	388	373	364	325	315	291	
490	466	456	441	426	417	407	392	377	368	328	319	294	
495	470	460	446	431	421	411	396	381	371	332	322	297	
500	475	465	450	435	425	415	400	385	375	335	325	300	
505	480	470	455	439	429	419	404	389	379	338	328	303	
510	485	474	459	444	434	423	408	393	383	342	332	306	
515	489	479	464	448	438	427	412	397	386	345	335	309	
520	494	484	468	452	442	432	416	400	390	348	338	312	
525	499	488	473	457	446	436	420	404	394	352	341	315	
530	504	493	477	461	451	440	424	408	398	355	345	318	
535	508	498	482	465	455	444	428	412	401	358	348	321	
540	513	502	486	470	459	448	432	416	405	362	351	324	
545	518	507	491	474	463	452	436	420	409	365	354	327	
550	523	512	495	479	468	457	440	424	413	369	358	330	
555	527	516	500	483	472	461	444	427	416	372	361	333	
560	532	521	504	487	476	465	448	431	420	375	364	336	
565	537	525	509	492	480	469	452	435	424	379	367	339	
570	542	530	513	496	485	473	456	439	428	382	371	342	
575	546	535	518	500	489	477	460	443	431	385	374	345	
580	551	539	522	505	493	481	464	447	435	389	377	348	
585	556	544	527	509	497	486	468	450	439	392	380	351	
590	561	549	531	513	502	490	472	454	443	395	384	354	
595	565	553	536	518	506	494	476	458	446	399	387	357	
600	570	558	540	522	510	498	480	462	450	402	390	360	

The leftmost column is labeled **LOAD IN POUNDS OR KILOGRAMS***

*Whenever possible, round down to the nearest 5 lb or 2.5 kg increment.

The 6RM test is very similar to the test for determining the 1RM; the main difference is that each testing set includes six repetitions (67). Since the number of repetitions is greater, the load changes across testing sets should be smaller (~50% of the amounts suggested for 1RM testing in chapter 11).

Once the client's 6RM has been determined, table 15.6 can be used to estimate the 1RM. The personal trainer will look at the row titled "Max repetitions" and move across that row until they find the notation for 6 repetitions, which is "~85% 1RM". Once this column is located, the trainer can move down this column looking for the number closest to (but not greater than) the client's 6RM. For example, if the client's 6RM for the leg press is 140 pounds (64 kg), the estimated 1RM will be 165 pounds (75 kg). This load will be used as the basis of the client's actual training loads.

The results of the RM test can also be used with prediction equations to determine the 1RM. A number of these equations, which use repetitions to failure to estimate 1RM, have been published (table 15.7) (1, 18, 27, 73, 74, 79, 80, 84). In general, the accuracy of these equations is greater when heavier loads are used (1). Therefore the recommendation is to use heavier loads performed for fewer repetitions than the 10RM with prediction equations (1, 17, 21, 81, 122). The phase of the training plan also affects the accuracy of these equations (9). If the client has been training with high volumes such as sets of 10 to 15 repetitions, the equations will become less accurate; conversely, a prediction equation becomes more robust if the client is using lower volumes and heavier weights.

Percent of Body Weight Testing

Another method for estimating strength in either core or assistance exercises is to test using a certain percentage of a client's body weight (%BWT) (10). This method of determining training loads is best suited for untrained or inexperienced clients because the loads are typically relatively light. The %BWT method should not be used with more experienced clients because they will have a greater strength to body weight ratio and thus their training loads will be grossly underestimated.

The %BWT method uses an exercise-specific numerical factor to determine a **trial load** for testing based on a percentage of the client's body weight (tables 15.8 through 15.10). Table 15.8 provides basic guidelines for performing an assessment based on %BWT. A maximum body weight of 175 pounds (79 kg) for male clients and 140 pounds (64 kg) for female should be used with this test. This accounts for individual differences in body composition and ensures test safety. The goal of this type of assessment is to derive a trial load that the client can lift for only 12 to 15 repetitions. Using the factors presented in tables 15.9 and 15.10 will accomplish this goal; but it is important to realize that individual differences, variations in technical proficiency, and the number of different types of equipment make it impossible to calculate the testing load perfectly. Nevertheless this method appears to be a valuable tool for establishing training loads.

As an example, to use the %BWT method to test a 130-pound (59.1 kg) female on the leg press on a pivot-based machine, one would use a trial load of 130 pounds (BWT × 1.0; table 15.9). After an appropriate warm-up, the client would perform as many repetitions as possible with the 130-pound load, which in theory should be somewhere between 12 and 15.

Repetition Maximum Testing

Another method for determining the client's capabilities is to decide on a number of **goal repetitions** for the client to perform in the actual training program. For example, if an advanced client will perform four repetitions of the back squat in the workout, the personal trainer uses a 4RM test.

While this is probably not the best method for determining training loads, it can be used to assess all core exercises, although higher RMs (i.e., eight or more repetitions) can result in a large amount of accumulated fatigue if multiple trial sets are performed (107). With assistance exercises, only an 8RM load or lighter should be used (10), for the same reasons these exercises should not be 1RM tested. Repetition maximum testing is usually appropriate for most intermediate to advanced clients, while

TABLE 15.7 Sample 1-Repetition Maximum Prediction Equations

Reference			Equation
Adams (2)	1RM	=	$\text{RepWt} / (1 - 0.02 \times \text{RTF})$
Brown (16)	1RM	=	$(\text{Reps} \times 0.0338 + 0.9849) \times \text{RepWt}$
Mayhew et al. (78)	1RM	=	$\text{RepWt} / (0.522 + 0.419\ e^{-0.055 \times \text{RTF}})$
O'Conner et al. (84)	1RM	=	$0.025\,(\text{RepWt} \times \text{RTF}) + \text{RepWt}$

1RM = 1-repetition maximum; RepWt = repetition weight, load <1RM to perform repetitions; RTF = repetitions to failure.

Adapted from Mayhew et al. 2008 (79).

TABLE 15.8 Protocol for Assessing Strength With a Percentage of a Client's Body Weight

Step	Action
1	In either table 15.9 or 15.10 (depending on gender), locate the exercise to be tested. There are two types of machines, the cam machine (CM) and the pivot machine (PM), that you must differentiate between.
2	Determine the client body weight (BWT), which will determine the training load. Remember that a maximum of 175 lb (79 kg) should be used for male clients and a maximum of 140 lb (64 kg) for female clients. If the client's weight is below these maximums, use actual body weight to determine the trial load.
3	Once the body weight has been determined, multiply it by the factor (i.e., the percentage expressed as a decimal point) and round down to the nearest 5-lb increment to determine the trial load. With weight stack machines, choose the resistance closest to the determined trial load.
4	Explain and demonstrate the exercise to the client and then allow the client to perform a few practice repetitions with the exercise using minimal or no resistance. While the client is familiarizing himself with the exercise, decide if his technique is good enough to enable him to perform the test. If technique is acceptable, instruct the client to warm up with one set of 10 repetitions with 50% of the trial load.
5	Allow 1 to 3 min rest after the warm-up set before starting the assessment. During this time, change the weight to the trial load. After the recovery, the client should perform as many repetitions as possible with the trial load. It is important that good technique be used throughout the test. If technique begins to fail or the client can no longer complete the repetitions, stop the assessment.
6	Once the assessment is competed, record the number of repetitions. This will serve as the base for establishing the training load for the plan.

Adapted from Baechle and Groves 1998 (10) and Earle and Baechle 2004 (26).

TABLE 15.9 Protocol for Percent Body Weight Strength Assessments for Women

Body part or muscle group	Exercise	BWT	Factor	Trial load	Repetitions completed	Adjustment	Training load
Chest							
	Bench press (FW)		× 0.35				
	Bent-arm fly (CM)		× 0.27				
	Chest press (PM)		× 0.27				
Back							
	Bent-over row (FW)		× 0.35				
	Seated row (CM)		× 0.20				
	Pullover (CM)		× 0.20				
	Seated row (PM)		× 0.25				
Shoulders							
	Standing press (FW)		× 0.22				
	Seated press (PM)		× 0.15				
	Shoulder press (CM)		× 0.25				
Biceps							
	Biceps (FW)		× 0.23				
	Preacher curl (CM)		× 0.12				
	Low pulley curl (PM)		× 0.15				
Triceps							
	Triceps extension (FW)		× 0.12				
	Triceps extension (CM)		× 0.13				
	Triceps pushdown (PM)		× 0.19				
Legs							
	Dual leg press (CM)		× 1.00				
	Leg press (PM)		× 1.00				
Abdominal muscles							
	Trunk curl (CM)		× 0.20				

The trial load is designed to allow 12 to 15 repetitions to be performed. FW = free weights; CM = cam-based machine; PM = pivot-based machine; BWT = body weight. To account for differences in body composition, use a maximum of 140 lb (64 kg) when determining testing loads for women.

Adapted from Baechle and Groves 1998 (10) and Earle and Baechle 2004 (26).

TABLE 15.10 Protocol for Percent Body Weight Strength Assessments for Men

Body part or muscle group	Exercise	BWT	Factor	Trial load	Repetitions completed	Adjustment	Training load
Chest							
	Bench press (FW)		× 0.60				
	Bent-arm fly (CM)		× 0.55				
	Chest press (PM)		× 0.55				
Back							
	Bent-over row (FW)		× 0.45				
	Seated row (CM)		× 0.40				
	Pullover (CM)		× 0.40				
	Seated row (PM)		× 0.45				
Shoulders							
	Standing press (FW)		× 0.38				
	Seated press (PM)		× 0.35				
	Shoulder press (CM)		× 0.40				
Biceps							
	Biceps (FW)		× 0.30				
	Preacher curl (CM)		× 0.20				
	Low pulley curl (PM)		× 0.25				
Triceps							
	Triceps extension (FW)		× 0.21				
	Triceps extension (CM)		× 0.35				
	Triceps pushdown (PM)		× 0.32				
Legs							
	Dual leg press (CM)		× 1.30				
	Leg press (PM)		× 1.30				
Abdominal muscles							
	Trunk curl (CM)		× 0.20				

The trial load is designed to allow 12 to 15 repetitions to be performed. FW = free weights; CM = cam-based machine; PM = pivot-based machine; BWT = body weight. To account for differences in body composition, use a maximum of 175 lb (79 kg) when determining testing loads for men.

Adapted from Baechle and Groves 1998 (10) and Earle and Baechle 2004 (26).

novice or untrained clients should be limited to lighter loads with higher repetitions (≥8RM). Regardless of the client's training status, it is important to monitor the client to help avoid excessive fatigue that could result in an increased risk of injury; the general recommendation is to limit testing to three sets.

Repetition maximum testing is very similar to assessment of the 1RM (see chapter 11), but the client performs the number of goal repetitions for each trial set with lower load ranges (~50-75% of 1RM) than recommended for a 1RM.

Guidelines for Assigning Loads

When determining the loads to be used in a program, the personal trainer must consider the primary goals of the client (muscular endurance, hypertrophy, muscular strength, or muscular power). Different load and repetition schemes can have different training effects (table 15.11). It is recommended that various loading schemes be employed in a program (4, 117) to avoid overtraining, allow for progression, and maximize training adaptations.

Assigning Load Based on 1-Repetition Maximum

The training load can be established directly based on the 1RM test or from an estimation of the client's 1RM. The repetition scheme will be based on the goals of the training phase—muscular endurance, hypertrophy, muscular strength, or muscular power (table 15.11). Having established the repetitions, the personal trainer can multiply the 1RM load (directly tested or estimated) by the percent of the 1RM associated with the goal repetitions to establish the training load.

If, for example, a client's goal is hypertrophy (increase in muscle size), he or she will perform 6 to 12 repetitions with a load between 67% and 85% of 1RM. If his or her 1RM back squat is 220 pounds (100 kg) and he or she is to perform 10 repetitions, the load could range from 147 to 187 pounds (220 × 0.67 = 147; 220 × 0.85 = 187). To properly load the barbell, he or she will set the resistance at 150 to 185 pounds (68 to 85 kg) depending on the focus of the workout. The load will be adjusted according to the goals for the individual training session and the targeted training intensity for the session.

Assigning Load Based on Percent Body Weight Testing

Another method for determining the training load is based on the %BWT assessment. Once the personal trainer has established the training plan and determined the repetition range (tables 15.9 and 15.10), he or she can compare the number of repetitions performed during the assessment with repetition ranges in table 15.11 Although the %BWT assessment is designed to produce 12 to 15 repetitions, it is possible that the client will perform less than 12 or more than 15 repetitions. Thus the trial load will need to be adjusted in order to better target the client's goals. Table 15.12 provides one possible

method for making this adjustment, increasing the load if the client performs too many repetitions or reducing the load if he or she performs too few. These adjustments are only guides and are not without error (e.g., multijoint exercises may require larger load adjustments), but they provide a valuable starting point for structuring the training plan.

For example, if a client wants to target muscular hypertrophy, a load and repetition scheme of 67% to 85% 1RM for 6 to 12 repetitions is recommended (table 15.11). If the client weighed 170 pounds (77 kg) and performed the %BWT assessment with 100 pounds on the bench press (BWT × 0.60 = 102 pounds or 46 kg) and completed 10 repetitions, the personal trainer could adjust the load according to the program goals. If the repetitions had been set at eight or nine, the load would have to be adjusted based on the information provided in table 15.12. The rows in table 15.12 show "Goal repetitions" and the columns show "Repetitions completed with the trial load." This client had a goal of eight or nine repetitions and completed 10 repetitions. The 8-9 goal repetition row and the 10-11 repetitions completed column intersect at the +5 cell, indicating that the trial load should be increased by 5 pounds (2.5 kg). Thus the assigned load would be 105 pounds

TABLE 15.11 Training Load and Repetition Schemes for Targeted Goals

Training emphasis	LOAD (%1RM)			REPETITIONS		
	Novice	Intermediate	Advanced	Novice	Intermediate	Advanced
Muscular endurance	≤65	≤70	≤75	10-15	10-15	10-25
Hypertrophy	67-80	67-85	67-85	8-12	6-12	6-12
Muscular strength*	≥70	≥80	≥85	≤6	≤6	≤6
Muscular power**	n/a	30-60	30-70	n/a	3-6	1-6

*These loads apply to core exercises; assistance exercise should use load ≤8RM.

**These loads are different than those noted in the repetition–load continuum.

Based on ACSM 2009 (4); Baechle, Earle, and Wathen 2008 (9); Earle and Baechle 2004 (26); Fleck and Kraemer 2004 (31); Kraemer et al. 2002 (66); Peterson, Rhea, and Alvar 2004 (86); Rhea et al. 2003 (95); Stone 1987 (111); Stone, Stone, and Sands 2007 (117).

TABLE 15.12 Adjusting the Trial Load to Allow the Goal Number of Repetitions

Goal repetitions	REPETITIONS COMPLETED WITH THE TRIAL LOAD									
	≥18	16-17	14-15	12-13	10-11	8-9	6-7	4-5	2-3	<2
14-15	+10	+5		−5	−10	−15	−15	−20	−25	−30
12-13	+15	+10	+5		−5	−10	−15	−15	−20	−25
10-11	+15	+15	+10	+5		−5	−10	−15	−15	−20
8-9	+20	+15	+15	+10	+5		−5	−10	−15	−15
6-7	+25	+20	+15	+15	+10	+5		−5	−10	−15
4-5	+30	+25	+20	+15	+15	+10	+5		−5	−10
2-3	+35	+30	+25	+20	+15	+15	+10	+5		−5

Load increase (+) or decrease (−).

Adapted from Baechle and Earle 1989 (7) and Earle and Baechle 2000 (26).

(100 + 5 = 105 pounds = 48 kg). This method can be used to determine the training loads for each of the exercises listed in table 15.9 and 15.10, where they can be recorded.

An additional option is to use this adjustment to modify the training load during a workout session. For example, if the client cannot complete two or more sets of eight or nine repetitions with the 105-pound load in the bench press, the load can be adjusted according to the information in 15.12; if the client can perform only six repetitions with the 105-pound load, the load could be reduced by 5 pounds. Although this method is easy to apply, it should be used with caution. The use of repetition ranges with this type of loading can create an overtraining scenario due to a lack of intensity variation. Conceptually this type of model requires the client to train to failure on each set to achieve the prescribed repetition ranges, and training to muscular failure has been clearly established as a poor way to train (86, 105).

Assigning Load Based on Repetition Maximum Testing

Another method sometimes used to assign training load is the RM method. There are no calculations, and the load established in the RM test is used as the training load. The number of repetitions used in the RM test is identical to that in the actual training plan; therefore the RM is the training load.

For example, in table 15.11, six or fewer repetitions with loads ≥85% of 1RM are suggested for improving strength with advanced clients. If the personal trainer assessed a 4RM for the bench press and the client was able to bench press only 200 pounds (91 kg) for four repetitions, the load would then be established as 200 pounds. While this method is straightforward, it involves training to muscular failure, which as noted earlier is a poor method of developing strength and in fact has been shown to mute strength gains when compared to not training to failure (86, 105). If clients are directed to always use maximal loads (RMs) to establish their training loads, overtraining and increased occurrence of injuries are possible. A far better approach to loading is to use percentages of 1RM and to vary intensity within the training week.

> Training to muscular failure is a poor method for assigning training loads; RM target and RM zones appear to be suboptimal methods for determining training load; and using percentage of maximum is a superior method.

Training Volume: Repetitions and Sets

Volume in resistance training is best defined as the *volume load* (112, 117), which is calculated as follows:

$$\text{Volume load} = \text{Total repetitions} \times \text{Load}$$

where total repetitions = sets × reps.

The volume load is a reasonable indicator of the amount of work that is accomplished during resistance training (83). The inclusion of the load in the calculation of volume is important because it contributes to the total amount of work performed. If only repetitions are used to determine volume, the depiction of work will be inaccurate. For example, three sets of 10 repetitions and five sets of six repetitions both total 30 repetitions. This might suggest that the work accomplished in the two set and repetition schemes is identical, but it is not. A client whose maximum back squat is 300 pounds (136 kg) would be able to perform 10 repetitions with 225 pounds (102 kg) and 255 pounds (116 kg) for six repetitions (table 15.6). It is easy to see that the volume is substantially higher for five sets of six repetitions with 255 pounds (7,650 pounds or 3,477 kg) than for three sets of 10 repetitions with 225 pounds (6,750 pounds or 3,068 kg).

Influential Factors

Many factors can affect the volume of training. The targeted goal of the client or training plan exerts a primary influence on the number of sets (series of repetitions linked together) or repetitions placed into the plan. For example, if the client wants to develop muscular endurance, higher repetitions (≥12 repetitions) should be planned. Conversely, if muscular strength is targeted, lower repetition schemes would be employed (six repetitions or less). The personal trainer can also manipulate the training volume by modifying the number of sets used for a particular exercise.

Single-set protocols have been shown to be inferior to multiple-set protocols (4, 87, 95) in untrained individuals (94, 95) and trained populations (86, 95, 129). Single-set protocols may be effective with the novice or untrained client when employed in the initial stages of the training program; but as the client becomes more trained it is essential that volume of training be increased, and this is probably best accomplished with use of a multiple-set training plan (4).

Guidelines for Assigning Volume

The volume of training that clients undertake is dependent on their training goals and more importantly on their training status.

Resistance Training Goals

The ability to induce specific adaptations is dependent on the ability to induce an overload and on targeting the specific training outcomes by manipulating volume and intensity of training (tables 15.11 and 15.13). Additionally, it is essential that progression and variation be structured into the training plan to facilitate the adaptive responses necessary to achieve the client's goals. The design of the training plan must address one of four goals: muscular endurance, hypertrophy, muscular strength, or muscular power (table 15.13).

- *Muscular endurance:* The plan generally uses more repetitions (i.e., ≥10 repetitions per set) with varying numbers of sets depending on training status (4, 9, 26, 31, 66, 86, 95, 111, 117).
- *Hypertrophy:* The plan uses a higher training volume (i.e., 6-12 repetitions) with moderate to high loads (67-85% 1RM) depending on training status (4, 9, 26, 31, 66, 86, 95, 111, 117).
- *Muscular strength:* For core exercises, the plan uses six or fewer repetitions with multiple sets (three or more) per exercise. For assistance exercises, it uses eight or more repetitions with one to three sets (4, 9, 26, 31, 66, 86, 95, 111, 117).
- *Power exercises:* Power exercises should not be used with untrained or novice clients. These clients should target the development of strength before focusing on training for power (66). With intermediate clients, programs that target power development should use one to three sets of three to six repetitions, while advanced clients should use three

to six sets of one to six repetitions (4, 9, 26, 31, 66, 86, 95, 111, 117).

Resistance Training Status

The training status of the client can affect the number of sets he or she can perform with a resistance training exercise. Generally, untrained or novice clients will perform fewer sets than either intermediate or advanced clients (4, 66). Initially it may be acceptable for novice clients to use a single-set program, but a multiple-set training plan is eventually necessary in order for them to progress (4). Table 15.13 presents a volume progression that can be used as the client moves from a novice to intermediate or advanced training status (4, 66).

Rest Intervals

The time period between multiple sets, or **rest interval,** can exert a strong impact on the physiological responses to a training session (4, 8, 9). The term *rest interval* can also refer to the time period between exercises. Overall the rest interval, whether between sets or exercises, is largely predicated on the goals of the client and the structure of the training plan.

Influential Factors

In general, there is a direct relationship between the load and the need for rest between sets; the heavier the load, the longer the rest needed between sets or exercises (9, 31, 77, 107). An additional consideration is the client's training status; untrained or novice clients may require longer times between sets and exercises in order to achieve adequate recovery to maintain exercise technique.

Guidelines for Establishing Rest Intervals

The overall goals of the client play a large role in dictating assignment of the resistance training loads

TABLE 15.13 Training Volume Schemes for Targeted Goals

Training emphasis	REPETITIONS			SETS		
	Novice	Intermediate	Advanced	Novice	Intermediate	Advanced
Muscular endurance	10-15	10-15	10-25	1-3	≥3	≥3
Hypertrophy	8-12	6-12	6-12	1-3	≥3	≥3
Muscular strength*	≤6	≤6	≤6	1-3	≥3	≥3
Muscular power**	n/a	3-6	1-6	n/a	1-3	3-6

*These loads apply to core exercises; assistance exercise should use load ≤8RM.
*These loads are different than those noted in the repetition–load continuum.

Based on ACSM 2009 (4); Baechle, Earle, and Wathen 2008 (9); Earle and Baechle 2004 (26); Fleck and Kraemer 2004 (31); Kraemer et al. 2002 (66); Peterson, Rhea, and Alvar 2004 (86); Rhea et al. 2003 (95); Stone 1987 (111); Stone, Stone, and Sands 2007 (117).

and volumes, both of which exert a large influence on the rest intervals chosen.

Resistance Training Status

Table 15.14 presents recommended rest interval lengths, but it is important to note that these are merely recommendations. Typically they will not work for novice or untrained clients, who will require twice as much rest as a more trained individual. With these clients it may be best to use a rest interval of 2 to 5 minutes to facilitate recovery between sets and exercises. This is particularly important when the client is learning new exercises or attempting to master a technical exercise (4). As the client becomes more trained and has mastered the technical aspects of each lift, the recommendations presented in table 15.14 may become more appropriate.

Resistance Training Goal

To tailor the training plan to the individual client's goals, the personal trainer must craft a program that allows enough rest between sets and exercises to allow the client to lift the selected loads for the assigned number of repetitions. The basic rest interval lengths for muscular endurance, hypertrophy, power, and strength, presented in table 15.14, are as follows:

- *Muscular endurance:* A relatively short rest interval, typically ≤30 seconds, is recommended for circuit-based training with exercises using dissimilar muscle groups (96, 126), while up to 3 minutes' rest may be warranted between exercises using similar muscle groups (126).
- *Muscular hypertrophy:* Rest intervals for hypertrophy should be short to moderate in duration (4, 126), ranging from 30 seconds to 1.5 minutes (49, 85, 119). Longer rest intervals with multijoint large-muscle exercises may be warranted because of their high metabolic demands (107).
- *Muscular power:* Longer rest intervals on the order of 2 to 5 minutes are warranted (107, 126) between maximal-effort sets.
- *Muscular strength:* Longer rest intervals are necessary for exercises targeting strength development (126). This is especially true for lower body or whole-body exercises (4, 128). The general recommendation is 2 to 5 minutes (69, 75, 85, 92).

Variation

Regardless of how effective or individualized a training program is, it will eventually need to be varied to ensure continued adaptation (4, 117). The concept of variation involves the appropriate alteration of training variables to produce adaptations over the long term (65, 72, 112, 113, 117). One key component of variation is a purposeful sequencing of training factors (45, 90, 117). If training is sequenced correctly, the adaptations stimulated by one period of training can exert a powerful effect on the next period of training, resulting in a summation of training effect (45, 58, 59). If the resistance training plan includes appropriate and correctly sequenced variation, it will be incrementally more effective.

Much less training variation is needed with novice or untrained clients, as any reasonable training plan will produce results (117). As clients become more trained, their progress may begin to slow if the plan does not include variation and progression. Maintenance of the same training plan without variation can induce what has been termed "monotonous overtraining" (106). If the training stimulus is unvaried for a long period of time (i.e., several months), even more experienced or trained clients can show decreases in muscular strength and neuromuscular activation (40, 41, 42, 43, 45) and an increased occurrence of overtraining symptoms (32, 33, 45, 106).

The best way to avoid stagnation is to include purposeful variation of the program design variables used to expose the client to training stimuli (23, 117). The many levels at which the personal trainer can alter the training stimulus include frequency, intensity, and volume of training, as well as the rest intervals between sets and exercises (23, 29, 45, 85, 90, 108, 109, 117). Variation in the training plan can occur within a workout, during a week, or over a period of several weeks. Only a few of the possible

TABLE 15.14 Rest Interval Recommendation Based on Training Goals

Training goal	Rest interval length
Muscular endurance	≤30 s
Muscular hypertrophy	30 s to 1.5 min
Muscular power	2 to 5 min
Muscular strength	2 to 5 min

These rest intervals are only guidelines and should be used with caution. The maintenance of technique is of primary importance; if the rest interval length selected results in a reduction in technical proficiency, increase the rest interval. Also consider the rest interval length as a function of the total amount of work (volume load) encountered in a training set; the more work completed in a set, the longer the rest interval needs to be.

Based on ACSM 2009 (4); Baechle, Earle, and Wathen 2008 (9); Fleck and Kraemer 2004 (31); Stone and O'Bryant 1987 (107).

methods for introducing variation into the training plan are presented here. (See chapter 23 for a detailed discussion of periodization, or a systematic method for inducing training variation.)

Within-Session Variation

During an individual training session, there are a number of ways to vary the training stimulus. One often employed method is to vary the intensity at which individual exercises are performed—some exercises are performed at higher intensities and others at lower intensities (117). A single session may employ some longer rest intervals and some shorter rest intervals. Typically, longer rest intervals are used with core exercises and shorter rest intervals are used with assistance exercises (4, 65, 88, 97, 127).

Another way to vary the training stimulus during a session is to alter the set configuration (36, 37, 39). Traditionally sets are performed in a continuous fashion with little or no rest between each repetition. Recent research suggests that one can modify the focus of a set by altering the interrepetition rest interval to construct what has been termed a "cluster set" (39). A cluster set uses a rest interval of 5 to 45 seconds between each repetition (36). For example, if endurance or conditioning is the focus, a shorter rest interval may be employed (~5 seconds). If power generation is the main focus, rest intervals may be longer (~45 seconds). When using the cluster set paradigm, the personal trainer can add an additional layer of variation by introducing changes to the loading used during each repetition of the set. There are three categories of cluster sets: (1) the standard cluster set, in which the load is not altered across the set; (2) the undulating cluster, in which the load is increased and then decreased within the set; and (3) the ascending cluster, in which the load increases

across the set (table 15.15) (36, 37, 39). Cluster sets offer another level of variation that can affect the focus of an individual training session.

Within-Week Variation

One of the best ways to incorporate variation into a training plan is to vary the intensity of exercises selected across the week (117). It may be difficult for clients to undertake high training loads across an entire week. As the week progresses, the client's cumulative stress (i.e., training, work, home, personal, etc.) is likely to increase steadily and his or her ability to tolerate the training stress will decline (107, 117); this increases the potential for overtraining (106). One strategy to combat this is to use light and heavy days of training; the light days allow the client to recover, thereby reducing the risk of overtraining.

There are a multitude of strategies for varying the training load, but one that is particularly easy to employ is to vary the percentages of 1RM during the sessions across the week. For example, if a client's maximum back squat is 300 pounds (136 kg) and the targeted number of repetitions for the training day is five, a very heavy load for this client would be around 260 pounds (118 kg), which would be roughly a 5RM. Let's say the client is squatting two days a week (Monday and Thursday). Monday would be the heaviest day, in this case 240 pounds (109 kg, ~92% of 260 pounds), and Thursday would be around 208 to 220 pounds (95 to 100 kg, ~80-85% of 260 pounds). The second session would use ~10% to 15% less resistance, thus accounting for the cumulative fatigue associated with the training week, while still supplying adequate training stimulus to induce adaptive responses. As mentioned previously, training to failure (100% of RM values) is not necessary (105), produces suboptimal results (60,

TABLE 15.15 Sample Within-Cluster Set Structures

Type of cluster	Sets	x	Repetitions	Interrepetition rest interval (seconds)	Sample cluster set repetition loading structures									
Standard	1-3	×	10/1	5	80/1	80/1	80/1	80/1	80/1	80/1	80/1	80/1	80/1	80/1
	1-3	×	10/2	10	80/2	80/2	80/2	80/2	80/2					
	1-3	×	10/5	15	80/5	80/5								
Undulating	1-3	×	10/1	5	75/1	80/1	82.5/1	85/1	85/1	82.5/1	80/1	77.5/1	75/1	80/1
	1-3	×	10/2	10	77.5/1	80/1	85/1	80/1	77.5/1					
Ascending	1-3	×	10/1	5	55/1	60/1	65/1	70/1	75/1	85/1	90/1	95/1	100/1	105/1
	1-3	×	10/2	10	70/2	75/2	80/2	85/2	90/2					

10/1 = 10 total repetitions broken into 10 clusters of one; 10/2 = 10 total repetitions broken into five clusters of 2; 10/5 = 10 total repetitions broken into two clusters of five.

All weights based on a max power clean of 100 kg (80 kg = 80% of 1-repetition maximum). Each set has an average intensity of 80 kg or 80% of 1-repetition maximum. Rest interval lengths can be increased to 45 s depending on the goal of the training structure.

Adapted from: Haff et al. 2003 (37), Haff et al. 2008 (38), and Haff et al. 2008 (39).

TABLE 15.16 Sample Daily and Weekly Variations

Day	Exercises	TARGET ZONE Sets	TARGET ZONE Reps	INTENSITIES (POUNDS) Week 1	Week 2	Week 3	Week 4
Monday	Back squat	3	10	200	210	220	205
	One-leg squat	3	10	135	140	145	135
	Leg curl	3	10	120	125	130	120
	Leg extension	3	10	150	155	160	150
	Abdominal exercises	3	25				
Tuesday	Bench press	3	10	180	185	190	180
	Bent-over row	3	10	150	155	160	150
	Shoulder press	3	10	130	135	140	130
	Lat pulldown	3	10	140	145	150	140
	Triceps press-down	3	10	100	105	110	100
	Biceps curl	3	10	95	100	105	95
Thursday	Back squat	3	10	180	185	190	185
	One-leg squat	3	10	120	125	130	125
	Leg curl	3	10	105	110	115	110
	Leg extension	3	10	135	140	145	130
	Abdominal exercises	3	25				
Saturday	Bench press	3	10	160	165	170	160
	Bent-over row	3	10	135	140	145	135
	Shoulder press	3	10	115	120	125	115
	Lat pulldown	3	10	125	130	140	125
	Triceps press-down	3	10	90	95	100	90
	Biceps curl	3	10	85	90	95	85

	Monday			Tuesday			Thursday			Saturday			Weekly		
Microcycle	Reps	VL	TI	Reps	VL	TI	Reps	VL	TI	Reps	VL	TI	Reps	VL	TI
1	120	18,150	151	180	23,850	133	120	16,200	135	180	21,300	118	600	79,500	134
2	120	18,900	158	180	24,750	138	120	16,800	140	180	22,200	123	600	82,650	140
3	120	19,650	164	180	25,650	143	120	17,400	145	180	23,250	129	600	85,950	145
4	120	18,300	153	180	23,850	133	120	16,500	138	180	21,300	118	600	79,950	135

Reps = repetitions; VL = volume load (reps × sets × pounds); TI = volume load / total repetitions.

87), and increases the risk of overtraining (32). A far superior strategy is to plan specific load variations while maintaining the targeted repetitions. Table 15.16 offers an example of how intensity could be varied across a training week and across a period of four weeks. Another example of weekly variation is presented in table 15.17. In this example, the client achieves a 225-pound (102 kg) back squat during the 1RM test. This value can be used in conjunction with table 15.6 to estimate the 5RM (195 pounds or 89 kg) or 10RM (170 pounds or 77 kg). The estimated 10RM can then be used to determine percentage zones, which can be used for creating light and heavy days. This is an excellent method for programming and has been shown to be very effective in maximizing training adaptations while decreasing the risks of overtraining.

> When planning light days, the personal trainer should reduce the loading and leave the repetitions the same. If the volume is reduced in conjunction with an increase in repetitions, the cumulative workload will increase and the light day will actually become a heavy day.

Between-Week Variation

The training program should vary between weeks, through alterations in volume, intensity, frequency, exercise selection, and training focus. For example,

TABLE 15.17   Sample Loading Classification and Weekly Variation

LOADING CLASSIFICATION*					
Intensity		% Initial RM	% Initial 1RM	% Estimated 5RM	% Estimated 10RM
Very heavy	(VH)	95–100	214–225	185–195	162–170
Heavy	(H)	90–95	203–214	176–185	153–162
Moderately heavy	(MH)	85–90	191–203	166–176	145–153
Moderate	(M)	80–85	180–191	156–166	136–145
Moderately light	(ML)	75–80	169–180	146–156	128–136
Light	(L)	70–75	158–169	137–146	119–128
Very light	(VL)	65–70	146–158	127–137	111–119

WEEKLY VARIATION**							
Week	Monday	Tuesday	Wednesday	Thursday	Friday	Saturday	Sunday
1	VL (111-119)			VL (111-119)			
2	L (119-128)			VL (111-119)			
3	ML (128-136)			L(119-128)			
4	L (119-128)			L (119-128)			

*225 lb was determined as the 1RM in testing of the back squat. Table 15.7 shows that the 5RM is estimated at 195 lb and the 10RM is estimated at 170 lb.

**In this example, the back squat is performed on Monday and Thursday with three target sets of 10 repetitions.

Adapted from Stone and O'Bryant 1987 (107) and Stone et al. 2006 (110).

if a four-week period of training targets muscular endurance, the plan may call for three sets of 12 repetitions based on the information presented in table 15.11. According to the principles of periodization, the average intensity could be increased for three weeks and then reduced during the fourth week, creating what is termed a 3:1 loading paradigm (table 15.16) (15, 90). In table 15.16, the weekly volume load (e.g., week 1 = 79,500 pounds; week 2 = 82,650 pounds; week 3 = 85,950 pounds; week 4 = 79,950 pounds) and average training intensity (i.e., week 1 = 134 pounds; week 2 = 140 pounds; week 3 = 145 pounds; week 4 = 135 pounds) increase across the first three weeks. This type of loading is considered the most basic loading structure for resistance training, but there are other possibilities, for example, a 2:1, 4:1, 3:2, or 4:2 structure. If these types of loading are coupled with daily variations as discussed previously, the client will be able to maximize training adaptations while minimizing the chances of overtraining.

Another way to incorporate variation between training weeks is to alter the training density. For example, week 1 may include four resistance training sessions, two high-intensity interval training sessions, and two aerobic training sessions. In this week, the main focus is the resistance training. In the second week, the resistance training sessions could be reduced to three, the high-intensity interval training sessions increased to three, and the frequency of aerobic training maintained, thus changing the focus of the week to interval training. By playing with the various training modes over the training week, one can selectively target specific outcomes and manage fatigue more efficiently, ultimately allowing the client to experience greater training adaptations.

> Training to failure (100% of RM values) is not necessary, produces suboptimal results, and increases the risk of overtraining. A far superior strategy is to plan specific training load variations while maintaining the targeted repetitions.

Sequencing Training

One of the classic mistakes made in the design of a resistance training program is not appropriately sequencing the training factors (45, 90, 117). Appropriately sequenced training programs result in superior adaptations and performance gains (45). Conversely, an inappropriately sequenced training plan will mute the physiological and performance adaptations that are expected from the training plan.

It appears that traditionally, personal trainers have targeted only the primary training goals (i.e., muscular endurance, hypertrophy, muscular strength, or muscular power) when designing a program. While at first glance this seems logical based on the principles of specificity, scientific evidence strongly supports the idea of interdependence among the goals. For example, when maximal strength is the main desired training outcome, a period of training that targets hypertrophy should precede training that targets maximal strength.

> Training sequence targeting maximal strength
> = Hypertrophy training → Maximal strength training

By sequencing training in this fashion, greater levels of strength can be developed because of the underlying muscular adaptations stimulated by increasing muscle cross-sectional area.

Similarly, it is very clear that if maximal power-generating capacity is the target outcome, one needs to first develop overall strength levels.

> Training sequence targeting power development
> = Hypertrophy training → Maximal strength training
> → Muscular power training

The increases in muscle cross-sectional area would thus increase the ability to increase maximal strength, which would then contribute to maximizing muscular power development when the training focus shifts to power-based training.

As a general rule, all clients should begin resistance training with a plan based on either muscular endurance or hypertrophy. These phases are important because they establish the training base, which lays the foundation for the development of other targeted goals (90, 107). Most clients can tolerate these phases of training for two to four weeks with appropriate variations in volume and intensity. After about four weeks of this type of training, the client's adaptive responses become asymptotic and training adaptations will slow dramatically. At this time the personal trainer should alter the training goals to obviate the problem by shifting the focus of the program toward the development of muscular strength, typically targeting strength development for two to five weeks. Most clients would then shift back to a muscular endurance or hypertrophy focus, but athletes would likely progress toward a muscular power–based plan. Regardless of the goals, the sequencing of training appears to result in a phase potentiation effect, whereby the attributes developed in one phase facilitate the physiological and performance adaptations seen in the subsequent phase (15, 58, 59, 107). When sequencing training, the personal trainer should consider the basic guidelines for the length of each phase presented in table 15.18.

The client's overall training goals, as established early on by the personal trainer and client, will determine the sequence of the training plan. As noted previously, the goals will also help the personal trainer establish the basic volume and loading parameters. However, no client can keep targeting the same goals indefinitely. Therefore the program should vary the targeted goals by periodically alter-

TABLE 15.18 Training Factor Sequencing Guidelines

Phase of training	Length (weeks)	Ratio of heavy to light weeks (heavy/light)
Muscular endurance	2-4	2-3/1
Hypertrophy	2-4	2-3/1
Muscular strength	2-5	2-4/1
Muscular power	2-4	2-3/1

2-3/1: Two or three weeks with increasing loads followed by one unloading week. 2-4/1: two to four weeks with increasing loads followed by one unloading week.

Adapted from Stone & O'Bryant 1984 (107).

ing the training target. For example, a client who is targeting muscular hypertrophy might perform a four-week period of hypertrophy training (e.g., three sets of 10) followed by three weeks of muscular strength work, then return to four weeks of hypertrophy training. Alternating between muscular strength and hypertrophy will produce greater increases in hypertrophy and strength (91). Three of many methods for sequencing training are shown in figure 15.1.

> Sequencing the training emphasis is critical to achieving specific training outcomes. A periodic shifting of targeted training goals in a sequential fashion avoids stagnation and overtraining while encouraging physiological and performance adaptations.

Progression

An essential component of any training program is the concept of progression. Progression is a process in which the client continues to move toward a predetermined goal (4), while maintenance is a time point at which the goal has been achieved and the client is attempting to maintain a specific level of fitness (4, 66). Progression should be considered a general training principle and is a function of training variation. Progression can be accomplished through increasing loads, volume, or frequency or making any number of alterations that modify the training stimulus. The most frequently used method for progressing clients is to change the load and volume lifted in each exercise.

The best method for determining when to increase training load is to schedule periodic RM assessments. These assessments can use any of the methods previously described to either directly measure or estimate the client's capabilities. If, for example, the client is assessed on the back squat

Muscular Endurance Focus

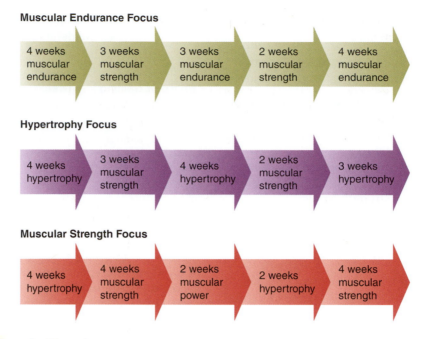

Hypertrophy Focus

Muscular Strength Focus

FIGURE 15.1 Example 16-week program sequences.

for a 10RM and lifts a 165-pound (75 kg) load, the personal trainer can use table 15.6 to estimate the 1RM (i.e., 220 pounds or 100 kg) and then determine the training loads by taking percentages of this value. It is easy to integrate this method into the weekly and daily variation schedules described previously in this chapter. This appears to be the best way to establish training loads because of the inferiority of training to failure as a method of loading (95, 105). Generally, when progressing training loads, one can use a conservative increase in load of 2.5% to 10%, depending on the type of exercise, client training status, and the part of the body being trained (table 15.19) (9).

Another method that is somewhat popular is the **2-for-2 rule** (8, 9, 10), which is based on the achievement of goal repetitions for a training session. The rule states that if the client can complete two more repetitions than the repetition goal in the final set of an exercise for two consecutive training sessions, the load in all of the sets for that exercise during subsequent training sessions can be increased (see table 15.20 for example). While some find this method effective, it may not be the best because it requires consistently training to muscular failure.

Sample Programs for Targeted Training Outcomes

Numerous combinations of training programs can be constructed based on the sequential approach

to designing training plans. Remember that before focusing on strength development, the client should complete a muscular endurance or hypertrophy phase. Additionally, a strength phase should precede a phase of training that focuses on muscular power. Each program should be individualized to meet the client's needs and should meet all the general principles of training addressed at the beginning of this chapter. There are numerous possibilities; the programs presented in tables 15.21 through 15.24 on pages 377 to 383 are simply examples rather than plans to apply to all clients.

Table 15.21 presents a plan that targets **muscular endurance training** for a novice client. This program uses the body weight method for determining training loads because the client is a beginner. The methods are primarily machine based, and the rest intervals are short to facilitate the development of muscular endurance. This program can be used for a short period of time until a training base has been established; at this point the program should be modified so that training intensities can be based on percentages of either predicted or actual maximal lifts in order to maximize the client's adaptive responses. After completing this program, the client should enter into a two- to four-week phase that targets muscular strength. Subsequently the focus can be reoriented toward muscular endurance, and more advanced training techniques can be employed.

The program presented in table 15.22 is a four-week training block that targets muscular hypertrophy. This example is based on the client's stated

TABLE 15.19 Sample Load Increases for a Training Session in Which Increases in Intensity Are Planned

Resistance training status	Body area	Type of exercise	APPROXIMATE LOAD INCREASE	
			Absolute increase (weight)	Relative increase (% of previous load)
Beginner	Upper body	Core	2.5 to 5 lb 1 to 2 kg	2.5%
		Assistance	1.25 to 2.5 lb 0.6 to 1 kg	1-2%
	Lower body	Core	10 to 15 lb 4 to 7 kg	5%
		Assistance	5 to 10 lb 2 to 4 kg	2.5-5%
Intermediate or advanced	Upper body	Core	5 to 10+ lb 2 to 4+ kg	2.5-5+%
		Assistance	5 to 10 lb 2 to 4 kg	2.5-5%
	Lower body	Core	15 to 20+ lb 7 to 9+ kg	5-10+%
		Assistance	10 to 15 lb 4 to 7 kg	5-10%

These load increases should be considered only guidelines and are best for programs with volumes of three sets of 5 to 10 repetitions. Periodic testing should be used to determine actual training load demands of a client.

Adapted from Baechle and Earle 2000 (8) and Baechle et al. 2008 (9).

TABLE 15.20 Using the 2-for-2 Rule to Increase the Training Load (an Example)

EXAMPLE: BEGINNER CLIENT WHOSE REPETITION GOAL FOR THE BACK SQUAT EXERCISE IS 10				
Training session 1	**Set 1**	**Set 2**	**Set 3**	
Weight	135 lb	135 lb	135 lb	
Repetitions completed	10	10	11	Exceeded goal by one repetition
Training session 2	**Set 1**	**Set 2**	**Set 3**	
Weight	135 lb	135 lb	135 lb	
Repetitions completed	12	11	10	Did not exceed repetition goal
Training session 3	**Set 1**	**Set 2**	**Set 3**	
Weight	135 lb	135 lb	135 lb	
Repetitions completed	12	12	12	Exceeded goal by two repetitions
Training session 4	**Set 1**	**Set 2**	**Set 3**	
Weight	135 lb	135 lb	135 lb	Exceeded goal by two repetitions in two consecutive
Repetitions completed	12	12	12	training sessions
Next training session	**Set 1**	**Set 2**	**Set 3**	
Weight	145 lb	145 lb	145 lb	10 lb added to all three sets
Repetition goal	10	10	10	

Adapted from Baechle and Earle 2000 (26).

goals of muscular hypertrophy, a fitness evaluation that uses a 10RM test to estimate the individual's 1RM, and the client's training status (table 15.1). From this 1RM, the actual training loads are used to determine the client's training zones (based on table 15.17). Training takes place four times per week, with most of the exercises targeting multijoint movements performed on free weights. The program employs inter- and intraintensity variation as indicated by the inclusion of heavy and light training days. The overall block exhibits a 3:1 loading paradigm: The load increases over the first three weeks, while the fourth week is an unloading week as indicated by the overall decrease in training intensity.

A sample training program that targets muscular strength is presented in table 15.23. This example includes a four-week block of training. The plan is for an advanced client who is targeting the maximization of muscular strength. Based on the client's level of development and experience, the plan calls for a frequency of four times per week (based on table 15.2). The majority of the exercises are performed with free weights, with three sets of five repetitions for core exercises and three sets of 10 repetitions for assistance exercises. Intensities are determined based on 1RM and 10RM testing, which is used to estimate 5RM loads. From these loads training zones are established. The program has a 3:1 loading structure, with heavy and light days to facilitate recovery and adaptation.

Finally, table 15.24 presents a sample muscular power training plan for an advanced client. This program uses training intensities based on estimated 1RM and 3RM loads for the core exercises. The majority of the exercises are free weight exercises. Because this client is advanced, the training fre-quency is set at four days per week. In keeping with the recommendations presented in tables 15.13 and 15.14, the client will perform three sets of three repetitions with 3 minutes' rest between sets. Additionally, the power clean and power snatch will use ascending or traditional clusters as shown in table 15.15. A 3:1 loading paradigm with daily and weekly fluctuations in training intensity is used (table 15.17 and 15.19).

Conclusion

Designing a resistance training program requires the personal trainer to understand the concepts of specificity of training, overload, variation, progression, and sequencing. Many training factors can be altered, such as the exercises selected, frequency of training, overload, volume, intensity, rest interval, and sequence, to optimize outcomes. Once the program is established, the personal trainer must vary and advance the plan in order to continue to help clients achieve their training goals.

TABLE 15.21 Sample Muscular Endurance Program: Alternating Upper and Lower Body Exercises

WORKOUT (TUESDAYS AND FRIDAYS)			TRAINING LOADS		
Exercises	Exercise type	Sets	Repetitions	Weight	Rest interval
Bench press	Free weights	2	15	50	30 s
Leg press	Pivot machine	2	15	150	30 s
Seated row	Cam machine	2	15	30	30 s
Leg (knee) curl	Cam machine	2	15	15RM	30 s
Shoulder press	Cam machine	2	15	20	30 s
Leg (knee) extension	Cam machine	2	15	15RM	30 s
Biceps curl	Free weights	2	15	25	30 s
Seated heel raise	Pivot machine	2	15	15RM	30 s
Triceps press-down	Pivot machine	2	15	20	30 s
Abdominal muscles		2	25		30 s

Explanation of program

Initial Consultation	Initial training status and experience based on table 15.1	Beginner
	Fitness evaluation	% Body weight and 15RM test
	Primary resistance training goal	Muscular endurance
Exercises	Exercise choices	Mixture of free weights, cam machine, and pivot machine exercise
	Core exercises	Bench press, leg press, seated row, and shoulder press
	Assistance exercises	Leg (knee) curl, leg (knee) extension, biceps curl, seated heel raise, triceps press-down, abdominal crunch
	Number of exercises per muscle group	1 exercise per muscle group
Frequency	Frequency of training (table 15.2)	2 or 3 times per week spaced evenly throughout the week
Order	Exercise order	Alternate between upper and lower body exercises
		Complete one set of each exercise, then repeat

Determining load*

Percent body weight testing (tables 15.8 and 15.9)

Determine training load based on client's body weight. 140-lb female client.

Exercise		Calculation	Trial load	Number of repetitions completed
Bench press	Free weights	140 × 0.35	49 lb (round to 50 lb)	15
Leg press	Pivot machine	140 × 1.00	140 lb	20
Seated row	Cam machine	140 × 0.20	28 lb (round to 25 lb)	16
Shoulder press	Cam machine	140 × 0.25	35 lb	8
Biceps curl	Free weights	140 × 0.23	32 lb (round to 30 lb)	12
Triceps press-down	Pivot machine	140 × 0.19	26.6 lb (round to 25 lb)	13

Assigning load**

Based on %BWT testing: goal repetitions 15.

Adjust the loads from %BWT testing to assign loads (table 15.8, 15.9 and 15.10).

Assign training load based on body weight. 140-lb female client.

Exercise		Load adjustment	Equation	Assigned training load
Bench press	Free weights	None needed	n/a	50 lb
Leg press	Pivot machine	+10	140 + 10 = 150	150 lb
Seated row	Cam machine	+5 lb	25 + 5 = 30	30 lb
Shoulder press	Cam machine	−15 lb	35 − 15 = 20	20 lb
Biceps curl	Free weights	−5 lb	30 − 5 = 25	25 lb
Triceps press-down	Pivot machine	−5 lb	25 − 5 = 20	20 lb

*15RM testing for these exercises (conservative testing to avoid client fatigue; limited to three testing sets): leg (knee) curl, leg (knee) extension, and seated heel raise.

**Based on RM testing (note that the RM loads may have to be decreased due to the multiple assigned sets): Assign loads from 15RM testing for leg (knee) curl, leg (knee) extension, and seated heel raise.

TABLE 15.22   Sample Hypertrophy Program: Four Times Per Week Split Routine

Day	Exercise	Sets	Repetitions	TRAINING LOADS Week 1	Week 2	Week 3	Week 4
Monday	Back squat	3	10	ML	M	MH	ML
	Lunge	3	10	ML	M	MH	ML
	Romanian deadlift	3	10	ML	M	MH	ML
	Leg curl	3	10	ML	M	MH	ML
	Standing heel raise + seated heel raise	3	10	ML	M	MH	ML
	Bent-knee sit-up	3	25				
Tuesday	Bench press	3	10	ML	M	MH	ML
	Dumbbell incline press	3	10	ML	M	MH	ML
	Bent-over row	3	10	ML	M	MH	ML
	Shoulder press	3	10	ML	M	MH	ML
	Shoulder shrug	3	10	ML	M	MH	ML
	Biceps curl	3	10	ML	M	MH	ML
	Triceps extension	3	10	ML	M	MH	ML
	Abdominal crunch	3	25				
Thursday	Back squat	3	10	L	ML	M	L
	Lunge	3	10	L	ML	M	L
	Romanian deadlift	3	10	L	ML	M	L
	Leg curl	3	10	L	ML	M	L
	Standing heel raise + seated heel raise	3	10	L	ML	M	L
	Bent-knee sit-up	3	25				
Saturday	Bench press	3	10	L	ML	M	L
	Dumbbell incline press	3	10	L	ML	M	L
	Bent-over row	3	10	L	ML	M	L
	Shoulder press	3	10	L	ML	M	L
	Shoulder shrug	3	10	L	ML	M	L
	Biceps curl	3	10	L	ML	M	L
	Triceps extension	3	10	L	ML	M	L
	Abdominal crunch	3	25				

All sets and exercises have rest intervals of 1.5 min or 90 s. Only the superset of triceps press-down and biceps curl and the compound set of standing and seated heel raise do not follow this recommendation.

Explanation of program

Initial consultation	Initial training status and experience based on table 15.1	Intermediate
	Fitness evaluation	10RM testing (to estimate 1RM)
	Primary resistance training goal	Hypertrophy
Exercises	Exercise choices	Primarily free weights; machines for assistance exercises
	Core exercises	Back squat, lunge, Romanian deadlift, bench press, shoulder press, bent-over row
	Assistance exercises	Biceps curl, triceps press-down, leg curl, standing heel raise, seated heel raise, shoulder shrug
	Number of exercises per muscle group	1 or 2 exercises per muscle group
Frequency	Frequency of training (table 15.2)	3 or 4 times per week spaced evenly throughout the week
Order	Primary methods	Core exercise and then assistance exercises Exercises that train large muscle groups first and then exercises that train small muscle groups Multijoint exercises first, then single-joint exercises
	Secondary methods	Exercises performed in a compound set: heel raise, seated heel raise

Determining load	Determine the training load using RM testing.		10RM testing is used to estimate a 1RM (protocol in chapter 11, but modified; see tables 15.5 and 15.6)					
	Exercise	**10RM**		**Estimated 1RM**				
	Bench press	165 lb		220 lb				
	Dumbbell incline press	40 lb (each hand)		55 lb (each hand)				
	Bent-over row	80 lb		110 lb				
	Shoulder press	90 lb		120 lb				
	Shoulder shrug	160 lb		215 lb				
	Biceps curl	90 lb		120 lb				
	Triceps extension	100 lb		135 lb				
	Back squat	225 lb		300 lb				
	Lunge	75 lb		100 lb				
	Romanian deadlift	150 lb		200 lb				
	Leg curl	120 lb		160 lb				
	Seated heel raise	110 lb		145 lb				
	Standing heel raise	120 lb		160 lb				

Repetitions	Based on table 15.13 and the client's targeted goals.
	Repetition range is set based on client's classification: intermediate, 6 to 12 repetitions; in this case, sets of 10 were chosen.

Sets	Based on table 15.13 and the client's classification: intermediate, three or more sets; in this case, three sets were chosen. The set structure presented is for the target sets and does not include warm-ups; two or three or more warm-up sets may be needed.

Rest periods	Rest periods are based on table 15.14. All sets and exercises have rest intervals of 1.5 min or 90 s. Only the superset of triceps press-down and biceps curl and the compound set of standing and seated heel raise do not follow this recommendation.

Assigning load*	Assign training load based on RM testing.				10RM testing is used to determine specific training zones with table 15.17.			
	Exercise	**10M**	**VH**	**H**	**MH**	**M**	**ML**	**L**	**VL**
	Bench press	165 lb	165-157	157-149	149-140	140-132	132-116	116-107	107-99
	Dumbbell incline press	40 lb (each hand)	40-38	38-36	36-34	34-32	32-30	30-28	28-26
	Bent-over row	80 lb	80-76	76-72	72-68	68-64	64-60	60-56	56-52
	Shoulder press	90 lb	90-86	86-81	81-77	77-72	72-68	68-63	63-59
	Shoulder shrug	160 lb	160-152	152-144	144-136	136-128	128-120	120-112	112-104
	Biceps curl	90 lb	90-86	86-81	81-77	77-72	72-68	68-63	63-59
	Triceps extension	100 lb	100-95	95-90	90-85	85-80	80-75	75-70	70-65
	Back squat	225 lb	225-214	214-203	203-191	191-180	180-169	169-158	158-149
	Lunge	75 lb	75-71	71-68	68-64	64-60	60-56	56-53	53-49
	Romanian deadlift	150 lb	150-143	143-135	135-128	128-120	120-113	113-105	105-98
	Leg curl	120 lb	120-114	114-108	108-102	102-96	96-90	90-84	84-78
	Seated heel raise	110 lb	110-105	105-99	99-94	94-88	88-83	83-77	77-72
	Standing heel raise	120 lb	120-114	114-108	108-102	102-96	96-90	90-84	84-78

*Estimated 10RM values will be used to calculate the training zones for specific training sessions based on table 15.17.

TABLE 15.23 Sample Muscular Strength Program: Within- and Between-Week Variation

Day	Exercise	Sets	Repetitions	TRAINING LOADS			
				Week 1	Week 2	Week 3	Week 4
Monday	Power clean	3	5/1	M	MH	H	M
	Back squat	3	5	M	MH	H	M
	Bench press	3	5	M	MH	H	M
	Biceps curl	3	10	M	MH	H	M
	Triceps press-down	3	10	M	MH	H	M
	Abdominal crunch	3	25				
Tuesday	Deadlift	3	5	ML	M	MH	ML
	Bent-over row	3	5	ML	M	MH	ML
	Shoulder shrug	3	5	ML	M	MH	ML
	Romanian deadlift*	3	5	ML	M	MH	ML
	Lat pulldown	3	10	ML	M	MH	ML
	Abdominal crunch	3	25				
Thursday	Power clean	3	5/1	ML	M	MH	ML
	Back squat	3	5	ML	M	MH	ML
	Bench press	3	5	ML	M	MH	ML
	Biceps curl	3	10	ML	M	MH	ML
	Triceps press-down	3	10	ML	M	MH	ML
	Abdominal crunch	3	25				
Saturday	Deadlift	3	5	M	MH	H	M
	Bent-over row	3	5	M	MH	H	M
	Shoulder shrug	3	5	M	MH	H	M
	Romanian deadlift*	3	5	M	MH	H	M
	Lat pulldown	3	10	M	MH	H	M
	Abdominal crunch	3	25				

Rest interval between sets and exercises is set at 3 min. 5/2 = cluster set with 30 s rest between repetitions.

*Load for the Romanian deadlift is based on the power clean maximum.

Explanation of program

Initial consultation	Initial training status and experience based on table 15.1	Advanced
	Fitness evaluation	1RM and 10RM testing (to estimate 1RM)
	Primary resistance training goal	Muscular strength
Exercises	Exercise choices	Primarily free weights, but some machines for assistance exercises
	Core exercises	Power clean, back squat, bench press, deadlift, bent-over row, Romanian deadlift
	Assistance exercises	Biceps curl, triceps press-down, shoulder shrug, lat pulldown
	Number of exercises per muscle group	1 or 2 exercises per muscle group
Frequency	Frequency of training (table 15.2)	3 or 4 times per week spaced evenly throughout the week
Order	Primary methods	Core exercise and then assistance exercises
		Exercises that train large muscle groups first and then exercises that train small muscle groups
		Multijoint exercises first, then single joint exercises

Determining load	Determine the training load based on RM testing.		1RM testing for specific core exercises		
			10RM testing is used to estimate a 1RM (protocol in chapter 11, but modified; table 15.5) for assistance exercises and those core exercises that are not safe to max out.		

1RM TEST RESULTS		
Exercise	1RM	Estimated 5RM
Power clean	225 lb	196 lb
Back squat	375 lb	326 lb
Bench press	300 lb	261 lb
Deadlift	325 lb	283 lb

10RM TEST RESULTS			
Exercise	10RM	Estimated 5RM	Estimated 1RM
Bent-over row	140 lb	161 lb	185 lb
Lat pulldown	175 lb	300 lb	230 lb
Biceps curl	105 lb	122 lb	140 lb
Triceps press-down	105 lb	122 lb	140 lb

EXERCISES ESTIMATED FROM THE POWER CLEAN MAXIMUM		
Exercise	1RM	Estimated 5RM
Shoulder shrug	225 lb	196 lb
Romanian deadlift	225 lb	196 lb

Repetitions	Based on table 15.13 and the client's targeted goals.
	Repetition range is set based on client classification: advanced, six or fewer repetitions; in this case, sets of six were chosen.
Sets	Based on table 15.13 and the client's classification: advanced, three or more sets; in this case, three sets were chosen.
	The set structure presented is for the target sets and does not include warm-ups; two or three more warm-up sets may be needed.
Rest periods	Rest periods are based on table 15.14.
	All sets and exercises have rest intervals of 3 min or 180 s. Only the superset of triceps press-down and biceps curl and the compound set of standing and seated heel raise do not follow this recommendation.
Assigning load*	Assign the training load based on RM testing. 1RM and 10RM testing is used to determine specific training zones with table 15.17.

Exercise	5RM	VH	H	MH	M	ML	L	VL
Power clean	196 lb	196-186	186-176	176-167	167-157	157-147	147-137	137-127
Back squat	326 lb	329-310	310-293	293-277	277-261	261-245	245-228	228-212
Bench press	261 lb	261-248	248-235	235-222	222-209	209-196	196-183	183-170
Deadlift	283 lb	283-269	269-255	255-241	241-226	226-212	212-198	198-184
Bent-over row	161 lb	161-153	153-145	145-137	137-129	129-121	121-113	113-105
Shoulder shrug	196 lb	196-186	186-176	176-167	167-157	157-147	147-137	137-127
Romanian deadlift	196 lb	196-186	186-176	176-167	167-157	157-147	147-137	137-127

Exercise	10RM	VH	H	MH	M	ML	L	VL
Lat pulldown	175 lb	175-166	166-158	158-149	149-140	140-131	131-123	123-114
Biceps curl	105 lb	105-100	100-95	95-89	89-84	84-79	79-74	74-68
Triceps press-down	105 lb	105-100	100-95	95-89	89-84	84-79	79-74	74-68

*1RM and 10RM values will be used to calculate the training zones for specific training sessions based on table 15.17.

TABLE 15.24 Sample Muscular Power Program: Within- and Between-Week Variation

| Day | Exercise | Sets | Repetitions | TRAINING LOADS | | | |
				Week 1	Week 2	Week 3	Week 4
Monday	Power clean	3	3/1 ascending clusters	M	MH	H	ML
	Speed squat	3	3	M	MH	H	ML
	Push press	3	3	M	MH	H	ML
	Biceps curl	3	10	M	MH	H	ML
	Triceps press-down	3	10	M	MH	H	ML
	Abdominal exercises	3	25				
Tuesday	Snatch grip shrug	3	3	ML	M	MH	L
	Power snatch	3	3/1 traditional clusters	M	MH	H	ML
	Snatch grip Romanian deadlift	3	3	ML	M	MH	L
	Lat pulldown	3	10	ML	M	MH	L
	Abdominal exercises	3	25				
Thursday	Power clean	3	3/1 traditional clusters	ML	M	MH	L
	Jump squat	3	3	ML	M	MH	L
	Push press	3	3	ML	M	MH	L
	Biceps curl	3	10	ML	M	MH	L
	Triceps press-down	3	10	ML	M	MH	L
	Abdominal exercises	3	25				
Saturday	Snatch grip shrug	3	3	L	ML	M	VL
	Power snatch	3	3/1 ascending clusters	L	ML	M	VL
	Snatch grip Romanian deadlift*	3	3	L	ML	M	VL
	Lat pulldown	3	10	L	ML	M	VL
	Abdominal exercises	3	25	L	ML	M	VL

Rest interval between sets and exercises is set at 3 min. 3/1 = ascending clusters with weight increasing each rep of the cluster according to table 15.14 with 45 s rest between repetitions.
*Load for the snatch grip Romanian deadlift is based on the power snatch maximum.

Explanation of program

Initial consultation	Initial training status and experience based on table 15.1	Advanced
	Fitness evaluation	1RM and 10RM testing (to estimate 1RM)
	Primary resistance training goal	Muscular power
Exercises	Exercise choices	Primarily free weights, but some machines for assistance exercises
	Core exercises	Power clean, speed squat, push press, jump squat, Romanian deadlift
	Assistance exercises	Biceps curl, triceps press-down, snatch grip shoulder shrug, lat pulldown
	Number of exercises per muscle group	1 or 2 exercises per muscle group
Frequency	Frequency of training (table 15.2)	3 or 4 times per week spaced evenly throughout the week
Order	Primary methods	Core exercises and then assistance exercises
		Exercises that train large muscle groups first, then exercises that train small muscle groups
		Multijoint exercises first, then single-joint exercises

Determining load	Determine training load based on RM testing.		1RM testing for specific core exercises					
			10RM testing is used to estimate a 1RM (protocol in chapter 11, but modified; table 15.5) for assistance exercises and those core exercises that are not safe to max out.					

1RM TEST RESULTS

Exercise	1RM	Estimated 3RM
Power clean	255 lb	235 lb
Power snatch	200 lb	185 lb
Back squat	300 lb	280 lb
Push press	220 lb	205 lb

10RM TEST RESULTS

Exercise	10RM	Estimated 3RM	Estimated 1RM
Lat pulldown	175 lb	219 lb	230 lb
Biceps curl	105 lb	130 lb	140 lb
Triceps press-down	105 lb	130 lb	140 lb

EXERCISES ESTIMATED FROM THE POWER SNATCH MAXIMUM

Exercise	1RM	Estimated 3RM
Snatch grip shoulder shrug	240 lb	223 lb
Snatch grip Romanian deadlift	255 lb	235 lb

EXERCISES ESTIMATED FROM THE BACK SQUAT MAXIMUM

Speed squat	165 lb	150 lb
Jump squat	135 lb	126 lb

Based on table 15.13 and the client's targeted goals.

Repetition range set based on client's classification: advanced.

Sets	Based on table 15.13 and the client's classification: advanced, three or more sets; in this case, three sets were chosen.
	The set structure presented is for the target sets and does not include warm-ups; two or three more warm-up sets may be needed.
Rest periods	Rest periods are based on table 15.14.
	All sets and exercises have rest intervals of 3 min or 180 s.
Assigning load*	Assign the training load based on RM testing. 1RM and 10RM testing is used to determine specific training zones with table 15.17.

Exercise	3RM	VH	H	MH	M	ML	L	VL
Power clean	235 lb	235-223	223-212	212-200	200-188	188-176	176-165	165-153
Power snatch	185 lb	185-176	176-167	167-157	157-148	148-148	139-130	130-120
Push press	205 lb	205-195	195-185	185-174	174-164	164-154	154-144	144-133
Snatch grip Romanian deadlift	235 lb	235-223	223-21	212-200	200-188	188-176	176-165	165-153
Snatch grip shoulder shrug	223 lb	223-212	212-201	201-190	190-178	178-167	167-156	156-145
Speed squat	150 lb	150-143	143-135	135-128	128-120	120-113	113-105	105-98
Jump squat	126 lb	126-120	120-113	113-107	107-101	101-95	95-88	88-82
Exercise	**10RM**	**VH**	**H**	**MH**	**M**	**ML**	**L**	**VL**
Lat pulldown	175 lb	175-166	166-158	158-149	149-140	140-131	131-123	123-114
Biceps curl	105 lb	105-100	100-95	95-89	89-84	84-79	79-74	74-68
Triceps curl	105 lb	105-100	100-95	95-89	89-84	84-79	79-74	74-68

*1RM and 10RM values will be used to calculate the training zones for specific training sessions based on table 15.17.

Study Questions

1. Which of the following exercise orders is recommended when using a push/pull exercise arrangement method?

   A. bench press, shoulder press, lying triceps extension, biceps curl, and bent-over row

   B. shoulder press, biceps curl, lying triceps extension, bench press, bent-over row

   C. bent-over row, shoulder press, bench press, biceps curl, lying triceps extension

   D. bench press, bent-over row, shoulder press, biceps curl, lying triceps extension

2. Which of the following is the load for the bench press exercise on a "moderately light day" if the client is performing sets of five repetitions and his 1RM is 200 pounds (91 kg)?

   A. 174 to 165 pounds (79 to 75 kg)

   B. 113 to 122 pounds (51 to 56 kg)

   C. 157 to 148 pounds (71 to 67 kg)

   D. 139 to 131 pounds (63 to 59 kg)

3. Which of the following programs is ideal for an intermediate client targeting muscular strength with her training program?

   A. 3 sets of 10 repetitions

   B. 5 sets of 15 repetitions

   C. 5 sets of 5 repetitions

   D. 1 set of 4 repetitions

4. An intermediately-trained client was able to perform 17 repetitions during a 15RM test of the bench press exercise. Which of the following relative load adjustments would allow the client to achieve the desired 15 repetitions?

   A. +5%

   B. +10%

   D. −10%

   D. −5%

5. Which of the following rest interval ranges is used for muscular hypertrophy training?

   A. 10 to 20 seconds

   B. 30 to 90 seconds

   C. 2 to 3 minutes

   D. 4 to 6 minutes

Applied Knowledge Question

Based on the following initial consultation and fitness testing information, fill in the empty spaces to determine the client's training loads for selected exercises.

Initial consultation and fitness evaluation	Initial training status and experience	Intermediate	
	Fitness evaluation	10RM testing to estimate a 1RM	
	Primary resistance training goal	Hypertrophy	
Assessing load capabilities	**10RM LOADS AND THEIR ESTIMATED 1RMS FOR THESE SELECTED EXERCISES**		
	Exercises (all are cam machines)	**10RM (pounds)**	**Estimated 1RM (pounds)**
	Vertical chest press	60	
	Seated row	50	
	Shoulder press	45	
	Biceps curl	35	
	Triceps extension	30	
	Leg (knee) extension	70	
	Leg (knee) curl	60	
Assigning loads	Repetition range to match training goal:_____ to _____ per set		
	Goal repetitions: eight		
	Loading (%1RM) range to match training goal: _____ % to _____%1RM		
	%1RM associated with eight goal repetitions: _____%1RM		

Calculating training loads from the estimated 1RM	Exercises (all are cam machines)	Estimated 1RM (pounds)	x	%1RM associated with 8 goal repetitions (in decimal form)	=	Calculated training load	Assigned training (round down)
	Vertical chest press		x		=		
	Seated row		x		=		
	Shoulder press		x		=		
	Biceps curl		x		=		
	Triceps extension		x		=		
	Leg (knee) extension		x		=		
	Leg (knee) curl		x		=		

References

1. Abadie, B.R., and M. Wentworth. 2000. Prediction of 1-RM strength from a 5-10 repetition submaximal test in college aged females. *Journal of Exercise Physiology* (Online) 3: 1-5.

2. Adams, G.M. 1998. *Exercise Physiology Laboratory Manual,* 3rd ed. Boston: McGraw-Hill.

3. Aján, T., and L. Baroga. 1988. *Weightlifting: Fitness for All Sports.* Budapest: International Weightlifting Federation.

4. American College of Sports Medicine. 2009. Position stand. Progression models in resistance training for healthy adults. *Medicine and Science in Sports and Exercise* 41: 687-708.

5. Atha, J. 1981. Strengthening muscle. *Exercise and Sport Sciences Reviews* 9: 1-73.

6. Baechle, T.R., and R.W. Earle. 1989. *Weight Training: A Text Written for the College Student.* Omaha, NE: Creighton University Press.

7. Baechle, T.R., and R.W. Earle. 1995. *Fitness Weight Training.* Champaign, IL: Human Kinetics.

8. Baechle, T.R., and R.W. Earle, eds. 2000. *Essentails of Strength Training and Conditioning,* 2nd ed. Champaign, IL: Human Kinetics.

9. Baechle, T.R., R.W. Earle, and D. Wathen. 2008. Resistance training. In: *Essentials of Stength Training and Conditioning,* T.R. Baechle and R.W. Earle, eds. Champaign, IL: Human Kinetics. pp. 381-412.

10. Baechle, T.R., and B.R. Groves. 1998. *Weight Training: Steps to Success,* 2nd ed. Champaign, IL: Human Kinetics.

11. Baker, D., and S. Nance. 1999. The relation between running speed and measures of strength and power in professional rugby league players. *Journal of Strength and Conditioning Research* 13: 230-235.

12. Bastiaans, J.J., A.B. Van Diemen, T. Veneberg, and A.E. Jeukendrup. 2001. The effects of replacing a portion of endurance training by explosive strength training on performance in trained cyclists. *European Journal of Applied Physiology* 86: 79-84.

13. Behm, D.G., G. Reardon, J. Fitzgerald, and E. Drinkwater. 2002. The effect of 5, 10, and 20 repetition maximums on the recovery of voluntary and evoked contractile properties. *Journal of Strength and Conditioning Research* 16: 209-218.

14. Berger, R.A. 1962. Effect of varied weight training programs on strength. *Research Quarterly* 33: 168-181.

15. Bompa, T.O., and G.G. Haff. 2009. *Periodization: Theory and Methodology of Training,* 5th ed. Champaign, IL: Human Kinetics.

16. Brown, H.L. 1992. *Lifetime Fitness,* 3rd ed. Scottsdale, AZ: Gorsuch Scarisbrick.

17. Bryzychi, M. 1993. Strength testing: Predicting a one rep max from reps to fatigue. *Journal of Physical Education, Recreation and Dance* 64: 88-90.

18. Bryzychi, M. 2000. Assessing strength. *Fitness Manage* (June), 4-37.

19. Candow, D.G., and D.G. Burke. 2007. Effect of short-term equal-volume resistance training with different workout frequency on muscle mass and strength in untrained men and women. *Journal of Strength and Conditioning Research* 21: 204-207.

20. Caserotti, P., P. Aagaard, J. Buttrup Larsen, and L. Puggaard. 2008. Explosive heavy-resistance training in old and very old adults: Changes in rapid muscle force, strength and power. *Scandinavian Journal of Medicine and Science in Sports* 18:773-782.

21. Chapman, P., J.R. Whitehead, and R.H. Binkert. 1998. The 225-lb reps-to-failure test as a submaximal estimation of 1-RM bench press performance in college football players. *Journal of Strength and Conditioning Research* 12: 258-261.

22. Coyle, E.F., D.C. Feiring, T.C. Rotkis, R.W.D. Cote, F.B. Roby, W. Lee, and J.H. Wilmore. 1981. Specificity of power improvements through slow and fast isokinetic training. *Journal of Applied Physiology* 51: 1437-1442.

23. Craig, B.W. 2000. Variation: An important component of training. *Strength and Conditioning Journal* 22: 22-23.

24. Craig, B.W., J. Lucas, R. Pohlman, and H. Schilling. 1991. The effect of running, weightlifting and a combination of both on growth hormone release. *Journal of Applied Sport Science Research* 5: 198-203.

25. Dudley, G.A., P.A. Tesch, B.J. Miller, and P. Buchanan. 1991. Importance of eccentric actions in performance adaptations to resistance training. *Aviation, Space, and Environmental Medicine* 62: 543-550.

26. Earle, R.W., and T.R. Baechle. 2004. Resistance training program design. In: *NSCA's Essentials of Personal Training,* T.R. Baechle and R.W. Earle, eds. Champaign, IL: Human Kinetics. pp. 361-398.

27. Epley, B. 1985. Poundage chart. In: *Boyd Epley Workout.* Lincoln, NE: University of Nebraska.

28. Epley, B. 2004. *The Path to Athletic Power.* Champaign, IL: Human Kinetics. p. 318.

29. Fleck, S.J. 1999. Periodized strength training: A critical review. *Journal of Strength and Conditioning Research* 13: 82-89.

30. Fleck, S.J., and W.J. Kraemer. 1997. *Designing Resistance Training Programs,* 2nd ed. Champaign, IL: Human Kinetics.

31. Fleck, S., and W.J. Kraemer. 2004. *Designing Resistance Training Programs,* 3rd ed. Champaign, IL: Human Kinetics. p. 375.

32. Fry, A.C., W.J. Kraemer, F. Van Borselen, J.M. Lynch, J.L. Marsit, E.P. Roy, N.T. Triplett, and H.G. Knuttgen. 1994. Performance decrements with high-intensity resistance exercise overtraining. *Medicine and Science in Sports and Exercise* 26: 1165-1173.

33. Fry, R.W., A.R. Morton, and D. Keast. 1991. Overtraining in athletes. An update. *Sports Medicine* 12: 32-65.

34. Gillam, G.M. 1981. Effects of frequency of weight training on muscle strength enhancement. *Journal of Sports Medicine* 21: 432-436.

35. Graves, J.E., M.L. Pollock, S.H. Leggett, R.W. Braith, D.M. Carpenter, and L.E. Bishop. 1988. Effect of reduced training frequency on muscular strength. *International Journal of Sports Medicine* 9: 316-319.

36. Haff, G.G., S. Burgess, and M.H. Stone. 2008. Cluster training: Theoretical and practical applications for the strength and conditioning professional. *Professional Strength and Conditioning*. 12: 12-17.

37. Haff, G.G., R.T. Hobbs, E.E. Haff, W.A. Sands, K.C. Pierce, and M.H. Stone. 2008. Cluster triaining: A novel method for introducing training program variation. *Strength and Conditioning* 30: 67-76.

38. Haff, G.G., W.J. Kraemer, H.S. O'Bryant, G. Pendlay, S. Plisk, and M.H. Stone. 2004. Roundtable discussion: Periodization of training-part 1. *National Strength and Conditioning Association Journal* 26: 50-69.

39. Haff, G.G., A. Whitley, L.B. McCoy, H.S. O'Bryant, J.L. Kilgore, E.E. Haff, K. Pierce, and M.H. Stone. 2003. Effects of different set configurations on barbell velocity and displacement during a clean pull. *Journal of Strength and Conditioning Research* 17: 95-103.

40. Häkkinen, K. 1994. Neuromuscular adaptations during strength training, aging, detraining, and immobilization. *Critical Reviews in Physical Rehabilitation Medicine* 6: 161-198.

41. Häkkinen, K., M. Alen, and P.V. Komi. 1985. Changes in isometric force- and relaxation-time, electromyographic and muscle fibre characteristics of human skeletal muscle during strength training and detraining. *Acta Physiologica Scandinavica* 125: 573-585.

42. Häkkinen, K., and P.V. Komi. 1983. Electromyographic changes during strength training and detraining. *Medicine and Science in Sports and Exercise* 15: 455-460.

43. Häkkinen, K., and P.V. Komi. 1985. Effect of explosive type strength training on electromographic and force production characteristics of leg extensor muscles during concentric and various stretch-shortening cycle exercises. *Scandinavian Journal of Sports Science* 7: 65-76.

44. Häkkinen, K., A. Pakarinen, M. Alen, H. Kauhanen, and P.V. Komi. 1988. Neuromuscular and hormonal responses in elite athletes to two successive strength training sessions in one day. *European Journal of Applied Physiology* 57: 133-139.

45. Harris, G.R., M.H. Stone, H.S. O'Bryant, C.M. Proulx, and R.L. Johnson. 2000. Short-term performance effects of high power, high force, or combined weight-training methods. *Journal of Strength and Conditioning Research* 14: 14-20.

46. Hazell, T., K. Kenno, and J. Jakobi. 2007. Functional benefit of power training for older adults. *Journal of Aging and Physical Activity* 15: 349-359.

47. Henwood, T.R., S. Riek, and D.R. Taaffe. 2008. Strength versus muscle power-specific resistance training in community-dwelling older adults. *Journals of Gerontology Series A: Biological Sciences and Medical Sciences* 63: 83-91.

48. Henwood, T.R., and D.R. Taaffe. 2006. Short-term resistance training and the older adult: The effect of varied programmes for the enhancement of muscle strength and functional performance. *Clinical Physiology and Functional Imaging* 26: 305-313.

49. Herrick, A.R., and M.H. Stone. 1996. The effects of periodization versus progressive resistance exericse on upper and lower body strength in women. *Journal of Strength and Conditioning Research* 10: 72-76.

50. Hickson, R.C., B.A. Dvorak, E.M. Gorostiaga, T.T. Kurowski, and C. Foster. 1988. Potential for strength and endurance training to amplify endurance performance. *Journal of Applied Physiology* 65: 2285-2290.

51. Hickson, R.C., K. Hidaka, and C. Foster. 1994. Skeletal muscle fiber type, resistance training, and strength-related performance. *Medicine and Science in Sports and Exercise* 26: 593-598.

52. Hoeger, W.W.K., S.L. Barette, D.F. Hale, and D.R. Hopkins. 1987. Relationship between repetitions and selected percentages of one repetition maximum. *Journal of Applied Sport Science Research* 1: 11-13.

53. Hoeger, W.W.K., D.R. Hopkins, S.L. Barette, and D.F. Hale. 1990. Relationship between repetitions and selected percentages of one repetition maximum: A comparison between untrained and trained males and females. *Journal of Applied Sport Science Research* 4: 47-54.

54. Hoffman, J.R., C.M. Maresh, L.E. Armstrong, and W.J. Kraemer. 1991. Effects of off-season and in-season resistance training programs on a collegiate male basketball team. *Journal of Human Muscle Performance* 1: 48-55.

55. Hori, N., R.U. Newton, W.A. Andrews, N. Kawamori, M.R. McGuigan, and K. Nosaka. 2008. Does performance of hang power clean differentiate performance of jumping, sprinting, and changing of direction? *Journal of Strength and Conditioning Research* 22: 412-418.

56. Humphries, B., E. Dugan, and T.L. Doyle. 2006. Muscular fitness. In: *ACSM's Resource Manual for Guidelines for Exercise Testing and Prescription*, L.A. Kaminsky, ed. Baltimore: Lippincott Williams & Wilkins. pp. 206-224.

57. Hunter, G.R., J.P. McCarthy, and M.M. Bamman. 2004. Effects of resistance training on older adults. *Sports Medicine* 34: 329-348.

58. Issurin, V. 2008. *Block Periodization: Breakthrough in Sports Training*, M. Yessis, ed. Muskegan, MI: Ultimate Athlete Concepts. p. 213.

59. Issurin, V. 2008. Block periodization versus traditional training theory: A review. *Journal of Sports Medicine and Physical Fitness* 48: 65-75.

60. Izquierdo, M., J. Ibanez, J.J. Gonzalez-Badillo, K. Häkkinen, N.A. Ratamess, W.J. Kraemer, D.N. French, J. Eslava, A. Altadill, X. Asiain, and E.M. Gorostiaga. 2006. Differential effects of strength training leading to failure versus not to failure on hormonal responses, strength, and muscle power gains. *Journal of Applied Physiology* 100: 1647-1656.

61. Jung, A.P. 2003. The impact of resistance training on distance running performance. *Sports Medicine* 33: 539-552.

62. Kemmler, W.K., D. Lauber, A. Wassermann, and J.L. Mayhew. 2006. Predicting maximal strength in trained postmenopausal women. *Journal of Strength and Conditioning Research* 20: 838-842.

63. Kemmler, W., J. Lauber, J. Weineck, J. Mayhew, W.A. Kalender, and K. Engelke. 2005. Trainingssteuerung in gesundheitssport. Lastvorgabe versus subjektive intensitatswahl impraventivsportlichen krafttraining. *Deutsche Zeitschrift für Sportmedizin*. 56: 165-170.

64. Korhonen, M.T., A. Cristea, M. Alen, K. Häkkinen, S. Sipila, A. Mero, J.T. Viitasalo, L. Larsson, and H. Suominen. 2006. Aging, muscle fiber type, and contractile function in sprint-trained athletes. *Journal of Applied Physiology* 101: 906-917.

65. Kraemer, W.J. 1997. A series of studies: The physiological basis for strength training in American football: Fact over philosophy. *Journal of Strength and Conditioning Research* 11: 131-142.

66. Kraemer, W.J., K. Adams, E. Cafarelli, G.A. Dudley, C. Dooly, M.S. Feigenbaum, S.J. Fleck, B. Franklin, A.C. Fry, J.R. Hoffman, R.U. Newton, J. Potteiger, M.H. Stone, N.A. Ratamess, and T. Triplett-McBride. 2002. American College of Sports Medicine position stand. Progression models in resistance training for healthy adults. *Medicine and Science in Sports and Exercise* 34: 364-380.

67. Kraemer, W.J., and A.C. Fry. 1995. Strength testing: Development and evaluation of methodology. In: *Physiological Assessment of Human Fitness*, P.J. Maud and C. Foster, eds. Champaign, IL: Human Kinetics. pp. 115-138.

68. Kraemer, W.J., D.L. Hatfield, and S.J. Fleck. 2007. Types of muscle training. In: *Strength Training*, L.E. Brown, ed. Champaign, IL: Human Kinetics. pp. 45-72.

69. Kraemer, W.J., B.J. Noble, M.J. Clark, and B.W. Culver. 1987. Physiologic responses to heavy-resistance exercise with very short rest periods. *International Journal of Sports Medicine* 8: 247-252.

70. Kraemer, W.J., and N.A. Ratamess. 2004. Fundamentals of resistance training: Progression and exercise prescription. *Medicine and Science in Sports and Exercise* 36: 674-688.

71. Kraemer, W.J., J.L. Vingren, D.L. Hatfield, B.A. Spiering, and M.S. Fragala. 2007. Resistance training programs. In: *ACSM's Resources for the Personal Trainer*, W.R. Thompson et al., eds. Baltimore: Lippincott Williams & Wilkins. pp. 372-403.

72. Kramer, J.B., M.H. Stone, H.S. O'Bryant, M.S. Conley, R.L. Johnson, D.C. Nieman, D.R. Honeycutt, and T.P. Hoke. 1997. Effects of single vs. multiple sets of weight training: Impact of volume, intensity, and variation. *Journal of Strength and Conditioning* 11: 143-147.

73. Kravitz, L., C. Akalan, K. Nowicki, and S.J. Kinzey. 2003. Prediction of 1 repetition maximum in high-school power lifters. *Journal of Strength and Conditioning Research* 17: 167-172.

74. Lander, J.E. 1985. Maximum based on reps. *National Strength and Conditioning Association Journal.* 6: 60-61.

75. Larson, G.D., and J.A. Potteiger. 1997. A comparison of three different rest intervals between multiple squat bouts. *Journal of Strength and Conditioning Research* 11: 115-118.

76. Lesuer, D.A., J.H. McCormick, J.L. Mayhew, R.L. Wasserstein, and M.D. Arnold. 1997. The accuracy of prediction equations for estimating 1-RM performance in the bench press, squat, and deadlift. *Journal of Strength and Conditioning Research* 11: 211-213.

77. Lombardi, V.P. 1989. *Beginning Weight Training.* Dubuque, IA: Brown.

78. Mayhew, J.L., T.E. Ball, M.E. Arnold, and J.C. Bowen. 1992. Relative muscular endurance performance as a predictor of bench press strength in college men and women. *Journal of Applied Sport Science Research* 6: 200-206.

79. Mayhew, J.L., B.D. Johnson, M.J. Lamonte, D. Lauber, and W. Kemmler. 2008. Accuracy of prediction equations for determining one repetition maximum bench press in women before and after resistance training. *Journal of Strength and Conditioning Research* 22: 1570-1577.

80. Mayhew, J.L., J.L. Prinster, J.S. Ware, D.L. Zimmer, J.R. Arabas, and M.G. Bemben. 1995. Muscular endurance repetitions to predict bench press strength in men of different training levels. *Journal of Sports Medicine and Physical Fitness* 35: 108-113.

81. Mayhew, J.L., J.S. Ware, K. Cannon, S. Corbett, P.P. Chapman, M.G. Bemben, T.E. Ward, B. Farris, J. Juraszek, and J.P. Slovak. 2002. Validation of the NFL-225 test for predicting 1-RM bench press performance in college football players. *Journal of Sports Medicine and Physical Fitness* 42: 304-308.

82. Mayhew, J.L., J.R. Ware, and J.L. Prinster. 1993. Using lift repetitions to predict muscular strength in adolescent males. *National Strength and Conditioning Association Journal* 15: 35-38.

83. McBride, J.M., G.O. McCauley, P. Cormie, J.L. Nuzzo, M.J. Cavill, and N.T. Triplett. 2009. Comparison of methods to quantify volume during resistance exercise. *Journal of Strength and Conditioning Research* 23: 106-110.

84. O'Conner, B., J. Simmons, and P. O'Shea. 1989. *Weight Training Today.* St. Paul, MN: West. pp. 26-33.

85. Pearson, D., A. Faigenbaum, M. Conley, and W.J. Kraemer. 2000. The National Strength and Conditioning Association's basic guidelines for the resistance training of athletes. *Strength and Conditioning Journal* 22: 14-27.

86. Peterson, M.D., M.R. Rhea, and B.A. Alvar. 2004. Maximizing strength development in athletes: A meta-analysis to determine the dose-response relationship. *Journal of Strength and Conditioning Research* 18: 377-382.

87. Peterson, M.D., M.R. Rhea, and B.A. Alvar. 2005. Applications of the dose-response for muscular strength development: A review of meta-analytic efficacy and reliability for designing training prescription. *Journal of Strength and Conditioning Research* 19: 950-958.

88. Pincivero, D.M., W.S. Gear, N.M. Moyna, and R.J. Robertson. 1999. The effects of rest interval on quadriceps torque and perceived exertion in healthy males. *Journal of Sports Medicine and Physical Fitness* 39: 294-299.

89. Plisk, S.S. 1991. Anaerobic metabolic conditioning: A brief review of theory, strategy and practical application. *Journal of Applied Sport Science Research* 5: 22-34.

90. Plisk, S.S., and M.H. Stone. 2003. Periodization strategies. *Strength and Conditioning* 25: 19-37.

91. Poliquin, C. 1988. Five steps to increasing the effectiveness of your strength training program. *National Strength and Conditioning Association Journal* 10: 34-39.

92. Ratamess, N.A., M.J. Falvo, G.T. Mangine, J.R. Hoffman, A.D. Faigenbaum, and J. Kang. 2007. The effect of rest interval length on metabolic responses to the bench press exercise. *European Journal of Applied Physiology* 100: 1-17.

93. Reynolds, J.M., T.J. Gordon, and R.A. Robergs. 2006. Prediction of one repetition maximum strength from multiple repetition maximum testing and anthropometry. *Journal of Strength and Conditioning Research* 20: 584-592.

94. Rhea, M.R., B.A. Alvar, and L.N. Burkett. 2002. Single versus multiple sets for strength: A meta-analysis to address the controversy. *Research Quarterly for Exercise and Sport* 73: 485-488.

95. Rhea, M.R., B.A. Alvar, L.N. Burkett, and S.D. Ball. 2003. A meta-analysis to determine the dose response for strength development. *Medicine and Science in Sports and Exercise* 35: 456-464.

96. Richardson, T. 1993. Circuit training with exercise machines. *National Strength and Conditioning Association Journal* 15: 18-19.

97. Robinson, J.M., M.H. Stone, R.L. Johnson, C.M. Penland, B.J. Warren, and R.D. Lewis. 1995. Effects of different weight training exercise/rest intervals on strength, power, and high intensity exercise endurance. *Journal of Strength and Conditioning Research* 9: 216-221.

98. Rydwik, E., C. Karlsson, K. Frandin, and G. Akner. 2007. Muscle strength testing with one repetition maximum in the arm/shoulder for people aged 75+ - test-retest reliability. *Clinical Rehabilitation* 21: 258-265.

99. Shaw, C.E., K.K. McCully, and J.D. Posner. 1995. Injuries during the one repetition maximum assessment in the elderly. *Journal of Cardiopulmonary Rehabilitation* 15: 283-287.

100. Shimano, T., W.J. Kraemer, B.A. Spiering, J.S. Volek, D.L. Hatfield, R. Silvestre, J.L. Vingren, M.S. Fragala, C.M. Maresh, S.J. Fleck, R.U. Newton, L.P. Spreuwenberg, and K. Häkkinen. 2006. Relationship between the number of repetitions and selected percentages of one repetition maximum in free weight exercises in trained and untrained men. *Journal of Strength and Conditioning Research* 20: 819-823.

101. Siff, M.C. 2003. *Supertraining,* 6th ed. Denver: Supertraining Institute. p. 496.

102. Siff, M.C., and Y.U. Verkhoshansky. 1999. *Supertraining,* 4th ed. Denver: Supertraining International.

103. Simao, R., T. Farinatti Pde, M.D. Polito, A.S. Maior, and S.J. Fleck. 2005. Influence of exercise order on the number of repetitions performed and perceived exertion during resistance exercises. *Journal of Strength and Conditioning Research* 19: 152-156.

104. Stone, M.H., and R.A. Borden. 1997. Modes and methods of resistance training. *Strength and Conditioning* 19: 18-23.

105. Stone, M.H., T.J. Chandler, M.S. Conley, J.B. Kramer, and M.E. Stone. 1996. Training to muscular failure: Is it necessary? *Strength and Conditioning* 18: 44-51.

106. Stone, M.H., R. Keith, J.T. Kearney, G.D. Wilson, and S.J. Fleck. 1991. Overtraining: A review of the signs and symptoms of overtraining. *Journal of Applied Sport Science Research* 5: 35-50.

107. Stone, M.H., and H.O. O'Bryant. 1987. *Weight Training: A Scientific Approach*. Edina, MN: Burgess.

108. Stone, M.H., H.S. O'Bryant, B.K. Schilling, R.L. Johnson, K.C. Pierce, G.G. Haff, A.J. Koch, and M. Stone. 1999. Periodization: Effects of manipulating volume and intensity. Part 1. *Strength and Conditioning Journal* 21 (2): 56-62.

109. Stone, M.H., H.S. O'Bryant, B.K. Schilling, R.L. Johnson, K.C. Pierce, G.G. Haff, A.J. Koch, and M. Stone. 1999. Periodization: Effects of manipulating volume and intensity. Part 2. *Strength and Conditioning Journal* 21 (3): 54-60.

110. Stone, M.H., K. Pierce, W.A. Sands, and M. Stone. 2006. Weightlifting: Program design. *Strength and Conditioning* 28: 10-17.

111. Stone, M.H., K. Pierce, G.D. Wilson, and R. Rozenek. 1987. Heart rate and lactate levels during weight-training exercise in trained and untrained men. *Physician and Sportsmedicine* 15: 97-101.

112. Stone, M.H., S. Plisk, and D. Collins. 2002. Training principles: Evaluation of modes and methods of resistance-training – a coaching perspective. *Sports Biomechanics* 1: 79-104.

113. Stone, M.H., J.A. Potteiger, K.C. Pierce, C.M. Proulx, H.S. O'Bryant, R.L. Johnson, and M.E. Stone. 2000. Comparison of the effects of three different weight-training programs on the one repetition maximum squat. *Journal of Strength and Conditioning Research* 14: 332-337.

114. Stone, M.H., K. Sanborn, H.S. O'Bryant, M. Hartman, M.E. Stone, C. Proulx, B. Ward, and J. Hruby. 2003. Maximum strength-power-performance relationships in collegiate throwers. *Journal of Strength and Conditioning Research* 17: 739-745.

115. Stone, M.H., W.A. Sands, K.C. Pierce, J. Carlock, M. Cardinale, and R.U. Newton. 2005. Relationship of maximum strength to weightlifting performance. *Medicine and Science in Sports and Exercise* 37: 1037-1043.

116. Stone, M.H., W.A. Sands, K.C. Pierce, R.U. Newton, G.G. Haff, and J. Carlock. 2006. Maximum strength and strength training: A relationship to endurance? *Strength and Conditioning Journal* 28: 44-53.

117. Stone, M.H., M.E. Stone, and W.A. Sands. 2007. *Principles and Practice of Resistance Training*. Champaign, IL: Human Kinetics. p. 376.

118. Tan, B. 1999. Manipulating resistance training program variables to optimize maximum strength in men: A review. *Journal of Strength and Conditioning Research* 13: 289-304.

119. Tesch, P. 1993. Training for bodybuilding. In: *Strength and Power in Sports,* P.V. Komi, ed. London: Blackwell Scientific.

120. Verkhoshansky, Y.U. 2006. *Special Strength Training: A Practical Manual for Coaches*. Muskegan, MI: Ultimate Athlete Concepts. p. 137.

121. Verkhoshansky, Y.U. 2007. Theory and methodology of sport preparation: Block training system for top-level athletes. *Teoria i Practica Physicheskoj Culturi* 4: 2-14.

122. Ware, J.S., C.T. Clemens, J.L. Mayhew, and T.J. Johnston. 1995. Muscular endurance repetitions to predict bench press and squat strength in college football players. *Journal of Strength and Conditioning Research* 9: 99-103.

123. Wathen, D. 1994. Load assignment. In: *Essentials of Strength Training and Conditioning,* T.R. Baechle and R.W. Earle, eds. Champaign, IL: Human Kinetics. pp. 435-446.

124. Westcott, W.L. 1982. *Strength Fitness*. Boston: Allyn & Bacon.

125. Whisenant, M.J., L.B. Panton, W.B. East, and C.E. Broeder. 2003. Validation of submaximal prediction equations for the 1 repetition maximum bench press test on a group of collegiate football players. *Journal of Strength and Conditioning Research* 17: 221-227.

126. Willardson, J.M. 2006. A brief review: Factors affecting the length of the rest interval between resistance exercise sets. *Journal of Strength and Conditioning Research* 20: 978-984.

127. Willardson, J.M., and L.N. Burkett. 2005. A comparison of 3 different rest intervals on the exercise volume completed during a workout. *Journal of Strength and Conditioning Research* 19: 23-26.

128. Willardson, J.M., and L.N. Burkett. 2006. The effect of rest interval length on the sustainability of squat and bench press repetitions. *Journal of Strength and Conditioning Research* 20: 400-403.

129. Wolfe, B.L., L.M. Lemura, and P.J. Cole. 2004. Quantitative analysis of single- vs. multiple-set programs in resistance training. *Journal of Strength and Conditioning Research* 18: 35-47.

130. Young, W.B., R. James, and I. Montgomery. 2002. Is muscle power related to running speed with changes of direction? *Journal of Sports Medicine and Physical Fitness* 42: 282-288.

131. Zatsiorsky, V.M., and W.J. Kraemer. 2006. *Science and Practice of Strength Training,* 2nd ed. Champaign, IL: Human Kinetics. p. 251.

Aerobic Endurance Training Program Design

Patrick Hagerman, EdD

After completing this chapter, you will be able to

- design aerobic endurance training programs based on the principle of specificity and individual client goals;

- select the appropriate mode of aerobic exercise;

- determine aerobic endurance training intensity, frequency, and duration and understand their interactions and effects on the training outcome;

- determine training intensity using calculated target heart rate zones, ratings of perceived exertion, or metabolic equivalents;

- design programs with proper warm-up, cool-down, and exercise progression; and

- apply long slow distance, pace/tempo, interval training, cross-training, arm exercise, and combination training in accord with client goals.

Aerobic endurance training is an essential component of any general exercise program. Health clubs and fitness centers dedicate large sections of their facilities to aerobic endurance training equipment, and the majority of athletic competitions for the general public are designed around aerobic endurance exercise (10K and 5K runs, marathons, cycling tours, and sprint triathlons). To underscore the importance of aerobic endurance activities, the 1996 Surgeon General's report on physical activity and health emphasized the recommendation that everyone engage in some form of aerobic exercise on most days of the week (89). Additionally, in its *Healthy People 2010,* the U.S. Department of Health and Human Services listed lack of physical activity and obesity as the top two major health issues facing the nation (90). As a result, the goals for Healthy People 2010 included increasing (1) "the proportion of adults who engage regularly, preferably daily, in moderate physical activity for *at least* 30 minutes per day" and (2) "the proportion of adolescents who engage in vigorous physical activity that promotes cardiorespiratory fitness 3 or more days per week for 20 or more minutes per occasion" (90). There can be no doubt as to the importance of proper aerobic endurance training.

Aerobic endurance training is often referred to as *aerobic exercise, cardiovascular exercise,* or *cardiorespiratory exercise.* These terms should be considered synonymous because they all refer to exercise that involves the cardiovascular and respiratory systems, including the heart, blood vessels, and lungs.

Designing an aerobic endurance training program necessitates an examination of the client's present level of fitness, exercise history, and fitness goals. One of the more common health-related goals among the general population is fat loss (often incorrectly referred to as "weight loss"), and a well-designed aerobic endurance training program should be a part of workouts for clients with this goal. Likewise, clients who wish to compete in a 10K race or complete a marathon will need specific training guidelines in order to meet their goals.

Previous chapters have dealt with determining fitness level and appropriateness of exercise levels. This chapter is devoted to putting together proper aerobic exercise programs for a variety of clients.

Specificity of Aerobic Endurance Training

The same principle of specificity that applies to resistance training applies to aerobic endurance training. The principle of specificity states that the results of a training program will be directly related to the type of training performed (23). The results of a resistance training program will be specific to resistance training, and the results of aerobic endurance training will be specific to aerobic endurance training. In other words, resistance training does not significantly improve maximal aerobic power ($\dot{V}O_2$max) (41, 44, 58). In addition, training that involves one mode of aerobic exercise will not guarantee equal improvement with a different aerobic exercise mode (10, 101). For instance, a person who has achieved a high level of aerobic conditioning through cycling will not necessarily be able to produce the same aerobic performance, as measured by peak $\dot{V}O_2$ capability, during a running workout (74, 86, 99). The muscle activation patterns and oxygen requirements among exercise modes are not equal, so the responses and adaptations are not equal (12, 71, 101). Even though improvements in $\dot{V}O_2$ elicited from one exercise mode will help in other exercise modes, they will not do so to the same extent (11, 62, 92).

Components of an Aerobic Endurance Training Program

An aerobic endurance training program consists of several components that can be manipulated in a variety of ways to produce a number of particular outcomes. These components include the mode of exercise, intensity of training during each session, frequency of exercise sessions, and duration of each exercise session. A personal trainer needs to consider each component in relation to the client's personal goals, as well as in terms of how each component interacts with the other components.

Two hypothetical clients will serve throughout the remainder of this chapter to highlight some practical examples of integrating the components into an overall aerobic endurance training program. The first client, Becky, has a goal of completing a local 10K race in less than 50 minutes. The second client is Floyd, who wants to lose about 30 pounds (14 kg) of body fat. Neither client has any musculoskeletal dysfunction, and each has received physician clearance for exercise. Client example 16.1 provides the initial status and goals of these two hypothetical clients.

Exercise Mode

The first step in designing aerobic endurance training programs is to decide on the mode of exercise. Exercise **mode** refers simply to what exercise or activity will be performed. As discussed in chapter 14, aerobic exercise modes include machine and nonmachine exercises. Athletes should choose the exercise mode that most closely mimics their specific sport or the movement that they perform during competition. The same goes for a client who wishes to compete in an amateur event such as a 5K run or 25-mile (40 km) cycling tour. The decision about which exercise mode to use depends on several factors, including equipment availability, personal preference, the client's ability to perform the exercise, and the client's goals.

The machine exercise modes use aerobic endurance training equipment and depend on what is available at the facility where the training will take place. Most fitness centers have a variety of aerobic endurance training equipment that typically includes treadmills, elliptical machines, stair climbers, stationary bikes, cross-country ski simulators, rowing ergometers, upper body ergometers, semirecumbent bikes, rotating climbing walls, and others.

If aerobic endurance training equipment is not available, nonmachine exercises can provide a variety of options as well. Nonmachine exercises comprise anything that allows the person to move freely and independently of equipment. This includes walking, jogging, running, swimming, water-resisted walking or running, skating, cycling, cardio kickboxing, and aerobic dance or step classes.

Machine exercise modes that appear similar to nonmachine exercise modes may not elicit the same cardiorespiratory response or provide the same abil-

Client Example 16.1

Initial Client Status and Goals

Client: Becky

Age: 30

Height: 5 feet 5 inches (165 cm)

Weight: 120 pounds (55 kg)

Goal: Complete 10K race in less than 50 minutes

Training status: Intermediate. Has run 3 to 5 miles (4.8-8.1 km) an average of two times a week for the past three years, at a pace and speed that is comfortable and not strenuous for her. Her 10K personal best is 53 minutes.

Other activities: Works as a receptionist, mostly sitting from 8 a.m. to 5 p.m. No other structured exercise or activities.

Client: Floyd

Age: 52

Height: 6 feet 0 inches (183 cm)

Weight: 230 pounds (105 kg)

Goal: Lose about 30 pounds (14 kg) of body fat

Training status: Beginner (untrained), former college baseball player. Has not been involved in a regular exercise program since college.

Other activities: Works long hours as bank officer. Walks throughout the office during the day, but no more than 40 feet (12 m) at a time, and is usually sitting in his office. Teaches at the community college at night. No structured exercise or activity.

---

ity to help clients reach their goals. For instance, running on a treadmill requires different motor patterns and muscle use than running on a track or trail. The propulsion is provided by the moving belt, so running on the treadmill does not require use of the muscles of the leg and hip to push the client forward. Likewise, riding a stationary bike uses the same muscles to turn the crank as a regular bike, but does not require the muscles to provide balance; nor is there a headwind or friction between the ground and tires on a stationary bike. The mode of exercise used should match the needs and goals of the client, especially if the client is training for a running or cycling event.

Clients' personal preferences on exercise mode have a great influence on how well they will adhere to the program (5, 73, 76). Selecting activities or exercises that clients enjoy will help them complete the training program as it was designed, rather than cutting corners to shorten the exercise session or decrease the intensity.

The mode of exercise must also be matched to the client's physical abilities. Clients with lower body orthopedic concerns may be limited in their ability to perform certain exercises because of impact strain on the foot, knee, or hip. These clients would be better served by a nonimpact form of exercise.

Clients who have limitations in joint range of motion need an exercise that works within their capacity. For instance, a client with diagnosed shoulder impingement may not be able to use an upper body ergometer (arm bike).

The initial exercise mode must also be within the client's current $\dot{V}O_2$ capacity. In many cases clients have not had a graded exercise test to determine their $\dot{V}O_2$max. Without data to help determine what a client is capable of, it is always prudent to begin with an enjoyable exercise mode. A client who used to walk or ride a bike might begin a new exercise program by resuming those activities. This method will prevent situations in which clients are instructed to perform an activity that is inappropriate for them. For instance, if a running program is assigned to a client who does not have the fitness capacity to complete a brisk walk, he or she will not be able to participate in an exercise session of sufficient duration to elicit any improvement. A different, less demanding exercise mode is needed instead.

Finally, exercise mode should match the client's ultimate goals for specificity of training. For instance, Becky, who wishes to complete a 10K race, will spend a good deal of time running on an outdoor track or trail, or indoors using a treadmill during inclement weather. In a different approach, Floyd, who is interested in losing body fat, will need to purposely expend calories, which does not necessitate any particular piece of equipment or mode of exercise; so several different modes of exercise could be used to provide variety in his workouts.

> The decision about which exercise mode to use depends on several factors, including equipment availability, personal preference, the client's ability to perform the exercise, and the client's goals.

Exercise Intensity

The **intensity** of exercise sessions is the main determinant of both exercise frequency and training duration. The intensity level required to reach the client's goal must be ascertained before the frequency and duration of exercise sessions are determined.

Regulating and monitoring exercise intensity are key to prescribing the correct aerobic endurance training program and preventing over- or undertraining. A certain threshold of $\dot{V}O_2$ or **heart rate reserve (HRR)**, which is the difference between a client's maximal heart rate and his or her resting heart rate, must be attained during an aerobic exercise session before improvements in the cardiorespiratory system are seen (38, 47, 55, 70, 80, 97). Oxygen uptake reserve ($\dot{V}O_2R$ = difference between $\dot{V}O_2$max and resting $\dot{V}O_2$) has been shown to equate fairly evenly to the HRR. Since it is not common to have laboratory-assessed $\dot{V}O_2$max or $\dot{V}O_2R$ data for a personal training client, the use of HRR for determining exercise intensity is acceptable (3, 55, 67, 85).

Ultimately, the necessary aerobic exercise threshold depends on a client's initial fitness level, but for the apparently healthy adult it is generally considered to be approximately 50% to 85% of HRR (4, 84, 85). Extremely deconditioned clients may need to begin at an intensity of 30% of HRR (4). Depending on their fitness level, some may find 50% of HRR strenuous, while more advanced clients may find 85% of HRR insufficient to elicit cardiorespiratory system improvements. If the exercise intensity is too high, overtraining and injury may result. If the intensity is too low, the physiological stimulus to improve will be insufficient, and it will take longer to reach the goals that have been set. The key to knowing where to begin lies in examining the client's exercise and medical history and in the results of any recent exercise testing. It is always smart to begin conservatively and increase the intensity as needed, rather than beginning too high and risk overtraining and poor adherence.

Target Heart Rate

Heart rate and oxygen consumption ($\dot{V}O_2$) are closely related. During exercise, heart rate increases with increases in workload, and an increase in workload necessitates an increase in oxygen consumption. Therefore, as heart rate nears a client's **maximal heart rate (MHR)**, a greater percentage of $\dot{V}O_2$max is being used. Table 16.1 illustrates a range of percent $\dot{V}O_2$max and the related percent HRR and percent of maximal heart rate (%MHR). This relationship has been shown to be consistent across age, sex, coronary artery disease status, fitness level, training status, muscle groups exercised, and testing mode (29, 81, 82, 98). Because of this relationship, heart rate is often used as a quick and easy way to measure exercise intensity.

The only way to determine a client's true MHR is to perform a graded exercise test that takes the client to the point where the heart rate does not increase with an increase in workload. At this point the heart has reached its maximal beat per minute (beat/min) capacity. For safety's sake, it may be recommended that a physician be present during a maximal graded exercise test on a client (67). Refer to chapter 9 for discussion on the conditions warranting the presence of a physician during exercise testing. Instead of performing a maximal graded exercise test, the personal trainer can use an estimate of a client's MHR in most cases. The most commonly used **age-predicted maximal heart rate (APMHR)** equation is as follows:

$$APMHR = 220 - Age \qquad (16.1)$$

This is only an estimate, with an error range of ±10 to 15 beats/min (42, 94). This error range is important to note when calculating target heart rate training zones. For example, a 20-year-old client with

TABLE 16.1 Relationship Between $\dot{V}O_2$max, HRR, and MHR

%$\dot{V}O_2$max	%HRR	%MHR
50	50	66
55	55	70
60	60	74
65	65	77
70	70	81
75	75	85
80	80	88
85	85	92
90	90	96
95	95	98
100	100	100

%$\dot{V}O_2$max = percent of maximal oxygen uptake; %HRR = percent of heart rate reserve; %MHR = percent of maximal heart rate.

an APMHR of 200 may actually have an estimated MHR as low as 185 (200 − 15) or as high as 215 (200 + 15) when the error range is taken into account. The APMHR will therefore actually be maximal for some, unattainable for others, and submaximal for the rest (56). However, a client should never reach his or her MHR during the course of submaximal aerobic endurance training, so the age-predicted estimate provides a close approximation that is acceptable for designing aerobic exercise programs (94). An exception to using APMHR exists for clients who are taking medications such as beta blockers that blunt the heart rate response to exercise. In these clients, the medication prevents heart rate from rising above a certain point independent of the exercise intensity or workload. Before using APMHR to prescribe exercise intensity, the personal trainer must determine that the client is not taking any heart rate–altering medications; if the client is doing so, use of alternative intensity prescriptions not based on heart rate is necessary. Refer to chapter 20 for discussion of heart rate–altering medications.

If the use of APMHR is appropriate and this value has been calculated, an appropriate exercise intensity "training zone" or **target heart rate range (THRR)** can be determined through one of two different calculations.

Percent of Age-Predicted Maximal Heart Rate

Once the APMHR is known, a range of exercise intensities based on known relationships between percentages of the APMHR and $\dot{V}O_2max$ can be used. For the apparently healthy adult, 55% to 75% of $\dot{V}O_2max$ approximates to 70% to 85% of the APMHR, which provides the appropriate stimulus to improve aerobic function (97). Other ranges may be calculated depending on the client's medical history, any complications present, and physician recommendations. Because initial fitness level greatly affects the minimal threshold for cardiorespiratory improvement, for clients who are very deconditioned, a lower range of 55% to 65% of APMHR may be more appropriate (2, 49, 59, 77).

To determine the intensity training zone using a percent of APMHR for an apparently healthy adult, multiply the client's APMHR by 70% and 85% (called the **percent of APMHR method**). The results provide the lower and upper limits of exercise heart rate needed for improving cardiorespiratory function (table 16.2).

$$\text{Target heart rate (THR)} = \text{APMHR} \times \text{Exercise intensity} \qquad \textbf{(16.2)}$$

Percent of Heart Rate Reserve: The Karvonen Formula   The **Karvonen formula** is related to the percent of APMHR formula but allows for differences in **resting heart rate (RHR)** (47, 48). To use this formula, you will need to obtain the client's RHR. The best time for people to measure RHR is first thing in the morning upon waking but before getting out of bed. Clients should be taught how to take their resting heart rate using a radial pulse palpitation (index and forefinger over the radial pulse) for 1 minute. To obtain the HRR, subtract the RHR from the APMHR:

$$\text{HRR} = \text{APMHR} - \text{RHR} \qquad \textbf{(16.3)}$$

TABLE 16.2   Aerobic Endurance Training Exercise Heart Rates

Age	APMHR* (beats/min)	PERCENT OF APMHR METHOD		KARVONEN FORMULA METHOD**	
		70%	85%	50%	85%
80	140	98	119	105	130
75	145	102	123	108	134
70	150	105	128	110	138
65	155	109	132	113	142
60	160	112	136	115	147
55	165	116	140	118	151
50	170	119	145	120	155
45	175	123	149	123	160
40	180	126	153	125	164
35	185	130	157	128	168
30	190	133	162	130	172
25	195	137	166	133	176
20	200	140	170	135	181
15	205	144	174	138	185

*APMHR = Age-predicted maximal heart rate.
**Assumes a resting heart rate of 70 beats/min.

The HRR is the available increase in heart rate over the RHR, up to the APMHR. In other words, the HRR is the number of beats per minute that the heart rate can increase from resting up to maximal. For instance, a 40-year-old client has an APMHR of 180; if he or she has an RHR of 70, then his or her HRR is 110 beats/min (an APMHR of 180 minus an RHR of 70). As mentioned earlier, 50% to 85% of HRR is needed to improve cardiorespiratory function. To determine the target training zone, multiply the HRR by 50% and 85%, and then add the RHR back to each answer to obtain the lower and upper heart rate limits. Failure to add the RHR back to the answer will result in an underestimated training zone that will not provide the desired improvements. In the case of this client, his or her HRR of 110 beats/min × 0.50 = 55 and × .85 = 94. When we add his RHR of 70 to these values, we get a THRR of 125 to 164.

$$\text{Low end of THR} =$$
$$(\text{HRR} \times \text{Lower exercise intensity value})$$
$$+ \text{RHR} \qquad (16.4)$$

$$\text{High end of THR} =$$
$$(\text{HRR} \times \text{Higher exercise intensity value})$$
$$+ \text{RHR}$$

The benefit to using HRR is that it is specific to the client because it is based on that client's baseline RHR. As a client becomes more fit and the RHR decreases, the HRR will increase; this represents a greater "reserve" to draw from.

As shown in table 16.2, in most situations, using the Karvonen formula provides slightly larger training ranges than the percent of APMHR formula (28, 67). To calculate exercise heart rate range, use 70% to 85% of APMHR or 50% to 85% of HRR. Both will provide a heart rate range that produces an appropriate exercise stimulus to improve cardiorespiratory fitness (4, 47, 54). Note that untrained or beginning clients probably should begin with a THR based on the lower half of the APMHR intensity range (e.g., 70% to 80% of APMHR) and more trained clients typically can tolerate intensities in the upper half of the HRR range (e.g., 70% to 85% of HRR). See "Exercise Intensity Calculations Using Heart Rate" for exercise intensity formulas and sample calculations for both methods.

> To calculate exercise heart rate range, assign an exercise intensity of 70% to 85% of APMHR or 50% to 85% of HRR.

Exercise Intensity Calculations Using Heart Rate

Percent of APMHR Method

Formula: Age-predicted maximal heart rate (APMHR) = 220 − age

Target heart rate (THR) = (APMHR × exercise intensity)

Do this calculation twice for the lower and upper limits to determine the target heart rate range (THRR).

Example: *30-year-old client; 70% to 85% of APMHR*

APMHR = 220 − 30 = 190 beats/min
THR (70%) = 190 × 0.70 = 133 beats/min
THR (85%) = 190 × 0.85 = 162 beats/min
THRR = 133 to 162 beats/min

Karvonen Method

Formula: Age-predicted maximal heart rate (APMHR) = 220 − age

HRR = APMHR − RHR

Target heart rate (THR) = (HRR × exercise intensity) + RHR

Do this calculation twice for the lower and upper limits to determine the target heart rate range (THRR).

Example: *30-year-old client; 50% to 85% of HRR; RHR = 70 beats/min*

APMHR = 220 − 30 = 190 beats/min
HRR = 190 − 70 = 120 beats/min
THR (50%) = (120 × 0.50) + 70 = 130 beats/min
THR (85%) = (120 × 0.85) + 70 = 172 beats/min
THRR = 130 to 172 beats/min

Percent of Functional Capacity

If a client's **functional capacity** (measured as $\dot{V}O_2$max) has been determined through a physician-supervised graded exercise test, the true MHR will be known. In this situation, it is best to use the measured MHR rather than an estimate. Either the Karvonen formula or the percent of APMHR formula (using the actual MHR in place of the APMHR) can be used to determine the aerobic exercise training zone.

Ratings of Perceived Exertion

An additional method, to be used along with heart rate calculation methods, is known as a **rating of perceived exertion (RPE)** scale. An RPE scale is designed to help clients monitor their exercise intensities using a rating system that accounts for all of the body's responses to a particular exercise intensity. A client must be taught to quantify the stress of the exercise session in terms of both physiological and psychological factors, based on the mode of exercise; environment (temperature, humidity, etc.); intensity of the effort; and extent of strain, discomfort, or fatigue (27, 57, 75). An RPE is not just a measure of how fast the heart is beating, but is meant to include exertion, respiration, and emotional responses to exercise.

Often during graded exercise testing, clients are asked to give an RPE during each successive workload. These RPEs are paired with the $\dot{V}O_2$ of that workload so that when the test is completed, any given workload and $\dot{V}O_2$ has a known RPE. Because the personal trainer now knows what exertion rating corresponds to a given workload, he or she can use the RPE to determine approximate $\dot{V}O_2$ during exercise without the need to directly measure $\dot{V}O_2$. For example, if it is known that a particular $\dot{V}O_2$ elicited an RPE of 7 on a 1 to 10 scale during the YMCA cycle ergometer test (see chapter 11), during the next exercise session the personal trainer can approximate that same $\dot{V}O_2$ intensity with a different exercise mode by simply adjusting the intensity of the exercise to the point where the client rates the exercise at an RPE of 7. Figure 16.1 shows an example of an RPE scale.

The numerical ratings on the RPE scale are associated with adjectives that describe the effort needed to maintain the given exercise level. These ratings range from "Nothing at all" to "Maximum effort." Teaching a client to differentiate between exertion levels may take some time. The lowest level of each scale can be compared to lying still and not exerting any effort at all, while the highest level of each scale is the maximal amount of effort the client is capable of producing. The difficulty in using RPE is that very few clients will have ever actually reached the upper levels of effort and therefore cannot per-

Rating	Description
1	Nothing at all (lying down)
2	Extremely little
3	Very easy
4	Easy (could do this all day)
5	Moderate
6	Somewhat hard (starting to feel it)
7	Hard
8	Very hard (making an effort to keep up)
9	Very very hard
10	Maximum effort (can't go any further)

FIGURE 16.1 Rating of perceived exertion (RPE) scale.

ceive what a 10 actually feels like. The RPE will have a greater degree of subjectivity in clients who have not completed a maximal stress test. To untrained, deconditioned clients, an exercise level that produces a heart rate of 60% HRR may seem maximal because they are unaccustomed to exercise and do not really know what a maximal effort is. Only through training and changes in exercise intensities will such clients learn the true meaning of the rating adjectives and how to accurately report their RPE.

A downside to using RPEs is that they vary between clients and between exercise modes for any given heart rate (64). Rating of perceived exertion scales should be used along with heart rate measurements so that over time, a pattern of exercise intensity for a given client can be established. Combining THHR and RPE in an exercise prescription will allow the personal trainer to determine the different effects a mode of exercise has on the client. For instance, while riding a stationary bike, a client may be working at 80% of his or her THR and report an RPE of 7, whereas the same client running on a treadmill at 80% of his or her THR may report an RPE of 9. Differences in mode of exercise will often include different amounts of muscle use and energy expenditure, which will change %THR, RPE, or both. Therefore, the personal trainer should avoid general exercise prescriptions based simply on an RPE, as they do not take individual differences into account.

The strength of RPE scales is that they allow for more than just a measurement of heart rate. These scales can be used when traditional heart rate intensity prescriptions are inaccurate due to the influence of medications or illness. When combined with heart rate, RPE allows assessments of whether the exercise intensity is providing enough of a stimulus for a particular client. For instance, if an advanced client is exercising at 80% of HRR and indicates an RPE of

4 on a 1 to 10 scale, an increase in exercise intensity is appropriate. In contrast, if a new client indicates a rating of 9 but has an actual exercise heart rate equal to 70% of HRR, the personal trainer should reduce exercise intensity until the client becomes better trained. The personal trainer must remember that an RPE is an indicator of overall effort, not just heart rate; so the client may be including feelings of fatigue, respiratory effort, pain, and mental effort or stress among other factors.

Metabolic Equivalents

Exercise intensity can also be prescribed in terms of **metabolic equivalents (METs)**. One MET is equal to $3.5 \text{ ml} \cdot \text{kg}^{-1} \cdot \text{min}^{-1}$ of oxygen consumption and is considered the amount of oxygen required by the body to function when at rest (60). Therefore, any given MET level is an indication of how much harder than rest a particular activity is. For example, an activity that has a 4-MET rating is four times harder than rest, meaning that it requires the body to work four times harder than at rest. In order to accurately prescribe an exercise intensity based on METs, the personal trainer or physician must perform a maximal graded exercise test on a client to obtain the maximal MET level possible for that client (i.e., $\dot{V}O_2$max divided by 3.5). Without this information, assigning a percentage of maximal METs is not possible.

There are published MET approximations as shown in table 16.3. These approximations can be used to prescribe a variety of activities for the client's total exercise program and to compare the energy requirements of one activity to another. Client example 16.2 provides updated information for the hypothetical clients with sample intensity prescriptions based on various methods.

TABLE 16.3 Estimated Metabolic Equivalents for Various Activities

METs	Activity	METs	Activity
1.0	Lying or sitting quietly, doing nothing, lying in bed awake, listening to music, watching a movie	6.0	Resistance training (free weight, Nautilus or Universal type), powerlifting or bodybuilding, vigorous effort
2.0	Walking, <2 miles per hour (<3.2 km/h), level surface	6.3	Stair stepping (with a 12-in. [30 cm] step height), 20 steps per minute
2.5	Stretching, hatha yoga	6.3	Walking, 4.5 miles per hour (7.2 km/h), level surface
2.5	Walking, 2 miles per hour (3.2 km/h), level surface	6.9	Stair stepping (with an 8-in. [20 cm] step height), 30 steps per minute
3.0	Resistance training (free weight, Nautilus or Universal type), light or moderate effort	7.0	Aerobic dance, high impact
3.0	Stationary cycling, 50 watts, very light effort	7.0	Badminton, competitive
3.0	Walking, 2.5 miles per hour (4 km/h)	7.0	Cross-country skiing, 2.5 miles per hour (4 km/h), slow or light effort, ski walking
3.3	Walking, 3 miles per hour (4.8 km/h), level surface	7.0	Rowing machine, 100 watts, moderate effort
3.5	Calisthenics, home exercise, light or moderate effort	7.0	Stationary cycling, 150 watts, moderate effort
3.5	Golf, using a power cart	7.0	Swimming laps, freestyle, slow, moderate or light effort
3.5	Rowing machine, 50 watts, light effort	8.0	Basketball, game
3.5	Stair stepping (with a 4-in. [10 cm] step height), 20 steps per minute	8.0	Calisthenics (e.g., pushups, sit-ups, pull-ups, jumping jacks), vigorous effort
3.8	Walking, 3.5 miles per hour (5.6 km/h), level surface	8.0	Circuit training, including some aerobic stations, with minimal rest
4.0	Water aerobics, water calisthenics	8.0	Cross-country skiing, 4.0 to 4.9 miles per hour (6.4-7.9 km/h), moderate speed and effort
4.5	Badminton, social singles and doubles	8.0	Outdoor cycling, 12 to 13.9 miles per hour (19.3-22.4 km/h)
4.5	Golf, walking and carrying clubs	8.0	Tennis, singles
4.8	Stair stepping (with a 4-in. [10 cm] step height), 30 steps per minute	8.0	Walking, 5 miles per hour (8.4 km/h)
4.9	Stair stepping (with an 8-in. [20 cm] step height), 20 steps per minute	8.5	Rowing machine, 150 watts, vigorous effort
5.0	Aerobic dance, low impact	8.5	Step aerobics (with a 6- to 8-in. [15 to 20 cm] step)
5.0	Tennis, doubles	9.0	Cross-country skiing, 5 to 7.9 miles per hour (8.1-12.7 km/h), brisk speed, vigorous effort
5.0	Walking, 4 miles per hour (6.4 km/h), level surface		
5.5	Stationary cycling, 100 watts, light effort		
6.0	Basketball, nongame		
6.0	Outdoor cycling, 10 to 11.9 miles per hour (16.1-19.2 km/h)		

METs	Activity	METs	Activity
9.0	Running, 5.2 miles per hour (8.4 km/h) (11.5-min mile)	12.0	Rowing machine, 200 watts, very vigorous effort
9.0	Stair stepping (with a 12-in. [30 cm] step height), 30 steps per minute	12.5	Running, 7.5 miles per hour (12.1 km/h) (8-min mile)
10.0	Outdoor cycling, 14 to 15.9 miles per hour (22.5-25.6 km/h)	12.5	Stationary cycling, 250 watts, very vigorous effort
10.0	Running, 6 miles per hour (9.7 km/h) (10-min mile)	13.5	Running, 8 miles per hour (12.9 km/h) (7.5-min mile)
10.0	Step aerobics (with a 10- to 12-in. [25 to 30 cm] step)	14.0	Cross-country skiing, >8 miles per hour (>12.9 km/h), racing
10.0	Swimming laps, freestyle, fast, vigorous effort	14.0	Running, 8.5 miles per hour (13.7 km/h) (7-min mile)
10.5	Stationary cycling, 200 watts, vigorous effort	15.0	Running, 9 miles per hour (14.5 km/h) (6-min, 40-s mile)
11.0	Running, 6.7 miles per hour (10.8 km/h) (9-min mile)	16.0	Outdoor cycling, >20 miles per hour (>32.2 km/h)
11.5	Running, 7 miles per hour (11.3 km/h) (8.5-min mile)	16.0	Running, 10 miles per hour (16.1 km/h) (6-min mile)
12.0	Outdoor cycling, 16 to 19 miles per hour (25.7-30.6 km/h)	18.0	Running, 10.9 miles per hour (17.5 km/h) (5.5-min mile)
12.0	In-line skating, not coasting		

MET = metabolic equivalent.

Adapted from Ainsworth et al. 2000 (1) (consult this reference for a comprehensive list of the MET level for 605 specific activities) and ACSM 2010 (4).

Client Example 16.2

Exercise Intensity

A variety of intensities are provided for each client. The personal trainer should choose one based on the mode of exercise and the intensity monitoring tools that are available (e.g., heart rate monitor or RPE). (Refer to chapter 11 for illustrations and instructions on how to measure a client's heart rate manually.)

Becky

Age: 30

RHR: 65

APMHR: 190 beats/min

70% to 85% HRR = 153 to 171 beats/min

RPE = 5 to 6

METs = 12.5 (8 minute/mile pace)

Because Becky is somewhat trained, her THRR can be based on the upper half (e.g., 70% to 85%) of her HRR. Her current 10K personal best time is 53 minutes, which is about 8.5 minutes per mile. Although Becky's workouts may vary from day to day, to reach her goal time of under 50 minutes she needs to increase her average training pace to 8 minutes per mile. Her personal trainer can monitor her ability to tolerate this increase in exercise intensity by either an RPE or heart rate.

Floyd

Age: 52

RHR: 74

APMHR: 168 beats/min

70% to 80% APMHR = 118 to 134 beats/min

RPE = 3 to 4

METs = 3 to 3.8 (walking at 2.5-3.5 miles [4-5.6 km] per hour); 5.5 (stationary cycling at 100 watts; refer to chapter 11 to convert watts to an exercise work rate)

Because Floyd is untrained, his THRR can be based on the lower half (70% to 80%) of his APMHR. The MET intensities chosen for Floyd will allow him to exercise at a pace he can sustain as a beginner for weight-bearing exercises, and a little harder (5.5 METs) for non-weight-bearing exercises. Until Floyd becomes accustomed to exercise and can give accurate RPEs, his personal trainer should monitor his exercise intensity by regularly measuring his heart rate during the exercise session.

Training Frequency

Training frequency refers to how often the workouts are performed (e.g., the number of training sessions per week). The frequency of training sessions depends on the client's goals, current fitness level, duration, intensity, and recovery time required for the exercise.

As noted earlier, the U.S. Surgeon General has recommended that all people over the age of 2 years accumulate at least 30 minutes of aerobic endurance–type physical activity, of at least moderate intensity, on most—preferably all—days of the week (89). In a 1998 position stand, the American College of Sports Medicine stated that aerobic exercise should be done three to five days per week and that training for fewer than two days per week is generally not a sufficient stimulus for developing and maintaining fitness (2). So a minimum of two days per week, up to five days per week, is suggested for general fitness goals. Some advanced clients may be able to tolerate more than five days per week if the rest between sessions is sufficient to prevent overuse injury.

Beginning clients (e.g., no participation in a regular aerobic exercise program for the past six months) should start with the minimum number of sessions per week, spaced out evenly (table 16.4). As fitness levels improve, the frequency of training can increase. As the number of exercise sessions per week increases, the frequency should not exceed the frequency that a client is willing to adopt and maintain (3). For example, despite the common examples shown, some clients may have only the weekdays (or just the weekends) to exercise, so the personal trainer will need to design an exercise schedule around when the client is available. Most desirably, however, the client's rest days should be placed in between exercise days to space them evenly throughout the week.

In the case of Becky, because she is already running twice a week, her exercise prescription can begin at three or four days per week. Floyd, on the other hand, as a nonexerciser, will begin with two days per week, although he reports that he has the flexibility and desire to exercise in the morning before work and during his lunch hour (not on the weekends, though).

Ultimately, the frequency of exercise must be balanced with the duration and intensity of exercise. In general, exercise sessions of longer duration or higher intensity require more recovery time and are therefore performed less frequently, whereas exercise sessions of shorter duration or less intensity do not require as much recovery time and can be performed more often (69).

> Exercise sessions of long duration and high intensity require longer recovery times and therefore cannot be performed very often; short-duration exercise at low intensity does not require as much recovery time and can be performed more frequently.

Exercise Duration

Exercise **duration** is a measure of how long an exercise session lasts. Along with training frequency, exercise duration depends on the client's goals, current fitness levels, and the intensity of the exercise. The greater the intensity of an aerobic exercise session, the greater the $\dot{V}O_2$ requirement and the less time a client will be able to spend exercising at that level (78).

The National Institutes of Health Consensus Development Panel on Physical Activity and Cardiovascular Health agrees with the Surgeon General's report in stating that duration of aerobic endurance training should be at least 30 minutes (66). The American Heart Association recommends between 30 to 60 minutes for the purposes of health promotion and cardiovascular disease prevention (24). Finally, the American College of Sports Medicine recommends 20 to 60 minutes of continuous or intermittent bouts accumulated throughout the day (4).

TABLE 16.4   Sample Exercise Frequency Options

Day	BEGINNER		INTERMEDIATE		ADVANCED
	5 days rest 2 days exercise	4 days rest 3 days exercise	3 days rest 4 days exercise	2 days rest 5 days exercise	1 day rest 6 days exercise
Sunday	Rest	Rest	Rest	Rest	Exercise
Monday	Exercise	Exercise	Exercise	Exercise	Exercise
Tuesday	Rest	Rest	Exercise	Exercise	Exercise
Wednesday	Rest	Exercise	Rest	Rest	Rest
Thursday	Exercise	Rest	Exercise	Exercise	Exercise
Friday	Rest	Exercise	Exercise	Exercise	Exercise
Saturday	Rest	Rest	Rest	Exercise	Exercise

If time constraints prevent a client from dedicating a block of time large enough to meet exercise duration needs, or if the client is very deconditioned, shorter **intermittent exercise** bouts can be substituted. If the intensity is moderate to high, intermittent exercise bouts of at least 10 minutes each can improve the aerobic fitness of all but the most advanced clients (19, 33, 65). Intermittent bouts have also been shown to improve adherence to exercise in people who are unaccustomed to exercise (54). For clients who are severely deconditioned and unable to complete even a 10-minute exercise bout, several shorter bouts of exercise with rest periods in between will allow them to build up to a continuous bout.

Beyond the recommended minimum of 30 minutes, the human body is capable of withstanding hours of aerobic endurance exercise, as is evident in athletes who complete iron-distance triathlons, 24-hour ultra-marathons, or cycling races of 100 miles (160 km) or more. The total duration of a given client's program is ultimately determined by that client's personal goals, the intensity level of a given workout, and the client's ability to fit the training session into his or her schedule. In the case of Becky, she has been running 3 to 5 miles (4.8-8.1 km) at about a 8.5 minute/mile pace for an exercise duration of 25 to 42 minutes. Since her goal of completing a 10K in less than 50 minutes requires a continuous exercise bout, intermittent training throughout the day will not offer her sufficient training specificity; therefore, she must adjust her schedule (e.g., exercise before or after work) to allow for longer exercise sessions. In contrast, Floyd's goal of weight loss does not require sustained bouts of exercise; and although he will be able to eventually sustain a longer exercise bout, he may begin with two 10- to 15-minute sessions each exercise day.

> **Exercise duration is inversely related to exercise intensity.**

Progression

One of the keys to designing a proper aerobic endurance training program is exercise **progression**. For purposes of training the general population, aerobic endurance training programs can be divided into two distinct types: *improvement* and *maintenance*. The type of program the personal trainer designs for a client depends on the client's initial fitness level and training background. The untrained beginner will always start with an improvement program; a client who has been exercising but wants to improve will also use an improvement program; and a client who just wishes to maintain his or her current level of aerobic endurance will use a maintenance program.

Improvement in aerobic endurance training can be measured as an increase in $\dot{V}O_2$ capacity, or an increased tolerance for longer durations or higher intensities. Following an improvement program requires making periodic, progressive increases in exercise frequency, duration, or intensity. As a general rule, increases in frequency, intensity, or duration should be limited to 10%, and increases should be made only after the body has adjusted to the new program. Constraints on a client's available training time, along with the fact that there are only seven days in a week, often mean that exercise frequency and duration reach their upper limits before exercise intensity does, after which improvements in aerobic capacity will have to result from increases in intensity. In other words, the client will have only so much time available to exercise, but he or she can continually (albeit gradually) increase exercise intensity. Client example 16.3 updates the information on the sample clients and illustrates options for progression of their workouts.

The maintenance program is reserved for clients who want to maintain their current level of fitness or who have progressed through the improvement program and have reached the upper limits of how intensely they wish to train. Maintenance of aerobic capacity requires significantly less effort than trying to improve (raise) it. Over the long term, clients can maintain improvements from an aerobic endurance training program if they reduce the frequency of training to no fewer than two sessions per week but maintain the duration and (especially) the intensity during the exercise sessions they do perform (38, 39, 40). Additionally, to keep a client motivated during a maintenance program and to facilitate continued adherence, the personal trainer can design the program to use a variety of exercise modes (5, 32). Another use of a maintenance program is for a client who wishes to take some time off from training (or needs to because of a business trip or vacation); this person can decrease the total volume of aerobic exercise for a few weeks by as much as 70% without negatively affecting $\dot{V}O_2max$ (61).

> **As a general rule, increases in frequency, intensity, or duration should be limited to 10%.**

Warm-Up and Cool-Down

Regardless of which program a client is using, appropriate warm-up and cool-down procedures should be integrated into the exercise sessions. The purpose of a warm-up is to increase blood flow to the muscles that will be used during the workout, slowly increase heart rate so that oxygen debt is

Client Example 16.3

Six-Week Progression

Becky

Becky indicated that she can work out only three days a week. Since she has been running 3 to 5 miles (4.8-8.1 km) at about a 8.5 minute/mile pace (25-42 minutes) twice a week, her six-week program will concentrate on gradually increasing the distance she runs while maintaining the faster training pace (8 minutes per mile) needed to prepare her for running a 10K in her goal time.

Week 1: Three days (Mon, Wed, Fri): running 3 miles (4.8km) in 24 minutes

Week 2: Three days (Sun, Tue, Thu): running 4 miles (6.4 km) in 32 minutes

Week 3: Three days (Mon, Wed, Fri): running 4.5 miles (7.2 km) in 36 minutes

Week 4: Three days (Sun, Tue, Thu): running 5 miles (8 km) in 40 minutes

Week 5: Three days (Mon, Wed, Fri): running 5.5 miles (8.9 km) in 44 minutes

Week 6: Three days (Sun, Tue, Thu): running 6 miles (9.7 km) in 48 minutes

Floyd

Floyd indicated that he can begin with working out two days a week (although he has each weekday available), in two 15-minute sessions each exercise day. His six-week program will concentrate on increasing the number of days and the duration of exercise while keeping him within his APMHR training zone of 118 to 134 beats/min.

Week 1: Two days (Mon, Thu), two times each day (in the morning before work and during the lunch hour)—walking on a treadmill at 2.5 to 3.5 miles (4-5.6 km) per hour for 10 to 15 minutes

Week 2: Three days (Tue, Thu, Sat), two times each day: in the morning before work—riding the stationary bike at 100 watts for 10 to 15 minutes; during the lunch hour—walking on a treadmill at 2.5 to 3.5 miles (4-5.6 km) per hour for 10 to 15 minutes

Week 3: Four days (Mon, Tue, Thu, Fri), once each day—riding the stationary bike at 100 watts for 20 to 25 minutes

Week 4: Four days (Mon, Tue, Thu, Fri), once each day—walking on a treadmill at 2.5 to 3.5 miles (4-5.6 km) per hour for 15 to 20 minutes

Week 5: Five days (Mon, Tue, Wed, Thu, Fri), once each day (Floyd can decide when)—three times a week (Mon, Wed, Fri), walking on a treadmill at 2.5 to 3.5 miles (4-5.6 km) per hour for 20 to 25 minutes; two times a week (Tue, Thu)—riding the stationary bike at 100 watts for 25 to 30 minutes

Week 6: Five days (Mon, Tue, Wed, Thu, Fri), once each day (Floyd can decide when)—walking on a treadmill at 2.5 to 3.5 miles (4-5.6 km) per hour for 25 to 30 minutes

minimized, prepare the nervous system for action, and increase muscle core temperature to cause more complete unloading of oxygen from the blood to the muscles (30, 79, 91). Proper warm-up involves a slow progression from small, simple movements to the larger, more complicated movements that mimic those used during the exercise session (22, 51). For instance, if a client will be running, a proper warm-up will include progression from normal walking with the arms at the sides, to slow jogging with a swinging of slightly bent arms, to running with full pumping of the arms at a 90° bend in the elbows. The client should allow enough time in each activity for the heart rate to increase to meet metabolic demands before progressing further.

The cool-down uses the same progression in reverse. The client progresses from running to jogging to walking, allowing the heart rate to decrease and reach a lower steady state before slowing down. Clients can do additional flexibility exercises after the cool-down. See chapter 12 for more information on warm-up, cool-down, and flexibility exercises.

Types of Aerobic Endurance Training Programs

There are many ways to design aerobic endurance training programs, but all will contain the components previously discussed. As mentioned earlier, the first step is deciding which mode or modes of exercise to use. Sometimes choosing more than one mode is appropriate. For instance, outdoor running, cycling, and swimming are all dependent on the weather. Combining machine and nonmachine exercises that mimic each other can provide a continued training stimulus when the environment is not conducive to outdoor workouts. Running outside or on a treadmill, cycling or riding a stationary bike, and swimming in a lake or in a pool can all provide the stimulus needed for improvement if adjustments for duration and intensity are made. The exercise mode must be one that the client will enjoy and can perform without any problems or pain, and one that provides enough of a challenge to stimulate improvement.

After exercise modes have been selected, the frequency, duration, and intensity can be combined in a number of ways, each of which will produce a different effect. The final program may take the form of long slow distance training, pace/tempo training, interval training, circuit training, or cross-training. The most important determinant of how to combine these components is the goal of the client.

Long Slow Distance

In long slow distance (LSD) training, exercise sessions should be performed at an intensity less than that normally used so that the duration of the workout can be longer. For example, during LSD, a client capable of running at a 6 minute/mile pace may exercise at an 8 minute/mile pace for a longer distance. A client who normally rides a stationary bike for 30 minutes at 150 watts may ride for 1 hour at 100 watts. The basic premise of LSD is to increase exercise duration at a lower intensity than normal. A good indicator of proper intensity other than percent of HRR is whether the client can carry on a conversation during the exercise session. The idea is not to speak at length, but to be able to talk without becoming short of breath. The goals of LSD include improvements in the anaerobic threshold, development of endurance in supporting musculature, and fat utilization with corresponding glycogen sparing. Typical training sessions last between 30 minutes and 2 hours and, to prevent overtraining, should not take place more than twice a week (18, 93).

Once target intensity is achieved, the exercise can continue as long as the client is able to maintain his or her heart rate within the prescribed zone and as long as energy is available. When heart rate increases beyond the training zone, the anaerobic systems begin to provide energy at the expense of carbohydrate and glycogen stores, and volitional fatigue will quickly follow. Once the client's heart rate begins to increase without an increase in workload, the exercise session is complete. For the beginning exerciser, this may occur after only a brief period of time (10 to 15 minutes). With subsequent exercise sessions, the client can increase the duration of exercise as cardiorespiratory system improvements allow for greater perfusion of oxygenated blood, delivery of energy substrates, and removal of waste products.

Personal trainers should note that not all clients will initially be able to achieve the 50% to 85% HRR training zone or be able to continue the exercise for more than a short time period. Seriously deconditioned clients will require a lower starting point and a slower increase in both intensity and duration.

Pace/Tempo Training

For clients who wish to improve their cardiorespiratory endurance and who are capable of working at the highest percentages of their heart rate range, **pace/tempo training** can help improve $\dot{V}O_2$max. Pace/tempo training allows clients to train for short periods of time at their goal pace, which will be higher than their current pace. Pace/tempo training sessions typically last between 20 and 30 minutes and require clients to exercise at their lactate threshold (16, 18). The workout can be performed either intermittently or steadily. *Intermittent pace/tempo training* involves work bouts of 3 to 5 minutes with rest periods of 30 to 90 seconds, repeated until the desired pace cannot be maintained. During the rest period, clients may engage in very light (slow) walking to prevent any blood pooling in the legs. Intermittent pace/tempo training is best suited for clients who typically do not tolerate an intensity at their lactate threshold for very long. Over time, these clients will increase their tolerance and can progress to steady pace/tempo training. *Steady pace/tempo training* involves one bout of exercise lasting 20 to 30 minutes, sustained at the desired pace. Because pace/tempo training requires that a higher intensity be achieved during a workout session, the duration of the workout is reduced. Pace/tempo training should be performed only one or two times a week. Client example 16.4 provides a sample intermittent pace/tempo workout.

Interval Training

Interval training programs get their name from the alternating periods of high- and low-intensity exercise they include. Interval training can involve short periods of exercise at intensities at or above the lactate threshold and $\dot{V}O_2$max, alternated with longer periods of lesser intensities. Interval training

Client Example 16.4

Sample Intermittent Pace/ Tempo Workout for Becky

Overall Parameters

Intervals: 3 to 6 minutes

Intensity: 80% to 85% HRR or 8 METs

Rest between intervals: 60 seconds

Mode: Elliptical machine

Elliptical Machine

Warm-up

    Three minutes at level 8 (on a machine with 1-10 levels), 60 seconds rest

    Four minutes at level 8, 60 seconds rest

    Five minutes at level 8, 60 seconds rest

    Six minutes at level 8, 60 seconds rest

    Five minutes at level 8, 60 seconds rest

    Four minutes at level 8, 60 seconds rest

    Three minutes at level 8

Cool-down

    Total time completed at goal pace/intensity: 30 minutes

can also involve high-intensity exercise (90-100% HRR) with periods of rest in between. The benefit of interval training is that with the correct spacing of work and rest, clients can accomplish a great amount of work at higher intensities that are normally not possible with a continuous program. For instance, exercising at such a high intensity (90-100% HRR) will cause a client to tap into the anaerobic energy systems and fatigue quickly. With interval training, fatigue will result; but the length of time spent exercising is kept relatively short, and the rest periods are lengthened to allow for more complete recovery between exercise intervals. Thus complete fatigue is delayed. If a client attempts to maintain an intensity of 90% to 100% HRR for as long as possible, fatigue will set in within a few minutes and the exercise intensity must be lowered. However, during the course of an interval program, a client may train at the high intensity for several short periods of time, with rest in between, which allows for a greater total amount of time spent at the highest intensity. For instance, clients who want to increase their running or cycling speed may use intervals of faster running or cycling that push their HRR limits, alternated with rest periods in which they continue moving at a pace that is at the lower end of their HRR. A client who wishes to burn the maximum number of

calories in a set amount of time could employ interval training also. In this case, alternating high and low intensities, instead of using one set intensity, allows the client to burn a greater number of calories during a workout (6, 7, 13).

Properly adjusting the **work-to-rest ratio** is essential to allow the client to complete the prescribed exercise session. High-intensity intervals should last between 3 and 5 minutes, with a rest period of 1:1 to 1:3 depending on the ability of the client to perform successive high-intensity intervals. As the client fatigues, the rest interval can be lengthened to allow for greater recovery between work bouts. Extending the rest interval beyond 1:3 reduces the amount of time that can be spent in high-intensity work bouts during a fixed-length exercise session, and thus reduces the total amount of work done and improvement made. The 1:1 to 1:3 work-to-rest ratios cause improvements in cardiorespiratory endurance mainly through raising the lactate threshold and enhancing the body's ability to clear lactate from the bloodstream (20, 93).

Clients should use interval training only after they have established a firm aerobic base and are able to maintain exercise intensity within their HRR training zone for a period of time roughly equal to the total time that will be spent on interval training (52). As an example, a client who is able to maintain a steady-state HRR training zone for 60 minutes could perform interval training for up to 60 minutes (exercise and rest time combined).

Almost any aerobic endurance exercise can be selected for an interval training workout. If the intensity can be adjusted quickly and easily, aerobic endurance training machines can be used in the same way that outdoor exercises are used for interval training. For variety, the high-intensity bouts can be done on one machine and the rest bouts performed with another exercise. For example, an interval training program could involve using the stair climber for the work period and the treadmill for the rest period. Client example 16.5 provides a sample training program with LSD, interval, and pace/tempo routines.

> Long slow distance, interval, and pace/tempo programs are advanced aerobic endurance exercise programs that should be used only after an initial aerobic endurance training program has been completed.

Circuit Training

Circuit training combines resistance training with aerobic endurance training. The client performs

Client Example 16.5

Sample Training Programs With Long Slow Distance, Interval, and Pace/Tempo

Because LSD, interval, and pace/tempo programs require a firm aerobic base, these sample programs should be viewed as a progression to be used after some tolerance for exercise has been established through consistent and regular aerobic endurance training.

Becky (Rest Days: Tuesday, Thursday, Friday, Sunday)

	Monday	Wednesday	Saturday
Type of training	Long slow distance	Interval	Pace/tempo
Activity	Outdoor running	Treadmill	Outdoor running
Distance or duration	15K to 20K (9.3-12.4 miles)	60 min	30 min steady
Pace or intensity	9 to 10 min/mile pace	5-min work period at a 6 min/mile pace (10 miles per hour [16.1 km/h]) alternated with a 5-min rest period at a 12 min/mile pace (5 miles per hour [8.1 km/h])	8 min/mile pace

Floyd (Rest Days: Sunday, Saturday)

	Monday and Thursday	Tuesday and Friday	Wednesday
Type of training	Interval	Long slow distance	Pace/tempo
Activity	Stationary cycle	Treadmill	Stationary cycle
Distance or duration	30 min	60 min	20 min intermittent
Pace or intensity	5-min work period at 150 watts alternated with a 5-min rest period at 75 watts	3 miles [4.8 km] per hour	Four 5-min work periods at 80% to 85% HRR alternated with a 1-min rest period

short intervals of aerobic endurance training between resistance training sets. The goal is to increase heart rate to the training zone and keep it there for the duration of the exercise session, thus inducing improvement in cardiorespiratory endurance and muscular endurance at the same time. Unfortunately, most investigations on variations of circuit training have shown that although strength increased, $\dot{V}O_2$max did not significantly improve compared to values for participants in an aerobic exercise–only program or a combined circuit training and aerobic program (31, 63, 88). Those research studies that did show small improvements in $\dot{V}O_2$max due to circuit training required the subjects to train at heart rates close to 90% HRR (17). However, although circuit training has not been shown to significantly increase $\dot{V}O_2$ in many cases, there is no evidence that $\dot{V}O_2$ decreases during a circuit training program. Therefore, it may be a useful tool in a maintenance program. Circuit training can also be used with beginning clients as a means of introducing them to both resistance and aerobic endurance training when their available time for training is short.

Cross-Training

Cross-training is a method of combining several exercise modes for aerobic endurance training. In order for cross-training to be effective in maintaining or improving $\dot{V}O_2$max, the intensity and duration of each exercise must be of sufficient quantity with respect to the client's fitness level (95, 96). For clients who wish to do cross-training, the personal trainer must prescribe the intensity and duration of each mode of exercise individually while keeping the combined volume of exercise within the client's capabilities. The benefit of cross-training is that it distributes the physical stress of training to different muscle groups during the different activities and increases the adaptations of the cardiorespiratory and musculoskeletal systems (51, 68, 102).

The result of cross-training is that it overcomes the limitations of specificity of training. That is, when a client has a goal that cannot be met with use of one particular exercise, competing in a triathlon for instance, cross-training is a way of obtaining that goal.

Aerobic endurance cross-training can be accomplished by two different means: (1) using different modes of exercise each training period, rotating through two or more modes within a week; or (2) using several different exercise modes within the same workout. With the first option, a client may train on the treadmill one day, cycle outdoors the next, and then finish the week on a rowing machine. The second option entails setting up a series of exercise modes that can be completed back to back. For example, instead of doing 30 minutes on the treadmill, the client may complete 10 minutes each on the treadmill, elliptical trainer, and arm ergometer.

The key to making cross-training effective is ensuring that clients work within their prescribed training zone with each exercise mode. Different exercises may elicit different heart rates for a given workload or speed, so individualization of the program for each mode is necessary. Client example 16.6 provides some sample cross-training workouts.

Client Example 16.6

Sample Cross-Training Workouts

Cross-training workouts should be designed around the total volume or duration of exercise that the client is capable of. The following examples are progressions to be used after some tolerance for exercise duration has been established through consistent and regular aerobic endurance training.

Becky

Monday: 60 minutes on the treadmill

Wednesday: 60 minutes on the stationary bike

Friday: 30 minutes on the stair climber

Floyd

Monday: 10 minutes on the treadmill, 10 minutes on the stationary bike, 10 minutes on the stair climber

Tuesday: 10 minutes on the rowing machine, 10 minutes on the elliptical trainer, 10 minutes on the treadmill

Thursday: 30 minutes on the stationary bike

Saturday: 20 minutes walking outdoors, 15 minutes on the rowing machine

---

Arm Exercise

Many aerobic endurance activities primarily involve the major muscles of the lower body. However, arm exercises are becoming more popular, are often part of cardiac rehabilitation programs, and are a contributing source of power for swimming. To prescribe a THRR based on a percent of APMHR, the personal trainer must make downward adjustment of 10 to 13 beats/min when calculating the APMHR because heart rate is higher during arm exercise than during leg exercise for any given workload (21, 25, 26, 46, 87). Additionally, the $\dot{V}O_2$max for arm exercise is significantly lower than that for leg exercise (21, 46). The result is that the lactate threshold is reached at lower intensities than during leg exercise (72).

Upper body ergometers (UBEs or arm bikes) are the most common type of arm-specific equipment found in fitness centers. Many stationary bicycles, elliptical trainers, and some stair climbers have an attachment that allows the arms to work in a push–pull motion and may be used in an arms-only mode for upper body aerobic endurance exercise. Likewise, the arm portion of a rowing machine may be isolated if the feet are placed on the floor so that the body does not slide back and forth.

Arm exercise is probably the most underused type of aerobic endurance exercise. To increase variety, arm work can be added to current programs that mainly use lower body exercises. Arm exercise is especially helpful in providing some aerobic endurance exercise to clients who have orthopedic problems with their lower body, such as an injury to the foot, knee, or hip.

Combined Aerobic and Resistance Training

Quite often, clients undertake aerobic endurance and resistance training programs simultaneously. While the benefits of both are clear and there is no doubt that both should be part of a complete training program, there is a downside to combining these two different types of training. Research has shown that when properly designed resistance training and aerobic endurance training programs are combined, the increase in strength gains will be blunted while $\dot{V}O_2$ increases normally. Clients will see increases in aerobic endurance similar to those they would have seen if they had done only aerobic endurance training, but the increases in strength from the resistance training portion of their program will be smaller than if they had done only resistance training (9, 15, 34, 35, 43). Along with reduced maximum strength gains, combined programs result in reductions in

Sample Combined Aerobic and Resistance Training Programs

Goal: Increased Muscular Strength, Maintenance of Aerobic Endurance

1. Perform initial aerobic endurance training for 8 to 10 weeks: three to four days a week, 50% to 85% HRR, 30 to 60 minutes.
2. Reduce aerobic endurance training to two days per week, 50% to 85% HRR, 30 minutes, and begin resistance training.

Goal: Increased Aerobic Endurance, Maintenance of Muscular Strength

1. Perform 8 to 10 weeks of initial resistance training.
2. Reduce resistance training to two days per week and begin aerobic endurance training three to four days per week, 50% to 85% HRR, 30 to 60 minutes.

the amount of muscle girth gains and in specific speed- and power-related performances (17, 35, 53). On the other hand, the addition of anaerobic resistance training to an aerobic endurance training program seems to improve low-intensity aerobic endurance (37, 41, 83).

A relatively sedentary client who is just beginning to exercise will show improvements from both aerobic and resistance training when using both programs within a total workout. However, for more advanced clients who are reaching plateaus in improvement, it is doubtful that they will obtain the full benefits of both programs at the same time because there will be little to no recovery time (days off to rest).

To remedy this problem, the personal trainer can design a program to allow the client to complete the aerobic endurance training program before beginning the resistance training program. For instance, a client could perform eight weeks of aerobic endurance training only, followed by eight weeks of resistance training with only the minimal amount of aerobic endurance training needed for maintenance. This would allow the client to increase $\dot{V}O_2max$ and establish an aerobic base first, then work on increasing muscular fitness (e.g., strength) while maintaining the improved $\dot{V}O_2$ (8, 14, 36). After the initial 16 weeks, the client could begin alternating periods of aerobic endurance training and minimal resistance training for maintenance of strength with periods of resistance training and minimal aerobic endurance

training for maintenance of aerobic endurance (38). This style of program provides continued increases in both aerobic endurance and muscular strength, although at a reduced rate in comparison to training only for one or the other, but also allows for changes in program variables such as mode and intensity to enhance variety. See the "Sample Combined Aerobic and Resistance Training Programs" for combined training programs based on differing training goals.

Conclusion

Designing aerobic endurance training programs that meet clients' goals and improve the working capacity of the cardiovascular and cardiorespiratory systems requires careful thought and accurate calculations. Because of individual differences in exercise preference, long-term goals, and current training status, the personal trainer must take care when manipulating the components of intensity, duration, and frequency. When program components are properly aligned, improvements in $\dot{V}O_2max$ for an individual are limited only by genetics. Incorporation of different training methods such as long slow distance, pace/tempo training, interval training, circuit training, cross-training, arm exercises, and the combination of aerobic and resistance training will allow clients to continue making improvements in aerobic capacity and overall fitness.

Study Questions

1. A client is preparing for his first half-marathon and wants to complete the 13.1-mile (21 km) distance in 2 hours. Which of the following would be an appropriate long slow distance workout?

   A. cycling 13.1 miles (21 km) at a pace of 7 miles per hour (11.3 kph)

   B. stair climbing for 2 hours

   C. running 15 miles (24 km) at a pace of 5 miles per hour (8.0 kph).

   D. freestyle swimming for 1 hour

2. The personal trainer is designing an aerobic exercise program for a 43-year-old client who has a resting heart rate of 75 beats/min. Using the Karvonen method, which of the following is the target heart rate range if the personal trainer assigns an intensity of 60% to 70% of the client's HRR?

   A. 106 to 123 beats/min

   B. 136 to 146 beats/min

   C. 123 to 137 beats/min

   D. 154 to 165 beats/min

3. Which of the following exercise modes would be most appropriate for a 52-year-old female client with no medical or physical contraindications whose goal is to ride in a 50-mile cycling event?

   A. walking on a treadmill

   B. riding a bicycle

   C. using an elliptical machine

   D. using a rowing machine

4. A sedentary 35-year-old client is morbidly obese and would like to lose weight. The personal trainer selected the semirecumbent bike as the exercise mode. Which of the following is an appropriate exercise program for the first exercise session?

   A. three 5-minute bouts with rest in between at 50% to 65% HRR

   B. 20 minutes continuous at 75% HRR

   C. 25 minutes of intervals at 90% HRR and 70% HRR

   D. 30 minutes of LSD at 65% HRR

Applied Knowledge Question

Fill in the chart to describe the types of aerobic endurance training programs.

Type	Intensity	Duration	Frequency	Goals
LSD				
Pace/tempo: intermittent				
Pace/tempo: steady				
Interval				

References

1. Ainsworth, B.E., W.L. Haskell, M.C. Whitt, M.L. Irwin, A.M. Swartz, S.J. Strath, W.L. O'Brien, D.R. Bassett, K.H. Schmitz, P.O. Emplaincourt, D.R. Jacobs, and A.S. Leon. 2000. Compendium of physical activities: An update of activity codes and MET intensities. *Medicine and Science in Sports and Exercise* 32 (9 Suppl): S498-S516.

2. American College of Sports Medicine. 1998. The recommended quantity and quality of exercise for developing and maintaining cardiorespiratory and muscular fitness, and flexibility in healthy adults. *Medicine and Science in Sports and Exercise* 30 (6): 975-991.

3. American College of Sports Medicine. 2001. Appropriate intervention strategies for weight loss and prevention of weight regain for adults. *Medicine and Science in Sports and Exercise* 33 (12): 2145-2156.

4. American College of Sports Medicine (ACSM). 2010. *Guidelines for Exercise Testing and Prescription,* 8th ed. Philadelphia: Lippincott Williams & Wilkins.

5. Annesi, J.J., and J. Mazas. 1997. Effects of virtual reality-enhanced exercise equipment on adherence and exercise-induced feeling states. *Perceptual and Motor Skills* 85: 835-844.

6. Åstrand, I., P.O. Åstrand, E.H. Christensen, and R. Hedman. 1960. Intermittent muscular work. *Acta Physiologica Scandinavica* 48: 443.

7. Åstrand, P.O., and K. Rodahl. 1986. *Textbook of Work Physiology.* New York: McGraw-Hill.

8. Bell, G.J., S.R. Petersen, J. Wessel, K. Bagnall, and H.A. Quinner. 1991. Adaptations to endurance and low velocity resistance training performed in a sequence. *Canadian Journal of Sport Science* 16 (3): 186-192.

9. Bell, G.J., S.R. Petersen, J. Wessel, K. Bagnall, and H.A. Quinner. 1991. Physiological adaptations to concurrent endurance training and low velocity resistance training. *International Journal of Sports Medicine* 12: 384-390.

10. Ben-Ezra, V., C. Lacy, and D. Marshall. 1992. Perceived exertion during graded exercise: Treadmill vs step ergometry. *Medicine and Science in Sports and Exercise* 24 (5 Suppl): S136.

11. Ben-Ezra, V., and R. Verstraete. 1991. Step ergometry: Is it task-specific training? *European Journal of Applied Physiology* 63: 261-264.

12. Bressel, E., G.D. Heise, and G. Bachman. 1998. A neuromuscular and metabolic comparison of forward and reverse pedaling. *Journal of Applied Biomechanics* 14 (4): 401-411.

13. Christensen, E.H., R. Hedman, and B. Saltin. 1960. Intermittent and continuous running. *Acta Physiologica Scandinavica* 50: 269.

14. Chtara, M., K. Chamari, M. Chaouachi, A. Chaouachi, D. Koubaa, Y. Feki, G.P. Millet, and M. Amri. 2005. Effects of intra-session concurrent endurance and strength training sequence on aerobic performance and capacity. *British Journal of Sports Medicine* 39 (8): 555-560.

15. Chtara, M., A. Chaouachi, G.T. Levin, M. Chaouachi, K. Chamari, M. Amri, and P.B. Laursen. 2008. Effect of concurrent endurance and circuit resistance training sequence on muscular strength and power development. *Journal of Strength and Conditioning Research* 22 (4): 1037-1045.

16. Costill, D.L. 1986. *Inside Running: Basics of Sports Physiology.* Indianapolis: Benchmark Press.

17. Craig, B.W., J. Lucas, R. Pohlman, and H. Stelling. 1991. The effects of running, weightlifting and a combination of both on growth hormone release. *Journal of Applied Sport Science Research* 5 (4): 198-203.

18. Daniels, J. 1989. Training distance runners—a primer. *Gatorade Sports Science Exchange* 1: 1-5.

19. Ebisu, T. 1985. Splitting the distance of endurance running: On cardiovascular endurance and blood lipids. *Japanese Journal of Physical Education* 30: 37-43.

20. Esfarjani, F., and P.B. Laursen. 2007. Manipulating high-intensity interval training: Effects on VO2max, the lactate threshold and 3000 m running performance in moderately trained males. *Journal of Science and Medicine in Sport* 10 (1): 27-35.

21. Eston, R.G., and D.A. Brodie. 1986. Responses to arm and leg ergometry. *British Journal of Sports Medicine* 20 (1): 4-6.

22. Faigenbaum, A., and J.E. McFarland Jr. 2007. Guidelines for implementing a dynamic warm-up for physical education. *Journal of Physical Education, Recreation and Dance* 78 (3): 25-28.

23. Fleck, S.J., and W.J. Kraemer. 2004. *Designing Resistance Training Programs,* 3rd ed. Champaign, IL: Human Kinetics.

24. Fletcher, G.F., G. Balady, S.N. Blair, J. Blumenthal, C. Caspersen, B. Chaitman, S. Epstein, E.S. Sivarajen Froelicher, V.F. Froelicher, I.L. Pina, and M.L. Pollock. 1996. Benefits and recommendations for physical activity programs for all Americans. A statement for health professionals by the Committee on Exercise and Cardiac Rehabilitation of the Council on Clinical Cardiology, American Heart Association. *Circulation* 94: 857-862.

25. Franklin, B.A. 1983. Aerobic requirements of arm ergometry: Implications for testing and training. *Physician and Sportsmedicine* 11: 81.

26. Franklin, B.A. 1989. Aerobic exercise training programs for the upper body. *Medicine and Science in Sports and Exercise* 21: S141.

27. Glass, S.C., R.G. Knowlton, and M.D. Becque. 1994. Perception of effort during high-intensity exercise at low, moderate, and high wet bulb globe temperatures. *European Journal of Applied Physiology* 68: 519-524.

28. Goldberg, L., D.L. Elliot, and K.S. Kuehl. 1988. Assessment of exercise intensity formulas by use of ventilatory threshold. *Chest* 94 (1): 95-98.

29. Green, J.H., N.T. Cable, and N. Elms. 1990. Heart rate and oxygen consumption during walking on land and in deep water. *Journal of Sports Medicine and Physical Fitness* 30: 49-52.

30. Gutin, B., K. Stewart, S. Lewis, and J. Kruper. 1976. Oxygen consumption in the first stages of strenuous work as a function of prior exercise. *Journal of Sports Medicine and Physical Fitness* 16 (1): 60-65.

31. Haennel, R., K.K. Teo, A. Quinney, and T. Kappagoda. 1989. Effects of hydraulic circuit training on cardiovascular function. *Medicine and Science in Sports and Exercise* 21 (5): 605-612.

32. Hanson, J.M. 1994. *The Relationship Between Personal Incentives for Exercise and the Selection of Activity Among Patrons of Fitness Centers and Recreation Centers.* Microform Publications. Eugene, OR: University of Oregon, International Institute for Sport and Human Performance.

33. Hardman, A.E. 2001. Issues of fractionization of exercise (short vs long bouts). *Medicine and Science in Sports and Exercise* 33 (6 Suppl): S421-S427.

34. Hennessy, L.C., and A.W.S. Watson. 1994. The interference effects of training for strength and endurance simultaneously. *Journal of Strength and Conditioning Research* 8 (1): 12-19.

35. Hickson, R.C. 1980. Interference of strength development by simultaneous training for strength and endurance. *European Journal of Applied Physiology* 45: 255-263.

36. Hickson, R.C., B.A. Dvorak, E.M. Gorostiaga, T.T. Kurowski, and C. Foster. 1988. Potential for strength and endurance training to amplify endurance performance. *Journal of Applied Physiology* 65 (5): 2285-2290.

37. Hickson, R.C., B.A. Dvorak, E.M. Gorostiaga, T.T. Kurowski, and C. Foster. 1988. Strength training and performance in endurance-trained subjects. *Medicine and Science in Sports and Exercise* 20: S86.

38. Hickson, R.C., C. Foster, M.L. Pollock, T.M. Galassi, and S. Rich. 1985. Reduced training intensities and loss of aerobic power, endurance, and cardiac growth. *Journal of Applied Physiology* 58 (2): 492-499.

39. Hickson, R.C., C. Kanakis Jr., J.R. Davis, A.M. Moore, and S. Rich. 1982. Reduced training duration effects on aerobic power, endurance, and cardiac growth. *Journal of Applied Physiology* 53: 225-229.

40. Hickson, R.C., and M.A. Rosenkoetter. 1981. Reduced training frequencies and maintenance of increased aerobic power. *Medicine and Science in Sports and Exercise* 13: 13-16.

41. Hickson, R.C., M.A. Rosenkoetter, and M.M. Brown. 1980. Strength training effects on aerobic power and short-term endurance. *Medicine and Science in Sports and Exercise* 12 (5): 336-339.

42. Howley, E.T. 2000. You asked for it: Question authority. The equation "220 - age" is used to estimate maximal heart rate, but there is potential error in the estimate. Where did that

equation come from, and are better equations available? *ACSM's Health & Fitness Journal* 4 (4): 6-18.

43. Hunter, G., R. Dement, and D. Miller. 1987. Development of strength and maximum oxygen uptake during simultaneous training for strength and endurance. *Journal of Sports Medicine and Physical Fitness* 27: 269-275.

44. Hurley, B.F., D.R. Seals, A.A. Ehsani, L.-J. Cartier, G.P. Dalsky, J.M. Hagberg, and J.O. Holloszy. 1984. Effects of high-intensity strength training on cardiovascular function. *Medicine and Science in Sports and Exercise* 16 (5): 483-488.

45. Jakicic, J.M., R.R. Wing, B.A. Butler, and R.J. Robertson. 1995. Prescribing exercise in multiple short bouts versus one continuous bout: Effects on adherence, cardiorespiratory fitness, and weight loss in overweight women. *International Journal of Obesity* 19: 893-901.

46. Kang, J., E.C. Chaloupka, M.A. Mastrangelo, and J. Angelucci. 1999. Physiological responses to upper body exercise on an arm and a modified leg ergometer. *Medicine and Science in Sports and Exercise* 31 (10): 1453-1459.

47. Karvonen, M., K. Kentala, and O. Mustala. 1957. The effects of training on heart rate: A longitudinal study. *Annales Medicinae Experimentalis et Biological Fennial* 35: 307-315.

48. Karvonen, J., and T. Vuorimaa. 1988. Heart rate and exercise intensity during sports activities. Practical application. *Sports Medicine* 5 (5): 303-311.

49. Kearney, J.T., A.G. Stull, and J.L. Ewing. 1976. Cardiorespiratory responses of sedentary college women as a function of training intensity. *Journal of Applied Physiology* 41: 822-825.

50. Kohrt, W.M., D.W. Morgan, B. Bates, and J.S. Skinner. 1987. Physiological responses of triathletes to maximal swimming, cycling, and running. *Medicine and Science in Sports and Exercise* 19: 51-55.

51. Kraemer, J. 2002. Performance benefits of the warm-up. *Olympic Coach* 12 (4): 8-9.

52. Lamb, D.R. 1995. Basic principles for improving sport performance. *Sports Science Exchange* 8: 1-5.

53. Levin, G.T., M.R. Mcguigan, and P.B. Laursen. 2009. Effect of concurrent endurance and resistance training on physiologic and performance parameters of well-trained endurance cyclists. *Journal of Strength and Conditioning Research* 23 (8): 2280-2286.

54. Liang, M.T.C., J.F. Alexander, H.L. Taylor, R.C. Serfass, and A.S. Leon. 1982. Aerobic training threshold: Intensity, duration and frequency of exercise. *Scandinavian Journal of Sports Sciences* 4 (1): 5-8.

55. Londeree, B.R., and S.A. Ames. 1976. Trend analysis of the %VO2max-HR regression. *Medicine and Science in Sports* 8: 122-125.

56. Londeree, B.R., and M.L. Moeschberger. 1982. Effect of age and other factors on maximal heart rate. *Research Quarterly in Exercise and Sport* 53 (4): 297-304.

57. Mahon, A.D., K.O. Stolen, and J.A. Gay. 2001. Differentiated perceived exertion during submaximal exercise in children and adults. *Journal of Pediatric Exercise Science* 13: 145-153.

58. Marcinik, E.J., J. Potts, G. Schlabach, S. Will, P. Dawson, and B.F. Hurley. 1991. Effects of strength training on lactate threshold and endurance performance. *Medicine and Science in Sports and Exercise* 23 (6): 739-743.

59. Marigold, E.A. 1974. The effect of training at predetermined heart rate levels for sedentary college women. *Medicine and Science in Sports* 6: 14-19.

60. McArdle, W.D., F.I. Katch, and V.L. Katch. 2009. In: *Exercise Physiology: Energy, Nutrition, and Human Performance,* 7th ed. Philadelphia: Lippincott Williams & Wilkins.

61. McConell, G.K., D.L. Costill, J.J. Widrick, M.S. Hickey, H. Tanaka, and P.B. Gastin. 1993. Reduced training volume and intensity maintain aerobic capacity but not performance in distance runners. *International Journal of Sports Medicine* 14 (1): 33-37.

62. McKenzie, D.C., E.L. Fox, and K. Cohen. 1978. Specificity of metabolic and circulatory responses to arm or leg interval training. *European Journal of Applied Physiology* 39: 241-248.

63. Monteiro, A.G., D.A. Alveno, M. Prado, G.A. Monteiro, C. Ugrinowitsch, M.S. Aoki, and I.C. Picarro. 2008. Acute physiological responses to different circuit training protocols. *Journal of Sports Medicine and Physical Fitness* 48 (4): 438-442.

64. Moyna, N.M., R.J. Robertson, C.L. Meckes, J.A. Peoples, N.B. Millich, and P.D. Thompson. 2001. Intermodal comparison of energy expenditure at exercise intensities corresponding to perceptual preference range. *Medicine and Science in Sports and Exercise* 33: 1404-1410.

65. Murphy, M.H., and A.E. Hardman. 1998. Training effects of short and long bouts of brisk walking in sedentary women. *Medicine and Science in Sports and Exercise* 30: 152-157.

66. National Institutes of Health: Consensus Development Panel on Physical Activity and Cardiovascular Health. 1996. Physical activity and cardiovascular health. *Journal of the American Medical Association* 276: 214-246.

67. Nieman, D.C. 2003. *Exercise Testing and Prescription,* 5th ed. Boston: McGraw-Hill.

68. O'Toole, M.L., P.S. Douglas, and W.D.B. Hiller. 1989. Applied physiology of a triathlon. *Sports Medicine* 8: 201-225.

69. Potteiger, J.A. 2000. Aerobic endurance exercise training. In: *Essentials of Strength Training and Conditioning,* 2nd ed., T.R. Baechle and R.W. Earle, eds. Champaign, IL: Human Kinetics. pp. 495-509.

70. Powers, S.K., and E.T. Howley. 2008. *Exercise Physiology: Theory and Application to Fitness and Performance,* 7th ed. New York: McGraw-Hill.

71. Raasch, C.C., and F.E. Zajac. 1999. Locomotor strategy for pedaling: Muscle groups and biomechanical functions. *Journal of Neurophysiology* 82 (5): 515-525.

72. Reybrouck, T., G.F. Heigenhauser, and J.A. Faulkner. 1975. Limitations to maximum oxygen uptake in arms, leg, and combined arm-leg ergometry. *Journal of Applied Physiology* 38 (5): 774-779.

73. Rhodes, R.E., A.D. Martin, J.E. Taunton, E.C. Rhodes, M. Donnelly, and J. Elliot. 1999. Factors associated with exercise adherence among older adults: An individual perspective. *Sports Medicine* 28 (6): 397-411.

74. Riddle, S., and C. Orringer. 1990. Measurement of oxygen consumption and cardiovascular response during exercise on the Stairmaster 4000PT versus the treadmill. *Medicine and Science in Sports and Exercise* 22 (2 Suppl): S65.

75. Robertson, R.J., and B.J. Noble. 1997. Perception of physical exertion: Methods, mediators, and applications. *Exercise and Sport Sciences Reviews* 25: 407-452.

76. Ryan, R.M., C.M. Frederick, D. Lepes, N. Rubio, and K.M. Sheldon. 1997. Intrinsic motivation and exercise adherence. *International Journal of Sport Psychology* 28 (4): 335-354.

77. Saltin, B., L. Hartley, A. Kilbom, and I. Åstrand. 1969. Physical training in sedentary middle-aged and older men. *Scandinavian Journal of Clinical and Laboratory Investigation* 24: 323-334.

78. Sharkey, B.J. 1970. Intensity and duration of training and the development of cardiorespiratory fitness. *Medicine and Science in Sports* 2: 197-202.

79. Shellock, F.G., and W.E. Prentice. 1985. Warming-up and stretching for improved physical performance and prevention of sports-related injuries. *Sports Medicine* 2: 267.

80. Shepard, R.J. 1969. Intensity, duration, and frequency of exercise as determinants of the response to a training regime. *Internationale Zeitschrift fur Angewandte Physiologie* 26: 272-278.

81. Skinner, J.S., S.E. Gaskill, T. Rankinen, A.S. Leon, D.C. Rao, J.H. Wilmore, and C. Bouchard. 2003. Heart rate versus %VO2max: Age, sex, race, initial fitness, and training response - HERITAGE. *Medicine and Science in Sports and Exercise* 35 (11): 1908-1913.

82. Springer, C., T.J. Barstow, K. Wasserman, and D.M. Cooper. 1991. Oxygen uptake and heart rate responses during hypoxic exercise in children and adults. *Medicine and Science in Sports and Exercise* 23: 71-79.

83. Stone, M.H., S.J. Fleck, W.J. Kraemer, and N.T. Triplett. 1991. Health and performance related adaptations to resistive training. *Sports Medicine* 11 (4): 210-231.

84. Swain, D.P., K.S. Abernathy, C.S. Smith, S.J. Lee, and S.A. Bunn. 1994. Target heart rates for the development of cardiorespiratory fitness. *Medicine and Science in Sports and Exercise* 26: 112-116.

85. Swain, D.P., and B.C. Leutholtz. 1997. Heart rate reserve is equivalent to VO2 reserve, not % VO2 max. *Medicine and Science in Sports and Exercise* 29: 837-843.

86. Thomas, T., G. Ziogas, T. Smith, Q. Zhang, and B. Londeree. 1995. Physiological and perceived exertion responses to six modes of submaximal exercise. *Research Quarterly in Exercise and Sport* 66 (3): 239-246.

87. Tulppo, M.P., T.H. Makikallio, R.T. Laukkanen, and H.V. Huikuri. 1999. Differences in autonomic modulation of heart rate during arm and leg exercise. *Clinical Physiology* 19 (4): 294-299.

88. Turcotte, L., W. Byrnes, P. Frykman, P. Freedson, and F. Katch. 1984. The effects of hydraulic resistive training on maximal oxygen uptake and anaerobic threshold. *Medicine and Science in Sports and Exercise* 16: S183.

89. U.S. Department of Health and Human Services. 1996. *Physical Activity and Health: A Report of the Surgeon General.* Atlanta: U.S. Department of Health and Human Services, Centers for Disease Control and Prevention, National Center for Chronic Disease Prevention and Health Promotion.

90. U.S. Department of Health and Human Services. 2000. *Healthy People 2010: Understanding and Improving Health,* 2nd ed. Washington, DC: U.S. Government Printing Office. P.26

91. Van de Graff, K.M., and S.J. Fox. 1989. *Concepts of Human Anatomy and Physiology,* 2nd ed. Dubuque, IA: Brown.

92. Velasquez, K.S., and J.H. Wilmore. 1993. Changes in cardio-respiratory fitness and body composition after a 12-week bench step training program. *Medicine and Science in Sports and Exercise* 24 (Suppl): S78.

93. Wells, C.L., and R.R. Pate. 1995. Training for performance of prolonged exercise. In: *Perspectives in Exercise Science and Sports Medicine,* D.R. Lamb and R. Murray, eds. Indianapolis: Benchmark Press. pp. 357-388.

94. Whaley, M.H., L.A. Kaminsky, G.B. Dwyer, L.H. Getchell, and L.A. Norton. 1992. Predictors of over- and under-achievement of age-predicted maximal heart rate. *Medicine and Science in Sports and Exercise* 24 (10): 1173-1179.

95. White, L.J., R.H. Dressendorfer, S.M. Muller, and M.A. Ferguson. 2003. Effectiveness of cycle cross-training between competitive seasons in female distance runners. *Journal of Strength and Conditioning Research* 17 (2): 319-323.

96. Wilber, R.L., R.J. Moffatt, B.E. Scott, D.T. Lee, and N.A. Cucuzzo. 1996. Influence of water run training on maintenance of aerobic performance. *Medicine and Science in Sports and Exercise* 28: 1056-1062.

97. Wilmore, J.H., and D.L Costill. 2007. *Physiology of Sport and Exercise,* 4th ed. Champaign, IL: Human Kinetics.

98. Yamaji, K., M. Greenley, D.R. Northey, and R.L. Houghson. 1990. Oxygen uptake and heart rate responses to treadmill and water running. *Canadian Journal of Sport Science* 15: 96-98.

99. Zeni, A., M. Hoffman, and P. Clifford. 1996. Energy expenditure with indoor exercise machines. *Journal of the American Medical Association* 275: 1424-1427.

100. Zeni, A., M. Hoffman, and P. Clifford. 1996. Relationships among heart rate, lactate concentration, and perceived effort for different types of rhythmic exercise in women. *Archives of Physical Medicine and Rehabilitation* 77: 237-241.

101. Zimmerman, C.L., T.M. Cook, M.S. Bravard, M.M. Hansen, R.T. Honomichl, S.T. Karns, M.A. Lammers, S.A. Steele, L.K. Yunker, and R.M. Zebrowski. 1994. Effects of stair-stepping exercise direction and cadence on EMG activity of selected lower extremity muscle groups. *Journal of Occupational and Sports Physical Therapy* 19 (3): 173-180.

102. Zupan, M.F., and P.S. Petosa. 1995. Aerobic and resistance cross-training for peak triathlon performance. *Strength and Conditioning* 17: 7-12.

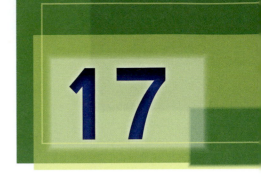

Plyometric and Speed Training

Vanessa van den Heuvel Yang, MS, Kevin Messey, MS,
Stacy Peterson, MA, and Robert Mamula

After completing this chapter, you will be able to

- explain the mechanics and physiology of plyometric and speed-enhancing exercises,

- identify the phases of the stretch–shortening cycle,

- understand the different roles of plyometric and speed training,

- recommend proper equipment for use during plyometric exercise performance,

- design safe and effective plyometric and speed training programs, and

- provide instruction in correct plyometric and speed training technique and recognize common errors.

In an effort to improve sport performance, athletes at all levels want an advantage that allows them to outplay their opponent. Athletes are looking for ways to become quicker and more explosive, for ways to jump higher and sprint faster. Plyometric and speed training are two training techniques that allow athletes of all ages and abilities to accomplish these goals. Although not typically emphasized in the design of programs for personal training clients, plyometric and speed training are important components of a well-balanced plan to improve not only sport performance, but also job

performance and activities of daily living. Exercises designed to train clients to jump higher and run faster are arguably essential program components. Further, because so many injuries occur as the result of an inability to control decelerative forces, the use of both plyometric and speed training, with their emphasis on the efficient production and use of ground reaction forces, should be considered an integral part of any program whose goal is injury prevention. Additional benefits of incorporating plyometric and speed training components include overall enhanced coordination, increased agility, and improved anaerobic and general conditioning (69).

A plyometric movement is a quick, powerful movement consisting of an eccentric muscle action, also known as a countermovement or prestretch,

The authors would like to acknowledge the contribution of David H. Potach, who wrote this chapter for the first edition of *NSCA's Essentials of Personal Training*.

followed by an immediate powerful concentric muscle action (115). Speed is simply the ability to achieve high velocity. Both plyometrics and speed rely heavily on the **stretch–shortening cycle** (SSC) to elicit the desired outcome. Since all functional activities are composed of a series of repetitive SSCs, it is essential to incorporate exercises that strengthen clients in these areas (30). The purpose of plyometric exercise is to use the stretch reflex and natural elastic components of both muscle and tendon to increase the power of subsequent movements and strengthen the muscles and tendons functionally (19, 30, 69, 78, 120). Speed training exercises are designed to use these same mechanical and neurophysiologic components, in concert with technique and muscular strength, to produce larger ground forces, thereby allowing clients to run faster. This chapter describes how to use plyometric and speed training exercise effectively as part of an overall training program.

Plyometric Mechanics and Physiology

Successful, goal-directed movements—athletic, job related, and functional—depend on all active musculotendinous structures working in concert at appropriate velocities. The term used to define this force–speed relationship is *power* (see chapter 4 for a definition of power). When used correctly, plyometric training has consistently demonstrated the ability to improve the production of muscle force and power (6, 58, 69, 93, 107). This increased production of muscular power is best explained by two proposed models as discussed in this section—mechanical and neurophysiological (116). The function of each model is then summarized by a description of the SSC.

Mechanical Model of Plyometric Exercise

In the *mechanical model,* elastic energy is stored following a rapid stretch and then released during a subsequent concentric muscle action, thereby increasing the total force production (2, 16, 59). A common model presents the function of the musculotendinous unit as a relationship between three mechanical components, the series and parallel elastic components and the contractile component (CC) (figure 17.1, row 2). While the **series elastic component (SEC)**—a primary contributor to force production during plyometric exercises—includes some muscular components (actin and myosin), it is composed mainly of tendon (19). When the musculotendinous unit is stretched,

as during an eccentric muscle action, the SEC acts as a spring and is lengthened, storing elastic energy. If the muscle then *immediately* begins a concentric muscle action, the stored energy is released, contributing to the total force production by naturally returning the muscles and tendons to their resting configuration. If a concentric muscle action does not occur immediately following the eccentric action, or if the eccentric phase is too long or requires too great a motion about the given joint, the stored energy dissipates and is lost as heat. Consequently, no plyometric effect will occur (19, 78).

Neurophysiological Model of Plyometric Exercise

The *neurophysiological element* involves a change in the force–velocity characteristics of the muscle's contractile components caused by stretch (40); concentric muscle force is increased with the use of the stretch reflex (figure 17.1, row 3) (9, 10, 11, 12). The **stretch reflex** is the body's involuntary response to an external stimulus that causes a rapid stretching of the muscle. In response to this rapid stretch, a signal is sent to the spinal cord, which in turn sends a message back, resulting in a concentric contraction of the same overstretched muscle (78). The stretch reflex responds to the rate at which the muscle is stretched (22, 54, 76). An example of the stretch reflex in action is the quick knee jerk reaction that occurs when the patellar tendon is hit by an external stimulus such as a reflex hammer. A quick stretch of the patellar tendon occurs when the reflex hammer comes in contact with the tendon. The quadriceps muscle then senses this stretch and responds with an involuntary concentric contraction, resulting in the knee jerk as seen by the observer (22, 78).

This reflexive component of plyometric exercise is composed primarily of muscle spindle activity. Muscle spindles are organs located within the muscle near the musculotendinous junction. They are sensitive to the rate and magnitude of a stretch; when a quick stretch is detected, muscular activity reflexively increases (54, 76, 78). This reflexive response increases the activity in the agonist muscle, thereby increasing the force the muscle produces (9, 10, 11, 12, 64). Although response time of the reflex does not really change with training, the strength of the response in terms of the muscle contraction elicited does increase with training, resulting in power gains. The faster a muscle is stretched, the greater the concentric force following the stretch, resulting in increased power output (22). As with the mechanical model, if a concentric muscle action does not immediately follow a stretch (e.g., due to an

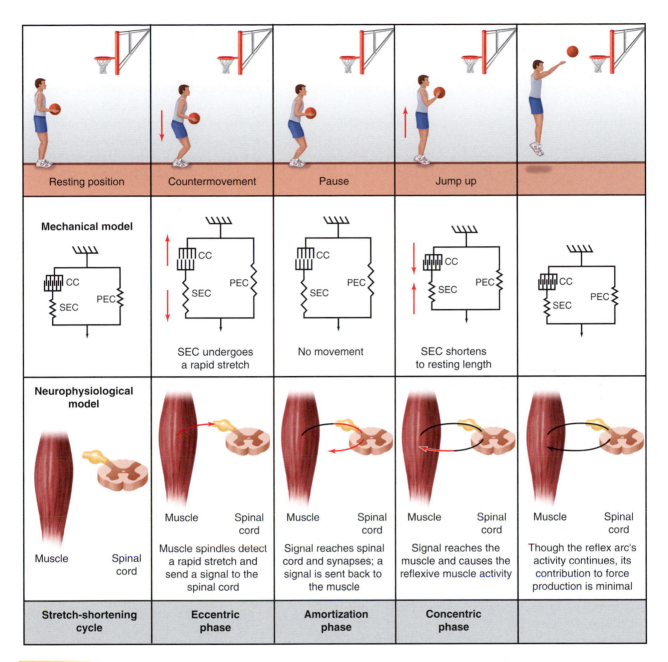

	Resting position	Countermovement	Pause	Jump up	
Mechanical model		SEC undergoes a rapid stretch	No movement	SEC shortens to resting length	
Neurophysiological model	Muscle Spinal cord	Muscle Spinal cord — Muscle spindles detect a rapid stretch and send a signal to the spinal cord	Muscle Spinal cord — Signal reaches spinal cord and synapses; a signal is sent back to the muscle	Muscle Spinal cord — Signal reaches the muscle and causes the reflexive muscle activity	Muscle Spinal cord — Though the reflex arc's activity continues, its contribution to force production is minimal
Stretch-shortening cycle	**Eccentric phase**	**Amortization phase**	**Concentric phase**	

FIGURE 17.1   Illustration of the stretch–shortening cycle (SSC) with the events of the mechanical model (row 2) and neurophysiological model (row 3) that occur during each of its three phases (row 4). For example, during the eccentric phase of the SSC (column 2)—that is, the client's countermovement—the series elastic component (SEC) undergoes a rapid stretch that the muscle spindles detect, which then send a signal to the spinal cord

Reprinted by permission from Albert 1995.

excessive delay between the stretch and concentric action or with a movement occurring over too large a range), the **potentiation,** or enhancement, of the stretch reflex is negated (19, 78).

Stretch–Shortening Cycle

The SSC is a model explaining the energy-storing capabilities of the SEC and stimulation of the stretch reflex that facilitate a maximal increase in muscle recruitment over a minimal amount of time. The SSC involves three distinct phases (table 17.1). While these phases outline the individual mechanical and neurophysiological events of the SCC, it is important to remember that all the events listed do not necessarily occur within the given phase, as some events may last longer or require less time than the given phase allows. The eccentric phase—the **deceleration**

TABLE 17.1   Stretch–Shortening Cycle

Phase	Action	Physiological event
I—Eccentric	Stretch of the agonist muscle	■ Elastic energy is stored. ■ Muscle spindles are stimulated. ■ Signal is sent to spinal cord.
II—Amortization	Pause between phases I and III	■ Nerves synapse (meet) in spinal cord. ■ Signal is sent to stretched muscle.
III—Concentric	Shortening of agonist muscle fibers	■ Elastic energy is released from the SEC. ■ Stretched muscle is stimulated by nerve.

SEC: series elastic component.

phase—involves preloading the agonist muscle group(s). During this phase, the SEC stores elastic energy and the muscle spindles are stimulated (7, 55). To visualize the eccentric phase, think about a basketball jump shot. The eccentric phase is the countermovement, beginning at the initiation of the half-squat motion and continuing until the bottom of the movement (figure 17.1, column 2).

The **amortization,** or transition, **phase** is the time between the eccentric and concentric phases—the time from the end of the eccentric phase to the initiation of the concentric muscle action. This is the turn-around time from landing to takeoff and is the most important part of the plyometric exercise, as it is critical for power development (78). There is a delay between the eccentric and concentric muscle actions during which the spinal cord begins to transmit signals to the agonist—stretched—muscle group. For a period of milliseconds, an isometric contraction occurs as the body prepares to change direction. This phase must be kept short in duration. If the amortization phase lasts too long, the energy stored during the eccentric phase will be dissipated as heat, and the stretch reflex will not increase muscle activity during the concentric phase (14, 78). Consider again the basketball jump shot. Once the person's downward half squat has stopped, the amortization phase has begun. As soon as upward movement begins, the amortization phase has ended (figure 17.1, column 3).

The concentric phase is the body's response to the events occurring during the eccentric and amortization phases. During this final phase of the SSC, the energy stored in the SEC during the eccentric phase is either used to increase the force of the subsequent movement or is dissipated as heat. Use of the stored elastic energy increases the force produced during the concentric phase movement to a level above that of an isolated concentric muscle action (15, 107, 112). In addition, the agonist muscle group performs a reflexive concentric muscle action as a result of the stretch reflex. Again visualize the jump shot. Following the half squat movement, as soon as movement begins

in an upward direction, the concentric phase of the SSC has begun and the amortization phase has ended (figure 17.1, column 4). In this example, one of the agonist muscles is the quadriceps femoris. During the countermovement, the quadriceps femoris undergoes a rapid stretch (eccentric phase); there is a delay in movement (amortization phase); then the muscle acts concentrically to extend the knee, allowing the person to push off the ground (concentric phase) (figure 17.1, columns 2, 3, and 4, respectively).

> The stretch–shortening cycle describes the stretch reflex and stored elastic energy–induced increases in concentric force production that follow a rapid eccentric muscle action.

When to Use Plyometric Exercise

It should seem obvious that plyometric training offers significant benefits to athletic clients in that most sporting movements rely on quick, powerful movements to be successful (3, 78). Which other populations may benefit from use of these types of movements is less clear. This bias has allowed plyometric exercise to become an ignored training modality for the general population. Many nonathletic clients, however, may benefit from the increases in muscular power production that plyometric training provides. The ability of the personal trainer to identify nonathletic clients who may benefit from plyometrics, as well as those for whom plyometrics are not necessary, is an essential skill for designing individualized exercise programs.

Plyometric Training and Sport Performance

When training clients whose goals include becoming more explosive in their sport, components of the training regimen must include exercises that mimic the movements occurring in that sport. Being able to train clients to produce greater muscular force (power) at a faster speed will provide them the edge in performance they are looking for. Increased production of muscular power is an established outcome of participation in a plyometric training program (2, 16, 57, 58, 59, 75, 78, 86, 96, 107, 117). The ability to produce more muscular power has been associated with improved sport performance (including increased jump performance, decreased sprint times, and increased strength) (4, 5, 33, 70, 77, 106). Plyometric training, then, is an ideal exercise mode when the goal is to improve muscular power production (77, 78, 96). In addition, plyometric training prepares athletes for the deceleration–acceleration and change-of-direction requirements in most sports by improving their ability to perform these types of tasks. An additional benefit of moderate plyometric training in average-distance runners was an improved "running economy" (the distance run per amount of oxygen consumed) (108).

Plyometric Training and Work Performance

In addition to sport performance, participation in a plyometric training program has the potential to improve performance at work (68). Though this has not been sufficiently examined in the literature, an analysis of some job requirements indicates that the production of muscular power is a key to movement efficiency and may improve job output. For example, police officers, firefighters, or clients preparing for military training must be able to run quickly, change direction effectively, and jump onto or over objects (e.g., fences) in preparation for their occupational demands.

Plyometric Exercise and Injury Prevention

Decreasing the incidence of injury, especially in populations who are at a greater risk of injury than others, is an important consideration when one is designing an exercise training program. There is great interest in the utility of plyometric training in decreasing risk of injury. Studies have shown that athletic injury rates decrease following participation in a plyometric training program (8, 18, 57, 58, 121). Research has also shown that proper plyometric training improves bone mineral content, muscle recruitment, strength, body control, and balance (19, 82, 120). The increased bone mineral content development could lead to a decreased risk of osteoporosis later in life.

Since plyometric training teaches the neuromuscular system to quickly perform an SSC while also focusing on proper technique and biomechanics, the client develops the ability to control all joints in the kinetic chain. This results in an improved stability of the entire body (121). These results suggest that the plyometric program should focus on proper jumping and landing mechanics, which will carry over into the client's athletic or work activity. When the client engages in the activities in either work or play that incorporate jumping and landing components, he or she will do so correctly, which will decrease the risk of injury. Plyometric training improves dynamic joint stability (18) and the ability to control the body during activities (e.g., controlled knee positioning during landing). This can help decrease the chances of knee injuries like patellofemoral pain syndrome and anterior cruciate ligament injuries (18, 82, 104). Also, the increased ability to control the body has the potential to reduce the risk of falls that could result in fractures (120).

It is difficult, however, to extrapolate the results of these studies to different populations. A component of plyometric training is eccentric control of movement, which research has shown may decrease the risk of injury (101). Eccentric training may therefore be a compromise for clients who wish to engage in injury prevention activities but for whom plyometric training is not appropriate. Eccentric training can consist of normal weight training with a focus on the eccentric phase of the lift. The personal trainer can guide clients to perform a lift with both the concentric and eccentric phases but to perform the eccentric phase more slowly. Even more effective is having the client perform the eccentric phase on his or her own and the personal trainer assist with the concentric phase. This technique allows clients to resist more weight than they would without the assistance. For example, although plyometric training may not be appropriate for a 75-year-old female client, this client would benefit from eccentric training to lessen her chance of falling.

Safety Considerations

There has been no research to delineate populations for whom plyometric training is contraindicated, though analysis of a client's age, experience, and current training level may help identify clients who are and are not ready for plyometric training. To reduce the risk of injury and to improve the performance of plyometric exercises, the client must understand proper plyometric technique and possess a sufficient base of strength, speed, and balance. In addition, the client must be sufficiently mature both physically and psychologically to participate in a plyometric training program.

Plyometric exercise is not inherently dangerous; however, as with all modes of exercise, injury risk is present. Injuries may occur following an accident, but they more typically occur when training procedures are violated. Improper program design, inadequate instruction and supervision, or an inappropriate training environment can contribute to increased injury risk. Often these injuries occur when the muscles are fatigued, since fatigue affects the body's proprioceptive ability. Ankle and knee sprains are the most common injuries that occur with plyometrics due to breaks in form resulting from muscular fatigue (22). In addition, anytime the client adds more difficult exercises or movements or trains at an increased intensity level, there is an increased risk of injury until the client becomes proficient at the exercise (69). Personal trainers must understand and address these and other risk factors to improve the safety of the client performing plyometric exercise. The following evaluative items will help determine whether these conditions have been met.

Age and Maturity

Plyometric training places great stress on the body, so it is important to consider all factors to ensure that the client's health is not compromised. Plyometrics at certain intensities are safe for the majority of populations; however, modifications to intensity and volume must also be made based on age.

Current research shows that plyometrics are safe and beneficial for youth (42). Guidelines indicate that as soon as the client is mature enough to accept and follow directions, one can safely integrate plyometrics into the training program (42, 43). In fact, this is an ideal time to implement plyometrics with a comprehensive training program, including resistance and flexibility training, as a youth's body is very moldable and adept at learning these motor skills (43, 66). In addition to improving running velocity and vertical jump, plyometrics will improve bone mass and decrease sport injury rate (42, 66, 119) in young clients. The client must be careful because the addition of high-intensity lower body plyometrics could place the client at an increased risk for bone injury as the epiphyseal plates (growth plates) of the bones of prepubescent children have yet to close (63, 72). Therefore, it is important that a plyometric program is implemented following the recommended guidelines.

When developing a plyometric program for youth, it is important to focus on teaching the proper technique, especially jumping and landing techniques, described later in the chapter (42, 43, 52, 66). Young clients should not focus on competing with or outperforming others, but rather on improving self-performance and mastering the skill. The exercises should be low-intensity plyometrics performed at the beginning of a session, before the client is fatigued (69). This ensures that the client has proper neuromuscular and postural control to perform the exercises correctly. Increased errors and injuries are likely to occur if the client is learning these exercises tired. Incorporating plyometric exercises into a dynamic warm-up is ideal. The exercises should take the form of fun and creative activities that resemble structured play and games so that the actual training goal is not apparent to the child (92, 98). Examples include having the child react to balls, run obstacle courses, perform jumping jacks, hopscotch, or pretend he or she is being chased (42, 43, 92).

For adolescent clients, it is appropriate to incorporate low-intensity plyometric exercise into the training regimen as long as the client has met all of the safety conditions outlined later (97, 98, 102, 120). The personal trainer should emphasize proper technique as well, since adolescents are still developing neuromuscular control. It is safe to perform low-intensity plyometrics at small volumes, incorporating them into warm-up activities. Once these low-intensity exercises have been mastered, the client may perform moderate-intensity exercises (22, 104). Benefits of adding plyometric exercises to an adolescent client's workout exceed just the increase in performance. Plyometrics have also been shown to help adolescents develop bone strength, balance, and coordination (49, 102, 120).

The other population of concern is the aging population. Due to decreasing bone strength as one ages as well as the possibility of degenerative joint conditions, high-intensity plyometrics may need to be avoided for this population. However, it is very beneficial for older people to continue training the SSC (98) by integrating low- to moderate-intensity plyometrics into their training program. The older client should begin with low-intensity exercises and progress to moderate-intensity plyometrics only when the personal trainer has ensured the client is able to safely and correctly perform the exercises (80). A recent study found that properly performed, high-intensity resistance training had positive results for people older than 60 (34). This outcome suggests that the addition of plyometrics may be beneficial, so long as the client is medically cleared and has met all of the safety conditions listed in the next section.

For all ages, physical maturity should not be the sole determinant of plyometric preparedness. Psychological maturity as well as mental maturity and acuity are necessary before someone begins plyometric training. The client must respond positively to the personal trainer's instructions to proceed with plyometric training. If he or she does not, plyometric training should be postponed. Injury, overtraining, or undertraining may result if the client is inattentive to instructions.

Posture, Flexibility, and Stability

Many lower body plyometric drills require the client to move in nontraditional movement patterns (e.g., double-leg zigzag hops and backward skips) or on a single leg (e.g., single-leg tuck jump and single-leg hops). These types of drills necessitate a solid base of support on which the client can safely and correctly perform the exercises. Even lower-intensity drills performed by clients just beginning a plyometric program require sufficient balance to prevent injury. As a result, it is essential that the personal trainer assess whether the client can safely meet the demands of plyometric training. The fundamental position that all lower body plyometric exercises originate from and end in is the partial, or half-squat position. Therefore, it is essential the personal trainer begin by assessing the client's ability to hold this position (104) in order to determine his or her potential to land properly with each exercise.

For both the partial squat position and the squat movement itself, the client's feet should be approximately shoulder-width apart. The chin should be tucked in slightly. The scapulae should be slightly retracted. The trunk should be parallel to the tibias. The knees should be directly over or slightly posterior to the toes, and the heels should remain on the ground. The client's body weight should be centered over a stable base of support (104), and the client must maintain this position in proper form.

Once the client can hold this position, the client should perform a body weight squat. The personal trainer should have the client stand with his or her feet approximately shoulder-width apart. To initiate the squat movement, the client should anteriorly rotate the pelvis, then flex at the ankles, knees, and hips while keeping the trunk parallel to the tibias throughout the entire range of motion. Also, the knees should remain either posterior to the toes or directly over them, and the feet should remain flat on the ground, avoiding liftoff of the heels if possible. Common errors include rounded shoulders, a forward head, a flexed thoracic spine, a posterior pelvic tilt, and a heel liftoff (104).

Once clients can both hold a proper double-leg squat position and perform a proper body weight squat, they may begin low-intensity plyometric exercises. When performing low-intensity beginning plyometrics, they must learn to maintain the proper alignment, providing a strong base for dynamic action (104). Errors in alignment will not only lead to potential injury but also cause increased ground contact time during the amortization phase, resulting in less than optimal concentric force (104, 121).

Before the personal trainer increases the level of exercises, the client should be able to hold a single-leg squat position as described for the balance tests shown in table 17.2. These are divided into level of difficulty; each test position must be held for 30 seconds (111). For example, a client doing plyometric training with double-leg drills for the first time must balance on one leg for 30 seconds without falling. This indicates that the client has enough leg strength to do double-leg drills. An experienced client beginning an advanced plyometric training program involving single-leg drills must maintain a single-leg half squat for 30 seconds without falling. The added dimension of the half squat indicates the client has enough strength on the leg to do single-leg plyometric exercises. The surface on which the balance testing is performed must be the same as that for the plyometric drills.

Strength

Before adding plyometrics to a client's workout program, the personal trainer must also take the client's level of strength into consideration. Clients who have never participated in a resistance training program should be precluded from taking part in a plyometric training program. Plyometric training requires significant strength and muscle control, especially during the eccentric phase. For this reason,

TABLE 17.2 Balance Tests

Level*	Position**	Drill variation***
Beginning	Standing	Double leg Single leg
Intermediate	Quarter squat	Double leg Single leg
Advanced	Half squat	Double leg Single leg

*Each of these levels corresponds with a drill's intensity level (e.g., beginning-level balance corresponds with low-intensity plyometric drills).

**The client is required to maintain each position with each variation for 30 s before attempting plyometric exercises of the same intensity and the more difficult balance test.

***The type of balance test (i.e., how many legs are used) needs to match the intended type of plyometric drill (e.g., the beginning client has to pass the standing single-leg balance test to qualify to perform single-leg plyometric drills).

clients should be encouraged to perform a resistance training program that includes standard exercises (e.g., squat, bench press, deadlift) before beginning a plyometric training program.

If the client does not possess sufficient muscular strength, plyometrics should be delayed until certain standards—originally intended for athletes—are met. Because research has yet to define a prerequisite level of strength, the following are the only published recommendations available for personal trainers to use when determining a client's readiness to participate in a plyometric training program:

- For lower body plyometrics, the client's 1-repetition maximum (1RM) squat should be at least 1.5 times his or her body weight (17, 38, 60, 69, 84, 114).

- For upper body plyometrics, clients weighing more than 220 pounds (100 kg) should have a bench press 1RM of at least 1.0 times their body weight; those under 220 pounds should have a bench press 1RM of at least 1.5 times their body weight (60, 84, 114).

- An alternative measure of prerequisite upper body strength is the ability to perform five clap push-ups in a row (84, 114).

These guidelines ensure that the client has sufficient strength to engage in plyometric exercises.

Although these guidelines provide a good rule of thumb, it is not necessary for clients to possess this level of strength to engage in low to moderate levels of plyometric activity, like simple jumps in place, as long as they can tolerate moderate loading during a resistance program and have proper landing technique (19, 78). When moving a client to more advanced levels of plyometric exercises, such as depth jumps, it is recommended that the personal trainer follow the strength guidelines listed (97). However, personal trainers should recognize that it is possible to modify even high-intensity plyometric exercises to make them appropriate for a client's strength level so that he or she can perform them safely and still achieve similar gains.

Another aspect of strength that is very important to assess is core strength (78, 98). Core strength is the body's ability to control its center of mass in response to forces on the trunk generated by other parts of the body, including upper and lower extremities (83, 98, 121). In other words, the core is responsible for maintaining balance and postural stability during all activities (83, 98). Core strength directly affects all other aspects of strength. A strong core provides a solid base for all other muscles and joints to work from, therefore allowing them to function in an optimal manner. A weak core will negatively affect the manner in which muscles and joints function since the base of support is weak and therefore, unstable. A direct effect of a weak core is an increased amortization phase time, which will compromise the plyometric effect (78). Overall, proper form will be compromised, performance will be hindered, and the chance of injury will increase with poor core strength (121).

Speed

Perhaps a more specific requirement for plyometric training participants is speed of movement. Because plyometric exercise relies on quick movements, the ability to move rapidly is essential before a client begins a plyometric program. In the absence of research specifying the level of speed necessary for plyometric exercise, personal trainers can use the following guidelines. For lower body plyometrics, the client should be able to perform five repetitions of a squat with 60% body weight in 5 seconds or less (84, 114). To satisfy the speed requirement for upper body plyometrics, the client should be able to perform five repetitions of the bench press with 60% body weight in 5 seconds or less. Like the strength guidelines presented previously, these speed requirements were originally intended for athletic populations. Should a client lack the speed of movement described here, he or she may begin a plyometric training program that starts with lower-intensity drills that do not rely as heavily on speed (e.g., two-foot ankle hop, standing long jump, double-leg vertical jump).

Landing Position

For lower body plyometrics, proper landing technique is essential to maximize the effectiveness of the exercise and minimize the risk of injury. This is especially true for depth jumps. If the center of gravity is offset from the base of support, performance will be hindered and injury may occur (104). If the earlier squat assessment reveals proper posture, flexibility, and stability, the personal trainer should begin assessing and training landing technique.

During the landing, the shoulders should be over the knees; the knees should be over or slightly posterior to the toes, with the ankles, knees, and hips flexed and the feet approximately shoulder-width apart (figure 17.2). Clients should land softly and maintain a dorsiflexed position of the ankle with the feet in full contact with the ground. Clients should

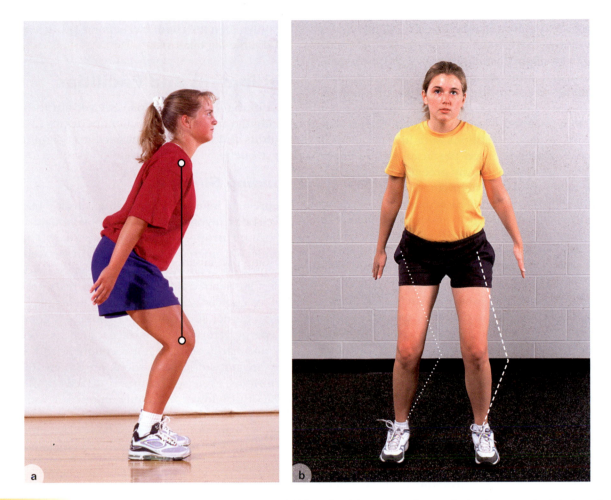

FIGURE 17.2   Proper plyometric landing position. (*a*) The shoulders are in line with the knees, which helps place the center of gravity over the body's base of support. (*b*) The knees are in line with the feet. There is no valgus (dotted line) or varus (dashed line) deviation.

also keep their weight more on the ball of the foot and not on the heel. This position allows a quick turn-around on the landings so that the client spends as little time as possible on the ground, achieving maximum power output (22). Instilling a proper landing technique will also teach the client to control the body's center of gravity within the base of support (104).

Landings can be taught during several exercises, including a vertical jump followed by a freeze in the landing position to allow proper analysis of the landing position, a forward or backward jump followed by a freeze in the landing position, or even a lateral jump followed by a freeze in the landing position. It is important for the personal trainer to provide constant feedback during and after each drill or exercise in order to instill proper technique.

For plyometric jumps, hops, leaps, bounds, skips, and quick foot drills, clients should concentrate on keeping their knees and their thumbs up. This will help with balance by keeping the workload centered around the hips and legs. Normally, when the knees are brought up quickly, as is the case with these exercises, the tendency is for the shoulders to drop forward. To prevent this, clients should focus on holding their hands in a position in which the thumbs are pointing up toward the sky, which forces the torso to remain in a more upright position. This also helps with maintaining balance (98). Also, the arms should be brought behind the midline of the body so they can move forward and up rapidly to help increase the strength of the muscle action (22, 98).

Medical History

As with other forms of exercise, joint structure, posture, body type, and previous orthopedic injuries must be examined and reviewed before the start of a plyometric training program. Previous injuries or abnormalities of the spine, lower extremities, or upper extremities may increase a client's risk of injury during performance of plyometric exercise. Specifically, clients with a history of muscle strains, pathological joint laxity, or spinal dysfunction (including vertebral disc dysfunction or compression injuries) (48, 49) should exercise caution when beginning plyometric training (60, 99). Clients with a history of such conditions should have medical clearance from a licensed physician before beginning plyometric activity. Any preexisting injury may require modifications to plyometric activity. For example, a client with patellofemoral pain may not be able to squat without pain and thus should not be doing high-intensity plyometric exercises like depth jumps. Before beginning any plyometric training, the client should be able to tolerate activities of daily living without pain or joint swelling (19).

Certain medical conditions, such as illnesses, osteoporosis, arthritis, or diabetes, may not respond well to plyometric activities. Therefore, personal trainers should require formal medical clearance before starting a client on plyometric activities. They should be well informed of the client's medical history and should ensure that the client has had a recent physical examination from a licensed physician (104).

Physical Characteristics

A specific characteristic warranting caution is client size. Clients weighing more than 220 pounds (100 kg) may be at increased risk for injury when performing plyometric exercises (84, 104, 114). Because greater weight increases joint compressive forces, these clients are at higher risk of injuring lower extremity joints. Therefore, clients weighing over 220 pounds (100 kg) should avoid high-volume, high-intensity plyometric exercises. For the same reason, clients weighing over 220 pounds should not perform depth jumps from heights greater than 18 inches (46 cm) (84, 104, 114). Lower-intensity plyometrics such as submaximal footwork patterns are a good alternative to the high-intensity plyometrics. Plyometric exercises should be limited to those involving double-leg takeoffs and progress to single

leg only when the client has become proficient with the double-leg takeoffs.

Equipment and Facilities

In addition to the participant's level of fitness and health, the area where the client performs plyometric drills and the equipment used may significantly affect safety.

Landing Surface

To prevent injuries, the landing surface used for lower body plyometrics must have adequate shock-absorbing properties but not be so soft that it significantly increases the transition between the eccentric and concentric phases. A grass field, field turf, a suspended floor, and rubber mats are good surface choices (22, 60, 78, 104). Clients may progress to harder surfaces that encourage higher rates of energy return (62). Surfaces such as concrete, tile, and hardwood are not recommended because they are not sufficiently shock absorbent (60, 78). Performing exercises on these surfaces can lead to a variety of lower extremity injuries. Excessively thick (greater than or equal to 6 inches [15 cm]) exercise mats and mini-trampolines may extend the amortization phase, thus preventing efficient use of the stretch reflex.

Training Area

The amount of space needed depends on the drill. Most bounding and running drills require at least 33 yards (30 m) of straightaway, though some drills may require a straightaway of 109 yards (100 m). For most standing, box, and depth jumps, only a minimal surface area is needed; but adequate height—9.8 to 13.2 feet (3-4 m)—is required.

Equipment

Boxes used for box jumps and depth jumps must be sturdy, should have a nonslip top, and should be closed on all sides. Boxes should also have few, if any, sharp or abrupt edges. Box heights should range from 6 to 42 inches (15-107 cm) (3, 26, 50, 65,

Minimum Requirements for Participation in a Plyometric Training Program

- Proper technique for each drill
- At least three months of resistance training experience
- Sufficient strength, speed, and balance for the level of drill used
- No current injuries to involved body segments

73) with landing surfaces of at least 18 by 24 inches (46 by 61 cm) (22). The box should be constructed of sturdy wood (e.g., 3/4-inch [1.9 cm] plywood) or heavy-gauge metal. To further reduce injury risk, ways to make the landing surface nonslip are to (1) add nonslip treads, (2) mix sand into the paint used on the box, or (3) affix rubberized flooring to the top of the box (22).

Plastic cones of varying heights (from 8 inches up to 24 inches [20-60 cm]) can be used as items to jump over during plyometric exercises. Since the cones are flexible, they are less likely to cause injuries if the client lands on them (22). Stairways, bleachers, and stadium steps also provide a plyometric training area. One must make sure they are safe for jumping on before the client begins the activities. Concrete steps are not a preferred surface since the concrete surface is unyielding, as mentioned in the previous paragraph(22). Medicine balls can be used for upper extremity plyometric exercises as well as in conjunction with some lower body exercises. They should be easy to grip, durable, and of varying weights (22).

Proper Footwear

Plyometrics require footwear with good ankle and arch support, good lateral stability, and a wide, nonslip sole (84, 114). Shoes with a narrow sole and poor upper support (e.g., running shoes) may invite ankle problems, especially with excessive lateral movements.

Supervision

In addition to the safety considerations already mentioned, clients must be closely monitored to ensure proper technique. Plyometric exercise is not intrinsically dangerous when performed correctly; but as with other forms of training, poor technique may unnecessarily predispose a client to injury. It is especially important for personal trainers to monitor client jumping and landing technique for lower extremity drills. In particular, personal trainers must instruct clients to avoid extremes of lateral knee motion (i.e., valgus and varus movements; see figure 17.2) and to minimize time spent on the ground. Knees should line up with the second and third toes while not passing ahead of them (anteriorly), and the amortization phase should be kept as short as possible. If the client deviates from these norms, drill intensity should be lowered to allow successful completion of each drill. Common technique errors are provided for each drill at the end of this chapter.

Plyometric Program Design

Plyometric exercise prescription is similar to resistance and aerobic exercise prescriptions (46). After an evaluation of the client's needs, the mode, intensity, frequency, duration, recovery, progression, and a warm-up period must all be included in the design of a sound program. Unfortunately, there is little research demarcating optimal program variables for the design of plyometric exercise programs. Therefore, in addition to the available research, personal trainers must rely on the methodology used during the design of resistance and aerobic endurance training programs and on practical experience when prescribing plyometric exercise. When in doubt about volume, frequency, or intensity, it is best to err on the side of caution (62). The guidelines that follow are based in part on Chu's work (20, 21, 22, 23, 25, 26) and the National Strength and Conditioning Association's position statement (84).

Needs Analysis

As with other training modalities, when incorporating plyometric exercise into a training program the personal trainer must perform a needs analysis to evaluate a client's current abilities. Specifically, the personal trainer determines the client's needs and the requirements of the client's activities and lifestyle. A combination of the following factors helps in the analysis of a client's needs:

- **Age**—Does the client's age predispose the client to injury and therefore preclude plyometric training?
- **Training experience and current training level**—Has the client been resistance training? If so, what types of exercises has he or she been performing? Has he or she participated in a plyometric training program? If so, when?
- **Injury history**—Is the client currently injured? Has he or she experienced an injury that might affect his or her ability to participate in a plyometric training program?
- **Physical testing results**—What are the client's current abilities as they relate to muscular power production (e.g., vertical and standing long jump results)?
- **Training goals**—What does the client want to improve? A specific movement (e.g., throwing)? A particular skill (e.g., volleyball hitting)? An on-the-job activity (e.g., loading a truck)?

- **Incidence of injury in a client's job or chosen activity**—What is the risk of injury in the client's chosen activity? Is the activity relatively sedentary (e.g., student or office worker)? Does the activity require constant change of direction (e.g., racquetball player or construction worker)? If the activity is dynamic, is the client prepared for it physically?

Client example 17.1 illustrates one form of the plyometric needs analysis. Near the end of this discussion of program design are sample programs for each of these six clients, illustrating the "how" of program design.

Mode

The *mode* of plyometric training is determined by the general part(s) of the body that are performing the given exercise. For example, a depth jump is a *lower body* plyometric exercise, whereas a medicine ball chest pass is an *upper body* exercise.

Lower Body Plyometrics

Lower body plyometrics are appropriate for clients involved in virtually any sport—including soccer, volleyball, basketball, and baseball—as well as in nonathletic activities or occupations that require muscular power production or quick changes of direction. These types of activities require participants to produce a maximal amount of force in a minimal amount of time. Soccer and basketball require quick, powerful movements and changes of direction from competitors. A client who plays basketball is an example of one who would benefit greatly from a plyometric training program, as basketball players must jump repeatedly for rebounds.

Lower body plyometric training allows the client's muscles to produce more force in a shorter amount of time, thereby allowing the person to jump higher. There are a wide variety of lower body plyometric drills with various intensity levels and directional movements. Descriptions of different types of lower body plyometric drills are provided in table 17.3 and in general are listed from lower to higher intensities.

Upper Body Plyometrics

Rapid, powerful upper body movements are requisites of several sports and activities, including golf, baseball, softball, and tennis. As an example, a baseball pitcher routinely throws a baseball at 80 to 100 miles per hour (129-161 km/h). To reach velocities of this magnitude, the pitcher's shoulder joint must move at over 6,000° per second (36, 44, 47, 90). Plyometric training of the shoulder joint would not only increase pitching velocity but may also prevent injury to the shoulder and elbow joints, although further research is needed to substantiate the role of plyometrics in injury prevention.

Plyometric drills for the upper body are not used as often as those for the lower body and have been studied less thoroughly. Nonetheless, they are essential to athletes requiring upper body power (87) and may help clients who need greater levels of upper body strength. Plyometrics for the upper body include medicine ball throws, catches, and push-up variations.

Intensity

Plyometric *intensity* refers to the amount of effort exerted by the muscles, connective tissues, and joints during performance of an exercise and is controlled both by the type of drill and by the distance covered (e.g., height of a jump) (table 17.4) (19, 22, 43). The intensity of plyometric drills ranges from low-level skipping that places less stress on the joints to high-level depth jumps that apply significant stress to the agonist muscles and joints (table 17.4). Intensity should be determined by both the ability of the body to handle the load and the ability of the client to maintain proper technique while performing the exercise (19). If technique suffers, the personal trainer should drop the intensity until the client can perform the exercise while maintaining the proper technique.

Intensity should be kept at a low level for those just beginning a plyometric program. Double-leg jumps in place, double-leg standing jumps, and simple skips are appropriate for such clients. Youth and adolescent clients should begin with one or two sets of six to eight repetitions to ensure quality reps in each set (42, 43). When in doubt, it is better to underestimate the physical ability of youth clients and have them do fewer repetitions. Rather than concentrating on advancing intensity, efforts should focus on ensuring proper technique to prevent injury when the client is ready for more advanced drills. Intensity can be increased by raising the platform height for box jumps or depth jumps, increasing the distance of bounds, and incorporating more advanced exercises like those involving single-leg takeoffs—and for the very advanced client, adding light weights or weighted vests (see table 17.5). It is important to remember that if intensity is too high because of excessive loading during the eccentric phase, an increase in the amortization phase may result, negating the plyometric benefit of the exercise (19, 78).

Needs Analysis for Plyometric Exercise

Sport client A. A healthy 30-year-old male has been fairly active all of his life and has joined a YMCA basketball league. He is currently in a resistance training program and performed plyometrics two years ago. He is 6 feet (183 cm) tall, weighs 200 pounds (91 kg), and has a 16-inch (40 cm) vertical jump and an 180-pound (82 kg) 1RM squat. He wants to

1. increase his vertical jump to improve his ability to rebound the basketball and
2. run up and down the court faster as well as change directions quickly.

Sport client B. A healthy, 28-year-old female fast-pitch softball player has played first base for the past five years but is transitioning to an outfield position. She trains with weights one or two times a week with a circuit weight training program for both the upper and lower body. She is 5 feet, 3 inches (160 cm) tall and weighs 125 pounds (57 kg). Her testing session reveals a 60-pound (27 kg) 1RM bench press and an 11-inch (28 cm) vertical jump. She requests help in improving her

1. ability to cover right field and
2. arm strength to help throw the ball to the infield.

Work client A. A 35-year-old firefighter participates in a resistance training program five days a week with both upper and lower body exercises. He was in a plyometric training program six months ago. He is 6 feet, 2 inches (188 cm) tall and weighs 225 pounds (102 kg). He has a 5.3-second 40-yard (37 m) dash time, 225-pound (102 kg) squat, and 20-inch (51 cm) vertical jump. In addition to the necessary cardiovascular training, he has requested help in improving his

1. lifting ability and
2. speed while carrying the hose.

Work client B. A 40-year-old female warehouse worker has had difficulty the past two months lifting boxes up and onto shelves at or above shoulder level. She has no complaints of pain and has been cleared by the company physician of any musculoskeletal dysfunction. She is 5 feet, 10 inches (178 cm) tall and weighs 150 pounds (68 kg). Her estimated 1RM bench press is 70 pounds (32 kg); estimated 1RM squat is 135 pounds (61 kg); and vertical jump is 13 inches (33 cm). She has never participated in a resistance training program. She has come to a personal trainer to assist her in improving her

1. arm strength, especially when pushing boxes onto a shelf, and
2. leg strength to assist her in lifting the heavier boxes.

Injury prevention client A. A healthy 14-year-old female soccer player is preparing to try out for her high school soccer team. She is 5 feet, 7 inches (170 cm) tall and weighs 110 pounds (50 kg). She has not performed 1RM testing, but her vertical jump is 12 inches (30 cm). Her parents are concerned that she will get hurt playing with girls who are so much older than she. She has been involved in a general resistance training program for the past six months but has never participated in a plyometric training program. The parents have requested help for their daughter to

1. reduce her risk of injury and
2. "get in shape."

Injury prevention client B. A 55-year-old female master's-level tennis player is returning to play following a yearlong layoff and is concerned about "losing a step" and injuring herself. She has not had any serious injuries. She is 5 feet, 6 inches (168 cm) tall and weighs 150 pounds (68 kg). Physical testing reveals an estimated 1RM squat of 140 pounds (64 kg), vertical jump of 10 inches (25 cm), and 40-yard (37 m) dash of 7.0 seconds. She has been resistance training for the past four months. She would like to

1. improve her speed when coming to the net and
2. reduce her risk of injury.

TABLE 17.3 Lower Body Plyometric Drills

Type of jump	Definition	Examples
Jump in place	Jumping and landing in the same spot, performed repeatedly, without rest between jumps	Squat jump, tuck jump, split squat jump
Standing jump	Maximal-effort jumps involving either vertical or horizontal components Recovery between repetitions required	Double-leg vertical jump, standing long jump, front barrier hop
Multiple hops and jumps	Drills involving repeated movements Commonly viewed as a combination of jumps in place and standing jumps	Double-leg hop, front barrier hop
Bounds	Drills that involve exaggerated movements with greater horizontal speed than other drills Volume for bounding typically measured by distance; normally greater than 98 ft (30 m)	Skip and alternate-leg bound, lateral bounding
Box drill	Multiple hops and jumps using a box to jump on or off Height of the box dependent on the size of the client, the landing surface, and goals of the program	Jump to box, jump from box
Depth jump	Drills in which the client assumes a position on a box, steps off, lands, and immediately jumps vertically, horizontally, or to another box	Depth jump, depth jump to second box

TABLE 17.4 Plyometric Exercises Listed by Intensity

Low intensity	Medium intensity	High intensity
Ankle flip	Double-leg tuck jump	Depth jump
Skip	Double leg hop	Single-leg jump
Standing long jump	Split squat jump	Lateral bounding
Double-leg vertical jump	Alternate-leg bounding	
Chest pass	Front barrier hop	
Jump to box	Jump from box	
	Depth push-up	
	Degree sit-up	

TABLE 17.5 Factors Affecting the Intensity of Lower Body Plyometric Drills

Factor	Methods to increase plyometric drill intensity
Points of contact	Progress from double- to single-leg support.
Speed	Increase the drill's speed of movement.
Multiple response added	Decrease the amortization phase by moving from pausing on landing into multiple responses on the ground.
Height of the drill	Raise the body's center of gravity by increasing the height of a drill (e.g., depth jump).
Participant's weight	Add weight (in the form of weight vests, ankle weights, and wrist weights).
Distance of the drill	Add a horizontal component to the drill to increase intensity as well.

Frequency

Frequency is the number of plyometric training sessions per week and depends on the client's age, ability, and goals (22). Often frequency and intensity are inversely proportional (19). Frequency increases as intensity decreases and vice versa. A low number of repetitions of low-intensity plyometric exercises can be performed multiple times per week. As for moderate-intensity plyometric training, current research shows that training two times per week is best and results in improved jumping ability, jump contact times, maximal concentric and isometric strength, and 22-yard (20 m) sprint time at the greatest training efficiency (19, 33). For youth and adolescent clients, plyometric training may be performed up to two times per week on nonconsecutive days.

Recovery

Rather than concentrating on the *frequency*, many personal trainers rely more on the *recovery time* (the time between repetitions, sets, and workouts) between plyometric training sessions (21, 22, 23, 25). Since plyometric drills often involve maximal efforts to improve anaerobic power, a complete, adequate recovery is required (19, 84, 114). The time between sets is determined by a proper work-to-rest ratio (i.e., a range of 1:5 to 1:10) (22, 39, 104) and is specific to the volume and type of drill being performed. That is, the higher the intensity of a drill, the more rest the client requires. For example, rest between sets of a plyometric skip will be shorter than the rest between sets of a depth jump (22). Recovery for depth jumps may range from 5 to 10 seconds of rest between single repetitions to 2 to 3 minutes between sets.

Shorter recovery periods between sets do not allow for maximum recovery and will thus compromise the potential benefits. Plyometrics is an anaerobic activity designed specifically to improve neuromuscular reactions, explosiveness, quickness, and the ability to generate forces in certain directions (22, 97). Each plyometric repetition requires a maximum, quality effort in order to be effective (104). Generally speaking, rest times of 60 to 120 seconds between drills should allow for full or nearly full recovery (98). Forty-eight to 72 hours between plyometric sessions (i.e., recovery time) is a typical guideline when one is prescribing plyometrics (21, 22, 23, 25, 104). This is especially applicable to beginners, who should have at least 48 hours of rest time (22). Using these typical recovery times, most clients should perform one to three plyometric sessions per week.

Volume

Plyometric *volume* is the total work performed during a single workout session (19, 22) and is typically expressed as the number of repetitions and sets performed during a session. Often plyometric volume is expressed as the number of contacts (each time a foot, feet together, or hand contact the surface) per workout (1, 19, 21, 22, 23, 25), but may also be expressed as distance, as with plyometric bounding. For example, a client beginning a plyometric training program may start with a double-arm bound for 33 yards (30 m) per repetition but advance to 109 yards (100 m) per repetition for the same drill (22). Lower body plyometric volumes vary for clients of different needs (i.e., client age and goals; resistance training and plyometric experience); suggested volumes are provided in table 17.6. Upper body plyometric volume is typically expressed as the number of throws or catches per workout. As for the number of repetitions, it is suggested that sets be kept to 8 to 12 repetitions each, with fewer repetitions for exercises that are more intense and more repetitions for exercises that are less intense (98).

The entire plyometric exercise session for beginners should never exceed 30 minutes. Adequate warm-up and cool-down should be included. Advanced clients may do longer workouts that may require a longer recovery (22). The effectiveness of the plyometric workout should not be determined by the level of fatigue the client feels. Using fatigue as a guideline often results in overtraining, pain, and overuse injuries. It is the quality of the exercise, not the quantity, that produces the most increases in power (22, 104). The volume of the plyometric session must relate inversely to the intensity of the drill. If the level of the plyometrics is considered low to moderate, the total number of foot contacts can be higher. Volume should increase only if technique is maintained without any adverse effects such as pain (19).

TABLE 17.6 General Plyometric Volume Guidelines Based on Age and Experience

Age	No resistance training experience	More than 3 months general resistance training experience	More than 3 months resistance training experience, including power exercises	More than 1 year general resistance training experience	More than 1 year resistance training experience, including power exercises	Resistance training but no plyometric training experience	Resistance training and plyometric training more than 1 year ago	Resistance training and plyometric training within past year
≤13	Nr*	Nr	Nr	Nr	Nr	Nr	Nr	Nr
14-17	Nr	40-60	40-60	60-80	80-100	40-60	60-80	80-100
18-30	Nr	60-80	60-80	80-100	100-120	80-100	100-120	120-140
31-40	Nr	40-60	60-80	60-80	80-100	60-80	80-100	100-120
41-60	Nr	40-60	40-60	60-80	60-80	40-60	60-80	80-100

Volume is expressed as number of foot contacts (lower body plyometrics) or throws and catches (upper body plyometrics). Beginning plyometric training volume may be based on a variety of factors. The volumes included in this table may be modified according to individual client goals and abilities.

*Nr = not recommended (i.e., no plyometric training for a client in this situation).

If plyometric exercises are being incorporated into a workout, they should be performed before any other exercise. In order to get maximum benefits, they must be done accurately. The client will benefit only from the number of reps performed well (22, 97). Also, previously fatigued muscles and tendons can become overstressed by the high demands placed upon them during a plyometric workout if it is performed after other activities. This can lead to overtraining and injury (98).

The guidelines of mode, intensity, frequency, and volume can now be applied to the sample clients introduced in client example 17.1. See client example 17.2 for sample plyometric programs designed for these clients.

Progression

Plyometric exercise is a form of resistance training and thus must follow the principles of progressive overload—a systematic increase in training frequency, volume, and intensity through the use of various combinations. Typically, as intensity increases, volume decreases, progressing from low to moderate volume for low-intensity plyometrics and to low to moderate volumes for moderate to high intensity. Plyometric progression should take place systematically, with proper landing position as the beginning point. Once proper landing technique is established, one can advance clients by adding horizontal or vertical components. They should progress slowly and focus on form during their low-intensity plyometric program, which could include such drills as skipping, 8-inch (20 cm) cone double-leg hops, squat jumps, and split jumps (22, 98). All plyometric activities should be double leg until the client has fully adjusted to the stress of plyometric training. A client considered to be at an intermediate level, including high school clients who have been exposed to weight training, can begin moderately intense plyometric exercises such as split jumps or bounding. Once the client has matured, become proficient at moderately intense plyometric exercises, and has a strong resistance training background, high-intensity plyometrics including one-legged plyometrics, depth jumps, and exercises with external resistance and vertical or horizontal components may be incorporated into the workout regimen (22).

Warm-Up

As with any training program, the plyometric exercise session must begin with general and specific warm-ups (refer to chapter 12 for discussion of warm-up). The general warm-up may consist of light

TABLE 17.7 Plyometric Warm-Up Drills

Dynamic warm-up drill	Description
Lunging	■ Performed to improve the client's readiness to move into a variety of positions ■ May be performed in a variety of directions (e.g., forward, diagonal, backward)
Toe jogging	Jogging while not allowing the heels to touch the ground
Straight-leg jogging	Jogging while maintaining an extended (or nearly extended) knee
Butt kicker	Jogging and allowing the heel to touch the buttocks through knee flexion
Skipping	Exaggerated mode of reciprocal upper and lower body movements
Footwork	A variety of drills that require changes in direction (e.g., shuffling, sliding, carioca, backward running)

jogging or using a stationary bicycle at low intensity, while a specific warm-up for plyometric training should consist of low-intensity, dynamic movements similar in style to those performed during plyometric exercises. Refer to table 17.7 for a description of dynamic warm-up drills that are generally appropriate for most clients.

> Plyometric programs must include the many elements essential to effective training program design. Following a needs analysis, the variables to be included in the program design are mode, intensity, frequency, recovery, volume, program length, progression, and warm-up.

Starting Levels for Plyometric Exercises

If the client is deemed ready for plyometric exercises, several tests can be performed to help determine the level at which the client should complete vertical jumps, depth jumps, box jumps, and the medicine ball toss (97, 98).

A vertical jump is performed with the client standing next to a wall with both feet flat on the ground. The client fully reaches and touches the wall, the point that will be used as the baseline measurement. The client should jump off both feet and touch the wall at the highest point of the jump. The distance between the initial reach mark and the mark made at the highest point of the jump is the client's vertical jump height. The client should perform five trials,

Client Example 17.2

Sample Plyometric Programs for Client Examples

Client	Mode	Intensity*	Frequency (sessions per week)*	Volume*	Activity-specific drills**
Sport client A	Lower body	Medium	2	100 contacts	Double-leg tuck jump Standing long jump Double-leg vertical jump Double-leg hop Jump to box Jump from box
Sport client B	Lower and upper body	Low	1	60 contacts 20 throws for UB	Standing long jump Double-leg hop Skip Jump to box Chest pass
Work client A	Lower and upper body	Medium-high	2	100 contacts for LB 20 throws for UB	Split squat jump Standing long jump Double-leg vertical jump Single-leg jump Jump to box Chest pass Depth push-up
Work client B	Though this client would benefit from plyometrics eventually, because she has not previously participated in a resistance training program she must begin there and can progress to plyometric training after three months.				
Injury prevention client A	Lower body	Low	1	40 contacts	Split squat jump Double-leg vertical jump Skip
Injury prevention client B	Lower and upper body	Low to medium	1	40 contacts	Split squat jump Standing long jump Single-leg jump Lateral bound

LB: lower body; UB: upper body.

*The values for these variables represent beginning levels; each will be advanced according to client tolerance and performance. (See client example 17.1 for descriptions of these clients.)

**The drills provided for each client are examples of exercises that are appropriate based on the client's background, goals, and experience. The client is not expected to include all of the listed drills in the program.

---

taking the best three jumps (97, 98). The result will be used in evaluating the height of the box used for the depth jump.

To perform a depth jump, the client steps off boxes of varying heights onto a firm or grass surface. Clients should begin with a 12-inch (30 cm) box. After stepping off the box and landing, the client immediately jumps up in an attempt to reach or surpass the mark placed on the wall during the vertical jump test. The height of the box should increase by 6 inches (15 cm) until the client can no longer jump to the vertical jump height. Rest between each jump should be about 1 to 2 minutes. The box height at which the max vertical jump height was attained is

the height the client should train at for this exercise. If a client cannot reach the vertical jump height from the 12-inch box, either the height of the box should be decreased or the client should avoid depth jumps until he or she gets strong enough (22, 97, 98).

The personal trainer can use a box jump test to determine the maximum height of the box for box jump plyometric training. The client stands flat-footed directly in front of a box, about arm's length away. The client jumps up on the box and lands cleanly and softly. After each successful attempt, the box height may be increased until the client finds it very difficult to jump up on it. The greatest height at which the client can land successfully should be the height the client trains box jumps at. Mats should be placed around the box and trained spotters should be present to catch the client in an unsuccessful attempt (97).

To determine the weight of the medicine ball to use for chest passes, the personal trainer should have the client sit in a straight-back chair strapped in with a belt. The client performs a chest pass with a weighted medicine ball with as much force as possible. If the ball travels more than 12 feet (3.7 m), the client should try again with a heavier ball. If the ball travels less than 10 feet (3 m), the client should use a lighter medicine ball for medicine ball chest passes (97).

Speed Training Mechanics and Physiology

Most sports depend on the speed of execution; for example, whether a client is a sprinter, cross country runner, or swimmer, success depends on the ability to perform a given task in the shortest time possible. Speed training has been classically considered a modality used to improve sport function. Indeed, many of the concepts discussed in the paragraphs that follow are difficult to incorporate into personal training programs for those uninvolved in sport. For example, the appropriateness of training to improve speed in soccer and base running in baseball should seem obvious. Training to improve speed in a work setting is more challenging to envision and difficult to defend as an appropriate exercise mode for the personal trainer to choose. The paragraphs that follow, then, use primarily athletic settings and situations as examples. Some nonsporting applications, however, are provided as appropriate.

Speed Training Definitions

The basis of speed training, accomplished in a variety of ways, is the application of maximal force in a minimal amount of time. This simply means that if clients are to move more quickly, they must *explode* when their feet are on the ground. **Speed-strength** is this application of maximum force at high velocities (109, 110). People improve speed-strength in essentially the same way they improve muscular power production, by performing rapid movements both with and without resistance. Examples include weightlifting-type movements (e.g., power clean, hang clean, snatch) and plyometric exercise; each of these exercise modes is performed quickly to potentiate muscle force through the release of stored elastic energy and the stretch reflex. Therefore, to improve speed-strength, the exercise prescription should rely on powerful exercises and avoid those requiring slow movement (105).

Speed-endurance is the ability to maintain running speed over an *extended duration* (typically longer than 6 seconds) (37). The development of speed-endurance helps prevent a client from slowing down during a maximal-speed effort. Consider a soccer player caught from behind on a breakaway or a police officer on foot who is unable to keep up with a fleeing suspect. Each of these illustrates poor speed-endurance; that is, each person either slowed down or was unable to accelerate due to fatigue.

Sprinting Technique

Technique evaluation is an important tool to use when assessing movement efficiency and, ultimately, in training to improve speed. The basic techniques of running are presented in chapter 14; running for speed, or sprinting, though similar, is a considerably different form of training. Like running, sprinting is a somewhat natural activity, though it may be performed in a variety of ways. Because of this relative normalcy, technique training should initially focus on optimizing form and correcting faults (24); developing completely new movement patterns is typically unnecessary. The form and faults that characteristically need correction center on posture and action of the legs and arms. Maximizing sprinting speed, therefore, depends on a combination of optimal body posture, leg action, and arm action (figure 17.3, *a* and *b*) (35, 51, 61, 74, 92, 103).

Posture

During the acceleration phase, the body should lean forward approximately 45° for 13 to 16 yards (12 to 15 m). When one is looking at a client who is accelerating, the angle between the lower leg and the foot will be much greater than when he or she is running at maximum speed. After the 13 to 16 yards of acceleration, the client should quickly move upright to a less than 5° lean during maximal speed (with the lean coming from the ground up, not the waist up). With the body maintained in a relaxed, upright position, the head, torso, and legs should be aligned at all times. Although commonly viewed as a controlled fall (13), sprinting may be more accurately described as a series of "ballistic strides where the body is repeatedly launched forward as a projectile" (95). The head should be relaxed and show minimal movement, and eyes should be focused straight ahead.

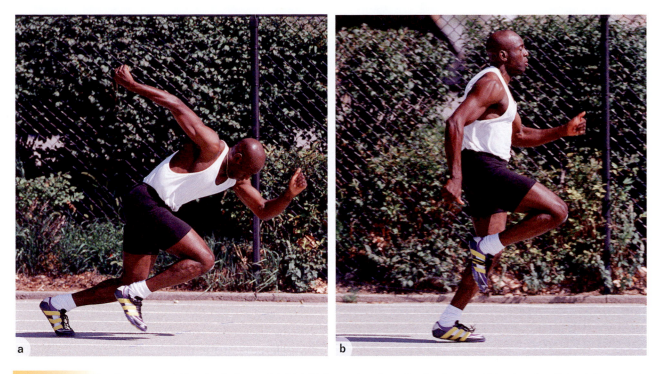

FIGURE 17.3 Proper sprinting technique. *(a)* At initial acceleration, the body should be leaning forward approximately 45°, and *(b)* should then quickly move upright to a less than 5° lean.

Leg Action

Two main phases of the sprint technique are outlined in the literature: the driving phase and the recovery phase (28). During the driving phase, or support phase, the lead foot, driven by the hip extensors (gluteals), lands on the lateral aspect of the forefoot, just in front of the client's center of gravity. At foot strike, the quadriceps muscles must contract to prevent excessive knee flexion resulting in the loss of elastic energy. The ankle should remain dorsiflexed and the great toe extended. The gluteals and hamstrings should then contract so the client pulls himself over the body's center of mass. The client should begin plantarflexing the foot once the hip crosses over the foot until the completion of toe-off. Ground contact time should be minimal while allowing explosive leg movement.

The recovery phase begins the moment the client's foot completely leaves the ground. As soon as the client enters the recovery phase of the sprint, he or she must immediately dorsiflex the ankle and extend the great toe. This places the leg in proper position so that, upon contact with the ground, the ground can push back against the body. The client can then utilize the ground's reactive force to propel forward. Leaving the foot on the ground too long causes the foot to absorb too much of the ground's force that would otherwise be used to help the client move more efficiently and effec-

tively (91). He or she must also flex the knee, driving the foot directly toward the buttocks. This helps to shorten the lever, which allows the leg to swing forward more quickly (28, 91). As the heel moves toward the buttocks, the leg swings forward as if the client is attempting to step over the opposite knee. The knee then extends to an approximately 90° position and then becomes nearly straight as the foot moves down and forward, driven toward the ground by the hip extensors. Increasing sprinting speed should increase the height the foot moves toward the buttocks (the heel kick).

Running heel-to-toe instead of landing on the lateral aspect of the forefoot is a common error. This causes balance issues as well as improper absorption of ground forces by the lower extremity structures, leading to hamstring injuries over time (28). Also, clients lacking good flexibility may have trouble bringing the heel toward the buttocks.

Arm Action

Remaining relaxed, each elbow should be flexed to approximately 90° (28, 91). Movement must be an aggressive front-to-back action originating from the shoulder with minimal frontal plane motion. The arm movement must be an aggressive backward hammering or punching motion and occur opposite to the leg motion in order to assist in balance and provide momentum for the legs (28, 91).

Also, if the client is aggressive with driving the arms back, the stretch reflex at the shoulder will activate and automatically force the arms forward. Hands should rise to shoulder level during anterior arm swing and should pass the buttocks when moving posteriorly.

Common errors for arm swing include (a) locking the upper arm into place and moving only the lower arm rather than having the action created at the shoulder, (b) allowing the arm to cross the midline of the body, (c) improper arm swing distance, and (d) emphasizing a forward motion of the arm swing rather than a backward motion (28, 91). If a client allows the arm to cross the body's midline, upper body rotation will occur, slowing him or her down. As for the arm swing distance, clients tend to either bring the hand past the shoulders or not bring the hand back far enough, stopping short of their hips.

Acceleration

In general, it will take the client approximately 13 to 16 yards (12 to 15 m) of acceleration to achieve the proper technique (27). During these first yards, the client focuses on increasing both velocity and stride length. Initially, foot strike will occur behind the body, rather than in front of the center of gravity, but this changes quickly over the 13 to 16 yards. Also, the client will have increased body lean and be focused more on the driving phase and less on the recovery phase of the sprint technique (27, 28). This increased body lean positions the client so he or she can place stronger emphasis on front-side running mechanics (i.e., high knee punch, dorsiflexion) and minimal emphasis on backside mechanics (i.e., plantarflexion, heel-to-hip contact).

> During a sprint, support time should be kept brief while braking forces at ground contact are minimized and the backward velocity of the lower leg and foot at touchdown is maximized. Maximizing sprinting speed depends on a combination of optimal body posture, leg action, and arm action.

Speed Training Program Design

As with plyometric exercise prescription, research on program design for speed training is sparse and therefore practical experience must be the guide. Speed training exercise prescription uses typical program design variables to provide a safe and effective plan to improve a client's speed.

Mode

The *mode* of speed training is determined by the speed characteristics that the given drill is designed to improve. Speed training focuses on three areas: form, stride frequency, and stride length. Improving sprinting technique may be accomplished in a number of ways, including sprint performance, stride analysis, and specific form drills. Drills designed to improve form are provided at the end of this chapter. Since form drills are performed at a slower speed, they should not substitute for actual sprint training. Form drills are great to include in the warm-up (28).

Within an analysis of running speed, stride frequency and stride length have an intimate relationship. In general, as both the stride frequency (the number of strides performed in a given amount of time) and stride length (the distance covered in one stride) increase, running speed improves. During the start, speed is highly dependent on stride length. Stride length drills help improve the rhythm of the sprinter's stride (29). The personal trainer should first measure the client's leg length from the greater trochanter to the floor, then multiply this measurement 2.3 to 2.5 times for females and 2.5 to 2.7 times for males. This is the client's optimal stride length. For example, if a client has a leg length of 36 inches (90 cm), since 2.5 x 36 is 90 inches (230 cm), the client's optimal stride length is 90 inches. Drills should be performed anywhere from 60% to 105% of optimal stride length, but the personal trainer should mark the distances of the optimal stride length so the client has a foot placement target during the drill (29). Using the 90-inch optimal stride length example, 60% of 90 is 54 inches (137 cm), and 105% of 90 inches is 94.5 inches (240 cm). Therefore, stride length drills should use between 54 and 94.5 inches per stride.

As sprinting speed increases, frequency becomes the more important variable (79, 88, 89, 104, 119). Of the two components, stride frequency is likely the more trainable, as stride length is highly dependent on body height and leg length (79, 81). Stride frequency is typically increased through the use of fast leg drills, **sprint-assisted training** (running at speeds greater than a client is able to independently achieve [31]), and resisted sprinting (29). With sprint-assisted training, the supramaximal speed forces clients to take more steps than they are accustomed to taking during a typical sprint. Assuming that stride length remains the same as during normal sprinting, increasing the frequency of strides will help them run faster. Methods used to accomplish sprint-assisted training include downgrade sprinting (3-7°), high-speed towing, and use of a high-speed treadmill. Regardless of the method used, sprint-assisted training should not increase speed by more than 10% of the client's maximal speed.

Sprint-assisted training is an advanced technique that requires careful instruction and demonstration on the part of the personal trainer and clear understanding on the part of the client. Sprint-assisted training may cause clients to alter their technique, which will affect running without assistance. Further, a proper warm-up to each session should be considered mandatory.

Resisted sprinting is used to help a client increase stride length, as well as speed-strength, by increasing the client's ground force production during the support phase (32, 35, 40, 51, 56, 61, 67, 71, 100), which is arguably the most important determinant of speed (105). Again, while maintaining proper form, clients may use uphill sprinting; running in sand or in water; or sprinting while being resisted by a sled, elastic tubing, a partner, or a parachute (29, 31, 80). Resisted sprinting is used especially to improve the acceleration of the sprint (32). Resisted towing and uphill running are two exercises that work well to improve the acceleration of the sprint as they increase trunk lean, stance duration, and horizontal force production during the propulsive phase of the stance (32, 53). Resisted sprinting should not increase external resistance by more than 10% (95). The personal trainer should use heavier resistance when the goal is to improve the acceleration phase and lighter resistance when the goal is to improve maximum velocity (32). Too much external resistance may alter running mechanics (i.e., increase ground contact time, decrease stride length, or decrease hip extension), thereby compromising performance outcomes (29). Another measure for gauging the amount of resistance is to use an external load that is equal to or less than 15% of the client's body mass. Again, another way to gauge the resistance level is to look at performance. If performance decreases by more than 10%, the load being used is too heavy and will have detrimental effects on sprinting technique. Resisted sprinting should be performed over relatively short distances, anywhere from 11 to 33 yards (10 to 30 m) (85).

As with most other speed training techniques, resisted sprinting targets clients wanting to improve speed-strength. Adding resistance to a nonathletic client's gait, however, may also improve function. For example, attaching elastic tubing to provide resistance to a 70-year-old client during walking may improve his or her ability to walk up hills or may

increase confidence during walking, thereby reducing the risk of injury from a possible fall. Providing resistance to a construction worker by having the individual push a weighted implement or sled may improve his or her ability to push a wheelbarrow filled with cement.

Although nearly all clients may perform form drills, sprint-assisted and -resisted training may be too advanced for some. A more general mode of speed training that most clients can easily perform is interval sprinting. The client sprints (or runs or walks, depending on abilities) as fast as possible over a given distance or for a predetermined amount of time, then rests. Following the rest period, the client repeats the bout. In performing interval training, clients are able to maintain higher-intensity work periods (i.e., sprint/run/walk) by interspersing them with times of rest (45).

Intensity

Speed training *intensity* refers to the physical effort required during execution of a given drill, and is controlled both by the type of drill performed and by the distance covered. The intensity of speed training ranges from low-level form drills to sprint-assisted and -resisted sprinting drills that apply significant stress to the body. Sprinting should be performed at close to maximum speed to ensure proper sprinting mechanics, stride length, and stride frequency (29). Distance is determined according to the goals of the client. Training acceleration requires covering short distances, whereas training maximum velocity requires covering longer distances (29).

Frequency

Frequency, the number of speed training sessions per week, depends on the client's goals. As with other program variables, research is limited on the optimal frequency for speed training sessions; again, personal trainers must rely on practical experience when determining the appropriate frequency. For clients who are athletes participating in a sport, two to four speed sessions per week is common; nonathletic clients may benefit from one or two speed sessions per week.

Recovery

Because speed training drills involve maximal efforts to improve speed and anaerobic power, a complete, adequate *recovery* (the time between repetitions and sets) is required to ensure maximal effort with each repetition (84, 114). The time between repetitions is determined by a proper work-to-rest ratio (i.e., a range of 1:5 to 1:10) and is specific to the volume and type of drill. That is, the higher the intensity of a drill, the more rest a client requires. Recovery for form training may be minimal, whereas rest between repetitions of downgrade running may last 2 to 3 minutes. Although near-full recovery is optimal for ensuring maximum effort with each repetition, having clients work on speed drills when they are less than 100% recovered may actually be beneficial as well, because it may be more specific to the type of tasks they will have to accomplish. However, consistently training for speed in a fatigued state will not yield optimal results (113). In fact, consistently training in a fatigued state may slow the client down, as this is teaching the client's body to run at slower speeds. It also interferes with body coordination, which results in training poor speed technique (28, 29). Recovery from sessions should last 24 to 48 hours depending on the intensity of the previous sprint training session.

Volume

Speed training *volume* typically refers to the number of repetitions and sets performed during a session and is normally expressed as the distance covered. For example, a client beginning a speed training program may start with a 33-yard (30 m) sprint but advance to 109 yards (100 m) per repetition for the same drill. As with intensity, speed training volume should vary according to the client's goals.

Progression

Speed training must follow the principles of progressive overload—a systematic increase in training frequency, volume, and intensity through various combinations. Typically, as intensity increases, volume decreases. The program's intensity should progress from

1. low to high volume of low-intensity speed drills (e.g., stationary arm swing) to
2. low to high volumes of moderate intensity (e.g., front barrier hop) to
3. low to high volumes of moderate to high intensity (e.g., downhill sprinting).

Warm-Up

As with any training program, the speed training session must begin with both general and specific warm-ups (refer to chapter 12 for a discussion of warm-up). The specific warm-up for speed training should consist of low-intensity, dynamic movements. Once mastered, many of the form drills provided at the end of this chapter may be incorporated into warm-up drills.

Speed Training Safety Considerations

While not inherently dangerous, speed training—like all modes of exercise—places the client at risk of injury. Injuries during speed training commonly occur because of insufficient strength or flexibility, inadequate instruction or supervision, or an inappropriate training environment.

Pretraining Evaluation

To reduce the risk of injury during participation in a speed training program, the client must understand proper technique and possess a sufficient base of strength and flexibility. In addition, the client must be sufficiently prepared to participate in a speed training program. The following evaluative elements will help determine whether a client meets these conditions.

Physical Characteristics

As with other forms of exercise, it is necessary to examine and review joint structure, posture, body type, and previous injuries before a client begins a speed training program. Previous injuries or abnormalities of the spine, lower extremities, and upper extremities may increase a client's risk of injury during participation in a speed training program. An area of concern is hamstring flexibility and strength; as the swing leg—the leg not on the training surface—transitions from an eccentric muscle action to concentric, the hamstring must be prepared to undergo extreme amounts of stretch (during the eccentric phase of the movement) followed by nearly instantaneous concentric muscle action. If this muscle is not prepared (through both strength and flexibility training), injury becomes likely.

Technique and Supervision

When a client will be performing speed training drills, it is essential that the personal trainer demonstrate and monitor proper movement patterns and sprint technique—as previously described—to maximize the drill's effectiveness and to minimize the risk of injury. Proper technique will ensure efficient and faster running, whereas poor technique will not only slow the client down, but also predispose him or her to injuries due to overloading of tissues (28). Posture and proper arm and leg actions are especially important characteristics for the personal trainer to watch. Should the client not demonstrate correct technique, intensity must be lowered to allow successful completion of each drill. Common technique errors are listed for each drill at the end of this chapter.

Exercise Surface and Footwear

In addition to proper participant fitness, health, and technique, the area where the client performs speed training drills may significantly affect safety. To prevent injuries, the landing surface used for speed training drills must possess adequate shock-absorbing properties, but must not be so absorbent as to significantly increase the transition between the eccentric and concentric phases of the SSC. Grass fields, suspended floors, and rubber mats are good surface choices (60). Avoid excessively thick exercise mats (6 inches [15 cm] or more) because they may lengthen the amortization phase, thus not allowing efficient use of the stretch reflex. In addition, footwear with good ankle and arch support and a wide, nonslip sole is required (84, 114).

Combining Plyometrics and Speed Training With Other Forms of Exercise

Plyometrics and speed training are just parts of a client's overall training program. Many sports and activities use multiple energy systems or require other forms of exercise to properly prepare athletes for their competitions or to help them reach their goals. A well-designed training program must address each energy system and training need.

Resistance, Plyometric, and Speed Training

Combining plyometric and speed training with resistance training requires careful consideration to optimize recovery while maximizing performance. The following list and table 17.8 provide appropriate guidelines for developing a program that com-

bines these different, but complementary, modes of training:

- In general, clients should perform *either* lower body plyometric training, speed training, *or* lower body resistance training on a given day, but not more than one of these types of training on the same day.

- It is appropriate to combine lower body resistance training with upper body plyometrics, and upper body resistance training with lower body plyometrics.

- Performing heavy resistance training and plyometrics on the same day is not usually recommended (17, 56). However, some athletes may benefit from **complex training**—a combination of resistance and plyometric training—by performing plyometrics followed by high-intensity resistance training. If an individual is engaging in this type of training, adequate recovery between the plyometrics and other high-intensity lower body training, including speed training, is essential.

- Traditional resistance training exercises may be combined with plyometric movements to further enhance gains in muscular power (117, 118). For example, performing a squat jump with approximately 30% of one's 1RM squat as an external resistance further increases performance (117, 118). This is an advanced form of complex training that should be performed only by clients with previous participation in high-intensity plyometric training programs.

Plyometric and Aerobic Exercise

Many sports and activities require both a power and an aerobic component. It is necessary to combine multiple types of training to best prepare clients for these types of sports. Because aerobic exercise may have a negative effect on power production during

TABLE 17.8 Sample Schedule for Resistance, Plyometric, and Speed Training

Day	Resistance training	Plyometric training	Speed training
Monday	Upper body	Lower body	Rest
Tuesday	Lower body	Upper body	Rest
Wednesday	Rest	Rest	Technique and sprint-assisted drills
Thursday	Upper body	Lower body	Rest
Friday	Lower body	Upper body	Rest
Saturday	Rest	Rest	Technique and sprint-resisted drills
Sunday	Rest	Rest	Rest

a given training session (17), it is advisable to perform plyometric exercise prior to the longer, aerobic endurance–type training. The design variables do not change and should complement each other to most effectively train the athlete for competition or help a client meet his or her goals. Recent studies actually indicate that plyometrics may improve long-distance running performance and decrease incidence of injury (30, 106, 115); therefore adding low-intensity bounding-type drills to non-running days may improve long-distance running performance.

> Plyometric exercise should be incorporated into an overall training program, including both strength and aerobic exercise. Speed training may be combined with plyometric and resistance training, but this requires careful planning to optimize recovery while maximizing performance.

Conclusion

The ability to apply force quickly and provide an overload to the agonist muscles is the major goal of plyometric training, a benefit to most sporting activities and many occupations. Further, because the ability to move rapidly is needed in sport, speed training may be another important component to include for clients active in competitive and recreational sports. Necessary during performance of each of these forms of exercise is the proper application of force to the ground in a minimal amount of time. If the force used is insufficient or takes too long to generate, the ability to effectively accelerate, change direction, or overtake an opponent is lost.

In addition to improving the potential to succeed in sport, speed and especially plyometric training may improve function on the job or may reduce the risk of injury. Many occupations require employees to lift or move large objects, move quickly, or otherwise perform explosive movements. Using the plyometric and speed training principles outlined is an ideal method of improving the speed-strength quality important to so many activities. In addition, the ability to decelerate efficiently and under control is indispensable to any attempt to reduce a client's risk of injury. Proper performance of plyometric drills helps clients learn how to decelerate when landing from a jump or when changing directions. Plyometric training and speed training should not be considered ends in themselves, but as parts of an overall program (in addition to resistance, flexibility, and aerobic endurance training and proper nutrition). Clients possessing adequate levels of strength perform plyometric and speed training drills more successfully. Further, combining these modes of exercise with others allows clients to optimize performance, regardless of sport or activity requirements.

Plyometric and Speed Drills

Lower Body Plyometric Drills

Ankle Flip

Intensity level: Low

Direction of jump: Vertical

Beginning position: Stand, feet shoulder-width apart. Body should be upright.

Arm action: Double arm

Preparatory movement: None

Upward movement: Pushing off using only ankles, hop up in place, plantarflexing ankles fully with each jump.

Downward movement: Land in starting position. Repeat the motion.

Common Errors

- Adding a countermovement
- Not fully plantarflexing ankles
- Landing and jumping asynchronously

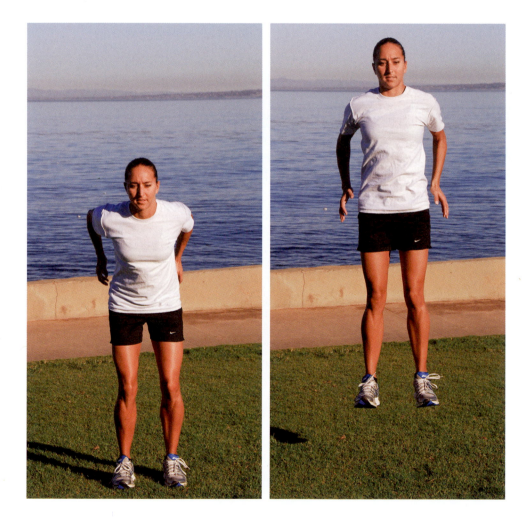

Skip

Intensity level: Low

Direction of jump: Horizontal and vertical

Beginning position: One leg is lifted to 90° of hip and knee flexion.

Arm action: Reciprocal (as one leg is lifted, the opposite arm is lifted)

Preparatory movement: Begin with a countermovement.

Upward movement: Jump up and forward on one leg. The opposite leg should remain in the starting position until landing. Drive toes of lead leg up, knee forward and up, and keep heel under hips.

Downward movement: Land in the starting position with the same leg. Repeat the motion with the opposite leg.

Advanced variation: This drill may also be performed backward. Jump up and backward on one leg. Land in the starting position with the same leg. Repeat the motion with the opposite leg.

Common Error

- Incoordination, that is, difficulty coordinating the transition from one leg to the other

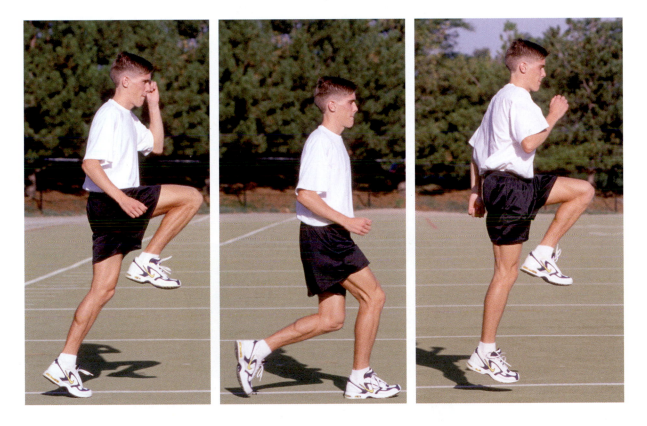

Standing Long Jump

Intensity level: Low

Direction of jump: Horizontal

Beginning position: Half squat position with feet shoulder-width apart

Arm action: Double arm

Preparatory movement: Begin with a countermovement.

Upward movement: Explosively jump forward as far as possible with both feet. Use the arms to assist with the jump.

Downward movement: Land in the starting position and repeat jump. Allow complete rest between repetitions.

Advanced variation: Progress to multiple jumps without a pause between jumps. Immediately, upon landing, jump forward again. Keep landing time short. Use quick double-arm swings when performing repetitions. This changes the intensity to medium.

Common Error

- Clients jump and land asynchronously; that is, feet neither leave nor contact the floor or ground at the same time.

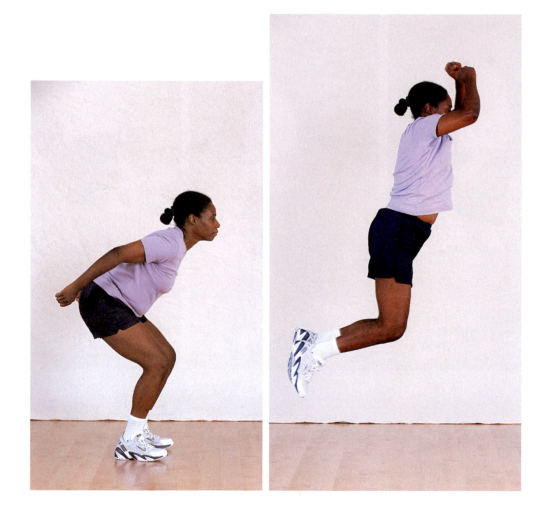

Double-Leg Vertical Jump

Intensity level: Low

Direction of jump: Vertical

Beginning position: Assume a comfortable upright stance with feet shoulder-width apart.

Arm action: Double arm

Preparatory movement: Begin with a countermovement.

Upward movement: Explosively jump up with both legs, using both arms to assist and reach for a target.

Downward movement: Land in the starting position and repeat the jump. Allow complete recovery between jumps.

Advanced variation: Increase the intensity of the double-leg vertical jump by performing the jump without a rest between jumps. Immediately upon landing, begin the jump again. Ground contact time between jumps should be minimal. This changes the intensity to medium. One can further progress the jump using one leg only. This changes the drill's intensity to high.

Common Errors

- Clients do not jump and land in the same place.
- Countermovement is too deep.
- Countermovement is too shallow.

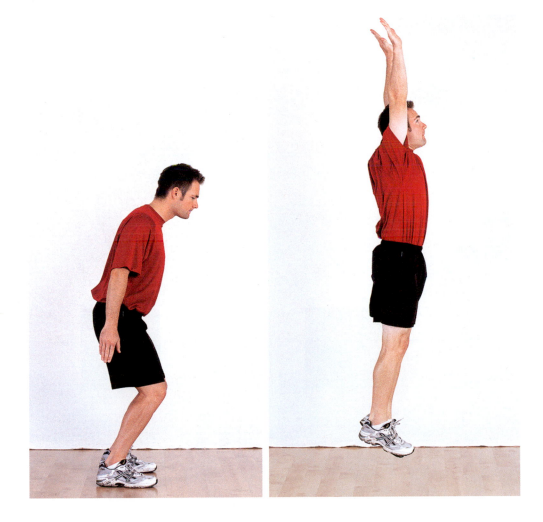

Jump to Box

Intensity level: Low

Equipment: Plyometric box, 6 to 42 inches (15 to 107 cm) high

Direction of jump: Vertical and slightly horizontal

Beginning position: Facing the plyometric box, assume a comfortable upright stance with feet shoulder-width apart.

Arm action: Double arm

Preparatory movement: Begin with a countermovement.

Upward movement: Jump onto the top of the box using both feet.

Downward movement: Land on both feet in a semi-squat position; step down from the box and repeat.

Advanced variation: Increase the intensity of this jump by clasping the hands behind the head or increasing the box height.

Common Errors

- Knees and feet separate in an effort to clear the barrier.
- Countermovement is too deep.
- Box is too tall for client's height or abilities.

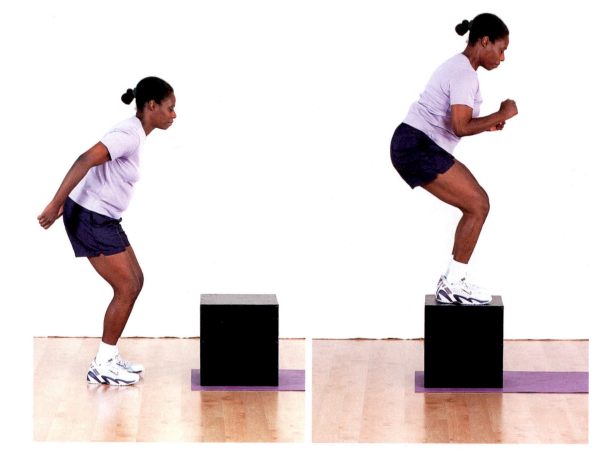

Double-Leg Hop

Intensity level: Medium

Direction of jump: Horizontal

Beginning position: Assume a comfortable upright stance with feet shoulder-width apart, knees slightly bent and arms at side.

Arm action: Double arm

Preparatory movement: Begin with a quick countermovement.

Upward movement: Extend hips, and tuck toes, knees, and heels as soon as vertical height is achieved. Jump forward. Immediately upon landing, repeat the hop forward. Ground contact time between jumps should be minimal.

Downward movement: Land in the beginning position with hips and knees slightly flexed.

Advanced variation: Progress to perform the hop with one leg only. This changes the drill's intensity from medium to high.

Common Errors

- Amortization phase (i.e., time on the floor or ground) between hops is too long.
- Proper posture is not maintained.
- Hopping too far forward so quickness of jumps is compromised.

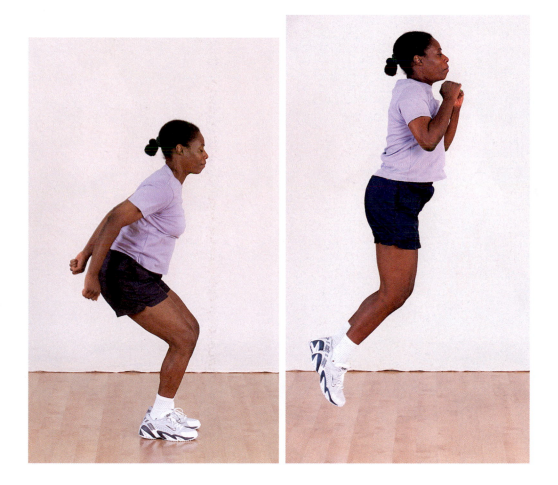

Alternate-Leg Bound—Double Arm

Intensity level: Medium

Direction of jump: Horizontal and vertical

Beginning position: Assume a comfortable upright stance with feet shoulder-width apart.

Arm action: Double arm

Preparatory movement: Jog at a comfortable pace; begin the drill with the left foot forward.

Upward movement: Push off with the left foot as it contacts the ground. During push-off, bring the right leg forward by flexing the thigh to a position parallel with the ground and the knee at 90°. During this flight phase of the drill, reach forward with both arms.

Downward movement: Land on the right leg and *immediately* repeat the sequence with the opposite leg upon landing.

Note: A bound is an exaggeration of the running gait; the goal is to cover as great a distance as possible during each stride.

Alternate variation: Instead of reaching forward with both arms during the flight phase, reach with a single arm while the opposite leg is in the flight phase.

Common Error

- Clients do not have appropriate balance between the horizontal and vertical components of the bound.

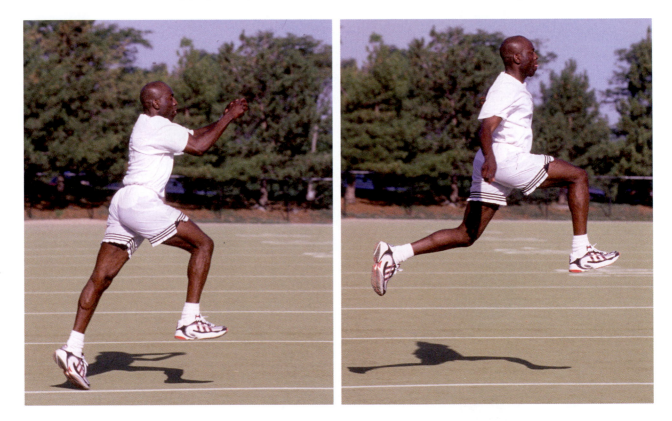

442

Split Squat Jump

Intensity level: Medium

Direction of jump: Vertical

Beginning position: Lunge position with one leg forward (hip and knee joints in approximately 90° of flexion with knee directly over foot) and the other behind the midline of the body

Arm action: Double or none

Preparatory movement: Begin with a countermovement.

Upward movement: Explosively jump up, using the arms to assist as needed. Maximum height and power should be emphasized.

Downward movement: When landing, maintain the lunge position (same leg forward) and *immediately* repeat the jump.

Note: After completing a set, rest and switch front legs.

Advanced variation: While off the ground, switch the position of the legs so the front leg is in the back and the back leg is in the front. When landing, maintain the lunge position (opposite leg forward) and immediately repeat the jump.

Common Errors

- The lunge position is too shallow.
- Amortization phase (i.e., time on the floor or ground) is too long.
- Clients do not jump and land in the same place; lateral and anterior or posterior movement are excessive.
- Shoulders do not remain back and in line with the hips, leading to decreased stability.

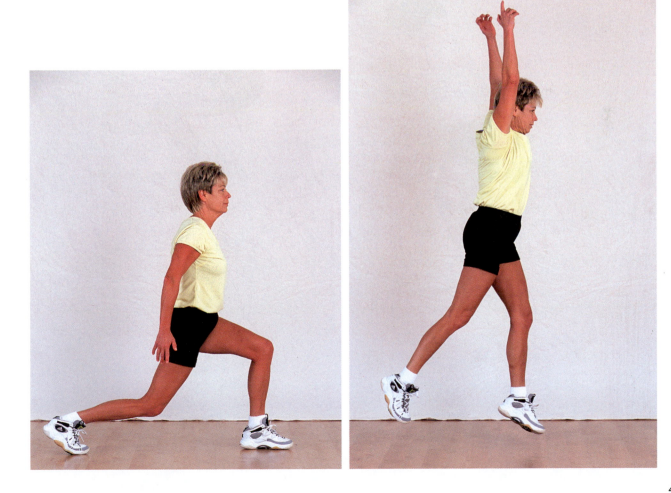

Double-Leg Tuck Jump

Intensity level: Medium

Direction of jump: Vertical

Beginning position: Assume a comfortable upright stance with feet shoulder-width apart, knees slightly bent, chest out, and shoulders back. Hands should be at chest height with palms facing down.

Arm action: Double arm

Preparatory movement: Begin with a quick countermovement.

Upward movement: Explosively jump up, driving knees to chest. Pull the knees to the chest and quickly grasp the knees with both hands and release before landing.

Downward movement: Land in the starting position and *immediately* repeat the jump. Ground contact time between jumps should be minimal.

Advanced variation: Progress from single jumps to multiple jumps with pauses in between each jump to multiple jumps without a pause in between jumps to jumps with one leg only (high intensity).

Common Errors

- Amortization phase (i.e., time on the floor) is too long.
- Clients do not jump and land in the same place; there is excessive lateral and anterior or posterior movement.

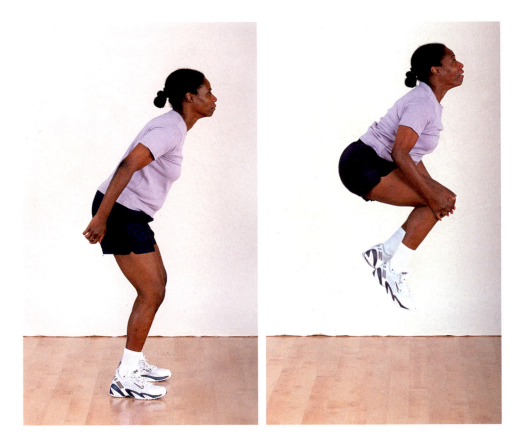

Front Barrier Hop

Intensity level: Medium

Direction of jump: Horizontal and vertical

Beginning position: Assume a comfortable upright stance facing a barrier, with feet shoulder-width apart.

Arm action: Double arm

Preparatory movement: Begin with a countermovement.

Upward movement: Jump over a barrier with both legs, using primarily hip and knee flexion to clear the barrier. Keep the knees and feet together without lateral deviation.

Downward movement: Land in the starting position and *immediately* repeat the jump over the next barrier.

Alternate variation: This drill may also be performed laterally. Stand to either side of the barrier; jump over the barrier with both legs. Land in the starting position and immediately repeat the jump to the starting side.

Advanced variation: To increase the intensity of barrier hops, progressively increase the height of the barrier (e.g., from a cone to a hurdle) or perform the hops with one leg only. This changes the drill's intensity from medium to high.

Common Errors

- Amortization phase (i.e., time on the floor) between hops is too long.
- Knees and feet separate in an effort to clear the barrier.

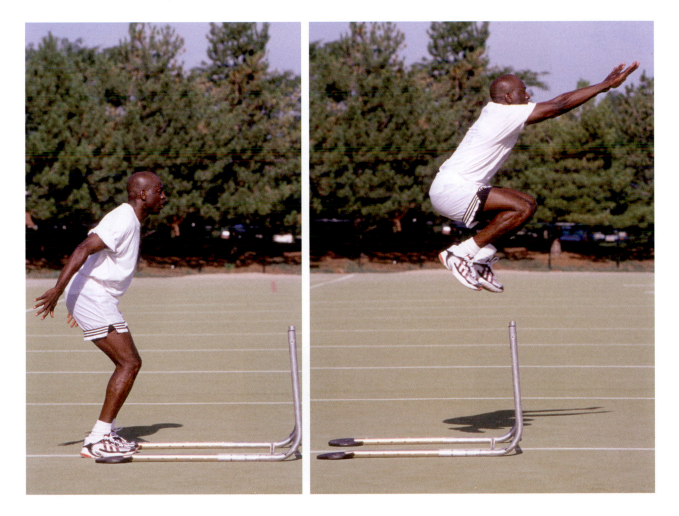

Jump From Box

Intensity level: Medium

Equipment: Plyometric box, 12 to 42 inches (30 to 107 cm) high

Direction of jump: Vertical

Beginning position: Assume a comfortable upright stance with feet shoulder-width apart on the box.

Arm action: None

Preparatory movement: Step from box.

Downward movement: Land on the floor with both feet quickly absorbing the impact upon touchdown. The lateral aspect of the midfoot should hit first; then quickly roll onto the medial edge of the forefoot. Step back onto box and repeat.

Common Errors

- Clients land asynchronously; that is, feet do not contact the floor or ground at the same time.
- Box is too tall for client's height or abilities.

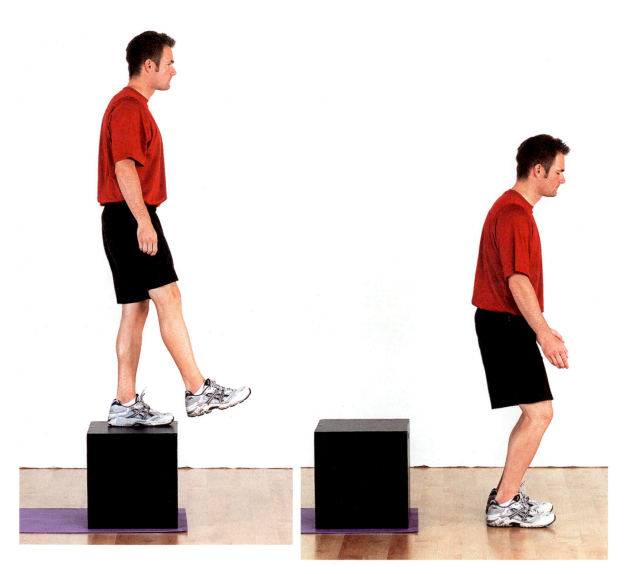

Depth Jump

Intensity level: High

Equipment: Plyometric box, 12 to 42 inches (30 to 107 cm) high

Direction of jump: Vertical

Beginning position: Assume a comfortable upright stance with feet shoulder-width apart on the box; toes should be near the edge of the box.

Arm action: Double arm

Preparatory movement: Step from box.

Downward movement: Land on the floor with both feet.

Upward movement: Upon landing, *immediately* jump up as high as possible.

Note: Time on the ground should be kept to a minimum.

Note: Vary the intensity by increasing the height of the box. Begin with height of 12 inches (30 cm).

Common Errors

- Amortization phase (i.e., time on the floor) is too long.
- Clients do not jump and land in the same place; there is excessive lateral and anterior–posterior movement after landing.
- Box is too tall for client's height or abilities.

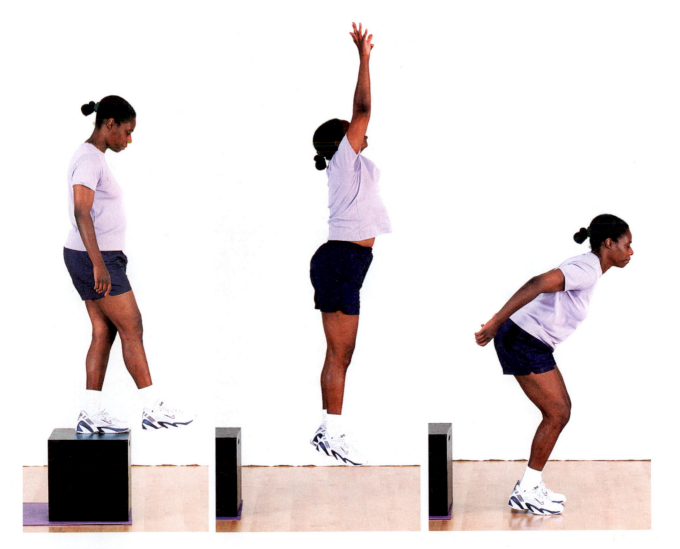

Lateral Bounding

Intensity level: High

Direction of jump: Lateral

Beginning position: Stand on one leg.

Arm action: Double arm

Upward movement: Begin by driving the non-stance leg and upper extremities in the direction of the jump (toward the non-stance leg). Then, push off the stance leg and jump laterally as far as possible to the side of the non-stance leg.

Downward movement: Land on ground on opposite foot from starting leg. Immediately upon landing, jump back in the opposite direction to starting leg. Repeat, with minimal rest time between bounds.

Common Errors

- Amortization phase (i.e., time on the floor) too long
- Jumping outside the lateral plane motion
- Unbalanced landing

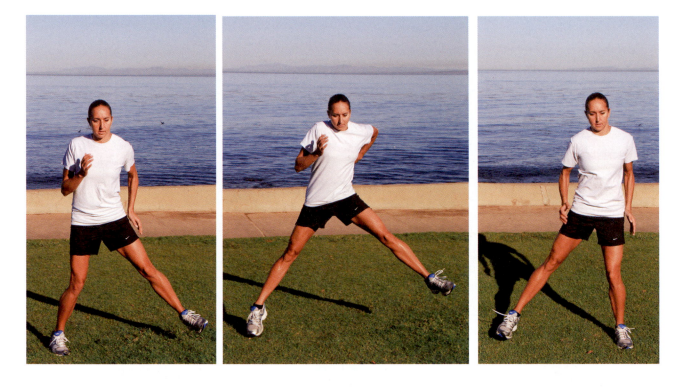

Upper Body Plyometric Drills

Chest Pass

Intensity level: Low

Equipment: Medicine or plyometric ball (weight 2-8 pounds [1-3.6 kg])

Direction of throw: Forward

Beginning position: Assume a comfortable upright stance with feet shoulder-width apart; face the personal trainer or a partner approximately 10 feet (3 m) away. Raise the ball to chest level with elbows flexed.

Preparatory movement: Begin with a countermovement. (With plyometric throws, a countermovement requires the performer to "cock" the arm(s), that is, move the arms slightly backward before the actual throw.)

Arm action: Using both arms, throw (or push) the ball to the partner by extending the elbows. When the partner returns the ball, catch it, return to the beginning position, and *immediately* repeat the movement.

Note: Increase intensity by increasing the weight of the medicine ball. Begin with a 2-pound (1 kg) ball.

Common Errors

- Amortization phase (i.e., time ball is in hands) is too long.
- Ball is too heavy.

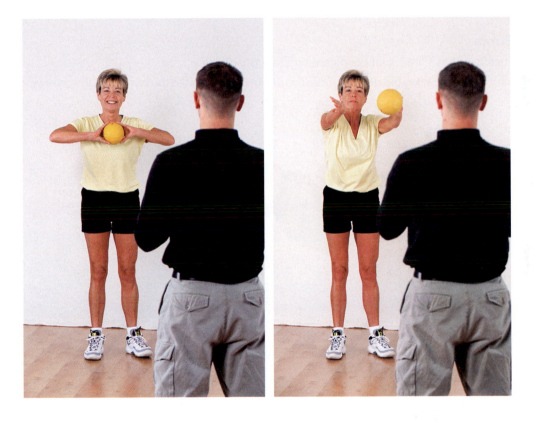

Depth Push-Up

Intensity level: Medium

Equipment: Medicine ball

Direction of movement: Vertical

Beginning position: Lie in a push-up position, with the hands on the medicine ball and elbows extended.

Preparatory movement: None

Downward movement: Quickly remove the hands from the medicine ball and drop down. Contact the ground with hands slightly more than shoulder-width apart and elbows slightly flexed. Allow the chest to almost touch the medicine ball.

Upward movement: Immediately and explosively push up by extending the elbows to full extension. Quickly place the palms on the medicine ball and repeat the exercise.

Note: When the upper body is at maximal height during the upward movement, the hands should be higher than the medicine ball.

Note: Increase intensity by increasing the size of the medicine ball. Begin with a 5-pound (2.3 kg) ball.

Advanced variation: To increase the intensity of this drill, perform it as described with the feet placed on an elevated surface (e.g., a plyometric box).

Common Errors

- Amortization phase (i.e., time hands are on the ground) is too long.
- Ball is too big, increasing the distance from the beginning position to the bottom of the downward movement.

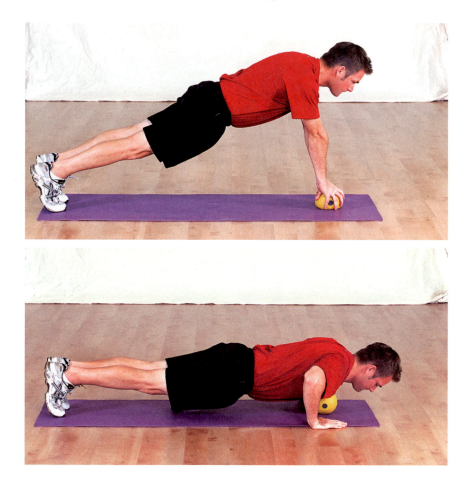

45-Degree Sit-Up

Intensity level: Medium

Equipment: Medicine or plyometric ball

Beginning position: Sit on the ground with the trunk approximately at a 45° angle to the ground. The personal trainer or partner should be in front with the medicine ball.

Preparatory movement: The partner throws the ball to outstretched hands.

Downward action: Once the partner throws the ball, catch it using both arms, allow some trunk extension, and *immediately* return the ball to the partner.

Note: Increase the intensity by increasing the weight of the medicine ball. Begin with a 2-pound (1 kg) ball.

Note: The force used to return the ball to the partner should be predominantly derived from the abdominal muscles.

Common Errors

- Eccentric phase (i.e., amount of trunk extension) is too long.
- Ball is too heavy.

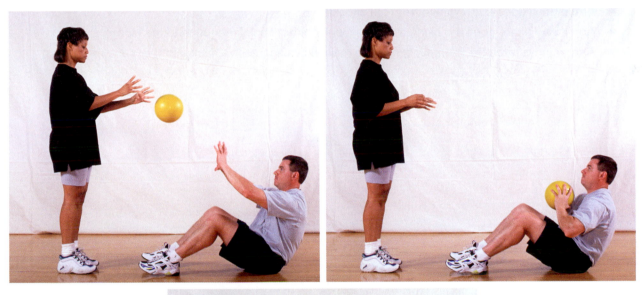

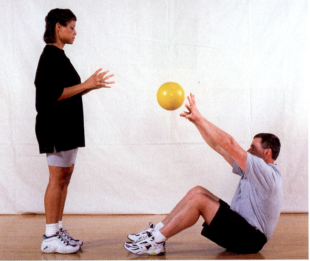

Stride Frequency Speed Drills

Stationary Arm Swing

Intensity level: Low

Equipment: None

Purpose: Teaches proper arm swing technique and upper body control.

Beginning position: Initial position is seated, progressing to kneeling, standing, walking, and finally jogging. Assume a seated position, sitting tall. Elbows should be at about 90° of flexion with right hand next to right hip and left hand in front of left shoulder.

Movement: Maintaining elbows approximately 90° and keeping hands relaxed, drive arms forward and back in a sprinting-type motion. The hands' arc of motion should be from shoulder level anteriorly to just past the hips posteriorly.

Advanced variation: Progression moves from seated to kneeling to standing to walking and finally to jogging. Each progression appropriately challenges the ability to stabilize the core and control the body, which leads to good form when jogging.

Common Errors

- Arms often cross the line of the body; arm swing should be maintained in the sagittal plane.
- Arm motion does not originate from the shoulder.
- Arm swing either goes too high past the shoulder or not back far enough to the hips.
- Arm swing is often not forceful; be sure to maintain an aggressive hammering or punching motion.

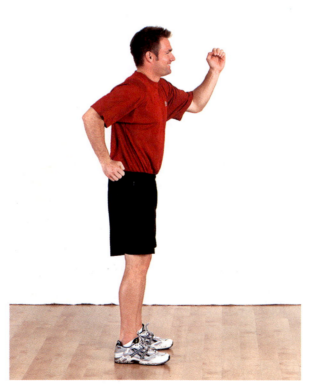

Ankling

Intensity level: Low

Equipment: None

Purpose: Teaches how to lift the feet off the ground and how to properly place them back on the ground during sprinting. Proper position of the foot will minimize the amount of time spent on the ground, minimize power lost into the ground, and minimize injuries due to the additional stress absorbed by the body with the increased ground time.

Beginning position: Start in a neutral, upright position, with feet hip-width apart. Focus on one leg at a time. Keep legs stiff.

Beginning Movement: Move forward until hips have passed over the feet. As soon as the right heel begins to lift off the ground, dorsiflex the ankle approximately 90° and extend the great toe, picking the foot up off the ground. The leg should move forward slightly (approximately one-fourth the length of the foot) with this movement initiated from the hips. As this is occurring, quickly plantarflex the right foot and make contact with the ground with the lateral forefoot and ball of the foot, pulling the body over the foot. Immediately repeat this action. Make sure the legs remain stiff throughout the drill. Focus on the movement at the ankle as well as getting the foot off the ground as quickly as possible. Repeat this dorsiflexion–plantarflexion action with just the right foot over the course of 3 feet (10 m), making as many foot contacts with the ground as possible. Steps should be no greater than one-fourth of foot length. Switch legs.

Advanced variations: (1) alternating feet while walking; (2) straight-leg bounding while ankling, focusing on one leg at a time; (3) straight-leg bounding while ankling, alternating legs; (4) running while ankling, alternating legs.

Common Errors

- Difficulty getting to 90° dorsiflexion with great toe extension and maintaining that position until foot contact
- Running on toes rather than landing on forefoot and having the foot pull body's center of gravity
- Not keeping legs stiff
- Taking steps greater than one-fourth the length of the foot
- Ball of foot spending too much time on the ground between each contact

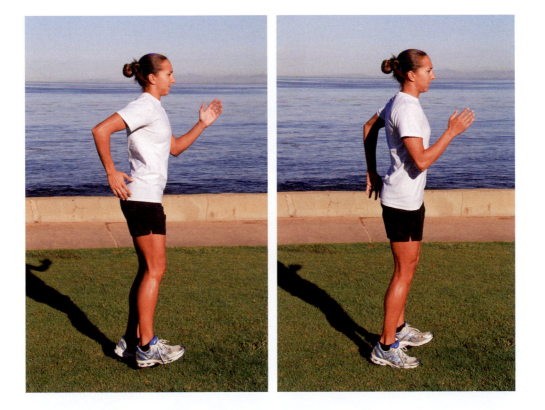

Butt Kicker

Intensity level: Low

Equipment: None

Purpose: Builds on the ankling drill. Teaches to bring heel to buttocks immediately following plantarflexion of the ankle during the sprinting motion.

Beginning position: Assume a comfortable, upright stance with feet shoulder-width apart. Begin to jog.

Movement: Pull the heel toward the buttocks contracting the hamstring, swinging the lower leg back. Allow the heel to "bounce" off the buttocks.

Advanced variation: Imagine a wall right behind you. Perform a butt kicker, but instead of having the heel drive posterior to the hips, bring the heel up along the imaginary wall to reach the buttocks, forcing the heel of the recovery leg to stay anterior to the buttocks. This variation improves knee lift during the flight phase of sprinting. This shortens the lever so the mass of the leg is closer to the axis of rotation, allowing the leg to be cycled forward more quickly during sprinting.

Common Errors

- Forcing the heel toward the buttocks; instead, "allow" the heel to elevate toward the buttocks.
- Excessive thigh motion; the thigh should not move too much—concentrate on moving at the knee versus the hip joint.

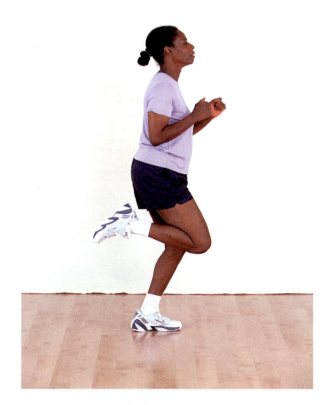

High Knee Drill

Intensity level: Low to moderate

Equipment: None

Purpose: Trains hip flexors and reinforces foot positioning taught during ankling drill; reinforces front-side mechanics while reinforcing dorsiflexion and conditioning the hip flexors.

Beginning position: Assume a comfortable, upright stance with feet shoulder-width apart. Begin to walk, focusing on one leg at a time.

Movement: Right ankle plantarflexes as hips move over foot. As soon as heel lifts off ground, immediately draw ankle into dorsiflexed position and extend great toe as in ankling drill. At the same time, flex right hip until thigh is parallel to ground. Keeping ankle dorsiflexed and toe extended, drive foot to ground, using hips, placing lateral aspect of forefoot slightly in front of hips.

Advanced variations: (1) walking, focusing on one leg at a time, no arm swing; (2) repeat, adding arm swing; (3) walking, alternating legs, no arm swing; (4) repeat, adding arm swing; (5) skipping, focusing on one leg, no arm swing; (6) repeat, adding arm swing; (7) skipping, alternating legs, no arm swing; (8) repeat, adding arm swing; (9) running, alternating legs, no arm swing; (10) repeat, adding arm swing.

Common Errors

- Inability to stand tall during this drill due to weak hip flexors and core; trunk will flex as the hip flexes
- Inability to keep ankle dorsiflexed and great toe extended when flexing hip

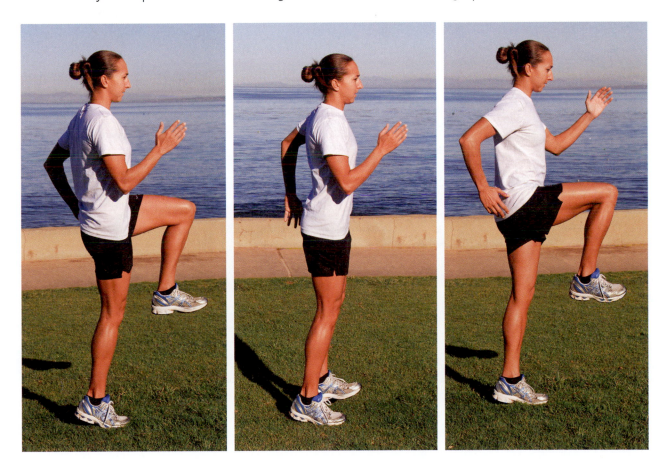

Fast Leg Drill

Intensity level: High

Equipment: None

Purpose: Move lower extremities at a faster speed than during normal running

Beginning position: Perform at a walk, beginning with right foot.

Movement: After the third step, perform a fast sequence of the following motions: heel to hip with ankle dorsiflexed and great toe extended as in butt kicker; bring right knee forward as if stepping over opposite foot; flex hip so that thigh is parallel to ground, then unfold leg and drive foot to ground as in high knee drill. Repeat every third step.

Advanced variations: (1) ankling for three steps, then fast leg motion one step, focusing on one leg at a time; (2) ankling for three steps, then fast leg motion one step, alternating legs; (3) ankling for two steps, then fast leg motion one step, alternating legs; (4) straight-leg bounding for three steps, then fast leg one step, focusing on one leg at a time; (5) straight-leg bounding for two steps, then fast leg one step, alternating legs; (6) straight-leg bounding one step, then fast leg one step, focusing on one leg at a time; (7) continuous fast leg for distance.

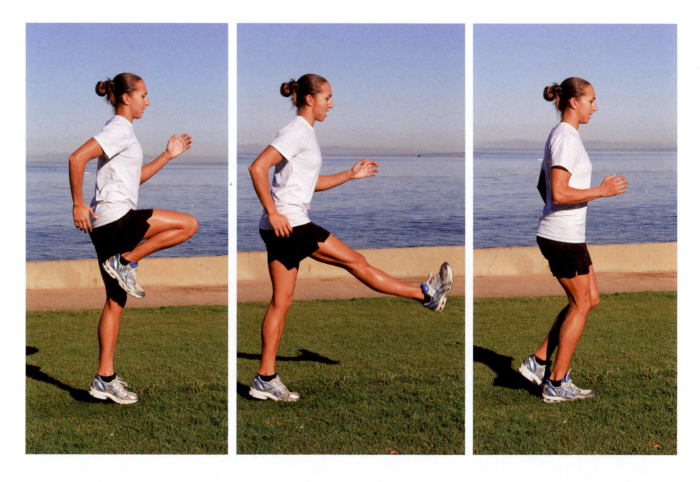

Uphill Sprint

Intensity level: High

Equipment: A 3° to 7° uphill sprinting surface

Beginning position: At the bottom of the downhill area, assume a comfortable, upright stance with feet shoulder-width apart.

Movement: Maintaining correct posture and technique, sprint 33 to 55 yards (30 to 50 m) uphill.

Common Errors

- Sprinting speed slows more than 10%; do not exceed a 7° slope, and decrease the slope if slowdown continues.
- Proper form is not maintained; decrease the slope until proper technique returns.

Partner-Resisted Sprinting

Intensity level: High

Equipment: 11 to 22 yards (10 to 20 m) of rubber tubing

Purpose: Works on increasing stride length, achieving full hip extension, and spending minimal time in contact with the ground.

Beginning position: With the client in front, the personal trainer or a partner attaches one end of the tubing or bungee to the client, then holds the other end. The client moves approximately 5.5 yards (5 m) ahead while the partner maintains the beginning position.

Movement: With the beginning distance maintained, the client begins sprinting while the partner resists. The partner should resist only enough for the client to slow speed by 10%. The client should sprint for a distance of only 11 to 16 yards (10 to 15 m).

Common Errors

- Sprinting speed slows more than 10%; the resistance should be decreased until proper technique returns.
- Proper form is not maintained; distance should be decrease until proper technique returns.

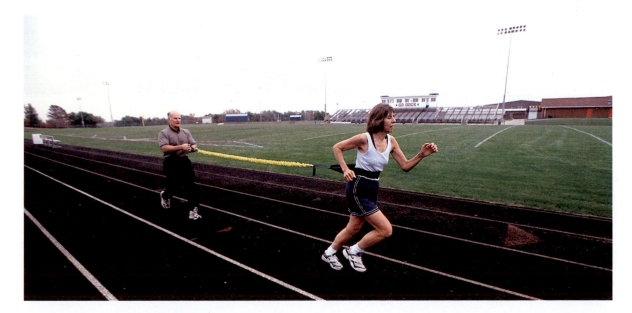

457

Stride Length Speed Drills

Downhill Sprint

Intensity level: High

Equipment: A 3° to 7° downhill angled sprinting surface

Purpose: Running at a greater velocity than one is normally capable of. This allows the body to learn how to run at greater stride frequencies, which will then transfer to nonresisted running or flat sprinting.

Beginning position: At the top of the downhill area, assume a comfortable, upright stance with feet shoulder-width apart.

Movement: Maintaining correct posture and technique, sprint 33 to 55 yards (30 to 50 m) downhill. Do not run at speeds greater than 106% to 110% of maximum speed.

Common Errors

- Excessive braking or deceleration; do not exceed a 7° slope, and decrease the slope if braking continues.
- Proper form is not maintained; decrease the slope until proper technique returns.

Partner-Assisted Towing

Intensity level: High

Equipment: 11 to 22 yards (10 to 20 m) of rubber tubing or bungee

Purpose: Running at a greater velocity than one is normally capable of. This allows the body to learn how to run at greater stride frequencies, which will then transfer to nonresisted running or flat sprinting.

Beginning position: The tubing or bungee is attached to both the client and the personal trainer or a partner, with the partner in front. The partner moves approximately 5.5 yards (5 m) ahead while the client maintains the beginning position.

Movement: The partner initiates the running with the client beginning almost immediately after. The client should run with a slight lean in an upright position,

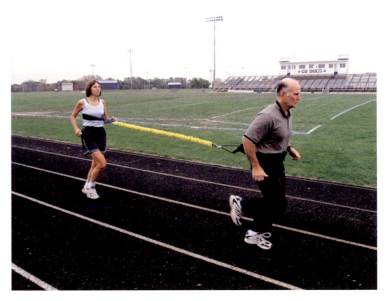

focusing on stepping up and over the other knee, dorsiflexing feet when in the air, making contact with the ground on the ball of the foot, and maintaining a good powerful arm drive.

Common Errors

- Insufficient assistance; the partner must be at least as fast as the client.
- Proper form is not maintained with increased speed. The client begins to brake to slow him- or herself down, which results in his or her leaning back and making contact with the heel instead of ball of the foot. In turn, the client spends too much time in contact with the ground, decreasing the stride length, getting slowed down, and over time predisposing him- or herself to overuse injuries. The partner should decrease the sprinting speed until proper technique returns.

Study Questions

1. Which of the following exercises benefits the most from the advantages of the stretch shortening cycle (SSC)?

   A. push press

   B. deadlift

   C. back squat

   D. front squat

2. Which of the following is a requirement to participate in a plyometric training program?

   A. at least 18 years of age

   B. more than one year performing power exercises

   C. at least three months of general resistance training exercises

   D. less than 50 years of age

3. Which of the following adjustments is most appropriate for a client having difficulty performing a depth jump correctly due to the amortization phase being too long?

   A. Discontinue the depth jump.

   B. Have the client try the jump using just one leg.

   C. Focus on absorbing the landing.

   D. Decrease the height of the box.

4. The personal trainer notices that a client takes short, choppy steps while sprinting. Which of the following types of training will help this client improve stride length the most?

   I. resisted sprinting

   II. assisted sprinting

   III. technique training

   IV. plyometric training

   A. I and III only

   B. II and IV only

   C. I, III, and IV only

   D. I, II, and III only

Applied Knowledge Question

A healthy, 35-year-old female who is a part-time aerobics instructor wants to begin a training program to compete in an aerobic fitness (sport aerobics) event. She has been resistance training since college and is familiar with how to perform plyometric drills. She is 5 feet, 5 inches (165 cm) tall, weighs 130 pounds (59 kg), and has a 195-pound (87 kg) 1RM back squat. During one of the weekly classes she teaches, she performs depth jumps and push-ups off an aerobic step. Fill in the chart to describe a sample plyometric training program based on the description and goals of the client.

Mode	
Activity-specific drills and their intensity	
Frequency	
Volume (table 17.6)	

References

1. Allerheiligen, B., and R. Rogers. 1995. Plyometrics program design. *Strength and Conditioning* 17: 26-31.

2. Asmussen, E., and F. Bonde-Peterson. 1974. Storage of elastic energy in skeletal muscles in man. *Acta Physiologica Scandinavica* 91: 385-392.

3. Aura, O., and J.T. Vitasalo. 1989. Biomechanical characteristics of jumping. *International Journal of Sport Biomechanics* 5 (1): 89-97.

4. Berg, K., R.W. Latin, and T.R. Baechle. 1990. Physical and performance characteristics of NCAA division I football players. *Research Quarterly for Exercise and Sport* 61: 395-401.

5. Berg, K., R.W. Latin, and T.R. Baechle. 1992. Physical fitness of NCAA division I football players. *National Strength and Conditioning Association Journal* 14: 68-72.

6. Blattner, S., and L. Noble. 1979. Relative effects of isokinetic and plyometric training on vertical jumping performance. *Research Quarterly* 50 (4): 583-588.

7. Bobbert, M.F., K.G.M. Gerritsen, M.C.A Litjens, and A.J. Van Soest. 1996. Why is countermovement jump height greater than squat jump height? *Medicine and Science in Sports and Exercise* 28: 1402-1412.

8. Borkowski, J. 1990. Prevention of pre-season muscle soreness: Plyometric exercise (abstract). *Athletic Training* 25 (2): 122.

9. Bosco, C., A. Ito, P.V. Komi, P. Luhtanen, P. Rahkila, H. Rusko, and J.T. Vitasalo. 1982. Neuromuscular function and mechanical efficiency of human leg extensor muscles during jumping exercises. *Acta Physiologica Scandinavica* 114: 543-550.

10. Bosco, C., and P.V. Komi. 1979. Potentiation of the mechanical behavior of the human skeletal muscle through pre-stretching. *Acta Physiologica Scandinavica* 106: 467-472.

11. Bosco, C., P.V. Komi, and A. Ito. 1981. Pre-stretch potentiation of human skeletal muscle during ballistic movement. *Acta Physiologica Scandinavica* 111: 135-140.

12. Bosco, C., J.T. Vitasalo, P.V. Komi, and P. Luhtanen. 1982. Combined effect of elastic energy and myoelectrical potentiation during stretch shortening cycle exercise. *Acta Physiologica Scandinavica* 114: 557-565.

13. Brown, L.E., V.A. Ferrigno, and J.C. Santana. 2000. *Training for Speed, Agility, and Quickness.* Champaign, IL: Human Kinetics.

14. Cavagna, G.A. 1977. Storage and utilization of elastic energy in skeletal muscle. In: *Exercise and Sport Science Reviews,* vol. 5, R.S. Hutton, ed. Santa Barbara, CA: Journal Affiliates. pp. 80-129.

15. Cavagna, G.A., B. Dusman, and R. Margaria. 1968. Positive work done by a previously stretched muscle. *Journal of Applied Physiology* 24: 21-32.

16. Cavagna, G.A., F.P. Saibere, and R. Margaria. 1965. Effect of negative work on the amount of positive work performed by an isolated muscle. *Journal of Applied Physiology* 20: 157-158.

17. Chambers, C., T.D. Noakes, E.V. Lambert, and M.I. Lambert. 1998. Time course of recovery of vertical jump height and heart rate versus running speed after a 90-km foot race. *Journal of Sports Sciences* 16: 645-651.

18. Chimera, N.J., K.A. Swanik, C.B. Swanik, and S.J. Straub. 2004. Effects of plyometric training on muscle-activation strategies and performance in female athletes. *Journal of Athletic Training* 39 (1): 24-31.

19. Chmielewski, T.L., G.D. Myer, D. Kaufman, and S. M. Tillman. 2006. Plyometric exercise in the rehabilitation of athletes: Physiological responses and clinical application. *Journal of Orthopaedic and Sports Physical Therapy* 36 (5): 308-319.

20. Chu, D. 1983. Plyometrics: The link between strength and speed. *National Strength and Conditioning Association Journal* 5 (2): 20-21.

21. Chu, D. 1984. Plyometric exercise. *National Strength and Conditioning Association Journal* 5 (6): 56-59, 61-64.

22. Chu, D. 1998. *Jumping Into Plyometrics,* 2nd ed. Champaign, IL: Human Kinetics.

23. Chu, D., and F. Costello. 1985. Jumping into plyometrics. *National Strength and Conditioning Association Journal* 7 (3): 65.

24. Chu, D., and R. Korchemny. 1989. Sprinting stride actions: Analysis and evaluation. *National Strength and Conditioning Association Journal* 11 (6): 6-8, 82-85.

25. Chu, D., and R. Panariello. 1986. Jumping into plyometrics. *National Strength and Conditioning Association Journal* 8 (5): 73.

26. Chu, D., and L. Plummer. 1984. Jumping into plyometrics: The language of plyometrics. *National Strength and Conditioning Association Journal* 6 (5): 30-31.

27. Cissik, J. 2002. Technique and speed development for running. *NSCA Performance Training Journal* 1(8): 18-21.

28. Cissik, J.M. 2004. Means and methods of speed training: Part I. *Strength and Conditioning Journal* 26 (4): 24-29.

29. Cissik, J. 2005. Means and methods of speed training: Part II. *Strength and Conditioning Journal* 27 (1): 18-25.

30. Clark, M.A., and T. Wallace. 2003. Plyometric training with elastic resistance. In: *The Scientific and Clinical Application of Elastic Resistance,* P. Page and T.S. Ellenbecker, eds. Champaign, IL: Human Kinetics. pp. 119-129.

31. Costello, F. 1985. Training for speed using resisted and assisted methods. *National Strength and Conditioning Association Journal* 7 (1): 74-75.

32. Cronin, J., and K.T. Hansen. 2006. Resisted sprint training for the acceleration phase of sprinting. *Strength and Conditioning Journal* 28 (4): 42-51.

33. de Villarreal, E.S.S., J.J. González-Badillo, and M. Izquierdo. 2008. Low and moderate plyometric training frequency produces greater jumping and sprinting gains compared with high frequency. *Journal of Strength and Conditioning Research* 22 (3): 715-725.

34. de Vos, N.J., N.A. Singh, D.A. Ross, T. M. Stavrinos, R. Orr, and M.A.F. Singh. 2005. Optimal load for increasing muscle power during explosive resistance training in older adults. *Journal of Gerontology* 60A (5): 638-647.

35. Dick, F.W. 1987. *Sprints and Relays.* London: British Amateur Athletic Board.

36. Dillman, C.J., G.S. Fleisig, and J.R. Andrews. 1993. Biomechanics of pitching with emphasis upon shoulder kinematics. *Journal of Orthopaedic and Sports Physical Therapy* 18 (2): 402-408.

37. Dintiman, G.B., R.D. Ward, and T. Tellez. 1998. *Sports Speed.* Champaign, IL: Human Kinetics.

38. Dursenev, L., and L. Raeysky. 1979. Strength training for jumpers. *Soviet Sports Review* 14 (2): 53-55.

39. Ebben W., 2007. Practical guidelines for plyometric intensity. *NCSA's Performance Training Journal.* 6(5): 12-16.

40. Enoka, R.W. 1994. *Neuromechanical Basis of Kinesiology.* Champaign, IL: Human Kinetics.

41. Faccioni, A. 1994. Assisted and resisted methods for speed development (part II). *Modern Athlete Coach* 32 (3): 8-11.

42. Faigenbaum A. 2006. Plyometrics for Kids: Facts and Fallacies. *NSCA's Performance Training Journal.* 5(2): 13 – 16.

43. Faigenbaum A., W. Kraemer, C.J.R. Blimkie, I. Jeffreys, L.J. Micheli, M. Nitka, and T.W. Rowland. 2009. Youth resistance training: Updated position statement paper from the National Strength and Conditioning Association. *Journal of Strength and Conditioning Research.* Supplement to 23(5): S60-S79.

44. Feltner, M., and J. Dapena. 1986. Dynamics of the shoulder and elbow joints of the throwing arm during a baseball pitch. *International Journal of Sport Biomechanics* 2: 235.

45. Fleck, S. 1983. Interval training: Physiological basis. *National Strength and Conditioning Association Journal* 5 (5): 40, 57-63.

46. Fleck, S., and W. Kraemer. 1997. *Designing Resistance Training Programs.* Champaign, IL: Human Kinetics.

47. Fleisig, G.S., S.W. Barrentine, N. Zheng, R.F. Escamilla, and J.R. Andrews. 1999. Kinematic and kinetic comparison of baseball pitching among various levels of development. *Journal of Biomechanics* 32 (12): 1371-1375.

48. Fowler, N.E., A. Lees, and T. Reilly. 1994. Spinal shrinkage in unloaded and loaded drop-jumping. *Ergonomics* 37: 133-139.

49. Fowler, N.E., A. Lees, and T. Reilly. 1997. Changes in stature following plyometric drop-jump and pendulum exercises. *Ergonomics* 40: 1279-1286.

50. Gambetta, V. 1978. Plyometric training. *Track and Field Quarterly Review* 80 (4): 56-57.

51. Gambetta, V., G. Winckler, J. Rogers, J. Orognen, L. Seagrave, and S. Jolly. 1989. Sprints and relays. In: *TAC Track and Field Coaching Manual,* 2nd ed., TAC Development Committees and V. Gambetta, eds. Champaign, IL: Leisure Press. pp. 55-70.

52. Gamble, P. 2008. Approaching physical preparation for youth team-sports players. *Strength and Conditioning Journal* 30 (1): 29-42.

53. Gottschall, J.S. and Kram, R. 2005. Ground reaction forces during downhill and uphill running. *Journal of Biomechanics* 38:445-452.

54. Guyton, A.C., and J.E. Hall. 1995. *Textbook of Medical Physiology,* 9th ed. Philadelphia: Saunders.

55. Harman, E.A., M.T. Rosenstein, P.N. Frykman, and R.M. Rosenstein. 1990. The effects of arms and countermovement on vertical jumping. *Medicine and Science in Sports and Exercise* 22: 825-833.

56. Harre, D., ed. 1982. *Principles of Sports Training.* Berlin: Sportverlag.

57. Hewett, T.E., T.N. Lindenfeld, J.V. Riccobene, and F.R. Noyes. 1999. The effect of neuromuscular training on the incidence of knee injury in female athletes. A prospective study. *American Journal of Sports Medicine* 27: 699-706.

58. Hewett, T.E., A.L. Stroupe, T.A. Nance, and F.R. Noyes. 1996. Plyometric training in female athletes. *American Journal of Sports Medicine* 24: 765-773.

59. Hill, A.V. 1970. *First and Last Experiments in Muscle Mechanics.* Cambridge: Cambridge University Press.

60. Holcomb, W.R., D.M. Kleiner, and D.A. Chu. 1998. Plyometrics: Considerations for safe and effective training. *Strength and Conditioning* 20 (3): 36-39.

61. Jarver, J., ed. 1990. *Sprints and Relays: Contemporary Theory, Technique and Training,* 3rd ed. Los Altos, CA: Tafnews Press.

62. Judge, L.W. 2007. Developing speed strength: In-season training program for the collegiate thrower. *Strength and Conditioning Journal* 29 (5): 42-54.

63. Kaeding, C.C., and R. Whitehead. 1998. Musculoskeletal injuries in adolescents. *Primary Care* 25 (1): 211-23.

64. Kilani, H.A., S.S. Palmer, M.J. Adrian, and J.J. Gapsis. 1989. Block of the stretch reflex of vastus lateralis during vertical jump. *Human Movement Science* 8: 247-269.

65. Korchemny, R. 1985. Evaluation of sprinters. *National Strength and Conditioning Association Journal* 7 (4): 38-42.

66. Kotzamanidis, C. 2006. Effect of plyometric training on running performance and vertical jumping on prepubertal boys. *Journal of Strength and Conditioning Research* 20 (2): 441-445.

67. Kozlov, I., and V. Muravyev. 1992. Muscles and the sprint. *Soviet Sports Review* 27 (6): 192-195.

68. Kraemer, W.J., S.A. Mazzetti, B.C. Nindl, L.A. Gotshalk, J.S. Volek, J.A. Bush, J.O. Marx, K. Dohi, A.L. Gomez, M. Miles, S.J. Fleck, R.U. Newton, and K. Häkkinen. 2001. Effect of resistance training on women's strength/power and occupational performances. *Medicine and Science in Sports and Exercise* 33 (6): 1011-1025.

69. LaChance, P. 1995. Plyometric exercise. *Strength and Conditioning* 17: 16-23.

70. Latin, R.W., K. Berg, and T.R. Baechle. 1994. Physical and performance characteristics of NCAA division I male basketball players. *Journal of Strength and Conditioning Research* 8: 214-218.

71. Lavrienko, A., J. Kravstev, and Z. Petrova. 1990. New approaches to sprint training. *Modern Athlete Coach* 28 (3): 3-5.

72. Lipp, E.J. 1998. Athletic epiphyseal injury in children and adolescents. *Orthopaedic Nursing* 17 (2): 17-22.

73. Luhtanen, P., and P. Komi. 1978. Mechanical factors influencing running speed. In: *Biomechanics VI-B,* E. Asmussen, ed. Baltimore: University Park Press. pp. 23-29.

74. Mach, G. 1985. The individual sprint events. In: *Athletes in Action: The Official International Amateur Athletic Federation Book on Track and Field Techniques.* London: Pelham Books. pp. 12-34.

75. Matavulj, D., M. Kukolj, D. Ugarkovic, J. Tihanyi, and S. Jaric. 2001. Effects of plyometric training on jumping performance in junior basketball players. *Journal of Sports Medicine and Physical Fitness* 41 (2): 159-164.

76. Matthews, P.B.C. 1990. The knee jerk: Still an enigma? *Canadian Journal of Physiology and Pharmacology* 68: 347-354.

77. McBride, J.M., G.O. McCaulley, and P. Cormie. 2008. Influence of preactivity and eccentric muscle activity on concentric performance during vertical jumping. *Journal of Strength and Conditioning Research* 22 (3): 750-757.

78. McNeely, E. 2005. Introduction to plyometrics: Converting strength to power. *NSCA Performance Training Journal* 6 (5): 19-22.

79. Mero, A., P.V. Komi, and R.J. Gregor. 1992. Biomechanics of sprint running: A review. *Sports Medicine* 13 (6): 376-392.

80. Miller, J.M., S.C. Hilbert, and L.E. Brown. 2001. Speed, quickness, and agility training for senior tennis players. *Strength and Conditioning Journal* 23 (5): 62-66.

81. Moravec, P., J. Ruzicka, P. Susanka, E. Dostal, M. Kodejs, and M. Nosek. 1988. The 1987 International Athletic Foundation/IAAF scientific project report: Time analysis of the 100 metres events at the II World Championships in athletics. *New Studies Athletics* 3 (3): 61-96.

82. Myer, G.D., K.R. Ford, S.G. McLean, and T.E. Hewett. 2006. The effects of plyometric versus dynamic stabilization and balance training on lower extremity biomechanics. *American Journal of Sports Medicine* 34 (3): 445-455.

83. Myer, G.D., M.V. Paterno, K.R. Ford, and T.E. Hewett. 2008 Neuromuscular training techniques to target deficits before return to sport after anterior cruciate ligament

reconstruction. *Journal of Strength and Conditioning Research* 22 (3): 987-1014.

84. National Strength and Conditioning Association. 1993. Position statement: Explosive/plyometric exercises. *National Strength and Conditioning Association Journal* 15 (3): 16.

85. Newman, B. 2007. Speed development through resisted sprinting. *NSCA Performance Training Journal* 6 (3): 12-13.

86. Newton, R.U., W.J. Kraemer, and K. Häkkinen. 1999. Effects of ballistic training on preseason preparation of elite volleyball players. *Medicine and Science in Sports and Exercise* 31 (2): 323-330.

87. Newton, R.U., A.J. Murphy, B.J. Humphries, G.J. Wilson, W.J. Kraemer, and K. Häkkinen. 1997. Influence of load and stretch shortening cycle on the kinematics, kinetics and muscle activation that occurs during explosive upper-body movements. *European Journal of Applied Physiology* 75: 333-342.

88. Ozolin, E. 1986. Contemporary sprint technique (part 1). *Soviet Sports Review* 21 (3): 109-114.

89. Ozolin, E. 1986. Contemporary sprint technique (part 2). *Soviet Sports Review* 21 (4): 190-195.

90. Pappas, A.M., R.M. Zawacki, and T.J. Sullivan. 1985. Biomechanics of baseball pitching: A preliminary report. *American Journal of Sports Medicine* 13: 216-222.

91. Phelps, S. 2001 Speed training. *Strength and Conditioning Journal* 23(2): 57-58.

92. Piper, T., and T. Teichelman. 2003. Organizational and motivational strategies for prepubescent athletes. *Strength and Conditioning Journal* 25 (4): 54-57.

93. Plattner, S., and L. Noble. 1979. Relative effects of isokinetic and plyometric training on vertical jumping performance. *Research Quarterly* 50 (4): 583-588.

94. Plisk, S.S. 1995. Theories, concepts and methodology of speed development as they relate to sports performance. Presented at the NSCA Certification Commission's Essential Principles of Strength Training and Conditioning Symposium, Phoenix, June.

95. Plisk, S.S. 2002. Personal communication, March 2002.

96. Potteiger, J.A., R.H. Lockwood, M.D. Haub, B.A. Dolezal, K.S. Almuzaini, J.M. Schroeder, and C.J. Zebas. 1999. Muscle power and fiber characteristics following 8 weeks of plyometric training. *Journal of Strength and Conditioning Research* 13 (3): 275-279.

97. Radcliffe, J.C., and R.C. Farentinos. 1985. *Plyometrics.* Champaign, IL: Human Kinetics.

98. Radcliffe, J.C., and R.C. Farentinos. 1999. *High-Powered Plyometrics.* Champaign, IL: Human Kinetics.

99. Radcliffe, J.C., and L.R. Osternig. 1995. Effects on performance of variable eccentric loads during depth jumps. *Journal of Sport Rehabilitation* 4: 31-41.

100. Romanova, N. 1990. The sprint: Nontraditional means of training (a review of scientific studies). *Soviet Sports Review* 25 (2): 99-102.

101. Sandler, R., and S. Robinovitch. 2001. An analysis of the effect of lower extremity strength on impact severity during a backward fall. *Journal of Biomechanical Engineering* 123 (6): 590-598.

102. Santos, E.J.A.M., and M.A.A.S. Janeira. 2008. Effects of complex training on explosive strength in adolescent male basketball players. *Journal of Strength and Conditioning Research* 22 (3): 903-909.

103. Schmolinsky, G., ed. 2000. *Track and Field: The East German Textbook of Athletics.* Toronto: Sport Books.

104. Shiner, J., T. Bishop, and A.J. Cosgarea. 2005. Integrating low-intensity plyometrics into strength and conditioning programs. *Strength and Conditioning Journal* 27 (6): 10-20.

105. Siff, M.C. 2000. *Supertraining,* 5th ed. Denver: Supertraining Institute.

106. Sinnett, A.M., K. Berg, R.W. Latin, and J.M. Noble. 2001. The relationship between field tests of anaerobic power and 10-km run performance. *Journal of Strength and Conditioning Research* 15 (4): 405-412.

107. Svantesson, U., G. Grimby, and R. Thome. 1994. Potentiation of concentric plantar flexion torque following eccentric and isometric muscle actions. *Acta Physiologica Scandinavica* 152: 287-293.

108. Turner, A.M., M. Owings, and J.A. Schwane. 2003. Improvement in running economy after 6 weeks of plyometric training. *Journal of Strength and Conditioning Research* 17 (1): 60-67.

109. Verkhoshansky, Y. 1969. Perspectives in the improvement of speed-strength preparation of jumpers. *Yessis Review of Soviet Physical Education and Sports* 4 (2): 28-29.

110. Verkhoshansky, Y., and V. Tatyan. 1983. Speed-strength preparation of future champions. *Soviet Sports Review* 18 (4): 166-170.

111. Voight, M.L., P. Draovitch, and S. Tippett. 1995. Plyometrics. In: *Eccentric Muscle Training in Sports and Orthopaedics,* M. Albert, ed. New York: Churchill Livingstone. pp. 61-88.

112. Walshe, A.D., G.J. Wilson, and G.J.C. Ettema. 1998. Stretch-shorten cycle compared with isometric preload: Contributions to enhanced muscular performance. *Journal of Applied Physiology* 84: 97-106.

113. Warpeha, J.M. 2007. Principles of speed training. *NSCA Performance Training Journal* 6 (3): 6-8.

114. Wathen, D. 1993. Literature review: Plyometric exercise. *National Strength and Conditioning Association Journal* 15 (3): 17-19.

115. Wilk, K.E., and M. Voight. 1993. Plyometrics for the overhead athlete. In: *The Athletic Shoulder,* J.R. Andrews and K.E. Wilk, eds. New York: Churchill Livingstone.

116. Wilk, K.E., M.L. Voight, M.A. Keirns, V. Gambetta, J.R. Andrews, and C.J. Dillman. 1993. Stretch-shortening drills for the upper extremities: Theory and clinical application. *Journal of Orthopaedic and Sports Physical Therapy* 17: 225-239.

117. Wilson, G.J., A.J. Murphy, and A. Giorgi. 1996. Weight and plyometric training: Effects on eccentric and concentric force production. *Canadian Journal of Applied Physiology* 21: 301-315.

118. Wilson, G.J., R.U. Newton, A.J. Murphy, and B.J. Humphries. 1993. The optimal training load for the development of dynamic athletic performance. *Medicine and Science in Sports and Exercise* 25: 1279-1286.

119. Wilt, F. 1968. Training for competitive running. In: *Exercise Physiology,* H.B. Falls, ed. New York: Academic Press. pp. 395-414.

120. Witzke, K.A., and C.M. Snow. 2000. Effects of plyometric jump training on bone mass in adolescent girls. *Medicine and Science in Sports and Exercise* 32 (6): 1051-1017.

121. Zazulak, B., J. Cholewicki, and N.P. Reeves. 2008. Neuromuscular control of trunk stability: Clinical implications for sports injury prevention. *Journal of the American Academy of Orthopaedic Surgeons* 16 (9): 497-505.

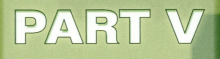
PART V

Clients With Unique Needs

Clients Who Are Preadolescent, Older, or Pregnant

Wayne L. Westcott, PhD, and Avery D. Faigenbaum, EdD

After completing this chapter, you will be able to

- describe developmentally appropriate physical activity programs for preadolescents that demonstrate an understanding of age-specific needs and concerns,

- explain the health benefits of senior exercise and outline exercise guidelines for older adults, and

- discuss exercise recommendations and precautions for pregnant women.

The purpose of this chapter is to present general training considerations and specific exercise guidelines for three groups of people who typically need modified workouts to maximize their conditioning benefits and minimize their injury risk. Preadolescent youth, older adults, and pregnant women can safely perform aerobic endurance exercise for improved cardiorespiratory fitness, as well as resistance training for increased musculoskeletal fitness. However, because each of these special populations has particular characteristics, personal trainers must incorporate a number of recommendations into exercise programs for them.

Preadolescent Youth

Preadolescence refers to a period of time before the development of secondary sex characteristics (e.g.,

pubic hair and reproductive organs) and corresponds roughly to ages 6 to 11 years in girls and 6 to 13 years in boys. Preadolescent youth (also referred to as children in this chapter) should be encouraged to participate regularly in a variety of physical activities that enhance endurance, strength, flexibility, and skill-related fitness abilities (i.e., agility, balance, coordination, reaction time, speed and power). Regular participation in physical activity programs can improve health- and skill-related components of physical fitness and have been found to enhance psychosocial well-being in school-age youth (139, 153, 165). Furthermore, increasing opportunities for regular physical activity during physical education classes and out-of-school time may support academic achievement (165). Health and fitness organizations support and encourage children's participation in physical activity programs that are consistent with the needs and abilities of the participants (30, 45, 133, 142).

The promotion of physical activity among youth has become a major public health concern because childhood overweight and obesity continue to increase worldwide, and the physical activity level of most boys and girls is down (28, 31, 146, 179). The percentage of overweight boys and girls has more than doubled during the past two decades, and many children who are overweight have one or more risk factors for cardiovascular disease (66, 135). The amount of time children spend with electronic media (e.g., television, video games, and computers) has grown considerably over the past few years, and less than 15% of children walk to or from school (25, 31). Nowadays, due to the unprecedented access to the Internet and cellular phones, children do not have to leave their homes to communicate with their friends outside of school hours.

The negative health consequences of childhood obesity and physical inactivity include the appearance of atherosclerosis and type 2 "adult-onset" diabetes in children and teenagers (92). The increasing incidence of type 2 diabetes in youth is particularly troubling because conditions related to uncontrolled diabetes such as kidney failure, blindness, and limb amputation will occur earlier in life. These findings have led some researchers to predict that the overall life expectancy observed in the modern era may soon decrease due to the increased prevalence of obesity-related comorbidities such as heart disease, diabetes, and cancer (136).

Since both positive and negative behaviors established during childhood tend to carry over into adulthood (46, 95, 116), the key is to value the importance of physical activity and help children develop healthy habits and behavior patterns at an early age. Personal trainers who model and support participation in developmentally appropriate fitness activities that are safe, fun, and supported by cultural norms can have a powerful influence on a child's health and activity habits. Well-organized personal training sessions that give boys and girls the opportunity to experience the mere enjoyment of physical activity can have long-lasting effects on their health and well-being. Thus, the goal of youth fitness programs is not only to engage boys and girls in a variety of age-appropriate games and activities, but also for youth to become aware of the intrinsic value and benefits of physical activity so they become adults who participate regularly in exercise and sport. Regular physical activity for children age 6 and older is recognized as one of the most important steps that can be taken to improve their health and fitness (45, 139).

Youth Physical Activity

Because youth have different needs than adults and are active in different ways, adult exercise guidelines and training philosophies should not be imposed on children. Watching boys and girls on a playground supports the contention that the natural activity pattern of children is characterized by sporadic bursts of moderate- to vigorous-intensity activity with brief periods of low-intensity activity or rest as needed. While adults often exercise within a predetermined target heart rate zone (5), children are intermittently active and often choose to exercise in an interval-type pattern characterized by haphazard increases and decreases in exercise intensity (9). Thus personal trainers should not expect preadolescents to exercise in the same manner as adults. The assumption that children are inactive simply because they do not perform continuous physical activity is inaccurate.

This does not mean that exercising continuously for 30 minutes or more within a predetermined target heart rate range (e.g., 70% to 85% predicted maximal heart rate) is not beneficial for children. Rather it means that this is not the most appropriate method for training preadolescents because most children do not see the benefit of prolonged periods of aerobic endurance training. Furthermore, because cardiorespiratory adaptations such as increased aerobic capacity are less noticeable in children compared to older adults (143), prolonged periods of vigorous activity can decrease rather than increase motivation for future activity. As children enter their teenage years, some may want to adhere to the adult target heart rate model depending on their needs, goals, and abilities.

Personal trainers also need to be aware of physiological differences between children and adults. Children have a higher breathing frequency and a lower tidal volume than adults at all exercise intensities (153). Thus it is normal for healthy children to breathe rapidly during a fitness workout. Children also exhibit a lower stroke volume and higher heart rate at all exercise intensities (153). Maximal heart rates do not change much during childhood, and it is not uncommon for a child's heart rate to exceed 200 beats/min during a vigorous fitness workout. Clinicians have also observed that children tend to be "metabolic nonspecialists" with regard to fitness performance (12). Unlike what is seen in adults who tend to specialize in sports such as weightlifting or long-distance running, the strongest child in class is likely to be the best at endurance events too. Personal trainers should appreciate the lack of metabolic specialization in children and should expose boys and girls to a variety of sports and activities during this developmental period.

Although the absolute level of physical activity required to achieve and maintain fitness in youth has not yet been determined, over the past few years several organizations and committees have developed youth physical activity guidelines (30, 45, 165). It has been recommended that children participate daily in 60 minutes or more of moderate to vigorous physical activity that is developmentally appropriate, is enjoyable, and involves a variety of activities (165). In addition to participation in structured programs such as physical education classes, personal training sessions, and team sports, lifestyle physical activities including playground games, walking or biking to and from school, and physical chores around the home (e.g., yard work) can contribute to the amount of time children engage in physical activity. Reducing the amount of time children spend watching television, viewing video games, or surfing the Internet can considerably increase the time they have available for physical activity (71).

Most children can remain physically active for 30 minutes or more provided that the exercise intensity varies throughout the session and that they are given the opportunity to take short breaks when needed. Even sedentary children can perform relatively large volumes of physical activity by alternating moderate to vigorous physical activity with brief periods of rest and recovery. Instead of a 30-minute jogging workout, the personal trainer can create a circuit of 8 to 12 stations that includes jumping rope, body weight exercises (e.g., jumping jacks, push-ups, and squats), medicine ball activities, balancing drills, and shuttle runs. As fitness levels improve, it becomes possible to decrease the rest period between stations and make the activities at each station more challenging. With qualified instruction, enthusiastic leadership, and adherence to safety issues, children can safely enhance their fundamental movement abilities and be better prepared for successful and enjoyable participation in recreational activities and sport.

> Youth should be encouraged to participate daily in 60 minutes or more of physical activity as part of play, games, sport, transportation, and school activities.

Resistance Training for Youth

For many years, youth fitness programs focused primarily on aerobic activities such as jogging, swimming, dance, and tag games. However, a compelling body of evidence now indicates that resistance training can be a safe, effective, and worthwhile method of conditioning for preadolescents provided that appropriate guidelines are followed (53, 57, 63, 117). Despite the traditional belief that resistance training was inappropriate or unsafe for children, the qualified acceptance of youth resistance training by medical and fitness organizations is becoming widespread (2, 5, 14, 22, 55).

The traditional concern that resistance training could damage the epiphyseal plates of children or impede the statural growth of young weight trainers caused some people to recommend that children not participate in resistance training. Over the past decade, however, scientific reports and public health recommendations have been aimed at increasing the number of children who regularly participate in physical activities that enhance and maintain muscle strength (45, 53, 175). For example, the U.S. Department of Health and Human Services recommends that children participate in "muscle strengthening" and "bone strengthening" activities as part of their 60 minutes or more of daily physical activity (45).

Current observations indicate no evidence of decrease in stature in preadolescent boys and girls who resistance train in supervised programs, and epiphyseal plate fractures have not been reported in any prospective youth resistance training study published to date (62). There is no scientific evidence to suggest that the risks associated with competently supervised and well-designed youth resistance training programs are greater than those of other recreational activities that children regularly participate in (57, 79, 117). However, children should not resistance train on their own without guidance from a qualified professional. It has been reported that children are more likely to be injured from home exercise equipment than older age groups due, in part, to unsafe behavior, equipment malfunction, and lack of adult supervision (98, 132). These findings underscore the importance of providing close supervision and safe training equipment for all youth resistance training programs.

Muscle Strength Gains and Other Benefits

Many studies have convincingly shown that children can increase muscular strength above and beyond that accompanying growth and maturation by participating in a well-designed resistance training program (53, 63, 117). Strength gains of roughly 30% to 40% have been observed in children following short-term (8-12 weeks) resistance training programs. Various combinations of sets and repetitions and different training modalities—including child-size weight machines, free weights (barbells and dumbbells), medicine balls, elastic bands, and body weight exercises—have proven to be safe and effective methods of conditioning for healthy children (32, 60, 123).

Since children lack sufficient levels of circulating androgens to stimulate increases in muscle hypertrophy, it appears that neural adaptations are primarily responsible for training-induced strength gains in preadolescents (140, 149). Intrinsic muscle adaptations (i.e., changes in excitation–contraction coupling, myofibrillar packing density, and muscle fiber composition), as well as improvements in motor skill performance and the coordination of the involved muscle groups, could also contribute to gains in strength (149). Longer training periods and more precise measuring techniques (e.g., computerized imaging) may uncover the potential for training-induced muscle hypertrophy in preadolescent youth.

In addition to increasing muscle strength, regular participation in strength-building activities can positively influence several measurable indexes of health and fitness (53). Reports indicate that regular participation in youth resistance training programs may increase bone mineral density (37, 130), enhance cardiorespiratory fitness (181), develop motor performance skills (e.g., vertical jump and sprint speed) (114), and lower elevated blood lipids (182). Others have noted significant improvements in mood and self-appraisal factors in children who participated in a physical activity program that included resistance training and aerobic games (6).

More recently, it has been reported that overweight youth can benefit from participation in resistance training activities (59). Overweight youth seem to enjoy resistance training because it is characterized by short periods of physical activity interspersed with brief rest periods between sets. Although resistance training may not result in a high caloric expenditure, this type of training has proven to be an important component of weight management programs for overweight youth, who often lack the motor skills and confidence to be physically active (16, 157, 162, 180). Clearly, an important first step in encouraging overweight youth to exercise is to increase their confidence in their ability to be physically active, which in turn may lead to an increase in physical activity and hopefully an improvement in body composition. This is particularly important in that overweight youth typically have limited experience participating in structured exercise programs.

Reducing Sport-Related Injuries

Since many sports have a significant strength or power component, it is attractive to assume that a stronger and more powerful child will perform better. Although more applied research regarding the effects of resistance training on youth sport performance is needed, it appears that young athletes who resistance train are more likely to experience success and are less likely to drop out of sport due to frustration, embarrassment, failure, or injury than those who do not (1, 75, 83).

In a growing number of cases, it seems that aspiring young athletes are not prepared for the demands of sport practice and competition (50, 127). On the basis of accelerometer measures, research findings indicate that only 42% of youth age 6 to 11 years achieve the recommended physical activity levels (169). To better prepare boys and girls for sport training and competition, children who have been physically inactive for the past two to three months (e.g., no regular participation in recreational physical activities or sport) should be encouraged to participate in a "preseason" conditioning program (two or three times per week) that includes strength-building activities; aerobic conditioning; flexibility exercises; and drills that enhance agility, balance, coordination, and power. In some cases, youth may need to spend less time practicing sport-specific skills and more time enhancing fundamental fitness abilities in order to establish a sound fitness base prior to sport training. As children gain confidence and competence in their physical abilities and begin to genuinely appreciate the potential health and fitness benefits of physical activity, they may be more likely to participate in sport in later years (151).

Comprehensive conditioning programs that include resistance training have proven to be an effective strategy for reducing sport-related injuries in adolescent athletes, and it is possible that similar effects would be observed in children (82, 84, 118). Although the total elimination of youth sport injuries is an unrealistic goal, an estimated 15% to 50% of acute and overuse injuries associated with youth sport could be prevented if more emphasis were placed on the development of fundamental fitness abilities (i.e., strength, power, aerobic endurance, and agility) than on sport-specific skills (127). This concern may be particularly important for young female athletes who appear to be particularly susceptible to knee injuries (150). Although additional clinical trials are needed to determine the best method for reducing sport-related injuries, it seems prudent for personal trainers to encourage inactive youth to participate in at least six to eight weeks of preparatory fitness conditioning before sport participation.

Guidelines for Youth Resistance Training

The belief that resistance training is unsafe or inappropriate for children is not consistent with the needs of children and the documented benefits associated with this type of training (53, 57, 117). While there is no minimum age for participation in a youth resistance training program, all participants should have the emotional maturity to accept and follow directions and should understand the benefits and risks associated with this type of training. In general, if a child is ready for recreational or sport activities (generally age 7 or 8), he or she should be ready for some type of resistance training. Although a medical examination prior to participation in a resistance training program is not mandatory for apparently healthy children, it is recommended for youth with signs or symptoms suggestive of disease and for youth with known disease (2).

It is important for youth to begin at a level commensurate with their physical abilities. Too often, the volume and intensity of training exceed a child's capabilities, and the prescribed rest periods between workouts are too short for an adequate recovery. This approach may undermine the enjoyment of the resistance training experience and may increase the risk of injury. When introducing preadolescents to resistance training activities, it is always better to underestimate their abilities than to overestimate their abilities and risk an injury. A light to moderate weight that can be lifted for 10 to 15 repetitions appears to be a safe and effective training resistance for children to begin with when they are participating in an introductory resistance training program (54, 61). The following are generally accepted guidelines for youth resistance training:

- Qualified adults should provide supervision and instruction.
- The training environment should be safe and free of hazards.
- Resistance training should be preceded by a 5- to 10-minute dynamic warm-up.
- One to three sets of 6 to 15 repetitions should be performed on a variety of exercises.
- Include exercises for the upper body, lower body and midsection.
- Increase resistance gradually (e.g., about 5% to 10%) as strength improves.
- Resistance train two or three nonconsecutive days per week.
- Children should cool down with less intense calisthenics and static stretching.
- Vary the resistance training program over time to optimize gains and prevent boredom.

Personal trainers working with a group of children should individually prescribe workloads and ask children to do the best they can within the allotted time period instead of setting one workload for all children in the group (e.g., 10 push-ups or 20 pounds [9 kg] on the chest press exercise). Personal trainers and children should work together to determine the workload that is most appropriate for each child's needs and abilities. Although some children may want to see how much weight they can lift during the first workout, their energy and enthusiasm should be redirected toward developing proper form and technique on a variety of exercises. In addition, basic education on fitness room etiquette, realistic outcomes, and safety concerns including appropriate spotting and proper storage of equipment should be part of all youth resistance training programs.

No matter how big or strong a child is, adult resistance training guidelines and training philosophies should not be imposed on young resistance training clients. Parents, teachers, coaches, and personal trainers who work with children should not overlook the importance of having fun and developing a more positive attitude toward resistance training and all types of physical activity. The importance of creating an enjoyable exercise experience for all participants should not be overlooked, since enjoyment has been shown to mediate the effects of youth physical activity programs (47). Long-term adherence to any type of exercise program is more probable when children are internally driven to do their best and when they feel good about their performances. If qualified supervision is present and if age-specific training guidelines are followed, resistance training can be a safe, effective, and enjoyable method of conditioning for preadolescent boys and girls.

Teaching Preadolescent Youth

Although boys and girls should be aware of the potential health- and fitness-related benefits associated with regular physical activity, enthusiastic leadership, creative programming, and age-specific teaching strategies are more likely to get youth "turned on" to physical activity. Personal trainers need to respect children's feelings while appreciating the fact that their thinking is different from that of adults. Personal trainers should not forget about the importance of play, which is one of the ways children learn (24). If personal trainers display physical vitality, relate to children in a positive manner, understand how children think, and participate in activities with children, their efforts are likely to be worthwhile and long lasting. The list on page 470 provides general recommendations for personal trainers who work with children.

Recommendations for Personal Trainers Who Train Children

- Provide close supervision and listen to each child's concerns.
- Speak to children using words they understand.
- Greet each child by name on arrival.
- Praise children for doing a good job.
- Realize that children are active in different ways than adults.
- Design activities that ensure equal participation and enjoyment.
- Gradually progress the fitness program.
- Play down competition and focus on skill improvement, personal successes, and having fun.
- Remind children that it takes time to learn a new skill and get in shape.
- Offer a variety of activities and avoid regimentation.
- Emphasize the importance of adequate hydration.
- Inform parents about the benefits of regular physical activity.

Of note, getting children ready for a fitness workout is not just about low-intensity aerobic exercise and static stretching. A well-designed warm-up can set the tone for the training session and establish a desired tempo for the upcoming activities. If a warm-up is slow and monotonous, then performance during the main physical activities that follow may be less than expected. However, if the warm-up is up-tempo, exciting, and possesses variety, performance during the fitness lessons will likely meet or exceed expectations. Moreover, dynamic warm-up activities that are active, engaging, and challenging and that provide an opportunity for children to gain confidence in their abilities to perform fundamental movement skills are more enjoyable than traditional "stretch and hold" activities (56). A reasonable suggestion is to perform dynamic activities during the warm-up and static stretching during the cool-down.

Since a major objective of youth fitness programs is for physical activity to become a habitual part of children's lives, personal trainers must strive to increase each participant's self-efficacy or self-confidence regarding his or her physical abilities. To achieve this objective, personal trainers should provide clear instructions and demonstrations so that participants can learn new exercises, experience success, and develop a sense of mastery of specific skills. Thus, the focus of personal training sessions should be on positive experiences instead of stressful competitions in which most children fail. It is unlikely that children will continue in a fitness program if they do not understand the instructions or are unable to perform the exercises. The development of successful youth programs requires preparation, coordination, and an awareness of individual differences in stress tolerance.

When children have fun, make friends, and experience success, they are more likely to engage in physical activities as a lifestyle choice.

Older Adults

Men and women 50 years of age and older, typically referred to as *seniors* or *older adults*, may begin sensible conditioning programs, including aerobic endurance training for improved cardiorespiratory fitness and resistance training for increased muscular fitness (3, 5). However, various medical conditions common among older adults call for physician approval and appropriate modifications to the exercise protocols. These include cardiovascular disease, cancer, diabetes, osteoporosis, low back pain, arthritis, depression, obesity, and general frailty.

Benefits of Aerobic Training

Perhaps no other age group can experience more health benefits from exercise than those over 50 years old (144, 189). Because the numerous health benefits associated with aerobic activity are better known, this section summarizes these relationships and then presents more detailed information on the equally important health benefits associated with resistance training.

It is well established that aerobic endurance exercise such as walking, jogging, and cycling is effective for increasing calorie utilization and improving cardiorespiratory fitness (3, 5, 52). An excellent review of cardiorespiratory research revealed that six months of standard endurance exercise may be sufficient to increase older adults' aerobic capacity ($\dot{V}O_2$max) by about 17% (158). Training at higher intensity levels (70% to 80% $\dot{V}O_2$peak) for three months increased $\dot{V}O_2$max by nearly 25%. In addition, aerobic endurance exercise is an excellent means for increasing calorie utilization, and reduced body weight may lessen the risk of high blood pressure, type 2 diabetes, and obesity (3, 5). Other benefits of aerobic fitness include reduced risk of cardiovascular disease, stroke, osteoporosis, certain types of cancer, and psychological stress, as well as improved sleep, digestion, and elimination (144, 189). Researchers have recently discovered that regular aerobic activity increases the volume of both gray and white matter in various regions of the brain after six months of training (35).

Benefits of Resistance Training

Although less well known, the health benefits of resistance exercise are equally impressive especially for older men and women. This section considers some recent research studies showing that resistance training may reduce the risk of many diseases and debilitating conditions frequently experienced by older adults.

Cardiovascular Disease

Coronary artery disease, the leading medical problem in the United States, is particularly prevalent among senior men and women. For most post-coronary patients, resistance training appears to be a safe and productive means of improving muscular fitness and physical performance, as well as for maintaining desirable body weight and positive self-concept. Numerous studies support resistance training for postcoronary patients (26, 58, 68, 77, 86, 101, 120, 163, 173). With respect to prevention, resistance exercise has been shown to reduce the risk of cardiovascular disease (21), as well as to lower the probability of premature all-cause mortality (91, 154).

There are four ways in which resistance training lowers the risk of cardiovascular disease. Foremost among these, regular resistance exercise reduces body fat (27, 88, 121, 147, 183), which may be a major preventive factor in both type 2 diabetes and cardiovascular disease. Due to the positive impact on resting metabolic rate, resistance exercise may have a greater effect on fat loss than aerobic activity (27, 76, 88, 144, 147).

Second, resistance training decreases resting blood pressure (systolic, diastolic, or both) (39, 80, 89, 102, 103). Reductions in diastolic blood pressure average about 4% after several weeks of regular resistance exercise. Reductions in systolic blood pressure average about 3% over a similar training period (102), and two months of circuit resistance training may reduce systolic blood pressure by up to 7 mmHg (millimeters of mercury) (185). In fact, some studies have shown that circuit-type resistance training may be as effective as aerobic exercise for reducing resting blood pressure (18, 160).

The third way in which resistance training benefits cardiovascular health is by improving blood lipid profiles. Although some studies have not shown significant changes in blood lipid levels (109, 110, 160), other research has revealed significantly decreased low-density lipoprotein cholesterol (LDL-cholesterol) in 40- to 55-year-old men (90). Several researchers have reported improved blood lipid profiles following various programs of resistance training (20, 104, 164, 170, 172), and other investigators have found that resistance training produces effects on blood lipids similar to those seen with aerobic exercise (17, 96, 160).

Fourth, resistance exercise enhances vascular condition (137), which facilitates circulation and arterial blood flow. Although the underlying mechanisms are not completely understood, strength training has been shown to improve endothelial function and peak flow-mediated dilation in the brachial artery, which represents an important cardiovascular adaptation. Taken together, the beneficial cardiovascular adaptations associated with appropriate resistance exercise provide significant risk reduction for metabolic syndrome (99, 188) and cardiovascular disease (21).

Research reveals that older adults can significantly improve their cardiorespiratory health by performing regular resistance exercise.

Colon Cancer

Because a slow gastrointestinal transit speed appears to be associated with an increased risk of colon cancer (89), moving food more quickly through the gut should lessen the probability of this disease. Running (38) and resistance training (108) have both been shown to speed up gastrointestinal transit. Therefore, resistance training may be an effective means for addressing age-related gastrointestinal modality disorders, as well as for reducing the risk of colon cancer.

Type 2 Diabetes

As our society becomes more sedentary, type 2 diabetes becomes more prevalent among men and women of all ages. Exercise promotes glucose utilization, and aerobic activity has traditionally been recommended for enhancing glucose uptake (40). However, research on resistance training suggests that resistance exercise may be equally effective for enhancing glucose utilization (48, 86, 129). Resistance training has been shown to improve insulin response (42, 128, 155), improve glycemic control (10, 29, 51), and increase glucose utilization (64, 90) in older men. In addition to stimulating more muscle glucose uptake (115), resistance training may be beneficial for preserving lean body mass (11) and addressing muscle myopathy (49), thereby lessening the severity and even reducing the risk of type 2 diabetes (70).

Osteoporosis

Osteoporosis is a degenerative disease of the skeletal system resulting in a progressive loss of bone proteins and minerals. Several studies have shown that resistance training is effective for maintaining a strong and functional musculoskeletal system that resists deterioration and osteoporosis (15, 36, 112, 156, 161). In fact, research with older men (126) and postmenopausal women (134, 167) indicates that bone loss can be changed to bone gain through regular resistance training.

Low Back Pain

Although not life threatening, low back pain is the most prevalent medical problem in the United States, affecting four out of every five adults during their lifetime. Research (97) has demonstrated a strong positive relationship between weak low back muscles and low back pain. Strengthening the low back (trunk extensor) muscles may alleviate or even eliminate low back pain in some patients (152). With respect to prevention, strong low back muscles provide better musculoskeletal function, support, control, and shock absorption, which should reduce the risk of both low back injury and structural degeneration (72, 131).

Arthritis

Studies (119, 148) indicate that stronger muscles may improve joint function and reduce arthritic discom-

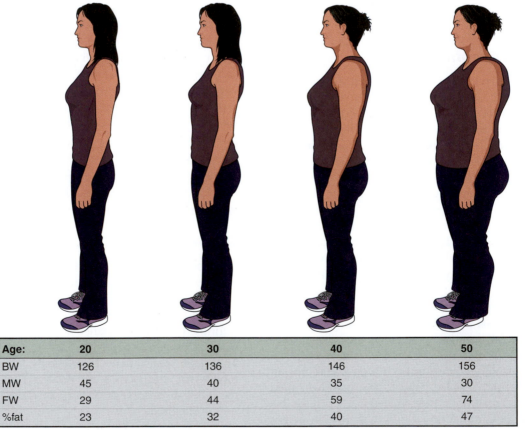

Age:	20	30	40	50
BW	126	136	146	156
MW	45	40	35	30
FW	29	44	59	74
%fat	23	32	40	47

Abbreviations: BW, body weight; FW, fat weight; MW, muscle weight; %fat, percent fat.

FIGURE 18.1 Body weight and body composition change throughout the life of an adult.
Reprinted by permission from Westcott 2003.

fort. In fact, researchers have found that patients with advanced knee osteoarthritis can experience substantial gains in strength (107), and that resistance training actually eases the pain of osteoarthritis and rheumatoid arthritis (94, 111, 171).

Depression

Depression in older individuals may be associated with decreased functionality. In one study (159), senior subjects experienced significant reductions in depression after 10 weeks of resistance training. Although more research is needed in this area, resistance training appears to be beneficial for enhancing self-confidence and counteracting depression in older adults (7, 8).

Muscle Loss and Metabolic Rate Reduction

In addition to reducing the risk of various degenerative diseases, resistance training offers even greater benefits for seniors with respect to replacing muscle tissue and recharging their metabolism. These are probably the most fundamental problems affecting men and women as they age. Adults lose about a half pound (0.22 kg) of muscle per year during their 30s and 40s; this process of muscle loss is referred to as *sarcopenia* (52, 73). Even more disturbing, there is evidence that the rate of muscle loss may double to 1 pound (0.45 kg) per year in people past 50 years of age (134). Figure 18.1 illustrates this insidious process, masked in most adults by their gradually increasing body weight due to progressively greater fat accumulation.

Although the average aging American adds about 10 pounds (4.5 kg) of body weight each decade of adult life, this actually represents approximately 5 to 10 pounds (2-4.5 kg) less muscle and 15 to 20 pounds (7-9 kg) more fat. Moreover, the loss of muscle may be partly responsible for the gain in fat. Researchers (52, 106) have found a 2% to 4% per decade reduction in resting metabolic rate attributed to decreased amounts of muscle tissue. A slower resting metabolism means that some calories previously used by high-energy muscle tissue are no longer needed and are therefore stored as fat.

Clearly, it would be highly desirable for people to perform some basic resistance exercises to prevent muscle loss and metabolic slowdown. Resistance training can help maintain muscle tissue that enables physical activity and enhances energy utilization throughout the senior years. In fact, resistance training is the only type of exercise that can maintain muscle and metabolism as people age and should therefore be an essential component of every senior fitness program. Numerous studies (65, 67, 74, 78, 85, 93, 122, 168, 177, 183, 186) have demonstrated significant increases in muscle mass following several weeks of standard strength training, and many studies (23, 27, 88, 113, 147, 174) have shown significant elevations in resting metabolic rate. Increases in resting energy expenditure average 7% and appear to take effect following the first few workouts (27, 76, 88, 124, 147, 174). Resistance training has also been shown to increase fat utilization during and after the exercise session (138).

Mitochondrial Function

Circuit strength training is a time-efficient protocol in which participants perform a set of exercise for one muscle group (e.g., quadriceps) followed (with minimal rest) by a set of exercise for a different muscle group (e.g., hamstrings), and so on for 8 to 12 exercises that cumulatively address the major muscle groups. Although each exercise set represents an anaerobic activity, the brief rest between successive exercises imparts an aerobic component to the circuit training session (typically completed in 20 to 30 minutes). Recent research has demonstrated that circuit strength training can increase the mitochondrial content and oxidative capacity of trained muscle tissue (141, 144, 166). Mitochondria serve as the powerhouse of each muscle cell. Aging is associated with genetic changes that cause various degrees of mitochondrial impairment with respect to energy production and muscle performance. One study has demonstrated a reversal in mitochondrial dysfunction following six months of progressive resistance exercise (125). The older adults in this study (mean age 68 years) experienced reversal of gene expression in 179 genes associated with age and exercise, resulting in mitochondrial characteristics similar to those of moderately active young adults (mean age 24 years). This would appear to be a compelling reason for senior men and women to engage in circuit strength training as well as in standard resistance exercise.

> Resistance training has been shown to reduce the risk of several degenerative problems that are common to older adults, including sarcopenia, osteopenia, high blood pressure, unfavorable blood lipid profiles, insulin insensitivity, delayed gastrointestinal transit, low back pain, and metabolic syndrome.

Functional Abilities

Many older adults experience a reduction in functional abilities that negatively affects their activities of daily living. Numerous studies have shown that resistance training can effectively reverse physical dysfunctions associated with sedentary aging by increasing muscle strength, power, and performance factors (13, 21, 87, 88, 100, 178).

Resistance Training Guidelines for Seniors

Generally speaking, seniors should perform resistance training two or three nonconsecutive days per week. Using both single- and multiple-joint movements, seniors may perform single or multiple sets for a variety of exercises that address at least the following major muscle groups: quadriceps, hamstrings, gluteals, pectoralis major, latissimus dorsi, deltoids, biceps, triceps, erector spinae, and rectus abdominis. Personal trainers should have seniors use controlled exercise speeds (typically 4 to 6 seconds per repetition) and full movement ranges (excluding positions in which discomfort is experienced).

Seniors may train with a wide range of repetitions depending on their experience and physical condition. Beginners and less fit seniors may start with relatively light weight loads that permit many repetitions, whereas more advanced seniors may perform fewer repetitions with higher resistance (5). As shown in figure 18.2, an acceptable resistance range may extend from 60% to 90% of maximum. Generally, older adults can perform about 16 repetitions with 60% of maximum resistance and about four repetitions with 90% of maximum resistance (184). Older adults are advised to begin their strength training program with exercise resistances that permit 10 to 15 repetitions, corresponding to approximately 75% to 60% of maximum resistance. When 15 repetitions can be completed, the resistance should be increased by about 5% (5).

The key to safe and successful senior resistance training experiences is competent instruction and careful supervision. With respect to teaching technique, we recommend the instructional model shown on page 475.

Aerobic Endurance Training Guidelines for Seniors

Adults of all ages are advised to perform aerobic endurance exercise for cardiorespiratory health and fitness (5). The recommended training frequency is two to five days per week, and the recommended exercise duration is 20 to 60 minutes per session. An exercise intensity of 60% to 90% of maximum heart rate is acceptable, but training at about 75% of maximum heart rate is generally prescribed (5). Because maximum heart rate decreases as people age (approximately 10 heartbeats per decade), the relative exercise intensity should be essentially the same for young, middle, and older adults. Of course, seniors who have limited cardiorespiratory fitness must begin with shorter exercise duration and lower training intensity. For some older adults, this may be only 5 to 10 minutes of physical activity at approximately 40% of maximum heart rate.

The recently revised recommendations from the American College of Sports Medicine and the American Heart Association (81) present two aerobic activity protocols that may be performed exclusively or alternated on different training days. The first calls for 30 minutes of moderate-intensity endurance exercise (e.g., walking) five days a week. The second calls for 20 minutes of vigorous-intensity endurance exercise (e.g., jogging) three days a week. We recommend that older adults who are beginning an exercise program perform lower-effort aerobic activities for a longer duration (e.g., 30 minutes of

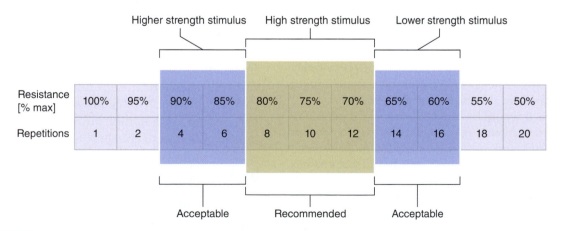

FIGURE 18.2 Resistance and repetition relationships for recommended resistance training protocols for older adults.
Reprinted by permission from Westcott and Baechle 2010.

Instructional Model for Teaching Seniors

A successful educational and motivational strategy for older adult exercisers should include

- understandable performance objectives,
- concise instruction with precise demonstration,
- attentive supervision,
- appropriate assistance,
- a request to perform one task at a time,
- gradual progression in complexity,
- positive reinforcement following correct performances,
- specific feedback,
- careful questioning, and
- pre- and postexercise dialogue (which should always involve the key phrases, such as Hello, Good-bye, Thank you, and the client's name).

Reprinted by permission from Westcott and Baechle 2010.

moderate-intensity activity) prior to progressing to higher-effort aerobic activities for a shorter duration (e.g., 20 minutes of vigorous-intensity activity). It is also advisable to combine these training protocols, for example by performing vigorous-intensity exercise sessions on Mondays and Fridays and moderate-intensity exercise sessions on Wednesdays and Saturdays.

Although the training protocol based on percentage of maximum heart rate is easy to monitor and generally appropriate for older adults, this method has certain limitations. For example, a senior with normal heart function could have a maximum heart rate up to 30 beats/min above or 30 beats/min below that predicted by the formula 220 minus age (187). Also, people taking certain medications, such as beta blockers, have lower maximum heart rates due to drug-induced bradycardia. Consequently, assessing the exercise intensity in older adults by both their heart rate response and their personal effort level is advised. The latter may be best assessed by means of the Borg scale of perceived exertion, which provides a subjective assessment to complement heart rate monitoring (19). Ideally, a healthy senior exercising at approximately 75% of maximum heart rate will report a perceived exertion rating of about 13 (range 12 to 14 on the original rating of perceived exertion [RPE] scale). However, a healthy senior exerciser whose heart rate is *above* 75% of age-predicted maximum but who reports a *low level* of perceived exertion (e.g., 10-11, "fairly light") should probably not be advised to reduce the training intensity. On the other hand, a senior exerciser whose heart rate is *below* 75% of age-predicted maximum but who reports a *high level*

of perceived exertion (e.g., 15-16, "hard") should definitely be advised to reduce the training intensity. (Refer to chapter 16 for more information on RPE scales.)

Another means of monitoring seniors' exercise effort is the talk test. Older adults who can talk in short- to medium-length sentences while they are exercising are probably performing their aerobic activity at the appropriate level of intensity. If they have difficulty carrying on a simple conversation during the activity, they are most likely exercising harder than necessary.

Screening and Program Design for Seniors

Resistance training is a vital physical activity for older adults. In addition to increasing muscle mass, muscle strength, and resting metabolism, resistance exercise provides benefits for the musculoskeletal system, cardiorespiratory system, gastrointestinal system, and endocrine system. Aerobic endurance training is equally important for senior men and women to enhance heart health and help with weight management. Unfortunately, some mature individuals may have already experienced physical or mental conditions that make it difficult for them to participate in standard resistance and aerobic exercise programs. The first step in every case is to check with the client's personal physician for specific exercise guidelines and training modifications. With this information the personal trainer can design an individualized program that is safe and appropriate for the older adult. When training seniors, of course, the personal trainer must be especially observant for any exercise contraindications or undesirable musculoskeletal or cardiorespiratory responses. The personal trainer should keep careful and detailed records of senior clients' exercise sessions and fitness assessments. Such information provides important educational material for future program design and serves as a powerful motivational tool for older clients.

Exercise Order

If seniors perform both resistance and aerobic exercise, they should begin with aerobic activity (including warm-up and cool-down phases), then do resistance training, and conclude with static stretches. If they do only resistance training, they should do 5 to 10 minutes of light aerobic activity before the resistance exercises. In both exercise sequences, the less strenuous aerobic activity provides a warm-up for the more strenuous resistance exercise. Flexibility exercises should be performed after the resistance exercises to provide a muscle-relaxing conclusion to the training session.

Safety and Comfort

Certain conditions common to seniors can affect the comfort and safety of exercise. Table 18.1 lists some of these conditions and the adjustments that clients or personal trainers can make to promote a safe exercise experience.

Pregnant Women

Women who are pregnant may seek out exercise programs for a number of reasons. They may feel self-conscious about their changing body, be concerned about having a healthy baby, want to stay in shape throughout their pregnancy, want to be able to handle the physical rigors of labor and delivery, or need additional social interactions and support during this new phase in their life. Healthy pregnant women without complications who exercise regularly may continue participating in appropriately adjusted sessions of physical activity, thereby maintaining cardiovascular and muscular fitness

TABLE 18.1 Conditions Common to Older Adults and Suggested Adaptations

Condition	Adaptations
Dry skin	Clients can apply lotion to elbows, knees, and contact points before exercising.
Poor balance	Clients should begin with weight-supporting machine exercises before progressing to weight-bearing free weight exercises and functional training.
	Clients should begin with weight-supporting aerobic endurance exercise such as stationary cycling before progressing to weight-bearing alternatives such as treadmill walking and stair climbing.
	Clients should avoid hard-to-control exercises such as lunges or step-ups.
	Clients can perform exercises in a seated or lying position instead of standing.
Propensity for injuries	Clients should train only in uncluttered facilities.
	Clients should use controlled movement speeds.
	Clients should emphasize proper posture and exercise positioning.
Susceptibility to colds and flu	Clients should drink plenty of fluids.
	Clients should obtain ample rest and sleep (at least 8 h a night).
	Clients should shower or wash face and hands after exercise session.
Reduced flexibility	Clients should warm up for 5 to 10 min prior to exercise.
	Clients should perform appropriate stretching exercises at end of training session.
	Clients should avoid exercises that require extreme movement ranges such as lunges.
Reduced tolerance to heat and humidity	Clients should train in climate-controlled facilities whenever possible.
	Clients should schedule training sessions earlier in the day.
	Clients should drink plenty of fluids, especially water.
	Clients should wear lightweight and light-colored exercise attire.
Difficulties seeing and hearing	Personal trainers should speak clearly and concisely with sufficient volume.
	Personal trainers should use large-print materials and workout cards.
	Personal trainers should give precise exercise demonstrations and manual assistance when necessary.
	Personal trainers should frequently ask clients if they understand instructions and exercise performance procedures.

throughout pregnancy and postpartum (4, 5).

Previously sedentary women may also benefit from regular exercise during pregnancy, although a program consistent with their physical capabilities should involve professional guidance, motivation, and a gradual increase in physical activity. Of note, some pregnant women prefer to start exercising during the second trimester after the nausea, vomiting, and fatigue from the first trimester subside (105). In any case, pregnant women should consult with their health care provider before initiating an exercise program or modifying a current program. In the presence of obstetric or medical complications, it may be necessary to alter the training program as determined by the client's obstetrician.

Benefits of Exercise During Pregnancy

Most pregnant women who follow their physician's recommendations can attain maternal health and fitness benefits while subjecting the developing fetus to minimal risk (5). The following are some of the benefits for pregnant women who engage in properly designed prenatal exercise programs (5, 145).

- Improved cardiorespiratory and muscular fitness
- Facilitated recovery from labor
- Faster return to prepregnancy weight, strength, and flexibility levels
- Reduced postpartum belly
- More energy reserve
- Fewer obstetric interventions
- Shorter active phase of labor and less pain
- Less weight gain
- Improved mood and self-concept
- Reduced feelings of stress, anxiety, and depression
- Increased likelihood of adopting permanent healthy lifestyle habits

Participation in an exercise program may also reduce the risk of developing conditions associated with pregnancy including **preeclampsia** (pregnancy-induced hypertension) and gestational diabetes mellitus (a form of diabetes first diagnosed during pregnancy) (44, 145). It appears that the physiological and psychological benefits associated with regular physical activity may play a role in reducing the risk of preeclampsia (145). Moreover, the favorable effects of regular physical activity on insulin secretion, insulin sensitivity, and glucose metabolism may improve glucose tolerance and thereby reduce a women's risk of developing gestational diabetes mellitus. Exercise training may also be beneficial in preventing or treating other conditions including low back pain, pelvic floor muscle dysfunction, pregnancy-related urinary incontinence, and chronic musculoskeletal conditions (145). In the absence of either medical or obstetric complications, exercise during pregnancy appears to be associated with many of the physical and psychosocial health benefits typically observed in nonpregnant women.

> **Healthy pregnant women should be encouraged to participate in daily physical activity throughout pregnancy.**

Fetal Response to Exercise

Some research has revealed reduced birth weight in babies whose mothers performed high-intensity exercise throughout their pregnancy (33). The lower birth weight was approximately 300 to 350 g (10-12 ounces) and apparently resulted from a decreased amount of subcutaneous fat in the newborn. More moderate exercise sessions may therefore be advisable for pregnant women.

Vigorous exercise during pregnancy is associated with a 5 to 15 beat/minute increase in fetal heart rate, but there are no documented adverse fetal effects related to exercise-induced fetal heart rate changes (4). With respect to preterm labor, the American College of Obstetricians and Gynecologists states that in the majority of healthy pregnant women without additional risk factors for preterm labor, exercise does not increase either baseline uterine activity or the incidence of preterm labor or delivery (4).

Accommodating Mechanical and Physiological Changes During Pregnancy

Medical and fitness organizations provide the following recommendations for accommodating the cardiovascular, respiratory, mechanical, metabolic, and thermoregulatory changes experienced during normal pregnancy (4, 5).

Cardiovascular Response

Although pregnancy alters the relationship between heart rate and oxygen consumption, general heart rate ranges that correspond to moderate-intensity exercise have been developed for pregnant women (43). For example, heart rate ranges of 135 to 150 beats/min and 130 to 145 beats/min have been recommended for women between ages 20 and 29 and between ages 30 and 39, respectively (5, 43). Personal trainers can also use the RPE scale to prescribe aerobic exercise intensity (19). Generally, an RPE rating on the original scale between 12 and 14 ("somewhat hard") seems appropriate for aerobic conditioning during pregnancy (5). At this intensity, pregnant women should be able to keep up a conversation while exercising. Of course, exercise programs need to be individually prescribed, and women may need to adjust the exercise intensity, duration, or both on any given day depending on how they feel.

After the first trimester of pregnancy, the back-lying (supine) position results in restricted venous return of blood to the heart because of the increasingly larger uterus. This position reduces cardiac output and may cause supine hypotensive syndrome. Consequently, exercises performed on the back should be phased out of the client's training program before the start of the second trimester. These include abdominal curls, bench presses, supine exercises on the stability ball, and stretching exercises with the back on the floor.

As an alternative, women can do curl-downs while splinting their abdomen for safety and support (see figure 18.3). Additionally, they can perform abdominal exercises in the crawling or side-lying position (see figures 18.4 and 18.5) and upper and lower body resistance training exercises in the seated position. For example, instead of performing the barbell bench press exercise to enhance upper body strength, pregnant women can use the vertical chest press machine or perform wall push-ups or a rubber cord exercise in the seated position to strengthen the same muscle groups.

Because of changes in the center of gravity later in pregnancy, it also may be advisable for some pregnant women to use weight machines, which provide more stability and support than the corresponding free weight exercises (e.g., machine biceps curl rather than standing dumbbell curl). This recommendation may be particularly important for previously sedentary women who want to resistance train.

Respiratory Response

Pregnant women may increase their minute ventilation by almost 50%, resulting in 10% to 20% more oxygen utilization at rest (4). Consequently, less oxygen is available for aerobic activity. Additionally, as the pregnancy progresses, the enlarging uterus interferes with diaphragm movement, increasing the effort of breathing and decreasing both subjective workload and maximum exercise performance. Personal trainers should adjust pregnant women's exercise program accordingly to avoid training at high

levels of fatigue or reaching physical exhaustion. Pregnant women should be cautioned to avoid the Valsalva maneuver because breath-holding during exertion places excessive pressure on the abdominal contents and pelvic floor. A general resistance training recommendation is to exhale on exertion or in the "lifting" phase of every exercise repetition. (See chapter 13 for additional breathing guidelines.)

Mechanical Response

As the uterus and breasts become larger during pregnancy, a woman's center of mass changes. This may adversely affect her balance, body control, and movement mechanics in some physical activities. Consequently, exercises requiring balance and agility should be carefully prescribed, with special attention to activity selection during the third trimester of pregnancy.

Although any activity that presents the potential for falling or even mild abdominal trauma should be avoided, some activities designed to enhance physical balance may be beneficial for pregnant women. For example, personal trainers may include "centering" activities, such as physical balance, deep abdominal breathing, and mental focus, that may help women achieve physical balance during pregnancy and help them become more aware of body movements during exercise (41). Because of joint laxity during pregnancy, exercises should be performed slowly and in a controlled manner to avoid damage to the joints. Furthermore, pregnant women should avoid participating in activities that present a high risk of falling or abdominal trauma. They should also avoid scuba diving because of the risk of decompression sickness to the fetus (4).

Although it is important to strengthen all the major muscle groups, personal trainers should emphasize abdominal and pelvic floor strength because these muscles provide the basis for postural support and prepare a woman for delivery (41). For example, strengthening the transverse abdominis, which is the deepest abdominal muscle located underneath the rectus abdominis and obliques, helps to support the lumbar spine and prepare a woman for the pushing stage of birth. Women can strengthen the transverse abdominis by blowing air out through the mouth while compressing the abdomen. A good image of this activity is that of shortening the distance between the navel and the spine by "sucking in" the abdomen. This exercise can be performed in the seated position or the crawling position on hands and knees.

Pelvic floor exercises **(Kegels)** are another important element of resistance training during pregnancy. These exercises involve tightening and

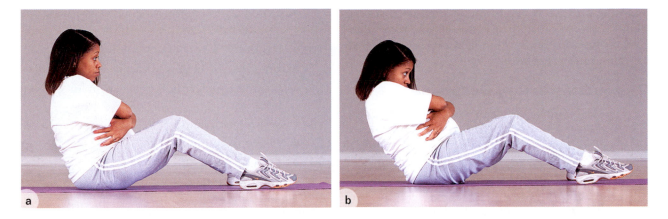

FIGURE 18.3 Curl-down exercise with the abdomen splinted: *(a)* beginning position and *(b)* final position.

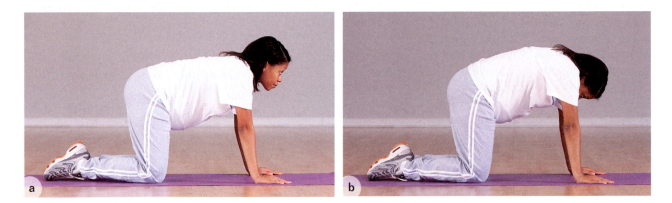

FIGURE 18.4 Abdominal exercise performed in crawling position: *(a)* beginning position and *(b)* final position.

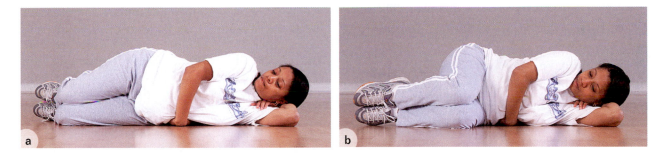

FIGURE 18.5 Abdominal exercise performed in side-lying position: *(a)* beginning position and *(b)* final position.

relaxing muscle groups in the pelvic region. With proper training, a woman can learn not only how to contract these muscles, but also how to relax them so that the baby can be delivered more easily (41). Specific guidelines for performing Kegel exercises are beyond the scope of this chapter but are available in most books on pregnancy.

Metabolic Response

The need for more oxygen during pregnancy is paralleled by the need for more energy substrate. Pregnant women typically use an extra 300 kilo-calories per day to meet the increased metabolic requirements for homeostasis of their expanded life functions. During exercise, pregnant women also use carbohydrates at a higher rate than women who are not pregnant (34). The obvious indication is for pregnant clients to attain an adequate intake of nutrient-dense foods and stay well hydrated through a balanced but expanded nutritional program. Of note, pregnant women should be sure to take in sufficient quantities of calcium, vitamin D, iron, and folic acid to achieve a healthy pregnancy outcome (176). Since the negative effects of poor maternal nutrition can be devastating, all pregnant women should receive nutritional counseling from a qualified professional to develop healthy habits that can be continued postpartum.

Thermoregulatory Response

Pregnancy elevates a woman's basal metabolic rate and heat production, which may be further increased by exercise. Exercise-associated rises in body temperature may be most likely in the first trimester of pregnancy. During this period, pregnant clients should be sure to facilitate heat dissipation through adequate hydration, appropriate clothing, and optimal environmental surroundings. If a client feels overheated or fatigued during an exercise session, the personal trainer should decrease the exercise intensity and begin the cool-down. Severe headaches, dizziness, and disorientation are indications of potential serious conditions that require referral to a client's health care provider. Clearly, pregnant women should be made aware of safe exercise guidelines and should know when to reduce the exercise intensity or stop exercising.

Contraindications for Exercise

Women without obstetric or medical complications can continue to exercise during pregnancy and derive related health and fitness benefits (4). However, certain conditions present absolute contraindications to exercise. These include the following:

- Pregnancy-induced hypertension (preeclampsia)
- Ruptured membranes
- Premature labor during the current pregnancy
- Persistent bleeding after 12 weeks
- A cervix that dilates ahead of schedule (incompetent cervix)
- Significant heart disease or restrictive lung disease
- Multiple-birth pregnancy that creates a risk of premature labor
- A placenta that blocks the cervix after 26 weeks

Adapted from the American College of Obstetricians and Gynecologists 2002 (4).

There are also relative contraindications to exercise that should be evaluated by the client's physician before participation in an exercise:

- Poorly controlled type 1 diabetes, seizures, hypertension, or hyperthyroidism
- Extreme morbid obesity

- Extremely low body weight (body mass index <12 kg/m^2)
- History of a very sedentary lifestyle
- Unevaluated maternal cardiac dysrhythmia
- Intrauterine growth restriction in current pregnancy
- Severe anemia
- Heavy smoking
- Chronic bronchitis
- Orthopedic limitations

Adapted from the American College of Obstetricians and Gynecologists 2002 (4).

Additionally, any of the following conditions is a reason to discontinue exercise and seek medical advice during pregnancy (5):

- Any signs of bloody discharge from the vagina
- Dyspnea before exertion
- Headaches or unexplained dizziness
- Chest pain
- Muscle weakness
- Calf pain or swelling
- Preterm labor
- Decreased fetal movement
- Amniotic fluid leakage

Exercise Guidelines

General exercise safety guidelines for pregnant women are outlined on page 481. Although additional clinical trials are needed to further examine the effects of different types, frequencies, and intensities of exercise on the maternal–fetal unit, the following exercise guidelines apply to healthy pregnant women without exercise contraindications (4, 5):

- Perform at least 15 minutes of moderate-intensity physical activity per day and gradually increase to 30 minutes per day of accumulated physical activity on at least three, if not all, days of the week.
- Resistance training for the major muscle groups can be performed provided that a resistance permitting multiple repetitions (e.g., 12-15) is used and isometric contractions are avoided.
- Avoid exercise in the supine position after the first trimester.
- Exercise should not continue past the point of fatigue and should never reach exhaustive levels.

General Exercise Safety Guidelines for Pregnant Women

- Check with your health care provider before you begin exercising.
- Exercise at a comfortable level at which you can maintain a conversation.
- Do not exercise if you have a fever.
- See your health care provider if you experience bleeding, a large amount of discharge, or swelling in your face and hands.
- Avoid lying on your back after the third month.
- Avoid straining or stretching to the point of discomfort.
- Wear proper footwear, and dress in layers.
- Use equipment in good condition.
- Drink 8 cups (2 L) of water a day and avoid exercising in hot, humid conditions.
- Avoid fatigue and overtraining.

Adapted from Cowlin (41).

- Dynamic, rhythmic physical activities such as stationary cycling or walking are favored for reducing injury risk and continuing the exercise program throughout pregnancy.
- Sports and activities that present the potential for even mild abdominal trauma or loss of balance should be avoided. Examples of sports and activities to avoid include soccer, basketball, horseback riding, scuba diving, in-line skating, outdoor cycling, and plyometric training.
- Large increases in body temperature should be minimized through adequate hydration, appropriate clothing, and optimal environmental surroundings during exercise.
- Because many of the physiologic and morphologic changes of pregnancy persist four to six weeks postpartum, women can gradually resume physical activity programs during the initial postpartum period until prepregnancy fitness levels are achieved.

Conclusion

Preadolescent youth, older adults, and pregnant women should be encouraged to participate regularly in physical activity programs that enhance and maintain cardiorespiratory and musculoskeletal fitness. Although the fundamental principles of exercise training are similar for individuals of all ages and abilities, there are unique considerations specific to each population. Personal trainers should understand and appreciate clients' individual needs and concerns so they can develop safe, effective, and enjoyable physical activity programs that are consistent with needs, abilities, and interests of preadolescent youth, older adults, and pregnant women.

Study Questions

1. Following eight weeks of regular strength training, a 10-year-old boy made significant gains in chest press and leg press performance. Which of the following is most responsible for his training-induced gains in muscle strength?

   A. muscle hypertrophy

   B. muscle hyperplasia

   C. neural adaptations

   D. enhanced body composition

2. Which of the following resistance training adaptations will lower the risk of cardiovascular disease in a 70-year-old client?

   I. reduced body fat

   II. decreased resting systolic blood pressure

   III. improved endothelial function

   IV. decreased high-density lipoprotein cholesterol

   A. I, II, and III only

   B. I, II, and IV only

   C. I, III, and IV only

   D. II, III, and IV only

3. Which of the following training protocols is the most appropriate goal for previously inactive older adults?

   A. aerobic exercise only, five days per week

   B. resistance exercise only, four days per week

   C. resistance exercise four days per week and aerobic endurance exercise two days per week

   D. resistance exercise two days per week and aerobic endurance exercise three days per week

4. Which of the following exercise recommendations is appropriate for a healthy pregnant client?

   I. Gradually increase to 30 minutes per day of accumulated physical activity on at least three days per week.

   II. Strength training for the major muscle groups can be performed provided a resistance that permits multiple repetitions (e.g., 12-15) is used.

   III. Activities such as horseback riding, in-line skating, and outdoor cycling can be performed provided the exercise intensity is moderate.

   IV. Avoid exercise in the supine position after the second trimester.

   A. I and IV only

   B. I and II only

   C. II and III only

   D. III and IV only

5. Which of the following chest exercises would be most appropriate for women in their second trimester of pregnancy?

   A. dumbbell bench presses

   B. standing cable crossovers

   C. dumbbell chest flys

   D. barbell bench presses

Applied Knowledge Question

Describe general resistance exercise guidelines, safety concerns, and exercise adherence strategies for an 8-year-old female, a 65-year-old male, and a healthy pregnant woman who are members at your fitness center.

References

1. Abernethy, L., and C. Bleakley. 2007. Strategies to prevent injury in adolescent sport: A systematic review. *British Journal of Sports Medicine* 41: 627-638.

2. American Academy of Pediatrics. 2008. Strength training by children and adolescents. *Pediatrics* 121: 835-840.

3. American Association of Cardiovascular and Pulmonary Rehabilitation. 2006. *AACVPR Cardiac Rehabilitation Resource Manual.* Champaign, IL: Human Kinetics.

4. American College of Obstetricians and Gynecologists. 2002. Exercise during pregnancy and the postpartum period. *International Journal of Gynecology and Obstetrics* 77: 79-81.

5. American College of Sports Medicine. 2010. *ACSM's Guidelines for Exercise Testing and Prescription,* 8th ed. Philadelphia: Lippincott Williams & Wilkins.

6. Annesi, J., A. Faigenbaum, W. Westcott, A. Smith, J. Unruh, and G. Franklin. 2007. Effects of the Youth Fit For Life protocol on physiological, mood, self-appraisal, and voluntary physical activity changes in African American preadolescents: Contrasting after-school care and physical education formats. *International Journal of Clinical and Health Psychology* 7: 641-659.

7. Annesi, J., and W. Westcott. 2007. Relations of physical self-concept and muscular strength with resistance exercise-induced feeling state scores in older women. *Perceptual and Motor Skills* 104: 183-190.

8. Annesi, J., W. Westcott, and S. Gann. 2004. Preliminary evaluation of a 10-week resistance and cardiovascular exercise protocol on physiological and psychological measures for a sample of older women. *Perceptual and Motor Skills* 98: 163-170.

9. Bailey, R., J. Olsen, S. Pepper, J. Porszasz, T. Barstow, and D. Cooper. 1995. The level and tempo of children's physical activities: An observational study. *Medicine and Science in Sports and Exercise* 27: 1033-1041.

10. Baldi, J., and N. Snowling. 2003. Resistance training improves glycemic control in obese type 2 diabetic men. *International Journal of Sports Medicine* 24: 419-423.

11. Ballor, D., V. Katch, M. Becque, and C. Marks. 1988. Resistance weight training during caloric restriction enhances lean body weight maintenance. *American Journal of Clinical Nutrition* 47: 19-25.

12. Bar-Or, O. 1983. *Sports Medicine for the Practitioner.* New York: Springer-Verlag.

13. Barry, B., and R. Carson. 2004. The consequences of resistance training for movement control in older adults. *Journals of Gerontology Series A: Biological Sciences and Medical Sciences* 59: 730-754.

14. Behm, D., A. Faigenbaum, B. Falk, and P. Klentrou. 2008. Canadian Society for Exercise Physiology position paper: Resistance training in children and adolescents. *Appl Physiol Nutr Metab* 33: 547-561.

15. Bell, N., R. Godsen, and D. Henry. 1988. The effects of muscle-building exercise on vitamin D and mineral metabolism. *Journal of Bone and Mineral Research* 3: 369-373.

16. Benson, A., M. Torade, and M. Fiatarone Singh. 2008. The effect of high-intensity progressive resistance training on adiposity in children: A randomized controlled trial. *International Journal of Obesity* 32:1016-1027.

17. Blessing, D., M. Stone, and R. Byrd. 1987. Blood lipid and hormonal changes from jogging and weight training of middle-aged men. *Journal of Applied Sport Science Research* 1: 25-29.

18. Blumenthal, J., W. Siegel, and M. Appelbaum. 1991. Failure of exercise to reduce blood pressure in patients with mild hypertension. *Journal of the American Medical Association* 266: 2098-2101.

19. Borg, G. 1998. *Borg's Perceived Exertion and Pain Scales.* Champaign, IL: Human Kinetics.

20. Boyden, T., R. Pamenter, S. Going, T. Lohman, M. Hall, L. Houtkooper, J. Bunt, C. Ritenbaugh, and M. Aickin. 1993. Resistance exercise training is associated with decreases in serum low-density lipoprotein cholesterol levels in premenopausal women. *Archives of Internal Medicine* 153: 97-100.

21. Braith, R., and K. Stewart. 2006. Resistance exercise training: Its role in the prevention of cardiovascular disease. *Circulation* 113: 2642-2650.

22. British Association of Exercise and Sport Sciences. 2004. BASES position statement on guidelines for resistance exercise in young people. *Journal of Sports Sciences* 22: 383-390.

23. Broeder, C., K. Burrhus, L. Svanevik, and J. Wilmore. 1992. The effects of either high-intensity resistance or endurance training on resting metabolic rate. *American Journal of Clinical Nutrition* 55: 802-810.

24. Burdette, H., and R. Whitaker. 2005. Resurrecting free play in young children. *Archives of Pediatric and Adolescence Medicine* 159: 46-50.

25. Bureau of Transportation Statistics. 2003. National household travel survey. www.bts.gov/programs/national_household_travel_survey. Accessed December 8, 2009.

26. Butler, R., W. Baierwalter, and F. Rogers. 1987. The cardiovascular response to circuit weight training in patients with cardiac disease. *Journal of Cardiopulmonary Rehabilitation* 7: 402-409.

27. Campbell, W., M. Crim, V. Young, and W. Evans. 1994. Increased energy requirements and changes in body composition with resistance training in older adults. *American Journal of Clinical Nutrition* 60: 167-175.

28. Carnethon, M., M. Gulati, and P. Greenland. Prevalence and cardiovascular disease correlates of low cardiorespiratory fitness in adolescents and adults. *Journal of the American Medical Association* 294: 2981-2988.

29. Castaneda, C., J. Layne, L. Munoz-Orians, P. Gordon, J. Walsmith, M. Foldvari, R. Roubenoff, K. Tucker, and M. Nelson. 2002. A randomized controlled trial of resistance exercise training to improve glycemic control in older adults with type 2 diabetes. *Diabetes Care* 25: 2335-2341.

30. Cavil, N., S. Biddle, and J. Sallis. 2001, Health enhancing physical activity for young people. Statement of the United Kingdom Expert Consensus Conference. *Pediatric Exercise Science* 13: 12-25.

31. Centers for Disease Control and Prevention. 2005. Participation in high school physical education – United States, 1991-2003. *Journal of School Health* 75: 47-49.

32. Chu, D., A. Faigenbaum, and J. Falkel. 2006. *Progressive Plyometrics for Kids.* Monterey, CA: Healthy Learning.

33. Clapp, J., and E. Capeless. 1990. Neonatal morphometrics after endurance exercise during pregnancy. *American Journal of Obstetrics and Gynecology* 163: 1805-1811.

34. Clapp, J., B. Seaward, R. Sleamaker, and J. Hiser. 1988. Maternal physiologic adaptations to early human pregnancy. *American Journal of Obstetrics and Gynecology* 159: 1456-1460.

35. Colcombe, S., K. Erickson, P. Scalf, J. Kim, R. Prakash, E. McAuley, S. Elavsky, D. Marquez, L. Hu, and A. Kramer. 2006. Aerobic exercise training increases brain volume in aging humans. *Journals of Gerontology Series A: Biological Sciences and Medical Science* 61: 1166-1170.

36. Colletti, L., J. Edwards, L. Gordon, J. Shary, and N. Bell. 1989. The effects of muscle-building exercise on bone mineral density of the radius, spine and hip in young men. *Calcified Tissue International* 45: 12-14.

37. Conroy, B., W. Kraemer, C. Maresh, S. Fleck, M. Stone, A. Fry, P. Miller, and G. Dalsky. 1993. Bone mineral density in elite junior Olympic weightlifters. *Medicine and Science in Sports and Exercise* 25: 1103-1109.

38. Cordain, L., R. Latin, and J. Behnke. 1986. The effects of an aerobic running program on bowel transit time. *Journal of Sports Medicine* 26: 101-104.

39. Cornelissen, V., and R. Fagard. 2005. Effect of resistance training on resting blood pressure: A meta-analysis of randomized controlled trials. *Journal of Hypertension* 23: 251-259.

40. Council on Exercise of the American Diabetes Association. 1990. Technical review: Exercise and NIDDM. *Diabetes Care* 13: 785-789.

41. Cowlin, A.F. 2002. *Women's Fitness Program Development.* Champaign, IL: Human Kinetics.

42. Craig, B., J. Everhart, and R. Brown. 1989. The influence of high-resistance training on glucose tolerance in young and elderly subjects. *Mechanisms of Ageing and Development* 49: 147-157.

43. Davies, G.L., M. Wolfe, F. Mottola, and C. MacKinnon. 2003. Society of Obstetricians and Gynecologists of Canada, SOGC Clinical Practice Obstetrics Committee. Joint SOGC/CSEP clinical practice guideline. Exercise in pregnancy in the postpartum period. *Canadian Journal of Applied Physiology* 28: 330-341.

44. Dempsey, J., C. Butler, and M. Williams. 2005. No need for a pregnant pause: Physical activity may reduce the occurrence of gestational diabetes and preeclampsia. *Exercise and Sport Sciences Reviews* 33: 141-149.

45. Department of Health and Human Services. 2008. *Physical Activity Guidelines for Americans.* Washington, DC: Author.

46. Dietz, W. Overweight in childhood and adolescence. 2004. *New England Journal of Medicine* 350: 855-857.

47. Dishman, R., R. Motl, R. Saunders, G. Felton, D. Ward, M. Dowda, and R. Pate. 2005. Enjoyment mediates effects of a school-based physical-activity intervention. *Medicine and Science in Sports and Exercise* 37: 478-487.

48. Durak, E. 1989. Exercise for specific populations: Diabetes mellitus. *Sports Training, Medicine and Rehabilitation* 1: 175-180.

49. Durak, E., L. Jovanovis-Peterson, and C. Peterson. 1990. Randomized crossover study of effect of resistance training on glycemic control, muscular strength, and cholesterol in Type I diabetic men. *Diabetes Care* 13: 1039-1042.

50. Emery, C., W. Meeuwisse, and J. McAllister. 2006. Survey of sports participation and sport injury risk in Calgary and area high schools. *Clinical Journal of Sports Medicine* 16: 20-26.

51. Eriksson, J., S. Taimela, K. Eriksson, S. Parvoinen, J. Peltonen, and U. Kujala. 1997. Resistance training in the treatment of non-insulin dependent diabetes mellitus. *International Journal of Sports Medicine* 18: 242-246.

52. Evans, W., and I. Rosenberg. 1992. *Biomarkers.* New York: Simon and Schuster.

53. Faigenbaum, A. 2007. Resistance training for children and adolescents: Are there health outcomes? *American Journal of Lifestyle Medicine* 1: 190-200.

54. Faigenbaum, A., R. Loud, J. O'Connell, S. Glover, J. O'Connell, and W. Westcott. 2001. Effects of different resistance training protocols on upper body strength and endurance development in children. *Journal of Strength and Conditioning Research* 15: 459-465.

55. Faigenbaum, A., W. Kraemer, C. Blimkie, I. Jeffreys, L. Micheli, M. Nitka, and T. Rowland. 2009. Youth resistance training: Updated position statement paper from the National Strength and Conditioning Association. *Journal of Strength and Conditioning Research* 23 (Suppl 5): S60-S79.

56. Faigenbaum, A., and J. McFarland. 2007. Guidelines for implementing a dynamic warm-up for physical education. *Journal of Physical Education, Recreation and Dance* 78: 25-28.

57. Faigenbaum, A., and G. Myer. 2010. Resistance training among young athletes: Safety, efficacy and injury prevention effects. *British Journal of Sports Medicine* 44: 56-63.

58. Faigenbaum, A., G. Skrinar, W. Cesare, W. Kraemer, and H. Thomas. 1990. Physiologic and symptomatic responses of cardiac patients to resistance exercise. *Archives of Physical Medicine and Rehabilitation* 70: 395-398.

59. Faigenbaum, A., and W. Westcott. 2007. Resistance training for obese children and adolescents. *President's Council on Physical Fitness and Sports Research Digest* 8: 1-8.

60. Faigenbaum, A., and W. Westcott. 2009. *Youth Strength Training*. Champaign, IL: Human Kinetics.

61. Faigenbaum, A., W. Westcott, R. Loud, and C. Long. 1999. The effects of different resistance training protocols on muscular strength and endurance development in children. *Pediatrics* 104: e5.

62. Falk, B., and A. Eliakim. 2003. Resistance training, skeletal muscle and growth. *Pediatric Endocrinology Reviews* 1: 120-127.

63. Falk, B., and G. Tenenbaum. 1996. The effectiveness of resistance training in children: A meta-analysis. *Sports Medicine* 22: 176-186.

64. Ferrara, C., A. Goldberg, H. Ortmeyer, and A. Ryan. 2006. Effects of aerobic and resistive exercise training on glucose disposal and skeletal muscle metabolism in older men. *Journals of Gerontology Series A: Biological Sciences and Medical Sciences* 61: 480-487.

65. Fiatarone, M., E. Marks, N. Ryan, C. Meredith, L. Lipsitz, and W. Evans. 1990. High-intensity strength training in nonagenarians. *Journal of the American Medical Association* 263: 3029-3034.

66. Freedman, D., W. Dietz, S. Srinivasan, and G. Berenson. 1999. The relationship of overweight to cardiovascular risk factors among children and adolescents: The Bogalusa heart study. *Pediatrics* 103: 1175-1182.

67. Frontera, W., C. Meredith, K. O'Reilly, H. Knuttgen, and W. Evans. 1988. Strength conditioning in older men: Skeletal muscle hypertrophy and improved function. *Journal of Applied Physiology* 64: 1038-1044.

68. Ghilarducci, L., R. Holly, and E. Amsterdam. 1989. Effects of high resistance training in coronary heart disease. *American Journal of Cardiology* 64: 866-870.

69. Goldberg, L., L. Elliot, R. Schultz, and F. Kloste. 1984. Changes in lipid and lipoprotein levels after weight training. *Journal of the American Medical Association* 252: 504-506.

70. Gordon, B., A. Benson, S. Bird, and S. Fraser. 2009. Resistance training improves metabolic health in type 2 diabetes: A systematic review. *Diabetes Research and Clinical Practice* 83: 157-175.

71. Gortmaker, S., A. Must, A. Sobol, K. Peterson, G. Colditz, and W. Dietz. 1996. Television viewing as a cause of increasing obesity among children in the United States, 1986-1990.

Archives of Pediatric and Adolescent Medicine 150: 356-362.

72. Graves, J., M. Pollock, and D. Foster. 1990. Effects of training frequency and specificity on isometric lumbar extension strength. *Spine* 15: 504-509.

73. Greenlund, L., and K. Nair. 2003. Sarcopenia-consequences, mechanisms, and potential therapies. *Mechanisms of Ageing and Development* 124: 287-299.

74. Grimby, G., A. Aniansson, M. Hedberg, G. Henning, U. Granguard, and H. Kvist. 1992. Training can improve muscle strength and endurance in 78 to 84 year old men. *Journal of Applied Physiology* 73: 2517-2523.

75. Grimmer, K., D. Jones, and J. Williams. 2000. Prevalence of adolescence injury from recreational exercise: An Australian perspective. *Journal of Adolescent Health* 27: 266-272.

76. Hackney, K., H. Engels, and R. Gretebeck. 2008. Resting energy expenditure and delayed-onset muscle soreness after full-body resistance training with an eccentric concentration. *Journal of Strength and Conditioning Research* 22: 1602-1609.

77. Haennel, R., H. Quinney, and C. Kappogoda. 1991. Effects of hydraulic circuit training following coronary artery bypass surgery. *Medicine and Science in Sports and Exercise* 23: 158-165.

78. Hagerman, F., S. Walsh, R. Staron, R. Hikida, R. Gilders, T. Murray, K. Toma, and K. Ragg. 2000. Effects of high-intensity resistance training on untrained older men. I. Strength, cardiovascular, and metabolic responses. *Journals of Gerontology Series A: Biological Sciences and Medical Sciences* 55: B336-346.

79. Hamill, B. 1994. Relative safety of weight lifting and weight training. *Journal of Strength and Conditioning Research* 8: 53-57.

80. Harris, K., and R. Holly. 1987. Physiological response to circuit weight training in borderline hypertensive subjects. *Medicine and Science in Sports and Exercise* 10: 246-252.

81. Haskel, W., I. Lee, R. Pate, K. Powell, S. Blair, B. Franklin, C. Macera, G. Heath, P. Thompson, and A. Bauman. 2007. Physical activity and public health: Updated recommendation for adults from the American College of Sports Medicine and the American Heart Association. *Circulation* 116: 1081-1093.

82. Heidt, R., L. Sweeterman, R. Carlonas, J. Traub, and F. Tekulve. 2000. Avoidance of soccer injuries with preseason conditioning. *American Journal of Sports Medicine* 28: 659-662.

83. Hewett, T., G. Myer, and K. Ford. 2005. Reducing knee and anterior cruciate ligament injuries among female athletes. *Journal of Knee Surgery* 18: 82-88.

84. Hewett, T., A. Stroupe, T. Nance, and F. Noyes. 1996. Plyometric training in female athletes. *American Journal of Sports Medicine* 24: 765-773.

85. Hikida, R., R. Staron, F. Hagerman, S. Walsh, E. Kaiser, S. Shell, and S. Hervey. 2000. Effects of high-intensity resistance training on untrained older men. II. Muscle fiber characteristics and nucleo-cytoplasmic relationships. *Journals of Gerontology Series A: Biological Sciences and Medical Sciences* 55: B347-354.

86. Holten, M., M. Zacho, M. Gaster, C. Juel, J. Wojaszewskil, and F. Dela. 2004. Strength training increases insulin-mediated glucose uptake, GLUT4 content, and insulin signaling in skeletal muscle in patients with type 2 diabetes. *Diabetes* 53: 294-305.

87. Hunter, G., J. McCarthy, and M. Bamman. 2004. Effects of resistance training on older adults. *Sports Medicine* 34: 329-348.

88. Hunter, G., C. Wetzstein, D. Fields, A. Brown, and M. Bamman. 2000. Resistance training increases total energy

expenditure and free-living physical activity in older adults. *Journal of Applied Physiology* 89: 977-984.

89. Hurley, B. 1994. Does strength training improve health status? *Strength and Conditioning* 16: 7-13.

90. Hurley, B., J. Hagberg, A. Goldberg, D. Seals, A. Ehsani, R. Brennan, and J. Holloszy. 1988. Resistance training can reduce coronary risk factors without altering VO2 max or percent body fat. *Medicine and Science in Sports and Exercise* 20: 150-154.

91. Hurley, B., and S. Roth. 2000. Strength training in the elderly: Effects on risk factors for age-related diseases. *Sports Medicine* 30: 249-268.

92. Institute of Medicine of the National Academies. 2005. *Preventing Childhood Obesity. Health in the Balance.* Washington, DC: National Academies Press. pp. 21-53.

93. Ivey, F., S. Roth, R. Ferrell, B. Tracy, J. Lemmer, D. Hurlbut, G. Martel, E. Siegel, J. Fozard, E. Metter, J. Fleg, and B. Hurley. 2000. Effects of age, gender, and myostatin genotype on the hypertrophic responses to heavy resistance strength training. *Journals of Gerontology Series A: Biological Sciences and Medical Sciences* 55: M641-648.

94. Jan, M., J. Lin, J. Liau, Y. Lin, and D. Lin. 2008. Investigation of clinical effects of high- and low-resistance training for patients with knee osteoarthritis: A randomized controlled trial. *Physical Therapy* 88: 427-436.

95. Janz, K., J. Dawson, and L. Mahoney. 2000. Tracking physical fitness and physical activity from childhood to adolescence: The Muscatine study. *Medicine and Science in Sports and Exercise* 32: 1250-1257.

96. Johnson, C., M. Stone, S. Lopez, J. Hebert, L. Kilgoe, and R. Byrd. 1982. Diet and exercise in middle-aged men. *Journal of the Dietetic Association* 81: 695-701.

97. Jones, A., M. Pollock, J. Graves, M. Fulton, W. Jones, M. MacMillan, D. Baldwin, and J. Cirulli. 1988. *Safe, Specific Testing and Rehabilitative Exercise for Muscles of the Lumbar Spine.* Santa Barbara, CA: Sequoia Communications.

98. Jones, C., C. Christensen, and M. Young. 2000. Weight training injury trends. *Physician and Sportsmedicine* 28: 61-72.

99. Jurca, R., M. LaMonte, T. Church, C. Earnest, S. Fitzgerald, C. Barlow, A. Jordan, J. Dampert, and S. Blaire. 2004. Associations with muscle strength and aerobic fitness with metabolic syndrome in men. *Medicine and Science in Sports and Exercise* 36: 1301-1307.

100. Kalapotharakos, V., M. Michalopoulos, S. Tokmakisis, G. Godolias, and V. Gourgoulis. 2005. Effects of heavy and moderate resistance training on functional performance in older adults. *Journal of Strength and Conditioning Research* 19: 652-657.

101. Kelemen, M., K. Stewart, R. Gillilan, C. Ewart, S. Valenti, J. Manley, and M. Kelemen. 1986. Circuit weight training in cardiac patients. *Journal of the American College of Cardiology* 7: 38-42.

102. Kelley, G. 1997. Dynamic resistance exercise and resting blood pressure in healthy adults: A meta-analysis. *Journal of Applied Physiology* 82: 1559-1565.

103. Kelley, G., and K. Kelley. 2000. Progressive resistance exercise and resting blood pressure: A meta-analysis of randomized controlled trials. *Hypertension* 35: 838-843.

104. Kelley, G., and K. Kelley. 2009. Impact of progressive resistance training on lipids and lipoproteins in adults: A meta-analysis of randomized controlled trials. *Preventive Medicine* 48: 9-19.

105. Kelly, A. 2005. Practical exercise advice during pregnancy. *Physician and Sportsmedicine* 33: 24-31.

106. Keys, A., H. Taylor, and F. Grande. 1973. Basal metabolism and age of adult man. *Metabolism* 22: 579-587.

107. King, L., T. Birmingham, C. Kean, I. Jones, D. Bryant, and J. Giffin. 2008. Resistance training for medial compartment knee osteoarthritis and malalignment. *Medicine and Science in Sports and Exercise* 40: 1376-1384.

108. Koffler, K., A. Menkes, R. Redmond, W. Whitehead, R. Pratley, and B. Hurley. 1992. Strength training accelerates gastrointestinal transit in middle-aged and older men. *Medicine and Science in Sports and Exercise* 24: 415-419.

109. Kokkinos, P., B. Hurley, M. Smutok, C. Farmer, C. Reece, R. Shulman, C. Charabogos, J. Patterson, S. Will, J. DeVane-Bell, and A. Goldberg. 1991. Strength training does not improve lipoprotein lipid profiles in men at risk for CHD. *Medicine and Science in Sports and Exercise* 23: 1134-1139.

110. Kokkinos, P., B. Hurley, P. Vaccaro, J. Patterson, L. Gardner, S. Ostrove, and A. Goldberg. 1998. Effects of low and high repetition resistive training on lipoprotein-lipid profiles. *Medicine and Science in Sports and Exercise* 20: 50-54.

111. Lange, A., B. Vanwanseele, and M. Fiatarone Singh. 2008. Strength training for treatment of osteoarthritis of the knee: A systematic review. *Arthritis and Rheumatism* 59: 1488-1494.

112. Layne, J., and M. Nelson. 1999. The effects of progressive resistance training on bone density: A review. *Medicine and Science in Sports and Exercise* 31: 25-30.

113. Lemmer, J., F. Ivey, A. Ryan, G. Martel, D. Hurlbut, J. Metter, J. Fozard, J. Fleg, and B. Hurley. 2001. Effect of strength training on resting metabolic rate and physical activity. *Medicine and Science in Sports and Exercise* 33: 532-541.

114. Lillegard, W., E. Brown, D. Wilson, R. Henderson, and E. Lewis. 1997. Efficacy of strength training in prepubescent to early postpubescent males and females: Effects of gender and maturity. *Pediatric Rehabilitation* 1: 147-157.

115. Lohmann, D., and F. Liebold. 1978. Diminished insulin response in highly trained athletes. *Metabolism* 27: 521-523.

116. Malina, R. 2001. Tracking of physical activity across the lifespan. *President's Council on Physical Fitness and Sports Research Digest* 3: 1-8.

117. Malina, R. 2006. Weight training in youth-growth, maturation and safety: An evidenced based review. *Clinical Journal of Sport Medicine* 16: 478-487.

118. Mandelbaum, B., H. Silvers, D. Watanabe, J. Knarr, S. Thomas, L. Griffin, D. Kirkendall, and W. Garrett. 2005. Effectiveness of a neuromuscular and proprioceptive training program in preventing anterior cruciate ligament injuries in female athletes. *American Journal of Sports Medicine* 33: 1003-1010.

119. Marks, R. 1993. The effects of isometric quadriceps strength training in mid-range for osteoarthritis of the knee. *Arthritis Care Research* 6: 52-56.

120. Marzolini, S., P. Oh, S. Thomas, and J. Goodman. 2008. Aerobic and resistance training in coronary disease: Single versus multiple sets. *Medicine and Science in Sports and Exercise* 40: 1557-1564.

121. Mason, C., S. Brien, C. Craig, L. Gauvin, and P. Katzmarzyk. 2007. Musculoskeletal fitness and weight gain. *Medicine and Science in Sports and Exercise* 39: 38-43.

122. McCartney, N., A. Hicks, J. Martin, and C. Webber. 1996. A longitudinal trial of weight training in the elderly—continued improvements in year two. *Journals of Gerontology Series A: Biological Sciences and Medical Sciences* 51: B425-B433.

123. Mediate, P., and A. Faigenbaum. 2007. *Medicine Ball for All Kids.* Monterey, CA: Healthy Learning.

124. Melby, C., C. Scholl, G. Edwards, and R. Bullough. 1993. Effect of acute resistance exercise on postexercise energy expenditure and resting metabolic rate. *Journal of Applied Physiology* 75: 1847-1853.

125. Melov, S., M. Tarnopolsky, K. Beckman, K. Felkey, and A. Hubbard. 2007. Resistance exercise reverses aging in human skeletal muscle. *PLoS ONE* 2: e465.

126. Menkes, A., S. Mazel, R. Redmond, K. Koffler, C. Libanati, C. Gunberg, T. Zizic, J. Hagberg, R. Pratley, and B. Hurley. 1993. Strength training increases regional bone mineral density and bone remodeling in middle-aged and older men. *Journal of Applied Physiology* 74: 2478-2484.

127. Micheli L. 2006. Preventing injuries in sports: What the team physician needs to know. In: *F.I.M.S. Team Physician Manual,* 2nd ed., K. Chan, L. Micheli, A. Smith, C. Rolf, N. Bachl, W. Frontera, and T. Alenabi, eds. Hong Kong: CD Concept. pp. 555-572.

128. Miller, J., R. Pratley, A. Goldberg, P. Gordon, M. Rubin, M. Treuth, A. Ryan, and B. Hurley. 1994. Strength training increases insulin action in healthy 50 to 65 year-old men. *Journal of Applied Physiology* 77: 1122-1127.

129. Miller, W., W. Sherman, and J. Ivy. 1984. Effect of strength training on glucose tolerance and post glucose insulin response. *Medicine and Science in Sports and Exercise* 16: 539-543.

130. Morris, F., G. Naughton, J. Gibbs, J. Carlson, and J. Wark. 1997. Prospective ten-month exercise intervention in pre-menarcheal girls: Positive effects on bone and lean mass. *Journal of Bone and Mineral Research* 12: 1453-1462.

131. Morrow, J. 1997. Relationship of low back pain to exercise habits. Paper presented at ACSM conference, Denver, May 31.

132. Myer G., C. Quatman, J. Khoury, E. Wall, and T. Hewett. 2009. Youth vs. adult "weightlifting" injuries presented to United States emergency rooms: Accidental vs. nonaccidental mechanisms. *Journal of Strength and Conditioning Research* 23: 2054-2060.

133. National Association for Sport and Physical Education. 2005. *Physical Education for Lifelong Fitness,* 2nd ed. Champaign, IL: Human Kinetics.

134. Nelson, M., M. Fiatarone, C. Morganti, I. Trice, R. Greenberg, and W. Evans. 1994. Effects of high-intensity strength training on multiple risk factors for osteoporotic fractures. *Journal of the American Medical Association* 272: 1909-1914.

135. Ogden, C., M. Carroll, and K. Flegal. 2008. High body mass index for age among US children and adolescents, 2003-2006. *Journal of the American Medical Association* 299: 2401-2405.

136. Olshansky, S., D. Passaro, R. Hershow, J. Layden, B. Carnes, J. Brody, L. Hayflick, R. Butler, D. Allison, and D. Ludwig. 2005. A potential decline in life expectancy in the United States in the 21st century. *New England Journal of Medicine* 352: 1138-1145.

137. Olson, T., D. Dengel, A. Leon, and K. Schmitz. 2006. Moderate resistance training and vascular health in overweight women. *Medicine and Science in Sports and Exercise* 38: 1558-1564.

138. Ormsbee, M., J. Thyfault, E. Johnson, R. Kraus, M. Choi, and R. Hickner. 2007. Fat metabolism and acute resistance exercise in trained men. *Journal of Applied Physiology* 102: 1767-1772.

139. Ortega, F., J. Ruiz, M. Castillo, and M. Sjostrom. 2008. Physical fitness in childhood and adolescence: A powerful marker of health. *International Journal of Obesity* 32: 1-11.

140. Ozmun, J., A. Mikesky, and P. Surburg. 1994. Neuromuscular adaptations following prepubescent strength training. *Medicine and Science in Sports and Exercise* 26: 510-514.

141. Parise, G., A. Brose, and M. Tarnopolsky. 2005. Resistance exercise training decreases oxidative damage to DNA and increases cytochrome oxidase activity in older adults. *Experimental Gerontology* 40: 173-180.

142. Pate, R., M. Davis., T. Robinson, E. Stone, T. McKenzie, and J. Young. 2006. Promoting physical activity in children and youth. *Circulation* 114: 1214-1224.

143. Payne, G., and J. Morrow. 1993. Exercise and VO2 max in children: A meta-analysis. *Research Quarterly for Exercise and Sport* 64: 305-313.

144. Phillips, S. 2007. Resistance exercise: Good for more than just Grandma and Grandpa's muscles. *Applied Physiology, Nutrition, and Metabolism* 32: 1198-1205.

145. Pivarnik, J., H. Chambliss, J. Clapp, S. Dugan, M. Hatch, C. Lovelady, M. Mottola, and M. Williams. 2006. Impact of physical activity during pregnancy and postpartum on chronic disease risk. *Medicine and Science in Sports and Exercise* 38: 989-1006.

146. Powell, K., A. Roberts, J. Ross, M. Phillips, D. Ujamma, and M. Zhou. 2009. Low physical fitness among fifth- and seventh-grade students, Georgia, 2006. *American Journal of Preventive Medicine* 36: 304-310.

147. Pratley, R., B. Nicklas, M. Rubin, J. Miller, A. Smith, M. Smith, B. Hurley, and A. Goldberg. 1994. Strength training increases resting metabolic rate and norepinephrine levels in healthy 50 to 65 year old men. *Journal of Applied Physiology* 76: 133-137.

148. Quirk, A., R. Newman, and K. Newman. 1985. An evaluation of interferential therapy, shortwave diathermy and exercise in the treatment of osteoarthritis of the knee. *Physiotherapy* 71: 55-57.

149. Ramsay, J., C. Blimkie, K. Smith, S. Garner, J. Macdougall, and D. Sale. 1990. Strength training effects in prepubescent boys. *Medicine and Science in Sports and Exercise* 22: 605-614.

150. Renstrom P., A. Ljungqvist, E. Arendt, B. Beynnon, T. Fukubayashi, W. Garrett, T. Georgoulis, T. Hewett, R. Johnson, T. Krosshaug, B. Mandelbaum, L. Micheli, G. Myklebust, E. Roos, H. Roos, P. Schamasch, S. Shultz, S. Werner, E. Wojtys, and L. Engebretsen. 2008. Non-contact ACL injuries in female athletes: An International Olympic Committee current concepts statement. *British Journal of Sports Medicine* 42: 394-424.

151. Reynolds, K., J. Killen, S. Bryson, D. Maron, C. Taylor, N. Maccoby, and J. Farquhar. 1990. Psychosocial predictors of physical activity in adolescents. *Preventive Medicine* 19: 541-551.

152. Risch, S., N. Norvell, M. Polock, E. Risch, H. Langer, M. Fulton, M. Graves, and S. Leggett. 1993. Lumbar strengthening in chronic low back pain patients. *Spine* 18: 232-238.

153. Rowland, T. 2005. *Children's Exercise Physiology,* 2nd ed. Champaign, IL: Human Kinetics. pp. 181-195.

154. Ruiz, J., X. Sui, F. Lobelo, J. Morrow, A. Jackson, M. Sjostrom, and S. Blair. 2008. Association between muscular strength and mortality in men: Prospective cohort study. *British Medical Journal* 337: a439.

155. Ryan, A., D. Hurlbut, M. Lott, F. Ivey, J. Fleg, B. Hurley, and A. Goldberg. 2001. Insulin action after resistance training in insulin resistant older men and women. *Journal of the American Geriatric Society* 49: 247-253.

156. Ryan, A., M. Treuth, M. Rubin, J. Miller, B. Nicklas, D. Landis, R. Pratley, C. Libanati, C. Grundberg, and B. Hurley. 1994. Effects of strength training on bone mineral density: Hormonal and bone turnover relationships. *Journal of Applied Physiology* 77: 1678-1684.

157. Shaibi, G., M. Cruz, G. Ball, M. Weigensberg, G. Salem, N. Crespo, and M. Goran. 2006. Effects of resistance training on insulin sensitivity in overweight Latino Adolescent males. *Medicine and Science in Sports and Exercise* 38: 1208-1215.

158. Shephard, R. 2009. Maximal oxygen intake and independence in old age, *British Journal of Sports Medicine,* 43: 342-346.

159. Singh, N., K. Clements, and M. Fiatarone. 1997. A randomized controlled trial of progressive resistance training in depressed elders. *Journal of Gerontology* 52A: M27-M35.

160. Smutok, M., C. Reece, P. Kokkinos, C. Farmer, P. Dawson, R. Shulman, J. De Vane-Bell, J. Patterson, C. Charabogos, A. Goldley, and B. Hurley. 1993. Aerobic vs. strength training for risk factor intervention in middle-aged men at high risk for coronary heart disease. *Metabolism* 42: 177-184.

161. Snow-Harter, C., M. Bouxsein, B. Lewis, D. Carter, and R. Marcus. 1992. Effects of resistance and endurance exercise on bone mineral status of young women. A randomized exercise intervention trial. *Journal of Bone and Mineral Research* 7: 761-769.

162. Sothern, M., M. Loftin, J. Udall, R. Suskind, T. Ewing, S. Tang, and U. Blecker. 1999. Inclusion of resistance exercise in a multidisciplinary outpatient treatment program for preadolescent obese children. *Southern Medical Journal* 92: 585-592.

163. Stewart, K., M. Mason, and M. Kelemen. 1988. Three-year participation in circuit weight training improves muscular strength and self-efficacy in cardiac patients. *Journal of Cardiopulmonary Rehabilitation* 8: 292-296.

164. Stone, M., D. Blessing, R. Byrd, J. Tew, and D. Boatwright. 1982. Physiological effects of a short term resistance training program on middle-aged untrained men. *National Strength Coaches Association Journal* 4: 16-20.

165. Strong, W., R. Malina, C. Blimkie, S. Daniels, R. Dishman, B. Gutin, A. Hergenroeder, A. Must, P. Nixon, J. Pivarnik, T. Rowland, S. Trost, and F. Trudeau. 2005. Evidence based physical activity for school-age youth. *Journal of Pediatrics* 146: 732-737.

166. Tang, J., J. Hartman, and S. Phillips. 2006. Increased muscle oxidative potential following resistance training induced fiber hypertrophy in young men. *Applied Physiology, Nutrition, and Metabolism* 31: 495-501.

167. Taunton, J., A. Martin, E. Rhodes, L. Wolski, M. Donnelly, and J. Elliot. 1997. Exercise for older women: Choosing the right prescription. *British Journal of Sports Medicine* 31: 5-10.

168. Trappe, S., D. Williamson, M. Godard, and P. Gallagher. 2001. Maintenance of whole muscle strength and size following resistance training in older men. *Medicine and Science in Sports and Exercise* 33: S147.

169. Troiano, R., D. Berrigan, K. Dodd, L. Masse, T. Tilert, and M. McDowell. 2008. Physical activity in the United States measured by accelerometer. *Medicine and Science in Sports and Exercise* 40: 181-188.

170. Tucker, L., and L. Silvester. 1996. Strength training and hypercholesterolemia: An epidemiologic study of 8499 employed men. *American Journal of Health Promotion* 11: 35-41.

171. *Tufts University Diet and Nutrition Letter.* 1994. Never too late to build up your muscle. 12 (September): 6-7.

172. Ulrich, I., C. Reid, and R. Yeater. 1987. Increased HDL-cholesterol levels with a weight training program. *Southern Medical Journal* 80: 328-331.

173. Vander, L., B. Franklin, D. Wrisley, and M. Rubenfire. 1986. Acute cardiovascular responses in cardiac patients: Implications for exercise training. *Annals of Sports Medicine* 2: 165-169.

174. Van Etten, L., K. Westerterp, F. Verstappen, B. Boon, and W. Saris. 1997. Effect of an 18-week weight-training program on energy expenditure and physical activity. *Journal of Applied Physiology* 82 (1): 298-304.

175. Vaughn, J., and L. Micheli. 2008. Strength training recommendations for the young athlete. *Physical Medicine and Rehabilitation Clinics of North America* 19: 235-245.

176. Vause, T., P. Martz, F. Ricjard, and L. Gramlich. 2006. Nutrition for healthy pregnancy outcomes. *Applied Physiology, Nutrition, and Metabolism* 31: 12-20.

177. Verdijk, L., B. Gleeson, R. Jonkers, K. Meijer, H. Savelberg, P. Dendale, and L. van Loon. 2009. Skeletal muscle hypertrophy following resistance training is accompanied by a fiber type-specific increase in satellite cell content in elderly men. *Journals of Gerontology Series A: Biological Sciences and Medical Sciences* 64: 332-339.

178. Vincent, K., R. Braith, R. Feldman, P. Magyari, R. Cutler, S. Persin, S. Lennon, A. Gabr, and D. Lowenthal. 2002. Resistance exercise and physical performance in adults aged 60 to 83. *Journal of the American Geriatric Society* 50: 1100-1107.

179. Wang, Y., and T. Lobstein. 2006. Worldwide trends in childhood overweight and obesity. *International Journal of Pediatric Obesity* 1: 11-25.

180. Watts, K., P. Beye, A. Siafarikas, E. Davis, T. Jones, G. O'Driscoll, and D. Green. 2004. Exercise training normalizes vascular dysfunction and improves central adiposity in obese adolescents. *Journal of the American College of Cardiology* 43: 1823-1827.

181. Weltman, A., C. Janney, C. Rians, K. Strand, B. Berg, S. Tippit, J. Wise, B. Cahill, and F. Katch. 1986. The effects of hydraulic resistance strength training in pre-pubertal males. *Medicine and Science in Sports and Exercise* 18: 629-638.

182. Weltman, A., C. Janney, C. Rians, K. Strand, and F. Katch. 1987. Effects of hydraulic-resistance strength training on serum lipid levels in prepubertal boys. *American Journal of Diseases in Children* 141: 777-780.

183. Westcott, W. 2009. ACSM strength training guidelines: Role in body composition and health enhancement. *ACSM's Health & Fitness Journal* 13: 14-22.

184. Westcott, W., and T. Baechle. 1999. *Strength Training for Seniors.* Champaign, IL: Human Kinetics. Updated as Baechle, T. and W. Westcott. *The Fitness Professional's Guide to Strength Training Older Adults,* 2nd ed. Champaign, IL: Human Kinetics.

185. Westcott, W., F. Dolan, and T. Cavicchi. 1996. Golf and strength training are compatible activities. *Strength and Conditioning* 18: 54-56.

186. Westcott, W., and J. Guy. 1996. A physical evolution: Sedentary adults see marked improvements in as little as two days a week. *IDEA Today* 14: 58-65.

187. Whaley, M., L. Kaminsky, G. Dwyer, L. Getchell, and J. Norton. 1992. Predictors of over- and underachievement of age-predicted maximal heart rate. *Medicine and Science in Sports and Exercise* 24: 1173-1179.

188. Wijndaele, K., N. Duvigneaud, L. Matton, W. Duquet, M. Thomis, G. Beunen, J. Lefevre, and R. Phillippaerts. 2007. Muscular strength, aerobic fitness, and metabolic syndrome risk in Flemish adults. *Medicine and Science in Sports and Exercise* 39: 233-240.

189. Wolfe, R. 2006. The underappreciated role of muscle in health and disease. *American Journal of Clinical Nutrition* 84: 475-482.

Clients With Nutritional and Metabolic Concerns

Douglas B. Smith, PhD, and Ryan Fiddler, MS

After completing this chapter, you will be able to

- delineate the scope of practice of the personal trainer working with people who have nutritional and metabolic concerns;

- discuss the appropriate exercise prescription and program design for individuals who are obese, are overweight, or have hyperlipidemia, eating disorders, or diabetes;

- describe general nutritional guidelines for individuals with these nutritional and metabolic concerns; and

- discuss lifestyle change strategies (diet, exercise, and behavior changes) that will improve the health status of people with these nutritional and metabolic concerns.

Advances in technology, industrialization, and automation have decreased the need for rigorous physical work, allowed more leisure time, and greatly increased food availability. These advances, which are positive in some respects, have negatively affected the population's health. Along with other factors, these societal changes have led to an increased prevalence of obesity, hyperlipidemia, and diabetes, as well as a trend toward disordered eating and eating disorders. Personal trainers are likely to encounter clients who have one or more of these nutritionally related conditions. Personal trainers should screen for these conditions as described in chapter 9 and obtain medical clearance when

needed (25). Clients with the conditions discussed in this chapter should be referred to their physician for medical care and to a dietitian for medical nutrition therapy, as a personal trainer's role is limited to exercise program design and execution along with lifestyle change support. Personal trainers should not diagnose or prescribe care for their clients nor accept or train clients who have medical conditions that may exceed their level of knowledge and experience. Instead, such clients should be referred to the appropriate health care professional (25).

> Personal trainers must not diagnose or prescribe care and should not train clients with medical conditions outside of their knowledge and experience; they should refer the client to an appropriate health care professional.

The authors would like to acknowledge the contributions of Christine L. Vega and Carlos E. Jiménez, who wrote this chapter for the first edition of *NSCA's Essentials of Personal Training*.

Chapter 19

Overweight and Obesity

Obesity and overweight, in both children and adults, has become a "global epidemic" (62). Recent surveys in the industrialized countries along with some of the developing countries show a growing proportion of children and adults who are overweight or obese (62). While the prevalence of obesity is 10% to 25% in most countries of Western Europe, 20% to 25% in some countries in the Americas, and over 50% in some island nations of the Western Pacific, the scope of the problem is even more alarming when the percentage of adults who are overweight (as opposed to obese only) is considered (62). The most recent U.S. National Health and Nutrition Examination Survey (NHANES 2007-2008) showed that 32.2% of U.S. men and 35.5% of U.S. women were obese (BMI ≥30). NHANES 2007-2008 showed that 68.0% of the adult population (ages 20 and older) were overweight (BMI ≥25) or obese (body mass index ≥30) (46).

These figures may increase even more in the future: National surveys in the United States have shown that the prevalence of obesity in childhood and adolescence has more than quadrupled among children ages 6 to 11 years and more than tripled among adolescents ages 12 to 19 years over the last four decades (37). The Office of the Surgeon General (61) has reported several important findings: (1) Risk factors for heart disease, such as high cholesterol and high blood pressure, occur with increased frequency in overweight children and adolescents compared to those with a healthy weight; (2) type 2 diabetes, previously considered an adult disease, has increased dramatically in children and adolescents; (3) overweight adolescents have a 70% chance of becoming overweight or obese adults, and this increases to 80% if one or more parent is overweight or obese; and

(4) the most immediate consequence of overweight, as perceived by children themselves, is social discrimination. Overweight and obesity are a public health problem of significant concern, as the condition of being overweight or obese raises the risk of morbidity from hypertension; hyperlipidemia; type 2 diabetes; coronary heart disease (CHD); stroke; gallbladder disease; osteoarthritis; sleep apnea and respiratory problems; and endometrial, breast, prostrate, and colon cancers (41, 62). Further, higher body weights are also associated with increases in all-cause mortality. Overweight and obesity have been designated as the second leading cause of preventable death in the United States (41, 42).

Definitions of Overweight and Obesity and Important Differences

Overweight is defined as a body mass index (BMI) of 25 to 29.9 kg/m², and obesity as a BMI of ≥30 kg/m² (41). The BMI describes relative weight for height and significantly correlates with total body fat content. The use of BMI has limitations with individuals who are very muscular (overestimates body fat) and with persons such as those of advanced age who have lost muscle mass (underestimates body fat) (42). The BMI should be used to assess overweight and obesity in addition to monitoring changes in body weight (41, 42, 62).

The BMI is calculated as weight (kg) divided by height squared (m²). To estimate BMI using pounds and inches, the calculation is (weight [pounds] divided by height squared [inches²]) × 703. See table 19.1 for the National Heart, Lung, and Blood Institute (NHLBI) agreed-on weight classifications by BMI. See "Calculating BMI" on page 491 for examples of how to calculate BMI using nonmetric and metric units.

TABLE 19.1 Classification of Overweight and Obesity by Body Mass Index (BMI), Waist Circumference, and Associated Disease Risk

	BMI (kg/m²)	Obesity class	Disease risk* relative to normal weight and waist circumference	
			Men ≤40 in. (≤102 cm), women ≤35 in. (≤88 cm)	Men >40 in. (>102 cm), women >35 in. (>88 cm)
Underweight	<18.5		–	
Normal**	18.5-24.9		–	–
Overweight	25.0-29.9		Increased	High
Obesity	30.0-34.9	I	High	Very high
	35.0-39.9	II	Very high	Very high
Extreme obesity	≥40.0	III	Extremely high	Extremely high

*Disease risk for type 2 diabetes, hypertension, and coronary heart disease.

**Increased waist circumference can also be a marker for increased risk even in persons of normal weight.

Reprinted from NIH and NHLBI 1998 (40).

Calculating BMI

Nonmetric Conversion

To calculate BMI using nonmetric units, use this formula:

$$\text{(Weight [pounds]} \div \text{Height squared [inches}^2\text{])} \times 703 \qquad \textbf{(19.1)}$$

For example, a person who weighs 164 pounds and is 68 inches (or 5 feet 8 inches) tall has a BMI of 25:

$$(164 \div 68^2) \times 703 = 25$$

Metric Conversion

To calculate BMI using metric units, use this formula:

$$\text{Weight (kilograms)} \div \text{Height squared (m}^2\text{)} \qquad \textbf{(19.2)}$$

For example, a person who weighs 78.93 kg and is 177 cm (1.77 m) tall has a BMI of 25:

$$78.93 \div 1.77^2 = 25$$

Remember that 100 cm = 1 m.

To select appropriate prevention strategies and design effective exercise programs, the personal trainer must understand the complex and important differences between overweight and obesity (16):

- People who are obese have a significantly greater excess of weight, particularly adipose tissue mass, than those who are overweight. Additionally, the percentage of adipose tissue as opposed to fat-free tissue is higher in persons who are obese. This means that people who are obese have significantly increased their fat stores without a concomitant increase in muscle mass (14).

- In general, persons who are obese are more likely to have had a larger positive energy balance over a longer period of time than those who are overweight. Contribution to the positive energy balance is not only from a decrease in physical activity, but also from an increase in food consumption (14). A neutral energy balance occurs when an individual is consuming as many calories as he or she expends, resulting in no change of body weight. A positive energy balance, or consuming more calories than are expended, will result in an increase in body weight; a negative energy balance, or the consumption of fewer calories than are expended, will result in a decrease in body weight.

- On the average, a person who is obese has a higher resting metabolic rate and expends more energy on activities than those who are overweight or normal weight. The reason is that moving a heavy mass around requires more energy (14).

A review of these differences and their implications would seem to indicate that a sedentary lifestyle or a low level of habitual activity appears to be the mechanism for a large proportion of adult overweight cases (13, 14). In other words, it is possible for an individual to become overweight by simply decreasing his or her activity level without consuming more food each day.

It is for this population, those who are overweight, that early intervention with an exercise program and increased physical activity are important. Hopefully, overweight individuals can be encouraged and convinced to start working with a personal trainer before they become obese. A return to previous activity levels or beyond would at least prevent a progression to obesity and possibly achieve significant weight loss, affording people the hope of returning to a normal weight classification without having to resort to moderate or severe caloric restriction.

On the other hand, individuals with severe obesity (i.e., BMI of 35 or more) have likely sustained a positive energy balance for long periods of time, that is, at least a few years. In most cases, this condition is achieved with an increase in energy intakes (increased consumption of food) and a decrease in energy expenditure (physical activity) (14). Therefore, it seems that in the case of people who are severely obese, inactivity is an important factor but is also coupled with increased consumption. Consequently, persons who are obese must have a strong emphasis on both cutting caloric intake and increasing activity.

Clients who are overweight may benefit simply by increasing physical activity along with some minor changes in their diets. Those who are obese should concentrate on both reducing caloric intake and increasing physical activity.

Causes and Correlates of Overweight and Obesity

No one theory completely answers the question of how and why obesity occurs. Although a positive energy balance due to the increased availability of calorie-rich food coupled with a sedentary lifestyle is a major factor in the worldwide increase in obesity, there are still other factors to consider (62). The Surgeon General's *Overweight and Obesity: Health Consequences* reported that "body weight is a combination of genetic, metabolic, behavioral, environmental, cultural, and socioeconomic influences" and that behavioral and environmental factors contribute largely to overweight and obesity. These two factors may also "provide the greatest opportunity for actions and interventions designed for prevention and treatment" (57).

Environmental factors can include food availability, socioeconomic status, and lack of access to exercise facilities such as a gym or a track. Behavioral factors include eating patterns determined by individual preferences and ethnic backgrounds, including overeating or binge eating, and activity patterns. Genetic and metabolic factors can include differences in resting metabolic rate, levels of lipoprotein lipase and other enzymes, sympathetic nervous system activity, and dietary-induced thermogenesis. Some of these variables serve as true predictors of body fat gain, allowing them to be considered risk factors. In other cases, researchers do not know whether the relationship is causal or whether the correlate is secondary to being obese. In most cases, the associations are in fact secondary and are a result of obesity (14).

Steffen and colleagues (57) recently examined the association between overweight in children and adolescents on the one hand and television viewing and parental weight on the other. The results were in agreement with previous research (16, 33, 19, 23, 31, 50, 58), showing TV viewing to be directly associated with children's becoming overweight. Furthermore, the authors reported that "1 additional hour of TV watching or total screen time per day increased the odds of being overweight by 20% to 30% in this population" and that obesity is familial (56). Another recent study by Yen and colleagues—also including

Internet use—presented similar results, showing that high TV viewing and high Internet use were associated with increased BMI in adolescents (63).

Fat Distribution

It is important not only to note whether a client falls into the overweight or obese category, but also to discern the pattern of fat distribution. There are two types of fat distribution, android obesity and gynoid obesity. Gynoid obesity (pear-shaped body) denotes the condition in which high amounts of body fat have been deposited in the hip and thigh areas. Android obesity (apple-shaped body) is characterized by high amounts of body fat in the trunk and abdominal areas. This presence of excess fat in the abdomen, out of proportion to total body fat, acts as an independent predictor of disease risk for type 2 diabetes, hypertension, and cardiovascular disease (CVD) (41, 42).

Measuring Abdominal Fat

Researchers have suggested that central obesity poses a more significant CVD risk than does total obesity and that waist circumference and waist/hip ratio may be better predictors of atherosclerosis and CVD risk than BMI (38). Furthermore, there is a positive correlation between abdominal fat content and the waist circumference measurement (41, 42, 63). The personal trainer can use this clinically acceptable measurement to assess the client's abdominal fat content before and during a weight loss program (41, 42). Proper measurement of the waist circumference is explained in chapter 11, page 214. For adult clients with BMIs between 25 to 34.9 kg/m², males whose waist circumference exceeds 40 inches (102 cm) and females whose waist circumference exceeds 35 inches (>88 cm) have an increased risk of developing type 2 diabetes, dyslipidemia, hypertension, and CVD (41, 42). Note that these waist circumference limits are not useful in terms of incremental risk prediction in clients with a BMI ≥35 kg/m², as these individuals will automatically exceed the cutoff points because of their higher weight. The following sidebar contains practical recommendations for conducting measurements of abdominal fat in clients who are overweight or obese.

Skinfold measurement of persons who are obese is very difficult; correctly placing the calibers requires a good deal of experience. Additionally, the process can be demeaning to a client who is obese because of the size of the skinfold. Because of the high acceptability of the BMI and waist circumference measurements, personal trainers are encouraged to use these measurements for both initial assessment

Assessing Abdominal Fat in Clients Who Are Overweight or Obese

- Use waist circumference and BMI measures in lieu of or in addition to skinfold measures.
- Conduct the assessment in a private setting and assure the client that no one else will see the results.
- Conduct the assessment in a matter-of-fact yet sensitive manner. Avoid uncomfortable humor.
- If the client is too embarrassed for someone to measure his or her waist, allow the client to conduct the measurement after having received instruction.
- Tell the client beforehand to wear thin clothing, and allow him or her to keep all clothes on during the measurement if he or she is uncomfortable about removing clothing. Although measurement will not be accurate, it will provide a starting point and avoid embarrassment.
- The following cutoffs indicate an increased risk for type 2 diabetes, dyslipidemia, hypertension, and CVD in individuals with a BMI between 25 and 34.9 kg/m^2 (19, 20):

  Men: >40 inches (>102 cm)

  Women: >35 inches (>88 cm)

and follow-up measurements. In fact, the demonstration of the loss of inches can have more meaning to a client. Circumference measurements can also be made of other parts of the body, for instance, the hips, arms, and thighs, to track progress in terms of weight loss. The use of dual-energy X-ray absorptiometry (DXA) has recently been investigated as a possible method to assess bone status and soft tissue composition in overweight individuals (15). Gately and colleagues (27) suggested that air displacement and DXA may be the most promising methods for body fat assessment in overweight and obese children. It appears, however, that further research is needed in this area to consider all limitations with this population. Furthermore, with regard to the use of DXA in this population, Brownbill and Ilich (15) mention that standard DXA equipment may not be able to accommodate some overweight or obese individuals due to insufficient scanning area.

Controlling Cardiovascular Risk Factors

Table 19.1 adds the disease risk of increased abdominal fat to the disease risk of BMI (41, 42). As is evident, the increased abdominal fat distribution moves an individual in the overweight or the class I obesity category to an even higher disease risk category. The categories in the table indicate *relative risk, not absolute risk* (41, 42). In other words, the comparison of risk is being made relative to a normal weight. This is in contrast to the calculation of absolute risk for disease, which is determined by a summation of risk factors (41, 42).

Personal trainers working with clients who are overweight should give as much emphasis to the control of cardiovascular risk factors as they do to

weight loss in their clients' overall programs (42). In other words, the client must understand that an increase in physical activity along with the cessation of smoking and the consumption of a heart healthy diet, with or without weight loss, will significantly improve his or her health status. In fact, even if clients do not change any of their other health habits but improve fitness to a moderate or high level, they will experience lower adjusted premature death rates from CVD and all-cause mortality (12). This allows one to measure the success of a client's program not only in weight loss, but also in positive behavior changes.

Benefits of Exercise in a Weight Reduction Program

The inclusion of physical activity in a weight reduction program provides physiological and psychological benefits. Although the exact mechanism by which physical activity affects weight loss and the degree to which it does so are not yet completely understood, exercise should be included in a weight loss program to ensure a better chance of success. A review of the literature showed that adults with obesity who participated in physical activity realized modest weight loss and a lowering of the risk factors for CVD (41).

It seems that some of the physiological benefits of exercise may not translate to weight loss as much as previously thought. For example, a person with obesity who is out of shape is often unable to perform exercise of sufficient duration or intensity to expend enough calories to meet the targeted daily caloric deficit. Hence, although the exercise session is important, a decrease in calories consumed would

Benefits of Exercise in a Weight Loss Program

- Increases energy expenditure
- Reduces the risk of heart disease more than weight loss alone can
- May help reduce body fat and prevent the decrease in muscle mass that often occurs during weight loss
- May decrease abdominal fat
- Decreases insulin resistance
- May contribute to better dietary compliance, including reduced caloric intake
- May not prevent the decline in resting metabolic rate associated with a low-calorie diet, but may minimize the decrease
- Improves mood and general well-being
- Improves body image
- Increases self-esteem and self-efficacy
- Serves as a coping strategy

Based on NIH and NHLBI 2000 (42); Baker and Brownwell 2000 (10).

have an even greater effect on weight loss. Still, an exercise program is important for its positive effects on lowering the risk factors for CVD along with the other general physiological and psychological benefits listed below.

While the area of the psychological and emotional benefits of exercise and their effects on increased motivation, commitment, and psychological resources deserves further research, the combination of the existing studies and experiential data indicates that those benefits do occur. The possible psychological outcomes of an exercise program that promotes these increases in motivation and commitment are increased well-being and mood, improved

body image, improved self-esteem and self-efficacy, and improved coping abilities (10). For example, the improved well-being and enhanced self-esteem produced by physical activity may generalize to other areas of life and lead to improved dietary adherence. In other words, the client feels more productive and more in control of his or her life and is therefore better able and more willing to make the proper choices of food and portion sizes. Figure 19.1 (10) provides an overview of the proposed mechanism and potential pathways that link exercise to success in weight control.

Although the results of research supporting the benefit of physical activity during the weight loss

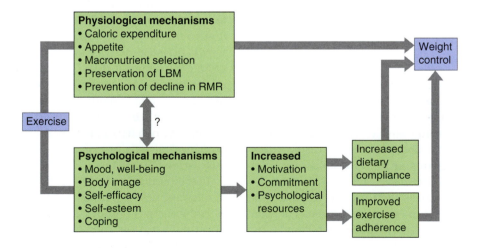

FIGURE 19.1 Proposed mechanisms linking exercise and weight control. LBM = lean body mass; RMR = resting metabolic rate.

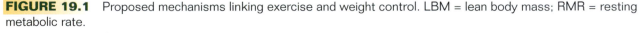

Reprinted by permission from Baker and Brownwell 2000.

phase of a weight management program are mixed, strong evidence supports the role of physical activity as a necessary factor for long-term weight maintenance (55). Regular physical activity not only helps to improve weight loss and physical fitness during the weight loss phase of a weight management program, but also is needed to ensure that the client maintains his or her target weight over time. One of the main goals of the personal trainer should be to help clients establish the habit of frequent exercise.

> While physical activity may or may not help a client lose weight, it reduces many obesity-related risk factors and is critical for long-term weight maintenance.

Lifestyle Change Program for Obesity

In general, the most successful weight management programs consist of a combination of diet modification, increased physical activity, and lifestyle change (41, 42). Personal trainers work with their clients not only to increase physical activity levels but also to provide lifestyle change support.

Diet Modification and the Low-Calorie Diet

The majority of clients who are overweight or obese need to make adjustments in their diets in order to achieve a caloric deficit resulting in weight loss. Personal trainers should refer these clients to a dietitian. The dietitian will most likely evaluate the client's diet, design an appropriate calorie-reduced yet nutrient-dense diet, offer follow-up to make adjustments in the diet, answer questions and concerns, and solve any problems. Referral to a dietitian is very highly recommended for clients who are obese and who have high cholesterol levels, and is necessary for clients with diabetes. (Diabetes is managed by a physician and normally in conjunction with a dietitian.)

To be effective, the diet must be designed in accordance with the client's cultural and ethnic background, should include the client's food preferences, should take into account the availability and cost of the food in the diet, should contain a selection of foods that will decrease the risk of other nutritionally related cardiovascular risk factors such as hyperlipidemia and high blood pressure, and should fit into the client's particular lifestyle (42). Additionally, the diet should ensure that all of the recommended dietary allowances are met, which may require the use of a dietary or vitamin supplement for those who are eating in the lower calorie

ranges (42). Once the diet is individualized to the client's needs and preferences, the personal trainer can be of great help in supporting and motivating the client to adhere to the diet.

Most weight loss in persons who are obese occurs primarily because of decreased caloric intake. The NHLBI guidelines recommend that a diet be individually planned to help create a deficit of 500 to 1,000 calories per day to facilitate a weight loss of 1 to 2 pounds (0.45-0.9 kg) per week. This moderate reduction in calories is recommended so as to achieve a slow yet progressive weight loss. Excess weight will gradually decrease with this level of caloric intake. (The target amount also depends on the amount of exercise the client performs on a daily basis. In other words, if the client expends 250 calories a day in an exercise session, the diet may have to be reduced by only 250 to 750 calories per day, which will make it easier to accomplish.)

The exact calorie load for each individual is determined through use of the calorie calculation formulas on page 113 of chapter 7 and trial-and-error adjustments. It is recommended that caloric intake be reduced only to the level required to maintain weight at a desired level.

In general, women should consume diets containing not less than 1,000 to 1,200 kilocalories (kcal)/day, and men should consume a diet no lower than 1,200 to 1,600 kcal/day (42). The higher intake of 1,200 to 1,600 kcal/day may also be appropriate for women who weigh 165 pounds (75 kg) or more or for women who exercise regularly (42). If a client consumes a 1,600 kcal/day diet and does not lose weight, it may be advisable to try the 1,200 kcal/day diet. On the other hand, if a client gets hungry on the lower-calorie diet or is without sufficient energy to make it through the day or to engage in physical activity, he or she may need to consume an additional 100 to 200 kcal/day (42).

Additionally, more lean body tissue will be spared if the client consumes a **low-calorie diet (LCD)** in comparison to the great losses that occur with the very low-calorie diets (VLCDs), which consist of less than 800 kcal/day. The use of VLCD is to be carried out only by physicians with specialized training and experience, as the diet requires special monitoring and supplementation and should be used only in limited circumstances with specific individuals (44). In actuality, clinical trials have demonstrated that LCDs have the same success rates as VLCDs in promoting weight loss after one year (61).

Refer to table 19.2 for the general dietary guidelines for an LCD as outlined in the Low-Calorie Step I Diet recommended by NHLBI. This diet also contains the nutrient composition that will decrease other

TABLE 19.2 Low-Calorie Step I Diet

Nutrient	Recommended daily intake
Calories[1]	Approximately a 500 to 1,000 kcal reduction from usual intake
Total fat[2]	30% or less of total calories
Saturated fatty acids[3]	8% to 10% of total calories
Monounsaturated fatty acids	Up to 15% of total calories
Polyunsaturated fatty acids	Up to 10% of total calories
Cholesterol[3]	<300 mg
Protein[4]	Approximately 15% of total calories
Carbohydrate[5]	55% or more of total calories
Sodium	No more than 100 mmol (approximately 2.4 g of sodium or approximately 6 g of sodium chloride)
Calcium[6]	1,000 to 1,500 mg
Fiber[5]	20 to 30 g

[1] A reduction in calories of 500 to 1,000 kcal/day will help achieve a weight loss of 1 to 2 pounds/week. Alcohol provides unneeded calories and displaces more nutritious foods. Alcohol consumption not only increases the number of calories in a diet but has been associated with obesity in epidemiologic studies as well as in experimental studies. The impact of alcohol calories on a person's overall caloric intake needs to be assessed and appropriately controlled.

[2] Fat-modified foods may provide a helpful strategy for lowering total fat intake but will be effective only if they are also low in calories and if there is no compensation by calories from other foods.

[3] Patients with high blood cholesterol levels may need to use the Step II diet to achieve further reductions in LDL-cholesterol levels; in the Step II diet, saturated fats are reduced to less than 7% of total calories, and cholesterol levels to less than 200 mg/day. All of the other nutrients are the same as in Step I.

[4] Protein should be derived from plant sources and lean sources of animal protein.

[5] Complex carbohydrates from different vegetables, fruits, and whole grains are good sources of vitamins, minerals, and fiber. A diet rich in soluble fiber, including oat bran, legumes, barley, and most fruits and vegetables, may be effective in reducing blood cholesterol levels. A diet high in all types of fiber may also aid in weight management by promoting satiety at lower levels of calorie and fat intake. Some authorities recommend 20 to 30 g of fiber daily, with an upper limit of 35 g.

[6] During weight loss, attention should be given to maintaining an adequate intake of vitamins and minerals. Maintenance of the recommended calcium intake of 1,000 to 1,500 mg/day is especially important for women who may be at risk of osteoporosis.

Reprinted from NIH and NHLBI 2000 (42).

risk factors for CVD such as high blood cholesterol levels and hypertension.

An initial and reasonable goal of a weight loss program is a 10% reduction in body weight. A reasonable time to achieve this goal is six months (42). After six months, the personal trainer along with the dietitian and physician can set new goals. Even if the client only reaches this initial 10% reduction and maintains it, he or she has accomplished a significant decrease in the severity of the obesity-associated risk factors (41, 42). In fact, the literature has shown that a reduction of only 3% to 5% of body weight is sufficient to achieve a reduction in health risk (6).

> Reducing body weight by 10% over six months is an appropriate initial goal; at this time, new goals can be set. It is much better to lose a moderate amount of weight relatively slowly than to lose a large amount quickly and then regain most of it.

Many clients may find it difficult to lose weight after the first six months because of decrease in their resting metabolic rates and increased challenge over time of continuing with the diet and exercise regime. Additionally, their energy requirements decrease as their weight decreases (less mass to move around means less workload). Thus an even larger increase in the dietary goals (further decrease in calories) and physical activity goals (further increase in activity levels) is needed in order to create an energy deficit at the lower weight (42).

After the initial weight goal of a 10% reduction in body weight has been achieved, the personal trainer and client can set new goals for weight loss, if appropriate. The benefits of achieving a moderate weight loss over a long period of time far outweigh benefits of losing a great deal of weight quickly only to gain most of it back. This situation of weight regain, especially when repeated a number of times, undermines the benefits of participating in a weight loss program in terms of time spent, financial costs, health determinants, and especially a possible decrease in self-esteem (42).

Although it is not within the scope of practice for personal trainers to offer dietary prescription and counseling to their clients, personal trainers can support their clients' efforts by offering nutrition education or orientation. Topics may include low-calorie food choices, low-fat food preparation techniques, food label reading, holiday eating strategies, the importance of adequate hydration, ways to include more fruits and vegetables in the diet, and so on.

> Dietary prescription or counseling is beyond the personal trainer's scope of practice; instead the personal trainer can offer nutrition education.

Physical Activity

Moderate levels of physical activity for at least 30 minutes, most days of the week, are recommended for clients who are overweight or obese and who are beginning an exercise program (45, 46). A moderate level of physical activity is defined as the amount of activity that uses approximately 150 kcal/day, with a total of approximately 1,000 kcal/week (41, 42). In fact, the Centers for Disease Control and Prevention, the American College of Sports Medicine (ACSM), the Surgeon General, and the National Institutes of Health (NIH)/NHLBI make the following recommendation as expressed in the NHLBI *Practical Guide:* "All adults should set a long term goal to accumulate at least 30 minutes or more of moderate-intensity physical activity on most, and preferably all, days of the week" (42, 48, 55). A review of the most current literature on this subject reinforces these guidelines.

The ACSM's *Guidelines for Exercise Testing and Prescription,* 8th edition, 2010, recommends a minimum of between 150 to 250 minutes per week of moderate-intensity (40-60% $\dot{V}O_2R$ or heart rate reserve [HRR]) to vigorous-intensity (50-75% $\dot{V}O_2R$ or HRR) physical activity to effectively *prevent weight gain* for individuals who are overweight or obese. Furthermore, the guidelines suggest that overweight and obese clients progress to a level of physical activity of 250 to 300 minutes per week or 50 to 60 minutes per day five days a week to enhance *long-term weight loss maintenance.* For the purposes of *weight loss,* some individuals may need to progress to 60 to 90 minutes per day of moderate- to vigorous-intensity physical activity. Examples of moderate amounts of physical activity are shown in table 19.3.

It is important to consider the concept of progression when designing a physical activity program for a client. Many clients who are obese may not be able to start with a moderate-level activity program. For these clients, the initial activities may have to be low in intensity or even simply a matter of focusing on increasing the tasks of daily living. For example, clients might

- take a walk after lunch,
- walk to a coworker's desk or office instead of using the phone,
- use stairs instead of an elevator or escalator,
- walk to pick up lunch instead of ordering a delivery,

TABLE 19.3   Examples of Moderate Amounts of Physical Activity

Common chores	Sporting activities	Less vigorous, more time*
Washing or waxing a car for 45 to 60 min	Playing volleyball for 45 to 60 min	↑
Washing windows or floors for 45 to 60 min	Playing touch football for 45 min	
Gardening for 30 to 45 min	Walking 1 3/4 miles in 35 min (20 min/mile)	
Wheeling self in wheelchair for 30 to 40 min	Basketball (shooting baskets) for 30 min	
Pushing a stroller 1 1/2 miles in 30 min	Bicycling 5 miles in 30 min	
Raking leaves for 30 min	Dancing fast (social) for 30 min	
Walking 2 miles in 30 min (15 min/mile)	Water aerobics for 30 min	
Shoveling snow for 15 min	Swimming laps for 20 min	
Stair walking for 15 min	Basketball (playing a game) for 15 to 20 min	
	Jumping rope for 15 min	↓
	Running 1 1/2 miles in 15 min (10 min/mile)	**More vigorous, less time**

Note: A moderate amount of physical activity is roughly equivalent to physical activity that uses approximately 150 calories of energy per day, or 1,000 calories per week.

*Some activities can be performed at various intensities; the suggested durations correspond to expected intensity of effort.
Reprinted from NIH and NHLBI 2000 (42).

- get off the bus or subway at least one stop early and walk the remainder of the way,
- park in a space at the mall that is farther from the entrance and requires more walking,
- walk to the neighborhood mini-mart to pick up milk instead of driving the block or two,
- walk the dog,
- do yard work, or
- play actively with children or grandchildren.

A well-designed, progressive program avoids the incidence of injury in addition to making the beginning exercise sessions comfortable and tolerable. Many people with obesity, because of their sedentary lifestyles, have very low functional capacities. What may seem like a moderate intensity or a moderate amount of physical activity to a personal trainer may actually be a great challenge to an obese individual. An exercise program that is too demanding may lead to soreness to which clients are not accustomed. These uncomfortable sensations may lead to a loss of motivation, discouraging a client from continuing with the program.

As the client loses weight and increases his or her functional capacity, exercise of increased intensity and increased duration can be programmed. Although longer sessions of moderate-intensity activities (such as fitness walking) can involve the same amount of activity and caloric expenditure as shorter sessions of higher-intensity exercises (such as running), it is best to go with the longer-duration, lower-intensity exercise (at least at the start of the program) in order to avoid injury and promote adherence to the program. Examples of appropriate exercises include fitness walking, fitness swimming, aqua fitness classes, cycling in and out of doors, rowing, hiking, square dancing, and aerobic dance in addition to resistance and flexibility training.

An additional 100 to 200 kcal/day spent in common chores and recreational activities will promote an even larger caloric deficit with a concomitant increase in fat loss, functional capacity, and lean body mass (42). All of this increased activity along with programmed exercise sessions will add up and contribute to the caloric deficit needed to ensure weight loss and subsequent weight maintenance.

> Longer sessions of moderate intensity can involve the same amount of activity and caloric expenditure as shorter sessions of higher intensity; but longer durations and lower intensities are advisable, at least at the beginning, to avoid injury and promote adherence.

Lifestyle Change Support

Lifestyle change support consists of various strategies that can help clients adhere to their physical activity and diet programs. Lifestyle change support helps clients identify the obstacles that are keeping them from following the program and then uses a problem-solving approach to design and implement strategies to overcome these obstacles. It is not easy for anyone to change well-established behaviors and to overcome the obstacles to those changes. Specifically, the techniques of self-monitoring, rewards, goal setting, stimulus control, and dietary behavior changes may help clients to see how continuing with their current weight loss or weight maintenance program and will allow them to make realistic, long-term lifestyle changes (46).

Self-Monitoring The practice of clients' taking note of their activity and diet behaviors and recording them is referred to as *self-monitoring*. Recording food and calorie intake, bouts of exercise and physical activity, moods when eating, where a food was eaten, weight lost or gained, and so forth can provide valuable information for both the personal trainer and the client. Further, in some cases, just self-monitoring a behavior can bring about positive changes as clients become keenly aware of what they are doing and can make immediate changes (42). The personal trainer can provide clients with specific self-monitoring forms such as the "Small Steps . . . Big Changes Diet and Activity Diary" on page 499. Self-monitoring can help the client and personal trainer

- identify behaviors that put the success of the program at risk,
- identify obstacles to engaging in physical activity or eating healthfully, and
- chart progress to both motivate the client and serve as a basis for the reward system.

As an example of identifying risky behaviors, a diet history form that notes the food consumed, time of food consumption, site of food consumption, and even the mood of the client at the time may bring forth the fact that the client tends to eat high-calorie snacks, in relatively large amounts, when sitting in front of the television. The client could be advised to prepare a bowl of cut, crisp fresh vegetables or a controlled amount of unbuttered popcorn to consume during a show. Or, clients may detect on their form that upon arrival home from work they make a trip directly to the refrigerator to eat whatever is available. They could solve this problem by eating a piece of fruit on the way home and then waiting until the planned dinner is prepared and on the table.

Small Steps . . . Big Changes Diet and Activity Diary

Name: _____   Day and date: _____

Time	Food eaten or activity performed	Time spent eating or doing activity	Place	Thoughts and feelings

Food

1. Record the time at which you ate a snack or meal. Also record the amount of time you spent eating.
2. List the foods that you ate and the amount that you ate.
3. Record where you were when you ate and whether or not you had any feelings or thoughts (positive, negative, or neutral).

Exercise and Activity

1. Record any formal exercise in which you participated (i.e., walking, aerobics class, biking, resistance training, aqua exercise, etc.).
2. Also record the time of day, the amount of time you spent exercising, and any accompanying feelings and thoughts (positive, negative, or neutral).
3. Record any other physical activities in which you engaged along with the time performed and time spent (i.e., walking up stairs, sweeping, mopping, yard work, washing windows).

From NSCA, 2012, *NSCA's essentials of personal training*, 2nd ed., J. Coburn and M. Malek (eds.), (Champaign, IL: Human Kinetics). ©2003 Christine L. Vega, MPH, RD, CSCS.

Self-monitoring of exercise behaviors also helps identify obstacles to engaging in the prescribed amount of physical activity. For example, the client and personal trainer may have agreed that they would meet twice a week for a weight training session and that the client would engage in a 30- to 45-minute walk on alternate days. Inspection of the exercise self-monitoring form may bring to light that the client did exercise on the days planned for an early morning walk before work. Conversely, when the client planned to walk in the afternoon, she never got around to it because of work constraints and finally was too tired to exercise upon arrival at home. This client would need to plan her exercise sessions in the morning.

Rewards Rewards can be used to encourage and acknowledge attainment of the client's behavioral goals or specific outcomes. An effective reward is something that is desirable to the client, awarded on a timely basis, and contingent upon meeting the goal (42).

Rewards can be big or small, tangible or intangible, awarded by the client's family or by the client, or awarded to the client by the personal trainer. Tangible rewards include items like a new blouse, an exercise outfit, or a book. Intangible rewards usually include some pleasant use of time such as a fishing excursion, an afternoon at the mall, quiet time to read a book, or a weekend getaway to a country inn. Usually, small rewards are given for attainment of steps within the goal or a short-term goal, while bigger awards are granted for attaining a long-term goal such as the target 10% reduction of body weight within a six-month period.

Goal Setting Goal setting is covered in chapter 8. When one is working with clients who are overweight or obese, it is especially important to set goals that are realistic and to set short-term goals within long-term goals. For example, a client may have the goal of losing 20 pounds (9 kg) over a six-month period. Breaking this down to 3 to 4 pounds (1.3-1.8 kg) per month enables the client to celebrate the attainment of each goal. Fortunately, if the client does not achieve the whole weight goal in the first six months but has achieved some of the smaller goals, he or she will most likely still feel motivated to continue the program (59).

However, focusing only on weight loss goals as opposed to behavior change can set clients up for failure. Using behavior change goals in addition to weight loss goals will help clients see the value in continuing the program, even when they experience plateaus in weight loss. For example, a goal may be to walk 40 minutes at least four times per week. If the client meets this goal, he or she is successful, regardless of the amount of weight lost.

Goal setting is to be used in conjunction with self-monitoring and rewards. Additionally, the client can commit to a self-contract. In a self-contract, the client usually outlines a desired goal or behavior (e.g., to lose half a pound [0.2 kg] per week for a total of 2 pounds [0.9 kg] per month, to walk 30 minutes at least four times per week). The client will also decide on the reward for achievement of the goal. The Activity and Exercise Contract on page 501 is an example of a self-contract.

Stimulus Control Stimulus control consists of identifying the social or environmental cues that seem to trigger undesired eating patterns or nonparticipation in physical activity and then modifying those cues (5). Sometimes the term "environmental trigger" is used in place of "stimulus," as triggering is exactly what happens. Something in the environment sets off an undesirable behavior, and the client starts engaging in unwanted eating patterns. For example, a client may find that he always eats popcorn and drinks a soda at a movie despite not being hungry, overeats at a buffet, overeats while working at his desk, or tends to have rich desserts when out with a particular friend.

Using the self-monitoring strategy, reflection, or both, the client may be able to identify these cues in the environment and problem solve ways to manage the situation. For example, clients who eat popcorn at the movies even when they are not hungry could either eat a smaller meal before going to the movies or a salad and then go to the movies and eat popcorn. If a client eats large amounts at a buffet, a solution could be to go only to restaurants where food is served from a menu. Clients who unwittingly overeat while working at their desks may be advised to make a rule to snack only away from the desk. Clients who tend to overeat or over-drink when they go out with a particular friend may need to decide to meet the friend for a nonfood activity like shopping or going to the movies. The problem-solving step either seeks to eliminate the cue or to manage it in a way that avoids overeating.

Food Consumption Behavior Changes Food consumption behavior changes may also help the client eat less without feeling deprived (42). Some clients should be encouraged to slow the rate of eating. Eating too fast does not allow the body time to identify the satiety signals that develop before the end of a meal. Clients can also use smaller plates to make portion sizes appear bigger. The use of smaller plates is also recommended at buffets to prevent

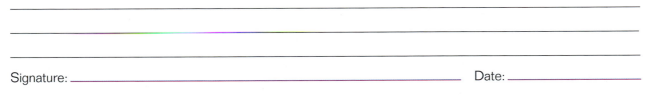

Activity and Exercise Contract

I, _____, will incorporate the following activity or exercise into my daily/weekly schedule for the week of _____.

Extra physical activities* I will incorporate into my daily routine:

Activity	Where	When	Number of times performed	Duration

Formal exercise sessions** in which I will participate:

Name of exercise or program	Where	When	Duration	Time per week

*Examples include taking the stairs at work and taking a 10-minute walk at lunch.

**Examples include a session with a personal trainer, a 30-minute walk, an aerobics class, or lap swimming.

If I fulfill this one-week contract, I will reward myself by:

_____

_____

_____

Signature: _____   Date: _____

From NSCA, 2012, *NSCA's essentials of personal training*, 2nd ed., J. Coburn and M. Malek (eds.), (Champaign, IL: Human Kinetics).

placing large amounts of food on the plate. Some clients do best by eating only three meals a day in order to avoid eating too many snacks, while others do better with four to six small meals, as they tend to overeat at a meal when they eat only three times per day. Clients who tend to skip or delay meals and overeat later because they are overly hungry must consider tightly scheduling their meals to avoid this problem. As every client is an individual, there is no recipe for eating patterns that will work best for each. Through trial and error, the personal trainer and client will find what works best.

Exercise Concerns of Clients Who Are Overweight or Obese

There are a number of physiological and biomechanical concerns to consider when one is working with individuals who are overweight or obese. The following concerns may affect the exercise program design, exercise selection, and instruction of the client (54): heat intolerance, movement restriction and limited mobility, weight-bearing stress, posture problems and low back pain, balance concerns, and hyperpnea and dyspnea.

Heat Intolerance

Heat intolerance is a result of the added insulation of excess fat. Compared to persons of normal weight, it is harder for individuals with obesity to thermoregulate, especially under hot and humid conditions (53). The personal trainer should encourage clients to wear cotton clothes, preferably shorts and a T-shirt, in moderate and hot temperatures. (Wearing shorts may be embarrassing to some clients, although they can cover up with a long T-shirt worn over bicycle pants or basketball-length shorts. If the client does not want to wear shorts, then the personal trainer should encourage lightweight, loose-fitting cotton pants.) On particularly hot or humid days, any of the following modifications should be considered: lowering the intensity of the workout to avoid discomfort and a possible heat emergency; training in a temperature-controlled environment; swimming or performing aqua exercise for the cardiovascular training component of the workout; conducting the resistance training in the pool; and water walking and jogging in the pool. Personal trainers must ensure that the client drinks enough cool water before, during, and after the exercise session. (See chapter 7 for recommendations.)

Movement Restriction and Limited Mobility

In people who are obese, movement restriction or limited mobility due to the excess fat mass may require the modification of various exercises (7). For example, excess fat on the thigh and calf may make it difficult for a client to perform a quadriceps stretch with the leg held behind and the foot pressed into the buttock. For a more suitable quadriceps stretch, one could have the client lower the back knee and press the hips forward from a calf stretch. Alternatively, the client could perform an active stretch of the quadriceps by using the hamstring muscles to bend the knee as far back as the fat mass allows while performing a pelvic tilt to put the hip into extension (see figure 19.2). Although these modifications would not allow a full stretch of the quadriceps, they would provide some flexibility training benefit.

As another example, a client may be unable to reach his or her leg (because of the restriction imposed by the abdominal fat mass) in order to move it toward the chest during a back-lying hamstring stretch. In this case, the client could be given a towel to wrap around the back of the thigh to perform the assisted passive stretch (see figure 19.3), or simply be instructed to perform an active stretch of the hamstrings by using the hip flexors to put the leg into the stretch position. The personal trainer needs to observe the client performing various stretches and exercises in order to make the modifications specific to the client's limitations (see figure 19.4).

Weight-Bearing Stress

Weight-bearing stress on the joints is definitely a concern for people who are overweight or obese, especially those who have osteoarthritis or musculoskeletal injuries (53). Low-impact activities, not necessarily low in intensity, will prevent some of this stress. For example, fitness walking provides less stress to the joints than jogging or running. Other low-impact activities include indoor and outdoor cycling; swimming; aqua aerobics; shallow-water walking, jogging, and aerobics; deep-water running; hiking; and rowing (not advised if the client has a movement restriction due to the fat mass). Activities that require sustained single-limb support (standing on one leg for an extended period of time while performing exercises with the other leg) can also impose an excessive weight-bearing stress on the involved joints, especially the hips. Many traditional aerobics classes and balance activities include such standing legwork. A way to avoid this situation is to alternate the supporting leg frequently when performing these exercises.

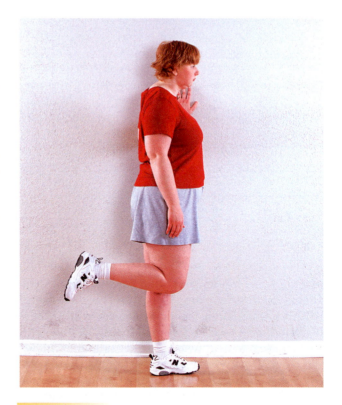

FIGURE 19.2 In the modified quadriceps stretch, the client performs an active stretch by flexing the right knee as much as possible and "rocking" or pressing the right hip forward while maintaining an erect posture.

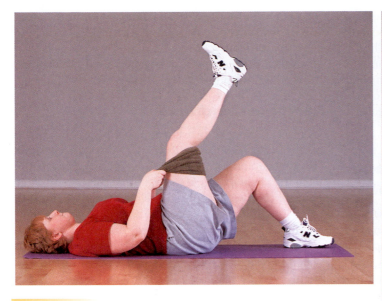

FIGURE 19.3 In the modified hamstrings stretch, the client pulls the right leg toward the chest with the help of a towel while trying to extend (not hyperextend) the knee.

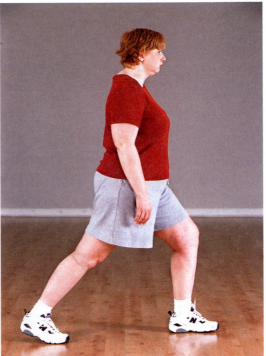

FIGURE 19.4 In the modified hip flexors stretch, the client takes a lunge stance with the ball of the right (rear) foot on the floor. The client then "rocks" or presses the right hip forward to actively stretch the hip flexors. The right knee can have a slight or a significant degree of flexion.

Posture Problems and Low Back Pain

Because of the stress of the abdominal fat mass on the spine and often inadequate strength of the muscles of the abdominal wall, posture problems and low back pain are not uncommon in persons who are obese. This situation may cause lordosis of the lower spine, with or without an accommodating kyphosis of the upper spine, along with other possible postural changes. Further, the hip flexors in persons with obesity can be quite strong owing to the repeated load of moving a large mass around; this further contributes to the muscular imbalance caused by weaker abdominal muscles. Therefore, the personal trainer must include a variety of exercises to strengthen the abdominal muscles along with flexibility exercises for the hip flexors (e.g., iliopsoas) in the training program. Because of the larger fat mass and weaker abdominal muscles, some of the abdominal exercises may have to be modified. Further, attention must be given to exercises to strengthen the muscles of the upper back and increase the flexibility of the chest muscles. Clients with significant or chronic low back pain should be referred to an orthopedist for an evaluation. The physician may refer the client to a physical therapist for a back education and rehabilitation program in addition to the personal training sessions.

Balance Concerns

Clients who are obese may have little experience in movement and sport and may not have had the chance to develop good balance. Unfortunately, when clients do start to fall because of lack of balance in a movement, the excess weight, lack of experience in proprioceptive adjustments, and lack of adequate strength can contribute to a greater difficulty in righting themselves. Therefore, the personal trainer should include balance training, but on a progressive basis, and needs to observe, correct, and spot the client during the various exercises that require good balance.

Hyperpnea and Dyspnea

Hyperpnea and dyspnea during exercise can be both uncomfortable and a source of anxiety to clients who are obese (53). Although some hyperpnea (increased respiratory rate) or dyspnea (labored or difficult breathing) is expected during an exercise session, persons with obesity may experience more because of their low functional capacity. This condition can be disquieting and uncomfortable enough to cause them to give up on the exercise training due to fear. The personal trainer can avoid problems in this area by ensuring that clients are working at the appropriate exercise intensity through use of a rating of perceived exertion scale (see chapter 16). The use of modified interval training, especially at the beginning of an exercise program, is highly recommended, as the rest intervals (active or inactive) will allow clients to bring their breathing into better control. With time, the work intervals can be increased and the rest intervals can be decreased.

Exercise Prescription and Program Design for Clients Who Are Overweight or Obese

The components of a well-rounded exercise program for those who are obese or overweight include aerobic conditioning, resistance training, and flexibility training (table 19.4). The personal trainer and client must first come to an agreement regarding how many days a week they will schedule and the content of the workout sessions. For example, they could decide that the personal training sessions will consist of all three of the components or only a warm-up followed by a resistance and flexibility training program. This would mean that the client would perform aerobic conditioning on days alternate to the personal training session days, before the personal training sessions, or both. The initial sessions should contain the aerobic conditioning phase so that the personal trainer can supervise, instruct, motivate, and ensure that

the client is working both correctly and efficiently on the cardiovascular training program. If the client has any difficulty complying with the cardiovascular program, this component should remain within the personal training session.

Aerobic Conditioning

A typical exercise prescription for a person who is overweight or obese calls for five days of participation in an aerobic conditioning program to ensure that the client expends the maximal calories possible during the week and establishes a regular physical activity habit. Some clients may not be able to start with the full cardiovascular component of the exercise program. In this case the beginning sessions need to be low in intensity, and the client would also be asked to work at increasing daily living activities as described earlier. Even when clients do achieve a full workout, it is important to encourage the daily activity levels so that they expend more calories, thereby enhancing weight loss.

Some individuals will be so out of shape that they will not be able to walk one lap of a track, or even less, without stopping to rest. In such a situation, the personal trainer should consider an interval training program. For example, the client would walk one-half of the track, stop to do a body weight calisthenic or exercise with a band, walk another half lap, stop to perform another exercise for 10 to 20 repetitions,

TABLE 19.4 Exercise Prescription for Clients Who Are Obese

Mode	Frequency, intensity, duration	Guidelines and concerns
Aerobic conditioning	<ul><li>Minimum recommendation = 30 min most days of the week (150 min/week)</li><li>≥5 days/week to maximize caloric expenditure</li><li>Eventual goal = 300 min/week</li><li>Moderate intensity (40 to 60% $\dot{V}O_2R$ or HRR) to vigorous intensity (50-75% $\dot{V}O_2R$ or HRR)</li><li>Intermittent exercise of at least 10 min in duration is an effective alternative to continuous exercise.</li></ul>	<ul><li>Use low-impact activities.</li><li>Take appropriate precautions due to increased risk of orthopedic injury, cardiovascular disease, and hyperthermia.</li><li>Initially emphasize increasing duration rather than increasing intensity to optimize caloric expenditure.</li><li>Modify equipment as necessary (e.g., wide seats on cycle ergometers and rowers).</li></ul>
Resistance training	<ul><li>2 or 3 days/week on nonconsecutive days</li><li>1 or more sets initially progressing to 2 to 4 sets, 10 to 15 reps per set</li><li>Training for each major muscle group (chest, shoulders, upper and lower back, abdomen, hips, and legs)</li><li>Gradual load increases</li></ul>	<ul><li>Can begin with body weight exercises.</li><li>Can intersperse with aerobic exercise.</li><li>Modify equipment as necessary (e.g., larger-framed machines).</li><li>Can complement aerobic conditioning (i.e., to maintain or gain lean body weight).</li></ul>
Flexibility training	<ul><li>2 or 3 days/week</li><li>≥4 reps per muscle group</li><li>Hold static stretches for 15 to 60 seconds</li></ul>	

Adapted from ACSM 2010 (2).

and so on until he or she has walked a mile. With time, the client would increase the length of the walk intervals until he or she can walk half a mile before stopping to do half of the resistance exercises, and then complete the next half-mile before performing the last half of the resistance exercises. Eventually the client will be able to walk a mile or two without stopping before doing the exercises.

Resistance Training

A recently updated position stand by the American College of Sports Medicine (5) states that "although the effects of resistance training on body weight and composition may be modest, resistance training has been associated with improvements in CVD risk factors in the absence of significant weight loss." Furthermore, the position stand cited research supporting the following benefits of resistance training: improvements in high-density lipoprotein cholesterol (HDL-C) (36), low-density lipoprotein cholesterol (LDL-C) (28, 32), and triglyceride levels (27); improvements in insulin sensitivity (22, 36); reductions in glucose-stimulated plasma insulin concentrations (32); and reductions in systolic and diastolic blood pressures (34, 45). The design of the resistance training program will depend on the available equipment along with the abilities and limitations of the client. It is recommended that the personal trainer check with the client for any orthopedic problems such as hip, back, or knee injuries and modify the program and specific exercises accordingly. Clients can start with body weight exercises (see figure 19.5 for example) and move on to machines or light free weights. The personal trainer must keep in mind that the client has a built-in workload with the excess body weight.

People who are obese are often quite strong in the lower body because of the adaptations the body makes to carrying the excess body weight. Hence, upper body strength should also be well addressed in a training session. Still, as the major goals of the resistance training session are to expend calories and increase muscle mass, emphasis should be on the core exercises, and the client should not spend a great deal of time on the smaller muscle groups. In general, one should follow the guidelines for resistance training presented in chapters 13 and 15.

Flexibility Training

Although stretching exercises typically do not result in large expenditures of energy, they are important to prevent injury and maintain range of motion around the joints. Light stretching can be included in the warm-up, while more intense stretches would be included at the end of an exercise session or after various resistance training exercises in order to develop flexibility. This timing ensures that the muscles are well warmed and thus more pliable. Stretches should be performed for all the major muscle groups.

Stretches are to be modified in accordance with the client's structural and physiological limitations. See pages 502 and 503 for examples of modifications. The personal trainer must be cognizant of the limited range of motion of clients who are overweight or obese. For instance, in a sitting toe touch, the client may only be able to reach just below the knees. The goal would not be to actually reach the toes. Instead, the goal would be to stretch until light tension is felt.

Eating Disorders

There is tremendous pressure in our society to be thin. Thin is in, and many of our young girls and women—and even some boys and men—are compromising their health to try to get there.

About 1% to 5% of adolescents and young adult women have eating disorders (40). Although cases have been reported in all social and racial groups, these disorders seem to predominately affect Caucasian upper-middle and middle-class females.

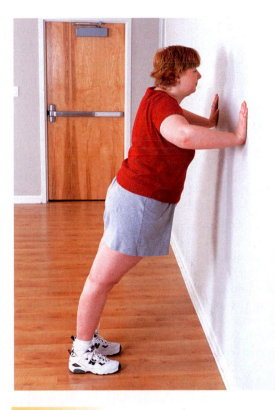

FIGURE 19.5 The wall push-up can be used for clients who cannot perform the standard push-up (i.e., on the floor).

Clinical samples have shown that only 5% to 10% of individuals with eating disorders are males (40). Given the current social and cultural environment, this number may increase in the future.

Personal trainers not only have a responsibility to educate clients about the risks of engaging in disordered eating; they also must be sure not to promote unnecessary or risky behaviors to lose weight and not to set unrealistic goals that may push a client into disordered eating patterns. Although a personal trainer would not be the sole cause of a client's eating disorder (the client would have to be already susceptible), an inappropriate comment or goal can serve as a trigger for someone to engage in disordered eating practices and possibly end up with an eating disorder.

Personal trainers need to orient their clients to the genetically determined differences in body types and the differences in body composition between men and women. Personal trainers need to be sure that they help each client set a goal that is realistic and in accordance with the client's genetic makeup, which has a significant effect on both the client's metabolism and body type. According to Dr. Carol Otis, "your ideal body weight is the range where you feel healthy and fit, have no signs of an eating disorder to maintain that weight, and have healthy, functioning immune and reproductive systems" (47).

> It is the responsibility of the personal trainer to educate clients about the risks of disordered eating and to avoid promoting risky weight loss behaviors or setting unrealistic goals.

Disordered Eating

The development of an eating disorder usually passes through the stages of dieting, disordered eating, and finally a full-blown eating disorder. Clients may start out by dieting to lose weight and become frustrated when the weight loss does not seem fast enough or significant. This frustration, even desperation, causes them to restrict their diet even further. When this does not work in their viewpoint, they start to experiment with even more dangerous disordered eating practices such as the use of diuretics (a medication that increases the rate of urination, hence increases water loss), diet pills, self-induced vomiting, food faddism (eating only one or a few specific foods or following fad diets such as the pineapple diet or the grapefruit diet), fasting, using saunas to sweat weight off, spitting out food that has been chewed, and using laxatives or even enemas (47). Unfortunately, these practices do not work. Although there may be a loss of weight according to the scale, the lost poundage can be attributed to water loss and probably lean tissue as opposed to fat.

There is a wide range in the frequency of disordered eating practices. Some people may engage infrequently in one of the techniques mentioned, while others may do so several times a day. Engaging in these disordered eating practices is the first step toward developing the eating disorders of anorexia nervosa and bulimia.

The key to preventing the development of an eating disorder is for the personal trainer, client, or both to recognize this common and complex condition. The personal trainer may be able to pick up on some of the disordered eating practices just by talking with the client about his or her diet or by having a client fill out a self-monitoring form for a few days to a week. Although many of the disordered eating practices may not be identifiable on the monitoring form, at least one could notice the types of foods consumed. The main point is that if the personal trainer offers good education, appropriate goal setting, and support, perhaps the client can be convinced to return to healthy eating before developing a full-blown eating disorder.

The concern is that individuals engaging in disordered eating practices can experience both the short- and long-term medical and psychological conditions characteristic of persons with anorexia and bulimia. These complications include depression, low self-esteem, stomach and digestive problems, menstrual irregularities, and heart problems and may even result in death from heart failure or suicide (47). The earlier an individual seeks help, the better chance he or she has at preventing and treating an eating disorder.

Anorexia Nervosa

Anorexia nervosa is characterized by extreme weight loss, a refusal to maintain body weight, an intense fear of gaining weight or becoming fat although the individual is underweight, distorted body image, and **amenorrhea** (loss of menses for at least three consecutive menstrual cycles) (8). The weight loss is usually facilitated through the restriction of food intake in conjunction with excessive exercise and may include the aforementioned disordered eating practices. The psychological and emotional problems associated with anorexia may include low self-esteem and a distorted body image, among others. Further, the condition of any extremely malnourished person may lead to symptoms of apathy, confusion, social isolation, and nonresponsiveness (40).

The two specific types of anorexia are the *restricting type* and the *binge eating and purging type* (40).

An individual with the restricting type of anorexia does not regularly engage in binge eating or purging behaviors such as self-induced vomiting or the misuse of laxatives, diuretics, or enemas during an episode, although he or she does severely restrict food intake in terms of the type and amount of food consumed (40). This is the most common type of anorexia. Alternatively, individuals with the binge eating and purging type of anorexia nervosa regularly engage in binge eating followed by purging behaviors (40).

If a personal trainer notes the signs listed in "Warning Signs for Anorexia," in a client, it becomes important to refer the client to a physician for a comprehensive treatment plan, which usually includes medical, dietary, and psychological or spiritual counseling from a team of professionals (physician, dietitian, psychologist, or religious or spiritual counselor). It may be hard for individuals with anorexia to acknowledge they have a problem. Therefore, the personal trainer should share this list with the client in the hopes of getting the person to seek help.

Bulimia Nervosa

Bulimia is a complicated disorder that consists of recurring episodes of binge eating followed by purging behaviors. During the bingeing phase the person eats large amounts of food over a short period of time. The purging behaviors may include self-induced vomiting; taking laxatives, diuretics, or enemas; and exercising excessively and obsessively in order to burn calories (40, 47). Whereas an individual with anorexia exhibits strict control of food intake, the individual with bulimia is experiencing a loss of control (40, 47).

The diagnosis of bulimia comes when the binge eating and purging behaviors occur on an average of at least twice a week for at least three months. The bingeing phase consists of eating large amounts of food within any 2-hour span and a feeling of lack of control to stop eating, lack of control over what or how much to eat, or both. Further criteria for the diagnosis of bulimia include the use of one or more purging methods or compensatory behaviors such as excessive exercise or fasting, and overconcern with body shape or weight (8). Even if the bingeing and purging behaviors are occurring with less frequency than just described, emphasis should be on prevention and breaking the cycle. Early detection and help in this condition to break the cycle will prevent further or permanent damage to the body, mind, and spirit.

It is not easy to recognize bulimia. In fact, it often goes undetected. Individuals with bulimia often try to hide the condition from their family and friends. People with bulimia can be of normal weight or slightly overweight, come from diverse backgrounds, and practice many types of eating behaviors. They frequently have weight fluctuations greater than 10 pounds (4.5 kg) due to alternate binges and fasts (40). It is important for personal trainers to be familiar with the signs, effects, and behaviors associated

Warning Signs for Anorexia

- Dramatic loss of weight (up to 15% or more below expected weight range)
- Denial; feelings of being fat even when thin; obsession with weight, diet, and appearance
- Use of food rituals or avoidance of social situations involving food
- Obsession with exercise; hyperactivity
- Sensitivity to cold
- Use of layers of baggy clothing to disguise weight loss
- Fatigue (in later stages)
- Decline in work, school, or athletic performance
- Growth of baby-fine hair over face and body (lanugo hair)
- Yellow tint to skin, palms, and soles of feet (from high levels of carotene)
- Hair loss, dry hair, dry skin, brittle nails
- Loss of muscle mass and tone
- No menstrual periods (amenorrhea)
- Slow pulse at rest, light-headedness on standing up quickly
- Constipation

Reprinted by permission from Otis and Goldingay 2000.

Warning Signs for Bulimia

- Self-induced vomiting (at least two times a week for at least three months)
- Laxative, diuretics, or enema use
- Excessive exercise
- Overconcern with body shape
- Weight fluctuations of more than 10 pounds (4.5 kg)
- Traces of odor of vomit on the breath
- Scabs or scars on knuckles
- Swollen, persistently puffy face and cheeks
- Broken blood vessels in the face and eyes
- Sore throat and dental problems
- Abdominal symptoms
- Rapid weight changes of 2 to 5 pounds (0.9-2.5 kg) overnight
- Erratic performance in work, sport, and academics
- Irregular or absent menstrual periods
- Lacerations of the oral cavity
- Diarrhea
- Constipation
- Fatigue
- Electrolyte disturbances
- Heart irregularities
- Ruptures in the stomach

Reprinted by permission from Otis and Goldingay 2000.

with bulimia so they may be able to identify the condition in a client and refer him or her for help (see "Warning Signs for Bulimia").

Female Athlete Triad

Eating disorders can result in the female athlete triad, composed of the following interrelated disorders (4):

- Disordered eating
- Amenorrhea
- Osteoporosis

The label includes the word "athlete" because this condition was first discovered in young female athletes. In actuality, the condition affects a wide range of women with different levels of activity, not just athletes (5). It is not the participation in exercise or sport that causes the triad, but the misguided goal of girls and women to become unrealistically thin, consequent to their thinking that this will improve sport performance or appearance (47).

The woman starts with disordered eating practices and consequently puts her body into an energy deficit, which results in amenorrhea over time. Amenorrhea (loss of menses) is a serious medical problem as the woman is now deficient in the hormones necessary for bone density accruement, which normally occurs from birth through the age of 30. Unfortunately, this condition leads to a lack of normal bone formation and irreversible loss in bone mass, resulting in osteoporosis and its subsequent complications (4, 49). Personal trainers should be alert to women who exhibit signs of the female athlete triad and refer such clients to a health care professional for evaluation.

The female athlete triad often begins with disordered eating, which leads to amenorrhea, which leads to osteoporosis. It occurs in a wide range of women, not just athletes.

Exercise Prescription and Program Design for Clients Recovering From an Eating Disorder

Clients with a diagnosed eating disorder should receive clearance from their physician before returning to an exercise program. An exercise program can be beneficial, both physically and emotionally, but the program must be designed so that it is safe and does not prompt a return to the use of exercise as a purging technique. The physician must determine whether and when it is medically safe for the client to start exercise.

When resuming a client's exercise program, the personal trainer needs to reassess the client. Some clients may have stress fractures due to the osteoporosis and will have to find alternative forms of exercise until healing occurs, such as swimming or deep-water aqua exercise, in which there is no impact. Yoga and Pilates classes could also be considered. Clients who have experienced complications of the eating disorder (abnormal electrolytes, an irregular heartbeat, having passed out at any time) will not be able to exercise until the problem is corrected or alleviated. Once a client with the triad returns to exercise, it is important to monitor heart rate and blood pressure.

An exercise program should deemphasize weight loss and emphasize exercise with a low energy demand (2). A return to high caloric expendi-

Program Design for Clients Recovering From an Eating Disorder

- Require the client recovering from an eating disorder to see a physician for a complete medical exam before returning to or continuing an exercise program.
- Do not prescribe a vigorous exercise program.
- Help the client to engage in a well-rounded program of aerobic conditioning, resistance training, and flexibility exercise.
- Ensure adequate hydration and rehydration.
- Encourage the client to ingest an adequate dietary intake.
- Encourage the client to consume 200 to 400 kcal of complex carbohydrates during the first 30 to 90 minutes following an exercise session.
- Schedule exercise sessions so that the client does not exercise every day and takes two to three days off a week.
- Check the client's blood pressure and pulse.
- Do not allow impact exercise if the client has a stress fracture.
- Maintain regular communication with the client's physician, dietitian, and other health care professionals.
- If a client experiences any of the following signs or symptoms, he or she should seek medical clearance before continuing the exercise program: light-headedness, irregular heartbeats, nausea, injuries, abnormal blood pressure levels or pulse.

ture exercise should be delayed until the client is cleared by a physician. Resistance exercise should be included in order to preserve lean body mass, although its effectiveness will be severely compromised if the client does not consume adequate calories and nutrients.

The personal trainer may encounter an individual who has an eating disorder but refuses to see a physician. Although the personal trainer, as one of very few people who may be in touch with the client, may be tempted to continue to train the client, the personal trainer should require a medical release before continuing. Should the client refuse to see a physician, the personal trainer cannot train the client.

Hyperlipidemia

Cardiovascular disease is the leading cause of death in the industrialized nations and is responsible for more than 1 million deaths a year in the United States. Blood lipid disorders are risk factors that play a significant role in the process of arteriosclerosis resulting in the clinical syndromes of coronary heart disease, angina pectoris, myocardial infarction, sudden cardiac death, and chronic heart failure.

Blood lipid disorders include hyperlipidemia and dyslipidemia. **Hyperlipidemia** is a general term for elevated concentrations of any or all of the lipids (fats) in the blood, such as cholesterol, **triglycer-**

ides, and lipoproteins. This term usually indicates high levels of **low-density lipoproteins (LDLs)** and **very low-density lipoproteins (VLDLs)**. The term **dyslipidemia** refers to abnormal lipid (fat) levels in the blood, lipoprotein composition, or both.

In 2001, the NIH released the National Cholesterol Education Program Adult Treatment Panel III (ATP III) guidelines for the detection, evaluation, and treatment of cholesterol (43). The guidelines set lower LDL goals, raised **high-density lipoprotein (HDL)** goals, and also lowered the triglyceride classification cut points. Refer to table 19.5 for this information.

These guidelines also recommend **therapeutic lifestyle change** or **TLC** as the first line of therapy for the majority of the disorders. Therapeutic lifestyle change includes diet, physical activity, and weight loss. Drug therapy may be necessary for higher-risk individuals or those who do not respond well to TLC. Personal trainers should become familiar with these and future NIH guidelines in order to be able to design an effective physical activity program and promote the other necessary lifestyle changes prescribed by the client's physician to improve the lipid profile and other risk factors for CVD.

Possible Causes of Hyperlipidemia

Substantial amounts of research have shown that an elevated LDL level is a major cause of coronary

TABLE 19.5 ATP III Classification of LDL, HDL, Total Cholesterol, and Triglycerides (mg/dl)

LDL-cholesterol	
<100	Optimal
100-129	Near optimal
130-159	Borderline high
160-189	High
≥190	Very high
Total cholesterol	
<200	Desirable
200-239	Borderline high
≥240	High
HDL-cholesterol	
<40	Low
≥60	High
Serum triglyceride levels	
<150	Normal
150-199	Borderline high
200-499	High
≥500	Very high

Reprinted from NIH and NHLBI 2001 (43).

heart disease (CHD) (43). Furthermore, clinical trials provide strong evidence that LDL-lowering therapy reduces risk for CHD. Hence, the ATP III guidelines identify elevated LDLs as the primary target of cholesterol-lowering therapy (43). The goal for the majority of adults who do not have diabetes or CVD is <130 mg/dl, while the goal for those who do have diabetes or CVD is <100 mg/dl.

The ATP III has also designated low HDLs, defined as a level <40 mg/dl, as a strong independent predictor of CHD. The possible causes of low HDL levels, which are also correlated to insulin resistance, include elevated triglycerides, overweight and obesity, physical inactivity, and type 2 diabetes. Other causes include cigarette smoking, high carbohydrate intakes (especially simple sugars), and certain drugs (e.g., beta blockers, anabolic steroids, progestational agents). Therapy to increase low HDL levels is twofold. The goal is to focus on lowering LDL levels with the diet, drug therapy, or both and to increase physical activity and weight loss for those who have the metabolic syndrome (as diagnosed by a physician when a client has three or more of the risk determinants listed on page 513 along with its increased risk of CVD and diabetes) (43).

Elevated triglycerides are an additional concern as they have been shown to be an independent CHD risk factor (43). Factors that can raise triglycerides to higher than normal levels in the general population include obesity and overweight, lack of physical activity, cigarette smoking, excess alcohol intake, and high-carbohydrate diets, as well as several diseases (type 2 diabetes, chronic renal failure, and nephritic syndrome along with certain drugs) and genetic disorders. (The personal trainer who is aware of some of these causes can encourage clients to make changes in their habits such as consuming less alcohol, eating less sweets and high-carbohydrate foods, and stopping smoking in addition to following the overall TLC program.)

Table 19.6 offers a review of the possible causes and treatment of unfavorable LDL, HDL, and triglyceride levels.

Because diet and weight loss play a major role in lowering LDL and triglyceride levels, clients with hyperlipidemia should see a registered dietitian in addition to visiting their physician regularly. The dietitian will provide the client with *medical nutrition therapy*, the term for the nutritional intervention and guidance provided by a registered dietitian. Medical nutrition therapy for blood lipid disorders is a process that includes assessing the client's current diet, using the ATP III guidelines to design a diet to lower LDL and triglyceride levels in addition to controlling weight, and offering behavior modification strategies to ensure that the client can adhere to the diet. Follow-up sessions are an important contributor to the success of the diet program.

The personal trainer can play an effective role in the implementation and success of a TLC program. As mentioned earlier, the multifaceted approach consists of diet, increased physical activity, and weight loss. The personal trainer will be the one to facilitate the exercise program with its positive effects on increasing HDLs, lowering triglycerides, and promoting weight loss. Additionally, the personal trainer can serve a supportive role in motivating the client to adhere to the TLC diet prescribed by the physician with subsequent dietary counseling from a registered dietitian.

Therapeutic Lifestyle Change Diet

The *major emphasis and most important* phase of TLC for high LDL levels is the consumption of an antiatherogenic diet (43). An antiatherogenic diet or TLC diet is referred to as a "heart healthy diet" in the lay literature as it tends to lower cholesterol

TABLE 19.6 Possible Causes of and Treatment Strategies for Unfavorable Lipid Levels

Lipid	Possible etiology (possible causes)	Possible treatment strategies*
High LDL levels	■ Abdominal obesity ■ Sedentary lifestyle ■ Overweight and obesity ■ Atherogenic diet** ■ Insulin resistance ■ Glucose intolerance ■ Genetic predisposition ■ Genetic disorders ■ Other diseases, such as hypothyroidism, obstructive liver disease, chronic renal failure ■ Certain drugs (e.g., progestins, anabolic steroids, corticosteroids)	■ Weight reduction ■ TLC diet including control of saturated fat and cholesterol intake ■ Reduced calorie consumption where appropriate ■ Increased consumption of (soluble) fiber (10-25 g/day) ■ Increased physical activity ■ Drug therapy ■ Control of other risk factors (such as smoking, hypertension)
Low HDL levels	■ Overweight and obesity ■ Sedentary lifestyle ■ Elevated trigycerides ■ Insulin resistance ■ Type 2 diabetes ■ Cigarette smoking ■ High carbohydrate intake (>60% of kilocalories) ■ Certain drugs (e.g., beta blockers, anabolic steroids, progestational agents)	■ Control of LDL level ■ Weight reduction ■ Physical activity ■ Smoking cessation ■ TLC diet, including control of caloric and carbohydrate intake ■ Drug therapy
Triglycerides	■ Overweight and obesity ■ Sedentary lifestyle ■ Cigarette smoking ■ Excessive alcohol intake ■ High carbohydrate intake (>60% of kilocalories) ■ Insulin resistance ■ Other diseases, such as type 2 diabetes, chronic renal failure, nephritic syndrome ■ Certain drugs (e.g., corticosteroids, estrogens, retinoids, higher doses of beta-adrenergic blocking agents) ■ Genetic disorders	■ Control of LDL level ■ Physical activity ■ Weight reduction ■ TLC diet including control of caloric and carbohydrate intake ■ Restriction of excessive alcohol intake ■ Drug therapy ■ Very low-fat diets for clients with *very high triglyceride levels* (≥500 mg/dl)

*The client's physician will decide on each client's specific treatment strategy in accordance with that person's specific condition and its severity.
**An atherogenic diet is high in fat, high in saturated fats, high in cholesterol, high in trans fatty acids, high in calories, or low in fruits and vegetables or any combination of these.
Data from NIH and NHLBI 2001 (43).

levels, especially if combined with physical activity and weight loss.

The mainstay of the TLC diet is the limited intake of saturated fats (<7% of total calories) and cholesterol (<200 mg/day). Table 19.7 shows the overall composition of the diet.

In practical terms, the recommendations in table 19.7 translate to eating a diet that is low in overall fat intake and in saturated fat; low in cholesterol; adequate in nutrients; and high in fruits, vegetables, and whole grains.

TLC Physical Activity: Exercise Prescription and Program Design for Clients With Hyperlipidemia

Physical inactivity is targeted for therapy by the ATP III guidelines as a major, underlying risk factor for CHD. Regular physical activity lowers risk by reducing VLDL levels with a subsequent decrease in triglycerides; raising HDLs; and in some individuals,

TABLE 19.7 Nutrient Composition of the TLC Diet

Nutrient	Recommended intake
Saturated fat*	<7% of total calories
Polyunsaturated fat	Up to 10% of total calories
Monounsaturated fat	Up to 20% of total calories
Total fat	25% to 35% of total calories
Carbohydrate**	50% to 60% of total calories
Fiber	20 to 30 g/day
Protein	Approximately 15% of total calories
Cholesterol	<200 mg/day
Total calories	Balance energy intake and expenditure to maintain desirable body weight and prevent weight gain***

*Trans fatty acids are another LDL-raising fat that should be kept at a low intake.
**Carbohydrate should be derived predominantly from foods rich in complex carbohydrates including grains, especially whole grains, fruits, and vegetables.
***Daily energy expenditure should include at least moderate physical activity (contributing approximately 200 kcal/day).
Reprinted from NIH and NHLBI 2001 (43).

lowering LDL levels (41). Other risk factors for CHD are also mitigated by physical activity, as it can also play a significant role in lowering blood pressure, reducing insulin resistance, and improving cardiovascular function. It is for these reasons that the ATP III recommends regular physical activity as a routine component in the management of high serum cholesterol (41, 48).

Although a single session of aerobic exercise produces beneficial lipoprotein changes, it is necessary to participate in a regular, long-term exercise program of at least a year and to continue thereafter in order to attain and sustain lasting results (11, 32). Furthermore, programs should involve a relatively high frequency of exercise sessions per week, as acute exercise has been shown to improve both insulin action and lipid profiles for up to 48 to 72 hours after each exercise session (21). The target exercise guidelines for improving lipid levels are listed in table 19.8.

Although the evidence is not conclusive, resistance training may have a positive effect on the lipid profile and other concomitant risk factors for CHD such as diabetes mellitus, obesity, and overweight (18, 49). A resistance training program would follow the recommendations in chapter 15. In light of these benefits, it is prudent for the personal trainer to provide clients with a well-rounded exercise program that includes aerobic, resistance, and flexibility training components.

TLC Weight Loss

Weight loss in conjunction with an exercise and diet program can bring about even larger decreases in LDLs, increase HDLs, and reduce total cholesterol (47). The personal trainer must educate clients about the importance of weight-loss management of hyperlipidemia. Information on safe weight loss is included at the beginning of this chapter.

Metabolic Syndrome

Magkos and colleagues (39) have described **metabolic syndrome** as "a clinical entity characterized by a constellation of metabolically related abnormalities and cardiovascular risk factors, including obesity, insulin resistance/glucose intolerance, dyslipidemia, and hypertension." However, there has been some controversy regarding the exact definition of metabolic syndrome. Most definitions have included abdominal obesity, hypertriglyceridemia, low HDL-cholesterol, hypertension, and elevated fasting glucose concentrations (41). This syndrome has also been referred to as *syndrome X*, *dyslipidemic hypertension*, and *insulin resistance syndrome*. People with the metabolic syndrome are at increased risk for developing diabetes mellitus and CVD, as well as increased mortality from CVD and other illnesses. The *Third Report of the Expert Panel on Detection, Evaluation, and Treatment of High Blood Cholesterol in Adults (Adult Treatment Panel III) Executive Summary* (47) provided a con-

TABLE 19.8 Exercise Prescription for Clients With Hyperlipidemia

Mode	Frequency, intensity, duration	Guidelines and concerns
Aerobic conditioning	■ ≥5 days/week to maximize caloric expenditure ■ 30 to 60 min/day ■ Eventual goal: 50 to 60 min/day to promote or maintain weight loss ■ 40 to 75% of $\dot{V}O_2R$ or HRR	■ Obesity may limit exercise type. ■ Initially emphasize increasing duration rather than increasing intensity to optimize caloric expenditure.

Adapted from ACSM 2010 (2).

sensus definition of this syndrome. Persons having three or more of the following criteria were defined as having the metabolic syndrome (26):

1. Abdominal obesity: waist circumference >102 cm (>40 inches) in men and >88 cm (>35 inches) in women

2. Hypertriglyceridemia: ≥150 mg/dl (1.69 mmol/L)

3. Reduced HDL-cholesterol: <40 mg/dl (1.04 mmol/L) in men and <50 mg/dl (1.29 mmol/L) in women

4. Elevated blood pressure: ≥130/85 mmHg

5. Elevated fasting glucose: ≥110 mg/dl (≥6.1 mmol/L)

The overall prevalence of the metabolic syndrome is approximately 27% in the U.S. adult population (38). The metabolic syndrome is associated with a two- to fourfold increase in cardiovascular morbidity and stroke (38). It has increased in prevalence over the last few decades and parallels the rise in obesity and type 2 diabetes (7), and it is now believed that these conditions are linked through underlying pathophysiological mechanisms (35). Poor blood glucose regulation, due to insulin resistance, has been proposed as the underlying cause of this syndrome. Insulin is an important hormone that stimulates the cells of the body to take in glucose from the blood. Insulin does this by binding with specific receptor sites on the cells' surfaces. People with the metabolic syndrome typically have **hyperinsulinemia,** which means high levels of insulin in the blood. Insulin levels appear to be high because of insulin resistance, which means that the cells are not responding appropriately to insulin. Insulin receptors become less numerous and less sensitive to insulin, so the insulin stays in the blood rather than binding to the cells. Meanwhile, blood glucose levels remain high as well, since the receptors are not letting insulin help the glucose get into the cells.

People with metabolic syndrome often have the "apple-shaped" or android body type, which is characterized by high amounts of fat in the trunk and abdomen. Researchers have found that abdominal fat cells deposit high amounts of triglycerides into the bloodstream. The nearby liver takes up this fat and produces VLDL molecules, which transport triglycerides to the cells of the body. Upon losing the triglycerides, VLDLs convert into LDLs. It is the LDL molecule that carries large amounts of cholesterol and deposits the cholesterol around the body. Therefore, high levels of LDLs are associated with an increased risk of coronary heart disease and stroke due to the progression of atherosclerosis. The

elevation in triglycerides is also believed to disrupt blood glucose regulation. The resulting rise in insulin levels may, in turn, stimulate sympathetic nervous system regulation, which increases blood pressure. The combination of these conditions results in the following unhealthy "total package" called *metabolic syndrome*: high blood glucose, high blood lipids, hypertension, and abdominal obesity.

Like coronary heart disease, the metabolic syndrome usually develops slowly and even over several years before the affected individual meets the criteria for medical intervention. Unfortunately, people with abnormal levels of glucose, blood pressure, fat, and blood lipids are at high risk for developing heart disease and stroke. People with abdominal obesity or a family history of diabetes should be especially vigilant for the early signs of metabolic syndrome development.

The metabolic syndrome has both a genetic and a behavioral component. Family history increases one's risk for developing this syndrome in addition to cigarette smoking, a sedentary lifestyle, alcohol consumption, a poor diet, and stress. Early intervention that includes weight loss through dietary modification and enhanced physical activity can significantly delay or prevent the development of this syndrome.

Exercise is the first line of treatment for the metabolic syndrome because it influences all components of this disorder. Regular physical activity helps reduce excess body fat. Exercise also improves the sensitivity of the cells to insulin, thus normalizing blood insulin levels and decreasing blood glucose levels. It helps to decrease blood pressure, in addition to increasing HDL-cholesterol levels. Ross and Despres (51) recently reported that leading health organizations now promote the use of physical activity as a therapeutic strategy for management of the metabolic syndrome. Personal trainers should be sure to work in conjunction with the client's physician and a registered dietitian to ensure the client's success in dealing with the various conditions of the metabolic syndrome (1, 22, 29, 30).

> Early intervention that effects weight loss through dietary changes and increased physical activity can significantly delay or prevent the onset of metabolic syndrome.

Diabetes Mellitus

Diabetes mellitus is a group of metabolic diseases characterized by an excessively high (or uncontrolled) blood glucose level. Some of the signs and symptoms of diabetes include

- increased frequency of urination,
- increased thirst,
- increased appetite, and
- general weakness.

The diagnosis of diabetes mellitus is based on two fasting glucose levels of 126 mg/dl or higher. Other options for diagnosis include two 2-hour postprandial (i.e., after a meal) plasma glucose measurements of 200 mg/dl or higher after a glucose load of 75 g or two casual glucose readings of 200 mg/dl. Chronic uncontrolled diabetes is associated with long-term damage to various body organs including the eyes, kidneys, nerves, heart, and blood vessels. Diabetes is the leading cause of blindness, renal failure, and lower extremity amputations.

Types of Diabetes

The major types of diabetes mellitus are type 1, type 2, and gestational. **Type 1 diabetes mellitus,** formerly known as *insulin-dependent diabetes mellitus (IDDM)*, is associated with pancreatic beta cell destruction by an autoimmune process, usually leading to absolute insulin deficiency. Approximately 10% of patients with diabetes have type 1, and most of these people develop the disease before the age of 25. Exogenous insulin by either injection or pump is required for survival. People with uncontrolled or newly diagnosed type 1 diabetes are prone to developing diabetic ketoacidosis. Diabetic ketoacidosis is a metabolic acidosis caused by the accumulation of **ketones** due to severely depressed insulin levels. The initial symptoms are frequent urination, nausea, vomiting, abdominal pain, and lethargy. Untreated individuals may progress to coma.

Type 2 diabetes mellitus was formerly referred to as *non-insulin-dependent diabetes mellitus* (NIDDM) and is characterized by insulin resistance in peripheral tissues and an insulin secretory deficit of the pancreatic beta cells. This is the most common form of diabetes mellitus (composing about 90% of cases of diabetes) and is highly associated with a family history of diabetes, older age, obesity, and lack of exercise. The treatment for type 2 diabetes usually includes diet modification, weight control, regular exercise, and oral hypoglycemic agents.

Gestational diabetes mellitus is a condition in which the glucose level is elevated and other diabetic symptoms appear during pregnancy in women who have not previously been diagnosed with diabetes. Gestational diabetes is not caused by a lack of insulin, but by insulin resistance. All diabetic symptoms usually disappear following delivery, but affected mothers are at increased risk of developing type 2 diabetes mellitus later in life. Approximately 2% to 5% of all pregnant women in the United States are diagnosed with gestational diabetes. Treatment for gestational diabetes includes special diet, exercise, and insulin injections.

Exercise Prescription and Program Design for Clients With Diabetes Mellitus

Exercise is an essential component of diabetic management. In both types of diabetes mellitus, exercise can increase insulin sensitivity and glucose utilization, thus lowering blood glucose levels. In addition, regular physical activity reduces other risk factors related to CVD such as hypertension, dyslipidemia, and obesity. Although exercise is highly beneficial for clients with diabetes, there are some potential complications, such as **hypoglycemia** (blood glucose level of 65 mg/dl or lower), that the personal trainer needs to keep in mind when designing and supervising an exercise program (17).

Before beginning an exercise program, clients with diabetes should have a medical evaluation to assess their glycemic control and to screen for any complications that may be exacerbated by exercise. Stress cardiac testing performed by a medical professional is also generally recommended for all clients with diabetes who are planning to engage in moderate-intensity exercise and are considered at risk for heart disease. This group includes clients who are older than 35 years, those with type 2 diabetes of more than 10 years' duration, those with type 1 diabetes of more than 15 years' duration, and those with evidence of microvascular disease (retinopathy or nephropathy) (17).

Individuals exhibiting organ damage from long-standing diabetes need to be careful and to abstain from certain exacerbating physical activities. For example, individuals with peripheral neuropathy are at an increased risk of ulceration and infection of the feet because of lack of sensation and decreased healing reaction. Therefore, in this condition, low-impact exercises, such as swimming and biking, may be preferable to walking and jogging. Also proper footwear—shoes that are comfortable and well fitted—is essential to prevent blisters and other foot injuries. Any dizziness, weakness, or shortness of breath should alert the personal trainer to the possibility of cardiac disease and the need for a medical evaluation. Contraindications to exercise for persons with diabetes are listed on page 515.

Contraindications to Exercise for Clients With Diabetes

- Blood glucose >250 mg/dl and ketones in urine for type 1 diabetes (7)
- Blood glucose >300 mg/dl without ketones for type 1 diabetes (7)
- Clients with type 2 diabetes may participate in exercise provided they are felling well and are hydrated
- Proliferative retinopathy—clients with this condition should avoid strenuous high-intensity activities
- Severe kidney disease
- Loss of protective sensation in the feet (peripheral neuropathy)—clients with this condition should avoid outdoor walking and jogging (swimming or biking is recommended)
- Acute illness, infection, or fever
- Evidence of underlying CVD that has not been medically evaluated

Glycemic Control

The principal risk of exercise among those who have diabetes is hypoglycemia (blood glucose level of 65 mg/dl or lower). This is of greater concern for patients who have type 1 diabetes than for those who have type 2.

Factors that predispose to hypoglycemia during exercise include

- increased exercise intensity,
- longer exercise time,
- inadequate caloric intake prior to exercise,
- excessive insulin dose,
- insulin injection into exercising muscle, and
- colder environmental temperatures.

The mechanism for exercise-induced hypoglycemia is related to the fact that exercise enhances the absorption of exogenous insulin, increases the muscle uptake of glucose, and impairs the mobilization of glucose in blood. Signs of hypoglycemia include apparent loss of concentration, shaking or shivering, sweating, tachycardia, and loss of consciousness. See the box below for a comprehensive

Hypoglycemia

Signs and Symptoms of Hypoglycemia

- Sweating
- Hunger
- Palpitations
- Headache
- Tachycardia
- Anxiety
- Tremor
- Dizziness
- Blurred vision
- Confusion
- Convulsion
- Syncope
- Coma

Responding to a Client Who Has Hypoglycemia

1. Consider dialing 911.
2. Immediate treatment with carbohydrate is essential.
3. Measure blood glucose level with glucose monitoring device (if available).
4. If the blood glucose level is below 70 mg/dl or the client is known to have diabetes and is having signs or symptoms of hypoglycemia, provide 15 g of carbohydrate, which is equivalent to any of the following:
   - About three or four glucose tablets
   - 1/2 cup of regular soft drink or fruit juice
   - About six saltine crackers
   - 1 tablespoon of sugar or honey
5. Wait about 15 minutes and remeasure glucose level. If the level remains under 70 mg/dl, provide another 15 g of carbohydrate. Repeat testing and giving food or tablets until blood glucose level rises above 70 mg/dl.

list of the signs and symptoms of hypoglycemia. Personal trainers working with clients who have diabetes should know how to recognize the signs of hypoglycemia and be able to manage hypoglycemia cases with glucose or fructose foods and drinks when affected individuals are unable to treat themselves. See page 515 for a recommended response to hypoglycemia. Clients with diabetes should always wear a medical alert identification bracelet where it can be easily seen in case of a hypoglycemic reaction (24).

Blood glucose measurements using portable glucose monitors are an essential part of the exercise prescription. Clients should monitor their blood sugar before and after exercise and also every 30 minutes during prolonged exercise. According to the American Diabetes Association, people with type 1 diabetes should not exercise if their glucose level is greater than 300 mg/dl or greater than 250 mg/dl with urinary ketones (7). The American College of Sports Medicine has recommended that individuals with type 2 diabetes can participate in exercise as long as they feel well and are adequately hydrated, though they should use caution if their blood glucose levels exceed 300 mg/dl without ketones (6). Exercising at these levels can worsen the hyperglycemia and promote ketosis and acidosis. On the other hand, individuals with preexercise glucose levels below 100 mg/dl are at risk of developing hypoglycemia during or after exercise; therefore they should ingest a carbohydrate snack before exercise.

Adjustment of medication dosage, either insulin or oral hypoglycemic drugs, as well as proper timing of meals, is the key for maintaining good glycemic control during physical activity. Exercise should generally be scheduled 1 to 2 hours after a meal, or when the hypoglycemic medication is not at its peak activity. After exercise, carbohydrate stores should be replenished according to the duration and intensity of the activity. The client's physician will direct the patient's insulin use. This is normally done in conjunction with a dietitian to ensure that a hypoglycemic event does not occur. The personal trainer is never to advise a client about the use of insulin or the timing of meals. Should a client experience regular episodes of lack of blood glucose control, the client should be sent back to his or her physician for care.

Finally, each client with diabetes has his or her own metabolic response to exercise. No general guideline can take the place of intelligent self-observation and regular glucose monitoring in developing an individualized plan to facilitate safe, enjoyable exercise. Guidelines for aerobic conditioning and resistance exercise are shown in table 19.9.

Aerobic Conditioning

Exercise prescription for clients with diabetes mellitus should include aerobic physical activity with a frequency of three to seven days a week, for 20 to 60 minutes per day at 50% to 80% of VO_2 reserve ($\dot{V}O_2R$) or HRR (2, 3). $\dot{V}O_2R$ is the difference between resting and maximal $\dot{V}O_2$ (2, 3). People who are unconditioned can perform exercise at a lower intensity level for a longer duration, at least until they achieve a higher level of fitness. Exercise sessions should

TABLE 19.9 Exercise Prescription for Clients With Diabetes

Mode	Intensity, frequency, duration	Guidelines and concerns
Aerobic conditioning	■ 3 to 7 days/week ■ 20 to 60 min/day (150 min/week) ■ Eventual goal: 300 min/week ■ 50% to 80% $\dot{V}O_2R$ or HRR (corresponding RPE of 12 to 16 on a 6 to 20 scale)	■ A snack may be needed before exercise. ■ Monitor blood glucose before and after exercise. ■ Include a 5- to 10-min warm-up and cool-down period. ■ Monitor intensity via RPE, especially if the client is taking a heart rate-altering medication.
Resistance training	■ 2 or 3 nonconsecutive days/week ■ 2 or 3 sets, 8 to 12 reps per set (60-80% 1RM) ■ Up to 8 to 10 multijoint exercises for all major muscle groups in the same session (whole body) or sessions split into selected muscle groups	■ Can begin with body weight exercises and progress to free weights and resistance machines. ■ Clients with well-controlled diabetes can progress to strength training (i.e., higher loads, fewer repetitions).
Flexibility training	■ >2 or 3 days/week* ■ ≥4 reps per muscle group	

*Hold static stretches for 15 to 60 s.
Adapted from ACSM 2010 (2).

begin with a low-intensity warm-up and stretching of the muscle to be exercised and should conclude with a cool-down period. These activities ease the cardiovascular transition between rest and exercise and help prevent muscle and joint injuries. Balducci and colleagues (9) recently reported the effects of regular aerobic exercise on type 2 diabetic patients; regular aerobic exercise improved glycemic control, lipoprotein and lipid control, body weight control, and increased insulin sensitivity. The authors also reported that exercising at a vigorous level may have a higher benefit than exercising at low-to-moderate levels. Clients should also be instructed to work to voluntary fatigue, not to exhaustion.

Resistance Training

The recommendation for resistance training is two to three days a week, with sessions including at least one set of each of 8 to 10 different exercises using the major muscle groups. Each set should consist of 8 to 12 repetitions, with the amount of weight increased when the individual can complete 12 or more repetitions. For clients with diabetes who are older than 50 or who have other health conditions such as hypertension, more repetitions (12 to 15)

at a lower weight may be more suitable (2, 48). Balducci and coworkers (9) reported that participation in a regular resistance training program offers the same benefits (improved glycemic control, increased insulin sensitivity, increased lean body mass, and increased overall functionality) as participating in a regular aerobic exercise program. Furthermore, they reported that participation in a mixed aerobic training and resistance training program may offer the optimal benefit for improvement of glycemic index control compared to either one alone.

Conclusion

Personal trainers play a valuable role in helping clients with obesity, eating disorders, hyperlipidemia, and diabetes achieve fitness and health goals through adherence to a healthy diet and a well-designed exercise program. Personal trainers should strongly consider the value of working in conjunction with the client's physician and with a dietitian in order to ensure the client's success. In so doing, they can play a significant role in the client's health care team.

Study Questions

1. Based on his calculated BMI, which of the following is the disease risk for a 69-inch (175 cm), 198-pound (90 kg) male client with a waist circumference of 41 inches (104 cm)?

   A. no risk

   B. increased

   C. high

   D. very high

2. All of the following are dietary goals that can apply to all clients who are overweight EXCEPT

   A. setting a weight loss goal of 10% of body weight over the first six months.

   B. changing food selections to decrease caloric and fat intake.

   C. aiming for a 1- to 2-pound (0.45-0.9 kg) weight loss per week.

   D. following a 1,200 kcal/day food plan.

3. Which of the following are undesirable blood lipid levels?

   I. total cholesterol: 250 mg/dl

   II. triglycerides: 200 mg/dl

   III. LDLs: 100 mg/dl

   IV. HDLs: 50 mg/dl

   A. I and IV only

   B. I and II only

   C. II and III only

   D. III and IV only

4. Which of the following describes a difference between type 1 and type 2 diabetes?

   A. Only clients with type 1 diabetes can have gestational diabetes.

   B. Clients with type 1 diabetes are more prevalent.

   C. Clients with type 2 diabetes can produce insulin.

   D. Only clients with type 2 diabetes can receive exogenous insulin.

Applied Knowledge Question

Provide dietary modifications, exercise program guidelines, and lifestyle change support suggestions for a client who is obese.

References

1. Alberti, K.G., P. Zimmet, and J. Shaw. 2006. Metabolic syndrome—a new world-wide definition. A consensus statement from the international diabetes federation. *Diabetic Medicine* 23: 469-480.

2. American College of Sports Medicine. 2010. *ACSM's Guidelines for Exercise Testing and Prescription.* 8th ed. Philadelphia: Lippincott Williams & Wilkin.

3. American College of Sports Medicine. 2010. *ACSM's Resource Manual for Guidelines for Exercise Testing and Prescription.* 8th ed. Philadelphia: Lippincott Williams & Wilkins.

4. American College of Sports Medicine. 2007. Position stand: The female athlete triad. *Medicine and Science in Sports and Exercise* 39 (10): 1867-1882.

5. American College of Sports Medicine. 2009. Position stand: Appropriate physical activity intervention strategies for weight loss and prevention of weight regain for adults. *Medicine and Science in Sports and Exercise* 41 (2): 459-471.

6. American College of Sports Medicine and American Diabetics Association. 2010. Position stand: Exercise and type 2 diabetes. *Medicine and Science in Sports and Exercise* 42 (12): 2282-2303.

7. American Diabetes Association. 2002. Position statement: Diabetes mellitus and exercise. *Diabetes Care* 25 (Suppl 1): S64.

8. American Psychiatric Association. 1994. *Diagnostic and Statistical Manual of Mental Disorders (DSMV IV),* 4th ed. Washington, DC: APA.

9. Balducci, S., S. Zanuso, F. Fernando, S. Falluccaa, F. Fallucca, and G. Pugliese. 2009. Physical activity/exercise training in type 2 diabetes. The role of the Italian diabetes and exercise study. *Diabetes Metabolism Research and Reviews* 25: S29-S33.

10. Baker, C., and K.D. Brownell. 2000. Physical activity and maintenance of weight loss: Physiological and psychological mechanisms. In: *Physical Activity and Obesity,* C. Bouchard, ed. Champaign, IL: Human Kinetics. pp. 311-328.

11. Berg, A., I. Frey, M.W. Baumstark, H. Halle, and J. Keul. 1994. Physical activity and lipoprotein lipid disorders. *Sports Medicine* 17 (1): 6-21.

12. Blair, S.N., J.B. Kampert, H.W. Kohl, C.E. Barlow, C.A. Macera, R.S. Paffenbarger, and L.W. Gibbons. 1996. Influences of cardiorespiratory fitness and other precursors on cardiovascular disease and all-cause mortality in men and women. *Journal of the American Medical Association* 276 (3): 205-210.

13. Blair, S., and M.Z. Nichaman. 2002. The public health problem of increasing prevalence rates of obesity and what should be done about it. *Mayo Clinic Proceedings* 77: 109-113.

14. Bouchard, C. 2000. Introduction. In: *Physical Activity and Obesity,* C. Bouchard, ed. Champaign, IL: Human Kinetics. pp. 3-19.

15. Brownbill, R.A., and J.Z. Ilich. 2005. Measuring body composition in overweight individuals by dual energy x-ray absorptiometry. *BMC Medical Imaging* 5: 1.

16. Caballero, B. 2004. Obesity prevention in children: Opportunities and challenges. *International Journal of Obesity and Related Metabolic Disorders* 28 (3S): S90-95.

17. Colberg, S.R., and D.P. Swain. 2000. Exercise and diabetic control. *Physician and Sportsmedicine* 28 (4): 63-81.

18. Conley, M.S., and R. Rozenek. 2001. National Strength and Conditioning Association position statement: Health aspects of resistance exercise and training. *Strength and Conditioning Journal* 23 (6): 9-23.

19. Delva, J., L.D. Johnston, and P.M. O'Malley. 2007. The epidemiology of overweight and related lifestyle behaviors: Racial/ethnic and socioeconomic status differences among American youth. *American Journal of Preventative Medicine* 33 (4S): S178-S186.

20. De Pietro, L., J. Dziura, C.W. Yeckel, and P.D. Neufer. 2006. Exercise and improved insulin sensitivity in older women: Evidence of the enduring benefits of higher intensity training. *Journal of Applied Physiology* 100: 142-149.

21. Despres, J.P., and B. Lamarche. 2000. Physical activity and the metabolic complications of obesity. In: *Physical Activity and Obesity,* C. Bouchard, ed. Champaign, IL: Human Kinetics. pp. 329-354.

22. Despres, J.P., I. Lemieux, and D. Prud'homme. 2001. Treatment of obesity: Need to focus on high risk abdominally obese patients. *British Medical Journal* 322: 716-720.

23. Dietz, W.H. Jr., and S.L. Gortmaker. 1995. Do we fatten our children at the television set? Obesity and television viewing in children and adolescents. *Pediatrics* 75: 807-812.

24. Drazin, M.B. 2002. Type 1 diabetes and sports participation. *Physician and Sportsmedicine* 28 (12): 49-66.

25. Eickhoff-Shemek, J. 2002. Scope of practice. *ACSM's Health and Fitness Journal* 6 (5): 28-31.

26. Ford, E.S., W.H. Giles, and W.H. Dietz. 2002. Prevalence of the metabolic syndrome among US adults: Findings from the Third National Health and Nutrition Examination Survey. *Journal of the American Medical Association* 287: 356-359.

27. Gately, P.J., D. Radley, C.B. Cooke, S. Carroll, B. Oldroyd, J.G. Truscott, W.A. Coward, and A. Wright. 2003. Comparison of body composition methods in overweight and obese children. *Journal of Applied Physiology* 95: 2039-2046.

28. Goldberg, L., D.L. Elliott, R.W. Schutz, and F.E. Kloster. 1984. Changes in lipid and lipoprotein levels after weight training. *Journal of the American Medical Association* 252: 504-506.

29. Grundy, S.M., H.B. Brewer Jr., J.I. Cleeman, S.C. Smith Jr., and C. Lenfant. 2004. Definition of metabolic syndrome: Report of the National Heart, Lung, and Blood Institute/American Heart Association conference on scientific issues related to definition. *Circulation* 109: 433-438.

30. Grundy, S.M., B. Hansen, S.C. Smith Jr., J.I. Cleeman, and R.A. Kahn. 2004. Clinical management of metabolic syndrome: Report of the American Heart Association/National Heart, Lung, and Blood Institute/American Diabetes Association conference on scientific issues related to management. *Circulation* 109: 551-556.

31. Hancox, R.J., and R. Poulton. 2006. Watching television is associated with childhood obesity: But is it clinically important? *International Journal of Obesity* 30: 171-175.

32. Hurley, B.F., J.M. Hagberg, A.P. Goldberg, et al. 2005. Resistive training can reduce coronary risk factors without altering VO2max or percent body fat. *Medicine and Science in Sports and Exercise* 20 (2): 150-154.

33. Ibanez, J., M. Izquierdo, I. Arguelles, et al. 2005. Twice-weekly progressive resistance training decreases abdominal fat and improves insulin sensitivity in older men with type 2 diabetes. *Diabetes Care* 28: 662-667.

34. Kelley, G. 1997. Dynamic resistance exercise and resting blood pressure in adults: A meta-analysis. *Journal of Applied Physiology* 82 (5): 1559-1565.

35. Klem, M.L., R.R. Wing, M.T. McGuire, H.M. Seagle, and J.O. Hill. 1997. A descriptive study of individuals successful at long-term maintenance of substantial weight loss. *American Journal of Clinical Nutrition* 66: 239-246.

36. Kokkinos, P.F., and B. Fernhall. 1999. Physical activity and high density lipoprotein cholesterol levels. *Sports Medicine* 28: 307-314.

37. Koplan J.P., C.T. Liverman, and V.I. Kraak. 2005. Preventing childhood obesity: Health in the balance: Executive summary. *Journal of the American Dietetic Association* 105 (1): 131-138.

38. Lavie, C.J., R.V. Milani, S.M. Artham, D.A. Patel, and H.O. Ventura. 2009. The obesity paradox, weight loss, and coronary disease. *American Journal of Medicine* 122 (12): 1106-1114.

39. Magkos, F., M. Yannakoulia, J.L. Chan, and C.S. Mantzoros. 2009. Management of the metabolic syndrome and type 2 diabetes through lifestyle modification. *Annual Review of Nutrition* 29: 223-256.

40. Magrann, S., and S. Radford Keagy. 2001. *Weight Control and Eating Disorders.* Eureka, CA: Nutrition Dimension.

41. National Institutes of Health and National Heart, Lung, and Blood Institute. 1998. *Clinical Guidelines on the Identification, Evaluation, and Treatment of Overweight and Obesity in Adults.* NIH Pub. No. 98-4083. www.nhlbi.nih.gov/guidelines/obesity/ob_gdlns.pdf. Accessed January 13, 2003.

42. National Institutes of Health and National Heart, Lung, and Blood Institute. 2000. *The Practical Guide: Identification, Evaluation, and Treatment of Overweight and Obesity in Adults.* NIH Pub. No. 00-4084. www.nhlbi.nih.gov/guidelines/obesity/prctgd_c.pdf. Accessed November 21, 2002.

43. National Institutes of Health and National Heart, Lung, and Blood Institute. 2001. *Third Report of the National Cholesterol Education Program (NCEP) Expert Panel on Detection, Evaluation, and Treatment of High Blood Cholesterol in Adults (Adult Treatment Panel III) Executive Summary.* NIH Pub. No. 01-3670. www.nhlbi.nih.gov/guidelines/cholesterol/atp3xsum.pdf. Accessed November 21, 2002.

44. National Task Force on the Prevention and Treatment of Obesity, National Institutes of Health. 1993. Very low-calorie diets. *Journal of the American Medical Association* 270: 967-974.

45. Norris, R., D. Carroll, and R. Cochrane. 1990. The effect of aerobic and anaerobic training on fitness, blood pressure, and psychological stress and well-being. *Journal of Psychosomatic Research* 34: 367-375.

46. Ogden, C.L., M.D. Carroll, M.A. McDowell, and M.K. Flegal. 2007. Obesity among adults in the United States--no statistically significant change since 2003-2004. *NCHS Data Brief* (1): 1-8.

47. Otis, C., and R. Goldingay. 2000. *The Athletic Woman's Survival Guide.* Champaign, IL: Human Kinetics.

48. Pate, R.R., M. Pratt, S.N. Blair, W.L. Haskell, C.A. Macera, C. Bouchard, D. Buchner, W. Ettinger, G.W. Heath, and A.C. King. 1995. Physical activity and public health: A recommendation from the Centers for Disease Control and Prevention and the American College of Sports Medicine. *Journal of the American Medical Association* 273: 402-407.

49. Pollock, M.L., B.A. Franklin, G.J. Balady, B.L. Chaitman, J.L. Fleg, B. Fletcher, M. Limacher, I. Pi-a, R.A. Stein, M. Williams, and T. Bazzarre. 2000. AHA Science Advisory. Resistance exercise in individuals with and without cardiovascular disease: Benefits, rationale, safety, and prescription. *Circulation* 101 (7): 828-833.

50. Proctor, M.H., L.L. Moore, D. Gao, et al. 2003. Television viewing and change in body fat from preschool to early adolescents: The Framingham Children's Study. *International Journal of Obesity and Related Metabolic Disorders* 27: 827-833.

51. Pronk, N.P., and R.R. Wing. 1994. Physical activity and long-term maintenance of weight loss. *Obesity Research* 2: 587-599.

52. Ross, R., and F.P. Despres. 2009. Abdominal obesity, insulin resistance, and the metabolic syndrome: Contribution of physical activity/exercise. *Obesity* 17: S1-S2.

53. Steffen, L.M., , S. Dai, J.E. Fulton, and D.R. Labarthe. 2009. Overweight in children and adolescents associated with TV viewing and parental weight. *American Journal of Preventative Medicine* 37: S50-S55.

54. Storlie, J., and H.A. Jordan, eds. 1984. *Behavioral Management of Obesity.* Champaign, IL: Human Kinetics.

55. U.S. Department of Health and Human Services. 1996. Historical background, terminology, evolution of recommendations, and measurement, Appendix B, NIH consensus conference statement. In: *Physical Activity and Health: A Report of the Surgeon General.* Atlanta: U.S. Department of Health and Human Services, Centers for Disease Control and Prevention, National Center for Chronic Disease Prevention and Health Promotion. p. 47.

56. U.S. Department of Health and Human Services. 2007. *Overweight and Obesity: At a Glance: The Surgeon General's Call to Action to Prevent and Decrease Overweight and Obesity.* Washington, DC: U.S. Department of Health and Human Services, Office of Surgeon General.

57. U.S. Department of Health and Human Services. 2007. *Overweight and Obesity: Health Consequences: The Surgeon General's Call to Action to Prevent and Decrease Overweight and Obesity.* Washington, DC: U.S. Department of Health and Human Services, Office of Surgeon General.

58. Vanderwater, E.A., and X. Haung. 2006. Parental weight status as a moderator of the relationship between television viewing and childhood overweight. *Archives of Pediatrics and Adolescent Medicine* 160: 622-627.

59. Vega, C.L. 1991. Taking small steps . . . to big changes. *IDEA Today* 2: 20-22.

60. Vega, C.L. 2001. Nutrition. In *Aquatic Fitness Instructor Fitness Manual.* Nokomis, FL: Aquatic Exercise Association.

61. Wadden, T.A., G.D. Forester, and K.A. Letizia. 1994. One-year behavioral treatment of obesity: Comparison of moderate and severe caloric restriction and the effects of weight maintenance therapy. *Journal of Consulting and Clinical Psychology* 621: 165-171.

62. World Health Organization. 1998. *Obesity: Preventing and Managing the Global Epidemic.* Report of a WHO Consultation on Obesity. Geneva: WHO.

63. Yen, C.F., R.C. Hsiao, C.H. Ko, J.Y. Yen, C.F. Huang, S.C. Liu, and S.Y. Wang. 2010. The relationships between body mass index and television viewing, internet use and cellular phone use: The moderating effects of socio-demographic characteristics and exercise. *International Journal of Eating Disorders* 43 (6): 565-571.

Clients With Cardiovascular and Respiratory Conditions

Moh H. Malek, PhD

After completing this chapter, you will be able to

- understand the pathophysiology and risk factors for hypertension, myocardial infarction, cerebrovascular accident, peripheral vascular disease, asthma, and exercise-induced asthma;

- understand the stages of the various diseases and how exercise can be used to enhance the client's quality of life; and

- know when it is appropriate to refer a client to a medical professional.

Cardiovascular and respiratory diseases present a challenge not only to the traditional health care provider, but also to the personal trainer. Although deaths related to cardiovascular and cerebrovascular diseases in the United States are declining, deaths related to lung disease, including chronic obstructive pulmonary disease (COPD), are on the rise (see figure 20.1) (33). Hypertension is a major risk factor for cardiovascular disease, with myocardial infarctions (heart attacks) and cerebrovascular accidents (strokes) the most common cardiovascular diseases that personal trainers will encounter. In addition to providing information about these common conditions, this chapter includes information about training clients with peripheral vascular disease, as such clients can benefit a great deal from light-intensity aerobic conditioning.

Respiratory disease in general is a topic well beyond the scope of this chapter. However, the chapter does address asthma and exercise-induced asthma, both of which are commonly seen in personal training clients. The rehabilitation and training programs of the chronic lung patient need to be overseen by a respiratory rehabilitation specialist, whose level of training is beyond that of a personal trainer.

To properly guide, educate, and train cardiovascular and respiratory patients, the personal trainer must understand the pathophysiology of the disease and be able to recognize the early signs of inadequate

The author would like to acknowledge the contributions of Robert Watine, who wrote this chapter for the first edition of *NSCA's Essentials of Personal Training*.

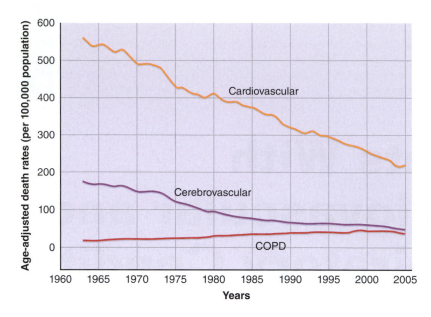

FIGURE 20.1 Age-adjusted death rates due to cardiovascular disease, cerebrovascular disease, and chronic obstructive pulmonary disease (COPD).

Based on data from U.S. National Center for Health Statistics 2006 (33).

blood circulation and labored breathing during training. This said, personal trainers can have a dramatic positive impact on the quality of life for their clients as long as they pay careful attention to them. Additionally, it is important for the personal trainer to approach the exercise regimen as part of a team, with the physician as the leader. Any client who has a medical condition or disease should receive clearance from his or her physician. Of course, liability waivers should be signed by all parties to provide as much protection as possible should issues of liability ever arise (see chapter 25).

Health Screening and Risk Stratification

The health screening process is a critical component prior to the start of any fitness assessment or training regimen. In addition, the personal trainer *must* have a physician's clearance before training clients with medical conditions. As discussed in chapter 9, clients should complete the Physical Activity Readiness Questionnaire (PAR-Q), and the personal trainer should document and complete a detailed health history. On the basis of the health history questionnaire, the client should then be stratified into either a low-, moderate-, or high-risk group. It is important to note that a personal trainer who intends to train clinical patients should receive additional training related to the mechanism of the disease and common signs and symptoms associated with it. For example,

personal trainers working with cancer patients must have a strong understanding of the side effects of various therapies (i.e., chemotherapy or radiation therapy) on such physiological functions as cardiovascular, respiratory, and musculoskeletal functions. This chapter focuses on clients who have known cardiovascular or respiratory conditions.

Hypertension

Hypertension is a disease of not just the old, but also of the young (26, 27, 28). Over 50 million Americans age 6 and above have this disease, defined by a systolic reading of 140+ mmHg (millimeters of mercury), a diastolic reading of 90+ mmHg, or both (2). Hypertension is an idiopathic disease, which means that it occurs without a known etiology (cause). This is why hypertension is considered the "silent killer." No person, not even a doctor, can look at 10 people in a room and pick out who has the disease and who does not. Ninety percent of cases are idiopathic. It is the other 10% that are curable because they are due to secondary causes, that is, other diseases.

Those secondary causes include hyperthyroidism, pheochromocytoma, hypercortisolism, hyperaldosteronism, and renal artery stenosis. Each of these diseases has subclassifications that are tangential to this discussion. However, the important point is twofold: (1) Anyone under the age of 35 with hypertension needs to be aggressively evaluated for one of these diagnoses (to be performed by a doctor); and (2) any client observed to be hypertensive must be referred to a doctor for further evaluation and treatment. It has been found that those newly diagnosed with hypertension who are under 35 years have a greater incidence of the secondary causes.

Elevated blood pressure puts an individual at risk for a heart attack, stroke, or both. Mildly elevated blood pressure (over time) can lead to kidney disease and generalized vascular disease. People cannot determine how high their blood pressure is based on how they feel. If a person truly were to perceive his or her blood pressure to be high, it would most likely be in the range of a hypertensive crisis with associated chest pains, visual blurring, neurologic deficits, or some combination of these.

Blood pressure risk stratification is shown in table 20.1. The stages are stratified into normal, prehypertension, and stage 1 and stage 2 hypertension. These stratifications are based on the presence of major risk factors (e.g., smoking, dyslipidemia, diabetes mellitus, age greater than 60, men and postmenopausal women, and a family history), as well as target organ damage (TOD) and clinical cardiovascular disease (CCD). Any client with stage 1 or greater readings should not begin an exercise program until a physician has his or her pressure controlled and has cleared him for exercise (4, 6).

Target organ damage includes cardiac, brain, kidney, peripheral vascular, and retinal disease. Target organ cardiac disease refers to left ventricular thickening or hypertrophy due to untreated or inadequately treated hypertension, a history of exertional chest pain or angina, having had a heart attack, having had reperfusion surgery (i.e., coronary bypass, stenting, or balloon angioplasty), and overall cardiac dysfunction (failure). Stroke and peripheral vascular disease have pathophysiology similar to that of coronary artery disease. Kidney disease results in glomerular dysfunction, leading to the kidneys' inability to cleanse the blood, as well as affecting blood flow to and from the kidney, which can lead to hypertension as well. Retinal disease is a function of hemorrhages from high blood pressure, thereby affecting eyesight with the potential for the development of blindness.

A client with high normal readings (no major risk factors; no TOD or CCD) is treated with lifestyle modification. The same applies to prehypertension (at least one major risk factor, not including diabetes; no TOD or CCD). Stage 1 and stage 2 have TOD/CCD, diabetes, or both, with or without other risk factors, thereby necessitating physician intervention for treatment and clearance.

> **Clients with stage 1 or greater readings (≥140/≥90) should not be trained until their blood pressure is controlled and a physician has cleared them for exercise.**

Management of Hypertension

Lifestyle modification for clients with hypertension includes nonpharmacologic interventions, for example proper exercise, weight loss, and dietary

TABLE 20.1   Classification and Management of Blood Pressure for Adults*

BP classification	SBP* mmHg	DBP* mmHg	Lifestyle modification	INITIAL DRUG THERAPY Without compelling indication	INITIAL DRUG THERAPY With compelling indications**
Normal	<120	and <80	Encourage	No antihypertensive drug indicated	Drug(s) for compelling indications‡
Prehypertension	120-139	or 80-89	Yes		
Stage 1 hypertension	140-159	or 90-99	Yes	Thiazide-type diuretics for most; may consider ACEI, ARB, BB, CCB, or combination	Drug(s) for the compelling indications‡ Other antihypertensive drugs (diuretics, ACEI, ARB, BB, CCB) as needed
Stage 2 hypertension	≥160	or ≥100	Yes	Two-drug combination for most† (usually thiazide-type diuretic together with ACEI, ARB, BB, or CCB)	

DBP, diastolic blood pressure; SBP, systolic blood pressure.

Drug abbreviations: ACEI, angiotensin converting enzyme inhibitor; ARB, angiotensin receptor blocker; BB, beta blocker; CCB, calcium channel blocker.

*Treatment determined by highest BP category.

**Compelling indications include heart failure, postmyocardial infarction, high coronary disease risk, diabetes, chronic kidney disease, and recurrent stroke prevention.

†Initial combined therapy should be used cautiously in those at risk for orthostatic hypotension.

‡Treat patients with chronic kidney disease or diabetes to BP goal of <130/80 mmHg.

Adapted from NIH and NHLBI 2003 (22).

changes. General lifestyle changes include adequate amount of sleep, reduction in daily sodium intake to 1 teaspoon (~2,300 mg) of salt daily, adequate potassium intake, weight loss if needed, limiting alcohol intake, increasing aerobic activity to 30 to 45 minutes four or more days per week, reducing dietary saturated fat and cholesterol, and the cessation of smoking.

The DASH diet has received a great deal of favorable publicity for lowering blood pressure. It entails reducing saturated fats, cholesterol, and total fat intake. Emphasis is on more fruits, vegetables, and low-fat dairy products; more whole grain products, fish, poultry, and nuts; reduction in red meat, sweets, and sugar-containing beverages; and an increase in foods rich in magnesium, potassium, calcium, protein, and fiber.

Clients with hypertension will be taking one or more of a multitude of medications. The classes of medications include **beta blockers, calcium channel blockers,** ACE (angiotensin converting enzyme) inhibitors, ARBs (angiotensin receptor blockers), diuretics, and **alpha blockers.** The exact mechanisms of action of these medications are beyond the scope of this chapter except for the fact that they all lower blood pressure. Diuretics cause volume depletion. However, the personal trainer should never restrict clients' use of fluids or worry about their use of electrolyte solutions. Alpha, beta, and calcium channel blockers cause vasodilation with the potential for blood pooling. Angiotensin converting enzyme inhibitors and the ARBs exert their effects on the kidneys' vasculature. These medications can cause blood pooling, which necessitates a longer period for cool-down, especially after treadmill walking, jogging, and circuit weight training. Additionally, beta blockers not only slow the heart rate but also prevent the heart rate from elevating as a normal response to exercise. This makes it difficult to use heart rate as a measure of intensity and necessitates use of the rating of perceived exertion (RPE) scale.

Safety Considerations for Clients With Hypertension

What is most promising for the client and exciting for the personal trainer is that the client with *controlled* hypertension can exercise with limited restrictions. Simple precautions need only to be maintained to allow for the application of all modalities. There are numerous benefits of exercise to the body, but exercise may be especially beneficial to clients with hypertension. Several studies have shown significant reductions in resting blood pressure after long-term

exercise. A review of the literature by meta-analysis revealed approximate decreases in systolic and diastolic pressures of 4.5/3.8 mmHg and 4.7/3.1 mmHg, respectively, due to long-term resistance and aerobic training (7, 9, 12, 13, 14, 15, 16, 17, 18). The questions now to be raised are as follows:

1. At what intensity level can a client be placed in order to cause the desired response?
2. Are any exercises contraindicated?
3. What exercises can be given to the client?

> Clients with *controlled* hypertension can exercise with limited restrictions.

Intensity

Since it has been shown that people can achieve a positive training adaptation to exercise, that is, lowered resting blood pressure, by training at intensities of 40% to 50% maximal oxygen uptake (5, 25), the personal trainer can design a program that will cause the adaptation without increasing the risk for the client. According to research, low-intensity exercise appears to be a more effective stimulus than moderate-intensity exercise training in reducing resting blood pressure and blood pressure responses to stress.

This is important because often a client comes with medical clearance for exercise but the personal trainer believes that the client is not in "condition" to embark on a strenuous program. Personal trainers can feel secure in beginning a low-intensity program with such a client because training at this level will not unduly stress the physiology or cause an increased risk of an acute cardiac or neurologic event (5).

Contraindications

As for which exercises are contraindicated, these include any type of activity that would increase intrathoracic pressure, thereby decreasing blood flow return to the heart, with a corresponding decrease in cardiac output. Essentially this means any exercise with an associated prolonged Valsalva maneuver (greater than 1 or 2 seconds). The burden is on the personal trainer to be certain not only that the client is performing the exercise in a technically correct manner, but also that he or she is breathing properly (see chapter 13 for more breathing guidelines).

Safe Exercises

Clients with controlled hypertension may participate in many types of training including, but not limited to, the use of free weights, weight machines, body weight, or elastic bands; aerobic exercise (walking, jogging, swimming); and circuit weight training. Essentially all exercises are permissible (3). If a client with hypertension has a comorbid condition, however, the choice of exercise may be altered or restricted (32).

Comorbid conditions include the following:

1. Musculoskeletal conditions or diseases: degenerative joint diseases, rheumatologic diseases

2. Neurologic disorders: stroke, myasthenia gravis, muscular dystrophy

3. Vascular diseases: carotid artery disease, cardiac conditions, aneurysms

Exercise Guidelines for Clients With Hypertension

If the blood pressure is stage 1 or above, it is imperative to cancel the exercise session and advise the client to speak with his or her doctor. If the client is typically **normotensive,** reschedule the session and recheck before the next exercise session as previously discussed.

Aerobic Conditioning

The goals of an aerobic program are to increase the $\dot{V}O_2$max as well as the ventilatory threshold (which will increase the time before "shortness of breath" is perceived) (29). Additionally, the client will see an increase in both maximal workload and endurance levels. Caloric expenditure will be greater, and this will facilitate greater weight reduction (if needed). In addition, a low- to moderate-intensity exercise program has been shown to lower blood pressure (21). It is advised that the intensity level begin at 40% to 50% $\dot{V}O_2$max, ultimately attaining 50% to 85% $\dot{V}O_2$max (2). The RPE initially should be 8 to 10 (on the 6-20 scale), with a goal range of 11 to 13 (on the 6-20 scale). Each session should last between 15 and 30 minutes with an eventual target of 30 to 60 minutes, and the frequency should be three to seven days per week. The weekly caloric expenditure will be between 700 and 2,000 kilocalories. The time necessary to achieve these goals is four to six months. However, as in all cases, each program must be individualized.

Resistance Training

As for the remainder of the program, it should include some form of resistance exercise (19). To maintain consistency, clients should begin with a repetition range from 16 to 20 per set. This would

Goals for Clients With Hypertension

- Increase $\dot{V}O_2$max and ventilatory threshold.
- Increase maximal work and endurance.
- Increase caloric expenditure.
- Control blood pressure.
- Increase muscular endurance.

yield about 50% to 60% of the 1RM (1-repetition maximum), thereby keeping the client within the same guidelines as for aerobic intensity (2).

The rest interval initially should be 2 to 3 minutes (or longer) to allow the client to fully recover between sets. This will allow for physiologic compensation from the exercise, which is especially necessary because of the potential use of prescription medications for hypertension control (20). The client can do as few as one set per exercise, with a maximum of three per exercise, at the beginning of the program. As for the types of exercise performed, large muscle, multijoint movements are the safest choice at the beginning.

Over time (i.e., four to six months), the number of repetitions can decrease to the 8- to 12-repetition range. Exercise frequency should be two or three times a week, with a duration between 30 and 60 minutes per session.

Myocardial Infarction, Stroke, and Peripheral Vascular Disease

Myocardial infarction (MI), stroke, and peripheral vascular disease (PVD) all have very serious ramifications for a client's physiology as well as his or her psychology (23, 24). Physiologically, known disease is present, and thus also are true deficiencies or deficits in the body. Beyond the physiologic effect, there are true psychological problems whether the client realizes them consciously or not. These can manifest themselves in many ways, from a fear of exercise (i.e., fear of the precipitation of another acute event) to the other end of the spectrum of fearlessness on the part of the client. The attitude of "I'll show you, I can beat this thing, I'll just push through the barriers" must also be watched out for when working with these clients. Thus the personal trainer must actively listen to clients and pay attention to the messages being relayed via nonverbal cues and innuendo.

Pathophysiology

The pathophysiology is essentially the same for all three diseases, since they represent the end result of vascular occlusive diseases at various levels of the body, that is, the heart, the brain, or the generalized vascular system (11). An atheromatous (lipid-cholesterol) plaque forms within the lumen of a blood vessel. Focal inflammation around the area of the plaque occurs, leading to its instability. Over time, a collagen cap develops to stabilize the area, with a subsequent overlaying by smooth muscle cells (the normal inside lining of the blood vessel) (figure 20.2). Depending on the time line, the outcomes can be very different.

If the collagen cap and smooth muscles grow to a point of stability, the diameter of the blood vessel is dramatically reduced. This results in decreased blood flow with the potential for eddy currents to develop, as well as sludging of the circulation and the development of a thrombus that can either occlude the lumen or break off and flow downstream to occlude a more distal site. While the collagen cap is still soft and unstable, it can rupture (figure 20.3) and then release all the material within to flow downstream and cause sudden occlusive disease. The situation of the "mature" collagen cap as described in the preceding paragraph makes it more difficult for a rupture to occur and thus is more stable, allowing the body to dissolve the thrombus and thereby prevent it from reaching critical mass. A homeostatic mechanism with antithrombin III provides this protection. The collagen cap rupture is more dangerous, since the sudden release of the intracap material sent flowing distally can cause a sudden event such as an acute MI or a cerebrovascular accident (CVA). The problems associated with the stable collagen cap typically affect peripheral circulation, but can also be seen in the coronary arteries, as in **angina** (chest pain).

Risk Factors

Risk factors include hypertension, hypercholesterolemia, diabetes, smoking, obesity, and family history. High blood pressure increases the systemic vascular resistance, which increases the intracardiac pressure within the left ventricle to allow for systole to occur. During systole there is a compression of the cardiac vessels that feed the heart. When the pressure exceeds a certain threshold, there is a decrease in or a lack of flow to the interior of the heart, and thus chest pain occurs. Of course, with corresponding high cholesterol and cap formation, a rupture can occur, causing the same end result. This also can take place in the coronary arteries.

Diabetes exerts an acceleration effect on the process of vascular disease and thus has an indepen-

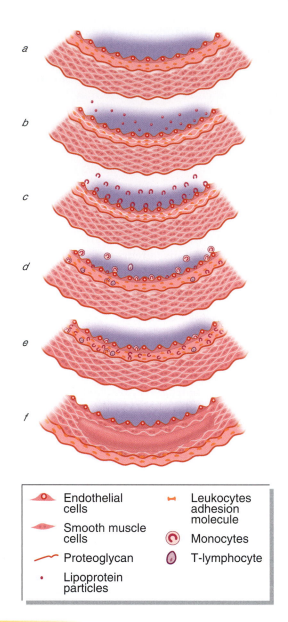

FIGURE 20.2 Development of a collagen cap. A normal artery (a) with the innermost layer of endothelial cells. As plaque (lipoprotein molecules) accumulates (b-e), a cap or layer of collagen is eventually created and covered by a layer of smooth muscle cells (fibers) (f).
Reprinted by permission from Fauci et al. 1998.

dent effect on the pathophysiology of heart attacks. Nicotine (i.e., smoking) increases systemic vascular resistance, that is, blood pressure, causing an effect similar to that described in the previous section. People who are obese require more blood vessels to feed the adipose tissue. This effectively increases the cardiac workload, affecting the circulatory efficiency of the heart's pumping action. Over time, this can lead to the development of one of the various types of cardiomyopathy and heart failure. As for family history, anyone who has a first-degree rela-

These reports give the personal trainer the needed information regarding where the doctor left off and thus where the personal trainer can begin (i.e., intensity level, among other parameters). The stress test provides the maximal oxygen uptake that enables one to determine the intensity level. It also becomes important to recognize that a subpopulation of clients have underlying coronary artery disease without associated chest pain during activity. These individuals are at risk for sudden death since they will exercise to the point of coronary artery spasm, acute heart attack, with a sudden stoppage of beating of the heart. Again, the stress test can reveal whether an individual is in this subclass. The personal trainer should not train these clients. These clients should exercise in a medically monitored setting.

> Personal trainers should not train clients who are post-MI and have existing coronary artery disease without associated chest pain. Such clients must be medically monitored while exercising.

Exercise Guidelines for Clients Postmyocardial Infarction

Post-MI clients are not to be trained until they have received clearance from their cardiologist, cardiovascular surgeon, or both (10). At that point, the medical professional must be able to provide an intensity level and training range for the personal trainer to work with. The medical professional should provide a metabolic equivalent (MET) level or $\dot{V}O_2$max for the personal trainer to use as a baseline for design of a program. The program should also be sent to the doctor for approval, or at the very least be placed in the client's medical file.

What is most important is for the personal trainer to be cognizant of and monitor for abnormal signs and symptoms. Some of these signs and symptoms are chest pain, palpitations, shortness of breath, diaphoresis, nausea, neck pain, arm pain (left or right), back pain, and a sense of impending doom.

One caveat is that many post-MI clients have comorbid diseases, such as diabetes and PVD. Peripheral vascular disease is discussed later in this chapter, and programming for clients with diabetes is addressed in chapter 19.

Exercise Program Components for Clients Postmyocardial Infarction

Once the client has been cleared by the physician(s), the goals are to increase $\dot{V}O_2$max, decrease blood pressure, and reduce the risk for further coronary artery disease events. The training intensity for

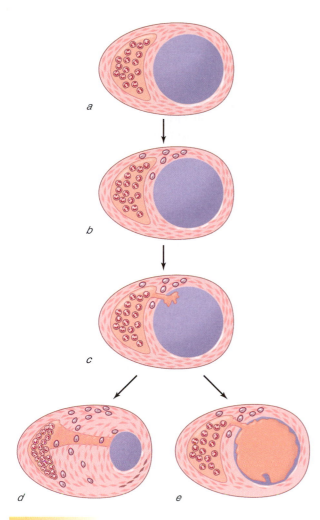

FIGURE 20.3 Rupture of immature collagen cap. If a normal artery (a) begins to develop a collagen cap (b) that ruptures (c), the artery can become partially (d) or fully (e) occluded.

Reprinted by permission from Fauci et al. 1998.

tive (parent or sibling) with known cardiac disease diagnosed before the age of 55 (male relative) or 65 (female relative) has an increased risk (1).

Myocardial Infarction

When an MI occurs, cardiac muscle potentially dies. Medical professionals intervene to try to salvage some of the damaged tissue or even reverse the entire process altogether. The personal trainer, however, will be working with a client who has had a heart attack, has gone through cardiac rehabilitation, and has been discharged from the physician to continue with an exercise program. This places the personal trainer in a most opportune position to get the most recent test data on the new client—exercise stress test results, echocardiogram results, and a letter of clearance and recommendations from the cardiologist.

Goals for Clients Who Have Had a Myocardial Infarction

- Increase aerobic capacity.
- Decrease blood pressure.
- Reduce risk of coronary artery disease.
- Increase ability to perform leisure, occupational, and daily living activities.
- Increase muscle strength and endurance.

aerobic conditioning typically begins at 40% of $\dot{V}O_2$max or an RPE of 9 to 11 (on the 6-20 scale). Sessions last between 15 and 40 minutes and take place three to four times per week. Additional time is devoted to warm-up and cool-down periods. There is not a definite time line for goal achievement, since the aim is to prevent further events as well as strengthen the heart muscle. Follow-up exercise stress tests performed by a cardiologist provide the necessary documentation regarding those endpoints.

Since many post-MI patients become fearful of simple activities of daily living, the goals are to rebuild their confidence to perform such tasks. Examples are lifting a milk carton, pouring from a bottle of orange juice, holding a handbag, or even pushing a grocery cart.

By performing resistance exercises, the client can receive immediate feedback as to his or her strength capabilities. This is more of a psychological boost than a reflection of actual strength increase. Programs should begin at 20 reps, one to three sets, two to three days per week. The personal trainer and the physician need to discuss the actual goals. The client is to be instructed to never perform a Valsalva maneuver.

> Clients who have had a myocardial infarction should never perform a Valsalva maneuver.

Cerebrovascular Accident

The client who has had a stroke, or cerebrovascular accident, has considerations other than the occlusive nature of the disease. Such clients typically have neurologic deficits and are often best served in a setting monitored by health care professionals. However, if a client has no neurological deficit and is released by his or her physician to exercise in an unmonitored setting, the personal trainer can follow the program design guidelines provided here and can help the client strive for improvements.

Exercise Guidelines for Post-Cerebrovascular Accident Clients

The post-CVA client faces many different challenges, all depending on which area of the brain has been affected. A good many individuals after CVA have difficulty with simple daily tasks because of a loss of motor function, often in the arm, leg, face, or mouth. Others have trouble hearing, speaking, or understanding spatial arrangements—or they may even ignore one side of their body. The discussion here is limited to the client who has experienced a left brain CVA, resulting in motor deficits of the right arm, leg, or both.

There is no question whatsoever that a properly instituted exercise program can significantly improve the life of people who have had a CVA. The program, however, must begin where the post-CVA rehabilitation left off. Therefore the personal trainer needs to have close contact with the rehabilitation team in order to ascertain the direction of the postrehabilitation training and the establishment of goals.

> Exercise can significantly improve the life of an individual who has had a stroke. Personal trainers may train post-CVA clients who have no neurological deficit and are released by their physicians to exercise in an unmonitored setting.

Exercise Program Components for Post-Cerebrovascular Accident Clients

Ergometers need to be the mainstay of aerobic conditioning for the post-CVA client. This is in contrast to the situation with the post-MI client, who can use a treadmill. With compromised limb function, not only is strength obviously affected; so too is the client's balance. The exercise intensity can begin as low as 30% peak $\dot{V}O_2$, since these clients become deconditioned rapidly after the CVA. Interestingly, this is why $\dot{V}O_2$max is undefined in patients after a CVA. They become so deconditioned that the $\dot{V}O_2$max cannot be determined, giving rise to the term *peak $\dot{V}O_2$* Post-CVA clients may eventually exercise at 40% to 70% peak $\dot{V}O_2$. Meanwhile, any activity will improve their capacity. The sessions can last between 5 and 60 minutes, depending on the individual, and the frequency is typically at least three times per week.

Not only will resistance training help to improve the overall sense of well-being; it will also help develop new neurologic pathways to the affected limbs via the recruiting of dormant channels. Additionally, resistance training of the healthy limb will have a crossover effect on the compromised limb. Regarding the amount of weight to be used, a 1RM cannot be determined; therefore slow and judicious evaluation of the client for starting loads is a responsibility of the personal trainer. Nonetheless, the personal trainer should eventually encourage the client to strive for three sets of 8 to 12 repetitions, two to three days per week. The purpose of flexibility training should be obvious for clients in this group. This type of activity will help to maintain mobility in the healthy limbs and hopefully improve the range of motion in an affected limb as well. Too often the post-CVA patient experiences joint contractures as a result of the lack of motion around the joint. The joint can be considered frozen; over time, bone remodeling by osteoclasts and osteoblasts will occur until the joint becomes calcified. Early range of motion training may prevent this from happening. Range of motion exercises should be performed before and after each training session (for as little as 5 minutes), as well as on nontraining days.

Coordination and balance exercises can also be added to the program. Standing on one foot, finger-to-nose activity, and finger to moving target activity are just a few examples. This is where the personal trainer can get creative in the design of a truly individualized program.

Peripheral Vascular Disease

A client with PVD presents a real challenge; but clients in this group have the potential to make very impressive gains in their capacities. Essentially, people with PVD have pain during walking. Typically they cannot walk for more than 2 to 5 minutes without having to stop and rest because of the searing pain in their calves. The goal is to increase the length of their activity to improve quality of life and possibly avoid the need for surgical intervention. See table 20.2 for more details about the symptoms of PVD.

Pharmacologic considerations for PVD are essentially the same as for persons with hypertension. The only notable addition is the use of physician-prescribed nitrates, that is, nitroglycerin, for chest pain. Nitroglycerin tablets or spray is applied under the tongue. If the medication is working, there will be a bitter taste and a soon-to-follow headache. If the client is experiencing anything suggestive of cardiac compromise (i.e., chest pain, ache, shortness of breath, etc.), he or she must stop immediately, sit down or even lie flat, and use the nitroglycerin as prescribed while someone calls emergency services (typically 911 in the United States). It is best if another person is available to either make the call or stay with the client; otherwise, the personal trainer must call before giving aid.

Exercise Guidelines for Clients With Peripheral Vascular Disease

Since the pathophysiology of PVD is present throughout the body, the personal trainer must be aware that exercise in a client with PVD may cause a cardiac event. Therefore, it is preferable for the client with PVD to be cleared from a cardiac viewpoint by

Goals for Clients Following Cerebrovascular Accident (Stroke)

- Increase daily living activities.
- Increase strength for both involved and uninvolved limbs.
- Increase range of motion of the involved side.
- Prevent joint contractures.

TABLE 20.2 Classification of Peripheral Vascular Disease

Fontaine scale			Rutherford scale		
Stage	Description	Grade	Category	Description
I	Asymptomatic	0	0	Asymptomatic
IIa	Mild pain while walking	I	1	Mild pain while walking
IIb	Moderate to severe pain while walking	I	2	Moderate pain while walking
		I	3	Severe pain while walking
III	Pain while resting	II	4	Pain while resting
IV	Tissue loss	III	5	Minor tissue loss
		IV	6	Moderate to severe tissue loss

Adapted from TASC 2000 (31).

Goals for Clients With Peripheral Vascular Disease

- Improve pain response; be active for increasingly longer periods.
- Reduce risk of coronary artery disease.
- Improve gait.
- Increase daily living activities.
- Increase work potential.
- Improve quality of life.

an exercise stress test before embarking on a training program. For the same reasons as in cardiac and stroke patients, aggressive lifestyle changes must occur along with hyperlipidemia management.

Generally, as the patient begins to exercise there is an increase demand for oxygen in the working muscle. Therefore, the patient's rating of pain may increase, however, it should be noted that each patient may respond differently depending on their level of pain tolerance. Nevertheless, the health fitness instructor needs to work in accordance with the patient's physician.

Exercise Program Components for Clients With Peripheral Vascular Disease

The reason the client needs aerobic conditioning is straightforward—to be able to walk greater distances pain free. The claudication or calf pain with walking is the rate-limiting factor. The pain is incapacitating. The client will not say that it hurts a little; it will hurt a lot. Clients will not be able to "walk through" the pain; rather they will need to stop, sit down, and rest. Some may be able to walk for only a minute before needing to stop. Therefore, program design becomes simple—walk until it hurts, stop, then do it again, and so on. The duration for walking should be between 10 and 30 minutes. The goal is to lengthen the time walking and shorten the rest interval until the exercise becomes one long continuous activity.

As for resistance training, including repetition ranges, sets, and rest periods, the same recommendations apply to clients with PVD as to clients who are hypertensive.

Finally, any discussion of the client with angina pectoris has been intentionally omitted from this chapter, since clients in this group are felt to be at too high a risk for the personal trainer who is functioning in the typical health club or home gym

setting. Such clients should be trained and thus monitored at a medical facility by appropriately trained personnel with the necessary emergency backup support systems.

Chronic Obstructive Pulmonary Disease

The term *chronic obstructive pulmonary disease (COPD)* is used to describe lung disease that becomes progressively worse and is not completely reversible (8). It should be noted that the term *chronic airflow limitation* has also been used instead of COPD. Chronic obstructive pulmonary disease, therefore, is an umbrella term encompassing a number of diseases that obstruct airflow, such as asthma, emphysema, and chronic bronchitis. It is the fourth leading cause of death in the United States and is projected to become the third leading cause of death for both men and women by 2020. Therefore, COPD is the only major disease that is continuing to grow rather than decline. One hallmark of COPD is skeletal muscle dysfunction that has resulted in a decreased activity level of COPD patients and consequently a poor quality of life. Muscle biopsies from the vastus lateralis of COPD patients indicate that this population has a loss of type I muscle fibers and reductions in oxidative enzymes such as succinate synthase.

Traditionally, individuals with COPD are assigned to pulmonary rehabilitation that includes various aerobic exercises. More recently, however, studies have shown that resistance training is also an important component of pulmonary rehabilitation. Furthermore, home-based exercise programs that combine aerobic exercise and weight training have been shown to strengthen motor and respiratory muscles and therefore improve quality of life.

> Patients with COPD should exercise in a formal pulmonary and respiratory rehabilitation facility and not under the direction of a personal trainer.

Asthma

By definition, asthma is a reversible airway disease with associated hyperreactivity, characterized by the ease of developing bronchospasm, constriction, or both. A very common subset of asthma is exercise-induced asthma (EIA) (30). Compared to the more common variety, exercise-induced asthma is usually self-limited; rarely results in hospitalization; begins

15 to 20 minutes (or as early as 5 minutes in some cases) into an exercise session; and has associated coughing, wheezing, or both. In addition, if left untreated, the client will recover and become symptom free within 10 to 30 minutes after cessation of exercise. Adult clients, compared to children, notice the onset of symptoms later in the exercise session, and the symptoms will last longer.

The two types of asthma clients experience similar symptomatology, the difference lying in the fact that the typical asthma client has symptoms during periods of rest or nonexercise. It is important to realize that there are more severe forms of asthma necessitating the use of medications beyond inhaled bronchodilators. These medications can include inhaled and oral steroids. Some people who have asthma experience emergencies due to acute mucus plugging of the airways (i.e., status asthmaticus); however, these people are under the care of a pulmonary doctor who is supervising the rehabilitation program.

In both asthma and EIA, the bronchospasm has an early and a late phase. The early phase is the result of bronchoconstriction, which responds favorably to inhaled bronchodilators. Prevention can be achieved through the use of a bronchodilator 15 to 20 minutes prior to the start of the exercise. The late phase is delayed in onset by 1 to 6 hours and is due to airway edema. It is best controlled with inhaled steroids. Clients with this late-phase component are best treated 2 to 3 hours after exercise.

Exercise Guidelines for Clients With Asthma

In working with clients who have asthma, the best way to monitor intensity is through RPE and the sense of shortness of breath. This is necessary because many clients are unable to achieve a "training" heart rate but will objectively show physiological gains. Clients who are taking systemic glucocorticoids (steroids) may have disease of the respiratory muscles, which can make breathing under stress more of a challenge.

Asthmatic clients do better with mid- to late-morning exercise sessions because of the natural daytime release of cortisol from the adrenal glands. They should avoid temperature extremes, since the ambient or inhaled air can precipitate bronchospasm. High humidity can have a similar effect. It is important to remember that the shortness of breath associated with the asthmatic client can lead to rather significant anxiety and depression, as well as fear over exercise.

> In the client with asthma, exercise intensity should be monitored with ratings of perceived exertion and sense of shortness of breath. Many clients with asthma are unable to achieve a training heart rate but will still exhibit physiological improvements.

Exercise Program Components for Clients With Asthma

Large muscle aerobic activity (i.e., walking, cycling, and swimming) helps to improve $\dot{V}O_2$max and thus aerobic capacity and endurance. There will be an associated increase in lactate and ventilatory thresholds, as well as a desensitization to dyspnea (shortness of breath). With a decrease in shortness of breath, an increase in activities of daily living can result as well.

An RPE of 11 to 13 (on the 6-20 scale) should be maintained, with continuous monitoring for dyspnea. Sessions should occur one to two times daily, three to seven days per week. Each session should last 30 minutes, although in the beginning clients may be able to perform for only 5 to 10 minutes. The emphasis is on the progression of duration versus intensity in order to desensitize the client to the dyspnea.

A general resistance training program is recommended. The objectives include increasing the maximal number of repetitions (to desensitize to shortness of breath), increasing the amount of training volume, and increasing lean body mass. The initial program should use lighter loads for more repetitions (≤16), two to three days per week.

Clients with asthma should follow a general flexibility program.

Conclusion

Working with clients who have cardiovascular and respiratory conditions poses unique challenges. The guidelines in this chapter have been presented with the idea of simplifying topics that can be very complex. The personal trainer must keep the need for finesse and true individualization of a program at the forefront during program design. It is always best to err on the side of conservativism. If in doubt, begin the program at a lower intensity than has been indicated. This way the client (who may already be fearful of exercise) has much room for improvement without the risk of injury or exacerbation of the underlying disease. With goals that are easy to attain, reaching goals will help clients psychologically to want to continue to train while limiting the risk of adverse effects.

Study Questions

1. A 44-year-old-male with history of high blood pressure (144/92) has never exercised before but would like to start an exercise program. His physician cleared him to participate. Which of the following is an example of the most appropriate beginning exercise intensity for this client?

    A. treadmill walking at an RPE of 14
    B. back squat at 75% of 1RM for 10 repetitions
    C. elliptical trainer at 65% $\dot{V}O_2$max
    D. dumbbell bench press at 50% 1RM for 16 repetitions

2. A 52-year-old-client had a heart attack three months ago and was recently cleared by his physician to begin a low-intensity exercise program. Which of the following combinations of exercise, intensity, and duration are most appropriate for this client?

	Mode	Intensity	Duration
A.	stationary bicycle,	RPE of 12,	15 minutes
B.	treadmill walking,	40% $\dot{V}O_2$max,	20 minutes
C.	stair stepper,	70% HRmax,	25 minutes
D.	elliptical trainer,	RPE of 8,	10 minutes

3. A 63-year-old client with peripheral vascular disease describes significant pain when walking for 5 minutes or more. Which of the following programs would best help her increase the amount of time she is able to walk pain free?

    A. Have the client "walk through" the pain for 2 minutes after the pain begins.
    B. Decrease the duration to 2 minutes at the same intensity.
    C. Have the client take a short rest break once the pain begins, and then continue walking until the pain returns.
    D. Discontinue walking as a form of exercise since it is too painful.

4. A client with exercise-induced asthma has been performing primarily resistance training exercises for the past year. He now requests help in improving his "stamina." Which of the following methods of monitoring aerobic intensity should be used for this client?

    I. target heart rate
    II. sense of dyspnea
    III. METs
    IV. RPE

    A. I and III only
    B. II and IV only
    C. I, II, and III only
    D. II, III, and IV only

Applied Knowledge Question

Fill in the chart to describe recommendations for a *beginning* exercise program and any exercise-related concerns that a personal trainer should be aware of with clients who have these conditions.

	BEGINNING EXERCISE PROGRAM				Exercise concerns
	Mode	Intensity	Frequency	Duration	
Hypertension					
MI					
Stroke					
PVD					
Asthma					

References

1. American College of Sports Medicine. 2010. *ACSM's Guidelines for Exercise Testing and Prescription,* 8th ed. Philadelphia: Lippincott Williams & Williams.

2. American College of Sports Medicine. 2003. *Exercise Management for Persons With Chronic Diseases and Disabilities,* 3rd ed. Champaign, IL: Human Kinetics.

3. American Heart Association. 2001. Exercise standards for testing and training: A statement for healthcare professionals from the American Heart Association. *Circulation* 104 (14): 1694-1740.

4. Arakawa, K. 1996. Effect of exercise on hypertension and associated complications. *Hypertension Research* 19 (Suppl 1): S87-S91.

5. Arakawa, K. 1999. Exercise, a measure to lower blood pressure and reduce other risks. *Clinical and Experimental Hypertension* 21 (5-6): 797-803.

6. Blumenthal, J.A., E.T. Thyrum, E.D. Gullette, A. Sherwood, and R. Waugh. 1995. Do exercise and weight loss reduce blood pressure in patients with mild hypertension? *North Carolina Medical Journal* 56 (2): 92-95.

7. Borhani, N.O. 1996. Significance of physical activity for prevention and control of hypertension. *Journal of Human Hypertension* 10 (Suppl 2): S7-S11.

8. CIBA-GEIGY Corporation. 1991. *Hazards of Smoking: A Patient Guide to COPD and Lung Cancer.* Peapack, NJ: Tim Peters and Company.

9. Conley, M., and R. Rozeneck. 2001. Health aspects of resistance exercise and training: NSCA position statement. *Strength and Conditioning Journal* 23 (6): 9-23.

10. Engstrom, G., B. Hedblad, and L. Janzon. 1999. Hypertensive men who exercise regularly have lower rate of cardiovascular mortality. *Journal of Hypertension* 17 (6): 737-742.

11. Fauci, A.S., E. Braunwald, K.J. Isselbacher, et al., eds. 1998. Disorders of the cardiovascular system. In: *Harrison's Principles of Internal Medicine,* 14th ed. New York: McGraw-Hill. pp. 1345-1352.

12. Hagberg, J.M., A.A. Ehsoni, and D. Goldring. 1984. Effect of weight training on blood pressure and haemodynamics in hypertensive adolescents. *Journal of Pediatrics* 104: 147-151.

13. Hagberg, J.M., J.J. Park, and M.D. Brown. 2000. The role of exercise training in the treatment of hypertension: An update. *Sports Medicine* 30 (3): 193-206.

14. Halbert, J.A., C.A. Silagy, R.T. Withers, P.A. Hamdorf, and G.R. Andrews. 1997. The effectiveness of exercise in lowering blood pressure: A meta-analysis of randomized controlled trials of 4 weeks or longer. *Journal of Human Hypertension* 11 (10): 641-649.

15. Harris, K.A., and R.G. Holly. 1987. Physiological responses to circuit weight training in borderline hypertensive subjects. *Medicine and Science in Sports and Exercise* 19: 246-252.

16. Kelley, G. 1997. Dynamic resistance exercise and resting blood pressure in adults: A meta-analysis. *Journal of Applied Physiology* 82 (5): 1559-1565.

17. Kelley, G.A., and K.A. Kelley. 2000. Progressive resistance exercise and resting blood pressure: A meta-analysis of randomized controlled trials. *Hypertension* 35 (3): 838-843.

18. Kokkinos, P.F., and V. Papademetriou. 2000. Exercise and hypertension. *Coronary Artery Disease* 11 (2): 99-102.

19. Majahalme, S., V. Turjanmaa, M. Tuomisto, H. Kautiainen, and A. Uusitalo. 1997. Intra-arterial blood pressure during exercise and left ventricular indices in normotension and borderline and mild hypertension. *Blood Pressure* 6 (1): 5-12.

20. Manolas, J. 1997. Patterns of diastolic abnormalities during isometric stress in patients with systemic hypertension. *Cardiology* 88 (1): 36-47.

21. Mughal, M.A., I.A. Alvi, I.A. Akhund, and A.K. Ansari. 2001. The effect of aerobic exercise training on resting blood pressure in hypertensive patients. *Journal of the Pakistan Medical Association* 51 (6): 222-226.

22. National High Blood Pressure Education Program. 2003 JNC 7 Express: The Seventh Report of the Joint National Committee on Prevention, Detection, Evaluation, and Treatment of High Blood Pressure (JNC 7). NIH Publication No .03-5233.

23. Papademetriou, V., and P.F. Kokkinos. 1996. The role of exercise in the control of hypertension and cardiovascular risk. *Current Opinion in Nephrology and Hypertension* 5 (5): 459-462.

24. Roberts, S. 1992. Resistance training: Guidelines for individuals with heart disease. *Conditioning Instructor* 2 (3): 4-6.

25. Rogers, M.W., M.M. Probst, J.J. Gruber, R. Berger, and J.B. Boone. 1996. Differential effects of exercise training intensity on blood pressure and cardiovascular responses to stress in borderline hypertensive humans. *Journal of Hypertension* 14 (11): 1369-1375.

26. Roos, R.J. 1997. The Surgeon General's report: A prime source for exercise advocates. *Physician and Sportsmedicine* 25 (4): 122-131.

27. Sallis, R.E., ed. 1997. *Essentials of Sports Medicine.* St. Louis: Mosby Year Book.

28. Sallis, R.E., M. Allen, and F. Massimino, eds. 1997. *Sports Medicine Review.* St. Louis: Mosby Year Book.

29. Seals, D.R., H.G. Silverman, M.J. Reiling, and K.P. Davy. 1997. Effect of regular aerobic exercise on elevated blood pressure in postmenopausal women. *American Journal of Cardiology* 80 (1): 49-55.

30. Storms, W., and D.M. Joyner. 1997. Update on exercise-induced asthma. *Physician and Sportsmedicine* 25 (3): 45-55.

31. TransAtlantic Inter-Society Consensus (TASC). 2000. Management of peripheral arterial disease (PAD). *J Vasc Surg* 31 (1): 1.

32. Tulio, S., S. Egle, and G. Greily. 1995. Blood pressure response to exercise of obese and lean hypertensive and normotensive male adolescents. *Journal of Human Hypertension* 9 (12): 953-958.

33. U.S. National Center for Health Statistics. 2006. *National Vital Statistics Reports* (June 28) 54 (19).

Clients With Orthopedic, Injury, and Rehabilitation Concerns

Kyle T. Ebersole, PhD, LAT, and David T. Beine, MS, LAT

After completing this chapter, you will be able to

- recognize common types of injury and orthopedic concerns;

- understand the impact of injury on physical function;

- describe the goals of each phase of tissue healing; and

- describe the personal trainer's role in relation to specific orthopedic, injury, and rehabilitation concerns.

The increased acceptance of the personal training profession and the limitations of health insurance coverage have created a unique practice opportunity for personal trainers with individuals recovering from an orthopedic injury. In many situations, the time needed for full restoration of function and movement and return to activity goals of the client following an orthopedic injury exceeds the reimbursement limits of the health care provider. Thus people frequently rely on the expertise of a personal trainer to design individualized, safe, and effective programs to support a full recovery and facilitate a return to activity. To successfully manage the needs of this clientele population, a personal trainer must understand the various types of orthopedic injury, time line for tissue healing, general psychophysiological factors that contrib-

ute to injury recovery, and considerations related to how injury may affect movement and function. Failure to recognize the framework of the healing process will unnecessarily slow the healing time line and ultimately interfere with the full restoration of client function.

This chapter is not intended to provide detailed rehabilitation protocols for specific injuries, nor is it designed to take the place of medical advice given by qualified health care professionals. Rather, the intent is to provide the personal trainer with a general framework to guide the delivery of personal training services to meet the unique needs of clients with orthopedic injuries or impairments. The information contained in this chapter should ultimately be augmented by collaborative communication and input from health care professionals to maximize client function and outcomes.

Chapter 21

Injury Classification

Musculoskeletal injuries are characterized and classified based on a variety of factors including onset and type of tissue damaged. Macrotrauma and microtrauma are mechanism-based terms used to classify injury onset. *Macrotrauma* refers to an injury with a sudden and obvious episode of tissue overload and subsequent damage. The acuteness of a macrotrauma differs from the insidious onset and frequently chronic nature of microtraumatic injuries (67). The lack of overt trauma suggests that microtrauma results from the accumulation of tissue damage across time; therefore microtrauma is often referred to as an "overuse injury." But it is important to note that unlike "overuse," the term *microtrauma* does not imply that the injury is due to repeated physical activity (30). Thus not all microtrauma injuries will recover from rest alone. For example, "overuse" injuries may be due to training errors (e.g., poor program design, progressing too early), suboptimal training surfaces (e.g., too hard or uneven), faulty biomechanics or technique during performance, insufficient motor control, decreased flexibility, or skeletal malalignment (29).

The type of injury (e.g., strain, **sprain**, fracture) is determined by the tissue involved (e.g., muscle, tendon, joint, bone). An understanding of common orthopedic injury classifications will provide an appreciation for the tissue healing time line and inform decisions relative to exercise program design and progression. Table 21.1 describes common musculoskeletal injuries.

Impact of Injury on Function

Injury often results in several physical impairments, including limitations to range of motion (ROM), strength, balance, and coordinated functional movement patterns. Additionally, it is important to recognize the possible psychological effects of injury on an individual and the subsequent recovery process and time line.

Range of motion can be especially affected since injury creates changes in all tissues. After trauma, injury by-products (i.e., exudate) and collagen cross-links (i.e., scar tissue) are deposited. Ground substance (gel-like material) decreases, resulting in fibrosis (a condition in which tissue becomes less supple and more dense, hard, and contracted), which limits the flexibility of connective tissue. Limitations in ROM can be even further complicated should a period of immobilization follow the onset of injury or if circulation is impaired due to age or a medical condition.

The progression of ROM or stretching exercises can depend on the type of tissue, severity of injury, stage of healing, and the person's motivation. If the injury is not too severe and motion is allowed shortly after the onset, active motion or ROM is primarily used and is preferred since it is not using outside assistance. If there is a period of reduced activity or immobilization following the injury, then collagen cross-linkage formation can be more significant and may require repeated lengthy stretches to regain as well as maintain ROM, even after full motion has been achieved. If the deposited collagen is new, it still should be supple and will respond reasonably well to active or passive short-term stretches. If it is a few or several months after the injury, the tissue may be less pliable and will require prolonged stretches if the ROM is still deficient.

The magnitude of the effect of injury on the expression of strength will depend on the extent of the injury, the area or type of tissue injured, the amount of time the person has been immobilized or disabled by the injury, or some combination of these. There can be damage to the muscle itself, or pain and swelling can contribute to the inhibition of a muscle or group of muscles (43, 47). Following injury, the rate of muscle loss is greater than the rate of gain; thus strength seems to be one of the most sought-after parameters following injury (49, 56, 67).

Injury-related deficits in neuromuscular control and proprioception are due to microscopic nerve damage in soft tissue, called *deafferentation*, and disruption in the sensory feedback pathways used for joint stabilization and neuromuscular coordination (67, 68, 90). More simply, this can affect the person's ability to normally interpret peripheral sensations and respond with the appropriate coordinated muscle action to protect the injured area. Thus, the injured tissue and associated structures (i.e., joint) are more prone to reinjury as well as to developing incorrect substitution patterns.

Much like the deficits in neuromuscular control after injury are the related compromises in balance and postural control. Although balance can be perceived to be a simple task, muscular weakness, proprioceptive deficits, and ROM deficits can alter the person's ability to appropriately sense the center of gravity over the base of support and result in a loss of balance (67). Injury causes damage to soft tissue and its neural tissue, resulting in impairments in adequate neural feedback in an injured extremity and contributing to decreased proprioceptive mechanisms to maintain balance (3, 25, 32).

Although injury is often associated with physiological impairments and function, the psychological effects must not be overlooked. The psychological

TABLE 21.1   Common Musculoskeletal Injuries

Injury	Description
Muscle contusion	Commonly referred to as a *bruise* and occurs from a sudden and forceful blow to the body. The result is formation of a hematoma (blood tumor) in tissues surrounding the injured muscle. Speed of healing depends on extent of damage and internal bleeding. Contusions may severely limit movement of the injured muscle.
Muscle strain	Often the result of an abnormal muscle action leading to a stretching or tearing of the muscle fibers. Strains are assigned grades or degrees (first, second, third) to indicate severity of injury. A first- or second-degree strain is a partial tear, whereas third degree reflects a complete tearing of the muscle tissue. Pain, strength limitations, and motion restrictions increase with an increase in the grade.
Tendinopathy	A more recently accepted term to describe the collective effects of tendinitis and tendinosis.
Tendinitis	Inflammation of a tendon. This microtrauma injury is frequently associated with obvious swelling and pain around the injured tendon. If left uncorrected or if the tissue is not allowed to fully heal, may lead to tendinosis.
Tendinosis	Represents a histological definition of tendinitis and involves further breakdown and structural degeneration of the injured tendon.
Ligament sprain	Trauma to the tissues that connect bones and contribute to joint stability. Ligament sprains occur when an excessive force (i.e., due to a change in movement direction) results in the joint moving beyond its anatomical limits and stretching the ligament. Ligament sprains are assigned grades (1, 2, 3) to indicate severity of injury. An increase in the grade is associated with greater pain and tenderness, swelling, joint instability, and loss of function.
Joint dislocation	A joint dislocation occurs when a synovial joint moves beyond its normal anatomical limits. Dislocations are divided into two categories: subluxation and luxation. A subluxation is a partial displacement or separation between two articulating bony surfaces. A luxation is a complete displacement resulting in a total disunion between two articulating bony surfaces.
Osteochondrosis	*Osteochondrosis* refers to degenerative changes in the epiphyses of bones, particularly during periods of significant growth in children. The exact cause(s) of osteochondrosis is not fully understood. Terms commonly used to describe variations of osteochondrosis are *osteochondritis dissecans* and *apophysitis*.
Osteoarthritis	Degeneration of the articular or hyaline cartilage in a joint. Can occur in any joint but is most common in weight-bearing joints such as the hip, knee, and ankle.
Bursitis	Bursae are small fluid-filled synovial membrane sacs designed to reduce friction between tissues such as tendon and bone. When irritated, the bursa becomes inflamed, resulting in bursitis. Bursitis commonly occurs in the hip, knee, elbow, and shoulder and is usually accompanied by swelling, pain, and partial loss of function.
Bone fracture	A partial or complete disruption of a bone due to a direct blow.
Bone stress fracture	A microtraumatic injury that may result from an abnormal muscle action, fatigue-related failure in the stress distribution across the bone, dramatic change in exercise or training ground surface (e.g., wood to grass), excessive training volume, or both. Recent literature has also suggested that nutrition may play a significant role in stress fractures.

reactions and adaptations can depend on the extent of the injury and rehabilitation (67). Short-term injuries and rehabilitation can be a mild inconvenience for the person, who may exhibit responses of impatience and even optimism to return to activity; but longer-term injuries and rehabilitation can create reactions of anger, frustration, fear, and even isolation, to name a few. The resultant behaviors may include loss of vigor, alienation, irrational thoughts, apprehension, and either independence or dependence on the therapist. All of these are influenced by an individual's personal coping skills, social support, experience with previous injury, and personality traits. That said, each person does not respond similarly or equally to an injury, and any recovery or training programs should be managed individually (72). Additionally, establishing a good rapport with the person and forming an authentic relationship can serve as a catalyst for optimal recovery (86).

Tissue Healing Following Injury

Despite the significant volume of literature and information available, there remain many unanswered questions concerning the specific aspects of the tissue healing process. It is generally agreed, however, that all tissues follow a pattern of healing that includes three phases: inflammation, proliferation, and remodeling. Although each phase is associated with known outcomes, tissue healing occurs across a continuum of considerable overlap with no definitive beginning or end time point. It is imperative to understand the tissue healing process, as introduction of a task or exercise prior to the injured tissues' readiness to tolerate the load or stress can ultimately impede full healing or cause additional injury (or both). Figure 21.1 summarizes and depicts the overlapping nature of the healing phases.

Inflammation Phase

Inflammation is the body's initial reaction to injury and is necessary in order for normal healing to occur. During the inflammatory phase, several events contribute to both tissue healing and an initial decrease in function. After tissues are damaged, several chemical mediators, including histamine and bradykinin, are released. These substances increase blood flow and capillary permeability, causing edema (the escape of fluid into the surrounding tissues), which inhibits contractile tissue function and significantly limits the injured client's activity level. In addition, the inflammatory substances may noxiously stimulate sensory nerve fibers, causing pain that may contribute to decreased function. Following an acute injury this phase typically lasts two to three days but may be as long as five to seven days in the presence of a compromised blood supply and more severe structural damage, as well as following surgery (67). Although the inflammatory phase is critical to tissue healing, if it does not end within a reasonable amount of time, further healing may not occur, thereby delaying the rehabilitation process.

The goal during the inflammatory phase is to prepare for the new tissue formation that occurs during the subsequent phases of tissue healing (66). A healthy environment for new tissue regeneration and formation is essential to prevent prolonged inflammation and disruption of the production of new blood vessels and collagen. To achieve these goals, relative rest and passive modalities, including ice, compression, and elevation, are the primary treatment options. While a rapid return to preinjury activity is important, the damaged tissue requires rest for protection from additional injury. Therefore, active treatment to the injured area, including exercise, is not recommended during this phase.

> Rest maximizes the natural physiological processes of the inflammatory phase and supports appropriate tissue healing.

Repair Phase

Though the inflammatory phase may continue, tissue repair begins within three to five days following injury, or potentially up to seven days in severe cases, and may last anywhere from a few weeks to up to two months. It is important to note that there is no definitive ending of the inflammation phase or definitive beginning of the repair phase; rather it is a transitional flow. The repair phase of healing allows for the replacement of tissues that are not viable following injury or surgery (67). In an attempt to improve tissue integrity, the damaged tissue is regenerated (i.e., scar tissue is formed). New capillaries and connective tissue form in the area, and collagen fibers (the structural component of the new tissue) are randomly laid down to serve as the framework on which the repair takes place (27). Collagen fibers are strongest when they are parallel and lie longitudinally to the primary line of stress, yet many of the new fibers are laid down transversely. This random alignment does not allow optimal strength of the new tissue and therefore limits its ability to transmit and accept force.

The goals during the repair phase are to prevent excessive muscle atrophy and joint degeneration of the injured area, promote collagen synthesis,

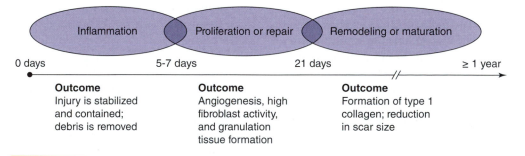

| 0 days | 5-7 days | 21 days | ≥ 1 year |

Outcome Injury is stabilized and contained; debris is removed

Outcome Angiogenesis, high fibroblast activity, and granulation tissue formation

Outcome Formation of type 1 collagen; reduction in scar size

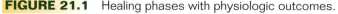

FIGURE 21.1 Healing phases with physiologic outcomes.

and avoid disruption of the newly formed collagen fibers (67). These cautions must be balanced with the gradual introduction of low-load stresses to promote increased collagen synthesis and prevent loss of joint motion. To protect the new, relatively weak collagen fibers, resistive exercises affecting the damaged tissue should be avoided. Specific exercises should be used during the repair phase only after consultation with the client's physician, athletic trainer, physical therapist, or more than one of these. Submaximal isometric exercise may be performed, provided that it is pain free and otherwise indicated. Submaximal isometric exercise allows strength gains to occur, but the intensity is low enough that newly formed collagen fibers are not disrupted.

Remodeling Phase

The weakened tissue produced during repair is strengthened during the remodeling phase of healing. Much like the previous phase transition from inflammation to repair, this repair to remodeling phase change is a gradual living transition with no definitive end or beginning. In the remodeling phase, production of collagen fibers has decreased significantly, allowing the newly formed tissue the opportunity to improve its structure, strength, and function. With increased loading, the collagen fibers of the newly formed scar tissue begin to hypertrophy (undergo enlargement or growth) and align themselves along the lines of stress, increasing the strength of the newly formed tissue and allowing for the injured client's return to function. Although strength of the collagen fibers improves significantly, the new tissue will likely never be as strong as the tissue it has replaced (1, 14, 27). Tissue remodeling can last up to two to four months or even beyond one year after injury depending on severity, type and location of tissue involved, previous injury, surgery performed, complications, age of client, and so on (48).

Optimizing tissue function is the primary goal during this final phase of healing. Clients improve function by continuing the exercises performed during the repair phase and by adding more advanced, activity-specific exercises that allow progressive stresses to be applied to the injured tissue. Progressive tissue loading allows improved collagen fiber alignment and fiber hypertrophy, optimizing the scar's tensile strength. Ultimately, rehabilitation and reconditioning exercises must be functional to facilitate a return to activity. Strengthening should transition from general exercises to activity-specific exercises designed to replicate movements common in given sports and activities.

> Full restoration of tissue function following injury can be optimized through careful alignment of activities with the physiologic phase of tissue healing.

Orthopedic Concerns and the Personal Trainer

It is not uncommon for a personal trainer to have a client presenting with an injury history. Therefore personal trainers should have a basic familiarity with common injuries and orthopedic conditions. However, it is important for personal trainers to understand their limitations and scope of practice, as it is not the personal trainer's responsibility to determine movement or exercise restrictions. Rather, personal trainers should be able to determine appropriate exercise strategies based on any movement restrictions or limitations commonly associated with an injury or established in consultation with the client's health care team including the physician, athletic trainer, or physical therapist. In many situations, a client's health care team may be augmented with additional professionals such as a nutritionist or sport psychologist. A personal trainer should establish effective communication across the entire health care team and frequently consult with the team members before making significant advancements in the exercise activities of a client with an orthopedic injury.

It can be somewhat difficult to determine the appropriate exercises and progression for a client with an injury concern. Selection of exercises and activities for an individual recovering from injury should be informed by the injury time line as well as monitoring of the client for signs and symptoms suggestive of ongoing injury complications. The most easily observable cardinal signs are pain, swelling, warmth and color, loss of ROM and flexibility, and decreased strength and function. The presence of any of these classic signs and symptoms may be a response to inappropriate exercise or to advancing the individual too quickly. It is good practice to increase only one exercise parameter at a time to make it easy to determine what may have triggered the negative response, should one occur. Table 21.2 should give readers an appreciation for the use of the physiology of healing to guide the selection of exercises.

The underlying pathophysiology for each type of orthopedic injury, surgical procedure, or disease process will be associated with specific exercise and movement guidelines based on indications,

TABLE 21.2   Integration of Rehabilitation Goals Across Healing Time Line

Rehabilitation goals	Inflammation phase	Proliferation phase	Remodeling phase
Control pain and inflammation (PRICE)	X		
ROM, flexibility		X	Maintain
Balance, proprioception, neuromuscular control		X	X
Strengthening		X	X
Functional strengthening			X
Return to activity			X

contraindications, and precautions. An **indication** is an activity that will benefit the injured client (66). For example, a client who recently had a knee replacement must maintain upper extremity function, so the personal trainer may design a program that allows the client to continue performing upper extremity strength training exercises during rehabilitation of the knee. A **contraindication** is an activity or practice that is inadvisable or prohibited because of the given injury (66). For example, during the rehabilitation from reconstruction of the knee's anterior cruciate ligament, a client must protect the anterior cruciate ligament graft, meaning that closed chain activities are more favored and open chain activities are contraindicated within a certain healing time line. Therefore, the final 30° of the leg extension exercise is contraindicated as it can place the graft in a compromised position. This is also an excellent example of a situation in which communication with the client's physician, athletic trainer, or physical therapist is essential to the outcome of the injury. A **precaution** is an activity that may be performed under supervision of a qualified personal trainer and according to client limitations and symptom reproduction (66). For example, while this is typically not advised, clients with anterior shoulder instability may perform the bench press provided that they avoid excessive shoulder horizontal abduction (i.e., the upper arms stay above parallel to the body) and use proper weight increases.

Because of the many different surgical procedures currently used, designing exercise programs for clients following surgery can be challenging. Typically these clients have undergone some form of formal rehabilitation or have been instructed in a home exercise program following the surgical procedure. Unfortunately, rehabilitation exercise programs often fail to allow the client's return to full function, whether due to limitations of insurance coverage or a lack of client compliance. This places the personal trainer in an ideal position to improve function through the use of both traditional and nontraditional exercise programs. Before designing these programs, however, it is important that the

personal trainer not only generally understand the surgical procedure but also understand and abide by the contraindications and precautions brought about by the surgery.

It is beyond the scope of this chapter to give an in-depth description of every injury, surgical procedure, or disease process. Likewise, it is difficult to provide all of the injury-specific possible exercise and movement guidelines. The sections that follow offer general descriptions for common orthopedic injuries and conditions, as well as guidelines to use when one is designing exercise programs for these clients. The information in the remaining sections of this chapter should not be considered a substitute for injury or postsurgical protocols. Nor should it replace the guidance of other health care providers. Rather, we provide a brief discussion of select injuries or other orthopedic conditions that is intended to augment the personal trainer's base of knowledge, thereby improving communication with health care providers and ultimately supporting recovery of the client's function in a safe, efficient manner. It is imperative that the personal trainer contact the client's physician, athletic trainer, or physical therapist for a description of the injury or surgery and obtain a list of acceptable movement and exercise guidelines prior to beginning an exercise program.

> An appreciation for the physiology of healing will allow for appropriate selection of exercises and support a client's full recovery.

Low Back

As one of the leading causes of pain and disability (5), low back pain has become a significant concern not only for health care providers, but also for personal trainers hired by clients with this diagnosis. "Low back pain" is a catch-all term involving several different diagnoses including, but not limited to, disc dysfunction, muscle strain, lumbar spinal stenosis (i.e., a narrowing of the spaces in the spine resulting in tissue compression), and spondylolisthesis. Each of these diagnoses presents differently and requires a different treatment approach; yet each can be logically treated through promotion and reinforcement of pain-reducing postures and movements, as well as avoidance of any movement that causes the back pain to increase or to radiate or spread over a larger area. For example, if a person has pain with bending forward, it would be recommended that he or she avoid this movement and maybe even perform extension exercises provided that these do not produce pain. Persons with disc herniation typically respond best to exercises involving lumbosacral extension, while those diagnosed with lumbar spinal stenosis tend to favor flexion (64). The aim of this section, then, is to apprise the personal trainer of appropriate and inappropriate movements and exercises for clients with given diagnoses. Figure 21.2 shows the basic anatomy of the lumbosacral spine and is referred to throughout this section.

Low Back Pain

Low back pain can be acute or chronic and can be caused by either a strain, a sprain, tight muscles or trigger points, hypomobility, hypermobility, or sacroiliac dysfunction, to name a few. In any case, there are often similar contributing factors associated with low back pain. Low back pain can cause a vicious cycle of pain, decreased function, and loss of muscular support that, if not properly regained,

can reappear frequently. Pain in the low back causes muscular inhibition, particularly in the multifidi, lumbar erector spinea, psoas, and transverse abdominis, all normally under automatic control and critical to providing segmental control and stabilization of the spine (71). Once inhibition occurs, the muscles become weak and function improperly. If the pain decreases, these muscles may still be weak, as their return to function is not automatic once pain ceases; and this may lead to future and repeated episodes of low back pain and dysfunction (39).

Movement and Exercise Guidelines

The low back or trunk has a functional muscular anatomy, frequently referred to as the *core*, that is important to performance. Likewise, nearby musculature can have a strong influence on proper low back function. Thus, it is not uncommon to have hypomobility in one segment and hypermobility in an adjacent segment of the low back. For example, the hamstring, even though it may be considered a lower extremity muscle group, can cause excessive forward flexion of the lumbar area due to the posterior pull on the pelvis, especially during movement, and can result in low back pain. Here, the recommendation may be as simple as stretches or exercises directed at increasing hamstring length.

Low back pain responds well to spinal stabilization exercise, posture correction(s), and flexibility exercises. Proper assessment for either tightness or weakness of contributing musculature is essential, and common culprits are located in the hip: hip flexors, hip lateral rotators (gluteals), and hamstrings (67). The extensors of the low back and abdominal muscles are essential in providing stability and support; thus strengthening these areas is necessary. Additionally, people without low back injury tend to stabilize or fulcrum about the ankle. Those with low back pain, however, tend to stabilize or fulcrum about the hips and low back to maintain an upright posture in balance tasks, thus increasing or making them more prone to difficulties in controlling postural sway and balance (60). Therefore, people with low back pain, especially those with hypermobility or instability problems, should have balance work incorporated into their programs (62).

In general, a proper assessment of flexibility or ROM and the contributing deficits should be conducted. Flexibility exercises to improve areas deficient in ROM may be done frequently and should not create pain, and may even need to be promoted in the opposite direction of painful motions. Establishing pain-free low back and pelvic neutral stabilization exercises and body mechanics should

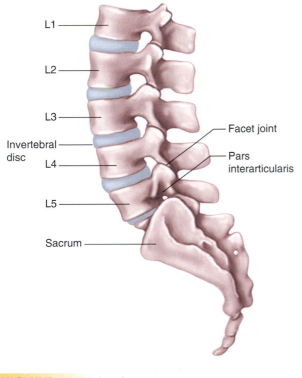

FIGURE 21.2 Lumbar spine anatomy.

L1
L2
L3
Invertebral disc
L4
L5
Sacrum
Facet joint
Pars interarticularis

be a primary strengthening goal, then progressing to trunk strengthening exercises and eventually more advanced stability and dynamic exercises (67). Should the client have a considerable history of low back pain or a low back injury or experience an increase of symptoms, or if the personal trainer is unclear about the condition or status, a consult with the medical providers (e.g., athletic trainer, physical therapist, or physician) is warranted.

Lumbar Disc Injury

In all sections of the vertebral column, the bodies of each vertebra are connected to each other by intervertebral discs (figure 21.3). These discs are designed to absorb shock and stabilize the vertebral column by preventing excessive shear. Each disc has essentially two layers; the annulus fibrosus is the tough outer layer that surrounds the nucleus pulposus, the gelatinous inner layer (65). In the lumbar region of the back, the annulus fibrosus is reinforced anteriorly by the strong anterior longitudinal ligament; because the posterior longitudinal ligament narrows in the lumbar region, the support it is able to provide the posterior aspects of the intervertebral discs is limited. This limited posterior support is one cause of posterolateral disc herniations, the most common type of disc herniation.

When an intervertebral disc herniates, part of the nucleus pulposus makes its way through the outer annulus fibrosus, resulting in inflammation; this inflammation subsequently irritates the spinal nerve roots (73). The irritation can manifest itself

in several ways. The client may feel pain in the back; or changes may occur in the lower extremities, including pain, abnormal sensation, and weakness. In addition to the weak posterior mechanical restraints to disc herniation, position is a significant contributor to lumbar disc dysfunction and injury. Excessive flexion (i.e., forward bending) tends to push the disc's nuclear material posteriorly, encouraging it to move beyond its normal confines toward the spinal canal and nerve roots. When a client has a herniated disc, he or she should seek treatment from a physician, whose treatment plan may include therapeutic exercise.

Movement and Exercise Guidelines

For the reasons just outlined, clients with herniated lumbar discs are generally encouraged to avoid lumbar flexion in favor of extension to prevent the posterior protrusion of the disc material (89). Therefore, they should avoid exercises involving significant lumbar flexion and should perform strengthening and stabilization activities in pelvic neutral. Resistance training contraindications may include full sit-ups, while precautions may include the squat, all rowing movements (e.g., seated row, bent-over row), and the deadlift. Aerobic exercise precautions may include bicycle riding (due to possible increased flexion with forward lean), use of the rowing ergometer, and flexion-based movements in aerobic dance. Flexibility is important with a client who has a herniated disc, but stretching exercises involving flexion should be used with caution; contraindicated flexibility exercises include hamstring stretches emphasizing lumbar flexion (e.g., standing toe touch) and other stretches requiring similar movements in the lumbar spine. Precautions may include gluteal, hip adductor, and upper back stretches.

Muscle Strain

As previously discussed, muscle strains are tears to muscle fibers. Strains to the muscles of the lumbosacral spine are quite common and may have a variety of causes, including direct trauma and overuse. Traumatic muscle strains require completion of the various phases of tissue healing in the affected muscle(s) with guidance from the client's health care practitioners. An overuse injury, on the other hand, requires the client to correct any improper posture and movement patterns. Retraining muscles to function in their intended manner will enable them to work more efficiently, thereby decreasing the abnormal stresses the affected muscle(s) experience.

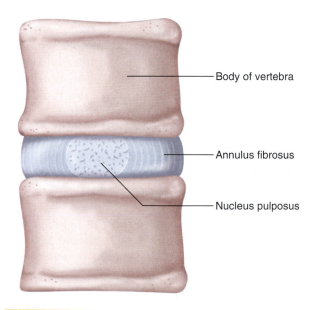

Body of vertebra

Annulus fibrosus

Nucleus pulposus

FIGURE 21.3 The components of the intervertebral disc.
Reprinted by permission from Watkins 2010.

Movement and Exercise Guidelines

Movement and exercise restriction following muscle strain is highly dependent on the muscle that has been strained. Once the medical provider has determined which muscle has been strained, exercises and movements that rely on that muscle should be avoided. For example, if the erector spinae muscles have been strained, lumbar extension exercises (e.g., hyperextension) and exercises requiring static maintenance of the normal lumbar lordosis (e.g., bent-over barbell row, use of elliptical trainer) should be avoided during the early phases of tissue healing; these and similar exercises may be included in exercise programming during the remodeling phase once the pain subsides in the injured muscle's primary actions.

Spondylolysis and Spondylolisthesis

Spondylolysis is a defect, or fracture, of the pars interarticularis region of a lumbar vertebra (an arched area of the vertebra that connects the superior and inferior facet joints—see figure 21.2) (37, 40). Spondylolisthesis is the possible progression of spondylolysis, a forward slippage of one vertebral body on another (46, 80). While causes vary, spondylolysis and spondylolisthesis commonly occur following lumbar extension injuries or in persons participating in activities requiring lumbar extension (e.g., divers and football linemen). Clients with spondylolysis and spondylolisthesis typically describe low back pain and possible lower extremity radicular pain, paresthesia, or muscle weakness. Complaints most often increase with lumbar extension and improve with flexion.

Movement and Exercise Guidelines

Like clients with lumbar spinal stenosis, clients with spondylolysis or spondylolisthesis should focus on strengthening the muscles surrounding the spine and should avoid exercises involving lumbar extension. Most abdominal exercises are appropriate, especially crunches and exercises for the obliques and transverse abdominis, as are stabilization-type exercises such as those performed on stability balls (provided that lumbar extension is not involved). In contrast to the situation with lumbar spinal stenosis, walking and other forms of standing cardiovascular exercise should not be considered contraindications for clients with spondylolysis or spondylolisthesis. Rather, it is a good idea to encourage these modes of exercise, though they may require modification to adapt to each client's needs. For example, if a client is unable to perform on a stair stepper for more than 10 minutes because of increased low back pain, exercise duration should be kept under that level and then gradually increased as tolerated. Additionally, rapid increases or changes in activity parameters (i.e., frequency, intensity, length of time, type of activity, surface, etc.) can produce symptoms, even in seemingly trained athletes. Table 21.3 provides a movement guide for clients with low back pain.

> Effective assessment for posture and movement impairments is essential for establishing appropriate pain-free low back and pelvic neutral stabilization and flexibility exercises.

TABLE 21.3 Low Back Pain Movement and Exercise Guidelines

Diagnosis	Movement contraindications	Exercise contraindications	Exercise indications
Disc injury	■ Lumbar flexion ■ Lumbar rotation	■ Sit-up ■ Knee-to-chest stretch ■ Spinal twist	■ Passive lumbar extension stretches ■ Isometric abdominal and extensor strengthening, progressing to lumbar stabilization program
Muscle strain	■ Passive lumbar flexion (during inflammatory phase) ■ Active lumbar extension (during inflammatory phase)	Knee-to-chest stretch	None during inflammatory phase, progressing to gentle flexion stretching, followed by extension strengthening
Spondylolysis and spondylolisthesis	■ Lumbar extension	■ Squat ■ Shoulder press ■ Push press	■ Knee-to-chest stretch ■ Abdominal crunch ■ Pelvic neutral stabilizations

Shoulder

Because of the inherent mobility of the shoulder and the need for dynamic muscular stability for proper function, the shoulder is an area where specific exercises following injury and surgery can have a tremendous influence on the client's overall function. The anatomy of the shoulder allows for great mobility of the joint, but this can also make it more susceptible to injury, whether acute, traumatic, atraumatic, or chronic or overuse. In the shoulder, it is necessary to consider posture, muscular balance, scapulothoracic control, ROM, and even the relationship to the trunk and hip for the joint to perform as a highly synchronous and balanced complex.

The trunk and hips are vital to shoulder function. The legs and trunk provide 51% to 55% of the total kinetic energy and total force for overhead activities (44). Consequently, a program for the shoulder should include strengthening exercises for the hip rotators, hip abductors, and hip extensors, as well as the abdominal and low back stabilizing muscles.

Another aspect that is essential to shoulder function is correct posture, and any person performing shoulder exercises or with a history of injury should have a posture assessment. Postures such as a head-forward or rounded shoulder **(kyphotic posture)** are common faults and cause medial rotation of the humerus and protraction of the shoulder, as well as weakness of the posterior aspect (scapular retractors and lateral rotators) and tightness of the anterior aspect (protractors and medial rotators) (67). This can prevent full elevation motion of the humerus and contribute to subacromial impingement as well as rotator cuff tendonitis and tears.

Muscle imbalance can contribute to shoulder injuries by affecting the force couples within the joint. In the glenohumeral joint, the external rotators form a force couple with the internal rotators, and the rotator cuff with the deltoid. This muscle balance is particularly important since the rotator cuff is assistive not only in producing shoulder motion, but also in compressing the humeral head into the glenoid fossa, promoting stability and proper joint movement. In the scapulothoracic region, the upper trapezius and levator scapulae elevate the scapula; the middle trapezius and rhomboids adduct the scapula; the lower trapezius adducts and depresses the scapula; the serratus anterior abducts and upwardly rotates the scapula; and the pectoralis minor depresses the scapula. The glenohumeral and scapulothoracic muscles act collectively to provide a synchronous and consistent relationship to produce shoulder movement (66). Common muscle imbalances can be a decreased external to internal

rotation ratio in strength, as well as increased activity of the upper trapezius and deltoid, decreased activity of the lower trapezius and rhomboids, and serratus anterior inhibition (67, 76). When considering these issues, it is important to note that rotator cuff strengthening should be done with lower loads of resistance. Increased loads produce activation of the deltoid that can be counterproductive to rotator cuff strengthening and create unwanted superior translation of the humeral head, thus counteracting the rotator cuff exercises and making the area more susceptible to impingement (12). Additionally, it has been noted that fatigue of the scapular muscles can affect shoulder performance; thus endurance activities, especially those in the closed chain that promote enhanced scapular stability, should be included (67). Again, should there be any uncertainty regarding the appropriate exercises and progressions, consultation with the medical care team should occur.

The following sections present an overview of each injury or surgical procedure, followed by specific exercise indications and contraindications. Included are estimates of the general time frames during which exercise can be most appropriately used. As with all of the conditions described in this chapter, the personal trainer should consult with the client's health care team including the physician, athletic trainer, or physical therapist before advising the client on any exercises.

Impingement Syndrome

Impingement syndrome is a "pinching" of the supraspinatus, the long head of the biceps tendon, or subacromial bursa under the acromial arch (figure 21.4). Impingement has many contributory factors;

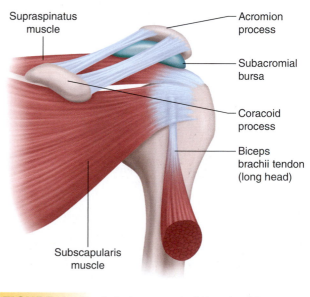

FIGURE 21.4   Anterior aspect of the shoulder.

some are changeable with conservative treatment, and others require surgical intervention (e.g., subacromial decompression). Causative factors that may necessitate surgery include anatomic or bony abnormalities (e.g., "hooked" acromion that compresses the subacromial structures). Factors that may be altered include muscle imbalances, poor posture and scapular control, and improper exercise technique or overuse of the shoulder, typically overhead (e.g., baseball pitchers, swimmers).

Many athletic trainers and physical therapists, after reducing inflammation, focus on exercises to improve muscular imbalance and endurance, ROM (if limited), scapular control, and posture. Once formal rehabilitation has ended, a personal trainer has the important responsibility of continuing the exercises performed during rehabilitation. After rotator cuff strength and scapular stability have returned, often as the client notes significantly decreased or absent shoulder pain, personal trainers gradually add typical resistance training exercises.

The rotator cuff muscles function to position the humeral head in the shallow glenoid, thereby resisting the upward migration of the humeral head into the acromion. Further, muscles attaching to the scapula—primarily the upper and lower trapezius, serratus anterior, and levator scapula muscles—must function properly to rotate the scapula during overhead movements. When any of these muscles become weak or fail to function properly, impingement may occur.

Movement and Exercise Guidelines

Figures 21.5 to 21.9 depict a series of rotator cuff exercises that elicit high levels of rotator cuff activation while minimizing compensation from other muscle groups (6, 67). These exercises are a staple of nonoperative and postoperative shoulder rehabilitation programs (18) and are indicated in postrehabilitation training programs to continue rotator cuff strengthening and maintain proper muscular balance. Because the rotator cuff muscles function primarily in an endurance role, these exercises are typically performed with light weights (seldom more than 4 pounds [1.8 kg]) and high repetitions (sets of 15 to 20 repetitions). The exercises are chosen for

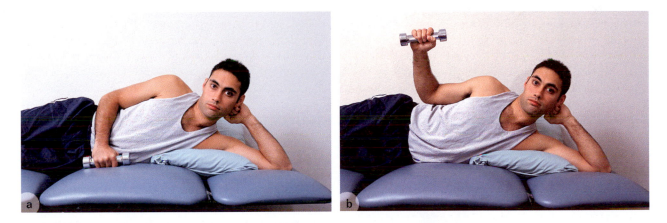

FIGURE 21.5 Side-lying external rotation: *(a)* beginning position; *(b)* end position.

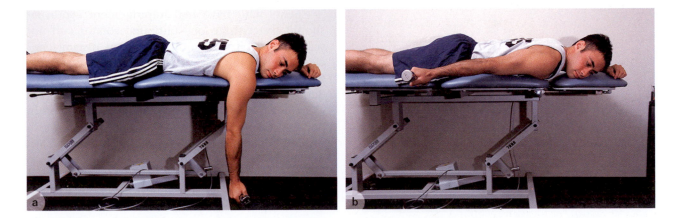

FIGURE 21.6 Prone shoulder extension: *(a)* beginning position; *(b)* end position.

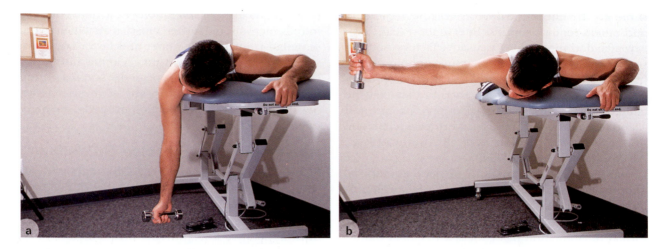

FIGURE 21.7 Prone horizontal abduction: (a) beginning position; (b) end position.

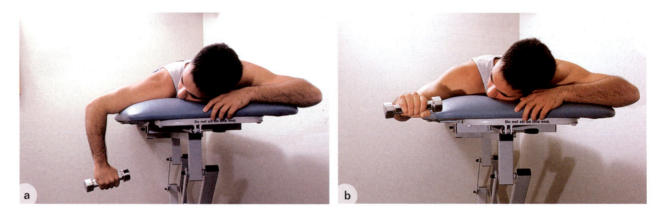

FIGURE 21.8 Prone 90°/90° external rotation: (a) beginning position; (b) end position.

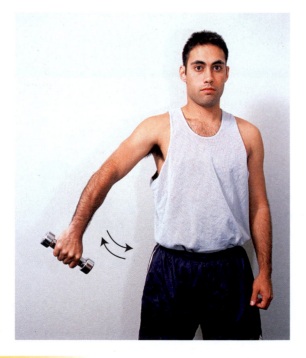

FIGURE 21.9 Standing empty can.

their muscle activation characteristics, as well as the positioning of the shoulder in safe, neutral environments below 90° of elevation and with the arm in a forward position relative to the body (anterior to the frontal plane). These positions minimize rotator cuff impingement and allow for pain-free exercise in most individuals.

Clients who have had impingement syndrome should concentrate on continued rotator cuff and scapular exercises. Multiple types of rowing exercise targeting the rhomboids and middle and lower trapezius, focusing on scapular retraction and depression, are recommended. Overhead pressing exercises (e.g., shoulder press) and all forms of the bench press exercise should be used cautiously; the decline bench press stresses this area the least and may therefore be an appropriate exercise choice in reintroduction of the bench press. The upright row should also be used with caution, as rowing too high (elbows up too high) may aggravate impingement-type pain. It is safe to apply exercises such as the lat pulldown by having the client pull the bar in front to the chest and focusing on activating the latissimus dorsi to depress the humeral head, rather than behind the neck.

Some cardiovascular exercises may also pose problems for the client recovering from shoulder impingement. Use of a VersaClimber should be considered a contraindication as it places the shoulder in prime position to be impinged (i.e., overhead), especially if strength of the rotator cuff muscles and scapular stabilizers has yet to return. Caution must be used with racket sports; again, placing the arm overhead, as with a tennis serve or racquetball smash, increases the likelihood of impinging structures within the shoulder.

Anterior Instability

In anterior shoulder (glenohumeral joint) instability, the head of the humerus moves too far forward, resulting in possible injury or dislocation (31). Management of individuals with this condition is one of the greatest challenges facing medical professionals in the orthopedic sports medicine area today. Because posterior instability occurs less frequently, the discussion here is limited to management of anterior instability, but guidelines for all directions of instability are listed in table 21.4.

Research has shown that, following an anterior dislocation of the shoulder, redislocation can occur in as many as 90% of young, active individuals while only 30% to 50% of middle-aged individuals redislocate their shoulders. In recent years, tremendous advances have been made in rehabilitative and surgical methodology to treat people with shoulder instability. Surgical management of shoulder instability has progressed to include procedures using primarily arthroscopy, as well as high-tech instruments that literally shrink the joint capsule (thermal capsulography) to assist in stabilizing the humeral head within the glenoid.

Movement and Exercise Guidelines

Exercise indications for instability (i.e., rotator cuff and scapular strengthening) are similar to those for impingement, since ultimately the rotator cuff is the primary dynamic stabilizer of the glenohumeral joint. Figures 21.5 through 21.9, as well as the contraindications listed in table 21.4, provide guidelines for performing exercises in a safe manner. Movements that involve greater than 90° of elevation, placing the hands and arms behind the plane of the shoulder (i.e., approximately 90° anterior to the frontal plane), are dangerous as they may place the shoulder in an unstable position. These criteria for shoulder exercises have led to the use of a safe zone that describes the position below 90° of elevation of the shoulder and arms anterior to the frontal plane of the body (figure 21.10) (19).

Clients with unstable shoulders may choose either a conservative, exercise-based approach or

TABLE 21.4 Shoulder Movement and Exercise Guidelines

Diagnosis	Movement contraindications*	Exercise contraindications*	Exercise indications
Impingement syndrome	Overhead with internally rotated shoulder or painful motions	■ Shoulder press ■ Lateral dumbbell raise with internally rotated shoulder ■ Upright row above shoulder level ■ Incline bench press	■ Rotator cuff strengthening exercises ■ Pain-free exercises
Instability	■ Anterior: combined external rotation with >90° abduction; horizontal abduction ■ Posterior: combined internal rotation, horizontal adduction, and flexion ■ Inferior: full elevation, dependent arm	■ Bench press** ■ Pec deck** ■ Push-up** ■ Behind-the-neck lat pulldown and shoulder press	■ Rotator cuff strengthening exercises ■ Scapular strengthening ■ Stabilization: static to dynamic
Rotator cuff pathology	Resisted overhead movements	Painful exercises and early quick eccentric actions	Rotator cuff strengthening exercises (beginning 4-6 weeks after surgery)*

*Consult with a medical professional to determine when or if these movements are no longer contraindicated for a specific client.
**Use close grip hand position, with hands no wider than shoulder width and avoid last 10° to 20° of shoulder extension.

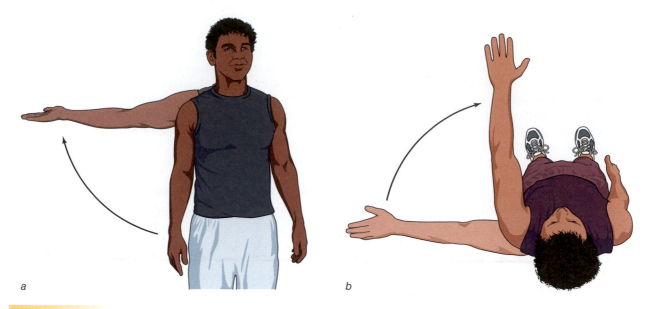

a   *b*

FIGURE 21.10   Safe zone exercise positions. Positions should be *(a)* below shoulder level and *(b)* in front of the body's frontal plane.

surgery as a remedy for instability. Individuals with unstable shoulders—both conservatively and surgically treated—frequently wish to return to traditional strength training or aerobic conditioning activities or both. It is imperative that exercise modifications be incorporated to protect the structures that were repaired during the surgical procedures. Following these exercise modifications may prove to be a permanent part of the individual's lifting program to ensure that shoulder stability is not compromised (figure 21.11) (31).

Once a client has completed treatment for an unstable shoulder, most aerobic training activities are generally safe to perform, with the exception of some aerobic dance steps, swimming (specifically the freestyle, backstroke, and butterfly), and some racket sport activities. Flexibility exercises that place the shoulder in a position outside the aforementioned safe zone are contraindicated (e.g., the hands-behind-back stretch and the behind-neck stretch, p. 267) because of the adverse stresses placed across an already unstable shoulder joint. Table 21.4 provides a movement guide for clients experiencing shoulder dysfunction.

Rotator Cuff Repair

A rotator cuff repair is typically carried out when damage to the rotator cuff tendons—most often the tendon of the supraspinatus muscle—includes a tear that is "full thickness," meaning that the rotator cuff is not merely frayed but has a tear that goes through its entirety. These tears cause significantly altered

joint mechanics (63) and are traditionally repaired using either sutures or suture anchors (fasteners that help reattach the torn tendon to its insertion), most often involving an open incision, in addition to arthroscopy.

Due to the additional open incision and greater extent of damage to the rotator cuff tendons, greater periods of immobilization in a sling are used following a rotator cuff repair. The exact amount of time spent in a sling without movement (commonly ranging from two days to six weeks) is determined by the surgeon and is dictated by factors such as the individual's age, tissue quality, and presence of additional injuries found at the time of surgery.

Movement and Exercise Guidelines

Overzealous client activity and inappropriate exercise introduction can lead to failure of the rotator cuff repair and disastrous results (9). Exercises for the scapular muscles and rotator cuff (figures 21.5 through 21.9) are also used with these clients, but often not for four to six weeks following surgery. People are often discharged from formal rehabilitation three to four months after the rotator cuff repair. The exercises in figures 21.5 through 21.9 should receive continued emphasis in the postrehabilitation programming to ensure continued activation of the rotator cuff musculature.

Contraindicated exercises for these clients are also listed in table 21.4. Overhead lifting and exercises such as push-ups and bench presses place the shoulder in a position of stress and can result in overload to the rotator cuff. Aerobic endurance

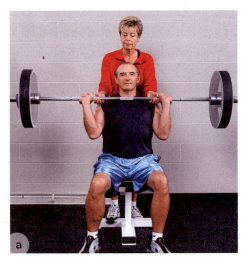
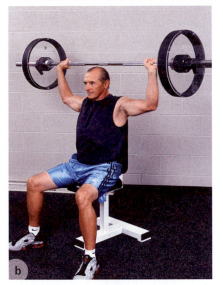
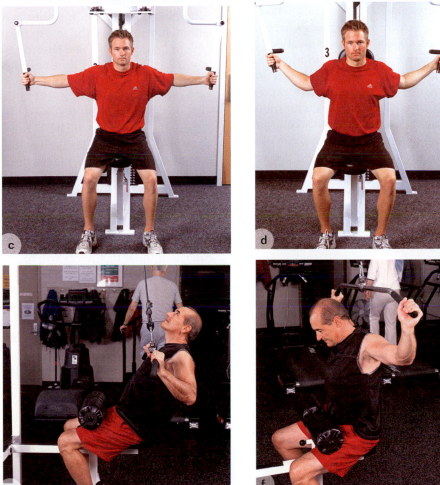

FIGURE 21.11 Exercise modification and anterior capsule stress. The photos in the left-hand column show exercises being performed correctly so as to not stress the anterior capsule. Harmful anterior capsule stress results when these exercises are performed incorrectly, as shown in the right-hand column. (*a*) Correct technique: front-of-face shoulder press. (*b*) Incorrect technique: behind-the-neck shoulder press. (*c*) Correct technique: pec deck. (*d*) Incorrect technique: excessive horizontal abduction with pec deck. (*e*) Correct technique: front-of-face lat pulldown. (*f*) Incorrect technique: behind-the-neck lat pulldown.

activities that cause discomfort or pain (e.g., swimming, VersaClimber) should be limited. Typically, aerobic endurance training using lower body exercises such as walking, running, and stair stepping is well tolerated and safe for inclusion during shoulder rehabilitation. Additionally, one complication following rotator cuff surgery is loss of ROM, the extent dependent on the amount of immobilization used after the surgery. The ROM loss usually includes the patterns of external rotation, internal rotation, and abduction. This finding further complicates the performance of traditional exercises, such as those that place the shoulder and arm posterior to (behind) the head.

Several of the types of shoulder conditions discussed in this section preclude performance of standard upper extremity strength training exercises. Responsible intervention by a personal trainer should include screening of individuals who may be at risk for the performance of these exercises. Table 21.5 describes appropriate modifications that can be made to common exercises and movements to reduce unwanted stress on the shoulder joint. Application of rotator cuff and scapular exercises as a "core" aspect of any upper extremity training program is recommended because of the important role these muscles play in providing movement and stabilization of the shoulder complex.

> Shoulder exercises should be anchored using an approach that ensures stability of the joint during functional activities through engagement of the scapular and rotator cuff muscles.

Ankle

The ankle sprain is one of the most common sport-related injuries, accounting for 10% to 28% of all athletic injuries (41, 73, 74). Ankle sprains are often linked to sports requiring sudden stops, changes of

Conditions Requiring Shoulder Exercise Modification

Exercise for clients with the following conditions is not contraindicated. Each condition, however, requires specific modifications to allow exercise participation.

- Rotator cuff repair
- Rotator cuff **tendinitis**
- Glenohumeral joint instability (prior dislocation or **subluxation**)
- Acromioclavicular joint injury (separation)
- Glenohumeral joint osteoarthritis

direction, and jumping such as soccer and basketball. An inversion sprain resulting in damage to the lateral ligaments is the most frequently reported type of ankle sprain. The lateral aspect of the ankle is primarily stabilized by three ligaments: anterior talofibular, posterior talofibular, and calcaneofibular ligament (figure 21.12) (41, 73, 74). Most lateral ankle sprains primarily involve the anterior talofibular ligament due to its relative weakness and susceptibility to not withstanding the force placed on the ankle in an inverted, plantarflexed, and internally rotated position. Although the posterior talofibular and calcaneofibular ligaments are likely to be damaged, it is generally believed that higher levels of inversion force are needed to sprain these ligaments. Thus a sprain involving the posterior talofibular or calcaneofibular ligaments will likely be quite severe. Perhaps due to the prevalence of the ankle sprain, many individuals choose to self-treat a sprain that results in minimal loss of function. Thus, the personal trainer may work with a client who is self-treating a mild ankle sprain or has been recently discharged from formal rehabilitation for a more severe sprain. An inappropriately managed ankle sprain, however,

TABLE 21.5   Shoulder Exercise Modifications

Exercise	Modification
Shoulder press	When lowering the barbell, allow the bar to pass in front of the client's head in order to minimize anterior shoulder stress.
Bench press	When lowering the bar, clients with shoulder dysfunction should not allow the bar to touch the chest at its lowest point in order to minimize anterior shoulder stress.
	Keep the upper arms near the body to limit horizontal abduction and decrease shoulder stress.
Pec deck	During the eccentric phase, clients with shoulder dysfunction should not allow the pads to pass behind the body at their most posterior position in order to minimize anterior shoulder stress.
Lat pulldown	When pulling down the bar, allow the bar to pass in front of the client's head in order to minimize anterior shoulder stress.
	Use a reverse (supinated) grip to reduce shoulder joint stress.

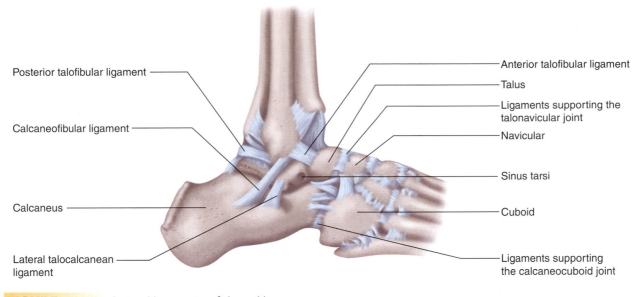

Posterior talofibular ligament

Calcaneofibular ligament

Calcaneus

Lateral talocalcanean ligament

Anterior talofibular ligament

Talus

Ligaments supporting the talonavicular joint

Navicular

Sinus tarsi

Cuboid

Ligaments supporting the calcaneocuboid joint

FIGURE 21.12 Lateral ligaments of the ankle.

Reprinted by permission from Watkins 2010.

can lead to chronic ankle instability. To minimize the potential for chronic problems with the ankle, it is important for the personal trainer to recognize the need to encourage the client to seek an evaluation by a doctor or clinician before establishing an exercise plan.

Movement and Exercise Guidelines

Vigorous exercise is generally discouraged in the initial phase of ankle rehabilitation, as the primary focus should be on controlling the pain and inflammation and protecting the joint to allow for ligament healing (43). The degree of allowed weight bearing will depend on the severity of the injury. In general, early ambulation, even if minimal, is encouraged, as it has been suggested that a small amount of stress promotes more complete tissue healing. During this early phase of recovery, the client will continue to experience muscle atrophy and loss of balance and postural control ability. As is the case with other musculoskeletal injuries, the magnitude of the functional deficits will depend on the severity of the injury. Once swelling and pain have subsided, exercises and activities can become more aggressive. In addition to maintaining cardiorespiratory endurance (e.g., stationary bike), emphasis should be placed on restoring ROM, strength, and proprioception and should progress to more functional (both simple and complex) tasks (43, 82).

Recent evidence has identified that incorporation of a planned balance training program can reduce the risk of ankle sprains (52, 84). Balance programs, like other training paradigms, should be progressive

in design and gradually incorporate a variety of more difficult and complex tasks. For athletes, the balance program should eventually transition to an in-season phase reflecting a lesser volume and frequency (84). Many of the balance and postural control tasks used as part of exercise protocols for other lower extremity injuries and conditions apply to the ankle as well. For example, single-leg balance on a stable and then advancing to an unstable surface (e.g., foam pad, Bosu ball) with and without eyes open, plyometric jumping and agility tasks, and running progressions (e.g., advancing from straight-line running to change-in-direction cuts) can be effective in restoring function to an injured ankle (13, 43, 69, 73, 74, 82). Table 21.6 provides movement guidelines for a lateral ankle sprain.

> Gradually progressing an injured ankle from non-weight-bearing to weight-bearing activities and subsequently incorporating strength, ROM, and balance activities will properly prepare the joint for more functional activities.

Knee

As with the shoulder, a variety of injuries and surgical procedures exist for the knee joint. Here we discuss three common conditions of the knee: anterior knee pain, anterior cruciate ligament injury, and total knee arthroplasty. Again, we do not give detailed descriptions of injury pathophysiology and surgical procedures. Rather we provide an overview

TABLE 21.6   Ankle Movement and Exercise Guidelines

Diagnosis	Movement contraindications	Exercise contraindications	Exercise indications
Inversion sprain*	Inversion with weight bearing	Activities requiring loaded or full weight bearing	Open chain ROM and strength activities until weight bearing is permitted

*Information presented based on an acute inversion ankle sprain and emphasizes early phases of recovery. Severity of sprain will determine the level of allowable activity. Once full weight bearing is allowed, closed chain and more functional activities can be incorporated.

of these procedures, discuss general rehabilitation, and outline exercise considerations (indications and contraindications) after discharge from formal rehabilitation. Figure 21.13 illustrates the ligaments of the knee.

Anterior Knee Pain

The term "anterior knee pain" is at times used interchangeably with "runner's knee," but it is referred to clinically as *patellofemoral pain syndrome (PFPS)* and is a common clinical diagnosis in young adults, associated with general anterior or retropatellar knee pain in the absence of other apparent pathology (17, 67, 88). Patellofemoral pain syndrome is a multifactorial condition with suggested etiologies associated with intrinsic factors such as malalignment of the lower extremity, quadriceps weakness, or neuromuscular inefficiencies of the thigh musculature

(or some combination of these) (17, 42, 88). Anterior knee pain, a common malady among personal training clients, can be associated with a variety of diagnoses (e.g., chondromalacia, iliotibial band friction syndrome, irritated plica, patellar tendinitis). Clients with anterior knee pain commonly describe pain with prolonged sitting and when walking up and down stairs. Consensus, however, is lacking in the literature regarding the cause and treatment of anterior knee pain. This lack of consensus is likely related to the multifactorial etiological nature of this condition, with proposed causes including overuse (particularly with running), overload, biomechanical faults, and muscular imbalance. Although the diagnosis of anterior knee pain is common, treatment demands an individualized approach based on the underlying precipitating factors and coexisting injuries that are specific to the client. That said, all diagnoses have several treatment commonalities, and rehabilitation frequently focuses on reducing pain and inflammation, correcting biomechanical faults, and optimizing tissue function.

Movement and Exercise Guidelines

Anterior knee pain has been referred to as the "miserable alignment syndrome," and the cause has been described as a combination of factors including femoral anteversion, patellar malalignment, increased quadriceps angle (Q-angle), and tibial external rotation (17). Overuse and training on unsuitable surfaces are common contributors to anterior knee pain and often occur with running, jumping, and bicycling activities. Collectively, these factors alter the tracking of the patella in the trochlear groove, resulting from tightness of surrounding tissues (e.g., lateral retinaculum, iliotibial band), imbalance in the forces acting on the patella, and possibly a change in foot biomechanics (e.g., excessive or improper pronation or supination) (17, 51). Thus education on proper running surfaces (concrete vs. asphalt vs. treadmill), appropriate footwear, and the benefits of cross-training is quite important in addressing overuse.

Muscular imbalances surrounding anterior knee pain commonly have to do with the relationship

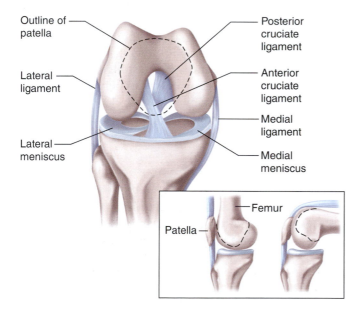

Outline of patella

Lateral ligament

Lateral meniscus

Posterior cruciate ligament

Anterior cruciate ligament

Medial ligament

Medial meniscus

Femur

Patella

FIGURE 21.13   Ligaments of the knee joint. Anterior aspect of the right knee, flexed at 90°, with patella removed to show the intracapsular cruciate ligaments and femoral condyles slightly raised to show the menisci. The collateral ligaments are located at the center of the joint but lie outside the joint cavity.

Reprinted by permission from Watkins 2010.

between the vastus lateralis and a portion of the vastus medialis, the vastus medialis obliquus (VMO). The common belief is that the vastus lateralis overpowers the VMO and pulls excessively on the patella, causing the patella to move laterally when the quadriceps muscles are active. Although it is possible that such an imbalance exists, its treatment is rather controversial. It would seem logical to strengthen the VMO to improve this balance, but research has yet to demonstrate that preferential VMO recruitment is possible. More recent research has suggested that in addition to the strength and function of the quadriceps, proximal muscle weakness (e.g., gluteus medius) may be a contributing factor to anterior knee pain. Specifically, weakness in the gluteus medius will allow the contralateral pelvis to drop, thereby forcing the stance limb into a position of internal femoral and tibial rotation (17, 42). This change in the alignment of the pelvis, femur, and tibia may also facilitate hyperpronation of the foot and exacerbate the already poor alignment pattern (17).

Because the quadriceps muscles help clients walk up stairs and assist deceleration of the body during walking on level surfaces and down steps, general quadriceps strengthening does improve patellofemoral function and reduces anterior knee pain. However, weakness in the proximal muscles will decrease an individual's general ability to stabilize the lower extremity, particular during dynamic movements. Thus, specific exercises emphasizing unilateral balance tasks and targeting hip strength are recognized as an essential component of treatment and prevention of anterior knee pain. Care must be taken, however, to use exercises that do not adversely stress the patellofemoral joint. No exercises are explicitly contraindicated for clients experiencing anterior knee pain, but some exercises require caution. Deep squats and other closed kinetic chain exercises requiring knee flexion of more than 90° must be prescribed with caution, as these increase compression between the patella and femur. Additionally, most open kinetic chain exercises, such as knee extension, in the last 30° increase patellofemoral joint load and should be avoided. Aerobic endurance activities such as high-impact aerobic dance or step aerobics, as well as aerobic endurance training that places the knee in positions such as a deep lunging or squatting position, would be contraindicated. Typically, cycling (provided seat height is appropriate) and water-based aerobic training activities are recommended to minimize impact and trauma to the knee joint and maintain an individual's aerobic condition during training. It is also common for clients with anterior knee pain to use a form of taping (e.g., McConnell), bracing, or orthotics to assist with stabilization of the patella and support proper mechanical alignment. Table 21.7 provides movement guidelines for anterior knee pain and other knee problems.

TABLE 21.7 Knee Movement and Exercise Guidelines

Diagnosis	Movement contraindications	Exercise contraindications	Exercise indications
Anterior knee pain*	Closed chain knee movements with >90° knee flexion	Full squat; full lunge	1/4 to 1/2 squat and leg press
	Open chain knee movements 0° to 30° knee flexion	End range of leg extension	Partial lunge; leg curl
		Stair stepper with large steps	Stair stepper with short, choppy steps
Anterior cruciate ligament reconstruction	Open chain knee movements <45° knee flexion	End range of leg extension	■ 3/4 squat and leg press ■ Step-up ■ Leg curl ■ Stiff-leg deadlift ■ Elliptical trainer
Total knee arthroplasty	■ Closed chain knee movements with >100° knee flexion ■ Kneeling	■ Full squat ■ Full lunge	■ 1/4 to 1/2 squat and leg press ■ Partial lunge ■ Leg extension and leg curl ■ Stationary bicycle ■ Aquatics, swimming

*Although these movement and exercise contraindications are commonly used, it should be remembered that individual clients react to anterior knee pain differently; therefore, for clients with this general diagnosis, the ranges of motion and exercises provided should be considered relative. Exercises and movements that cause anterior knee pain become absolute contraindications and should be eliminated from the client's exercise program.

Anterior Cruciate Ligament Reconstruction

The anterior cruciate ligament (ACL) is a major stabilizing structure of the knee. Injury to the ACL can lead to joint instability during landing and pivoting tasks (7, 16, 50). The ACL primarily limits anterior tibial translation and rotation relative to the femur (7, 16, 50). Because of these important functions, reconstruction is a common treatment choice for joint laxity and possible functional instability, especially with active, competitive people and those with high-demand occupations (e.g., firefighting, construction).

Advances in surgical technique and more aggressive and accelerated postoperative rehabilitation programs have allowed individuals to return to functional activities sooner and with fewer complications than in the past (78). Anterior cruciate ligament reconstruction techniques commonly use either the central third of the patellar tendon as the graft source or a hamstring graft (semitendinosus and gracilis muscles). There is conflicting evidence as to the relative strength of each graft (2, 4, 24), and each has its own set of advantages and disadvantages. In any case, exercises following ACL reconstruction are an extremely important part of a person's return to function and prevention of ACL injury.

Movement and Exercise Guidelines

For the most part, rehabilitation and postrehabilitation contraindications and precautions are the same for the two types of grafts. The primary difference between the grafts is the ability to use the hamstring muscles; semitendinosus and gracilis grafts preclude immediate postoperative active or resistive knee flexion exercise until approximately four to six weeks following surgery (regardless of the type of hamstring graft used). For either the patellar tendon or hamstring grafts, discharge from formal rehabilitation can now be as early as three to four months after surgery. Ideally, upon discharge individuals should have restored full ROM, strength of the lower extremity (particularly the musculature around the hip and knee), and reestablishment of static and dynamic balance ability (38).

During rehabilitation, both open and closed kinetic chain exercises are important parts of the overall program. **Open kinetic chain** exercises (figure 21.14) are exercises that have the distal aspect of the extremity terminating free in space (13, 20). Examples of open kinetic chain exercises include the straight-leg raise; leg curl; and hip flexion, extension, abduction, and adduction. The open kinetic chain leg extension exercise should be used with cau-

tion; research has shown that the greatest amount of anterior tibial translation—hence the greatest stress on the ACL graft—occurs in the final 30° of leg extension performed in an open kinetic chain (87). Therefore, open kinetic chain leg extension exercises should be performed using a ROM from 90° of knee flexion to only 45° of knee extension to decrease stresses placed on the ACL graft. Clients should adhere to this important modification, at a minimum, for the first six months to one year after surgery to protect the maturing graft and minimize damaging stress application.

Closed kinetic chain exercises (figure 21.15) are those that occur with the distal part of the extremity fixed to an object that is either stationary or moving (13, 20). Closed kinetic chain exercises include the leg press, squat, multidirection lunges, step-ups, and unilateral stance activities. Translation of the tibia relative to the femur is minimized because of the weight bearing and muscular cocontraction (quadriceps and hamstring muscles) during closed kinetic chain exercises; further, these exercises allow multiple joints and muscle groups to be trained simultaneously. Recent research (58) has shown that people with ACL reconstruction who perform bilateral closed kinetic chain exercise shield weight bearing away from the injured limb for up to a year following surgery, placing a greater percentage of weight bearing on the uninvolved or uninjured limb. They do this subconsciously and without volition. Therefore, reliance on only bilateral closed kinetic chain exercise activities for individuals following ACL reconstruction may result in inadequate training stimulus to the injured limb and suboptimal loading paradigms. Use of unilateral stance and exercise patterns such as single-leg squats and step-ups helps to ensure that this training compensation does not occur (13).

Incorporation of plyometric training is generally acceptable, as the development of explosive power and ability to rapidly change direction are necessary skills for most athletes recovering from ACL surgery (38, 69, 70). However, it is important that the personal trainer understand and establish proper landing mechanics before initiating or advancing a client to plyometric exercises.

The personal trainer should consider a dynamic warm-up to prepare these clients for an exercise session (70). Incorporation of a dynamic warm-up will promote posture, balance, stability, and flexibility across multiple planes of movement (70), all of which are essential to supporting the needs of a postsurgical ACL client. The dynamic warm-up can be tailored to meet the individual abilities and fitness levels of the client, but should include dynamic

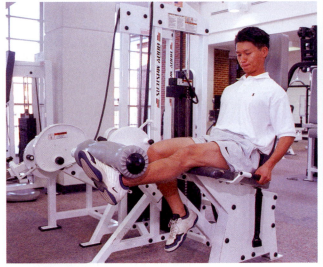

FIGURE 21.14 Example of open kinetic chain exercise for leg extension and leg flexion.

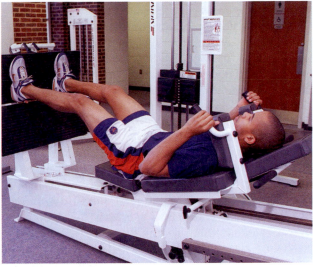

FIGURE 21.15 Example of closed kinetic chain exercise for quadriceps and gluteal muscles.

activities that emphasize full ROM across all major joints and require general and sport-specific motor skills. For example, Gambetta (28) has described a number of walking band exercises that direct the warm-up to hip function, a significant component of any ACL rehabilitation and prevention program.

To summarize from the information presented, specific contraindications for exercise following ACL reconstruction include full ROM open kinetic chain leg extension exercise, as well as closed kinetic chain exercise using greater than 90° of knee flexion. For ACL reconstructions using a semitendinosus or gracilis graft, active and resistive hamstring exercise is contraindicated for the first four to six weeks; this becomes a precaution for the personal trainer during postrehabilitation strength training and conditioning. Further, because both the patella and patellar tendon have become weakened with the patellar tendon graft, caution is warranted with activities that rely on significant quadriceps use (e.g., full squats and lunges, stair stepper using deep step movements). Bicycles, elliptical trainers, stair steppers using shallow steps, and swimming are all appropriate following ACL reconstruction, regardless of the type of graft used. Table 21.7 provides movement guidelines for ACL injury.

> A comprehensive ACL prevention program will emphasize proper mechanics and include strength, balance, and plyometric exercises targeting the development of neuromuscular control during all dynamic activities.

Total Knee Arthroplasty

Years of repetitive loading to the human knee can result in degeneration and degradation of the joint surfaces of the distal femur and proximal tibia. Often the degeneration is specifically located on either the medial or the lateral side of the knee joint, based on wear patterns and more specifically the individual's lower extremity alignment. People who are excessively bow-legged (genu varum) or knock-kneed (genu valgum), or who have had serious injury to the knee (such as extensive fractures through the joint, meniscal pathology, or instability of the knee due to unrepaired or failed repair of ligamentous structures), are often candidates for a total knee replacement.

Total knee arthroplasty (TKA) requires extensive exposure of the joint with a large central incision. Prosthetic components are selected and inserted to cover the worn areas at the ends of both the femur and tibia. Rehabilitation begins immediately with a ROM focus. Individuals perform open and closed kinetic chain exercises initially in the hospital and at home prior to formal outpatient rehabilitation.

Movement and Exercise Guidelines

Following discharge from formal rehabilitation, clients often have 100° to 120° of knee flexion and nearly complete knee extension. Indications for exercise include cycling, swimming, and endurance-based activities that minimize joint impact loading and improve muscular and cardiovascular function and fitness levels. Specific exercises such as leg press, multidirection hip strengthening, calf raises, and knee flexion and extension exercises using a low resistance and high repetition format are recommended. As an example, lunges onto a BOSU ball (figure 21.16) are not only a strategy for strengthening; they also benefit balance and proprioception for the entire kinetic chain.

Again, closed kinetic chain exercises that place the knee in greater than 100° of flexion are risky and impose added stresses on the knee. Further, because kneeling is generally contraindicated during the first few weeks following TKA, it is necessary for clients to avoid exercises requiring that position (e.g., kneeling lat pulldown, bent-over dumbbell row using a bench) or exercises that may cause them to kneel inadvertently (e.g., lunges performed too deeply). Exercises using less than 90° knee flexion postures are recommended in both open and closed kinetic chain exercises. Table 21.7 provides movement guidelines for clients experiencing knee pain.

> Each of the knee joint's structures requires a specific type of exercise to return the client to full function after injury or surgery; with anterior knee pain, for example, the focus is on reducing inflammation and pain, whereas after TKA the emphasis is on ROM. Quadriceps and hip strengthening is a common goal in nearly all knee injury rehabilitation and is a key to returning more normal function after injury.

Hip

Though hip dysfunction does occur, personal trainers will encounter relatively few hip injuries and surgical procedures in comparison to injuries to the knee and shoulder joints. The paucity of hip pathology is primarily due to the inherent stability of the hip; although it is the same type of joint as the shoulder, the hip has a much deeper acetabulum, or socket, which provides a much more stable articulation. This stability precludes many of the abnormal wear patterns and eliminates many of the traumas the other joints experience, resulting in fewer surgical procedures. Despite its generally good fit, however, the hip joint can experience injury and may be poorly aligned, with osteoarthritis and pain the result.

Hip Arthroscopy

The recent evolution of hip arthroscopy has revolutionized the management of hip injuries, particularly

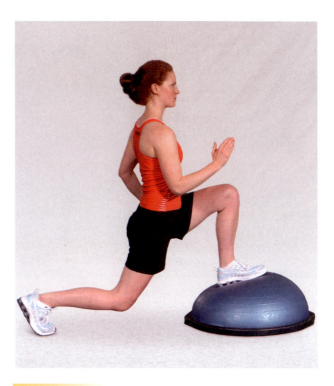

FIGURE 21.16 A lunge performed on a BOSU ball with the flat surface down will result in a greater challenge to the distal kinetic chain. An alternative method is to place the dome side of the BOSU down, resulting in a greater challenge to the proximal kinetic chain.

athletic hip injuries. Hip arthroscopy is minimally invasive and facilitates a quicker return to activity (10, 21). This surgical technique is frequently performed to remove intra-articular loose bodies or to repair a torn acetabular labrum (10). Although still considered a technique in development, current hip arthroscopic procedures have been informed by increased understanding of hip joint pathology and related pathomechanics. The development of the surgical technique has occurred far more rapidly than has the literature related to rehabilitation guidelines. However, the general approach to rehabilitation following hip arthroscopy remains consistent with that for other postsurgery rehabilitations in that it is quite important and should focus on restoration of ROM, strength, and gait (21, 79). In addition, rehabilitation protocols for athletes will emphasize development of power, speed, and agility along a progressively more challenging and difficult continuum (15).

Movement and Exercise Guidelines

Although a benefit of hip arthroscopy is the relatively rapid return to activity, strict adherence to tissue healing time lines must be maintained to minimize excess and deleterious stress on the repaired tissue and joint (10, 21, 79). It is generally reported that the total time for return to activity is approximately 16 to 32 weeks but is determined by the extent of the surgical procedure (i.e., loose bodies, labral tear, osteoplasty, microfracture) and the demands of the activity (10, 21, 79). However, in cases of a noncomplicated surgical procedure of a motivated individual, the time line may be much less. For example, discharge from supervised rehabilitation around 10 to 12 weeks is not unusual and will likely coincide with the initiation of sport-specific training. As with other injuries previously discussed, a personal trainer may play a significant role in contributing to the complete return to activity of post-hip arthroscopic clients. However, it is assumed that a personal trainer would likely work with a client upon discharge from rehabilitation. Thus, the client would likely present with full ROM and the ability to perform weight-bearing progressive resistance exercises. The sport-specific training phase of postoperative recovery should involve unilateral and bilateral balance and functional activities that continue to reestablish dynamic rotational stability, focus on activation and strength of the gluteus medius, and emphasize progressively more difficult, sport-specific skills challenging the client in all planes of motion (15, 21, 79). Examples of activities could include multidirectional lunges, lateral agility tasks, running progressions to include cuts and diagonal patterns, cariocas, and activities on unstable surfaces. Table 21.8 provides movement guidelines for hip arthroscopy.

> As tissue healing advances, hip arthroscopic rehabilitation must progressively address strength, balance, and sport-specific training for the entire lower extremity.

Total Hip Arthroplasty

Commonly termed *hip replacement*, total hip arthroplasty (THA) is the surgical treatment of choice if nonsurgical intervention (e.g., pharmaceutical and physical therapies) for hip osteoarthritis fails. More than 100,000 prosthetic hips are implanted each year, primarily to relieve osteoarthritic pain, with pain relief typically lasting more than 15 years. There are two primary prostheses: cemented and uncemented.

A variety of techniques (e.g., posterior, anterolateral, and transtrochanteric) are used during THA. Each has special movement and exercise indications and contraindications.

Cemented prostheses involve affixing the femoral and acetabular components with bone cement, whereas uncemented prostheses allow direct attachment of the prosthetic components to the bone. Each type of prosthesis has its advantages and disadvantages; one of the primary differences, however, is weight-bearing restriction following surgery. Cemented prostheses allow immediate postoperative weight bearing while uncemented prostheses require weight-bearing restrictions for anywhere from 6 to 12 weeks.

Like the options for prosthesis, each surgical approach has distinct advantages and disadvantages. Most importantly for the personal trainer are the movement restrictions following each method. Each technique approaches the hip joint from a different angle, thereby decreasing the strength of the hip joint's capsule at the point of entry. For example, the posterior approach—the most common approach in the United States—weakens the posterior aspect of the joint capsule, leaving the hip at increased risk of dislocation. Individuals typically adhere to the restrictions for a minimum of six weeks, though these depend on the surgeon's protocols.

Although varied across total hip arthroplasty surgical procedures, common movement restrictions during the first six weeks or when functional activities are introduced include the following:

- No hip flexion greater than 90°
- No hip adduction past neutral
- No hip internal rotation

Formal rehabilitation following THA is not prescribed as often as for the previously discussed surgical procedures. Postoperatively, individuals should progress to hip and lower extremity strengthening exercises (per surgeon's protocol) and should concentrate on improving their patterns of gait. A sample program might begin with aquatic therapy for gait training and then progress to land-based, weight-bearing activities once the incision has fully

TABLE 21.8 Hip Arthroscopy Movement and Exercise Guidelines

Diagnosis	Movement contraindications	Exercise contraindications	Exercise indications
Hip arthroscopy*	• Forceful hip flexion • Hip abduction and rotation (early phase of rehabilitation)	Ballistic or forced stretching	Aquatic walking

*Contraindications and indications will vary according to the specific arthroscopic procedure performed (i.e., labral repair, microfracture, etc.).

healed. This sequence will decrease joint load, fear of falling, and muscle guarding.

Movement and Exercise Guidelines

When working with clients who have undergone THA, personal trainers should contact the surgeon who performed the procedure to discuss any continued movement restrictions. When prescribing exercise, the personal trainer should avoid high-impact activities (e.g., running, step aerobics, plyometrics). Lower-impact activities (e.g., swimming, walking, stair stepping, use of elliptical trainer) are indicated following surgery to improve functions following THA. Weight training is not contraindicated after THA, but some specific exercises should be modified in accordance with the physical abilities and limitations of the client. Consulting with the surgeon should be considered mandatory when one is in doubt about movement and exercise choices. Table 21.9 provides a list of exercise indications and contraindications following THA.

Arthritis

Arthritis is a general term encompassing several different diseases. The two primary arthritis classifications are osteoarthritis and rheumatoid arthritis. Although both relate to the joint, these are two quite different diseases. Osteoarthritis (OA), commonly referred to as *degenerative joint disease*, is the progressive destruction of a joint's articular cartilage—the cartilage covering the surface of the given joint. Rheumatoid arthritis (RA), on the other hand, is a systemic inflammatory disease affecting not only the joint surface, but also connective tissue (e.g., joint capsules and ligaments). In the paragraphs that follow we provide a limited discussion of each form of arthritis and appropriate exercise choices.

Osteoarthritis

Osteoarthritis is a degenerative joint condition characterized by deterioration of the cartilaginous weight-bearing surfaces of articular joints, sclerotic changes in subchondral bone, and proliferation of new bone at the margins of joints (11, 22, 23, 53, 54). The proliferation of new bone, which often manifests itself as spurs or osteophytes, can interfere with normal joint function and cause both pain and limitation in ROM. Osteoarthritis is present in 15% of adult females and 11% of adult males, and some form of OA is present in some manner in the majority of people age 55 and older (8, 22, 53, 54).

The proposed pathophysiology of OA includes mechanical stresses that result in microfractures. This microfracturing leads to altered metabolism of chondrocytes, which then leads to a loss of cartilage, altered joint structure, and osteophyte production (11). Loss of cartilage at the joint leads to bone-on-bone contact, thereby causing inflammation.

The use of dietary supplements to improve joint function is currently recommended by physicians for nearly all forms of OA. The common oral over-the-counter supplements chondroitin sulfate, glucosamine, and hyaluronic acid have been recommended for treatment of OA in weight-bearing joints (11). Further research needs to be done to bring about better understanding of both the mechanism and the stage at which these supplements are most beneficial to individuals with OA.

Movement and Exercise Guidelines

Exercise indications for individuals with OA include low-resistance, high-repetition programs of exercise that minimize loading of articular surfaces. One application that is particularly helpful in clients with OA is aquatic exercise. The naturally buoyant properties of water allow individuals to exercise with significantly less joint loading than with other forms of activity (81, 83). Additional indications for exercise are the inclusion of cardiovascular training activities with limited weight bearing such as biking, use of the elliptical trainer, and swimming to protect the joint surfaces and minimize impact loading. Weight management, as well as muscular endurance gained via cardiovascular

TABLE 21.9 Hip Arthroplasty Movement and Exercise Guidelines

Surgical approach	Weight-bearing status	ROM limitations	Functional movement precautions
Posterolateral	Immediate full weight bearing	Flexion >90°, abduction, medial rotation	Moving in and out of a chair, hip flexion (putting shoes on)
Anterolateral	Restricted weight bearing for ≥6 weeks	Extension, adduction, lateral rotation	Turning away from surgical hip
Transtrochanteric	Restricted weight bearing for ≥6 weeks	Extension, adduction, lateral rotation	Turning away from surgical hip

TABLE 21.10 Osteoarthritis Movement and Exercise Guidelines

Movement contraindications	Exercise contraindications	Exercise indications
High-impact activities	■ Running ■ Snow skiing ■ Jogging	■ Bicycle ■ Stair stepper ■ Elliptical trainer ■ Aquatics, swimming

exercise, is of great benefit to the client with OA (table 21.10).

For the upper extremity, resistance exercise programs using predominantly open kinetic chain exercises are recommended. Closed kinetic chain exercises such as push-ups are contraindicated due to the compressive nature of the exercise at the glenohumeral joint. In the lower extremity, open kinetic chain exercises are typically indicated with the exception of full ROM leg extension exercises for the individual with patellofemoral OA. As discussed previously, modifications for this open kinetic chain leg extension exercise would include partial ROM arcs either from 90° to 45° or from 0° to 30° of knee motion, where patellofemoral compressive forces are the least damaging (51).

Clients can perform lightweight closed kinetic chain exercises for the lower extremities based on the presence of pain and the individual's general tolerance. Inclusion of balance training to enhance proprioception and motor control for the client with OA is another recommendation. This is particularly effective for training older individuals, who frequently have problems with balance.

Rheumatoid Arthritis

Rheumatoid arthritis is an inflammatory, autoimmune disease affecting many joints and often several body systems. Though it may be caused by a bacterial or viral precipitant, the etiology of RA is as of yet unknown. The most likely cause is the aberrant regulation of T-cells leading to the inflammation and destruction of joints (8, 22, 23, 61).

Rheumatoid arthritis involves the inflammation and proliferation of a joint's synovial lining. This proliferation, or thickening, increases joint pressure and, in concert with rheumatoid pannus (a tissue that dissolves collagen), leads to poor joint nutrition, joint swelling, and muscular inhibition. The inflammatory process, swelling, and lack of nutrition weaken the joint capsule and its ligamentous restraints; further, the joint surfaces (i.e., articular cartilage) deteriorate from the same causes. All of this can result in a hypermobile—or loose—and potentially unstable joint. A personal trainer who suspects that a client has an unstable joint should refer the client to his

or her primary medical provider for further evaluation and exercise programming. These changes are painful and typically cause a person with RA to limit movements to avoid pain, resulting in disuse atrophy (77, 85). The immobility contributes to continued cartilage degeneration, increasing the pain and further weakening the joint surface structure (33, 34). So, from the primary joint deterioration, the secondary impairments of RA include decreased strength, aerobic endurance, and flexibility (54).

Presentation of RA is variable, with cycles of exacerbation (flare-ups with increased pain, swelling, and stiffness) and remission (periods of relative comfort with no outward signs of inflammation). During RA exacerbation, clients typically describe warm, swollen joints and morning stiffness. In addition to these disease cycles, RA is considered progressive. Manifestations may include osteoporosis, muscle atrophy, periarticular nodules, joint deformity, and eventual joint ankylosis.

Areas commonly affected by RA include the neck, shoulders, and wrists and hands. The upper and midcervical regions of the neck are common sites of inflammation, resulting in the aforementioned tissue degeneration (45, 55). Degeneration or rupture of the ligaments supporting the first two cervical vertebrae may result in a life-threatening situation. For this reason, neck-specific exercises should be considered contraindicated or should be used only under supervision of a health care professional.

In addition to joints, RA affects muscles and bursae. Degeneration of the shoulder joints and associated structures (e.g., rotator cuff muscles and tendons) may lead to joint laxity resulting in abnormal movement patterns, possibly leading to an unstable shoulder joint. Rotator cuff tears occur in 30% to 40% of those with RA (26, 57). Ligamentous and capsular degeneration may result in unstable wrist joints; further, the joints of the fingers and thumb commonly swell, causing the client to lose grip strength.

Movement and Exercise Guidelines

As in OA, the pathology of RA cannot be prevented once started. However, it may be possible to slow the debilitating effects of RA's secondary impairments (i.e., decreased strength, aerobic endurance, and flexibility). Exercise goals for clients with RA focus on improving function during daily activities, improving general health, and providing protection to the affected joints. Maintaining muscular strength, aerobic endurance, joint and musculotendinous flexibility, functional balance, and body composition addresses these goals; and these are areas that personal trainers are well equipped to deal with.

Properly designed exercise programs that address these goals do not increase pain and may actually decrease the client's pain (53, 81). Resistance training is indicated for clients with RA. Both isometric and dynamic resistance training modes are appropriate (33, 34, 35, 59, 85), with isometric resistance training appropriate during periods of exacerbation (77). Further, and perhaps surprisingly, vigorous aerobic endurance exercise is not contraindicated. In fact, clients with RA not only tolerate high-intensity exercise; this type of exercise may actually be anti-inflammatory and pain relieving (22, 23, 36, 53, 85). A client who is experiencing joint inflammation, however, should avoid vigorous aerobic endurance exercise. Flexibility training is another form of exercise appropriate for clients with RA (53). While the personal trainer should emphasize not overstretching loose or unstable joints, clients with RA should perform flexibility exercises to maintain adequate joint movement (53, 59). They should perform stretching every day and can do so in a pain-free range during flare-ups.

The commonly affected areas (i.e., cervical spine, shoulders, and wrists) require modification of exercise programming. Exercises involving the cervical spine should be avoided (e.g., stretching and manually resisted neck strengthening exercises), as should exercises that place the shoulder in an impingement-prone position (e.g., upright row) or in a position outside the safe zone shown in figure 21.10 (e.g., behind-the-neck shoulder press). A last guideline is for exercises involving the wrists and hands; because the hands and wrists are affected,

clients with RA may need to have the diameter of the bar, dumbbell, or handle increased in an attempt to offset their weakened grip. For example, if a client has difficulty performing a dumbbell biceps curl, tape or padding may be applied to the dumbbell handle to "build up" the grip's diameter, thereby improving the client's ability to maintain his or her grasp on the dumbbell.

Because of the periods of changing pain and functional impairment, selection of exercises and intensities for clients with RA must be according to individual tolerances. Clients must be aware of the occurrence of periods of exacerbation and should adjust activity and exercise accordingly; specifically, if a joint is inflamed, rest is warranted (53, 54). Table 21.11 provides a list of appropriate and inappropriate exercises for clients diagnosed with RA.

> Clients with OA or RA both benefit from performing strengthening and aerobic exercise. The difference between the two is the body's response to activity. Exercise should not increase joint pain for either group. Particular care must be given to the client with RA during periods of exacerbation.

Conclusion

Personal trainers work with a wide variety of clients, many of whom have experienced injury or have undergone surgery necessitating a modified approach to exercise prescription. When designing exercise programs for this population, it is important to understand the basic types of injury and the stages of healing that all musculoskeletal tissues follow. In concert with communication between the personal trainer and other health care practitioners, familiarity with these stages of healing and with individual injury, surgical procedures, and disease processes will assist personal trainers in implementing safe and appropriate programs of exercise for their clients.

TABLE 21.11 Rheumatoid Arthritis Movement and Exercise Guidelines

Movement contraindications	Exercise contraindications	Exercise indications
■ High-impact cardiovascular exercise ■ Neck flexibility or strengthening in clients with history of neck instability ■ Movements outside the safe zone	■ Running or jogging ■ Upper trapezius stretch ■ Manually resisted neck strengthening ■ Behind-the-neck shoulder press	■ Moderate-intensity (60-80% maximal heart rate) (54) aerobic endurance exercise (e.g., stationary bicycle, elliptical trainer, stair stepper) ■ Range of motion and flexibility exercises ■ Isometric exercise (for the unstable joint) ■ Water aerobics ■ Stationary bicycling

Study Questions

1. Both forward lumbar and abdominal flexion exercises would be contraindicated for someone who has a history of which of the following?

   A. spondylolisthesis

   B. low back extensor strain

   C. posteriorly herniated disc

   D. spondylolysis

2. A client who participates in recreational softball has indicated that she has dislocated her shoulder in the past. Which of the following exercises is most appropriate for this client?

   A. rotator cuff strengthening

   B. push-up

   C. behind-the-neck lat pulldown

   D. overhead press

3. A client who plays basketball has a lateral ankle sprain. Assuming that he is ready to begin functional activities, all of the following are appropriate progressions EXCEPT

   A. balancing on floor with eyes closed, advancing to balancing with eyes open on an air pad.

   B. 12-inch (30 cm) box jumps advancing to 18-inch (45 cm) box jumps.

   C. diagonal and lateral running drills advancing to straight-line jogging drills.

   D. forward lunges on floor advancing to lateral lunges onto a domed device.

4. A 30-year-old client who is a runner is complaining of periodic knee pain. The personal trainer notices that her knee moves slightly medially when she runs. Which of the following exercises would be indicated, provided knee alignment with foot is maintained?

   A. deep squats

   B. forward 6-inch (15 cm) step-ups

   C. full ROM open kinetic chain leg (knee) extensions

   D. stair running

5. A 59-year-old male has successfully rehabilitated from a total hip arthroplasty. He is interested in doing cardiovascular exercises. All of the following are appropriate EXCEPT

   A. swimming.

   B. stair stepping.

   C. step aerobics.

   D. stationary cycling.

Applied Knowledge Questions

1. A firefighter is recovering from a sprained ankle. He has been cleared to return to work, but reports feeling unstable when climbing a ladder. Describe what exercises and activities you will implement to improve his strength and balance while climbing a ladder, as well as carrying heavy equipment.

2. A female soccer player recently completed a nine-month rehabilitation program following ACL surgery. She is preparing for the upcoming season and has asked for suggestions for exercises she could perform as part of an ACL injury prevention program. What kind of exercises will you suggest to develop neuromuscular control in the lower extremity?

References

1. Amadio, P.C. 1992. Tendon and ligament. In: *Wound Healing: Biochemical and Clinical Aspects,* I.K. Cohen, R.F. Diegelmann, and W.J. Lindblad, eds. Philadelphia: Saunders. p. 384.

2. Anderson, A.F., R.B. Snyder, and A.B. Lipscomb Jr. 2001. Anterior cruciate ligament reconstruction. A prospective randomized study of three surgical methods. *American Journal of Sports Medicine* 29 (3): 272-279.

3. Barrett, D. 1991. Proprioception and function after anterior cruciate reconstruction. *Journal of Bone and Joint Surgery (British)* 73: 833-837.

4. Barrett, G.R., F.K. Noojin, C.W. Hartzog, and C.R. Nash. 2002. Reconstruction of the anterior cruciate ligament in females: A comparison of hamstring versus patellar tendon autograft. *Arthroscopy* 18 (1): 46-54.

5. Berkowitz, M., and C. Greene. 1989. Disability expenditures. *American Rehabilitation* 15 (1): 7.

6. Blackburn, T.A., W.E. McLeod, B. White, and L. Wofford. 1990. EMG analysis of posterior rotator cuff exercises. *Athletic Training* 25: 40-45.

7. Boden, B.P., G.S. Dean, J.A. Feagin, and W.E. Garrett. 2000. Mechanisms of anterior cruciate ligament injury. *Orthopedics* 23 (6): 573-578.

8. Breedveld, F.C. 1998. New insights in the pathogenesis of rheumatoid arthritis. *Journal of Rheumatology* (Suppl) 53: 3-7.

9. Burkhart, S.S., D.L. Diaz Pagan, M.A. Wirth, and K.A. Athanasiou. 1997. Cyclic loading of anchor-based rotator cuff repairs. *Arthroscopy* 13 (2): 720-724.

10. Byrd, J.W.T. 2006. The role of hip arthroscopy in the athletic hip. *Clinics in Sports Medicine* 25: 255-278.

11. Carfagno, D., and T.S. Ellenbecker. 2002. Osteoarthritis of the glenohumeral joint: Nonsurgical treatment options. *Physician and Sportsmedicine* 30 (4, April): 19-32.

12. Clisby, E.F., N.L. Bitter, M.J. Sandow, M.A. Jones, M.E. Magarey, and S. Jaberzadeh. 2008. Relative contributions of infraspinatus and deltoid during external rotation with symptomatic subacromial impingement. *Journal of Shoulder and Elbow Surgery* 17 (1 Suppl): 87S-92S.

13. Cook, G. 2003. *Athletic Body in Balance*. Champaign, IL: Human Kinetics.

14. Curwin, S., and W. Stanish. 1984. *Tendinitis: Its Etiology and Treatment*. Lexington, MA: Collamore Press.

15. DePalma, B. 2001. Rehabilitation of the groin, hip, and thigh. In: *Techniques in Musculoskeletal Rehabilitation*, 1st ed., W.E. Prentice and M.L. Voight, eds. New York: McGraw-Hill.

16. Dodds, J.A., and S.P. Arnoczky. 1994. Anatomy of the anterior cruciate ligament: A blueprint for repair and reconstruction. *Arthroscopy* 10 (2): 132-139.

17. Earl, J.E., and C.S. Vetter. 2007. Patellofemoral pain. *Physical Medicine and Rehabilitation Clinics of North America* 18: 439-458.

18. Ellenbecker, T.S. 1995. Rehabilitation of shoulder and elbow injuries in tennis players. *Clinics in Sports Medicine* 14 (1): 87-110.

19. Ellenbecker, T.S. 2000. Postrehabilitation: Shoulder conditioning for tennis. *IDEA Personal Trainer* (March): 18-27.

20. Ellenbecker, T.S., and G.J. Davies. 2001. *Closed Kinetic Chain Rehabilitation*. Champaign, IL: Human Kinetics.

21. Enseki, K.R., R.L. Martin, P. Draovitch, B.T. Kelly, M.J. Philippon, and M.L. Schenker. 2006. The hip joint: Arthroscopic procedures and postoperative rehabilitation. *Journal of Orthopaedic and Sports Physical Therapy* 36 (7): 516-525.

22. Feldmann, M., F.M. Brennan, and R.N. Maini. 1996. Rheumatoid arthritis. *Cell* 85 (3): 307-310.

23. Feldmann, S.V. 1996. *Exercise for the Person with Rheumatoid Arthritis. Rehabilitation of Persons with Rheumatoid Arthritis*. Gaithersburg, MD: Aspen.

24. Feller, J.A., K.E. Webster, and B. Gavin. 2001. Early postoperative morbidity following anterior cruciate ligament reconstruction: Patellar tendon versus hamstring graft. *Knee Surgery, Sports Traumatology, Arthroscopy* 9 (5, September): 260-266.

25. Freeman, M., M. Dean, and I. Hanham. 1965 The etiology and prevention of functional instability of the foot. *Journal of Bone and Joint Surgery* 47B: 669-677.

26. Friedman, R.J. 1990. Total shoulder arthroplasty in rheumatoid arthritis. In: *Shoulder Reconstruction*. Philadelphia: Saunders. p. 158.

27. Galin, J.I., I.M. Goldstein, and R. Snyderman. 1988. *Inflammation: Basic Principles and Clinical Correlates*. New York: Raven Press.

28. Gambetta, V. 2007. *Athletic Development: The Art and Science of Functional Sports Conditioning*. Champaign, IL: Human Kinetics.

29. Giladi, M., C. Milgrom, A. Simkin, and Y. Danon. 1991. Stress fractures: Identifiable risk factors. *American Journal of Sports Medicine* 19 (6): 647-652.

30. Gregory, P.L. 2002. "Overuse" – an overused term. *British Journal of Sports Medicine* 36: 83-84.

31. Gross, M.L., S.L. Brenner, I. Esformes, and J.J. Sonzogni. 1993. Anterior shoulder instability in weight lifters. *American Journal of Sports Medicine* 21 (4): 599-603.

32. Guskiewicz, K.M., and D.H. Perrin. 1996. Effect of orthotics on postural sway following inversion ankle sprain. *Journal of Orthopaedic and Sports Physical Therapy* 23 (5): 326-331.

33. Häkkinen, A., K. Häkkinen, and P. Hannonen. 1994. Effects of strength training on neuromuscular function and disease activity in patients with recent-onset inflammatory arthritis. *Scandinavian Journal of Rheumatology* 23 (5): 237-242.

34. Häkkinen, A., T. Sokka, A. Kotaniemi, H. Kautiainen, I. Jappinen, L. Laitinen, and P. Hannonen. 1999. Dynamic strength training in patients with early rheumatoid arthritis increases muscle strength but not bone density. *Journal of Rheumatology* 26: 1257-1263.

35. Harkcom, T.M., R.M. Lampman, B.F. Banwell, and C.W. Castor. 1985. Therapeutic value of graded aerobic exercise training in rheumatoid arthritis. *Arthritis and Rheumatism* 28 (1): 32-39.

36. Hazes, J.M., and C.H.M. van den Ende. 1996. How vigorously should we exercise our rheumatoid arthritis patients? *Annals of Rheumatic Diseases* 55: 861-862.

37. Hensinger, R.N. 1989. Spondylolysis and spondylolisthesis in children and adolescents. *Journal of Bone and Joint Surgery* 71A: 1098-1107.

38. Hewett, T.E. 2007. *Understanding and Preventing Noncontact ACL Injuries,* T. Hewett, S. Shultz, and L. Griffin, eds. Champaign, IL: Human Kinetics.

39. Hides, J.A., C.A. Richardson, and G.A. Jeull. 1996. Multifidus muscle recovery is not automatic after resolution of acute, first-episode low back pain. *Spine* 21 (23): 2763-2769.

40. Hoshina, H. 1980. Spondylolysis in athletes. *Physician and Sportsmedicine* 8 (9): 75-79.

41. Hunter, S., and W.E. Prentice. 2001. Rehabilitation of the ankle and foot. In: *Techniques in Musculoskeletal Rehabilitation,* 1st ed., W.E. Prentice and M.L. Voight, eds. New York: McGraw-Hill.

42. Ireland, M.L., J.D. Willson, B.T. Ballantyne, and I.M. Davis. 2003. Hip strength in females with and without patellofemoral pain. *Journal of Orthopaedic and Sports Physical Therapy* 33 (11): 671-676.

43. Johansson, H., P. Sjolander, and P. Soljka. 1991. A sensory role for the cruciate ligaments. *Clinical Orthopedics and Related Research* 268: 161-178.

44. Kibler, W.B. 1995. Biomechanical analysis of the shoulder during tennis activities. *Clinics in Sports Medicine* 14: 79-85.

45. Kramer, J., F. Jolesz, and J. Kleefield. 1991. Rheumatoid arthritis of the cervical spine. *Rheumatic Diseases Clinics of North America* 17: 757.

46. Kraus, D.R., and D. Shapiro. 1989. The symptomatic lumbar spine in the athlete. *Clinics in Sports Medicine* 8: 59-69.

47. Kuland, D.N. 1983. The injured athletes' pain. *Current Concepts in Pain* 1: 3-10.

48. Leadbetter, W.B. 1992. Cell-matrix response in tendon injury. *Clinics in Sports Medicine* 11 (3): 533-578.

49. MacDougall, J.D., G.C.B. Elder, D.G. Sale, J.R. Moroz, and J.R. Sutton. 1980. Effect of strength training and immobilization on human muscle fibers. *European Journal of Applied Physiology* 43: 25-34.

50. Mandelbaum, B.R., H.J. Silvers, D.S. Watanabe, J.F. Knarr, S.D. Thomas, L.Y. Griffin, D.T. Kirkendall, and W. Garrett Jr. 2005. Effectiveness of a neuromuscular and proprioceptive training program in preventing anterior cruciate ligament injuries in female athletes: 2-year follow-up. *American Journal of Sports Medicine* 33 (7): 1003-1010.

51. McConnell, J. 2000. Patellofemoral joint complications and considerations. In: *Knee Ligament Rehabilitation,* 2nd ed., T.S. Ellenbecker, ed. Philadelphia: Churchill Livingstone.

52. McGuine, T.A., and J.S. Keene. 2006. The effect of a balance training program on the risk of ankle sprains in high school athletes. *American Journal of Sports Medicine* 34 (7): 1103-1111.

53. Minor, M.A., J.E. Hewett, R.R. Webel, S.K. Anderson, and D.R. Kay. 1989. Efficacy of physical conditioning exercises in patients with rheumatoid arthritis and osteoarthritis. *Arthritis and Rheumatism* 32: 1396-1405.

54. Minor, M.A., and D.R. Kay. 2003. Arthritis. In: *ACSM's Exercise Management for Persons with Chronic Diseases and Disabilities,* 2nd ed., J.L. Durstine and G.E. Moore, eds. Champaign, IL: Human Kinetics.

55. Moncur, D., and H.J. Williams. 1988. Cervical spine management in patients with rheumatoid arthritis. *Physical Therapy* 68: 509.

56. Muller, E.A. 1970. Influence of training and of inactivity on muscle strength. *Archives in Physical Medicine and Rehabilitation* 51: 449-462.

57. Neer, C.S., K.C. Weston, and F.J. Stanton. 1982. Recent experience in total shoulder replacement. *Journal of Bone and Joint Surgery* 64A: 319.

58. Neitzel, J.A., T. Kernozek, and G.J. Davies. 2002. Loading response following ACL reconstruction during parallel squat exercise. *Clinical Biomechanics* 17: 551-554.

59. Nieman, D.C. 2000. Exercise soothes arthritis joint effects. *ACSM's Health and Fitness Journal* 4: 20-27.

60. Nies-Byl, N., and P.L. Sinnott. 1991. Variations in balance and body sway in middle-aged adults: Subjects with healthy backs compared with subjects with low-back dysfunction. *Spine* 16: 325-330.

61. Panayi, G.S. 1997. T-cell-dependent pathways in rheumatoid arthritis. *Current Opinion in Rheumatology* 9 (3): 236-240.

62. Panjabi, M.M. 1992. The stabilizing system of the spine. Part I. Function, dysfunction, adaptation, and enhancement. *Journal of Spinal Disorders* 5: 383-389.

63. Parsons, I.M., M. Apreleva, F.H. Fu, and S.L. Woo. 2002. The effect of rotator cuff tears on reaction forces at the glenohumeral joint. *Journal of Orthopaedic Research* 20: 439-446.

64. Petersen, T., P. Kryger, C. Ekdahl, S. Olsen, and S. Jacobsen. 2002. The effect of McKenzie therapy as compared with that of intensive strengthening training for the treatment of patients with subacute or chronic low back pain: A randomized controlled trial. *Spine* 27 (16, August 15): 1702-1709.

65. Porterfield, J.A., and C. DeRosa. 1998. Mechanical low back pain. In: *Perspectives in Functional Anatomy,* 2nd ed. Philadelphia: Saunders.

66. Potach, D.H., and R. Borden. 2000. Rehabilitation and reconditioning. In: *Essentials of Strength Training and Conditioning,* 2nd ed., T.R. Baechle and R.W. Earle, eds. Champaign, IL: Human Kinetics.

67. Prentice, W.E. 2006. *Arnheim's Principles of Athletic Training,* 12th ed. New York: McGraw-Hill.

68. Rack, P.M.H., and D.R. Westbury. 1974. The short range stiffness of active mammalian muscle and its effect on mechanical properties. *Journal of Physiology* 240: 331-350.

69. Radcliffe, J.C. 1999. *High-Powered Plyometrics.* Champaign, IL: Human Kinetics.

70. Radcliffe, J.C. 2007. *Functional Training for Athletes at All Levels.* Berkeley, CA: Ulysses Press.

71. Richardson, C.A., C.J. Snijders, J.A. Hides, L. Damen, M.S. Pas, and J. Storm. 2002. The relationship between the transversus abdominis muscles, sacroiliac joint mechanics, and low back pain. *Spine* 27 (4): 399-405.

72. Rotella, R.J. 1985. Psychological care of the injured athlete. In: *The Injured Athlete,* 2nd ed., D. Kuland, ed. Philadelphia: Lippincott.

73. Saal, J. 1995. The role of inflammation in lumbar pain. *Spine* 20: 1821-1827.

74. Safran, M.R., R.S. Bendetti, A.R. Bartolozzi, et al. 1999. Lateral ankle sprains: A comprehensive review part 1: Etiology, pathoanatomy, histopathogenesis, and diagnosis. *Medicine and Science in Sports and Exercise* 31: S429-437.

75. Safran, M.R., R.S. Bendetti, A.R. Bartolozzi, et al. 1999. Lateral ankle sprains: A comprehensive review part 2: Treatment and rehabilitation with emphasis on the athlete. *Medicine and Science in Sports and Exercise* 31: S438-447.

76. Scovazzo, M.L., A. Browne, M. Pink, F.W. Jobe, and J. Kerrigan. 1991. The painful shoulder during freestyle swimming. An electromyographic cinematographic analysis of twelve muscles. *American Journal of Sports Medicine* 19 (6): 577-582.

77. Semble, E.L., R.F. Loeser, and C.M. Wise. 1990. Therapeutic exercise for rheumatoid arthritis and osteoarthritis. *Seminars in Arthritis and Rheumatism* 20: 32-40.

78. Shelbourne, K.D., and R.V. Trumper. 2000. Anterior cruciate ligament reconstruction: Evolution of rehabilitation. In: *Knee Ligament Rehabilitation,* 2nd ed., T.S. Ellenbecker, ed. Philadelphia: Churchill Livingstone.

79. Stalzer, S., M. Wahoff, and M. Scanlan. 2006. Rehabilitation following hip arthroscopy. *Clinics in Sports Medicine* 25: 337-357.

80. Standaert, C.J. 2002. Spondylolysis in the adolescent athlete. *Clinical Journal of Sport Medicine* 12 (2, March): 119-122.

81. Stenstrom, C. 1994. Therapeutic exercise in rheumatoid arthritis. *Arthritis Care Research* 7: 190-197.

82. Thacker, S.B., D.F. Stroup, C.M. Branche, J. Gilchrist, R.A. Goodman, and E.A. Weitman. 1999. The prevention of ankle sprains in sports. *American Journal of Sports Medicine* 27 (6): 753-760.

83. Thein, J.M., and L. Thein-Brody. 2000. Aquatic therapy. In: *Knee Ligament Rehabilitation,* 2nd ed., T.S. Ellenbecker, ed. Philadelphia: Churchill Livingstone.

84. Valovich-McLeod, T.C. 2008. The effectiveness of balance training programs on reducing the incidence of ankle sprains in adolescent athletes. *Journal of Sport Rehabilitation* 17: 1-8.

85. van den Ende, C.H.M., J.M.W. Hazes, S. le Cessie, W.J. Mulder, D.G. Belfor, F.C. Breedveld, and B.A. Dijkmans. 1996. Comparison of high and low intensity training in well controlled rheumatoid arthritis. Results of a randomized clinical trial. *Annals of Rheumatic Diseases* 55: 798-805.

86. Warner, M.J., and H.K. Amato. 1997. The mind: An essential healing tool for rehabilitation. *Athletic Therapy Today* (May): 37-41.

87. Wilk, K.E., and J.R. Andrews. 1990. The effects of pad placement and angular velocity on tibial displacement during isokinetic exercise. *Journal of Orthopaedic and Sports Physical Therapy* 17 (1): 24-30.

88. Wilk, K.E., G.J. Davies, and R.E. Mangine. 1998. Patellofemoral disorders: A classification system and clinical guidelines for non operative rehabilitation. *Journal of Orthopaedic and Sports Physical Therapy* 28: 307-322.

89. Williams, M.M., J.A. Hawley, R.A. McKenzie, and P.M. van Wijmen. 1991. A comparison of the effects of two sitting postures on back and referred pain. *Spine* 16 (10, October): 1185-1191.

90. Young, A., M. Stokes and J.F. Iles. 1987. Effects of joint pathology on muscle. *Clinical Orthopedics and Related Research* 47: 678-685.

Clients With Spinal Cord Injury, Multiple Sclerosis, Epilepsy, and Cerebral Palsy

Paul Sorace, MS, Peter Ronai, MS, and Tom LaFontaine, PhD

After completing this chapter, you will be able to

- understand the basic etiology and epidemiology of spinal cord injury, multiple sclerosis, epilepsy, and cerebral palsy;

- recognize the physiological, functional, and health-related impairments caused or exacerbated by spinal cord injury, multiple sclerosis, epilepsy, and cerebral palsy;

- understand the basic physiological responses to exercise among clients with these disorders compared to others;

- recognize abnormal physiological responses to exercise in clients with these disorders;

- take necessary precautions in planning and implementing exercise and physical activity programs for clients with these disorders; and

- understand the potential functional and health benefits of regular exercise in clients with these disorders.

The many benefits of regular exercise have been well defined in apparently healthy populations. In recent years, studies have demonstrated that persons with various chronic diseases and disabilities also derive significant health and fitness benefits from a regular, systematic exercise program. This chapter presents information on four chronic neuromuscular disorders: spinal cord injury, multiple sclerosis, epilepsy, and cerebral palsy. The chapter addresses the epidemiology and pathology

The authors would like to acknowledge the contributions of Tom LaFontaine, who wrote this chapter for the first edition of *NSCA's Essentials of Personal Training*.

of these diseases and disabilities, as well as the exercise responses, documented benefits of exercise, and exercise testing and training guidelines in these client populations.

Spinal Cord Injury

Spinal cord injury (SCI) results in the impairment or loss of motor function, sensory function, or both in the trunk or limbs due to irreversible damage to neural tissues within the spinal canal (32). The various grades of SCI may be classified as either complete or incomplete. In the complete form of paralysis, if the injury occurs between the highest thoracic (T-1) and highest cervical (C-1) segments of the spine, impairment of the arms, trunk, legs, and pelvic organs occurs (quadriplegia, also called tetraplegia). Injury to thoracic segments T-2 to T-12 causes impairment in the trunk, legs, or pelvic organs or in more than one of these (paraplegia). Paraplegia is also the result of irreversible SCI of the lumbosacral (cauda equina) segments of the spine.

In general, the higher the injury level, the more extensive the resulting deficits. If the SCI is incomplete, the injury to the spinal cord has been only partial. In comparison to the person with complete SCI, the person with incomplete SCI may have some sensation or motor function at least partially intact below the level of the injury. In these cases it is best to ask for a physician's statement regarding what muscle and sensory function remains for the individual.

Clinical Manifestations

Clinical manifestations of the acute phase of SCI are many and varied. The incidence of thrombo-embolic events and dysrhythmias is increased (73). Disruption of the autonomic nervous system leads to reduced vascular tone and unbalanced hyperactivity of the vagal system. Individuals with high lesions, T-3/T-4 and above, are prone to symptomatic brady-cardia (low heart rate), primary cardiac arrest, and serious cardiac conduction disturbances.

More relevant to the personal trainer are clinical manifestations associated with the chronic stage of SCI. Of particular importance are potential cardiovascular problems and events. The following are common cardiovascular problems observed in persons with chronic SCI.

- Orthostatic hypotension (i.e., baroreceptor insufficiency)
- Autonomic dysreflexia
- Impaired transmission of cardiogenic pain (T-4 lesion and above)

- Loss of reflex cardiac acceleration (T-1 through T-4 and above)
- Quadriplegic cardiac atrophy (loss of left ventricular mass)
- Atrial fibrillation and other cardiac conduction disorders
- Congestive heart failure
- Pseudomyocardial infarction (abnormal ST-wave changes)
- Sudden death due to asystole
- Atherosclerosis and its manifestations of angina pectoris and myocardial infarction

A relatively common manifestation of SCI that the personal trainer needs to be aware of is autonomic dysreflexia (AD). Spinal cord injury disrupts normal neural regulation of arterial blood pressure, particularly in persons with tetraplegia and lesions above the T-6 level (73). Autonomic dysreflexia results from noxious stimuli such as a distended bladder or bowel, constricted clothing, and infections that cause heightened sympathetic nervous system activity resulting in the sudden onset of hypertension. The sidebar on page 567 lists typical clinical manifestations and precipitators of AD (73).

Autonomic dysreflexia can be a life-threatening condition. To prevent AD, the personal trainer should ask clients with SCI each session if they have symptoms such as a headache, blurred vision, goose bumps, and anxiety; check blood pressure before and after the session; and be sure clients have emptied their bowel and bladder before beginning the session. One should look for untreated high blood pressure at rest or sustained high blood pressure during recovery from exercise. Diastolic blood pressure should be back to baseline within 15 minutes. In athletes, an increase in usual systolic blood pressure of 20 to 40 mmHg (millimeters of mercury) or greater could suggest "boosting" (voluntarily inducing AD during distance racing events to improve performance).

The personal trainer needs to be alert to sudden increases in blood pressure that could reflect AD. In addition, some athletic clients with SCI attempt to take advantage of this phenomenon by inducing it ("boosting") prior to competition. This practice has potentially hazardous consequences and must be discouraged. Clients with SCI generally demonstrate higher heart rates and lower blood pressures compared to others. To "boost" or maximize circulation during performance, some athletic clients with SCI attempt to increase their blood pressure by invoking AD through maneuvers such as holding their urine to distend their bladder or pinching themselves

Autonomic Dysreflexia

Autonomic dysreflexia can be life threatening. The personal trainer should look for signs of high blood pressure or boosting.

Signs and Symptoms of Autonomic Dysreflexia

- Sudden systolic blood pressure increase of >20 to 40 mmHg
- Pounding headache
- Profuse sweating and flushing of skin above level of injury, particularly of the head, neck, and shoulders
- Piloerection ("goose bumps")
- Blurred vision with spots in visual fields
- Nasal congestion
- Feelings of anxiety
- Cardiac dysrhythmias—atrial fibrillation, premature ventricular depolarizations, conduction abnormalities

Common Precipitators of Autonomic Dysreflexia

- Bladder distension, urinary tract infection, bladder or kidney stones
- Epididymis or scrotal compression
- Bowel distension or impaction
- Gallstones
- Gastric ulcers, gastritis, gastric or colonic irritation, appendicitis
- Menstruation, vaginitis, pregnancy
- Intercourse or ejaculation
- Deep vein thrombosis and pulmonary emboli
- Temperature fluctuations
- Pressure sores, in-grown toenail, sunburn, burn, blisters, insect bites
- Constrictive clothing, shoes, appliances
- Pain, fracture, other trauma
- Any pain or irritating stimuli below injury level

hard enough to cause a reflex response. One study showed that this practice can increase performance in track wheelchair and swimming events by 9.7% (69).

Preventing Injuries in Clients With Spinal Cord Injury

The most common exercise-induced injuries among persons with SCI occur at the shoulders, wrists, and elbows and are often overuse injuries. Among athletes in the National Wheelchair Athletic Association, 57% of reported injuries were to the shoulders and elbows (27). Carpal tunnel syndrome (CTS) is also common among wheelchair athletes, with 23% reporting CTS in one study (9). An excellent overview of medical and injury concerns in physically challenged athletes (82) emphasizes that although these types of injuries can be expected, many are preventable with adequate conditioning and training techniques, proper protective equipment, and excellent client–personal trainer communication. For example, stretching the anterior shoulder musculature and strengthening the posterior musculature can reduce shoulder injury and pain significantly (15).

Personal trainers working with persons with SCI need to be cognizant of these and other potential injuries. Adhering to appropriate exercise technique and exercise physiology principles regarding intensity, duration, frequency, balance in exercise choice, and progression and rest and recovery in particular is essential to injury prevention and optimal physiological adaptation in this population.

> Shoulder, wrist, and elbow overuse injuries are common in persons with SCI. These injuries may be prevented through an exercise program designed to stretch the anterior and strengthen the posterior muscle groups of the shoulder girdle.

Exercise Concerns in the Spinal Cord Injury Population

In addition to higher heart rate and lower blood pressure compared to others, several special concerns need to be addressed in the exercising SCI population, including temperature regulation and venous return. The personal trainer needs to be alert to potential adverse consequences of exercise in clients with SCI.

Temperature Regulation

Disorders of temperature regulation can be expected in persons with SCI, particularly those with lesions at T-6 or above. In extreme hot or cold environments, SCI clients with lesions at or above T-6 are unable to adequately thermoregulate through sweating or shivering (95). Adaptations that may be necessary for clients competing in these thermally challenging environments include wearing a wet suit in a cool pool or being splashed with cool water during track racing in hot, humid environments. Hot whirlpools and similar extreme temperature environments should be avoided. It is important to beware of freezer burn from cold packs or burns from heat packs.

It is crucial that persons with SCI who are exercising maintain adequate hydration and adapt gradually to environmental changes. Dehydration contributes greatly to the risk of hyper- or hypothermia. The personal trainer needs to pay special attention to ensuring good nutrition and fluid intake practices among these clients. Measures that the personal trainer can take to enhance exercise comfort include maintaining as constant an exercise environment as possible; having clients wear loose-fitting, lightweight, and breathable materials (Capilene, polypropylene, etc.); and ensuring access to cool water or sport drinks.

> Persons with SCI, particularly those with high lesions, are unable to increase skin blood flow in paralyzed areas; this impairs the ability to dissipate metabolic heat and places them at increased risk for heat-related injuries. The phenomenon also exposes them to increased risk for cold-related injuries.

Venous Return

Persons with SCI have poor venous return, particularly in the seated or upright posture, due to lower limb venous pooling secondary to lack of sympathetic tone and absence of the venous "muscle pump." This not only limits the degree of cardiovascular trainability but also can result in hypotension (low blood pressure) during exercise, with symptoms of light-headedness and faintness and inability to maintain stroke volume and cardiac output. Studies suggest that training persons with SCI in the supine posture may minimize this problem and improve the effectiveness of upper body arm exercise (33, 54). The use of gradient-style compression hosiery may be helpful as well to prevent swelling into the lower extremities. Monitoring blood pressure during exercise is recommended.

General Health Issues of Persons With Spinal Cord Injury

Persons with SCI are at risk for several metabolic disturbances. As a consequence of relative inactivity, decreased muscle mass, and increased adiposity, a high percentage of persons with SCI have abnormalities in oral carbohydrate processing resulting in insulin resistance and hyperinsulinemia (4). Persons with SCI also have frequencies of dyslipidemia, hypertension, and cardiovascular disease (CVD) that are slightly greater than in the non-SCI population (73).

A frequent consequence of tetraplegia is atrophy of cardiac muscle. This can result in cardiac dysfunction, further impairing exercise tolerance and increasing the risk for congestive heart failure. Such atrophy is probably related to neuromuscular dysfunction and inactivity that could possibly be lessened by electrical stimulation of paralyzed leg muscles and arm exercises (61).

Although the person with SCI may not perceive ischemic cardiac pain, other signs and symptoms such as unusual shortness of breath, excessive sweating, fatigue, light-headedness or sensation of fainting, and palpitations may occur. An exercise session should not be started, or should be terminated, if any of these symptoms are present, and medical follow-up should occur as soon as possible. In clients with suspected or known coronary heart disease, a physician-supervised clinical diagnostic exercise test should take place before the client starts a vigorous exercise program.

Exercise Testing and Training of Clients With Spinal Cord Injury

Persons with SCI can respond to exercise training in much the same way others do. However, problems associated with wheelchair use such as access to facilities, equipment, sidewalks, trails, and so on often make it challenging for people with SCI to engage in regular exercise. The personal trainer needs to be cognizant of these types of problems. In addition, a sound basic understanding of the acute and chronic responses to exercise in this population is critical to the implementation of a safe and effective exercise program.

The major pathophysiologic problems limiting the ability of persons with SCI to engage in and adapt to exercise training are extensive skeletal muscle paralysis (3, 4) and sympathetic autonomic nervous system impairment. These impairments in function reduce the capacity to support high rates of breathing frequency, heart rate, cardiac output, and metabolism. These factors, combined with the relatively sedentary lifestyle imposed by the neuromuscular disorder, result in markedly reduced cardiorespiratory and residual musculoskeletal fitness.

In a "sedentary lifestyle—loss of fitness model" that has been proposed for persons with SCI, impaired autonomic nervous system function and restricted physical activity lead to physical deconditioning and loss of musculoskeletal and cardiorespiratory fitness (20). Most persons with SCI have a markedly reduced physical fitness compared to apparently healthy age- and gender-matched peers. The sedentary lifestyle—loss of fitness model is useful for understanding the basis for this phenomenon and provides a clear recognition of the need for implementing exercise programs in clients with SCI.

Exercise Testing

The most common mode of exercise testing for persons with SCI is the arm crank ergometer. Because of the high risk of cardiovascular impairment in this group, maximal exercise testing should be administered *only* in medical settings. However, with proper screening and medical clearance, the competent personal trainer can safely administer submaximal cardiorespiratory fitness testing. Although beyond the scope of this discussion, protocols and norms for standardized arm ergometry testing in persons with SCI have been developed (19, 46).

A field test has been developed whereby the $\dot{V}O_2$peak of a person with paraplegia may be predicted from a 12-minute wheelchair propulsion distance test (35). However, this test requires significant skill, motivation, and a basic level of fitness on the part of the wheelchair user. There also is significant interindividual variability. In addition, these tests typically require a maximal effort that would be beyond the scope of practice of the personal trainer. Wheelchair ergometers also have been developed for exercise testing of persons with SCI, but the availability and practicality of these instruments are very limited.

> Maximal exercise testing of clients with SCI should be administered only in medical settings with appropriate professional and physician supervision.

Physical Activity and Fitness Levels in Persons With Spinal Cord Injury

The reduction in physical fitness in persons with SCI is due in part to the sedentary lifestyle imposed by the condition (20) but also may be related to the level of injury and degree of neuromuscular impairment. Several studies in the 1980s showed that there were few differences in physical performance, cardiorespiratory fitness, or muscular strength among persons with SCI who had lesions below T-6 when classified by the specific site (T-7, T-8, L-1, etc.) of SCI (46, 47, 93). However, those with lesions above T-6 (persons with tetraplegia) had markedly reduced cardiorespiratory fitness (as measured by $\dot{V}O_2$peak and muscle strength) compared to persons with lesions below T-6 (42).

Other researchers, however, have suggested that a significant proportion of variation in physical fitness could be attributed to neuromuscular impairment as defined by lesion level (8). One group reported that 46% of the variation in $\dot{V}O_2$peak could be explained by the level of injury, suggesting a moderate to strong relationship between neurological disruption and cardiorespiratory fitness (8).

As with other populations, there is a strong relationship between physical activity levels and both $\dot{V}O_2$peak and upper body muscle strength and endurance in persons with SCI; the greater the daily physical activity level, the greater the $\dot{V}O_2$peak and muscle strength and endurance (23, 25). Research evidence has also shown that physically active persons with SCI have 13% to 23% and 16% to 22% greater maximal cardiac outputs and stroke volumes, respectively, than their sedentary counterparts (21, 22). Thus, although there is controversy about the causes of the decreased cardiorespiratory and musculoskeletal fitness in persons with SCI, there appears to be a strong positive relationship between habitual physical activity levels and $\dot{V}O_2$peak, muscular strength, and other measures of physical fitness.

Particularly in people with tetraplegia, it is difficult to engage enough muscle mass to adequately stress the central circulation or the heart. For example, most of the cardiorespiratory improvements with arm crank training seen in persons with tetraplegia are peripheral (increased mitochondria density, aerobic enzymes, myoglobin, and capillary density) (30). In deconditioned persons with tetraplegia, however, the stimulus of upper body aerobic exercise may be sufficient to modestly improve maximal cardiac output and stroke volume (29).

Tetraplegia presents unique problems for cardiorespiratory training. Particularly in the upright posture, the hemodynamic responses to arm crank ergometry are markedly reduced. Peak heart rate is usually no greater than 120 to 130 beats/min; and cardiac output, stroke volume, and blood pressure are subnormal for given levels of oxygen uptake (32). Persons with SCI, particularly those with tetraplegia, have excessive lower limb and trunk venous pooling during exercise due to autonomic impairment and lack of lower limb and trunk muscle venous pump. In addition, upper body peripheral vasodilation during exercise is not compensated adequately by concomitant lower limb vasoconstriction (30). This reduces central circulatory volume and thereby limits hemodynamic responses to exercise. This dysfunctional syndrome has been referred to as "hypokinetic circulation" (24, 37, 38).

Forced vital capacity (total volume of air forcefully exhaled) is reduced by 50% in persons with high tetraplegia (51). A recent study demonstrated that resistive inspiratory muscle training (RIMT) can improve pulmonary function in people with tetraplegia (50). Thus RIMT may be of benefit and should be considered by the personal trainer who is planning an exercise training program for these clients (readers may refer to Liaw and colleagues [50] for more information on RIMT).

Exercise Prescription

In general, the principles of frequency, intensity, time, and type are as applicable in persons with SCI as in others. Initially, for cardiorespiratory training, intensity of 40% to 60% of maximal oxygen uptake, duration of 10 to 20 minutes, and frequency of three days per week or every other day is recommended. For resistance training, a suitable starting program is 8 to 12 exercises at 40% to 70% of 1-repetition maximum (1RM), performed for two or three sets of 8 to 12 repetitions with 1 to 2 minutes of rest between sets. The program should adhere to the principles of gradual progression, specificity, and

overload as for persons in other groups. See chapters 12 through 16 for general exercise technique and prescription.

People with SCI should eventually strive for a minimum of 30 minutes or more of physical activity on most, preferably all, days of the week. Goals for persons with SCI are no different than for others: increase functional capacity, improve health risk factors, enhance self-image and confidence, and so on. Clients with SCI are prone to **spasticity** (exaggerated muscle tone and reflexes), which can impair the ability to exercise. A gradual warm-up with a systematic, progressive increase in intensity and slow-paced muscle actions during resistance training, for example, can limit spasticity. Excessive, frequent spasticity warrants medical follow-up for possible adjustment in medical therapy.

In conclusion, it is clear that persons with SCI can benefit from a systematic and progressive comprehensive exercise program. Several publications provide more information on exercise for persons with SCI (5, 7, 49, 53, 94).

Exercise Guidelines for Clients With Spinal Cord Injury

Here are some guidelines that personal trainers should keep in mind when planning aerobic, flexibility, and resistance exercise for clients with SCI:

- Incorporate exercise that will restore or enhance balance around functional joints; in particular, strengthen muscle groups of the posterior shoulder and upper back areas, and stretch muscles of the anterior shoulder and chest areas.

- A conventional resistance training program of three sets of 8 to 12 repetitions performed for all functional muscle groups, two to three days per week, is recommended. Clients may also benefit, however, from a program of a single set to fatigue of 8 to 12 repetitions using 8 to 12 exercises, two to three days per week.

- As with all resistance exercise programs, full range of motion, proper exercise technique, avoidance of breath-holding, and controlled movement should be emphasized.

- Due to risk of shoulder, elbow, and wrist overuse injuries, caution in choice, intensity, and volume of exercise is necessary.

- Persons with SCI often have spasticity and may need to refrain from resistance training if the spasticity is severe (referral to medical team may be indicated) (31).

- Any exercise that triggers abnormal muscle tone must be stopped and avoided (31).

- In youth with SCI, precautions for resistance training include not overloading growing bones, as well as possibly limiting resistance training and emphasizing flexibility and aerobic training during periods of rapid growth (31).

- Standard guidelines for flexibility training apply, with particular attention paid to the shoulders, wrists, arms, trunk, and lower limbs (see chapter 12 on flexibility training).

- Aerobic exercise should begin at a moderate level and progress gradually in duration, frequency, and intensity with a goal of 30 minutes four or more days per week.

- Cardiorespiratory training modes may include arm cranking; wheelchair ergometry; wheelchair propulsion on a treadmill or rollers (in highly skilled clients in wheelchairs) or on accessible sidewalks, indoor or outdoor tracks, or trail surfaces; swimming; sports such as wheelchair basketball; ambulation with crutches and braces; arm-powered cycling; and functional electrical stimulation or facilitated support treadmill walking (generally in research and rehabilitative settings).

- Monitoring aerobic exercise intensity by heart rate in the SCI population can be problematic for various reasons (e.g., varying amount of active muscle mass, autonomic control of heart rate) (34). Rating of perceived exertion (RPE) is an appropriate alternative method to measure aerobic exercise intensity.

- Persons with SCI should be supervised during exercise and likely will need assistance with equipment adjustments, transfers, and so on.

- Most persons with SCI have their own bladder–bowel program and should empty both prior to exercise.

- Blood pressure should be monitored regularly at rest and frequently with exercise to avoid exercise-induced hypotension, particularly with exercise in the upright posture.

- Supine arm cranking may be preferred in clients with tetraplegia if equipment can be modified for this purpose.

- Avoid exercise within 2 to 3 hours after a meal. Digestion can impair the ability to shunt blood to the working muscles during exercise, creating competition between a limited cardiac output and blood flow, which can result in gastrointestinal disturbances during exercise.

- Because of loss of muscle function, loss of trunk control and balance, and loss of sensation in paralyzed areas, special equipment such as additional padding on equipment, gloves, elastic bandages, seat belts, and Velcro straps may be necessary.

- The client should avoid prolonged sitting and abrasions, particularly of the weight-bearing areas of the hip, ischium, sacrum, and coccyx, because of the risk of pressure sores, which do not heal easily.

- The client should avoid exercise during conditions such as cold, flu, bladder infection, constipation, and fever and should limit aerobic and resistance training during periods of increased spasticity (mild stretching may reduce spasticity but should be implemented by a personal trainer only with guidance and instruction from the client's personal physician).

- Transfers from wheelchair to exercise equipment should be minimal to reduce the risk of repetitive-strain injuries (89).

- Be aware of the client's regular medications and their side effects. See table 22.1 for common medications used for SCI.

- Thermoregulatory factors should always be considered (1); light and loose clothing, adequate hydration, cool exercise environments, and misting can enhance heat tolerance.

- The personal trainer needs to provide motivation and support for the client with SCI to promote exercise adherence and encourage increased daily physical activity, and have clients report these activities on a regular basis.

Multiple Sclerosis

Multiple sclerosis (MS) is an immune-mediated (autoimmune) disorder that occurs in genetically susceptible persons. Although the etiology of MS is uncertain, recent evidence suggests a viral origin such as Epstein-Barr virus (3). Multiple sclerosis is characterized by inflammation and progressive degeneration of the myelin sheath involving predominantly nerves of the eye, brain, periventricular gray matter, cerebellum, brain stem, and spinal cord (65).

Early symptoms of MS (sensory disturbances, fatigue and weakness, ipsilateral optical neuritis, gait ataxia, neurogenic bowel and bladder, and trunk and limb paresthesia evoked by neck flexion) are thought to be the result of axonal demyelination leading to a slowing or blockade of nerve conduction (65). Multiple sclerosis typically begins in early adulthood (ages 20 to 40 years) and has a variable clinical course and prognosis. Eighty percent of individuals have the relapsing–remitting type of MS while 20% have chronic (primary) progressive MS (65). The relapsing–remitting type can be further classified into benign, classical relapsing-remitting, and chronic-relapsing. Table 22.2 describes the clinical classifications of MS (41).

Multiple sclerosis is a devastating and potentially debilitating disease. Although there is no known cure, early diagnosis and treatment including rehabilitation, medical therapy, and exercise can improve the quality of life, functional status, and long-term outcomes in many persons with MS (16, 45, 52, 64, 71, 76, 77, 84).

Medical Management of Multiple Sclerosis

Essentially there are four aspects to the treatment of MS. The first involves education of the individual and family regarding the disease process, its progression, prognosis, and ways in which the disease can be managed. This aspect is primarily the responsibility of the client's physician and health care team. However, a knowledgeable personal trainer can reinforce the information and recommendations.

The second aspect of MS treatment involves the management of symptoms and secondary complications such as **dystonic spasms** (brief, recurring, painful posturing of one or more limbs), general spasticity, ataxia, incoordination, depression, other emotional disturbances, bladder and bowel dysfunction, and related pain syndromes.

The third aspect of treatment concerns the management of the disease process. Persons with MS will be on medication for managing the inflammation associated with the disease process and modifying the disease process (3, 4). Medical treatment for MS is very complex, and most individuals are under the care of a neurologist for this purpose. The personal trainer needs to be aware of medications that the person with MS may be taking and should seek the assistance of the client's medical team and resources such as *Physician's Desk Reference* (PDR) in order

TABLE 22.1 Common Medications Used by Individuals With Spinal Cord Injury

Drug type	Drugs	Purpose or action	Potential side effects
Spasmolytics	Baclofen, tizanidine, diazepam, clonidine, dantrolene	Decrease spasticity	Muscle weakness, fatigue in higher doses, hypotension, bradycardia, dizziness, sedation
Spasmolytics	Oxybutynin hydrochloride, phenoxybenzamine	Improve urinary bladder filling and emptying; prevent autonomic dysreflexia	Tachycardia, hypotension
Antithrombotics, anticoagulants	Warfarin, heparin sodium	Prevent and manage blood clots	Bruising, hemorrhage
Antibiotics	Sulfamethoxazole and trimethoprim	Prevent and treat infections (e.g., urinary tract)	None

TABLE 22.2 Major Clinical Classifications and Characteristics of Multiple Sclerosis

Classification	Characteristics
Relapsing-remitting MS (RRMS)	RRMS is characterized by relapse (attacks of symptom flare-ups) followed by remission (periods of recovery). Symptoms may vary from mild to severe, and relapses and remissions may last for days or months. More than 80 percent of people who have MS begin with relapsing-remitting cycles.
Secondary-progressive MS (SPMS)	SPMS often develops in people who have relapsing-remitting MS. In SPMS, relapses and partial recoveries occur, but the disability doesn't fade away between cycles. Instead, it progressively worsens until a steady progression of disability replaces the cycles of attacks.
Primary-progressive MS (PPMS)	PPMS progresses slowly and steadily from its onset. There are no periods of remission and symptoms generally do not decrease in intensity. About 15 percent of people who have MS have PPMS.
Progressive-relapsing MS (PRMS)	In this relatively rare type of MS, people experience both steadily worsening symptoms and attacks during periods of remission.

Reprinted from MayoClinic.org (www.mayoclinic.org/multiple-sclerosis/types.html).
For more information see Jackson and Mulchare 2009 (41).

TABLE 22.3 Common Medications Used to Manage Symptoms of Multiple Sclerosis

Drug type	Drugs	Purpose or action	Potential side effects
Corticosteroids	Prednisone, methylpred-nisolone	To reduce number, duration, and severity of MS attacks	Acne, weight gain, hypertension, osteoporosis, diabetes, increased infections
Beta interferons	Betaseron, Avonex, Rebif	To reduce number and severity of attacks and slow the disease progression	Fever, chills, sweating, muscle aches, fatigue, depression
Immunosuppresive agents Novantrone, methotrexate			Increased bacterial, and viral infections
Aminopyridine (fampridine)	Aminopyridine (fampridine)	Nerve impulse conduction enhancement, improved coordination and walking ability	
Synthetic myelin basic protein	Copolymer 1 (Copaxone)	To reduce the MS symptom relapse rate	Fewer side effects
Spasmolytics	Baclofen, tizanidine, diazepam, clonazepam, dantrolene	To treat spasticity	Muscle weakness, fatigue in higher doses, hypotension, dizziness
Antidepressants	Amantadine, pemoline, amitriptyline	To treat fatigue	Potential risk of seizures
Analgesics	Acetaminophen	To relieve pain	
Anti-inflammatories	Aspirin		
	Codeine		

Data from National Institute of Neurological Disorders and Stroke 2009 (62); Jackson and Mulcare 2009 (41).

to ensure the safety and efficacy of exercise therapy. Table 22.3 displays common medications used to manage symptoms of MS and potential side effects.

The fourth aspect of therapy for MS involves exercise. Persons with MS are generally sedentary, often because of the difficulties with movement and the associated fatigue and weakness. According to one study, an aerobic endurance training program can increase cardiorespiratory fitness by as much as 22% (70). Another researcher showed that aerobic endurance training in persons with MS may result in an increased aerobic capacity of 30%, but emphasized that the individual response to the same program over several weeks to months may vary by 2% to 54% (74). Exercise and behavioral therapy have been recommended as a management strategy for persons with MS who experience persistent fatigue (12). Regular stretching is essential to maintaining joint range of motion and tissue elasticity. Resistance training can increase muscle strength and endurance (16, 77, 92) and prevent muscle atrophy. Exercise modalities such as tai chi and yoga also may be beneficial.

Exercise Testing and Training of Clients With Multiple Sclerosis

The benefits of aerobic exercise for clients with MS seem clear. Aerobic endurance training in persons with MS can improve $\dot{V}O_2$peak, upper and lower body strength, body composition, and risk factors for CVD (16, 41, 56, 78, 84, 85). After 15 weeks of aerobic endurance training, a group of persons with MS showed significantly reduced levels of anger, depression, and fatigue (on the Profile of Mood States) and an improved total score on the Sickness Impact Profile, as well as on a number of its components (physical dimensions scale, social interaction, emotional behavior, and recreational pursuits) (70). In addition, exercise training can enhance general well-being while offsetting some of the psychological difficulties such as fatigue, stress, and depression that are common in persons with MS (84).

Many persons with MS experience heat sensitivity that is often associated with a transient increase in clinical signs and symptoms. This may preclude or deter persons with MS from participation in a regular exercise program in which metabolic heat is increased. Several studies have yielded positive results in this area, although, as with most studies on people with MS, few if any have included subjects over 55 years of age. Applying a precooling procedure (cool shower or whirlpool, cool wet neck wraps or cooling collars, or cool water sprays before and during exercise) to thermosensitive persons with MS prior to exercise may result in lower rectal temperature, heart rate, and perceived exertion than in exercisers who do not receive cooling treatment (91).

Persons with MS are prone to heat intolerance. Methods to precool the client and to ensure a cool, comfortable environment for exercise can enhance the physiological benefits and increase adherence. Proper hydration is critical to maintaining temperature balance during exercise in persons with MS.

Exercise Testing

Exercise testing of persons with MS should be administered with extreme caution. People with MS who have or who are at risk for CVD must be screened and administered a clinical exercise test with professional and physician supervision to rule out ischemia and coronary heart disease prior to starting an exercise program. However, with proper medical clearance, the personal trainer can safely administer a submaximal aerobic exercise test to establish a baseline for future comparisons. Because of incoordination and possible spasticity, leg or arm ergometry is the preferred modality. Flexibility tests such as the sit and reach can be safely administered with careful attention to technique. Little is known about the safety or efficacy of maximal 1RM or other forms of isotonic muscle strength or endurance testing for people with MS. The recommendation would be to use caution in administering maximal strength or muscular endurance testing to fatigue, but data to support the risks of these procedures, as well as the safety and efficacy, are limited.

Resistance Training

Although relatively few resistance training studies exist, newer evidence indicates that resistance training is a safe and effective form of exercise for persons with MS and mild and moderate disability (52, 77, 92). After engaging in an eight-week progressive resistance training program consisting of one set of 10 to 15 repetitions with 70% of maximal voluntary contractions (MVC), subjects improved knee extension, plantarflexion, and stepping performance by 7.4%, 52%, and 8.7%, respectively (92). After participating in a six-month randomized controlled exercise program consisting of one aerobic conditioning and three resistance training sessions per week, participants demonstrated significant improvements in walking speed, knee flexion strength, and upper extremity muscle endurance (77). In a recent pilot study, participants engaging in a three-month combined group and home strengthening program demonstrated significant improvements in exercise capacity, quality of life, and fatigue scores on standardized testing inventories (52). Field experience suggests that general resistance training program guidelines for people with MS should resemble those for untrained persons without MS (16, 41). A standard progressive resistance training program of 8 to 10 exercises, performed at 60% to 80% 1RM load for one to three sets of 8 to 15 repetitions (for all major muscle groups), results in beneficial outcomes in persons with MS with little or no risk. Goals of a resistance training program for persons with MS are to increase general muscle strength, improve muscle tone, equalize agonist–antagonist muscle strength, and reduce spasticity (41). Progression may need to occur at about 50% of the rate for persons without the disorder (i.e., increase loads every three to four instead of one to two weeks). In addition, daily stretching should be done to increase joint range of motion, counteract spasticity, and improve balance (16, 41).

Aerobic Conditioning

In the past, exercise training was not recommended for persons with MS because it was believed that exercise increased MS-associated fatigue. Exercise programs for people with MS should be carefully designed to adequately stimulate cardiorespiratory and musculoskeletal function in accordance with the principles of overload and progressive resistance. However, the overload must be presented gradually in order not to cause or exacerbate fatigue, nerve conduction block, or both.

The response of persons with MS to submaximal aerobic exercise appears to vary depending on the stage and severity of the disease process. In two studies, heart rate, ventilation, and oxygen uptake were higher and net energy expenditure was two to three times greater during submaximal treadmill walking in persons with MS than in age- and gender-matched peers (67, 68). However, a more recent study in moderately impaired persons with MS did not show a significant difference from age- and gender-matched controls in net energy expenditure at similar submaximal workloads (86). Additional studies have indicated that moderate-intensity aerobic exercises improve physical fitness (6), mobility (45, 81), walking speed and capacity (77), exercise tolerance (76) and also reduce fatigue (52) and decrease disability (45, 76). This research illustrates the need to carefully prescribe aerobic exercise intensity to ensure a light to moderate workload. The recommended aerobic intensity is 60% to 80% of heart rate peak or 50% to 70% of $\dot{V}O_2$peak (16, 41). Alternatively, intensity ranges between 40% and 60% of heart rate reserve (HRR) or $\dot{V}O_2$reserve may also be used. An initial exercise duration of 10 to 40 minutes is recommended depending on the disability level of the individual (16). During the first few months, progression should be achieved through increasing the training volume by either increasing training time or adding an extra training day (16). In most persons with MS, initiating exercise at 40% to 50% of $\dot{V}O_2$max or HRR is advised, with progression over three to six months to 50% to 70% as the client adapts. The goals of an aerobic conditioning program for persons with MS are to improve cardiovascular function, reduce the risks for CVD, and reduce activity-induced fatigue.

Clients with MS are prone to fatigue that can be disabling. Precautions must be taken to provide a systematic program that starts at the lower end of traditional recommendations and progresses at a rate that is 50% slower than for apparently healthy adults. For more information, readers may refer to published recommendations for physical activity in persons with MS (71).

Finally, although persons with MS are prone to heat intolerance, with the proper precautions, warm water aquatic therapy may benefit some without aggravating fatigue or increasing risk for heat-related problems (41, 62, 72).

> Exercise to exhaustion in clients with MS should be avoided. Persistent fatigue lasting more than two days should be a warning sign that an exercise program is excessive.

Exercise Testing and Training Guidelines for Clients With Multiple Sclerosis

Some precautions and guidelines for exercise testing and training of clients with MS are as follows:

- Complex skill-oriented exercises should be avoided in most persons with MS, partly because of the loss of proprioception, or ability to perceive muscle and joint position in space.

- The energy cost of walking may be two to three times higher than normal for people with MS, particularly those with advanced disease; thus adjustments in workloads to maintain a 60% to 75% maximal heart rate are necessary.

- Persons with MS are thermosensitive and therefore at increased risk for both heat- and cold-related injuries; this emphasizes the need to ensure adequate hydration and to have persons with MS exercise in thermoneutral environments. In addition, dehydration during exercise could be exacerbated in persons with MS who have bladder dysfunction (incontinence or sense of urgent need to urinate or both) and sometimes limit their fluid intake.

- It is important to be cautious with large muscle lower limb exercise, since muscle spasticity may be particularly predominant in the hip abductor and adductors.

- Sensory loss may preclude certain exercises such as free weights because of a client's inability to grasp the bars effectively, and may necessitate modification in other forms of exercise.

- Strapping may be necessary if more severe spasticity is present.

- Some evidence suggests that morning, when circadian body temperature is at its lowest, may be the preferred time for exercise.

- Recumbent bicycling may be preferred over upright cycling in clients with balance problems.

- Imbalances between agonist and antagonist muscles are common.

- Muscle weakness tends to be greatest in the lower limb and trunk muscles.

- Neuromuscular problems such as foot drop may be present in more advanced cases.

- Some clients may have cognitive deficits and are prone to depression; caution is warranted in education of these individuals, and constant reinforcement to enhance compliance is generally needed in clients with MS.

- The variable nature of MS symptoms and progression requires that the personal trainer adjust the exercise program on a daily basis.

- It is advisable to monitor heart rate before, during, and after aerobic exercise to ensure the appropriate metabolic intensity and stimulus.

- Regular follow-ups to monitor progress are highly recommended with persons who have MS in order to facilitate compliance and to adjust the exercise prescription appropriately.

- In the case of an exacerbation, exercise should be discontinued until complete remission.

- Since some individuals with MS have cognitive impairments, it may be necessary to provide information and instruction in both written and diagram formats. Frequent reminders of exercises, technique, and proper use of equipment may be necessary.

- If the client has incoordination in either the upper or the lower limbs, the use of a

TABLE 22.4 General Exercise Session Programming Guidelines for Clients With Multiple Sclerosis

Exercise component	Guidelines
AEROBIC TRAINING	
Mode(s)	Stationary cycling, recumbent cycling, recumbent stepping (NuStep), water aerobics, upper body ergometry, walking.
Intensity	Either 60% to 80% of peak heart rate, 40% to 60% of heart rate reserve, 50% to 70% of $\dot{V}O_2$peak, or 40% to 60% of $\dot{V}O_2$ reserve.
Duration	30 min/session, which might need initially to be accumulated in three 10-min sessions per day.
Frequency	2 to 3 days per week on nonresistance training days.
RESISTANCE TRAINING	
Mode(s)	Machines, free weights, resistance bands and tubing, pulleys, Pilates.
Muscle groups	8 to 10 exercises that emphasize all major muscle groups and attempt to establish balance in agonist–antagonist muscles.
Intensity	8 to 15 repetitions with 60% to 80% of 1RM.
Sets	One or more sets per muscle group as tolerated.
Rest periods	A minimum of 1 min rest between sets and exercises.
FLEXIBILITY TRAINING	
Mode(s)	Active range of motion, passive range of motion, yoga, tai chi.
Duration	Hold stretches between 30 and 60 s. Stretches should be held with mild to moderate tension but for a duration without discomfort.
Frequency	Perform gentle stretching one or two times a day.
Muscle groups	Stretch all major muscle groups. The hip flexors, hamstrings, hip adductors, plantarflexors, and anterior shoulder girdle muscles should receive high priority.

Data from Dalgas, Stenager, and Tingemann-Hansen 2008 (16); Jackson and Mulcare 2009 (41).

synchronized leg and arm ergometer may improve exercise performance by allowing the arms or legs to assist the weaker limbs.

- Resistance training should be performed on nonendurance training days to avoid fatigue.
- Resistance training should be done in the seated position initially if balance is impaired.
- Flexibility exercises should be performed from either a seated or a lying position (16, 41, 56).

General exercise session programming guidelines are listed in table 22.4.

Epilepsy

Epilepsy is defined medically as two or more unprovoked, recurring seizures (43). A **seizure** is an uncontrolled, paroxysmal electrical discharge within any part of the brain that causes physical or mental symptoms and may or may not be associated with convulsions. Seizures result in involuntary alteration in movement, sensation, perception, cognitive behavior, or loss of consciousness (LOC) or some combination of these. Table 22.5 defines classifications of seizures with characteristic signs and symptoms (13, 14). Epilepsy is as common as breast cancer in the United States, and although

it is often a misunderstood perilous condition, as many as 200,000 US citizens will be diagnosed with seizures or epilepsy (or both) each year (www.epilepsyfoundation.org). Thus is it is far from a benign condition.

Status epilepticus is defined as a seizure lasting more than 30 minutes or a series of seizures that occur so frequently that consciousness is not restored (43). Status epilepticus is a medical emergency, necessitating activation of emergency protocols including calling 911 or another local emergency number and transporting to a hospital emergency department.

It is important that the personal trainer understand and recognize common precipitants (causes or triggers) in clients with idiopathic or secondary seizures. Table 22.6 summarizes some known precipitants and recommendations for exercise session modification.

Anecdotal reports have suggested that physical activity may be a precipitant of seizure (48, 66, 79). However, systematic studies have shown that physical activity and sport have no adverse effects on seizure occurrence in the majority of clients with epilepsy and, in fact, may contribute to better seizure control (58, 59). As a cautionary note for the personal trainer working with clients who have epilepsy, however, these studies do suggest that exercise may be a seizure precipitant in approximately 10% of these individuals. This is particularly apparent

TABLE 22.5 Classification and Common Signs and Symptoms of Seizure Disorders and Approximate Percentage of Cases

Type of seizure	Signs and symptoms
PARTIAL SEIZURES—THE AFFECTED AREA OF THE BRAIN IS ON ONE SIDE	
Simple	These seizures don't result in loss of consciousness. They may alter emotions or change the way things look, smell, feel, taste or sound. They may also result in involuntary jerking of part of the body, such as an arm or leg, and spontaneous sensory symptoms such as tingling, vertigo and flashing lights.
Complex	These seizures alter consciousness, causing impaired awareness. Complex partial seizures often result in staring and nonpurposeful movements — such as hand rubbing, twitching, chewing, swallowing or walking in circles.
GENERALIZED SEIZURES—OCCUR ON BOTH SIDES OF THE BRAIN	
Absence (petit mal)	These seizures are characterized by staring and subtle body movement, and can cause a brief (2-15 s) loss of consciousness.
Myoclonic	These seizures usually appear as sudden, ultrashort jerks or twitches of your arms and legs.
Tonic-clonic (grand mal)	The most intense of all types of seizures, these are characterized by a loss of consciousness, body stiffening and shaking, and loss of bladder control.
Atonic	Also known as *drop attacks*, these brief (<15 s) seizures may cause clients to lose normal muscle tone and to suddenly collapse or fall down.

Adapted from MayoClinic.com (www.mayoclinic.com/health/epilepsy).

TABLE 22.6 Precipitants of Seizures and Exercise Modifications

Common precipitants of seizures	Suggested exercise modifications
Emotional stress	Modify intensity to lower level.
Hyperventilation	Teach breathing techniques and control.
Menstruation	Modify intensity to lower level.
Sleep deprivation	Avoid exercise.
Fever	Avoid exercise.
Photic stimulation (strobe lights, TV, etc.)	Avoid situations during exercise.
Alcohol excess or withdrawal	Modify intensity to lower level.

in clients with seizures secondary to trauma, infections, or stroke.

Many persons with epilepsy unnecessarily avoid physical activity and sport because of fear of seizure induction, seizure-related injury, or both. In general, studies suggest that persons with epilepsy are less active than the general population, but the results are equivocal. A Norwegian research group, for example, found no difference in physical activity levels among persons with epilepsy and the general population (59). The consensus of experts is that not only should exercise and sport participation in persons with epilepsy *not* be restricted; it should be encouraged (36, 83). The personal trainer needs to be aware of these issues and gently encourage clients with epilepsy to increase their physical activity levels.

In many persons with epilepsy, regular aerobic exercise may contribute to improved seizure control. However, in 10% of individuals, vigorous exercise may be a seizure precipitant.

Medical Management of Seizures

Medical management of seizures is completely effective in approximately 67% to 75% of cases (44). The choice of medication is determined by the client's physician based on the type of seizure and the client's tolerance of side effects. In the 25% to 33% of cases of epilepsy that are refractory to medical management, surgical options may be effective (44). It is beyond the scope of this chapter to expand on these procedures, and the reader is directed to the Epilepsy Foundation website (www.epilepsyfoundation.org) for more information. The sidebar briefly describes two of these procedures. The personal trainer needs to be aware of the medications a client may be on and consult a reference such as PDR for descriptions of the medications and their side effects. The personal trainer should be in communication with the client's personal physician regarding any exercise precautions or contraindications or possible negative interactions of medications or surgical procedures with exercise training. It needs to be emphasized that the discussion of exercise training in persons with epilepsy in this section clearly is applicable only to the perhaps 80% of those who are well controlled either medically, surgically, or with combined therapy. Table 22.7 provides a list of the most common medications used to treat epilepsy and their common side effects.

Exercise Testing and Training of Clients With Epilepsy

Most persons with epilepsy, unfortunately, live sedentary lives and therefore generally have low

physical fitness. This appears to be the case even though, most often, physical exercise and other leisure pursuits are not precipitators of seizures and do not increase the risk of seizure-related injuries (55, 60). In fact in the Norwegian study mentioned earlier, 36% of persons with epilepsy indicated that regular exercise contributed to better seizure control (59).

However, as mentioned earlier in this discussion, studies do suggest that exercise may precipitate seizures in a small percentage (~10%) of persons with epilepsy, particularly those with seizures secondary to infection, trauma, or stroke. Persons with epilepsy whose fitness level is low may be more prone to

TABLE 22.7 The Most Common Medications Used to Treat Epilepsy and Their Common Side Effects

Medication	Purpose	Common side effects
Tegretol or Carbatrol	First choice for partial, generalized tonic–clonic, and mixed seizures	Fatigue, vision changes, nausea, dizziness, rash
Zarontin	Used to treat absence seizures	Nausea, vomiting, decreased appetite, weight loss
Felbatol	Partial and some generalized seizures	Decreased appetite, weight loss, inability to sleep, headache, depression
Gabitril	Used usually in combination with other antiseizure medications for partial and some generalized seizures	Dizziness, fatigue, weakness, irritability, confusion, anxiety
Keppra	Used with other antiseizure medications for partial seizures	Tiredness, weakness, behavioral changes
Lamictal	Treats partial and some generalized seizures	Few side effects but possibly dizziness, rash, insomnia
Lyrica	Used to treat partial seizures	Dizziness, sleepiness, dry mouth, peripheral edema, blurred vision, weight gain, difficulty with concentration
Neurontin	Used with other antiseizure medications to treat partial and some generalized seizures	Few lasting side effects but possibly tiredness and dizziness during first weeks of treatment in particular
Phenytoin	Partial seizures and tonic–clonic seizures	Dizziness, fatigue, slurred speech, acne, rash, increased hair (hirsutism); in long run can be associated with bone thinning
Topamax	Used with other antiseizure medications to treat partial or generalized tonic–clonic seizures	Dizziness, fatigue, speech problems, nervousness, memory problems, vision problems, weight loss
Trileptal	Treats partial seizures	Tiredness, dizziness, headache, double vision
Depakote	Used to treat partial, absence, and tonic–clonic generalized seizures	Dizziness, nausea, vomiting, tremor, hair loss, weight gain, depression in adults, irritability in children, reduced attention, sometimes impaired cognition; has some serious long-term possible effects such as bone thinning, ankle edema, hearing loss, liver damage, decreased platelets, and pancreas problems
Zonegran	Used with other antiseizure medications to treat partial seizures	Drowsiness, dizziness, unsteady gait, kidney stones, abdominal discomfort, headache, and rash
Valium, Klonopin, Tranxene	Effective in short-term control of seizures as in an emergency department	Tiredness, unsteady gait, nausea, depression, loss of appetite; in children may see drooling, hyperactivity

Examples of Surgical Options for Refractory Epilepsy

The most common form of epilepsy surgery is a lobectomy or cortical resection. In this procedure, all or part of the left or right lobe—common sites of simple and complex partial seizures, some of which may generalize to the entire cerebral cortex—may be removed surgically.

Another option in selected patients in whom seizures are not controlled by medications is vagal nerve stimulation (VNS). This procedure involves implanting a flat, round battery about the size of a silver dollar into the patient's chest wall. Thin wires are threaded under the skin and wound around the vagus nerve in the neck. If the patient has an aura and feels a seizure coming on, the VNS unit can be activated by passing a small magnet over the battery, which then sends signals to the vagus nerve. The effectiveness of the VNS system is imperfect, with 33% of the 32,000 persons with this implant experiencing a major improvement, 33% some improvement, and 33% showing no benefit.

The personal trainer is directed to the Epilepsy Foundation (www.epilepsyfoundation.org) for more information on these and other epilepsy surgical procedures, their effectiveness, side effects, and so on.

exercise-induced seizures (59). The personal trainer needs to be aware of the type of seizure disorder a client has and be alert to signs and symptoms suggestive of a seizure. Many persons with epilepsy have an aura prior to a seizure. The personal trainer should know his or her client and be able to recognize signs and symptoms that suggest an impending seizure.

In general, there are no contraindications or restrictions to exercise in persons with well-controlled epilepsy. In fact, sport and regular exercise should be encouraged with minimal restrictions assuming that seizure management is optimal.

The personal trainer can apply the same exercise principles for persons with epilepsy as are recommended for apparently healthy populations. A gradual and progressive approach to physical activity and weight control is recommended. With proper medical clearance and adherence to standard guidelines, it is safe to administer submaximal exercise testing to establish baseline cardiorespiratory fitness, muscle strength and endurance, flexibility, and body composition. With regard to weight control, it is important to note that even a modest weight loss of 10 pounds (4.5 kg) may affect the biological availability of antiseizure medications and thus increase the risk of side effects. It also is important to note that some persons with epilepsy may be on a "ketogenic diet" (low carbohydrate, higher fat, adequate protein). A 2008 randomized trial demonstrated a clear benefit of this diet in treating refractory epilepsy in children, and there is limited evidence that it may be of benefit in adults also (63).

Finally, the personal trainer should know first aid for seizure, particularly the tonic–clonic (grand mal) type. "First Aid for Seizures" describes basic first aid steps to take during a seizure and the **postictal state** (the period immediately after the seizure).

First Aid for Seizures

1. Keep client prone—lying facedown if possible.
2. Remove eyeglasses and other items that may break and cause injury.
3. Loosen any tight clothing, particularly around the neck.
4. Do *not* restrain the client.
5. Keep objects out of client's path.
6. Do *not* place anything in the client's mouth.
7. After the seizure, turn the client to his or her side in recovery position (refer to CPR guidelines) to prevent aspiration.
8. Observe the client until he or she is fully awake.
9. Alert the client's physician and family.
10. The client may be able to return to exercise, but evaluate this with the client's physician on a case-by-case basis.

A weight loss of 10 pounds (4.5 kg) can increase the bioavailability of antiseizure medications and thus increase the risk of side effects.

Cerebral Palsy

Cerebral palsy (CP) is a term used to describe a group of chronic musculoskeletal deficits causing impaired body movement and muscle coordination. It is caused by damage to one or more areas of the brain during fetal development, or during or shortly after the birthing process, or in early infancy (88). Cerebral palsy is characterized by limitation in the ability to move, control balance and coordination, and maintain posture due to damage to the motor areas of the brain that control muscle function and spinal reflexes. It is not a progressive disease, as the brain damage does not worsen. However, secondary conditions such as spasticity can and often do worsen if not well managed, leading to further loss of joint motion and mobility and potential contractures (permanent shortening of muscles and tendons). See "Definitions of Cerebral Palsy–Related Terms" for definitions of related terms.

Characteristic signs and symptoms of CP include muscle tightness, spasticity, involuntary muscle movement, gait disturbances, muscle weakness, incoordination, and speech and swallowing impairments. Other signs and symptoms that may be noted are deficiencies in sensation and perception, impaired vision or hearing (or both), seizures, cognitive dysfunction and learning deficiencies, and breathing difficulty secondary to postural deformities.

Medically, CP can be classified by the specific type of muscle abnormalities noted. In addition, the type of muscle abnormality suggests the site of brain injury:

- A client with marked spasticity likely has had damage within the motor cortex of the cerebrum (10, 28).
- Athetosis suggests midbrain damage.
- Ataxia suggests damage to the cerebellum.
- Dyskinesis suggests damage to the basal ganglia.

In mixed forms, which also exist, damage has occurred to multiple areas (10, 28).

For more information on the classifications of CP for sports, please see the 10th edition of the CPISRA manual at www.cpisra.org. Although originally designed for sport participation, this classification system is a useful tool that can give the personal trainer insight into the range of functional abilities of persons with CP.

Although CP cannot be corrected, it can be managed to prevent complications and further loss of function and independence. Medical therapy focuses on reducing spasticity if present and on improving nerve and muscle coordination. Physical therapy and rehabilitation are essential for optimizing growth and development, preventing disability, and minimizing muscle and locomotor dysfunction. An ongoing exercise program can greatly assist persons with CP in becoming and remaining independent, productive members of society.

> Cerebral palsy is an irreversible condition, and medical and rehabilitative therapy focuses on controlling spasticity and athetosis and improving function and neuromuscular coordination.

Medical Management of Cerebral Palsy

The medical management of CP mostly involves managing the secondary complications of the irreversible lesion. Seizures or seizure tendencies occur in 60% of persons with CP. Thus persons with CP may be on antiseizure medications, antispasmodic medications, and muscle relaxants. In addition, many persons with CP have other secondary complications including joint pain, hip and back deformities, bladder and bowel dysfunction, and gastroesophageal reflux for which they may be

Definitions of Cerebral Palsy–Related Terms

apraxia—Inability to perform coordinated voluntary gross and fine motor skills.

ataxia—Uncoordinated voluntary movements; clients with ataxia often have a wide-based gait with genu recurvatum or "hyperextended knee" and may exhibit mild intention tremors.

athetosis—Slow, writhing, contortion-like motions of the appendicular musculature.

chorea—State of excessive, spontaneous movements, irregularly timed, that are nonrepetitive and abrupt; client is unable to maintain voluntary muscle contractions.

dyskinesis—Impairment of voluntary movement resulting in incomplete movements.

dystonia—Sustained muscle contractions that result in twisting and repetitive movements or abnormal posture.

myoclonus—Shock-like synchronous or asynchronous contractions of a portion of a muscle, an entire muscle, or a group of muscles.

spasticity—A state of increased tonus of a muscle characterized by heightened deep tendon reflexes.

on medications. Finally, persons with CP, in general, are sedentary and thus prone to several risk factors for CVD.

Exercise Testing and Training of Clients With Cerebral Palsy

Little research has examined the exercise responses and effects of exercise training in persons with CP. Historically, few persons with CP have participated in formal or informal physical activity programs. However, a recent survey of women with CP reported that a significant proportion of women with CP who lived independently engaged in regular exercise (43% of respondents indicated that they had done range of motion exercise or aerobic exercise in the past week) (87).

Exercise testing and training of persons with CP are complicated by the deformities, athetosis, ataxia, incoordination, and spasticity often associated with this disorder. However, there is no pathological basis for expecting persons with CP not to benefit from regular physical activity, which should be encouraged. Research in this area is increasing, and what is available clearly suggests that persons with CP can expect to derive benefits from a regular program of physical activity that are similar to those for people who do not have the disorder. Verschuren and colleagues recently reported the results of a randomized trial among children and adolescents with CP (90). Eighty-six youth with CP classified as Gross Motor Function Level I or II were randomized to either a combined aerobic and anaerobic exercise training group two times per week for 45 minutes per session or a control group. The project lasted eight months. Both anaerobic and aerobic capacity increased significantly more in the combined exercise training group compared to the control group. Scholtes and colleagues initiated a randomized trial of lower limb strengthening in children with CP, but these results have not been published at this time (80). The following list summarizes some of the findings from research concerning the trainability of persons with CP.

- Improved capacity to perform activities of daily life (28)
- Improved sense of wellness and body image, physical fitness, and quality of life (28, 90)
- Apparent lessening of severity of symptoms such as spasticity and athetosis (28)
- Improved peak oxygen uptake, ventilatory threshold, work rates at submaximal heart rates, range of motion, and coordination and skill of movement (28)

- Increased muscle strength and endurance including hypertrophy (17, 18)
- Increased skeletal bone mineral density of the femoral neck (11)
- Improved ventilatory capacities in children ages 5 to 7 (40)
- Higher gait velocity following resistance training with improved symmetry in muscle strength (17)
- Improved water orientation skills and self-concept after swimming exercise in kindergarten children (39)

All persons with CP should be screened properly for musculoskeletal abnormalities, CVD, and risk factors for chronic diseases such as atherosclerosis, diabetes, arthritis, and hypertension (2). High-risk clients with two or more risk factors for CVD (hypertension, dyslipidemia, tobacco use, sedentary lifestyle, age greater than 40, obesity, diabetes) or with symptoms (chest pain, dyspnea, increasing weakness or fatigue, palpitations) should undergo a clinical examination, including an electrocardiographically monitored graded exercise test supervised by a professional team including a physician. The client must obtain medical clearance before starting a moderate-intensity exercise program. Also many persons with CP will be on medications for spasticity, seizures, mood disturbances, and other problems associated with CP. Table 22.8 summarizes some of the common medications persons with CP may be prescribed, their purpose, and common side effects. Standardized submaximal fitness testing may then be recommended in persons with CP who are at low risk and in those at risk who have been properly screened and cleared medically. The competent personal trainer should be able to administer submaximal testing under these conditions.

In ambulatory persons with CP, the leg ergometer and the arm and leg ergometer are preferred modalities for exercise testing. The treadmill may be used in persons with CP who have good balance and coordination. Because of spasticity or athetosis, the client's feet may need to be strapped to the pedals, and sufficient practice is necessary to ensure good performance. In nonambulatory persons with CP, the arm crank ergometer and wheelchair ergometer, if available, are the preferred modalities for submaximal testing. Clients should wear gloves to prevent skin abrasions, particularly if they use a wheelchair. To assess aerobic endurance, the 6- to 12-minute walk or wheelchair push may be appropriate. These tests, however, assume maximal effort, as the objective is for clients to travel "as much distance as they can" in the timed period. Therefore, this test should

TABLE 22.8　Common Medications Used in the Management of Persons with Cerebral Palsy

Medication	Purpose	Common side effects
Baclofen	Antispasmodic, muscle relaxant	Sleepiness, nausea, headache, muscle weakness, light-headedness; most side effects are transient
Dantrium	Antispasmodic, muscle relaxant	Can cause liver damage, must be monitored medically; diarrhea, dizziness, drowsiness, fatigue, vague feeling of illness, weakness
Botox	Antispasmodic, given by injection	Headache or muscle aches after an injection
Flexeril	Antispasmodic, muscle relaxant	Drowsiness, dizziness, insomnia
Depakene	Antiseizure	Can cause liver damage, must be monitored medically; nausea, vomiting, indigestion
Valium	Sedative, anticonvulsant, muscle relaxant, antianxiety	Drowsiness, lethargy, depression, headache, confusion, dizziness, possible respiratory depression
Dilantin	Antiseizure	Drowsiness, dizziness, nausea, sleep disturbances, headache
Epival	Antiseizure	Can damage liver, must be monitored medically; caution in children under 10, never in children under 2; can cause blood disorders
Klonopin	Antiseizure	Can damage liver, must be monitored medically; drowsiness, behavior changes, salivation
Tegretol	Antiseizure, possibly for pain secondary to nerve damage and mood disorders	Swelling, increased blood pressure, slurred speech, leg cramps, dry mouth
Zarontin	Antiseizure, particularly petit mal	Dizziness, nausea, drowsiness, lethargy

be administered only to low-risk and properly screened clients.

Common tests of flexibility and muscle function such as the sit and reach and 1RM can be safely administered. Finally, skinfold thickness measurements can be taken at several sites, preferably on noninvolved body parts, and totaled for a score to establish a baseline for assessing changes in body composition. Although valid equations for predicting body fat percentage from skinfold measurements are limited in this population, the total thickness of seven to eight sites can be used for monitoring progress.

Persons with CP can expect a systematic program of physical exercise to yield health and fitness benefits similar to those obtained by persons without CP.

Guidelines for Exercise Testing and Training of Clients With Cerebral Palsy

Although research guidelines for exercise prescription in persons with CP are limited, there is no apparent reason to expect this group to respond differently than others do. The following is a list of some basic guidelines and precautions for exercise testing and training in persons with CP:

■ Because of the limitations of persons with CP, the personal trainer needs to be creative and often needs to modify equipment and exercises.

■ Most persons with CP will benefit most from a balanced approach addressing flexibility, muscle strength and endurance, and cardiorespiratory fitness.

■ As with other clients, standard guidelines for cardiorespiratory training can be applied; moderate to vigorous intensity of 50% to 85% of $\dot{V}O_2$max or HRR, 30 or more minutes per session, four or more days per week, should be the goal. Gradual progression is recommended as with sedentary persons without the disorder; in very deconditioned persons with CP, the recommendation is to begin with 5 to 10 minutes, twice per day, four or more days per week; increasing physical activity in daily life should be a goal as well.

■ People with CP can perform standard moderate resistance training of 8 to 12 exercises for one to three sets of 8 to 12 repetitions, two to three days per week at 40% to 60% of maximum, although some exercises will need to be modified. In general, maximal loads should not be used for most persons with CP.

■ In many persons with CP, athetosis and spasticity make the use of free weights inadvisable; if a client with CP does use free weights, extreme caution and careful spotting are necessary.

- All standard principles such as avoidance of breath-holding, 48 hours of rest between working the same muscle groups, full range of motion, and controlled movement should be carefully applied to persons with CP.

- It is important to give attention to muscle imbalances, with exercises chosen to improve any deficiencies.

- It is particularly important that persons with CP have a period of aerobic warm-up (10-15 minutes) and stretching before exercise and cool-down with additional stretching after resistance training. This is because of significant risk of loss of joint range of motion in persons with CP.

- Because of interference from spasticity, guidelines for flexibility training in this population include stretching all major muscle groups to the point of tension and holding for 60 to 120 seconds each. Special attention should be given to areas of limited range of motion; assisted stretching may be useful if performed cautiously; daily stretching of muscles that are causing the most problems with activities of daily living should be performed.

- The personal trainer must be aware of and sensitive to the fact that many persons with CP have cognitive, visual, hearing, and speech difficulties.

- Because of balance and coordination problems, supervision is recommended with the use of modes such as the treadmill, elliptical trainer, and cross-country ski machine.

- The personal trainer should emphasize proper nutrition in persons with CP, and in particular among clients who are overweight.

Conclusion

The scope of practice of personal trainers is expanding rapidly. Accumulating evidence supports the application of exercise training to numerous special populations, including persons with several neuromuscular disorders. Increasing and sustaining moderate to high levels of physical activity among persons with SCI, MS, CP, and epilepsy are strongly encouraged. The functional and health benefits of regular exercise for these populations are similar to those for other persons when the activities are performed safely and effectively. Many persons in these groups are at increased risk for chronic metabolic disorders, at least partially because of the high frequency of physical inactivity among these populations.

Personal trainers working under the guidance of health care professionals should make an effort to promote their services to populations with the disorders covered in this chapter. The intrinsic rewards of working with persons who have these neuromuscular disorders, as well as others such as Parkinson's disease, muscular dystrophy, and post-polio syndrome, are many and certainly as meaningful as those derived from working with other clients, both nonathletic and athletic. Finally, two key references that should become part of the library of any personal trainer working with special populations are *ACSM's Exercise Management for Persons with Chronic Diseases and Disabilities* and *ACSM's Resources for Clinical Exercise Physiology* (26, 57).

Study Questions

1. For reasons such as autonomic control of heart rate and varying amounts of active muscle mass, RPE is an appropriate method for monitoring aerobic exercise intensity in clients with which of the following?

    A. spinal cord injury

    B. multiple sclerosis

    C. epilepsy

    D. cerebral palsy

2. Your 38-year-old client diagnosed with multiple sclerosis is a civil engineer complaining of leg muscle fatigue while walking and climbing stairs at job sites. She performs 10 minutes each of recumbent stepping, combined arm–leg bicycle ergometry, and upper body ergometry at a heart rate range of 90 to 100 beats/min. She also performs two sets of 10 repetitions of lat pulldowns, seated rows, knee extensions, and chest presses at 70% of 1RM. Which of the following activities should be added during the next exercise session?

    A. jogging and jump squats

    B. rowing ergometry and seated hip adduction

    C. treadmill walking and leg presses

    D. jumping rope and box jumps

3. The personal trainer has been working with a client on weight loss who has a history of partial, complex seizures for the past three months. Her recommended weight loss was 22 pounds (10 kg). Upon completing a repeat body composition test, the personal trainer finds that she has lost 9.9 pounds (4.5 kg). Body composition results show that she has lost 8.8 pounds (4 kg) of body fat and 1.1 pounds (0.5 kg) of lean body mass. Which of the following is the personal trainer's primary concern?

   A. The rate of weight loss is too rapid.

   B. The weight loss may suggest she is dehydrated.

   C. The weight loss may increase the risk of antiseizure medication side effects.

   D. There are no particular concerns as a result of this weight loss.

4. A client diagnosed with cerebral palsy has functional use of his legs. Which of the following modes of exercise requires the LEAST amount of supervision?

   A. treadmill walking

   B. stairstepper

   C. stationary bicycle

   D. elliptical trainer

Applied Knowledge Question

Fill in the chart to describe the general exercise contraindications and safety concerns for clients with spinal cord injuries (SCI), multiple sclerosis (MS), epilepsy, and cerebral palsy (CP).

Condition	Exercise contraindications	Safety concerns
SCI		
MS		
Epilepsy		
CP		

References

1. American College of Sports Medicine. 2007. Position stand. Exertional heat illness during training and competition. *Medicine and Science in Sports and Exercise* 39 (3): 556-572.

2. Anderson, M.A., and J.J. Laskin. 2009. Cerebral palsy. In: *ACSM's Resources for Clinical Exercise Physiology,* 2nd ed., J. Myers and D. Nieman, eds. Baltimore: Lippincott Williams & Wilkins. Chapter 2, pp. 19-33.

3. Ascherio, A., K.L. Munger, E.T. Lennette, D. Spiegelman, M.A. Hernan, M.J. Olek, S.E. Hankinson, and D.J. Hunter. 2001. Epstein-Barr virus antibodies and risk of multiple sclerosis. *Journal of the American Medical Association* 286: 3083-3088.

4. Bauman, W.A., and A.M. Spungen. 2000. Metabolic changes in persons after spinal cord injury. *Physical Medicine and Rehabilitation Clinics of North America* 11: 109-140.

5. Birk, T.J., E. Nieshoff, G. Gray, J. Steeby, and K. Jablonski. 2001. Metabolic and cardiopulmonary responses to acute progressive resistive exercise in a person with C4 spinal cord injury. *Spinal Cord* 39: 336-339.

6. Bjarnadottir, O.H., A.D Konradsdottir, K. Reynisdottir, and E. Olasfsson. 2007. Multiple sclerosis and brief moderate exercise. A randomized study. *Multiple Sclerosis* 13 (6): 776-782.

7. Bradley-Popovich, G.E., K.R. Abshire, C.M. Crookston, and G.G. Frounfelter. 2000. Resistance training in paraplegia: Rationale and recommendations. *Strength and Conditioning Journal* 22: 31-34.

8. Burkett, L.N., J. Chisum, W. Stone, and B. Fernhall. 1990. Exercise capacity of untrained spinal cord injured individuals and the relationship of peak oxygen uptake and level of injury. *Paraplegia* 28: 512-521.

9. Burnham, R.S., and R.D. Steadrand. 1994. Nerve entrapment in wheelchair athletes. *Archives of Physical Medicine and Rehabilitation* 75: 519-524.

10. Cerebral Palsy International Sports and Recreation Association. 1991. *Classification and Sports Rules Manual,* 5th ed. Nottingham, England: CPISRA.

11. Chad, K.E., D.A. Bailey, H.A. McKay, G.A. Zello, and R.E. Snyder. 1999. The effect of a weight-bearing physical activity program on bone mineral content and estimated volumetric density in children with spastic cerebral palsy. *Journal of Pediatrics* 135: 115-117.

12. Comi, G., L. Leocani, P. Rossi, and B. Columbo. 2001. Physiopathology and treatment of fatigue in multiple sclerosis. *Journal of Neurology* 248: 174-179.

13. Commission on Classification and Terminology of the International League Against Epilepsy. 1981. Proposal for revised classification of epilepsies and epileptic seizures. *Epilepsia* 22: 389-399.

14. Commission on Classification and Terminology of the International League Against Epilepsy. 1989. Proposal for revised clinical and electroencephalopathic classification of epileptic seizures. *Epilepsia* 22: 489-501.

15. Curtis, K.A., T.M. Tyner, L. Zachary, G. Lentell, D. Brink, T. Didyk, K. Gean, J. Hall, M. Hooper, J. Klos, S. Lesina, and B. Pacillas. 1999. Effect of a standard exercise protocol on shoulder pain in long-term wheelchair users. *Spinal Cord* 37: 421-429.

16. Dalgas, U., E. Stenager, and T. Ingemann-Hansen. 2008. Multiple sclerosis and physical exercise: Recommendations for the application of resistance, endurance, and combined training. *Multiple Sclerosis* 14 (1): 35-53.

17. Damiano, D.L., and M.F. Abel. 1998. Functional outcomes of strength training in spastic cerebral palsy. *Archives of Physical Medicine and Rehabilitation* 79: 119-125.

18. Damiano, D.L., C.L. Vaughn, and M.F. Abel. 1995. Muscle response to heavy resistance training in spastic cerebral palsy. *Developmental Medicine and Child Neurology* 75: 658-671.

19. Davis, G.M. 1993. Exercise capacity of individuals with paraplegia. *Medicine and Science in Sports and Exercise* 25: 423-432.

20. Davis, G.M., and R.M. Glaser. 1990. Cardiorespiratory fitness following spinal cord injury. In: *Key Issues in Neurological Physiotherapy,* L. Ada and C. Canning, eds. Sydney: Butterworth-Heinemann. pp. 155-196.

21. Davis, G.M., and R.J. Shepard. 1988. Cardiorespiratory fitness in highly active versus less active paraplegics. *Medicine and Science in Sports and Exercise* 20: 963-968.

22. Davis, G.M., R.J. Shepard, and F.H.H. Leenen. 1987. Cardiac effects of short-term arm crank training in paraplegics: Echocardiographic evidence. *European Journal of Applied Physiology* 56: 90-96.

23. Davis, G.M., R.J. Shepard, and R.W. Jackson. 1981. Cardiorespiratory fitness and muscular strength in lower-limb disabled. *Canadian Journal of Applied Sport Sciences* 6: 159-165.

24. Davis, G.M., R.J. Shepard, and R.W. Jackson. 1991. Exercise capacity following spinal cord injury. In: *Cardiovascular and Respiratory Responses to Exercise in Health and Disease,* J.R. Sutton and R. Balnave, eds. Sydney: University of Sydney. pp. 179-192.

25. Davis, G.M., S.J. Tupling, and R.J. Shepard. 1986. Dynamic strength and physical activity in wheelchair users. In: *1984 Olympic Scientific Congress—Sports and Disabled Athletes,* C. Sherrill, ed. Champaign, IL: Human Kinetics. pp. 139-148.

26. Durstine, J.L. 2002. *ACSM's Exercise Management for Persons with Chronic Diseases and Disabilities,* 2nd ed. Champaign, IL: Human Kinetics.

27. Ferrara, M.S., W.E. Buelly, B.C. McCann, T.S. Limbird, J.W. Powell, and R. Robl. 1992. The injury experience of the competitive athlete with a disability: Prevention implications. *Medicine and Science in Sports and Exercise* 24: 184-188.

28. Ferrara, M., and J. Laskin. 1997. Cerebral palsy. In: *ACSM's Exercise Management of Persons with Chronic Diseases and Disabilities,* J.L. Durstine, ed. Champaign, IL: Human Kinetics. pp. 206-211.

29. Figoni, S.F. 1986. Circulorespiratory effects of arm training and detraining in one C5-6 quadriplegic man. *Physical Therapy* 66: 779.

30. Figoni, S.F. 1993. Exercise responses and quadriplegia. *Medicine and Science in Sports and Exercise* 25: 433-441.

31. Figoni, S.F. 1997. Spinal cord injury. In: *ACSM's Exercise Management for Persons with Chronic Diseases and Disabilities,* 1st ed., J.L. Durstine, ed. Champaign, IL: Human Kinetics. pp. 175-179.

32. Figoni, S.F., R.A. Boileau, B.H. Massey, and J.R. Larsen. 1988. Physiological responses of quadriplegics and able-bodied men during exercise at the same oxygen uptake. *Adapted Physical Activity Quarterly* 5: 130-139.

33. Figoni, S.F., C.G. Gupta, and R.M. Glaser. 1999. Effects of posture on arm exercise performance of adults with tetraplegia. *Clinical Exercise Physiology* 1: 74-85.

34. Figoni, S.F., B.J. Kiratli, and R. Sasaki. 2009. Spinal cord dysfunction. In: *ACSM's Resources for Clinical Exercise Physiology,* 2nd ed., J. Myers and D. Nieman, eds. Baltimore: Lippincott Williams & Wilkins. pp. 58-78.

35. Franklin, B.A., K.I. Swentek, K. Grais, K.S. Johnston, S. Gordon, and G.C. Timmis. 1990. Field test of maximum oxygen consumption in wheelchair users. *Archives of Physical Medicine and Rehabilitation* 71: 574-578.

36. Gates, J.R., and R.H. Spiegel. 1993. Epilepsy, sports, and exercise. *Sports Medicine* 15: 1-5.

37. Hjentnes, N. 1977. Oxygen uptake and cardiac output in graded arm exercise in paraplegics with low level spinal lesions. *Scandinavian Journal of Rehabilitation Medicine* 9: 107-113.

38. Hjentnes, N. 1984. Control of medical rehabilitation of para and tetraplegics by repeated evaluation of endurance capacity. *International Journal of Sports Medicine* 5: 171-174.

39. Hutzler, Y.A., A. Chacham, U. Bergman, and I. Reches. 1998. Effects of a movement and swimming program on water orientation skills and self-concept of kindergarten children with cerebral palsy. *Perceptual and Motor Skills* 86: 111-118.

40. Hutzler, Y., A. Chacham, U. Bergman, and A. Szeinberg. 1998. Effects of a movement and swimming program on vital capacity and water orientation skills of children with cerebral palsy. *Developmental Medicine and Child Neurology* 40: 176-178.

41. Jackson, K., and J. Mulcare. 2009. Multiple sclerosis. In: *ACSM's Resources for Clinical Exercise Physiology,* 2nd ed., J. Myers and D. Nieman, eds. Baltimore: Lippincott Williams & Wilkins. pp. 34-43.

42. Jackson, R.W., G.M. Davis, P.R. Kofsky, R.J. Shepard, and G.C.R. Keene. 1981. Fitness levels in lower limb disabled. *Transactions of the 27th Annual Meeting of the Orthopedic Society* 6: 12-14.

43. Kammerman, S., and L. Wasserman. 2001. Seizure diagnosis: Part 1. Classification and diagnosis. *Western Journal of Medicine* 175: 99-103.

44. Kammerman, S., and L. Wasserman. 2001. Seizure disorders: Part 2. Treatment. *Western Journal of Medicine* 175: 184-188.

45. Kilef, J., and A. Ashburn. 2005. A pilot study of the effect of aerobic exercise on people with moderate disability multiple sclerosis. *Clinical Rehabilitation* 19: 165-169.

46. Kofsky, P.R., G.M. Davis, G.C. Jackson, C.R. Keene, and R.J. Shepard. 1983. Field testing: Assessment of physically disabled adults. *European Journal of Applied Physiology* 15: 109-120.

47. Kofsky, P.R., R.J. Shepard, G.M. Davis, and R.W. Jackson. 1986. Classification of aerobic power and muscular strength for disabled individuals with differing patterns of habitual physical activity. In: *1984 Olympic Scientific Congress—Sports and Disabled Athletes.* Champaign, IL: Human Kinetics. pp. 147-156.

48. Korczya, A.D. 1979. Participation of epileptic patients in sports. *Journal of Sports Medicine* 19: 195-198.

49. Laskowski, E.R. 1994. Strength training in the physically challenged population. *Strength and Conditioning* 16: 66-69.

50. Liaw, M.Y., A.C. Lin, P.T. Cheng, M.K. Wong, and F.T. Tang. 2000. Resistive inspiratory muscle training: Its effectiveness in patients with acute complete cervical cord injury. *Archives of Physical Medicine and Rehabilitation* 81: 752-756.

51. Linn, W.S., A.M. Spungen, H. Gong Jr., R.H. Adkins, W.A. Bauman, and R.L. Waters. 2001. Forced vital capacity in two large outpatient populations with chronic spinal cord injury. *Spinal Cord* 39: 263-268.

52. McCullagh, R., A.P. Fitzgerald, R.P. Murphy, and G. Cooke. 2008. Long-term benefits of exercising on quality of life and

fatigue in multiple sclerosis patients with mild disability: A pilot study. *Clinical Rehabilitation* 22 (3): 206-214.

53. McLean, K.P., P.P. Jones, and J.S. Skinner. 1995. Exercise prescription for sitting and supine exercise in individuals with tetraplegia. *Medicine and Science in Sports and Exercise* 27: 15-21.

54. McLean, K.P., and J.S. Skinner. 1995. Effect of training position on outcomes of an aerobic training study on individuals with quadriplegia. *Archives of Physical Medicine and Rehabilitation* 76: 139-150.

55. Mellett, C.J., A.C. Johnson, P.J. Thompson, and D.R. Fish. 2001. The relationship between participation in common leisure activities and seizure occurrence. *Acta Neurologica Scandinavica* 103: 300-303.

56. Mulcare, J.A. 2002. Multiple sclerosis. In: *ACSM's Exercise Management for Persons with Chronic Diseases and Disabilities,* J.L. Durstine, ed. Champaign, IL: Human Kinetics. pp. 267-272.

57. Myers, J., W. Herbert, and R. Humphrey, eds. 2002. *ACSM's Resources for Clinical Exercise Physiology: Musculoskeletal, Neuromuscular, Neoplastic, Immunologic, and Hematologic Conditions,* 1st ed. Baltimore: Lippincott Williams & Wilkins.

58. Nakken, K.O. 1999. Physical exercise in outpatients with epilepsy. *Epilepsia* 40: 643-651.

59. Nakken, K.O., P.G. Bjorholt, S.L. Johannssen, T. Loyning, and E. Lind. 1990. Effect of physical training on aerobic capacity, seizure occurrence, and serum level of antiepileptic drugs in adults with epilepsy. *Epilepsia* 31: 88-94.

60. Nakken, K.O., and R. Lossius. 1993. Seizure-related injuries in multihandicapped patients with therapy-resistant epilepsy. *Epilepsia* 34: 846-850.

61. Nash, M.S., S. Bilsker, and A.E. Marcillo. 1991. Reversal of adaptive left ventricular atrophy following electrically stimulated exercise training in human tetraplegics. *Paraplegia* 29: 590-599.

62. National Institute of Neurological Disorders and Stroke (NINDS), National Institutes of Health. Multiple sclerosis: Hope through research. Updated July 1, 2010. www.ninds.nih.gov/disorders/multiple_sclerosis/detail_multiple_sclerosis.htm. Accessed October 20, 2010.

63. Neal, E.G., H. Chaffe, R.H. Schwartz, et al. 2008. The ketogenic diet for the treatment of childhood epilepsy: A randomized controlled trial. *Lancet Neurology* 7: 500-506.

64. Newman, M.A., H. Dawes, M. van den Berg, D.T. Ward, et al. 2007. Can aerobic treadmill training reduce the effort of walking and fatigue in people with multiple sclerosis: A pilot study. *Multiple Sclerosis* 13 (1): 113-119.

65. Noseworthy, J.H., C. Lucchinetti, M. Rodriguez, and B.G. Weinshenker. 2000. Multiple sclerosis. *New England Journal of Medicine* 343: 938-952.

66. Ogyniemi, A.O., M.R. Gomez, and D.K. Klass. 1988. Seizures induced by exercise. *Neurology* 38: 633-634.

67. Oligati, R., J.M. Burgunder, and M. Mumenthaler. 1988. Increased energy cost of walking in multiple sclerosis: Effect of spasticity, ataxia, and weakness. *Archives of Physical Medicine and Rehabilitation* 69: 846-849.

68. Oligati, R., J. Jacquet, and P.E. Di Prampero. 1986. Energy cost of walking and exertional dyspnea in multiple sclerosis. *American Review of Respiratory Disease* 134: 1005-1010.

69. Peck, D.M., and D.B. McKeag. 1994. Athletes with disabilities: Removing barriers. *Physician and Sportsmedicine* 24: 59-62.

70. Petajan, J.H., E. Gappmaier, A.T. White, M.K. Spencer, I. Mino, and R.W. Hicks. 1996. Impact of aerobic training on fitness and quality of life in multiple sclerosis. *Annals of Neurology* 39: 432-441.

71. Petajan, J.H., and A.T. White. 1999. Recommendations for physical activity in patients with multiple sclerosis. *Sports Medicine* 27: 179-191.

72. Peterson, C. 2001. Exercise in 94 degrees F water for a patient with multiple sclerosis. *Physical Therapy* 81: 1049-1058.

73. Phillips, W.T., B.J. Kiratli, M. Sarkarati, G. Weraarchakul, J. Myers, B.A. Franklin, I. Parkash, and V. Froelicher. 1998. Effect of spinal cord injury on the heart and cardiovascular fitness. *Current Problems in Cardiology* 23: 649-704.

74. Ponichtera-Mulcare, J.A. 1993. Exercise and multiple sclerosis. *Medicine and Science in Sports and Exercise* 25: 451-465.

75. Poser, C.M., D.W. Paty, and L. Scheinberg. 1983. New diagnostic criteria for multiple sclerosis: Guidelines for research protocols. *Annals of Neurology* 13: 227-231.

76. Rampello, A., M. Franceschini, M. Piepoli, R. Antenucci, et al. 2007. Effect of aerobic training on walking capacity and maximal exercise tolerance in patients with multiple sclerosis: A randomized crossover controlled study. *Physical Therapy* 5: 545-555.

77. Romberg, A., A. Virtanen, J. Ruutiainen, S. Aunola, et al. 2004. Effects of a 6-month exercise program on patients with multiple sclerosis: A randomized study. *Neurology* 63: 2034-2038.

78. Sadovnick, A.D., P.A. Baird, and R.H. Ward. 1988. Multiple sclerosis: Updated risks for relatives. *American Journal of Medical Genetics* 29: 533-541.

79. Schmitt, B., L. Thun-Hohenstein, L. Vontobel, and E. Boltshauser. 1994. Seizures induced by physical exercise: Report of two cases. *Neuropediatrics* 25: 51-53.

80. Scholtes, V.A., A.J. Dallmeijer, E.A. Rameckers, et al. 2008. Lower limb strength training in children with cerebral palsy: A randomized controlled trial protocol for functional strength training based on progressive resistance exercise principles. *BMC Pediatrics* 8: 41-48.

81. Snook, E.M., and R.W. Moti. 2009. Effect of exercise training on walking mobility in multiple sclerosis: A meta-analysis. *Neurorehabilitation and Neural Repair* 23 (2): 108-116.

82. Sopka, C. 1998. Sports medical concerns for conditioning athletes with disabilities. *Strength and Conditioning* 20: 24-31.

83. Spiegel, R.H., and J.R. Gates. 1997. Epilepsy. In: *ACSM's Exercise Management for Persons with Chronic Diseases and Disabilities,* J.L. Durstine, ed. Champaign, IL: Human Kinetics. pp. 185-188.

84. Sutherland, G.J., and M.B. Anderson. 2001. Exercise and multiple sclerosis: Physiological, psychological, and quality of life issues. *Journal of Sports Medicine and Physical Fitness* 41: 421-432.

85. Svenson, B., B. Gerdle, and J. Elert. 1994. Endurance training in patients with multiple sclerosis: Five case studies. *Physical Therapy* 74: 1017-1026.

86. Tantucci, C., M. Massucci, R. Piperno, V. Grassi, and C.A. Sorbini. 1996. Energy cost of exercise in multiple sclerosis patients with low degree of disability. *Multiple Sclerosis* 2: 161-167.

87. Turk, M.A., C.A. Geremski, P.F. Rosenbaum, and R.J. Weber. 1997. The health status of women with cerebral palsy. *Archives of Physical Medicine and Rehabilitation* 78: S10-17.

88. United Cerebral Palsy, UCP Net. Cerebral palsy – facts & figures. www.ucp.org/ucp_generaldoc.cfm/1/3/43/43-43/447. Accessed November 1, 2010.

89. Van Drongelen, S., L.H. van der Woude, T.W. Janssen, E.L. Angenot, E.K. Chadwiock, and D.H. Veeger. 2005. Glenohumeral contact forces and muscle forces evaluated in wheelchair-related activities of daily living in able-bodied

subjects versus subjects with paraplegia and tetraplegia. *Archives of Physical Medicine and Rehabilitation* 86 (7, July): 1434-1440.

90. Verschuren, O., M. Ketelaar, J.W. Gorter, et al. 2007. Exercise training program in children and adolescents with cerebral palsy: A randomized controlled trial. *Archives of Pediatrics and Adolescent Medicine* 161: 1075-1081.

91. White, A.T., T.E. Wilson, S.L. Davis, and J.H. Petajen. 2000. Effect of precooling on physical performance in multiple sclerosis. *Multiple Sclerosis* 6: 176-180.

92. White, L.J., S.C. McCoy, V. Castellano, G. Gutierez, et al. 2004. Resistance training improves strength and functional capacity in persons with multiple sclerosis. *Multiple Sclerosis* 10 (6): 668-674.

93. Winnich, J.P., and F.X. Short. 1984. The physical fitness of youngsters with spinal neuromuscular conditions. *Adapted Physical Activity Quarterly* 1: 37-51.

94. Wise, J.B. 1996. Weight training for those with physical disabilities at Idaho State University. *Strength and Conditioning* 18: 67-71.

95. Yamasaki, M., K.T. Kim, S.W. Choi, S. Muraki, M. Shiokawa, and T. Kurokawa. 2001. Characteristics of body heat balance of paraplegics during exercise in a hot environment. *Journal of Physiological Anthropology in Applied Human Sciences* 20: 227-232.

Additional Resources

Cerebral Palsy Research Foundation
5111 East 21st St.
Wichita, KS 67208
www.cprf.org

Epilepsy Foundation of America
8301 Professional Pl.
Landover, MD 20785
www.epilepsyfoundation.org

JAMA Patient Page: Multiple Sclerosis
Journal of the American Medical Association
http://jama.ama-assn.org/cgi/content/
full/293/4/514

Multiple Sclerosis: MedlinePlus Interactive Health Tutorial
www.nlm.nih.gov/medlineplus/tutorials/
multiplesclerosis/htm/index.htm

Multiple Sclerosis Association of America
706 Haddonfield Rd.
Cherry Hill, NJ 08002
webmaster@msaa.com
www.msassociation.org
856-488-4500
800-532-7667

National Institute of Neurological Disorders and Stroke
National Institutes of Health
Bethesda, MD 20892
www.ninds.nih.gov

National Multiple Sclerosis Society
733 Third Ave.
3rd Floor
New York, NY 10017-3288
nat@nmss.org
www.nationalmssociety.org
212-986-3240
800-344-4867 (FIGHTMS)

National Spinal Cord Injury Association
www.spinalcord.org

Neurology Patient Page: Multiple Sclerosis
www.neurology.org/content/68/9/E9.full

23

Resistance Training for Clients Who Are Athletes

David R. Pearson, PhD, and John F. Graham, MS

After completing this chapter, you will be able to

- understand how to apply overload and specificity to a resistance training program for a client who is training for a sport;

- understand the value, role, and application of a periodized training program;

- describe the cycles and phases of a periodized training program;

- understand how load and repetitions are manipulated in a linear and a nonlinear periodization model; and

- design a linear and a nonlinear periodization program.

Personal trainers have the opportunity to work with a large variety of client types. Many clients have sedentary lifestyles with limited recreational pursuits and are sometimes deconditioned to the extent that they develop cardiovascular or metabolic medical conditions. On the opposite end of the wellness continuum, some clients are very physically active, both in their jobs and in their personal time, and have competition-laced goals and aspirations. The training needs of these athletic clients are much different from those of the general population. Building upon the basic resistance training program design principles detailed in chapter 15, this chapter describes how to develop a more advanced periodized program that will help clients who are athletes meet their competitive goals.

Factors in Program Design

Resistance training programs have been used for many years as an integral part of a total exercise program to enhance athletic performance. During the past two decades, the effectiveness of carefully planned resistance training programs as a method of improving body development and sport performance has been accepted on the basis of the scientific literature (1, 2, 21, 22, 30, 35, 36). Significant benefits can

The text for this chapter has been adapted from D. Pearson, A. Faigenbaum, M. Conley, and W.J. Kraemer, 2000, "National Strength and Conditioning Association's Basic Guidelines for the Resistance Training of Athletes," *Strength and Conditioning Journal* 22 (4): 14-27; and J.F. Graham, 2002, "Periodization Research and an Example Application," *Strength and Conditioning Journal* 24 (6): 62-70.

be gained from the systematic and proper application of the overload and specificity principles, the two primary tenets of resistance training. Combined with the principles of periodization needed to optimize the exercise stimulus, resistance training provides one of the most potent and effective methods to increase muscular performance capabilities, improve sport performance, and help to prevent injury (9, 13, 35).

Overload Principle

The overload principle is based on the concept that the athlete must adapt to the demands of greater physiological challenges to the neuromuscular system. Thus, the training stress or loads placed on the muscles must be progressively increased for gains to occur (13, 30, 35). As explained in chapter 15, the personal trainer can apply overload by increasing the amount of weight lifted in an exercise, incorporating more workouts in a week, including more (or more difficult) exercises, or adding sets to one or more exercises in a workout.

Specificity of Training

Specificity refers to the fact that specific methods of training produce specific changes or results. In particular, the more similar the training activity is to the actual sport movement, the greater the likelihood of a positive transfer to that sport (3, 8, 14, 17, 18, 24, 34). Although athletes may enhance their speed and power with a non-sport-specific program (27), the most effective program will match the metabolic and biomechanical characteristics of the training program to the sport activity. This level of specificity will train the appropriate metabolic systems by including exercises that duplicate the joint velocities and angular movements of the sport. Therefore, the personal trainer should design the resistance training program to include at least one exercise that mimics the movement pattern of each primary skill of the athlete's sport (see table 23.1 for examples).

Although an increase in 1-repetition maximum (1RM) strength is a common outcome of all programs that involve lifting heavy loads, improving an athlete's ability to generate force at very rapid speeds requires training at high velocities (16). Thus, improving a 1RM by conventional slow-velocity heavy resistance training does not ensure the improvement of force development in ballistic sport movements (e.g., basketball jump shot, baseball pitch, volleyball spike). Instead, the personal trainer should select power exercises and assign

moderate loads to allow the athlete to perform the movements explosively (3).

> The more similar the training activity is to the actual sport movement, the greater the likelihood of a positive transfer to that sport. Therefore, the personal trainer should design the resistance training program to include at least one exercise that mimics the movement pattern of each primary skill of the athlete's sport.

Periodization of Resistance Training

One of the most important developments in the theory of sport training has been the advancement of concepts related to periodization. **Periodization** is the systematic process of planned variations in a resistance training program over a training cycle (12, 13, 30, 35). The primary goals of periodization are met by appropriately manipulating volume and intensity and by effectively selecting exercises. A significant amount of research has shown that this concept optimizes training adaptations (10, 20). One of the primary advantages of this training approach is the reduced risk of overtraining due to the purposeful time devoted to physical and mental recovery (13, 23, 30). Typically only core exercises are periodized, but all exercises can be varied for intensity and volume (13, 29, 30, 35).

> Periodization is the systematic process of planned variations in a resistance training program over a training cycle.

Cycles and Phases

Periodized programs are typically divided into three distinct cycles. The **macrocycle** is the largest division, which typically constitutes an entire training year but may also be a period of up to four years (e.g., for an Olympic athlete). Macrocycles typically comprise two or more **mesocycles** divided into several weeks to a few months. The number of mesocycles is dependent on the goals of the athlete and, if applicable, the number of sport competitions contained within the period. Each mesocycle is divided into **microcycles** that can range from one week to four weeks, which include daily and weekly training variations (5, 6, 7, 11, 13, 30, 32).

TABLE 23.1 Examples of Sport-Specific Exercises

Sport skill	Related sport-specific exercises*
Ball dribbling and passing	Chest pass, reverse curl, close-grip bench press, triceps pushdown, depth push-up
Ball kicking	Split squat, split squat jump, cable hip abduction, cable hip adduction, leg raise
Freestyle swimming	Lat pulldown, forward lunge, bent over lateral raise, standing long jump, double-leg vertical jump
Jumping	Power clean, jerk, back squat, power snatch, double-leg tuck jump, jump to box, front barrier hop
Racket stroke	Dumbbell fly, reverse fly, wrist curl, reverse wrist curl, wrist supination, wrist pronation
Rowing	Angled leg press, low pulley row, barbell bent-over row, double-leg tuck jump, bent knee sit-up, 45-degree sit-up
Running/Sprinting	Lunge, box step-up, single-leg straight-leg deadlift, power clean, butt kicker, stationary arm swing, downhill sprint, partner-assisted towing, uphill sprint, partner-resisted sprinting
Throwing/Pitching	Dumbbell pullover, triceps extension, front raise, shoulder internal/external rotation

*This is not an exhaustive list: Many sport-specific exercises can be included.

Adapted by permission from NSCA 2000.

In 1981, Stone and colleagues (31) in the United States developed an American model for strength and power sports by modifying the periodization program that had been created by the Soviet Union and Eastern European countries (35, 36). This approach divides a resistance training program into five mesocycles, each with a primary goal or focus:

- **Hypertrophy phase:** to develop a muscular and metabolic base for more intense future training using a resistance training program that includes sport-specific or non-sport-specific exercises performed at a high volume and a low intensity

- **Strength phase:** to increase maximal muscle force by following a resistance training program that focuses on sport-specific exercises of moderate volume and intensity

- **Strength/Power phase:** to increase the speed of force development and power by integrating sport-specific power/explosive exercises of low volume and high intensity

- **Competition or peaking phase:** to attain peak strength and power by performing a very high-intensity and very low-volume sport-specific resistance training program

- **Active rest phase:** to allow physiological and mental recovery through limited low-volume and low-intensity resistance training or the performance of physical activities unrelated to one's sport

It has been found that people can achieve greater strength and power gains by repeating this set of five mesocycles more than once per year (13, 30). The concept of variation is a vital factor that explains the advantage of performing the entire set of training phases *three* times in a single year instead of only once (13, 30).

Variation in Exercise Selection

Empirical evidence suggests that variations in exercise selection for the same muscle group result in greater increases in strength and power than a program with no variation in exercises. This does not mean that the personal trainer needs to vary the exercises performed in every training session or that all exercises must be changed when one change is made. However, changes in exercises may be made every two or three weeks, or some exercises can be varied on an every other training session basis (i.e., with two somewhat different training sessions performed alternately). Still, certain core exercises need to be maintained throughout the training program so that progress in the major exercises can be continuously made (25).

> Variations in exercise selection for the same muscle group result in greater increases in strength and power than a program with no variation in exercises.

Linear and Nonlinear Models of Periodized Resistance Training

The classic periodization model is generally a linear program; that is, training intensity gradually and continually increases, and training volume gradually and continually decreases from one mesocycle to the next. If there is variation in the loading within the week or microcycle, the number of sets and repetitions for a given exercise does not change across the workouts. A variation on the linear model involves within-the-week or microcycle vacillations in both the assigned training load and the training volume for most (or all) core exercises. This type of periodization model is referred to as **undulating** (or *nonlinear*) (4, 13, 28).

Linear Periodization Model

For the linear model, weekly fluctuations in the core exercises occur such that the repetition maximum level (RM) training (i.e., 100% of the assigned training load) is performed on one day (referred to as the *heavy day*). Subsequent training in the same week for the same exercise is performed at a light level (10-30% lighter loads than on the RM day), or a moderate or medium level (5-10% lighter loads than the RM day), or both (depending on whether there are two or three workouts in a week)—all with the same set and repetition assignments. (Refer to the section "Within-Week Variation" on p. 370 for further explanation.) An example of a linear program (although it shows only one week) is the "Sample Muscular Strength Program" in chapter 15 (table 15.23). The light day loads are only 80% of the full "heavy day" RM loads, but the number of sets and repetitions (i.e., volume) remains the same across the workouts. Advancing a linearly periodized program involves a gradual increase in intensity over multiple weeks (or microcycles) of training. Usually

the length of time devoted to a particular intensity load ranges from two to four weeks. The program ends with an active rest phase prior to the start of another complete training cycle or an in-season (competitive) period.

> A linear periodization program involves gradual and continual increases in training intensity and gradual and continual decreases in training volume from one mesocycle to the next, but no variation in the assigned number of sets and repetitions within each mesocycle.

Sample Linear Periodization Program

Before starting the periodized program, the personal trainer should recommend that the athlete complete a lower-intensity four- to six-week base training program. This introductory program will allow the athlete to learn exercise technique, gain an initial adaptation to resistance exercise stress, and prepare for the first training cycle. Loads are typically very light (e.g., 15-20RMs). This base program is especially important for beginners and may or may not be used with experienced, trained athletes. A summary of the parameters of the linear periodization phases is included in table 23.2, and a sample program is shown in table 23.3.

- **Hypertrophy/Endurance phase.** This two- to four-week phase formally starts a periodized program. The personal trainer should direct the athlete to perform three to five sets

TABLE 23.2 Summary of the Program Design of a Linear Periodization Program (Core Exercises)

Phase	Length (weeks)	Sets	Goal (repetitions)	Rest period (time)	Assigned load
Hypertrophy	2-3	3-5	8-12	1 to 2 min	~75% 1RM 80%-100% 8RM-12RM
Strength	2-3	3-5	5-6	3 to 5 min	~85% 1RM 80%-100% 5RM-6RM
Strength/Power	2-3	3-5	3-4	2 to 3* min	90%-93% 1RM 80%-100% 3RM-4RM**
Competition	2-3	3-4	1-2	3 to 5 min	≥95% 1RM 80%-90% 1RM-2RM**
Active rest	1	No resistance training	No resistance training	No resistance training	No resistance training

1RM, maximum weight for one repetition; RM, maximum weight for assigned repetition number.
*Some exercises or situations may require up to a 5-min rest.
**The loads for power exercises (e.g., push press, power clean) may need to be reduced to permit explosive and rapid movements (consult chapter 15 for details about assigning loads for power exercises).
Based on Pearson et al. 2000 (26) and Graham 2002 (15).

TABLE 23.3 Sample Three-Day Linear Program

Phase	Week	Sets	Goal reps*	Rest period length (minutes)	Monday Heavy day 100% of the assigned training load	Wednesday Light day 80% of the assigned training load***	Friday Medium day 90% of the assigned training load***
Hypertrophy	1	3	12	1	67% 1RM; 100% 12RM	54% 1RM; 80% 12RM	60% 1RM; 90% 12RM
	2	3	10	1.5	75% 1RM; 100% 10RM	60% 1RM; 80% 10RM	68% 1RM; 90% 10RM
	3	4	8	1.5	80% 1RM; 100% 8RM	64% 1RM; 80% 8RM	72% 1RM; 90% 8RM
Strength	4	3	6	3*	85% 1RM; 100% 6RM	68% 1RM; 80% 6RM	77% 1RM; 90% 6RM
	5	4	5	3*	87% 1RM; 100% 5RM	70% 1RM; 80% 5RM	78% 1RM; 90% 5RM
	6	5	5	3*	87% 1RM; 100% 5RM	70% 1RM; 80% 5RM	78% 1RM; 90% 5RM
Strength/Power	7	3	4	3*	90% 1RM; 100% 4RM**	72% 1RM; 80% 4RM	81% 1RM; 90% 4RM
	8	4	3	3*	93% 1RM; 100% 3RM**	74% 1RM; 80% 3RM	84% 1RM; 90% 3RM
	9	5	3	3*	93% 1RM; 100% 3RM**	74% 1RM; 80% 3RM	84% 1RM; 90% 3RM
Competition	10	3	2	5	95% 1RM; 100% 2RM**	76% 1RM; 80% 2RM	86% 1RM; 90% 2RM
	11	4	2	5	95% 1RM; 100% 2RM**	76% 1RM; 80% 2RM	86% 1RM; 90% 2RM
	12	4	1	5	100% 1RM; 100% 1RM**	80% 1RM; 80% 1RM	90% 1RM; 90% 1RM
Active rest	13			No resistance training			

1RM, maximum weight for one repetition; RM, maximum weight for assigned repetition number. These guidelines apply to core exercises only. For the load assignments, refer to chapter 15 for an explanation of the relationship between a percent of 1RM and the number of repetitions that typically can be performed.

*Some exercises or situations may require up to 5-min rest.

**The loads for power exercises (e.g., push press, power clean) need to be somewhat lighter to permit rapid and explosive movements (see chapter 15).

***The athlete should complete the same number of goal repetitions—not more simply because the loads are lighter. This applies also to the power exercises whose loads were lightened from the heavy day assignments. The %1RMs shown for the light and medium days were calculated by multiplying the %1RMs of the heavy day by 0.80 and 0.90 (respectively).

Based on Pearson et al. 2000 (26) and Graham 2002 (15).

of each exercise at an intensity that allows 8 to 12 repetitions (about 75% 1RM) per set with a 1- to 2-minute rest period between sets and exercises. This will create a higher-volume, lower-intensity stimulus.

- **Strength phase.** Using the same length cycle of two to four weeks, the athlete performs three to five sets of five to six repetitions per exercise with an intensity of about 85% 1RM. A 3- to 5-minute rest period is allowed between sets and exercises.

- **Strength/Power phase.** For the next two to four weeks, the athlete performs exercises that allow only three or four repetitions for three to five sets at 90% to 93% 1RM. The personal trainer also includes power exercises (e.g., push press, power clean) with somewhat lighter loads (3) to permit rapid and explosive movements. A longer rest period between sets is recommended for adequate recovery.

- **Competition phase.** During a two- or three-week time period, the personal trainer further increases the load so that it allows only one or two repetitions at ≥95% 1RM (slightly lighter loads for power exercises [3]). The athlete performs three or four sets of each exercise with a 3- to 5-minute rest period between sets and exercises. This phase allows for the peaking of strength and power abilities, which is especially important for sports that require maximal strength and rapid force development.

- **Active rest phase.** At this point, the athlete moves into the competitive season after a week of active rest or formally completes a one- to three-week active rest period before returning to the hypertrophy phase to repeat the periodized program.

Nonlinear Periodization Model

A nonlinear periodization model varies the intensity (load) and volume of the core exercises throughout the week. This is in contrast to the linear periodization model that modulates the load but keeps the volume intact. For example, the intensity of a four-day program could be Monday, heavy; Tuesday, light; Thursday, power; and Friday, moderate. (The remaining days of the week are rest days.) This continues for a given time period before the athlete begins a competition period or a one- or two-week active rest phase.

> A nonlinear or undulating periodization program involves within-week or microcycle vacillations in the assigned training load and volume.

Sample Nonlinear Periodization Program

As recommended prior to the start of the linear periodization program, the athlete may need to complete a four- to six-week base training program that incorporates many repetitions with light loads (e.g., 15-20RMs) to reinforce proper exercise technique and provide a foundation for later phases. A nonlinear program can use the same time period as a linear periodization model (i.e., 12-16 weeks). The different training sessions are sequenced or rotated within a seven-day (or longer) microcycle. The characteristics of nonlinear periodization workouts are listed in table 23.4, and a sample program is shown in table 23.5.

- **Monday (heavy day).** This workout emphasizes muscular strength by assigning three or four sets of each exercise with a 3- to 6RM load. To promote recovery, the personal trainer should allow a 3- to 5-minute rest period.

- **Tuesday (light day).** The lighter loads of this workout permit more repetitions, but they are still repetition maximums (e.g., 10-15RMs). The athlete performs two to four sets of each exercise with a 1- to 2-minute rest period between sets and exercises.

- **Thursday (power day).** There are two load and repetition schemes for this workout, depending on the exercise. For power exercises, the athlete performs three or four sets of two to four repetitions with 30% to 60% 1RM to allow higher movement velocities; all other core exercises are assigned the same number of sets but at 2- to 4RMs. In addition, the personal trainer can include plyometric power exercises (e.g., with a medicine ball) to develop the power component in the training program of trained and experienced athletes. A 2- to 3-minute rest period between sets is recommended to allow adequate rest for the power exercises, but the 2- to 4RM sets may require additional recovery time.

- **Friday (moderate day).** This session uses loads 5% to 10% lighter than on the heavy day, or at least a sufficiently reduced intensity that allows 8 to 10 repetitions for two to four sets

TABLE 23.4 Summary of the Program Design of a Nonlinear Periodization Program (Core Exercises)

Phase	Sets	Goal repetitions	Rest period length	Assigned load
Heavy	3-4	3-6	3 to 4 min	85%-93% 1RM 90%-100% 3RM-6RM
Light	2-4	10-15	1 to 2 min	63%-75% 1RM 70%-80% 10RM-15RM
Power	3-4	2-4	2 to 3 min*	**Power exercises** 30%-60% 1RM** 50%-80% 2RM-4RM **Other core exercises** 90%-95% 1RM** 90%-100% 2RM-4RM
Moderate	2-4	8-10	1 to 2 min	75%-80% 1RM 80%-90% 8RM-10RM***

1RM, maximum weight for one repetition; RM, maximum weight for assigned repetition number.
*Some exercises or situations may require up to a 5-min rest.
**For power exercises, the personal trainer should assign loads at 30% to 60% 1RM or 60% to 80% RM to allow the athlete to perform them explosively (consult reference 3 for details about assigning loads for power exercises). Other core exercises should be assigned 2- to 4RM loads.
***Or loads 5% to 10% less than the heavy day loads.
Based on Graham 2002 (15).

of each exercise. A 1- to 2-minute rest period is recommended between sets and exercises.

An example of a three-day nonlinear periodization program is to perform five sets with a 3RM load on the first training day of the week (i.e., the heavy day), three sets with a 10RM load on the next training day (the light day), and four sets with a 6RM load on the last training day (the moderate day). Again, both the load and volume are modified throughout the week.

Effectiveness of Linear and Nonlinear Periodized Programs

The effectiveness of a periodized program is attributed to the systematic variation that allows the athlete to adequately recover from the assigned loads and repetitions. Often the nonlinear method of periodization is used so that training can continue through the season. This is especially important for sports with long seasons (e.g., tennis, wrestling, basketball, hockey). Typically, during the in-season program, the frequency of training is reduced and the volume of exercise is modulated in relation to the amount of competition and volume of sport practice. The key element of this type of training is the variation and ability to allow rest after a training or competition period (25).

Further, although some sources suggest that there is no difference (4), it appears that the nonlinear model is more effective at promoting muscular strength gains than the linear model (20, 28, 33). A probable reason is that the athlete is not exposed to continually greater training intensities. Instead, a nonlinear periodized program applies a training stress that contributes less to accumulated neural fatigue (19). Alternatively, the personal trainer will need to monitor a well-trained athlete who is following a nonlinear program because of the high relative loading; for example, even the light day involves RM loads (3).

> During the in-season, training frequency is reduced and the volume of exercise is modulated in relation to the number of competitive events and the volume of sport practice.

Conclusion

Since one type of workout will not benefit every athlete in the same way, a training program should blend existing exercise science knowledge (e.g., adhering to the specificity and overload principles) with the practical requirements of administering an individualized exercise program. To this end, a personal trainer can design a periodized resistance training program that meets the needs of the athlete and attends to the specific demands of that individual's sport.

TABLE 23.5 Sample Four-Day Nonlinear Periodization Program

Week	Day 1 Heavy day				Day 2 Light day				Day 3 Power day					Day 4 Moderate day			
	Sets	Goal reps	Rest (min)	Load	Sets	Goal reps	Rest (min)	Load	Sets	Goal reps	Rest** (min)	Load* (power)	Load* (other)	Sets	Goal reps	Rest (min)	Load***
1	3	6	4	85% 1RM 90% 6RM	2	15	1	65% 1RM 70% 15RM	3	4	3	30% 1RM 50% 4RM	90% 1RM 90% 4RM	2	10	1.5	75% 1RM 80% 10RM
2	3	6	4	85% 1RM 95% 6RM	3	15	1	65% 1RM 72.5% 15RM	3	4	3	32.5% 1RM 52.5% 4RM	90% 1RM 92.5% 4RM	3	10	1.5	75% 1RM 82.5% 10RM
3	4	6	4	85% 1RM 100% 6RM	3	15	1	65% 1RM 75% 15RM	4	4	3	35% 1RM 55% 4RM	90% 1RM 95% 4RM	3	10	1.5	75% 1RM 85% 10RM
4	3	5	5	87% 1RM 92.5% 5RM	4	15	1	65% 1RM 77.5% 15RM	4	4	3	37.5% 1RM 57.5% 4RM	90% 1RM 97.5% 4RM	4	10	1.5	75% 1RM 87.5% 10RM
5	3	5	5	87% 1RM 95% 5RM	4	15	1	65% 1RM 80% 15RM	4	4	3	40% 1RM 60% 4RM	90% 1RM 100% 4RM	4	10	1.5	75% 1RM 90% 10RM
6	4	5	5	87% 1RM 97.5% 5RM	2	12	1.5	67% 1RM 70% 12RM	3	3	3	45% 1RM 65% 3RM	93% 1RM 90% 3RM	2	9	2	77% 1RM 80% 9RM
7	4	5	5	87% 1RM 100% 5RM	3	12	1.5	67% 1RM 72.5% 12RM	3	3	3	47.5% 1RM 67.5% 3RM	93% 1RM 92.5% 3RM	2	9	2	77% 1RM 82.5% 9RM
8	3	4	5	90% 1RM 92.5% 4RM	3	12	1.5	67% 1RM 75% 12RM	4	3	3	50% 1RM 70% 3RM	93% 1RM 95% 3RM	3	9	2	77% 1RM 85% 9RM

9	3	4	5	90% 1RM / 95% 4RM	4	12	1.5	67% 1RM / 77.5% 12RM	4	3	3	52.5% 1RM / 72.5% 3RM	4	9	2	77% 1RM / 87.5% RM
10	4	4	5	90% 1RM / 97.5% 4RM	4	12	1.5	67% 1RM / 80% 12RM	4	3	3	55% 1RM / 75% 3RM	4	9	2	77% 1RM / 90% 9RM
11	4	4	5	90% 1RM / 100% 4RM	2	10	1.5	75% 1RM / 70% 10RM	3	2	3	50% 1RM / 70% 2RM	2	8	2	80% 1RM / 80% 8RM
12	3	3	5	93% 1RM / 92.5% 3RM	3	10	1.5	75% 1RM / 72.5% 10RM	3	2	3	52.5% 1RM / 72.5% 2RM	3	8	2	80% 1RM / 82.5% 8RM
13	3	3	5	93% 1RM / 95% 3RM	3	10	1.5	75% 1RM / 75% 10RM	4	2	3	55% 1RM / 75% 2RM	3	8	2	80% 1RM / 85% 8RM
14	4	3	5	93% 1RM / 97.5% 3RM	4	10	1.5	75% 1RM / 77.5% 10RM	4	2	3	57.5% 1RM / 77.5% 2RM	4	8	2	80% 1RM / 87.5% 8RM
15	4	3	5	93% 1RM / 100% 3RM	4	10	1.5	75% 1RM / 80% 10RM	4	2	3	60% 1RM / 80% 2RM	4	8	2	80% 1RM / 90% 8RM
16	Active rest															

1RM, maximum weight for one repetition; RM, maximum weight for assigned repetition number. These guidelines apply to core exercises only. For the load assignments, refer to chapter 15 for an explanation of the relationship between a percent of 1RM and the number of repetitions that can typically be performed.

*For power exercises, the personal trainer should assign loads at 30% to 60% 1RM or 60% to 80% RM to allow the athlete to perform them explosively. (For further information about determining training loads for power exercises, refer to reference 3). Other core exercises should be assigned 2 to 4RM loads.

**Some exercises or situations may require up to a 5-min rest.

***Or loads 5% to 10% less than the heavy day loads.

Based on Pearson et al. 2000 (26) and Graham 2002 (15).

Study Questions

1. Which of the following is the most sport-specific resistance training exercise for a volleyball player?
    A. push press
    B. lateral shoulder raise
    C. seated shoulder press
    D. leg press

2. Which of the following is organized from shortest to longest?
    A. mesocycle, microcycle, macrocycle
    B. macrocycle, microcycle, mesocycle
    C. microcycle, mesocycle, macrocycle
    D. microcycle, macrocycle, mesocycle

3. Which of the following is the order of the phases of a periodized program?
    I. strength/power
    II. hypertrophy
    III. active rest
    IV. competition
    V. strength

A. I, II, III, V, IV
B. IV, III, II, I, V
C. III, IV, II, V, I
D. II, V, I, IV, III

4. A personal trainer includes the back squat exercise in an athlete's linearly periodized resistance training program. What is the load for a medium training day if the athlete's 1RM is 400 pounds (182 kg) and the number of goal repetitions is four per set?
    A. 360 pounds (164 kg)
    B. 325 pounds (148 kg)
    C. 285 pounds (130 kg)
    D. 255 pounds (116 kg)

5. An athlete who is able to perform 225 pounds (102 kg) on the back squat exercise for a maximum of five repetitions would use which of the following if the workout called for him or her to perform back squats with 80% of his 5 RM?
    A. 5 repetitions with 225 pounds (102 kg)
    B. 1 repetition with 225 pounds (102 kg)
    C. 5 repetitions with 180 pounds (82 kg)
    D. 1 repetition with 180 pounds (82 kg)

Applied Knowledge Question

Use table 23.3 as a guide to fill in the chart with the assigned loads for the bench press exercise for a well-trained athlete's linearly periodized resistance training program. His 1RM is 195 pounds. (Remember to round *down*.) Assume there are no increases in the athlete's strength across all of the training phases, despite the fact that the athlete's 1RM would certainly improve over time. Also, refer to table 15.5 to determine the relationship between a percent of a 1RM and the number of repetitions that typically can be performed.

Phase	Week	Goal reps	Tuesday Heavy day	Thursday Light day	Saturday Medium day
Hypertrophy/ Endurance	1	12			
	2	10			
	3	8			
Strength	4	6			
	5	6			
	6	5			
Strength/ Power	7	4			
	8	4			
	9	3			
Competition	10	2			
	11	2			
	12	1			

References

1. American College of Sports Medicine. 1998. Position stand: The recommended quantity and quality of exercise for developing and maintaining cardiorespiratory and muscular fitness, and flexibility in healthy adults. *Medicine and Science in Sports and Exercise* 30 (6): 975-991.

2. Atha, J. 1981. Strengthening muscle. *Exercise and Sport Science Reviews* 9: 1-73.

3. Baechle, T.R. and R.W. Earle. 2008. Resistance training. In: *Essentials of Strength Training and Conditioning,* 3rd ed., T.R. Baechle and R.W. Earle, eds. Champaign, IL: Human Kinetics.

4. Baker, D., G. Wilson, and R. Carlyon. 1994. Periodization: The effect on strength of manipulating volume and intensity. *Journal of Strength and Conditioning Research* 8: 235-242.

5. Chargina, A., M.S. Stone, J. Piedmonte, H.S. O'Bryant, W.J. Kraemer, V. Gambetta, H. Newton, G. Palmeri, and D. Pfoff. 1986. Periodization roundtable. *National Strength and Conditioning Association Journal* 8 (5): 12-23.

6. Chargina, A., M.S. Stone, J. Piedmonte, H.S. O'Bryant, W.J. Kraemer, V. Gambetta, H. Newton, G. Palmeri, and D. Pfoff. 1987. Periodization roundtable. *National Strength and Conditioning Association Journal* 8 (6): 17-25.

7. Chargina, A., M.S. Stone, J. Piedmonte, H.S. O'Bryant, W.J. Kraemer, V. Gambetta, H. Newton, G. Palmeri, and D. Pfoff. 1987. Periodization roundtable. *National Strength and Conditioning Association Journal* 9 (1): 16-27.

8. Coyle, E.F., D.C. Feiring, T.C. Rotkis, R.W. Cote, F.B. Roby, W. Lee, and J.H. Wilmore. 1981. Specificity of power improvements through slow and fast isokinetic training. *Journal of Applied Physiology* 51: 1437-1442.

9. DeLorme, P. 1945. Restoration of muscle power by heavy resistance exercises. *Journal of Bone and Joint Surgery* 27: 645-667.

10. Fleck, S.J. 1999. Periodized strength training: A critical review. *Journal of Strength and Conditioning Research* 13 (1): 82-89.

11. Fleck, S.J., and W.J. Kraemer. 1988. Resistance training: Exercise prescription. *Physician and Sportsmedicine* 16: 69-81.

12. Fleck, S.J., and W.J. Kraemer. 1996. *Periodization Breakthrough!* Ronkonkoma, NY: Advanced Research Press.

13. Fleck, S.J., and W.J. Kraemer. 1997. *Designing Resistance Training Programs,* 2nd ed. Champaign, IL: Human Kinetics.

14. Gardner, G. 1963. Specificity of strength changes of the exercised and nonexercised limb following isometric training. *Research Quarterly* 34: 98-101.

15. Graham, J.F. 2002. Periodization research and an example application. *Strength and Conditioning Journal* 24 (6): 62-70.

16. Häkkinen, K., P.V. Komi, M. Alen, and H. Kauhanen. 1987. EMG, muscle fibre and force production characteristics during a 1 year training period in elite weightlifters. *European Journal of Applied Physiology* 56: 419-427.

17. Kanehisa, H., and M. Miyashita. 1983. Specificity of velocity in strength training. *European Journal of Applied Physiology* 52: 104-106.

18. Knapik, J.J., R.H. Mawdsley, and M.U. Ramos. 1983. Angular specificity and test mode specificity of isometric and isokinetic strength training. *Journal of Orthopedic and Sports Physical Therapy* 5: 58-65.

19. Komi, P.V. 1986. Training of muscle strength and power: Interaction of neuromotoric, hypertrophic, and mechanical factors. *International Journal of Sports Medicine* 7 (Suppl): 101-105.

20. Kraemer, W.J. 1997. A series of studies: The physiological basis for strength training in American football: Fact over philosophy. *Journal of Strength and Conditioning Research* 11 (3): 131-142.

21. Kraemer, W.J., M.R. Deschenes, and S.J. Fleck. 1988. Physiological adaptations to resistance exercise: Implications for athletic conditioning. *Sports Medicine* 6: 246-256.

22. Kraemer, W.J., S.J. Fleck, and W.J. Evans. 1996. Strength and power: Physiological mechanisms of adaptation. *Exercise and Sport Science Reviews* 24: 363-397.

23. Kraemer, W.J., and B.A. Nindl. 1998. Factors involved with overtraining for strength and power. In: *Overtraining in Athletic Conditioning.* Champaign, IL: Human Kinetics.

24. Moffroid, M.T., and R.H. Whipple. 1970. Specificity of speed of exercise. *Physical Therapy* 50: 1693-1699.

25. Pearson, D. 1997. Weight training. In: *Physical Education Handbook,* 9th ed., N. Schmottlach and J. McManama, eds. New York: Prentice Hall.

26. Pearson, D., A. Faigenbaum, M. Conley, and W.J. Kraemer. 2000. National Strength and Conditioning Association's basic guidelines for the resistance training of athletes. *Strength and Conditioning Journal* 22 (4): 14-27.

27. Pearson, D., and G. Gehlsen. 1998. Athletic performance enhancement: A study with college football players. *Strength and Conditioning* 20 (3): 70-73.

28. Poliquin, C. 1988. Five steps to increasing the effectiveness of your strength training program. *National Strength and Conditioning Association Journal* 10 (3): 34-39.

29. Sale, D.G., J.D. MacDougall, A.R.M. Upton, and A.J. McComas. 1983. Effects of strength training upon motor neuron excitability in man. *Medicine and Science in Sports and Exercise* 15: 57-62.

30. Stone, M.H., and H.S. O'Bryant. 1987. *Weight Training: A Scientific Approach.* Minneapolis: Burgess.

31. Stone, M.H., H.S. O'Bryant, and J. Garhammer. 1981. A hypothetical model for strength training. *Journal of Sports Medicine and Physical Fitness* 21: 342-351.

32. Stone, M.H., H.S. O'Bryant, J. Garhammer, J. McMillan, and R. Rozenek. 1982. A theoretical model of strength training. *National Strength Coaches Association Journal* 4 (4): 36-40.

33. Stone, M.H., J. Potteiger, K.C. Pierce, C.M. Proulx, H.S. O'Bryant, and R.L. Johnson. 1997. Comparison of the effects of three different weight training programs on the 1RM squat: A preliminary study. Presentation at the National Strength and Conditioning Association Conference, Las Vegas, NV, June.

34. Thepaut-Mathieu, C., J. Van Hoecke, and B. Maton. 1988. Myoelectrical and mechanical changes linked to length specificity during isometric training. *Journal of Applied Physiology* 64: 1500-1505.

35. Wathen, D., T.R. Baechle, and R.W. Earle. 2008. Periodization. In: *Essentials of Strength Training and Conditioning,* 3rd ed., T.R. Baechle and R.W. Earle, eds. Champaign, IL: Human Kinetics.

36. Zatsiorsky, V. 1995. *Science and Practice of Strength Training.* Champaign, IL: Human Kinetics.

PART VI

Safety and Legal Issues

Facility and Equipment Layout and Maintenance

Shinya Takahashi, PhD

After completing this chapter, you will be able to

- understand the facility design and planning process, facility specification guidelines, the exercise equipment selection process, and spacing requirements of a health and fitness facility;

- understand the special considerations given to equipment layout needs for a home exercise facility; and

- identify the appropriate maintenance and cleaning guidelines for all aspects of an exercise facility and the exercise equipment.

Essential components of personal training involve health risk appraisal, proper selection of fitness assessments, accurate administration of assessments and interpretation of the results, designing appropriate exercise programs, and safe and effective instruction and coaching. In addition, personal trainers are frequently responsible for design of a health and fitness facility, as well as the maintenance of exercise equipment used within the facility. This chapter discusses the topics of facility design and equipment layout and maintenance.

Facility Design and Planning

An effective facility design requires painstaking effort and a well-organized plan. Designing and planning a facility includes four main phases: predesign, design, construction, and preoperation (8). Before any of these phases begin, a facility design committee should be formed. The committee should consist of various levels of professionals including, but not limited to, administrators, facility management personnel, an architect, a contractor, a lawyer, a representative number of prospective users of the facility, and a personal trainer (8). These phases are commonly identified whether the committee is considering building a new facility or adding to or updating an existing facility.

The author would like to acknowledge the contributions of Mike Greenwood, who wrote this chapter for the first edition of *NCSA's Essentials of Personal Training*.

A personal trainer should be involved in the four major phases of designing and planning a health and fitness facility: predesign, design, construction, and preoperation.

Predesign Phase

In the predesign phase, the committee conducts a needs analysis and a feasibility study. The committee also creates a master plan, selects an architect, and outlines possible future expansion and alternative uses of the areas within the facility.

When conducting a needs analysis, the committee should ask the following questions (8, 11):

- Who are or will be the clientele of the facility?
- What is the maximum number of prospective users? What is an expected number of users for the first year and beyond?
- Where should the facility be located? What are the geographic characteristics of the location (e.g., downtown, residential, close to a busy street, near competitors)?
- What programs and services are needed?
- What is the available budget?
- What are the specific needs of the potential clientele?
- What is the main focus of the facility?
- Who supervises and keeps up the facility?
- When is the facility to be constructed and functionally operational?
- What is the expected longevity of the facility?

When the committee finds that a need exists, the next step is to conduct a feasibility study, which will determine whether the project should be undertaken. As part of the feasibility study, the committee determines the cost, facility location, program needs, and projected usage of the facility. A **SWOT analysis**—an analysis of strengths, weaknesses, opportunities, and threats—is often conducted as part of a feasibility study (8).

If the results of the needs analysis and feasibility study are positive, the committee develops a master plan, which will explain in detail the project goals and the procedures needed to achieve those goals. The committee should state the major objective of the new facility (11) and write minor objectives such as equipment requirements—how many and what types of cardiovascular, free weight, selectorized, testing, and rehabilitation equipment will be needed. As part of this process, the group will need to gather and analyze information on currently available equipment and facilities (11). If facility expansion is a main goal, this information should be especially useful when updates are necessary.

An architect should be selected, and the selection should be based on a bid process in which the committee evaluates costs and experience. An architect with excellent credentials and a strong work record should be selected (8).

As part of the process, the committee should consider future expansion or alternative uses of the areas within the facility. This could be a part of the master plan and might include future expansion sites within or next to the facility as well as alternate future usage of the projected rooms. A common mistake is to plan the facility based on current needs and not consider and plan for future needs (8, 20).

Design Phase

The design phase may take several months, and the final result should be a detailed blueprint of the new facility. The committee will accomplish the detailed blueprint of the facility design by working closely with an architect from the committee, and other various facility management, facility design, and health and fitness professionals, including a personal trainer. The design should take into account equipment and facility spacing and local health, safety, and legal codes.

Construction Phase

The construction phase takes the majority of the time. Throughout the construction phase, the facility design committee should monitor to ensure that the master plan and project deadlines are being fulfilled in a timely manner and also oversee the construction (8).

Preoperation Phase

Staffing and staff development for a facility are the focus of the preoperation phase. The following questions may need to be considered (8):

- How many staff members will the facility need (professional staff, part-time staff, maintenance staff, interns, etc.)?
- What level of qualifications will the job positions require?
- How will positions be advertised and staff recruited?
- What interview process will be used?
- How will staff be scheduled?
- How will the staff be trained?

Facility Specification Guidelines

Personal trainers should be familiar with the structural specifications of a health and fitness facility. The following are guidelines for the design of a health and fitness facility, first for the facility as a whole and then for the resistance training room in particular.

General Health and Fitness Facility Guidelines

Many guidelines apply to the facility as a whole, including the cardiovascular machine area, resistance training room, stretching area, and other fitness areas or rooms.

- *Passageways.* According to the Americans with Disabilities Act (ADA), passageway width must be at least 36 inches (91 cm) to accommodate wheelchairs (8, 21). Hallways and circulation passages need to be at least 60 inches (152 cm) in width (21). The floor should remain level through door entrances (i.e., the door threshold on the floor should not be raised above floor level). If the threshold exceeds 0.5 inches (1.3 cm), the facility must have a ramp or lift with a slope of 1 foot (30 cm) for every inch (2.5 cm) of elevation change to accommodate access to the facility (8). Emergency exit signage must be free of obstructions and have clear visibility (e.g., sufficient lighting) (8).

- *Natural lighting and windows.* Natural lighting tends to increase an exerciser's motivation (19), so it is desirable to locate cardiovascular machines next to or facing windows. An open feeling and natural lighting are positives for people doing aerobic exercise. However, if higher windows or skylights are installed, it is essential to carefully evaluate their location (14). If glare is a problem, it can be significantly reduced by window tinting, shades, or blinds.

- *Repair and maintenance shop.* It is desirable to locate a repair and maintenance shop adjacent to or near a fitness room (14) for convenience when large, heavy equipment needs to be transferred to the shop.

- *Water fountain.* The recommendation is to have a water fountain installed close to the entrance of the main fitness rooms or other convenient locations for the users to access. However, it should not be located where it could be a distraction to clients or block the flow of traffic. The ADA requires that all water fountains be installed at a height that can be reached by a person in a wheelchair (21).

- *Emergency–first aid kit and **automated external defibrillator (AED)**.* It is desirable to install an emergency–first aid kit, as well as an AED, within or near fitness rooms for immediate access. The AEDs in a facility should be located within a 1.5-minute walk of a potential incident site (21). The ADA requires all AED devices to be at a height that can be reached by a person in a wheelchair (21).

- *Background music and noise.* It is recommended that health and fitness facilities be designed to maintain background noise levels below 70 decibels and never exceed 90 decibels (21). In addition, the recommended time-weighted average (TWA) exposure for occupational noise is 85 decibels per 8-hour time period (17). An exposure at or above this level is considered hazardous. To provide balanced sound distribution for music, speakers should be installed high in all corners of the rooms (18). When a room has a high ceiling and noise disturbance is prominent, sound panel installation to reduce this problem may be considered. In the resistance training room, another source of noise is the weights themselves. Urethane-coated free weights are more expensive than metal weights but may significantly reduce the noise.

- *Electrical requirements.* It is generally recommended that a fitness facility have both 110- and 220-volt outlets because some types of cardiovascular equipment require 220-volt outlets (14). To ensure meeting the electrical requirements, planners must consult with manufacturing companies before making a final decision on the equipment to purchase. Additional outlets around fitness rooms would be convenient for vacuuming, scrubbing, and other purposes. In addition, ground-fault circuit interrupters are essential safety devices for automatically shutting down power in the event of an electrical short due to water or insulation problems (14, 21).

- *Temperature and humidity control.* A recommended temperature range for the strength and conditioning facility is 72 °F to 78 °F (22-26 °C) (2). Other temperature recommendations range between 68 °F and 72 °F (20-22 °C) (21). Temperature can vary dramatically depending on the structure of the facility as well as usage level (e.g., windows, doors, insulation, and number of exercisers). In addition, the amount of motorized equipment being used at the same time may affect the temperature. Therefore, a zone heating and cooling system may be the most cost-effective and user friendly (14). The capacity of the ventilation systems should be at least 8 to 10 air exchanges per hour, and an optimal range is 12 to 15 air exchanges per hour (14). Further, it is desirable to have a sufficient mix of external fresh air and recirculated internal air moving through the facility (8). Optimal air circulation may be achieved by ceiling fans. For example, two or more fans can facilitate air circulation in a 1,200-square-foot (111 m²) facility. The optimal humidity level of a fitness area is 50% or less and no higher than 60% (21). In addition, air fresheners can be used where excessive odor is present.

■ *Signage.* Signage should be installed to clearly display operational policies, facility rules, safety guidelines, entrances, exits, rest rooms, and so on (20, 21).

■ *Communication boards.* Communication boards or display monitors can be used to display information on upcoming events, announcements, and educational materials. These should be located near the front entrance of the facility where people can view them without blocking the flow of traffic.

■ *Telephones.* Telephones should be located in the supervisor's office for emergency purposes. Additional phones may be installed at the front entrance and should be mounted at a maximum height of 4 feet (1.2 m) to accommodate persons in a wheelchair (21).

■ *Suggestion box.* A comment and suggestion box may be placed near the main entrance of a health and fitness facility.

Resistance Training Room Guidelines

Resistance training rooms have unique characteristics that require following guidelines specific to them.

■ *Location of resistance training room.* An ideal location of a resistance training room is on the ground floor near locker rooms and a service entrance so that delivery of equipment to and from the resistance training room is convenient (14). It is desirable to locate a resistance training room away from areas that require privacy and minimal noise, such as classrooms, laboratories, computer rooms, libraries, or hotel guest rooms.

■ *Space for supervisors.* A supervisor's office is ideally located in the resistance training room so that the supervisor can view the entire room, or at least in the proximity of the resistance training room so that he or she is easily accessible. If the supervisor's office is located in the resistance training room, large windows with an unobstructed view (e.g., no large exercise equipment in front of the windows) are recommended.

■ *Staff-to-client ratios.* The recommended ratio between fitness staff and exercisers in a resistance training room is around 1:10 (1, 9, 14). It is recommended that middle school strength and conditioning facilities not exceed a 1:10 staff-to-athlete ratio, secondary school facilities should not exceed a 1:15 ratio, and facilities that serve athletes or clients older than secondary school should not exceed a 1:20 ratio (2).

■ *Ceiling height.* The desirable ceiling height for a resistance training room ranges from 12 to 14 feet or 3.7 to 4.3 m (14). A common mistake when selecting a ceiling height for a resistance training room is not allowing sufficient space for heating and cooling air ducts, light fixtures, utility cables, wires, and plumbing structures (14).

■ *Windows.* Windows in the resistance training room should be a minimum of 20 inches (51 cm) above the floor (14). This will help to decrease the chance of breakage from a rolling barbell plate or dumbbell. If possible, it is best to avoid placing windows where spotters or exercisers would be likely to lean against them (14).

■ *Doors.* It is desirable to have double doors with removable center posts for more convenient transfer of large, heavy exercise equipment in a resistance training room (14). In addition, when a major deep cleaning is scheduled the large opening to the resistance training room facilitates moving cleaning and exercise equipment in and out from the resistance training room.

■ *Lighting.* It is desirable for lighting to be brighter than would be required for a classroom or office (i.e., 50 foot-candles or 538 lux) in a resistance training room. The recommendation for lighting in the resistance training room is 75 to 100 foot-candles or 807 to 1,076 lux (16, 21). The ADA requires all light switches to be at a height accessible by a person in a wheelchair (21).

■ *Storage area.* A resistance training room requires more storage space than one might expect (8). Storage may be needed for cleaning supplies and equipment, staff apparel, towels, small equipment, and exercise equipment accessories.

■ *Mirrors.* Mirrors in the resistance training room should be installed at least 20 inches (51 cm) above the floor so that they are not damaged by barbell plates or dumbbells rolling against them or barbell plates leaning against them (the diameter of a typical 45-pound Olympic barbell plate is approximately 18 inches or 46 cm) (14). Dumbbell racks and all other weight equipment should be placed at least

6 inches (15 cm) away from the mirrors to decrease the chance of breakage (14). If dumbbell racks are located close to mirrors and may tend to get moved, it may be necessary to secure them (i.e., bolt them down). Protective rails or special protective padding can be anchored to the base of the wall or floor to help protect the mirrors (2).

There are benefits to having mirrors in the resistance training room. A mirror provides a client with immediate feedback during an exercise. In addition, it provides feedback to a personal trainer on exercise technique via blind side viewing of a client's body during an exercise. Mirrors are also motivational because clients can see improvements and changes in their physical characteristics. Furthermore, mirrors enhance the looks of the resistance training room and make it appear more spacious.

However, mirrors have potential negative effects as well. Clients can become distracted watching the mirror and fail to concentrate on proper exercise technique. Also, some clients do not want to see themselves in a mirror.

■ *Floor.* For flooring material in the resistance training room, carpet is the most inexpensive choice; carpets also come in a wide range of colors and have an attractive appearance (5). Interlocking rubber mats usually provide more cushion and durability than carpet; however, dirt, sand, and other debris are more likely to become trapped in the interlocking spaces between mats (13). Darker colors are typically recommended for a floor because they are less likely to show dirt and stains (5). Although a poured rubber surface is the most expensive choice, it is the best flooring option because it is seamless and provides more cushion and durability (13).

A wood floor is the best flooring choice for Olympic platforms because the smooth, flat surface provides better foot contact (2). The surface of a floor should have the proper level of shock absorption and traction to minimize the risk of high-impact- or fall-related injuries. A suspended floor or rubber mats are appropriate for plyometric exercises. Hard surfaces, including concrete, asphalt, tile, and hardwood floors, are not proper surfaces for high-impact activities (10). If a resistance training room is not located on the ground floor, a load-bearing capacity of at least 100 pounds per square foot (488 kg/m²) is desirable to accommodate heavier exercise equipment and to avoid any structural damage from dropped heavy weights (18, 20).

■ *Walls.* The walls of a resistance training room with high traffic flow or high activity must be free of obstructions such as extended bars, cables, light bulbs, broken or unsecured mirrors, shelves, and other fixtures (7).

> In order to provide a safe and effective exercise environment, personal trainers should be familiar with all aspects of health and fitness facility specifications.

Selecting Exercise Equipment

Evaluating exercise equipment for a health and fitness facility involves three phases: developing functional criteria for the equipment, evaluating the specifications and the effectiveness of the equipment, and evaluating the manufacturers' business practices (12). In addition to this process, two other planning tools are used—a tentative floor plan and a priority list (13). The tentative floor plan reflects all major and minor objectives of the facility design. It should also specify the types and amounts of equipment needed (13). The priority list should be developed based on the facility's needs analysis. The highest priority in any health and fitness facility is safety and prevention of injuries.

> Personal trainers should be involved in all three phases of the exercise equipment selection process: developing functional criteria, evaluating specifications and effectiveness, and evaluating the manufacturers' business practices.

Phase 1: Develop Functional Criteria for the Equipment

The first step in selecting exercise equipment is to develop criteria that meet users' functional needs for the equipment. When selecting resistance exercise equipment, it is critical to understand the mechanics of the equipment (e.g., cam system; leverage system; resistance systems including water pressure, air pressure, weight stacks, barbell plates, springs, hydraulic and electromagnetic equipment). In addition, planners should analyze the types of movements that will be used (e.g., dynamic constant external resistance [DCER], isokinetic single plane vs. multiplane, and isolateral and bilateral) before making a final decision.

On the other hand, when selecting cardiovascular equipment it is essential to consider choosing the most versatile and popular types of equipment (e.g., a treadmill can be used for various speeds of walking and running; some elliptical machines can change the stride lengths) to meet the needs of a variety of targeted populations.

Phase 2: Evaluate Specifications and Effectiveness of the Equipment

Based on the facility's needs analysis, the following questions can be used in the exercise equipment selection process.

- What age groups and fitness levels characterize the individuals who will be using the equipment?

- Are there any priorities to be considered for purchasing the exercise equipment (e.g., cardiovascular versus resistance training equipment)?

- Are there any unique selling points of the facility to be considered?

- How can color coordination be achieved?

- How much should the equipment cost?

- What is the warranty on the equipment?

- Does the company provide maintenance training sessions?

- Does the company provide periodic maintenance services?

- How fast can replacement parts for the equipment arrive?

For resistance training equipment, the following four specification categories should be considered.

- Structural materials (i.e., size and gauge of the steel)

- Connecting materials (e.g., welds, bolts, nuts, sleeves, collars, gaskets, washers, clamps)

- Materials that affect functionality (e.g., bearings, bushings, rails, pulleys, cables, belts, handles, springs, insulators, lubricators, paint, upholstery, plating, grinding, and filing).

It is critical to estimate how many pieces of equipment a health and fitness facility needs before making purchasing decisions. In most cases, cardiovascular equipment is an essential component of a health and fitness facility, and the decision on how many pieces of cardiovascular equipment are needed should be a first priority. In the fitness industry, there are no specific standards or guidelines for estimating the correct amount of cardiovascular equipment, but it is common practice to follow several steps. The first step is to determine how many members will be using the facility during any given 2-hour period, by taking 25%

of the total membership (21). The second step is to determine the total number of members who will be daily users, by taking 33% of the 25% figure arrived at in step 1. The third step uses a previously established standard for how many pieces of equipment the facility will have for a given number of daily users. For example, if the facility has established a standard of one piece of cardiovascular equipment for every five daily users, a facility that has 2,000 members should have a total of 33 cardiovascular machines.

To maximize the use of floor space, cordless cardiovascular equipment may be advantageous. Whereas equipment with a power cord is limited as to location, cordless equipment can be installed anywhere in the facility. Several manufacturers make an attachable TV monitor for cardiovascular equipment. Some offer computer consoles that display TV channels, connect to the Internet, and so on; these of course are more expensive. One can keep expenses lower by installing multiple large TV monitors on walls or hanging them from the ceiling in front of a cardiovascular area. If the machine requires a cable to connect to cable or satellite TV, the location choices may be limited. If a computerized exercise tracking system is being considered for each weight training machine as well as the cardiovascular machines, additional wiring and outlets may be required.

While there are no standards or guidelines for how many or what types of resistance training equipment a facility should have, one can determine this based on the total facility space, the members' demographic characteristics (e.g., age, gender, physical abilities), the members' needs and preferences, and their patterns of usage. A common recommendation is to provide at least one circuit weight training area for each 1,000 users (21).

It is ideal to see and use equipment if possible before making a final decision. If the equipment under consideration as a top choice is used at a local facility, it is common practice to visit the facility to further evaluate the equipment. In some cases manufacturing companies, as well as local health and fitness dealers, are willing to provide a demo unit to try out. Attending exercise equipment trade shows or health fitness conferences is another way to see equipment and meet a company's sales representatives to obtain more information. There may be a special conference discount rate available. Most recently built health and fitness club facilities have budgeted approximately $15 to $25 per square foot for their exercise equipment (22).

It is also advisable to ask if an exercise equipment company or its dealer has a trade-in option to help lower the cost on a new purchase. A leasing option could also be considered.

Phase 3: Evaluate Manufacturers' Business Practices

The first step in evaluating exercise equipment manufacturers' business practices is to review the companies' business records, the quality of their products, their customer service, and overall reputation. To accomplish this, it is critical to contact as many sales representatives as possible from a variety of companies to find out about specific products and services. The manufacturers or dealers should be able to provide a list of facilities that have the specific equipment being considered. In addition, making calls to references for further evaluation of the equipment and services may be beneficial. Any equipment manufacturers or dealers with poor-quality products, poor customer service, or other unacceptable business practices should be eliminated from consideration (13).

If keeping expenses low is a priority it is ideal to purchase most, if not all, pieces of equipment from the same company, as a volume discount may be available. In addition, shipping costs can be lowered if a large quantity of equipment is ordered from one company since shipping costs are determined on a volume basis according to weight. However, since each manufacturer has its own specialties, it is almost impossible to purchase the best quality of all equipment that a facility needs from one manufacturer.

After specifications for all the equipment are determined, one should ask selected manufacturers, dealers, or both to provide bids. After all bids are obtained, one evaluates the bids and determines the best proposal (i.e., the best price for best quality of the equipment). A purchase order may be required. It is not uncommon to make a down payment of 50% at the time the order is placed (3). It is critical to have a clear understanding of a contract with the manufacturer or dealer including delivery date, installation obligations, and payment methods.

After Ordering New Exercise Equipment: Delivery and Arrival

After new exercise equipment is ordered, a definite delivery date and time should be established (20). It is common for the manufacturer to hire a shipping company to deliver the equipment, especially with large quantities. It is essential to contact both the manufacturer and the shipping company to confirm the delivery date and time. A shipping company's primary responsibility is delivering the equipment, not installing it. It is important to establish which party will be responsible for installation of new

equipment prior to its delivery. This should be clarified when the equipment is ordered.

Consideration needs to be given to the number of staff needed at the time of delivery, how the equipment will be transported to specific areas of the facility, whether the facility or part of the facility needs to be closed during the delivery process, and whether additional tools or equipment such as carts and pallet jacks will be required. As soon as the new equipment is installed, it should be inspected carefully; any defects should be documented and also photographed if possible. The manufacturer or dealer should be contacted as soon as possible regarding the appropriate actions for exchanging defective equipment. Recording and filing the serial and model numbers of the equipment for inventory is a good practice.

Floor Plan and Equipment Organization

Three general types of equipment are used in a health and fitness facility: equipment for resistance training, for aerobic training, and for stretching and body weight exercise. The following are methods of organizing equipment and relevant considerations:

- Arrange the facility so that the areas for cardiovascular machines, selectorized machines, free weights, Olympic lift platforms, stretching, body weight exercise, and rehabilitation are separate.

- Group the resistance training equipment in separate locations in the resistance training room based on the body part they target (e.g., chest, shoulders, back, arms, legs, abdomen). A color coding system (e.g., different upholstery colors) can help users easily identify which selectorized machines are for which muscles or muscle groups. In addition, a map can be displayed to show where particular resistance training machines are located.

- A circuit weight training area can be arranged so that all major muscles or muscle groups can be trained in a time-efficient way.

- Resistance training equipment and cardiovascular machines can be arranged based on brands or manufacturers. When a large quantity of equipment is purchased from more than two companies, this type of equipment arrangement may be preferable.

- Cardiovascular machines can be arranged based on the their types, such as treadmills, elliptical machines, bikes, rowing machines, and stair steppers. Arrangement options can be affected by whether a machine requires a power outlet or not.

- Special considerations, such as accessibility and an inclusive environment for persons with disabilities, should enter into organizing the equipment.

- Depending on the facility's size and targeted audience, organizing the exercise areas based on equipment type creates an efficient use of space (14). Larger facilities that serve more clients have more and a greater variety of equipment, so clustering equipment based on the body part targeted improves functionality and accessibility.

> Personal trainers should be familiar with all aspects of equipment placement and spacing guidelines in order to provide effective supervision as well as a safe exercise environment.

Equipment Placement

The following general guidelines should be followed for equipment placement in an exercise facility. More specific examples are listed in table 24.1, "Guidelines for Equipment User Space and Safety Cushion."

- Exercise equipment that requires a spotter should be located away from windows, mirrors, and doors to avoid distraction or collision with other clients; instead, they should be placed in areas that are easily supervised and accessible.

- Taller machines (e.g., lat pulldown, cable column) or pieces of equipment (e.g., squat racks, power racks) should be placed along the walls or pillars to allow better visibility. Also, they may need to be bolted to the walls or floors for increased stability and safety.

- Dumbbell racks and weight trees are typically placed against the walls. Shorter or smaller pieces of equipment should be placed in the middle of the room to improve visibility and maximize use of space. Single-tier and multi-tier dumbbell racks are available on the market. A decision should be made on how much space can be used for this purpose and how many dumbbells need to be available for the clients.

- For circuit weight training, resistance training machines are typically placed in an order such that large muscle groups are trained earlier and small muscle groups later (19). In addition, arranging the circuit in such a way that a user can train the muscles or muscle groups in an alternate fashion may minimize the length of breaks needed between the exercises (e.g., chest press, then leg press).

- A separate designated area for stretching should be created in a resistance training room. Typically the stretching area is located in an area that is quieter and has less traffic. In addition to the stretching area, in a larger facility it may be desirable to have individual stretching mats for convenience (e.g., a user may be able to take a mat and find another spot when the stretching area is too crowded).

- Cardiovascular machines that require clients to be in an upright position or that are taller (e.g., treadmills, stair climbers, elliptical trainers) should be placed behind the cardiovascular machines that require clients to be lower to the ground (e.g., rowing machines, stationary bikes, semirecumbent cycles). With this placement, the taller machines will not impair the visual field (e.g., for television watching) of clients using machines that are lower to the ground.

- Treadmills and any other cardiovascular machines with outside moving parts exposed should have sufficient surrounding room or safety reasons. In addition, treadmills should not be placed near or next to medicine balls or stability balls. A ball left on the floor can potentially be sucked under a treadmill belt and cause serious injury.

- All exercise equipment should be placed at least 6 inches (15 cm) from mirrors.

Equipment Spacing

Proper equipment spacing will allow easy access to the machines, better traffic flow, and safer execution of an exercise. Proper equipment spacing also allows for a personal trainer to supervise the facility and interact with the clients safely and effectively.

There are two major functions of proper equipment spacing. First, appropriate spacing of equipment improves the personal trainer's supervisory ability and provides sufficient room for clients to perform each exercise safely (called the **user space**). Second, proper spacing should also facilitate access between each piece of equipment (called the **safety space cushion**) and enhance the flow of traffic. The fitness area should provide between 25 and 50 square feet (7.6 and 15.2 m²) per piece of equipment on the floor (21). To effectively serve clients who use wheelchairs, more than 3 feet (91 cm) around the equipment may be needed. The ADA requires that each piece of equipment have an adjacent clear floor space of at least 30 by 48 inches (76 cm by 122 cm) (21).

Table 24.1 shows the total space requirements (i.e., the user space plus a safety space cushion) for various types of exercise equipment (14, 21). The following guidelines for equipment spacing are suggested by the National Strength and Conditioning Association (5, 8).

Facility Traffic Flow

- Sufficient traffic flow around the perimeter of resistance and cardiovascular machine areas is required to allow clients and personal trainers easy access to the equipment. Different colors or patterns of flooring or carpet can be used to identify walkways through the facility. To effectively serve clients who use wheelchairs, more than 3 feet (91 cm) of space may be needed.

- At least one walkway should bisect the room to provide quick and easy access in and out of the facility in an emergency.

- An unobstructed pathway of 3 feet (91 cm) wide should be maintained in the facility at all times as stipulated by federal, state, and local laws. No exercise machines or equipment should block or hinder the flow of traffic in the facility.

- Although ceiling height does not affect traffic flow on the floor, the ceiling should be free of all low-hanging items (beams, pipes, lighting, signs, etc.) and high enough to allow clients to perform overhead and jumping exercises. A minimum of 12 feet (3.7 m) is recommended.

Stretching and Body Weight Exercise Area

- An area for stretching that allows 40 to 60 square feet (12 to 18 m²) of space per user is reasonable (21), with 49 square feet considered optimal (7).

- A larger area may be needed if a personal trainer assists a client with stretching (e.g., proprioceptive neuromuscular facilitation exercises).

Resistance Training Machine Area

- All resistance training machines and equipment must be spaced at least 2 feet (61 cm), preferably 3 feet (91 cm), apart.

- If a free weight exercise will be performed in a resistance training machine area (e.g., a circuit training workout area), a 3-foot (91-cm) safety space cushion is needed between the ends of the barbell and all adjacent stations (14).

- Multistation machines may be a better choice for some facilities because of the shape of the resistance training room, arrangement of the equipment, and amount of space available. A variety of configurations can fit the different sizes and configurations of available space in a facility. If possible, more than the 3-foot (91-cm) spacing is recommended between multistation machines and single-station machines.

Resistance Training Free Weight Area

- The ends of all Olympic bars and fixed-weight barbells on racks should be spaced 3 feet (91 cm) apart.

- The area designated for free weights should be able to accommodate three or four exercisers.

- If resistance training equipment does not have weight racks (e.g., squat racks and power racks typically have weight racks), weight trees should be placed in close proximity to plate-loaded equipment and benches but not closer than 3 feet (91 cm).

- Dumbbell racks should be placed at least 6 inches (15 cm) away from a mirror to decrease the chance of breakage (14). The racks may need to be bolted down if they constantly shift toward the mirror. This shifting can occur when dumbbells are reracked by users.

Olympic Lifting Area

- Perimeter walkways around the platform area should be 3 to 4 feet (0.9-1.2 m) wide (8).

- Space needed for the Olympic lifting area is 36 square feet (3.3 m²) (15).

Aerobic Exercise Area

- An ideal safety space cushion of 3 feet (91 cm) should be provided on all sides of the aerobic exercise machines (placement too close to walls should be avoided) to allow clients and supervising personal trainers easy access as well as for safety reasons.

- Table 24.1 gives precise space guidelines, but common recommendations are 24 square feet (2.2 m²) for stationary bikes and stair machines, 6 square feet (0.6 m²) for skiing machines, 40 square feet (3.7 m²) for rowing machines, and 45 square feet (4.2 m²) for treadmills (6). These spacing recommendations include the safety space cushion between the machines.

TABLE 24.1   Guidelines for Equipment User Space and Safety Cushion

Type of exercise or equipment	Needed user space and safety cushion for stand-alone pieces of equipment
Supine and prone exercises (e.g., bench press, lying triceps extension)	**Formula** (Actual weight bench length [a user space length of 6 to 8 feet] + a safety space cushion of 3 feet on each side*) *multiplied by* (Actual bar length [a user space width of 4 to 7 feet] + a safety space cushion of 3 feet on each side*) **Example** If a client is using a 6-foot-long weight bench for the bench press exercise with an Olympic bar: (6 feet + 3 feet + 3 feet) × (7 feet + 3 feet + 3 feet) = 156 square feet
Standing exercises (e.g., biceps curl, upright row)	**Formula** (User space length for a standing exercise of 4 feet + a safety space cushion of 3 feet on each side*) *multiplied by* (Actual bar length [a user space "width" of 4 to 7 feet] + a safety space cushion of 3 feet on each side*) **Example** If a client is performing the (standing) biceps curl using a 4-foot-long bar: (4 feet + 3 feet + 3 feet) × (4 feet + 3 feet + 3 feet) = 100 square feet
Standing exercises from or in a rack (e.g., back squat, shoulder press)	**Formula** (User space length for a standing exercise [in a rack] of 4 to 6 feet + a safety space cushion of 3 feet on each side*) *multiplied by* (Olympic bar length [a user space width of 7 feet] + a safety space cushion of 3 feet on each side*) **Example** If a client is performing the back squat exercise in a 4-foot-square power rack using an Olympic bar: (4 feet + 3 feet + 3 feet) × (7 feet + 3 feet + 3 feet) = 130 square feet
Olympic lifting area (e.g., power clean, lunge**; step-up**)	**Formula** (Lifting platform length [a user space length of typically 8 feet] + a safety space cushion of 3 to 4 feet on each side*) *multiplied by* (Lifting platform width [a user space width of typically 8 feet]) + a safety space cushion of 3 to 4 feet on each side*) **Example** If a client is performing the power clean exercise on an Olympic lifting platform with a 4-foot safety space cushion: (8 feet + 4 feet + 4 feet) × (8 feet + 4 feet + 4 feet) = 256 square feet
Stretching and warm-up activities	**Formula** (A user space length of 7 feet) *multiplied by* (A user space width of 7 feet) **Example** If a client is performing a modified Hurdler's stretch: (7 feet) × (7 feet) = 49 square feet
Aerobic and resistance training exercise machines	**Formula** (see p. 611 for generic guidelines for aerobic equipment): (The length of the actual machine [a user space length of 3 to 8 feet] + a safety space cushion of 3 feet on each side*) *multiplied by* (The width of the actual machine [a user space length of 1 1/2 to 6 feet] + a safety space cushion of 3 feet on each side*) **Examples** If a client is running on a treadmill: (7 feet + 3 feet + 3 feet) × (3 feet + 3 feet + 3 feet) = 117 square feet If a client is performing the machine seated chest press exercise: (5 feet + 3 feet + 3 feet) × (4 feet + 3 feet + 3 feet) = 110 square feet
In a home exercise facility: Aerobic dance, kickboxing, calisthenics, body weight exercises	**Formula** (A user space length of 5 to 7 feet) *multiplied by* (A user space width of 5 to 7 feet) **Example** If a client is exercising to an aerobic dance videotape in a home facility: (6 feet) × (6 feet) = 36 square feet

*If this exercise or piece of equipment was placed in a group of similar equipment, then the safety space cushion would be only 3 feet on *one* side because the adjacent piece of equipment would provide the safety space cushion on the *other* side. Therefore, the space calculations would be (User space length + 3 feet) *multiplied by* (User space width + 3 feet).

**Although the lunge and step-up are not explosive or power exercises and therefore do not have to be performed on a platform, the "moving" or "traveling" nature of these exercises and others like them would benefit from the segregation provided by an Olympic platform. Thus, from a safety standpoint they are included in this row.

Adapted by permission from NSCA 2008.

Special Considerations for a Home Facility

In a home exercise facility, there are special considerations because of the smaller space available. Considerations that apply to the commercial setting, with respect to available space and equipment, also apply to a home exercise facility but typically on a smaller scale. It is still essential to provide sufficient space for effective instruction and a safe environment. In many cases, the client may look to a personal trainer for advice on purchasing home equipment. Clients and personal trainers need to address various aspects of potential hazards that may exist in a home exercise facility, such as environmental issues (e.g., lighting, temperature, humidity, etc.) and the safety of children and pets.

> A personal trainer should be familiar with home exercise equipment purchases, special considerations for home gym environment, and home gym space and equipment arrangements.

Home Exercise Equipment Purchases

The purchase of appropriate home exercise equipment is one of the greatest challenges the personal trainer and client face. A thorough analysis and evaluation of the equipment is necessary to make a final decision, and the following aspects of the home exercise equipment purchasing process should be taken into consideration.

Some critical decisions must be made before exercise equipment for a home environment is purchased. The first consideration is the needs of the client along with a predetermined budget. The next is the amount of available exercise space, including ceiling height, door width, and any other structural aspects of the home. Third, one examines the abundance of home exercise equipment available from reputable companies that provide attractive warranties. The Internet is an excellent way to find equipment, but it is a good practice to try out the equipment if it is available at a local store. Also, since most exercise equipment is heavy, the shipping and handling fees should enter into the a final decision. Fourth, cost is always an important factor, but variety, diversity, portability, and space efficiency are also necessary considerations. Some personal trainers warn against the purchase of exercise equipment that can be dismantled and stored out of sight because this practice can create

a barrier to accessing the equipment and reaching exercise goals.

Home Environment Issues

A home exercise facility presents additional safety concerns that revolve around the access to the exercise area by children and pets. Electrical concerns are another safety issue.

- In order to avoid serious injury, children and pets should be kept a safe distance away from electrical outlets and any exercise equipment.
- A see-through gate placed in the entryway can help promote a safer home exercise environment.
- If doors or windows provide access to the exercise area, they should be locked when the equipment is not in use. To ensure that the living environment is safe, it may be necessary to disable some types of equipment (i.e., unplug cords to treadmills, remove accessory attachments for resistance machines, remove weight pins from machines, remove weight plates from bars, place bars out of the flow of traffic).
- The client and personal trainer should also make sure that the home exercise facility has a sufficient electrical supply to accommodate the additional equipment (19).
- When possible, outlets should be **ground-fault circuit interrupter (GFCI)** protected with 110- and 220-voltage capabilities so that power is automatically shut down in the event of an electrical overload (14). Additional electrical outlets should be available for vacuum cleaners and other electric equipment and tools.
- The client should use a padded mat for floor exercises to help reduce perspiration accumulation on any permanent carpeted surface.

Home Equipment Layout

Because a home exercise facility is smaller, has less equipment, and serves fewer people than a commercial facility, all fixed equipment (e.g., aerobic exercise machines and dumbbell racks) is typically arranged along the perimeter of the room fairly close to the walls. Use common sense to avoid injuries and structural damage to the home facility (see figure 24.1).

- The space cushion around equipment is often reduced (e.g., 18 inches [46 cm] instead of 3 feet [91 cm]).

- The recommendation for space for activities such as aerobic dance, kickboxing, calisthenics, and body weight exercises is 25 to 49 square feet (2.4-4.6 m²) (21).

- Entertainment equipment such as televisions, VCRs, DVD players, radios, CD players, or newer technologies in the exercise area can be installed on a wall or the ceiling so the client can view instructional exercise videos and listen to music or news (21).

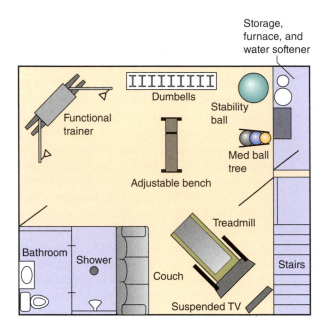

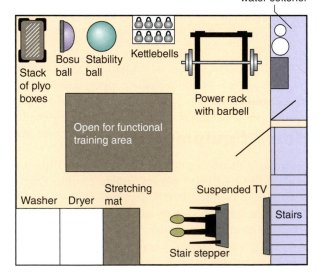

FIGURE 24.1 Two examples of home exercise facility floor plans.

Facility and Equipment Maintenance

Facility and equipment maintenance can easily become reactive rather than proactive. In order to provide a safe exercise environment, preventive maintenance procedures need to be a focus. Regular maintenance and cleaning procedures not only provide a safe environment but also increase the longevity of exercise equipment. A systematic daily, weekly, and monthly inspection, maintenance, and cleaning schedule should be established. This will ensure safety for clients and proper functioning of the equipment. Personal trainers must be familiar with all aspects of inspection, maintenance, and cleaning procedures for the equipment to safeguard their clients against potential injuries and avoid litigation.

> Proper facility and equipment maintenance not only promotes a safe exercise environment but also increases longevity of the facility and equipment.

Facility Maintenance

In many cases, a majority of members use a resistance training room for their main workouts; therefore the resistance training room becomes a representation of the entire facility. Areas such as those under and between equipment may be difficult to clean thoroughly. Therefore maintaining and cleaning health and fitness facilities should begin with an assessment of the types of surfaces that are present and the maintenance and cleaning difficulties that could arise in each area.

- Personal trainers should frequently assess the condition of walls, floors, and ceilings, as well as the accessibility and safe placement of equipment.

- Cleaning the commercial exercise facility is often handled not only by custodial staff but also by the personal training staff. Another option is to hire a professional cleaning company.

- Cleaning of the home facility can be handled by the owner of the house or by the personal trainer. If a personal trainer uses a client's home gym (on-site personal training), the cleaning obligations should be discussed and determined with the client.

Floor

- The personal trainer needs to inspect, maintain, and clean the floor regularly.

- Wooden flooring must be kept free of splinters, holes, protruding nails, uneven boards, and loose screws. Inspection of these potential problem areas should occur daily during regular cleaning.

- Tile flooring should be treated with antifungal and antibacterial agents, especially in the aerobic exercise area. Tile floors should also be resistant to slipping and moisture and should be free of chalk and dirt buildup.

- Resilient rubber flooring in the free weight and machine areas should be treated with antifungal and antibacterial agents in the same manner as the flooring in the aerobic exercise area. Rubber flooring must be kept free of large gaps, cuts, and worn spots.

- Interlocking mats must be secure, free from protruding tabs, and arranged so as not to pull apart or become wrinkled.

- The stretching area must be kept free of accumulated dust. Mats or carpets should be nonabsorbent and should contain antifungal and antibacterial agents.

- Carpeting must be kept free of tears, and walkways and high-traffic areas should be protected with additional mats. All areas must be swept and vacuumed or mopped according to designated cleaning schedules.

- Flooring must be kept glued and fastened down properly, and all fixed equipment must be attached (bolted) securely to the floor.

Walls

- The personal trainer needs to inspect, maintain, and clean walls regularly. Wall surfaces include mirrors, windows, exits, storage areas, and shelves. Wall surfaces should be cleaned two or three times a week or as needed.

Ceiling

- The personal trainer needs to inspect, maintain, and clean the ceiling. Maintenance and cleaning of ceilings in the exercise facility are often overlooked. This duty includes ceiling fixtures and attachments such as lights, air-conditioning units, heating units, air ducts, sprinkler heads and pipes, speakers, TV monitors, and ceiling fans.

- Tiled ceilings must be kept clean, and any damaged or missing tiles should be replaced as needed. Open ceilings with exposed pipes and ducts do not require regular dust removal but should be cleaned as needed.

Refer to the National Strength and Conditioning Association's (NSCA's) *Safety Checklist for Exercise Facility and Equipment Maintenance* for a list of facility maintenance tasks and cleaning schedule (p. 620).

Equipment Maintenance

Keeping the equipment functional, clean, and safe to use is a critical part of a personal trainer's daily duties. Equipment that is constantly used and not consistently cleaned or maintained is potentially dangerous to the client and the personal trainer.

- In a commercial exercise facility, the maintenance staff, personal trainers, and local equipment representatives should clean and maintain the exercise equipment regularly.

- Providing disposable cleaning towelettes and a cleaning solution bottle with rags near the exercise equipment may encourage users to clean the equipment before and after use. In addition, when bodily fluids such as sweat are cleaned off a machine, wearing disposable latex or latex-free gloves is recommended. These should be readily available at the facility. If this is not an option, hand washing with soap and water should be required after equipment has been cleaned of sweat or any other bodily fluids.

- Minor cleaning of exercise equipment in a health and fitness facility can be handled by a client; however, it is the personal trainer's responsibility to regularly and properly maintain and clean this equipment.

Refer to the NSCA's *Safety Checklist for Exercise Facility and Equipment Maintenance* for a list of equipment maintenance tasks and cleaning schedule (p. 620).

Stretching Area

Equipment commonly used for stretching includes padded mats, stretching sticks, elastic cords, and wall ladders.

- Mats in stretching areas should be cleaned and disinfected daily and in a timely manner.

- The mats should be free of cracks and tears.

- Areas between mats should be swept or vacuumed regularly to avoid dust and dirt buildup.

- The stretching area should be free of benches, dumbbells, and other equipment that may create clutter and may tear mat surfaces. All equipment should be stored after use, and elastic cords should be secured to a base, checked for wear, and replaced when necessary.

- Cleaning solution bottles and rags for cleaning mats after use may be considered. Such items should be in close proximity to the stretching mat but located so as not to represent a hazard.

Body Weight Exercise Area

Stability balls, medicine balls, plyometric boxes, ladders, cones, balance training equipment, utility benches, hyperextension benches, and jump ropes are typically used in the body weight exercise area.

- All mats and bench upholstery should be disinfected daily and should be free of cracks and tears.

- The tops and bottoms of plyometric boxes should have nonslip surfaces for safe use and should be inspected monthly for excessive wear.

- Other equipment and accessories should be inspected regularly for functional safety and should be cleaned on a regular basis to extend their life span.

Resistance Training Machine Area

A large variety of resistance training machines available on the market (e.g., cam, pulley, cable, belt, chain, plate loaded, selectorized, pneumatic, isokinetic) are available in both single-station or multistation designs.

- Bench upholstery and machine surfaces that come into contact with skin should be cleaned and disinfected daily and should be free of cracks and tears.

- Guide rods on selectorized machines should be cleaned and lubricated two or three times per week.

- No machine should have loose bolts, screws, cables, chains, or protruding or worn parts that need replacement or removal. In addition, if machines are bolted down to the floor or wall, the bolts should be inspected for safety monthly.

- Weight plates on resistance training machines should be inspected weekly for cracks.

- Extra L- or T-shaped pins designed for the selectorized machines and belts should be kept in stock so that clients do not try to improvise with unsafe substitutes.

- Chains, cables, belts, and pulleys should be adjusted for proper alignment, tension, and smooth function on a weekly basis, as even minor misalignments can cause premature wearing and damage to belts and cables.

Free Weight Resistance Area

Free weight resistance exercises involve the use of various types of bars, benches (with and without uprights or racks), squat or power racks, barbells, dumbbells, kettle bells, and weight trees for barbell plates.

- All equipment, including safety equipment (belts, straps, wraps, pads, chains, gloves, locks, safety bars, etc.), should be returned to proper storage areas after use to avoid pathway obstruction.

- All bench and rack welds should be inspected monthly or as needed.

- In and around squat and power racks, the floor should be nonslip and should be cleaned regularly.

- Dumbbells should be checked frequently for loose hex nuts or broken welds.

- An "Out of order" sign should be clearly posted on nonfunctional or broken equipment (even in a home facility), or a sheet can be placed over the nonfunctional equipment to prevent user access; or, more desirably, such equipment should be removed from the area or locked out of service.

- All protective padding and upholstery should be free of cracks and tears, and cleaned and disinfected daily.

Olympic Lifting Area

Not all facilities have an Olympic lifting area, but those that do commonly have a segregated wooden lifting platform, Olympic bars, bumper plates, racks, locks, and chalk bins. Maintenance and cleaning of this area should occur regularly.

- Olympic bars and curl bars should be properly lubricated and tightened to maintain the rotating bar ends.

- Any defective Olympic bars or curl bars should be replaced immediately.

- The knurling (rough area for hand placement) on Olympic bars should be kept free of debris and chalk buildup by means of occasional cleaning and brushing. A wire brush can be used to brush off the accumulated chalk residue on the knurling.

- The platform should be inspected for gaps, cuts, slits, and splinters (depending on the type of surface) and properly swept or mopped to remove chalk. A protective coating material (e.g., urethane) on a wooden platform may be reapplied if it is worn.

- The platform area should be free of benches, boxes, and other clutter to give the client sufficient room to safely perform power and explosive exercises.

Aerobic Exercise Area

Cardiovascular equipment is the second most popular type of equipment available at a health and fitness facility, and it is the most important priority for a facility expansion (21). A great variety of cardiovascular machines are available on the market, including stationary bikes, treadmills, rowing machines, semi-recumbent bikes, sprint machines, stair steppers, elliptical trainers, and skiing machines.

- Equipment surfaces that come into contact with skin should be cleaned and disinfected frequently. This is particularly true during and after periods of heavy use. Cleaning and disinfecting not only protects clients from unsanitary conditions, but also extends the life of equipment surfaces and maintains their appearance. There are commercially available holders for cleaning solution bottles. If heavy usage of exercise equipment is expected, it may be appropriate to install holders and supply rags so that people can clean the equipment after exercising. Placing floor mats or rugs to trap water, sand, dirt, and other unwanted debris in front of each entrance may help maximize the cleanliness and appearance of the facility.

- All moving parts (e.g., belts, chains, joints, flywheels) should be properly lubricated and cleaned two or three times weekly or when needed.

- During the cleaning process, straps, belts, connective bolts, and screws need to be checked for tightness or wear and replaced if necessary.

- Measurement devices such as revolutions per minute meters should be properly maintained; the manufacturer usually does this, but one can extend the life of the equipment by wiping off sweat and dirt regularly.

- Equipment parts such as seats and benches should be easy to adjust.

- If budget allows, keeping extra equipment parts for prompt replacement can be a good practice. This will eliminate the time for contacting a dealer or manufacturing company to order a part and waiting for the part to arrive.

Conclusion

Painstaking effort and systematic planning are the key elements to a successful facility design. The four main phases in designing the health and fitness facility are predesign, design, construction, and preoperation. Personal trainers should be familiar with all facility specification guidelines in order to design a safe and functional facility. Selecting exercise equipment for a facility is a multifaceted process. The three main phases of selecting exercise equipment are developing functional criteria, evaluating the specifications and the effectiveness of the equipment, and evaluating the manufacturers' business practices. A tentative floor plan and a priority list should be used to finalize the selection of the right equipment for a facility. Creating appropriate spaces between exercise equipment promotes better traffic flow, safer execution of exercises, more effective supervision of a facility, and better interaction with clients. Although a smaller scale of facility design and equipment arrangement applies to a home exercise facility, clients and personal trainers need to address various aspects of potential hazards that may exist, such as environmental issues and the safety of children and pets. Facility and equipment maintenance can easily become reactive rather than proactive. Proper facility and equipment maintenance can promote not only a sanitized and safe environment but also increased longevity of the facility and equipment.

Study Questions

1. A health and fitness facility has a total number of members of 3,000, and the facility's criterion for cardiovascular equipment is one cardiovascular machine for every four members. How many pieces of cardiovascular machines should the facility have based on the common practice used in the health and fitness industry?

   A. 56

   B. 62

   C. 72

   D. 81

2. Which of the following are appropriate guidelines for the use of mirrors in a fitness facility?

   I. 6 inches (15 cm) away from equipment

   II. 20 inches (51 cm) away from equipment

   III. 6 inches (15 cm) above the floor

   IV. 20 inches (51 cm) above the floor

   A. I and III only

   B. I and IV only

   C. II and III only

   D. II and IV only

3. When organizing exercise equipment in a health and fitness facility, which of the following guidelines should the personal trainer follow?

   I. Place taller resistance training machines in the middle of a resistance training room for better visibility.

   II. Equipment for exercises that require spotters should be located away from windows, mirrors, and doors.

   III. The ends of all Olympic bars should be spaced 3 feet (91 cm) apart.

   IV. All resistance training machines and equipment must be spaced at least 3 feet (91 cm), preferably 4 feet (121 cm), apart.

   A. I and III only

   B. I and IV only

   C. II and III only

   D. II and IV only

4. What is the minimum ceiling height sufficient for overhead exercises?

   A. 7 feet (212 cm)

   B. 9 feet (273 cm)

   C. 11 feet (334 cm)

   D. 12 feet (364 cm)

Applied Knowledge Question

Assuming stand-alone stations, calculate the recommended total area needed (in square feet) for these pieces of equipment or exercise areas:

A. A client is performing the seated shoulder press exercise (length: 4 feet; width: 3 feet).

B. A client is performing the upright row exercise using a 5-foot-long bar.

C. A client is using a 5-foot-long weight bench for the lying triceps extension exercise with a 4-foot "EZ curl" bar.

D. A client is performing the step-up exercise on an 8-foot Olympic lifting platform with a 3-foot safety space cushion.

E. A client is performing the front squat exercise in a 4 1/2 foot square power rack using an Olympic bar.

F. A client is exercising on a stair machine (length: 5 feet; width: 3 feet).

G. A client is performing a seated toe touch stretch.

References

1. Armitage-Johnson, S. 1989. Maintenance and safety: Maintaining a safe environment in the strength facility. *National Strength and Conditioning Association Journal* 11: 56-57.

2. Armitage-Johnson, S. 1994. Providing a safe training environment for participants, part I. *Strength and Conditioning* 16: 64-65.

3. Bates, M. 2008. Choosing the right equipment. In: *Health Fitness Management,* 2nd ed., M. Bates, ed. Champaign, IL: Human Kinetics.

4. Centers for Disease Control and Prevention. 2002. Nonfatal sports- and recreation-related injuries treated in emergency departments – United States, July 2000-June 2001. *Journal of the American Medical Association* 288: 1977-1979.

5. Coker, E. 1989. Weightroom flooring. *National Strength and Conditioning Association Journal* 11: 26-27.

6. Greenwood, M. 2000. Facility maintenance and risk management. In: *Essentials of Strength Training and Conditioning,* 2nd ed., T. Baechle and R. Earle, eds. Champaign, IL: Human Kinetics.

7. Greenwood, M. 2004. Facility and equipment layout and maintenance. In: *NSCA's Essentials of Personal Training,* R. Earle and T. Baechle, eds. Champaign, IL: Human Kinetics.

8. Greenwood, M. 2008. Facility organization and risk management. In: *Essentials of Strength Training and Conditioning,* 3rd ed., T. Baechle, and R. Earle, eds. Champaign, IL: Human Kinetics.

9. Hillman, A., and D. Pearson. 1995. Supervision: The key to strength training success. *Strength and Conditioning* 17: 67-71.

10. Holcomb, W., D. Kleiner, and D. Chu. 1998. Plyometrics: Considerations for safe and effective training. *Strength and Conditioning* 20: 36-41.

11. Kroll, B. 1989. Facility design: Developing the strength training facility. *National Strength and Conditioning Association Journal* 11: 53-55.

12. Kroll, B. 1990. Facility design: Evaluating strength training equipment. *National Strength and Conditioning Association Journal* 12: 56-65.

13. Kroll, B. 1990. Facility design: Selecting strength training equipment. *National Strength and Conditioning Association Journal* 12: 65-70.

14. Kroll, B. 1991. Facility design: Structural and functional considerations in designing the facility: Part II. *National Strength and Conditioning Association Journal* 13: 51-57.

15. Kroll, B. 1991. Structural and functional considerations in designing the facility: Part I. *National Strength and Conditioning Association Journal* 13: 51-58.

16. Kroll, W. 1991. Facility design: Aesthetics of the strength training facility. *National Strength and Conditioning Association Journal* 13: 55-58.

17. National Institute for Occupational Safety and Health. 1998. *Criteria for a Recommended Standard: Occupational Noise Exposure.* NIOSH Pub. No. 98-126. Cincinnati, OH: Author.

18. Patton, R., W. Grantham, R. Gerson, and L. Gettman. 1989. *Developing and Managing Health/Fitness Facilities.* Champaign, IL: Human Kinetics.

19. Polson, G. 1995. Weight room safety strategic planning - part IV. *Strength and Conditioning* 17: 35-37.

20. Sawyer, T., and D. Stowe. 2005. Strength and cardiovascular training facility. In: *Facility Design and Management for Health, Fitness, Physical Activity, Recreation, and Sports Facility Development,* 11th ed., T. Sawyer, ed. Champaign, IL: Sagamore.

21. Tharrett, S., K. McInnis, and J. Peterson. 2007. *ACSM's Health/Fitness Facility Standards and Guidelines,* 3rd ed. Champaign, IL: Human Kinetics.

22. Tharrett, S., and J. Peterson. 2006. *Fitness Management: A Comprehensive Resource for Developing, Leading, Managing, and Operating a Successful Health/Fitness Club.* Monterey, CA: Healthy Learning.

NSCA's Safety Checklist for Exercise Facility and Equipment Maintenance

Exercise Facility

Floor

- ☐ Inspected and cleaned daily
- ☐ Wooden flooring free of splinters, holes, protruding nails, and loose screws
- ☐ Tile flooring resistant to slipping; no moisture or chalk accumulation
- ☐ Rubber flooring free of cuts, slits, and large gaps between pieces
- ☐ Interlocking mats secure and arranged with no protruding tabs
- ☐ Nonabsorbent carpet free of tears; wear areas protected by throw mats
- ☐ Area swept and vacuumed or mopped on a regular basis
- ☐ Flooring glued or fastened down properly

Walls

- ☐ Wall surfaces cleaned two or three times a week (or more often if needed)
- ☐ Walls in high-activity areas free of protruding appliances, equipment, or wall hangings
- ☐ Mirrors and shelves securely fixed to walls
- ☐ Mirrors and windows cleaned regularly (especially in high-activity areas, such as around drinking fountains and in doorways)
- ☐ Mirrors placed a minimum of 20 inches (51 cm) off the floor in all areas
- ☐ Mirrors not cracked or distorted (replace immediately if damaged)

Ceiling

- ☐ All ceiling fixtures and attachments dusted regularly
- ☐ Ceiling tile kept clean
- ☐ Damaged or missing ceiling tile replaced as needed
- ☐ Open ceilings with exposed pipes and ducts cleaned as needed

Exercise Equipment

Stretching and Body Weight Exercise Area

- ☐ Mat area free of weight benches and equipment
- ☐ Mats and bench upholstery free of cracks and tears
- ☐ No large gaps between stretching mats
- ☐ Area swept and disinfected daily
- ☐ Equipment properly stored after use
- ☐ Elastic cords secured to base with safety knot and checked for wear
- ☐ Surfaces that contact skin treated with antifungal and antibacterial agents daily
- ☐ Nonslip material on the top surface and bottom or base of plyometric boxes
- ☐ Ceiling height sufficient for overhead exercises (12 feet [3.7 m] minimum) and free of low-hanging apparatus (beams, pipes, lighting, signs, etc.)

Resistance Training Machine Area

- ☐ Easy access to each station (a minimum of 2 feet [61 cm] between machines; 3 feet [91 cm] is optimal)
- ☐ Area free of loose bolts, screws, cables, and chains
- ☐ Proper selectorized pins used
- ☐ Securing straps functional
- ☐ Parts and surfaces properly lubricated and cleaned
- ☐ Protective padding free of cracks and tears
- ☐ Surfaces that contact skin treated with antifungal and antibacterial agents daily
- ☐ No protruding screws or parts that need tightening or removal
- ☐ Belts, chains, and cables aligned with machine parts
- ☐ No worn parts (frayed cable, loose chains, worn bolts, cracked joints, etc.)

Resistance Training Free Weight Area

- ☐ Easy access to each bench or area (a minimum of 2 feet [61 cm] between machines; 3 feet [91 cm] is optimal)
- ☐ Olympic bars properly spaced (3 feet [91 cm]) between ends
- ☐ All equipment returned after use to avoid obstruction of pathway
- ☐ Safety equipment (belts, collars, safety bars) used and returned
- ☐ Protective padding free of cracks and tears
- ☐ Surfaces that contact skin treated with antifungal and antibacterial agents daily
- ☐ Securing bolts and apparatus parts (collars, curl bars) tightly fastened
- ☐ Nonslip mats on squat rack floor area
- ☐ Olympic bars turn properly and are properly lubricated and tightened
- ☐ Benches, weight racks, standards, and the like secured to the floor or wall
- ☐ Nonfunctional or broken equipment removed from area or locked out of service
- ☐ Ceiling height sufficient for overhead exercises (12 feet [3.7 m] minimum) and free of low-hanging apparatus (beams, pipes, lighting, signs, etc.)

Olympic Lifting Platform Area

- ☐ Olympic bars properly spaced (3 feet [91 cm]) between ends
- ☐ All equipment returned after use to avoid obstruction of lifting area
- ☐ Olympic bars rotate properly and are properly lubricated and tightened
- ☐ Bent Olympic bars replaced; knurling clear of debris
- ☐ Collars functioning
- ☐ Sufficient chalk available
- ☐ Wrist straps, belts, and knee wraps available, functioning, and stored properly
- ☐ Benches, chairs, boxes kept at a distance from lifting area
- ☐ No gaps, cuts, slits, splinters in mat
- ☐ Area properly swept and mopped to remove splinters and chalk
- ☐ Ceiling height sufficient for overhead exercises (12 feet [3.7 m] minimum) and free of low-hanging apparatus (beams, pipes, lighting, signs, etc.)

Aerobic Exercise Area

- ☐ Easy access to each station (minimum of 2 feet [61 cm] between machines; 3 feet [91 cm] is optimal)
- ☐ Bolts and screws tight

- ☐ Functioning parts easily adjustable
- ☐ Parts and surfaces properly lubricated and cleaned
- ☐ Foot and body straps secure and not ripped
- ☐ Measurement devices for tension, time, and revolutions per minute properly functioning
- ☐ Surfaces that contact skin treated with antifungal and antibacterial agents daily

Frequency of Maintenance and Cleaning Tasks

Daily

- ☐ Inspect all flooring for damage or wear.
- ☐ Clean (sweep, vacuum, or mop and disinfect) all flooring.
- ☐ Clean and disinfect upholstery.
- ☐ Clean and disinfect drinking fountain.
- ☐ Inspect fixed equipment's connection with floor.
- ☐ Clean and disinfect equipment surfaces that contact skin.
- ☐ Clean mirrors.
- ☐ Clean windows.
- ☐ Inspect mirrors for damage.
- ☐ Inspect all equipment for damage; wear; loose or protruding belts, screws, cables, or chains; insecure or nonfunctioning foot and body straps; improper functioning or improper use of attachments, pins, or other devices.
- ☐ Clean and lubricate moving parts of equipment.
- ☐ Inspect all protective padding for cracks and tears.
- ☐ Inspect nonslip material and mats for proper placement, damage, and wear.
- ☐ Remove trash and garbage.
- ☐ Clean light covers, fans, air vents, clocks, and speakers.
- ☐ Ensure that equipment is returned and stored properly after use.

Two or Three Times per Week

- ☐ Clean and lubricate aerobic machines and the guide rods on selectorized resistance machines.

Once per Week

- ☐ Clean (dust) ceiling fixtures and attachments.
- ☐ Clean ceiling tile.

As Needed

- ☐ Replace light bulbs.
- ☐ Clean walls.
- ☐ Replace damaged or missing ceiling tiles.
- ☐ Clean open ceilings with exposed pipes or ducts.
- ☐ Remove (or place sign on) broken equipment.
- ☐ Fill chalk boxes.
- ☐ Clean bar knurling.
- ☐ Clean rust from floor, plates, bars, and equipment with a rust-removing solution.

From NSCA, 2012, *NSCA's essentials of personal training*, 2nd ed., J. Coburn and M. Malek (eds.), (Champaign, IL: Human Kinetics). Reprinted by permission from NSCA 2008.

Legal Aspects of Personal Training

David L. Herbert, JD

After completing this chapter, you will be able to

- appreciate and understand basic aspects of the law, particularly tort law, and the legal system as they are applicable to the delivery of personal training services;

- define negligence and delineate the four elements that an injured client must prove in a lawsuit against a personal trainer based on negligence;

- identify the professional and legal responsibilities of a personal trainer and understand the consequences of those responsibilities; and

- adopt risk management strategies to minimize the risks of claims and litigation in personal training.

This chapter explores the legal aspects of personal training. It concentrates on the expected **standard of care** owed to fitness clients by personal trainers, as well as service delivery issues for these professionals (1). The chapter also discusses concepts related to negligence and lawsuits against personal trainers. United States and state statutory law principles are reviewed, as are tort and contract law concepts as well as criminal law principles and requirements. (*Statutory laws* are those written by Congress or state legislatures.) Laws in place in other countries are different from those applicable in the United States. As a consequence, personal trainers providing services in other countries should seek out other legal information and advice as necessary. The chapter also addresses **risk management** strategies to avoid or minimize legal concerns for readers to

consider. The materials presented in this chapter or in other sources are no substitute for the professional legal advice that personal trainers should secure in individual situations and cases.

Risk management in this context is the identification of various risks applicable to personal training activities as obtained through internal or external audit, and then the use of such findings in efforts to eliminate, reduce, or transfer those risks to improve the safe delivery of services; reduce, eliminate, or transfer the chances of untoward events; and reduce, eliminate, or transfer related claims and lawsuits. Risk avoidance and minimization strategies focus on the safe and effective screening of fitness clients, the proper recommendation or prescription of activity, the appropriate provision and supervision of training exercises, and the effective delivery of emergency response when necessary—all in accordance with accepted standards and guidelines. Once personal trainers understand the legal requirements associated with their delivery of service to clients and once they appreciate the fact that their negligent acts or omissions may well lead to client harm and then claims and suits against them, they will be better equipped to minimize risks to their clients while reducing their own legal exposures arising out of professional activities (2).

Negligence concepts and principles are reviewed here so that personal trainers will be forearmed to appreciate and avoid or minimize their own risks arising out of these concepts. "Lines of defense" are also presented so that personal trainers may be able to protect themselves from untoward events and concomitant claims and suits. These lines of defense include adherence to professional standards and guidelines and the use of protective legal documents with clients, such as **assumption of risk** forms, prospectively executed waivers of liability or releases, or both. The protections provided by liability insurance are also of importance and represent yet another line of defense for personal trainers to protect or insulate them from client claims and lawsuits.

> Personal trainers should use the principles of risk management to ensure the safety of clients and to prevent costly lawsuits.

Claims and Litigation

Many personal trainers will never face a client claim or litigation related to their delivery of service. However, a good number of these professionals will be on the receiving end of such claims and lawsuits. As a consequence, it is important for personal trainers to understand the process through which such claims and lawsuits are determined, the manner and environment within which such matters are resolved, and the rules or legal concepts associated with the ultimate resolution of client claims and suits.

Claims and litigation are surely stressful for the party who asserts and institutes the proceedings. Professionals who must respond to and defend against such claims are also likely to be stressed by the mere receipt of a claim, not to mention by their defense against the filing and receipt of a lawsuit asserted against them related to a claim that is not resolved prior to its judicial determination.

While there is no hard, empirical evidence to clearly indicate that claims and litigation against fitness professionals and specifically personal trainers are increasing, it appears that this is indeed the case. This likely increase in claims and suits is probably due to a number of factors, not the least of which is the general tendency of the population to seek redress for everything or anything that may go wrong or astray in their lives. Such feelings may well include the concept "If something bad happens to me, it must be someone else's fault." In addition, there are more lawyers than ever before to assert claims and file lawsuits on behalf of clients. The "rules" regarding the appropriate provision of personal training services have also developed in recent times, so now it is somewhat clearer to members of the public what the expected level of personal training service should be and whether or not that level of service has been met in particular cases.

All of these factors and more, including the growth of the population, the aging of the population, and the increase in fitness activity participation for some segments of the population, lead to more activity involving a somewhat more "fragile" group of participants than ever before, more untoward events associated with the activity, and thus more claims and suits. However, if the personal training profession is adequately prepared, those professionals should be able to avoid, minimize, or adequately respond to and defend against relevant claims and suits.

Fitness Industry Response to Claims and Litigation

In an attempt to address the probable increase in claims and suits against fitness professionals and personal trainers in particular, based on their delivery of relevant services, the industry has mounted efforts to improve the delivery of such services. These efforts have taken at least three principal forms.

First, the industry has developed standards and guidelines applicable to the appropriate delivery of service. The American College of Sports Medicine (ACSM) and the National Strength and Conditioning Association (NSCA), among others, have been at the very forefront of this effort. The ACSM published its first statement in 1992 (3), while the NSCA developed its standards statement in 2001 (4). These two statements, along with similar documents developed by other professional groups and associations, have been put forth to raise the bar in the delivery of fitness services to clients. As of 2011, an effort by NSF International of Ann Arbor, Michigan, was under way to develop a comprehensive fitness industry standard that may lead to the accreditation of health and fitness facilities in the future, using the standard under development as a baseline for facility evaluation and then accreditation of such entities (5). The Medical Fitness Association (MFA) has already undertaken such efforts based on its own standards and guidelines for the accreditation of medically based health and fitness facilities (6). Since 1991, the ACSM has updated its industry standards and guidelines statement twice, and the NSCA updated its own standards and guidelines in 2009.

Secondly, the industry has moved forward to improve the education, training, and certification of fitness professionals, primarily personal trainers. The International Health, Racquet & Sportsclub Association (IHRSA) called together a number of prominent fitness organizations in 2002 to provide recommendations to improve the quality of fitness services offered by personal trainers in the United States. IHRSA initially brought together representatives of ACSM, NSCA, the American Council on Exercise (ACE), the Aerobic and Fitness Association of America (AFAA), and the Cooper Institute, to be joined later by other similar groups, to make recommendations to improve the delivery of such services to the public. As a consequence of IHRSA's efforts in this regard, IHRSA adopted a final resolution that became effective as of 2006, which made the following recommendations to its member club organizations:

> *Whereas, given the increasing importance of personal training in health, fitness and sports clubs, IHRSA recommends that, beginning January 1, 2006, member clubs hire personal trainers holding at least one current certification from a certifying organization/agency that has begun third-party accreditation of its certification procedures and protocols from an independent, experienced, and nationally recognized accrediting body.*
>
> *Furthermore, given the twenty-six year history of the National Organization for Competency Assurance (NOCA)[now known as the Institute for Credentialing Excellence (ICE)] as an organization dedicated to establishing quality standards for certifying agencies, IHRSA has identified the National Commission for Certifying Agencies (NCCA), the accreditation body of NOCA, as being an acceptable accrediting organization.*
>
> *IHRSA will recognize other, equivalent accrediting organizations contingent upon their status as an established accreditation body recognized by the Council for Higher Education Accreditation and/or the United States Department of Education for the pur-*

poses of providing independent, third-party accreditation.

Of the NCCA accredited organizations, the NSCA was the first to achieve this status in 1993.

Standards and **guidelines** establish the parameters of appropriate practice for professions such as personal training. *Certification* is the assessment of competence for a particular profession. *Accreditation* is the official recognition that an organization's educational program or certification test (or both) meets specified criteria.

Lastly, in addition to the two previously mentioned efforts, a number of legislators in a growing number of states have proposed legislation to regulate/license personal fitness trainers. Such proposals have been put forth in California, Massachusetts, Georgia, Maryland, New Jersey, and the District of Columbia. As of the end of the first quarter of 2009, no such proposal had yet resulted in any law. However, California's proposed law was favorably voted out of the California state Senate on April 23, 2009. Whether or not these efforts ever materialize in the form of state-mandated legislation, the fitness industry is otherwise moving toward decided improvement of the profession. If legislation is passed in any state, such action may well spur other states to move forward with similar proposals. If personal trainer licensing laws are adopted, such enactments may also clear up any lingering questions about the **duty of care** owed by fitness professionals to their clients. The duty owed by these professionals to their clients has created some inconsistent court rulings that have had a somewhat unsettling impact on the profession. We will consider this issue and these court decisions later in this chapter.

The effort to raise the professional standing of fitness professionals through any of these processes may also result in an increased expected legal standard of care, which may require the delivery of an enhanced level of service by fitness professionals to their clients. As a consequence, more rigorous professional and legal standards of care may well be applicable to personal trainers in the future and used in claims and litigation to judge professional conduct both in the short run and over the long term.

Licensure is a state-mandated and -approved process by which certain professionals who become licensed are authorized to provide defined services to others.

Claims in Health and Fitness Activities

Despite the provision of the best of care, untoward events and subsequent claims and litigation sometimes arise in the health and fitness industry, as with many other professions including medicine. Typically these claims are related to certain reoccurring subjects of concern. These areas relate to the following kinds of matters:

- The application of recommendations, standards, and guidelines to the delivery of particular fitness services
- Screening duties and responsibilities for clients
- Preexercise evaluation or functional testing of clients
- Exercise or fitness activity prescription or recommendations to clients
- Exercise activity supervision of clients
- Selection, assembly and installation, and maintenance of equipment and the design and maintenance of facilities for client use
- Emergency response
- Insurance
- Releases and waivers
- Records and ethics.

These broad subject areas account for nearly all of the claims and litigation involving health and fitness professionals. Occasionally other issues also arise, including those dealing with criminal law concerns. These latter issues are almost always related to thefts of client property, assaults or batteries of clients, or even inappropriate and criminally prohibited sexual misconduct of professionals with clients such as sexual imposition or rape. Similar relevant claims may also involve matters related to the unauthorized practice of medicine or some other health care provider practice reserved by law for provision by licensed individuals. Relevant claims in the fitness industry may also include those related to the unauthorized practice of dietetics or nutrition in those states where these practices are reserved for provision by specifically licensed individuals.

Typically, claims related to health and fitness professionals are evaluated in the **civil system** of American jurisprudence by judges and juries who are asked to examine and assess duty and liability. If duty and liability are determined, judges or juries are then asked to set the amount of compensation to be paid to redress such wrongs. On the criminal side of relevant issues, findings related to guilt or innocence and thus freedom or punishment are involved in criminal law charges and prosecutions. On the civil side, two broad legal concepts are involved—contract law and tort law.

Criminal Law

On the criminal side of the legal system, criminal laws are sometimes invoked to deal with issues related to conduct that is prohibited and made criminal by United States federal or state statutory laws or both. A criminal act is an unlawful act made so by Congressional or state legislative bodies, committed against society and punishable by fine, imprisonment, or death. For example, the provision of medical or dietetic services by personal trainers, when those services are reserved by state law for provision by licensed professionals, is made criminal by some state laws. Similarly, the provision of controlled drug substances by nonauthorized individuals to clients is made criminal by both federal and state laws. Consequently, it is important for personal trainers to avoid violations of any such criminal laws through their understanding of these laws, as well as their delivery of service only through authorized and nonprohibited scopes of practice.

Contract Law

Contracts, sometimes referred to as *agreements,* involve promises or performance negotiated and bargained for between at least two parties that are supported by some consideration—something of value. For example, the personal trainer's promise to deliver weekly services and the client's payment or promise to pay for those services is something of value sufficient to make a contract binding or, in other words, legally enforceable. The provision of services by personal trainers is generally provided pursuant to such agreements; and when agreements are not fulfilled or completed by the parties to those agreements, the civil judicial system is frequently called upon to resolve disputes. A breach of agreement would occur if a personal trainer did not provide services or if a client refused to pay for the services provided. In addition, contract law principles are relevant to the use of releases, waivers, informed consents, and a variety of other personal training documents.

Tort Law

Tort law concepts, on the other hand, apply to wrongful acts or omissions that occur between the relevant parties, namely the personal trainer and his or her clients. These acts or omissions often involve personal injury or even wrongful death claims. The word *tort* means *wrong*, and the tort system is that part of the judicial system designed to remedy wrongs. Fitness professionals and personal trainers have been ever increasingly involved with this system due to personal injury and wrongful death cases filed by or on behalf of clients against them.

Negligence Claims

In the fitness profession and industry, tort law claims generally involve claims of **negligence.** Negligence lawsuits require proof (evidence) of certain elements (like the ingredients of a recipe) by the party bringing such claims (the **plaintiff**) against the party defending from such claims (the **defendant**). These elements are established based on proof of

- duty,
- **breach of duty**,
- **proximate cause** (between an act or failure to act and some harm), and
- harm or damage.

> *Negligence* is the failure of one person to comply with a legally determined duty to protect another person, which failure proximately causes that other person harm.

Most such tort/negligence claims asserted against fitness professionals relate to injuries that are allegedly suffered by clients while receiving service from the professionals. These cases almost always deal with issues of whether or not a duty was owed by a professional to a client and if so, whether or not such a duty was breached. Judges, as opposed to juries, determine whether or not a duty to provide care by such professionals to their clients exists. If such a duty is determined to exist by a judge and thus to be applicable to the delivery of service by a professional to a client, then typically a jury is used to determine if the duty was breached and if so, the **damages**—the amount of money—to be awarded for such a breach.

In the determination of duty, judges look to state statutory laws, the overall mores of society, and concepts of justice and of right and wrong, as well as the relationship of one party to another party or parties. Judges also sometimes look to industry standards and guidelines to assess concepts of duty; and fact finders such as juries may also use these standards and guidelines to determine if duty—if first found to be applicable by a judge—has been breached, or in other words, not properly delivered by a professional to a client. If these determinations are made, awards of damages are then rendered in favor of the plaintiffs and against the defendants.

In the fitness and personal training industry, claims that have been filed as lawsuits have involved numerous fact patterns dealing with a variety of issues. Typically, claims against personal trainers revolve around alleged failures to screen, evaluate, or test clients before recommending activity; deficiencies in the exercise or fitness activity prescription or recommendation process; failures to properly supervise or instruct clients in activity; overuse injuries to clients; failures to refer clients to health care providers; failures to provide or secure appropriate emergency response for clients including failures to provide, or deficiencies in, the CPR process or the provision of automated external defibrillation (AED); inappropriate breaches of privacy or improper disclosure of private information; improper use of assumption of risk, waiver, or release documents; and a host of other claims. Claims and actual cases in these areas are reported with some regularity in at least one industry publication (7).

As of the end of 2009, the practice of personal training was not licensed or subject to regulation at the federal or state level in any state in the United States. As a consequence, there are no specific federal or state statutory laws or administrative regulations to look to in efforts to define what personal trainers can and cannot do as a matter of law in reference to their delivery of service to clients. However, health care provider practitioner laws and regulations in all states protect the public against the provision of defined health care services by those who are not licensed. As a consequence, personal trainers may not provide services that are included within those practice areas reserved for provision by licensed providers. Prohibited activities would include those related to the treatment of various illnesses. Under some such laws, even the provision of service that could be designated as preventive may be prohibited, for example recommending a particular activity or exercise to prevent the reoccurrence of an illness- or disease-related condition (8). Moreover, under many state statutes, nonlicensed individuals are not authorized to provide nutritional or dietary advice, which is reserved for provision by state-licensed dietitians (9). As a consequence, in each jurisdiction where personal trainers provide service, they need to ensure that the services they provide do not infringe upon those services that are reserved for provision by state-licensed professionals. Consultation with a lawyer may be necessary in this regard.

Courts sometimes struggle with the determination of legally required duties in health and fitness activities, including those carried on by personal trainers with clients. The lack of governmentally mandated licensure or regulation of personal trainers may well be one of the factors that affect this issue. While actual court decisions are discussed later in the chapter, when the assumption of risk defense is offered in response to a negligence action against a personal trainer, it is important to note the following additional matters:

- Personal trainers are ethically if not legally bound to follow and adhere to the standards and guidelines of their profession when delivering services to clients. Most fitness associations and fitness standards developers such as the National Strength and Conditioning Association (NSCA) have written and published both ethical codes and standards statements applicable to the delivery of personal training services. Even if some courts have not yet fully recognized the **legal duty** owed by a personal trainer to a client, or even where a duty has been judicially recognized but not fully specified, personal trainers may still suffer some adverse consequence if they fail to deliver appropriate services to clients. Professional associations that have certified personal trainers, companies that provide liability insurance to such trainers, employers of personal trainers and those allowing the provision of such services in their facilities, and professional groups of which personal trainers are members may all require adherence to ethical standards or written standards and guidelines (or both) as a condition of certification, as a prerequisite to the issuance or maintenance of liability insurance, as a requirement of employment, as a condition for securing or maintaining membership in a professional group, and so on.

- The judicial system is not in complete agreement on the specific duties owed by personal trainers to clients. Moreover, only a handful of published decisions have been issued to date to provide any guidance to the profession in this regard. In addition, the law develops and changes over time. Differing facts in particular cases may well cause a particular court response to the duty issue and potential liability when otherwise, in another case with a different fact pattern, it might not do so. State court decisions are not consistent among the various states, and no state supreme court—the highest court in a particular state—has issued any definitive decision on this particular subject. As a consequence, the law in this regard is unsettled.

- Needless injuries or deaths to clients of personal trainers have occurred in the past and unfortunately will probably occur in the future. Such events will undoubtedly create media attention, which may lead to legislative or judicial efforts (or both) to more strictly hold personal trainers to a particular duty and specific standard of care. For example, media attention focused on the personal training profession following the 1998 death of Anne Marie Capati in New York while she was working out under the supervision of a personal trainer. The personal trainer had allegedly recommended nutritional supplements to Capati that contained ephedra, now an FDA-banned substance. The story caused considerable media attention to be focused on the personal training profession and the fitness industry in general. Capati's death resulted in the filing of a $320 million lawsuit against a number of defendants, including the personal trainer in question and the fitness facility where he provided service (10). The case was thoroughly scrutinized by the media but settled before trial for a sum in excess of $4 million (11). The case may well have contributed to post-1998 industry efforts to move the profession forward.

Defenses to Negligence Actions

As previously stated, negligence cases against fitness personnel including personal fitness trainers are frequently filed and are based on a number of reoccurring negligence themes. In response to such lawsuits, fitness personnel including personal trainers generally raise a number of defenses. Those defenses typically include the following:

- Adherence to industry standards and guidelines
- Receipt of proper informed consent for testing
- Assumption of risk by the client
- Waiver or release of liability given by a client before activity

Adherence to Industry Standards and Guidelines

While the importance of industry standards and guidelines has already been discussed, in particular it is vitally important to the defense of client negligence actions that personal trainers be prepared to support their delivery of service in accordance with such standards. Since there are a number of such standards published in the industry, it would seem important for personal trainers to adhere to the standard that pertains most principally to their certification. If they are certified by the NSCA, they should adhere to and deliver client services in accordance with that standard. If they have more than one certification or similar credential, they should attempt to adhere to the most authoritative or the most conservative statement in their provision of client services. While adherence to such standards statements will not insulate a personal trainer from a client's filing of a lawsuit, the practice may well make the case legally defensible.

Securing Proper Informed Consent for Testing

While the provision of personal training services is not part of the traditional medical–health care model, the profession is moving toward becoming part of that model or at least toward affiliation with it. If licensure comes about and if duties and responsibilities are established for personal trainers by such laws, the medical or health care model may become more important to the profession. In any case, exercise testing services would inherently lend themselves to the need for personal trainers to secure informed consent from their clients prior to providing such service. **Informed consent** is a process, not just a piece of paper signed by a client. In fact, the signing a piece of paper labeled "Informed Consent" by a client is not a prerequisite to the process, although it is usually recommended. If the consent is properly written and secured during the process, the signed paper signifying the completion of the process is good evidence (proof) of adherence to that requirement.

> *Informed consent* in personal training is the process by which a particular procedure, usually exercise testing, is described to a client who will undergo the procedure with an explanation of the risks and benefits of such a procedure, whereby through this process, and with an opportunity to ask questions and receive answers, the client will determine to undergo or not undergo the procedure.

The informed consent process is part of the basic procedure required when participants are treated by health care providers. It applies to surgery as well as treatment and testing and should be part of the preexercise testing functions carried out by fitness providers with their clients. It should also be part of training program records. It is included in the established standards and guidelines from those professional associations that have developed and published standards and guidelines for the fitness industry.

The informed consent process consists of the provision of information as to what is to be done with a personal trainer's client—particularly with exercise testing, which has traditionally been the principal fitness-related activity for which consent is required. The process consists of the provision of sufficient information about what will be done to and with the client in the testing activity, what the risks of such testing or activity are, and what the available alternatives may be.

Once information about these matters is provided, the client should have an opportunity to ask questions of the professional and receive answers that address those concerns. After completion of this process, clients can then, in the exercise of good judgment, determine whether or not to undergo the given procedure. The question of whether or not the client had sufficient information to make the decision is determined in virtually all jurisdictions by reference to what a reasonable person would do in like circumstances and not by what the person in question would determine to do in hindsight, after the fact.

In the administration of the informed consent process, the disclosure of information, the client's questions and answers, and the client's decision should all be documented and noted not only on an informed consent document but in the client's records as well. An example of an informed consent for exercise testing and one for participation in a training program are included at the end of this chapter, on pages 635 and 637.

Assumption of Risk

By way of background, it is important to note that when a personal injury or wrongful death claim is filed, an assumption of risk defense may relieve a fitness professional of any obligation to adhere to any duty or responsibility toward the client other than avoiding an intentional or willful injury to the client. In other words, such a defense involves a mitigation of the duty requirement often owed by service provider such as a personal trainer to an individual such as a client. If there is no duty, then there can be no liability for an injury arising out of the activity.

Assumption of risk defenses to negligence actions are based on "a participant's voluntarily knowing, understanding and agreeing to assume those ordinary and reasonable risks associated with certain activities" (12). The doctrine has been frequently applied to sports and hazardous recreational activities but has also been asserted with mixed results in litigation against health and fitness professionals.

In the New York case of *Mathis v. New York Health Club, Inc.* (13), the plaintiff filed suit and claimed to have been injured on a weight training machine while under the care of a personal trainer who was supervising his activities. In response to the suit, the health club and trainer as defendants moved the court for the issuance of a summary judgment in their favor and contended that the plaintiff had assumed the risks associated with the activity that led to his injury. The trial court denied the motion, and an appeal ensued. On appeal the appellate court reviewed the allegations of the case and the law and ruled:

> *Defendants have moved to dismiss the complaint, claiming in support of their motion that plaintiff voluntarily assumed the risks that materialized in his injury. While it is clear that the plaintiff, who was not a novice to weight training, did assume those risks ordinarily entailed by properly supervised weight training, he cannot be said to have assumed risks in excess of those usually encountered in the activity, particularly unreasonably increased risks attributable to lapses in judgment by a personal trainer whose qualifications, plaintiff alleges, were not all they had been represented to be by defendant health club at the time plaintiff purchased the club's specialized training package. According to plaintiff, defendant trainer increased the weight on the training machine plaintiff had been using to 270 pounds and, despite plaintiff's repeatedly expressed doubts as to whether he could handle so much weight, urged plaintiff to continue with his repetitions. Given this scenario, factual issues are raised as to whether plaintiff's injury, which allegedly occurred in the course of the repetitions urged upon him by defendant trainer, was not the consequence of risks which, although inherent in weight training, were unreasonably augmented by culpable misjudgment as to plaintiff's capacity to bear so much weight. (14)*

Thus the appellate court determined that even though there were risks that could normally be assumed with weightlifting activities, those risks attributable to a personal trainer's "lapses in judgment" could not be taken on and thus assumed by a client so as to bar the client's claims based on such a defense. In essence, the court determined that there was a duty owed by the personal trainer to the client.

In another 2006 case from California, however, a different view was expressed by another appellate court. In this case, *Rostai v. Neste Enterprises* (15), during a client's first session with a personal trainer, the client suffered what he contended was a needless heart attack based on the trainer's alleged failure to screen and assess him and due to the aggressive workout the personal trainer provided for him. The personal trainer and the club asserted the assumption of risk doctrine as a defense to the suit. In response to this defense claim, the trial court granted the defendants' motion for summary judgment and the plaintiffs appealed. On appeal, the appellate court ruled:

> *In his complaint, plaintiff alleged that he had entered into an agreement with defendants to provide him with a customized physical fitness program; defendants owed plaintiff a duty to investigate his health history, including his current physical condition and cardiac risk factors; on September 11, 2002, plaintiff participated in his first training session at Gold's Gym with defendant Shoultz; defendant Shoultz knew plaintiff was not physically fit and was overweight; defendant Shoultz was aggressive in his training of plaintiff; near the end of the 60-minute training session, after complaining several times to defendant Shoultz that he needed a break, plaintiff suffered a heart attack; and defendants' negligence was a proximate cause of plaintiff's injury.*
>
> *In their answer to plaintiff's complaint, defendants asserted among other defenses that plaintiff's injury was the result of a risk inherent in strenuous physical activity; that defendants neither increased that risk nor concealed any of the inherent risks; and therefore the doctrine of primary assumption of the risk bars plaintiff's claim. . . . Defendants prevailed on summary judgment and plaintiff appeals. We will affirm for reasons we now explain. . . .*
>
> *The obvious purpose of working out with a personal trainer is to improve physical fitness and appearance. In order to accomplish that goal, the participant must engage in strenuous physical activity. The risks inherent in that activity include physical distress in general and in particular . . . muscle strains, sprains, tears and pulls, not only of obvious muscles such as those in the legs and arms, but also of less obvious muscles such as the heart. Stress on the cardiovascular system as a result of the*

physical exertion that is an integral part of fitness training with a personal trainer is a risk inherent in the activity. Eliminating that risk would alter the fundamental nature of the activity.

The court added the following:

Although plaintiff phrases his claim against defendant Shoultz in terms of failing to adequately assess plaintiff's physical condition and in particular his cardiac risk factors, the essence of plaintiff's claim is that Shoultz, in his capacity as plaintiff's personal fitness trainer, challenged plaintiff to perform beyond his level of physical ability and fitness. That challenge, however, is the very purpose of fitness training, and is precisely the reason one would pay for the services of a personal trainer. Like the coach in other sports or physical activities, the personal trainer's role in physical fitness training is not only to instruct the participant in proper exercise techniques but also to develop a training program that requires the participant to stretch his current abilities in order to become more physically fit. The personal trainer's function in the training process is, at bottom, to urge and challenge the participant to work muscles to their limits and to overcome physical and psychological barriers to doing so. Inherent in that process is the risk that the personal trainer will not accurately assess the participant's ability and the participant will be injured as a result.

Despite the plaintiff's claim, the California Court of Appeals, unlike the New York Court of Appeals in the Mathis case, reached its decision in favor of the personal trainer based on the assumption of risk defense even though there may have been no screening and no accurate assessment of the client's abilities and capacities for the prescribed exercise activity.

Regardless of the differences in these court decisions on this issue, the defense is readily available to personal trainers in almost all situations in which clients provide written assumption of risk documents in advance of activity. A client's provision of such a document demonstrates tangible evidence of the client's express assumption of risk. Such documents should be routinely included in personal trainer–client intake documents and should be part of that process. The use of written assumption of risk documents will be even more important to personal trainers in their defense of client negligence actions

when the personal trainer is located in a state that does not recognize the validity or enforceability of prospectively given client waivers or releases of liability. An example of an assumption of risk incorporating a release of liability form into one document is included at the end of this chapter, on page 639. In those states where prospectively executed releases are not recognized or are prohibited, the assumption of risk form should be a stand-alone document, and the release provisions should be removed from the forms.

Prospectively Given Waivers or Releases of Liability

Many years ago prospectively given **waivers** (or releases of liability) provided before exercise or recreational activity, to evidence a participant's waiver or release of others from potential liability for activity to then be engaged in, were often not recognized by courts in the United States judicial system. This determination was perhaps due to a number of concerns, some of them related to judicial notions of protectionism or paternalism, others related to state statutory prohibitions, and still others related to judicial determinations that society should not encourage negligent or reckless actions by giving judicial recognition to these releases. Today, however, a vast majority of states will give legal effect to properly worded, well-written, and properly administered waivers or releases of liability given in advance of activity—including health and fitness activities carried out by personal trainers for clients.

The use of prospectively executed waivers of liability has been upheld in certain states for the use of exercise machines (16), weight training routines (17), and even personal training activities (18). However, such documents are not valid in all states (19) and are not valid if signed by a minor (those under 18 years of age) since such individuals lack the legal capacity to contract (20), but may be valid in some states if signed by a parent on behalf of his or her minor child (21). Moreover, in some states these releases may not be legally valid so that they may be enforced on a person's spouse (22) or his or her estate or heirs if the person dies after signing a release document that attempts to prospectively apply to his or her spouse or in the event of death to his or her heirs or estate (23).

In some states, prospectively executed releases must state that such documents specifically release another from negligence (24), but not all states have such a requirement. Waivers that attempt to relieve another from gross negligence or willful, wanton, or criminal activities are generally not enforceable. Certain states, like Virginia (25) and some others, do not allow releases to be enforced as the courts have determined them to be against public policy.

Waivers and releases of liability need to be properly written and administered (read by or to the client, discussed with the client, and executed properly) to be lawful. An example of such a waiver/release incorporated into a document with an assumption of risk clause is included at the end of this chapter.

> In the context of personal training, *waivers* (or *releases of liability*) are contractual promises whereby one party agrees prospectively—in advance of activity—not to bring a claim or suit (or both) in the event she is injured during that activity.

Insuring Against Negligence Actions or Omissions

All personal trainers should secure and maintain adequate liability insurance that provides them with an insurance company–paid defense from client personal injury or wrongful death lawsuits or both. Moreover, such insurance needs to provide for indemnification of the insured from the payment of any settlement or judgment arising out of these lawsuits, at least up to and including the limits of the provided insurance.

Personal trainers need to consult with their insurance agents or personal legal advisors to make sure that the liability insurance they secure covers the activities they carry on in their professional practices. Some such insurance may not cover all trainer-provided services, and if this is the case it would be akin to not having insurance at all.

Many personal trainer certification associations and other professional membership groups offer the opportunity to secure liability insurance at established premium rates. Some companies even provide premium discounts to personal trainers who are trained and certified by certain of these groups. Liability insurance for this profession is a must.

> Insurance, in this context, is a contractual promise by which the insurer promises to defend and indemnify the insured, up to defined limits of liability, from certain defined liability risks at the insurer's cost in exchange for the payment of a premium.

Records and Documentation

Many lawyers who are involved in litigation where records are at issue have been trained to question the nonexistence of records that in accordance with appropriate practices should exist. These lawyers also question the poorly prepared and incomplete records associated with many professional endeavors that end up in court. Often these same legal practitioners believe "If it's not recorded, it didn't happen" or "If we can't see it, it doesn't exist" or "If no one bothered to write it down, they either didn't do it or didn't believe it was important." Such beliefs can affect the outcome of many lawsuits where records, recordings, or documentation of what turn out to be critical events are at issue.

To be sure, a good many people, including judges and juries, believe in tangible, written, recorded evidence. If paper records exist, the existence of such records can bolster and support claims or, conversely, help in the defense of lawsuits where such records demonstrate adherence to the proper standard of care. However, the absence of such records or incomplete or poorly prepared records may support plaintiff claims and lead to successfully prosecuted lawsuits. These concepts are particularly important in professions that provide service to people—to patients and to clients. This is particularly true in all the health care professions—medicine, dentistry, physical therapy, and other similar professions including personal training. While some of these professions, including certain medically based fitness programs, may be required as a matter of either federal or state law or both to generate and/or maintain certain records and in a particular manner, most personal training fitness programs have no such requirement (27).

Regardless of whether federal or state law mandates or does not mandate the confidentiality and privacy of fitness and personal trainer records, such records should be kept confidential. Many such records contain information that is personal, private, or related to medical issues. As a consequence, these records should be kept in secure storage. At the very least, personally identifiable information, like social security numbers and credit card information (other laws at the federal and state levels may apply to protect such information), screening information (PAR-Q), or health history documents and similar documents should be kept confidential. Disclosure of this kind of information may very well violate privacy expectations of clients or even contract type requirements and may needlessly lead to claims and lawsuits. Given the difference in state laws and in court interpretations as to when so-called statutes of limitations apply or don't apply so as to narrow or expand statutory limits on the time for the filing of lawsuits, records should be kept as long as possible and in accordance with individualized legal advice.

Ethical Codes

Most health and fitness/personal training certification and membership organizations have codes of ethics that certified or member trainers must agree to adhere to and to apply in their professional practices. The NSCA Code of Ethics is available at www.nsca.com/Publications/CodeofEthics.pdf. The four main points of this code are as follows:

1. Discrimination on the basis of gender, race, religion, nationality, or age is prohibited. All clients must be treated equally and their confidentiality must be protected.

2. Personal trainers should obey all relevant federal, state, and local laws; as well as all institutional guidelines and NSCA bylaws, policies, and procedures.

3. Personal trainers should not misrepresent their skills, training, or certification; and should provide only those services for which they are qualified.

4. Personal trainers should avoid professional or personal behavior that reflects negatively on the NSCA. For instance, they should never place their own financial gain over the well-being of a client and they should avoid substance abuse.

The NCSA Ethics Committee is responsible both for investigating potential violations of this code and for determining which disciplinary measures should be taken. Personal trainers who are found to have violated the code may be formally censured, may have their NSCA membership suspended or terminated, or may be removed from positions that require compliance with these principles.

As can be readily determined from a review of the NSCA Code of Ethics and similar codes of other groups, fitness personnel should take these statements seriously and follow the requirements established in those codes. Violations can lead to needless disciplinary proceedings; and as with all such matters, those violations, even if they don't lead to other kinds of legal controversies, should be avoided in the exercise of good professional practice.

Conclusion

A number of legal concerns affect the health and fitness profession and personal trainers in particular. In this regard, measures that will benefit professionals include compliance with authoritative standards and guidelines of prominent professional associations such as the NSCA; the use of protective legal documents as evidenced by written assumption of risk forms and prospectively executed waivers/releases of liability; the purchase of adequate liability insurance that covers the actual training activities performed by professionals for clients; the proper recording and maintenance of client and other professional records; adherence to applicable statutes, laws, and regulations; and adherence to professional ethical codes and rules of conduct. Such actions should improve the delivery of safe and effective services to clients while limiting personal trainers' exposure to claims and lawsuits.

Study Questions

1. The legal system decides personal injury and wrongful death cases in which of the following settings?

   A. the criminal justice system

   B. the civil justice system, focusing on tort law

   C. the civil justice system, focusing on contract law

   D. the civil justice system, focusing on equity

2. Personal trainers may lawfully and permissibly provide advice to clients in which of the following situations?

   A. the use of exercise equipment

   B. the use of various exercises to treat a client's medical conditions

   C. the use of particular exercises to lower a client's elevated blood pressure

   D. the use of medical procedures to prevent disease

3. An assumption of risk or a waiver/release of liability may be used by personal trainers

    A. in most states.

    B. only if authorized by statutory law.

    C. when approved by a judge prior to use.

    D. when the facility pays the participant to sign.

4. Professional standards of practice for personal trainers may be used for which of the following?

    A. to assist personal trainers in their delivery of service

    B. to help physicians provide diagnostic services for patients

    C. to qualify personal trainers to render physical therapy services for patients

    D. to qualify personal trainers to be licensed in particular states

Applied Knowledge Question

A 50-year-old sedentary male with type 2 diabetes responds to a health club solicitation to provide a membership and personal training services to him. He joins the club, but refuses to complete a PAR-Q form or to otherwise provide any information regarding his health status except the foregoing. He insists upon proceeding to receive instruction from a personal trainer in the use of various exercise machines at the facility. He also asks the personal trainer for advice to stop smoking, lose weight, and alleviate knee pain that he has had since high school even though his physician has recommended surgery to treat the condition and he has neglected to do so. Under these circumstances, how should the personal trainer respond to these requests?

Notes

1. Additional information on legal aspects of personal training can be found at D.L. Herbert and W.G. Herbert. 2002. *Legal Aspects of Preventive, Rehabilitative and Recreational Exercise Programs,* 4th ed. Canton, OH: PRC.

2. Risk management for personal trainers is also discussed in Eickhoff-Shemek, Herbert, and Connaughton. 2008. *Risk Management for Health/Fitness Professionals: Legal Issues and Strategies.* Philadelphia: Lippincott Williams & Wilkins. See also *The Exercise Standards and Malpractice Reporter,* published six times per year by PRC (Canton, OH). www.prcpublishingcorp.com.

3. *ACSM's Health/Fitness Facility Standards and Guidelines.* 1992. Champaign, IL: Human Kinetics.

4. www.nsca-lift.org/Publications/SCStandards.pdf

5. http://standards.nsf.org/apps/group_public/download.php?document_id=4126.

6. Medical Fitness Association. *Medical Fitness Association's Standards and Guidelines for Medical Fitness Center Facilities.* 2009. Monterey, CA: Author.

7. *The Exercise Standards and Malpractice Reporter,* published six times per year by PRC (Canton, OH). www.prcpublishingcorp.com.

8. See, e.g., *Stetino v. State Medical Licensing Board,* 513 N.E. 2d, 1234 (Ind. App. 2 Dist. K87); *State v. Winterich,* 157 Ohio St. 414 (1952).

9. See, e.g., Ohio Revise Code Adm. sect. 4759, 2006.

10. *Capati v. Crunch Fitness International, et al.,* analyzed in Herbert, 1999, "$320 million Lawsuit Filed Against Health Club," *The Exercise Standards and Malpractice Reporter* 13: 33-36.

11. *Capati v. Crunch Fitness International, et al.,* analyzed in Herbert, 2006, "Wrongful Death Case of Anne Marie Capati Settles for in Excess of $4 million," *The Exercise Standards and Malpractice Reporter* 20: 36.

12. Eickhoff-Shemek, Herbert, and Connaughton. 2009. *Risk Management for Health/Fitness Professionals.* Baltimore: Wolters Kluwer Health, Lippincott Williams & Wilkins.

13. 261 A.D. 2d 345 (NY App. Div., 1999).

14. Id.

15. *Rostai v. Neste Enterprises* (2006), 138 Cal.App.4th 326 (41 Cal.Rptr.3d 411).

16. *Neumann v. Gloria Marshall Figure Salon,* 500 N.E. 2d 1011 (Ill. App. Ct. 1964).

17. *Garrison v. Combined Fitness Center, Ltd.,* 201 Ill. App. 3d 581 (Ill. App. Ct. 1990).

18. *Avant v. Community Hospital* (2005), 826 NE 2d 7, analyzed in Herbert, 2006, "Personal Trainer's Fitness Routine Leads to Suit," *The Exercise Standards and Malpractice Reporter* 20 (6), 81, 85-86.

19. Cotton and Cotton. 1997. *Legal Aspects of Waivers in Sport, Recreation and Fitness Activities.* Canton, OH: PRC.

20. *Bowen v. Kil-Kare, Inc.,* 585 N.E. 2d 384 (Ohio 1992); but see *Byrd v. Matthews,* 571 So. 2d 258 (Miss. 1990).

21. *Dilallo v. Riding Safely, Inc.,* 687 So. 2d 353 (Fla. Dist. Ct. 1997).

22. *Zivich v. Mentor Soccer Club,* 82 Ohio St. 3d 367 (Ohio 1998).

23. See, e.g., *Kissinger v. Kissinger,* 2002-Ohio-3083; but see *Wade v. Watson,* 527 F. Supp. 1049 (N.D. Ga. 1981), *affirmed* 731 F. 2d 5890 (11th Ca. 1984).

24. D.L. Herbert and W.G. Herbert. 2002. *Legal Aspects of Preventive, Rehabilitative and Recreational Exercise Programs,* 4th ed. Canton, OH: PRC. pp. 348-349.

25. Cotton and Cotton. 1997. *Legal Aspects of Waivers in Sport, Recreation and Fitness Activities.* Canton, OH: PRC.

26. See, e.g., The Health Insurance Portability and Accountability Act (HIPAA) of 1996, Public Law 104-191.

Name _____

1. Purpose and Explanation of Test

I hereby consent to voluntarily engage in an exercise test to determine my circulatory and respiratory fitness. I also consent to the taking of samples of my exhaled air during exercise to properly measure my oxygen consumption. I also consent, if necessary, to have a small blood sample drawn by needle from my arm for blood chemistry analysis and to the performance of lung function and body fat (skinfold pinch) tests. It is my understanding that the information obtained will help me evaluate future physical activities and sports activities in which I may engage.

Before I undergo the test, I certify to the program that I am in good health and have had a physical examination conducted by a licensed medical physician within the last _____ months. Further, I hereby represent and inform the program that I have completed the pretest history interview presented to me by the program staff and have provided correct responses to the questions as indicated on the history form or as supplied to the interviewer. It is my understanding that I will be interviewed by a physician or other person prior to my undergoing the test who will in the course of interviewing me determine if there are any reasons which would make it undesirable or unsafe for me to take the test. Consequently, I understand that it is important that I provide complete and accurate responses to the interviewer and recognize that my failure to do so could lead to possible unnecessary injury to myself during the test.

The test I will undergo will be performed on a motor-driven treadmill or bicycle ergometer with the amount of effort gradually increasing. As I understand it, this increase in effort will continue until I feel and verbally report to the operator any symptoms such as fatigue, shortness of breath, or chest discomfort which may appear. It is my understanding and I have been clearly advised that it is my right to request that a test be stopped at any point if I feel unusual discomfort or fatigue. I have been advised that I should immediately upon experiencing any such symptoms, or if I so choose, inform the operator that I wish to stop the test at that or any other point. My wishes in this regard shall be absolutely carried out.

It is further my understanding that prior to beginning the test, I will be connected by electrodes and cables to an electrocardiographic recorder, which will enable the program personnel to monitor my cardiac (heart) activity. It is my understanding that during the test itself, a trained observer will monitor my responses continuously and take frequent readings of blood pressure, the electrocardiogram, and my expressed feelings of effort. I realize that a true determination of my exercise capacity depends on progressing the test to the point of my fatigue.

Once the test has been completed, but before I am released from the test area, I will be given special instructions about showering and recognition of certain symptoms that may appear within the first 24 hours after the test. I agree to follow these instructions and promptly contact the program personnel or medical providers if such symptoms develop.

2. Risks

I understand and have been informed that there exists the possibility of adverse changes during the actual test. I have been informed that these changes could include abnormal blood pressure, fainting, disorders of heart rhythm, stroke, and very rare instances of heart attack or even death. I have been told that every effort will be made to minimize these occurrences by preliminary examination and by precautions and observations taken during the test. I have also been informed that emergency equipment and personnel are readily available to deal with these unusual situations should they occur. I understand that there is a risk of injury, heart attack, or even death as a result of my performance of this test, but knowing those risks, it is my desire to proceed to take the test as herein indicated.

3. Benefits to Be Expected and Available Alternatives to the Exercise Testing Procedure

The results of this test may or may not benefit me. Potential benefits relate mainly to my personal motives for taking the test, that is, knowing my exercise capacity in relation to the general population, understanding my

(continued)

fitness for certain sports and recreational activities, planning my physical conditioning program, or evaluating the effects of my recent physical activity habits. Although my fitness might also be evaluated by alternative means, for example, a bench step test or an outdoor running test, such tests do not provide as accurate a fitness assessment as the treadmill or bike test, nor do those options allow equally effective monitoring of my responses.

4. Confidentiality and Use of Information

I have been informed that the information obtained in this exercise test will be treated as privileged and confidential and will consequently not be released or revealed to any person without my express written consent. I do, however, agree to the use of any information for research or statistical purposes so long as same does not provide facts that could lead to my identification. Any other information obtained, however, will be used only by the program staff to evaluate my exercise status or needs.

5. Inquiries and Freedom of Consent

I have been given an opportunity to ask certain questions as to the procedures. Generally these requests, which have been noted by the testing staff, and their responses are as follows:

_____

_____

_____

_____

_____

_____

I further understand that there are also other remote risks that may be associated with this procedure. Despite the fact that a complete accounting of all these remote risks has not been provided to me, I still desire to proceed with the test.

I acknowledge that I have read this document in its entirety or that it has been read to me if I have been unable to read same.

I consent to the rendition of all services and procedures as explained herein by all program personnel.

Date _____

Participant's signature _____

Witness' signature _____

Test supervisor's signature _____

The law varies from state to state. No form should be adopted or used by any program without individualized legal advice.

Informed Consent for Participation in a Personal Fitness Training Program of Apparently Healthy Adults (Without Known or Suspected Heart Disease)

Name _____

1. Purpose and Explanation of Procedure

I hereby consent to voluntarily engage in an acceptable plan of personal fitness training. I also give consent to be placed in personal fitness training program activities that are recommended to me for improvement of my general health and well-being. These may include dietary counseling, stress management, and health/fitness education activities. The levels of exercise I perform will be based on my cardiorespiratory (heart and lungs) and muscular fitness. I understand that I may be required to undergo a graded exercise test as well as other fitness tests prior to the start of my personal fitness training program in order to evaluate and assess my present level of fitness. I will be given exact personal instructions regarding the amount and kind of exercise I should do. I agree to participate 3 times per week in the formal program sessions. Professionally trained personal fitness trainers will provide leadership to direct my activities, monitor my performance, and otherwise evaluate my effort. Depending on my health status, I may or may not be required to have my blood pressure and heart rate evaluated during these sessions to regulate my exercise within desired limits. I understand that I am expected to attend every session and to follow staff instructions with regard to exercise, diet, stress management, and other health/fitness-related programs. If I am taking prescribed medications, I have already so informed the program staff and further agree to so inform them promptly of any changes my doctor or I make with regard to use of these. I will be given the opportunity for periodic assessment and evaluation at regular intervals after the start of my program. I have been informed that during my participation in this personal fitness training program, I will be asked to complete the physical activities unless symptoms such as fatigue, shortness of breath, chest discomfort, or similar occurrences appear. At that point, I have been advised that it is my complete right to decrease or stop exercise and that it is my obligation to inform the personal fitness training program personnel of my symptoms. I hereby state that I have been so advised and agree to inform the personal fitness training program personnel of my symptoms, should any develop.

I understand that while I exercise, a personal fitness trainer will periodically monitor my performance and perhaps measure my pulse and blood pressure or assess my feelings of effort for the purposes of monitoring my progress. I also understand that the personal fitness trainer may reduce or stop my exercise program when any of these findings so indicate that this should be done for my safety and benefit.

I also understand that during the performance of my personal fitness training program, physical touching and positioning of my body may be necessary to assess my muscular and bodily reactions to specific exercises, as well as to ensure that I am using proper technique and body alignment. I expressly consent to the physical contact for these reasons.

2. Risks

I understand and have been informed that there exists the remote possibility of adverse changes occurring during exercise including, but not limited to, abnormal blood pressure, fainting, dizziness, disorders of heart rhythm, and very rare instances of heart attack, stroke, or even death. I further understand and I have been informed that there exists the risk of bodily injury including, but not limited to, injuries to the muscles, ligaments, tendons, and joints of the body. I have been told that every effort will be made to minimize these occurrences by proper staff assessments of my condition before each exercise session, by staff supervision during exercise, and by my own careful control of exercise efforts. I fully understand the risks associated with exercise, including the risk of bodily injury, heart attack, stroke, or even death, but knowing these risks, it is my desire to participate as herein indicated.

3. Benefits to Be Expected and Available Alternatives to Exercise

I understand that this program may or may not benefit my physical fitness or general health. I recognize that involvement in the exercise sessions and personal fitness training sessions will allow me to learn proper ways to perform conditioning exercises, use fitness equipment, and regulate physical effort. These experiences should

(continued)

benefit me by indicating how my physical limitations may affect my ability to perform various physical activities. I further understand that if I closely follow the program's instructions, I will likely improve my exercise capacity and fitness level after a period of 3 to 6 months.

4. Confidentiality and Use of Information

I have been informed that the information obtained in this personal fitness training program will be treated as privileged and confidential and will consequently not be released or revealed to any person without my express written consent. I do, however, agree to the use of any information that is not personally identifiable with me for research and statistical purposes so long as same does not identify me or provide facts that could lead to my identification. I also agree to the use of any information for the purpose of consultation with other health/fitness professionals, including my doctor. Any other information obtained, however, will be used by the program staff in the course of prescribing exercise for me and evaluating my progress in the program.

5. Inquiries and Freedom of Consent

I have been given an opportunity to ask certain questions as to the procedures of this program. Generally, these requests have been noted by the interviewing staff with his/her responses as follows:

_____

_____

_____

_____

_____

_____

I further understand that there are also other remote risks that may be associated with this personal fitness training program. Despite the fact that a complete accounting of all these remote risks has not been provided to me, it is still my desire to participate.

I acknowledge that I have read this document in its entirety or that it has been read to me if I have been unable to read same.

I expressly consent to the rendition of all services and procedures as explained herein by all program personnel.

Date _____

Client's signature _____

By
Authorized representative _____

[Club name]
[Address]
[Address]

The law varies from state to state. No form should be adopted or used by any program without individualized legal advice.

User's Representations, Express Assumption of All Risks, and Release of Liability Agreement

Purpose of This Binding Agreement

By reading and signing this document, "You," the undersigned, sometimes also referred to as "User" or "I," will agree to release and hold [Club name] ("Club" or "We") harmless from, and assume all responsibility for, all claims, demands, injuries, damages, actions or causes of action to persons or property, arising out of or connected with your use of the Club's facilities, premises, or services. The agreement and release is for the benefit of the Club, its employees, agents, independent contractors, other users of the Club and all persons on the Club's premises. This agreement includes your release of these persons from responsibility for injury, damage, or death to yourself because of those acts or omissions claimed to be related to the ordinary negligence of these persons. This agreement also includes your representations as to important matters which the Club will rely upon.

A. Representations

The undersigned, You, represent: (a) that you understand that use of the Club premises, facilities, equipment, services and programs includes an inherent risk of injury to persons and property; (b) that you are in good physical condition and have no disabilities, illnesses, or other conditions that could prevent you from exercising and using the Club's equipment/facilities without injuring yourself or impairing your health; and (c) that you have consulted a physician concerning an exercise program that will not risk injury to yourself or impairment of your health. Such risk of injury includes, but is not limited to, injuries arising from or relating to use by you or others of exercise equipment and machines, locker rooms, spa and other wet areas, and other Club facilities; injuries arising from or relating to participation by you or others in supervised or unsupervised activities or programs through the Club; injuries and medical disorders arising from or relating to use of the Club's facilities including heart attacks, sudden cardiac arrests, strokes, heat stress, sprains, strains, broken bones, and torn muscles, tendons, and ligaments, among others; and accidental injuries occurring anywhere in the Club including lobbies, hallways, exercise areas, locker rooms, steam rooms, pool areas, Jacuzzis, saunas, and dressing rooms. Accidental injuries include those caused by you, those caused by other persons, and those of a "slip-and-fall" nature. If you have any special exercise requirements or limitations, you agree to disclose them to the Club before using the Club's facilities; and when seeking help in establishing an exercise program, you hereby agree that all exercise and use of the Club's facilities, services, programs, and premises are undertaken by you at your sole risk. As used herein, the terms "include," "including," and words of similar import are descriptive only, and are not limiting in any manner.

You also acknowledge and represent that you realize and appreciate that access to and use of the Club's facilities during nonsupervised times increases and enhances certain risks to you. You realize that if you use the Club during nonsupervised hours, any emergency response to you in the event of need for same may be impossible or delayed. While we encourage you to use the Club's facility with a partner during nonsupervised times, you may choose to do so without a partner, therefore enhancing and increasing the risks to you as to the provision of first aid and emergency response. You realize that a delay in the provision of first aid and/or emergency response may result in greater injury and disability to you and may cause or contribute to your death. Use of the Club with no one else present to supervise or watch your activities is not recommended and would not be allowed unless you agree to assume all risks of injury, whether known or unknown to you.

You do hereby further declare yourself to be physically sound and suffering from no condition, impairment, disease, infirmity, or other illness that would prevent your participation or use of equipment or machinery except as hereinafter stated. You do hereby acknowledge that you have been informed of the need for a physician's approval for your participation in an exercise/fitness activity or in the use of exercise equipment and machinery. You also acknowledge that it has been recommended that you have a yearly or more frequent physical examination and consultation with your physician as to physical activity, exercise, and use of exercise and training equipment so that you might have his recommendations concerning these fitness activities and equipment use. You acknowledge either that you have had a physical examination and have been given your physician's permission to participate, or that you have decided to participate in activity and use of equipment and machinery without the approval of your physician and do hereby assume all responsibility for your participation and activities, and utilization of equipment and machinery in your activities.

(continued)

YOU HAVE READ THE FOREGOING, ACKNOWLEDGE THAT YOU UNDERSTAND THE TERMS AND CONDITIONS SET FORTH IN THE PRECEDING PARAGRAPHS, AND AGREE TO SAME.

Initials: _____

B. Express Assumption of All Risks

You have represented to us and acknowledged that you understand and appreciate all of the risks associated with your participation in various activities at the Club and in the use of equipment/facilities at the Club, including the risks of injury, disability, and death. You have also acknowledged that there are greater, enhanced, and even other risks to you if you decide to use the Club's facility during nonsupervised times. Knowing and appreciating all of these risks and enhanced risks, you have knowingly and intelligently determined to expressly assume all risks associated with all of your activities and use of equipment/facilities at the Club.

You understand and are aware that strength, flexibility and aerobic exercise, including the use of equipment, is a potentially hazardous activity. You also understand that fitness activities involve the risk of injury and even death, and that you are voluntarily participating in these activities and using equipment and machinery with knowledge of the dangers involved. We have also reviewed the risks with you on the date when you signed this Agreement and answered any questions that you may have had. You hereby agree to expressly assume and accept any and all risks of injury or death including those related to your use of or presence at this facility, your use of equipment, and your participation in activity, including those risks related to the ordinary negligence of those released by this Agreement and including all claims related to ordinary negligence in the selection, purchase, setup, maintenance, instruction as to use, and use and/or supervision of use, if any, associated with all equipment and facilities.

YOU HAVE READ THE FOREGOING, ACKNOWLEDGE THAT YOU UNDERSTAND THE TERMS AND CONDITIONS SET FORTH IN THE PRECEDING PARAGRAPHS, AND AGREE TO SAME.

Initials: _____

C. Agreement and Release of Liability

In consideration of being allowed to participate in the activities and programs of the Club and to use its equipment/facilities and machinery in addition to the payment of any fee or charge, you do hereby waive, release, and forever discharge the Club and its directors, officers, agents, employees, representatives, successors and assigns, administrators, executors, and all others from any and all responsibilities or liability from injuries or damages resulting from your participation in any activities or your use of equipment/facilities or machinery in the above-mentioned activities. You do also hereby release all of those mentioned and any others acting upon their behalf from any responsibility or liability for any injury or damage to yourself, including those caused by the negligent act or omission of any of those mentioned or others acting on their behalf or in any way arising out of or connected with your participation in any activities of the Club. This provision shall apply to ordinary acts of negligence but shall not apply to gross acts/omissions of negligence, willful or wanton acts/omissions, or those of an intentional/criminal nature.

YOU HAVE READ THE FOREGOING, ACKNOWLEDGE THAT YOU UNDERSTAND THE TERMS AND CONDITIONS SET FORTH IN THE PRECEDING PARAGRAPHS, AND AGREE TO SAME.

Initials: _____

D. Loss or Theft of Property

The Club is not responsible for lost or stolen articles. You should keep any valuables with you at all times while using the facilities. Storage space or lockers do not always protect valuables. Consequently, by executing this Agreement and any accompanying documents, you do hereby agree to assume all responsibility for your own property and that of any dependent(s) and to insure that property against risk of loss as you see fit. By the execution hereof, you expressly, on behalf of yourself and any dependents, do hereby knowingly agree to forego, waive, release, and prospectively give up any right to institute any claim or action against the Club relating to lost or stolen property, including property lost or stolen due to the negligent act or omission of the Club. You agree to indemnify and save the Club and all of its personnel harmless from any action, claim, suit, or subrogated claim or suit instituted at any time hereafter against the Club related to the theft or loss of your or your dependents' property at the Club. The Club shall be indemnified by you for all costs, expenses, fees, including attorney fees, incurred by the Club or its personnel by reason of any such action.

YOU HAVE READ THE FOREGOING, ACKNOWLEDGE THAT YOU UNDERSTAND THE TERMS AND CONDITIONS SET FORTH IN THE PRECEDING PARAGRAPHS, AND AGREE TO SAME.

Initials: _____

User shall receive a copy of the foregoing Agreement at the time of its initialing and signing and hereby acknowledges User's receipt of same.

YOU HAVE READ THE FOREGOING, ACKNOWLEDGE THAT YOU UNDERSTAND THE TERMS AND CONDITIONS SET FORTH IN THE PRECEDING PARAGRAPHS, AND AGREE TO SAME.

Initials: _____

This Agreement shall be interpreted according to the laws of the State of _____. If any part of this Agreement should ever be determined by a court of final jurisdiction to be invalid, the remaining portions hereof shall be deemed to be valid and enforceable.

YOU HAVE READ THE FOREGOING, ACKNOWLEDGE THAT YOU UNDERSTAND THE TERMS AND CONDITIONS SET FORTH IN THE PRECEDING PARAGRAPHS, AND AGREE TO SAME.

Initials: _____

Acknowledgment

I have read and received a completed copy of this Agreement and all of its Exhibits, as well as any Rules and Regulations of the Club which are incorporated herein by reference. I agree to be bound by the terms and conditions of the Agreement and the Rules and Regulations of the Club, as same exist or as same may be amended from time to time hereafter. This Agreement shall be binding upon me and my spouse, my heirs, my estate, my executors, my administrators, and my successors and/or assigns. I realize that this Agreement is designed to prevent me and/or them from filing any personal injury or other lawsuit based upon ordinary negligence, including negligent battery, or even negligent wrongful death, loss of consortium, or any other similar lawsuit arising out of any injury to me which I or they may possess hereafter.

The undersigned, on behalf of myself and my heirs, executors, administrators, successors, and assigns hereby agree to indemnify the Club and all those hereby released and to hold them absolutely harmless if anyone, including the undersigned, should hereafter file suit against the Club or those released hereby for any matter intended to be released by this Agreement, including claims based upon ordinary negligence such as but not limited to personal injury, wrongful death, loss of consortium, or other similar actions.

Signature _____ Date: _____

Print name: _____

Address: _____

Phone number: (_____) _____

From NSCA, 2012, *NSCA's essentials of personal training,* 2nd ed., J. Coburn and M. Malek (eds.), (Champaign, IL: Human Kinetics).

Answers to Study Questions

CHAPTER 1
1. A; 2. C; 3. B; 4. B; 5. D

CHAPTER 2
1. B; 2. A; 3. D; 4. D; 5. D

CHAPTER 3
1. A; 2. A; 3. D; 4. A

CHAPTER 4
1. B; 2. A; 3. D; 4. C

CHAPTER 5
1. A; 2. B; 3. C; 4. D

CHAPTER 6
1. C; 2. B; 3. A; 4. C

CHAPTER 7
1. D; 2. B; 3. C; 4. C

CHAPTER 8
1. B; 2. C; 3. A; 4. B

CHAPTER 9
1. B; 2. B; 3. C; 4. D; 5. B

CHAPTER 10
1. D; 2. D; 3. C; 4. D

CHAPTER 11
1. C; 2. B; 3. C; 4. A

CHAPTER 12
1. C; 2. B; 3. B; 4. C

CHAPTER 13
1. C; 2. B; 3. C; 4. A

CHAPTER 14
1. D; 2. B; 3. D; 4. B

CHAPTER 15
1. D; 2. D; 3. C; 4. A; 5. B

CHAPTER 16
1. C; 2. B; 3. B; 4. A

CHAPTER 17
1. A; 2. C; 3. D; 4. C

CHAPTER 18
1. C; 2. A; 3. D; 4. B; 5. B

CHAPTER 19
1. C; 2. D; 3. B; 4. C

CHAPTER 20
1. D; 2. B; 3. C; 4. D

CHAPTER 21
1. C; 2. A; 3. C; 4. B; 5. C

CHAPTER 22
1. A; 2. C; 3. C; 4. C

CHAPTER 23
1. A; 2. C; 3. D; 4. B; 5. C

CHAPTER 24
1. B; 2. B; 3. C; 4. D

CHAPTER 25
1. B; 2. A; 3. A; 4. A

Suggested Solutions to Applied Knowledge Questions

Chapter 1

- When selecting exercises for aerobic fitness, choose weight-bearing exercises (walking, jogging, etc.).
- Include resistance training in the exercise program, and perform a variety of exercises for all the major muscle groups.
- Emphasize the eccentric phase (i.e., lowering of weight) during resistance training.

Chapter 2

This question tests the knowledge of the reader to use the Fick equation (2.6):

$\dot{V}O_2 = (HR \times SV) \times a{-}\bar{v}O_2$

Absolute $\dot{V}O_2$ = (160 beats/min $\times$ 100 ml/beat) $\times$ (13 ml O_2 ml/100 ml blood)

= (160 ml/min) $\times$ (13 ml O_2 ml/100 ml blood)

= 2,080 ml O_2/min

Relative $\dot{V}O_2$ = (absolute $\dot{V}O_2$) / (weight in kilograms)

= (2,080 ml O_2/min) / (77.10 kg)

= 26.97 ml $O_2 \cdot kg^{-1} \cdot min^{-1}$

Chapter 3

Activity	Carbohydrate	Fat
While the client is sitting in a chair listening to the personal trainer	Least	Most
The first few seconds of the treadmill test	Most	Least
During a stage when the client reached steady state	Least	Most (a shift toward fat)
At the end of the test as the client reaches maximum	Most (a shift toward carbohydrate)	Least

Chapter 4

Type of external resistance	Examples
Free weights	Barbells, dumbbells, body weight exercises
Constant-resistance machines	Pulleys, counterbalance machines
Variable-resistance machines	Machines with variable cams
Elastic materials	Elastic tubing, stretch bands, springs
Accommodating-resistance machines	Isokinetic dynamometers, flywheels, pneumatic equipment

Chapter 5

System	Two adaptations
Nervous	<ul><li>Increased EMG amplitude</li><li>Increased skill</li><li>Increased motor unit recruitment</li><li>Increased motor unit firing rate</li><li>Decreased cocontraction</li><li>Increased motor unit synchronization</li></ul>
Muscular	<ul><li>Increased cross-sectional area</li><li>Increased size</li><li>Fiber subtype shift from type IIx to type IIa</li></ul>
Skeletal	<ul><li>Increased bone formation/mass</li></ul>
Metabolic	<ul><li>Possibly increased concentration of ATP and CP</li><li>Possibly increased concentration of creatine kinase and myokinase</li></ul>
Hormonal	<ul><li>Increased concentration of testosterone</li><li>Altered epinephrine response</li><li>Increased sensitivity of receptor sites</li></ul>
Cardiorespiratory	<ul><li>Augmentation of the development of endurance and running efficiency</li><li>Increased capillarization</li><li>Decreased myoglobin and mitochondrial density</li></ul>

Chapter 6

System	Two adaptations
Respiratory	<ul><li>Decreased submaximal exercise pulmonary ventilation</li><li>Increased maximal exercise pulmonary ventilation</li><li>Increased respiratory muscle aerobic enzymes</li></ul>
Metabolic	<ul><li>Increased maximal aerobic power ($\dot{V}O_2max$)</li><li>Increased lactate threshold</li><li>Increased fat utilization during submaximal exercise</li><li>Decreased carbohydrate utilization during submaximal exercise</li></ul>
Skeletal muscle	<ul><li>Increased capillary density</li><li>Increased mitochondria density</li><li>Increased oxidative enzymes</li><li>Increased glycogen stores</li></ul>
Cardiovascular	<ul><li>Increased resting stroke volume</li><li>Increased submaximal exercise stroke volume</li><li>Increased maximal stroke volume</li><li>Increased maximal cardiac output</li><li>Decreased resting heart rate</li><li>Decreased submaximal exercise heart rate</li><li>Increased blood volume</li><li>Increased left ventricular end-diastolic chamber diameter</li></ul>
Endocrine	<ul><li>Reduced (smaller) rise in plasma levels of epinephrine and norepinephrine during submaximal exercise</li><li>Reduced (smaller) drop in plasma levels of insulin during submaximal exercise</li></ul>

Chapter 7

Nutrient	General daily requirements
Kilocalories	4,667-5,600 (from table 7.3, vigorous or vigorously active lifestyle)
Protein (grams)	131-218 (1.2 to 2 g/kg)
Carbohydrate (grams)	545-763 (5 to 7 g/kg; >7 g/kg would leave no room in calorie budget for fat and protein)
Fat (percent of total kilocalories)	20-30% (range based on calorie intake is 99 to 164 grams)
Monounsaturated fat (percent of total fat intake)	About 10%
Polyunsaturated fat (percent of total fat intake)	About 10%
Saturated fat (percent of total fat intake)	< 10%
Vitamin A	900 μ g/day
Vitamin E	15 mg/day
Calcium	1,000 mg/day
Iron	8 mg/day

Chapter 8

1. Make goals specific, measurable, and observable:
   - □ The client provided a *specific* goal of a 90-pound increase in his 1RM.
   - □ The goal increase is *measurable* (i.e., it is a certain load).
   - □ The goal is *observable* in that the client and the personal trainer can visually see that the leg press is loaded with the goal weight and a 1RM attempt is either successful or not successful; there is no "in between."

2. Clearly identify the time constraints:
   - □ The client stated a six-month time frame.

3. Use moderately difficult goals:
   - □ A 90-pound increase is very large and may have to be modified (although the client's training status is not mentioned; a relatively untrained healthy male client can probably attain this goal, but other client types may have difficulty).

4. Record goals and monitor progress:
   - □ The client can be retested every four to eight weeks to monitor progress.
   - □ A workout card or wall poster can be a valuable visual motivator.

5. Diversify process, performance, and outcomes:
   - □ If the client can tolerate it, a periodized resistance training program (see chapters 15 and 23) will be the most effective method.

6. Set short-range goals to achieve long-range goals:
   - □ If the client will be retested every eight weeks (two months), his short-term goals could be to reach a 1RM of 255 pounds in two months, 285 pounds in four months, then 315 pounds in six months.

7. Make sure goals are internalized:
   - □ Since the client provided his own goal, it is likely that he has internalized it.
   - □ The personal trainer should discuss the goal with the client to find out why he provided that particular goal; this will help the personal trainer determine what type of feedback or motivation is appropriate for the client (e.g., if the client's friend has a 1RM of 310 pounds, the client's stated goal of 315 pounds may indicate an ego-involved goal orientation).

Chapter 9

Based on comparisons to the coronary artery disease risk factor thresholds (table 9.1):

- Family history: no risk—his father's heart attack occurred after age 55 (his grandmother's heart attack is not a factor).
- Cigarette smoking: no risk—he is a nonsmoker.
- Hypertension: no risk—blood pressure is below the 140/90 mmHg reading.
- Hypercholesterolemia: at risk—his cholesterol is over the 200 mg/dl recommendation and his HDL level is at the 35 mg/dl cutoff.
- Fasting glucose: no risk—his reading is below the 110 mg/dl recommendation.
- Obesity: no risk—his BMI is less than 30 kg/m².
- Sedentary lifestyle: at risk—client is sedentary.

Based on the risk stratification categories (table 9.2), the client is at a "moderate" risk.

Chapter 10

Client	Description	Fitness component to be tested	Test 1	Test 2
27-year-old male	Has been participating in 5 km runs for three years	Cardiorespiratory endurance	1.5-mile run	12-min run
33-year-old female	Has been resistance training consistently for 10 years	Muscular strength	1RM bench press	1RM back squat
41-year-old female	Has been diagnosed as obese by her physician	Body composition	Girth measurements	BMI or waist-to-hip ratio
11-year-old male	Has no exercise experience or training	Muscular endurance	1-min sit-up test	Push-up test

Chapter 11

The fitness evaluation data suggest that the client's aerobic capacity is very poor. A ($\dot{V}O_2$max value of 26 ml · kg^{-1} · min^{-1} is below the 10th percentile in her age group.

Chapter 12

The training program could include the following exercises, all of which involve the hip extensors:

Static flexibility exercises

- Forward Lunge
- Lying Knee to Chest

Dynamic flexibility exercises

- Lunge Walk
- Reverse Lunge Walk
- Hockey Lunge Walk
- Walking Side Lunge
- Walking Knee Tuck

Body-weight exercises (for strengthening the hip extensors)
- Step-up

Stability ball exercises (for actively, or concentrically, training the hip extensors)
- Supine Leg Curl
- Supine Hip Lift
- Reverse Back Hyperextensions

Chapter 13

Starting Position
- Stand erect at opposite ends of the barbell with feet shoulder-width apart and the knees slightly flexed.
- Grasp the end of the barbell by cupping the hands together with the palms facing upward.
- At the client's signal, assist with lifting and balancing the barbell as it is moved out of the rack.
- Release the barbell smoothly in unison with the other spotter.
- Hold the hands 2 to 3 inches (5 to 8 cm) below the ends of the barbell.
- Move sideways in unison with the client as the client moves backward.
- Once the client is in position, assume a hip-width stance with the knees slightly flexed and the torso erect.

Downward Motion
- Keep the cupped hands close to—but not touching—the barbell as it moves downward.
- Slightly flex the knees, hips, and torso and keep the back flat when following the barbell.

Upward Motion
- Keep the cupped hands close to—but not touching—the barbell as it moves upward.
- Slightly extend the knees, hips, and torso and keep the back flat when following the barbell.

Chapter 14

	Walking	Running
Body position	■ The head should be held upright with the eyes looking straight ahead. ■ The shoulders should be relaxed but not rounded. ■ The upper body should be positioned directly over the hips. ■ Body should be upright with the torso positioned directly over the hips.	■ Same as for walking (see left column), plus; ■ The lower back should not be arched.
Foot strike	■ Heel strikes the ground and then the weight is immediately spread over the foot by a gentle rolling heel-to-ball action. ■ Primarily this heel-to-ball roll starts near the outer side of the heel and continues forward and slightly inward toward the middle of the ball of the foot at push-off.	■ Same as for walking (see left column), plus; ■ Bouncing with each step should be avoided Different from walking in this way: ■ Some elite runners run primarily ball-to-heel.

Arm action	■ The left arm swings forward when the right foot strides forward.	■ Same as for walking (see left column).
	■ The right arm swings forward when the left foot strides forward.	Different from walking in these ways:
	■ The arms swing naturally from relaxed shoulders.	■ Only some arm action occurs from the shoulders.
	■ The arms are held bent at the elbow at 90°.	■ Much of the arm movement comes from the lower arm.
	■ The elbows pass fairly close to the sides.	■ The elbow is unlocked.
	■ The arms and hands swing primarily in a forward and backward motion.	■ The angle at the elbow opens during the arm downswing and closes during the upswing.
	■ The hands should not cross the midline of the body.	■ The forearms are carried between the waist and chest.
	■ On the forward swing the hands come to the level of the chest at the nipple line.	
	■ On the backward swing the hands reach the hipbone at the side of the body.	
	■ The hands are cupped loosely.	

Chapter 15

Initial consultation and fitness evaluation	Initial training status and experience	Intermediate
	Fitness evaluation	10RM testing to estimate a 1RM
	Primary resistance training goal	Hypertrophy

Assessing load capabilities	10RM LOADS AND THEIR ESTIMATED 1RMS FOR THESE SELECTED EXERCISES		
	Exercises (all are cam machines)	10RM (pounds)	Estimated 1RM (pounds)
	Vertical chest press	60	80
	Seated row	50	65
	Shoulder press	45	60
	Biceps curl	35	45
	Triceps extension	30	40
	Leg (knee) extension	70	90
	Leg (knee) curl	60	80

Assigning loads	Repetition range to match training goal: _6_ to _12_ per set
	Goal repetitions: eight
	Loading (%1RM) range to match training goal: _67_ % to _85_ %1RM
	%1RM associated with eight goal repetitions: _80_ %1RM

Calculating training loads from the estimated 1RM	Exercises (all are cam machines)	Estimated 1RM (pounds)	x	%1RM associated with 8 goal repetitions (in decimal form)	=	Calculated training load	Assigned training (round down)
	Vertical chest press	80	x	80	=	64	60
	Seated row	65	x	80	=	52	50
	Shoulder press	60	x	80	=	48	45
	Biceps curl	45	x	80	=	36	35
	Triceps extension	40	x	80	=	32	30
	Leg (knee) extension	90	x	80	=	72	70
	Leg (knee) curl	80	x	80	=	64	60

Chapter 16

Type	Intensity	Duration	Frequency	Goals
LSD	Lower than normal; 50% to 85% HRR	Longer than normal; 30 min to 2 h	No more than twice a week	Improve anaerobic threshold; develop endurance in the involved muscles; promote fat use; improve glycogen sparing
Pace/tempo: intermittent	At lactate threshold; RPE of 13 to 14 (or 4-5, depending on the scale)	Repeated work intervals of 3 to 5 min alternated with rest intervals of 30 to 90 s	1 to 2 times per week	Improve $\dot{V}O_2$max
Pace/tempo: steady	At lactate threshold; RPE of 13 to 14 (or 4-5, depending on the scale)	One session of 20 to 30 min	1 to 2 times per week	Improve $\dot{V}O_2$max
Interval	At or above lactate threshold and $\dot{V}O_2$max; 90% to 100% of HRR	Repeated work intervals of 3 to 5 min alternated with rest intervals at 1:1 to 1:3 work:rest ratio	1 to 2 times per week	Complete more work at a higher level of intensity than in a continuous exercise session; enhance the body's ability to clear lactate form the blood

Chapter 17

Mode	■ Since her 1RM squat is 1.5 times her body weight, she can perform lower body plyometric drills. ■ Without knowing her 1RM bench press, one cannot be certain whether she can safely perform upper body plyometric drills.
Activity-specific drills and their intensity	Choose from these lower body drills; ■ Ankle flip (intensity level: low) ■ Double-leg vertical jump (intensity level: low) ■ Skip (intensity level: low) ■ Jump to box (intensity level: low) ■ Double-leg tuck jump (intensity level: medium) ■ Split squat jump (intensity level: medium) ■ Double-leg hop (intensity level: medium) ■ Jump from box (intensity level: medium) ■ Depth jump (intensity level: high) ■ Depth jump to second box (intensity level: high) If she is able to qualify to perform upper body plyometrics, she could include these exercises: ■ Depth push-up (intensity level: medium) ■ Power drop (intensity level: high)
Frequency	■ 2 or 3 per week (as long as this does not result in overtraining due to the frequency of teaching aerobic classes)
Volume (table 17.6)	■ 100 to 120 total (foot) contacts (since she is resistance trained and performs plyometric drills now during a class she teaches)

Chapter 18

Children, seniors, and women who are pregnant can benefit from resistance training provided the programs are well designed, sensibly progressed, and supervised by qualified professionals. Participants should wear proper attire, and the exercise room should be safe, free of hazards, and climate controlled whenever possible. All training sessions should begin with warm-up activities, and less intense calisthenics should be performed during the cool-down. Although resistance exercise guidelines will vary depending on individual needs, goals, and abilities, the following are general recommendations for children, seniors, and women who are pregnant.

Children

- Have children perform one to three sets of 6 to 15 repetitions on a variety of exercises.
- Increase resistance gradually (e.g., about 5% to 10%) as strength improves.
- Include exercises for the upper body, lower body, and midsection.
- Resistance train two or three nonconsecutive days per week.
- Focus on skill improvement, personal successes, and having fun.
- Praise children for doing a good job.
- Offer a variety of activities and avoid regimentation.

Seniors

- Check with the client's personal physician for specific exercise guidelines.
- Begin with 8 to 10 exercises and use a resistance that permits 10 to 15 repetitions.
- Include both single- and multiple-joint movements in the training program.
- Have seniors perform resistance exercises at a controlled movement speed.
- Clients with poor balance should begin with weight-supporting machine exercises before progressing to weight-bearing free weight exercises.
- Focus on the quality of each movement phase and the proper breathing pattern.
- Ask clients frequently if they understand instructions and exercise performance procedures.
- Provide positive reinforcement for correct technique with specific feedback and suggestions for improved performance.

Women Who Are Pregnant

- Check with the client's health care provider before having the client exercise.
- Use a resistance that permits multiple repetitions (e.g., 12-15) for the major muscle groups and avoid isometric contractions.
- Pelvic floor exercises (Kegels) are an important element of training during pregnancy.
- Women should avoid lying on their back after the third month.
- They should avoid the Valsalva maneuver while resistance training because breath-holding during exertion places excessive pressure on the abdominal contents and pelvic floor.
- Pregnant women should be made aware of safe exercise guidelines and should know when to reduce the exercise intensity or stop exercising.

Chapter 19

Dietary Modifications

- Refer to a registered dietician.
- Select foods that are aligned with the client's cultural and ethnic background.
- Select foods that help decrease risk of CVD risk factors (e.g., follow the TLC diet).
- Create a deficit of 500 to 1,000 kcal/day.

- Women: not less than 1,000 to 1,200 kcal/day (1,200-1,600 for women who weigh more than 165 pounds [75 kg] or for women who exercise regularly).
- Set a weight loss goal of 10% of body weight over the first six months, then set new goals.
- Aim for a 1- to 2-pound (0.45 to 0.9 kg) weight loss per week.
- Change food choices to lower caloric and fat intake.

Exercise Program Guidelines
- Increase expenditure to help contribute to the reduced food intake (deficit) of 500 to 1,000 kcal/day.
- Aim for a mode, intensity, and duration of activity that will expend at least 150 kcal/day (1,000 kcal/week); progress toward 300 kcal/day (2,000 kcal/week).
- Start all exercise at a low level.
- Aerobic conditioning:
  - Mode: low-impact activities
  - Frequency: five days per week (or daily)
  - Duration: can begin with two daily sessions of 20 to 30 minutes each; eventual goal is 40 to 60 minutes per day
  - Intensity: 40% or 50% to 70% $\dot{V}O_2$max
- Resistance training:
  - Begin with body weight exercises
  - Intersperse with aerobic exercise
- Flexibility training:
  - Frequency: daily (or at least five days per week)

Lifestyle Change Support Suggestions
- Self-monitoring:
  - Record activity and dietary behaviors, habits, and attitudes (e.g., use "Small Steps . . . Big Changes Diet and Activity Diary").
  - Identify the obstacles to regular exercise.
- Rewards:
  - Provide big or small, tangible or intangible rewards (from the personal trainer, the client, or the client's family or support group).
  - Small rewards are for reaching small goals; big rewards are for reaching big goals.
- Goal setting:
  - Set realistic, stepwise short-term goals to reach larger, long-term goals.
  - Fill out and sign an activity/exercise self-contract.
- Stimulus control:
  - Identify social or environmental cues that trigger undesired responses.
  - Modify those cues and determine ways to manage the situation.
- Encourage food consumption behavior changes:
  - Eat more slowly.
  - Use smaller plates.
  - Do not skip meals.
  - Develop techniques over time that work well for a specific client.

Chapter 20

	BEGINNING EXERCISE PROGRAM				Exercise concerns
	Mode	Intensity	Frequency	Duration	
Hypertension	Aerobic exercise ■ Walking ■ Jogging ■ Swimming Resistance exercise (multijoint exercises): ■ Weight machines ■ Elastic bands ■ Circuit training	Aerobic exercise: ■ 40% $\dot{V}O_2$max ■ 8 RPE on 6-20 scale ■ Expenditure of 700 kcal per week Resistance exercise: ■ 16 to 20 reps ■ 50% 1RM ■ 1 set	Aerobic exercise: ■ 3 days per week Resistance exercise: ■ 2 days per week	Aerobic exercise: ■ 15 min Resistance exercise: ■ 30 min	■ If the blood pressure is stage 1, cancel the exercise session and advise the client to speak with the doctor. ■ Avoid the Valsalva maneuver.
MI	Aerobic exercise: ■ Not limited, but include treadmill walking when possible	Aerobic exercise: ■ 40% $\dot{V}O_2$max ■ 9 RPE on 6-20 scale Resistance exercise: ■ 20 reps ■ 1 set	Aerobic exercise: ■ 3 days per week Resistance exercise: ■ 2 days per week	Aerobic exercise: ■ 15 min	■ Monitor client for angina, palpitations, shortness of breath, diaphoresis, nausea, neck pain, arm pain, back pain, or a sense of impending doom. ■ Avoid the Valsalva maneuver.
Stroke	Aerobic exercise: ■ Ergometer Resistance exercises Flexibility exercises Coordination and balance exercises	Aerobic exercise: ■ 30% $\dot{V}O_2$peak (not max) ■ 9 RPE on 6-20 scale Resistance exercise: ■ Eventually strive for 2 sets of 8-12 reps	Aerobic exercise: ■ 3 days per week Resistance exercise: ■ 2 days per week	Aerobic exercise: ■ 5 min Flexibility exercise: ■ Before and after each session (as little as 5 min)	■ Balance and strength are affected. ■ A 1RM cannot be determined; start with very light resistance training loads.
PVD	Aerobic exercise: ■ Walking Resistance exercise: ■ Same as for hypertensive clients	Aerobic exercise: ■ Walk until it hurts, stop, then do it again, and so on	Aerobic exercise: ■ Near daily	Aerobic exercise: ■ 10 min	■ PVD clients cannot walk for more than 2 to 5 min without having to stop and rest due to calf pain.

| Asthma | Aerobic exercise:
■ Walking
■ Jogging
■ Swimming
Resistance exercise:
■ General resistance training | Aerobic exercise:
■ 11 RPE on 6-20 scale
Resistance exercise:
■ 16-24 reps | Aerobic exercise:
■ 3 days per week
Resistance exercise:
■ 2 days per week | Aerobic exercise:
■ 5 min | ■ Monitor intensity via RPE and the sense of shortness of breath.
■ Avoid temperature extremes. |

Chapter 21

1. Confirm with the physician, physical therapist, or athletic trainer if there were any movement restrictions upon discharge. Most likely, this individual will be cleared to perform any activity that he tolerates. Lower extremity strength exercises should emphasize musculature around hip, knee, and ankle. Given that the ankle will serve as the base of support for climbing activities while supporting heavy equipment on the upper body, exercises that reinforce and further develop core trunk musculature will be important. Lastly, the exercise program should integrate functional activities to support the muscular strength and power needed for performing all firefighting-related tasks. This individual may benefit from integrating balance and plyometric activities that involve unilateral stance and movement patterns.

2. The personal trainer should talk with the physician to identify the surgical procedure (i.e., patellar tendon graft, hamstring graft, or other) that was performed and whether there were ongoing recovery concerns to be aware of at time of discharge. It would also be beneficial to obtain an assessment of current joint ROM, flexibility, and muscle strength across the lower extremity with particular emphasis on the hip and knee. Provided there are no residual deficiencies or asymmetrical movement patterns, this client should be prepared to participate in a progressively designed functional prevention program. An effective prevention program will incorporate strength, balance, and plyometric activities that emphasize unilateral and bilateral multidirectional patterns with proper movement mechanics, technique, and control. It may also be beneficial to consider whether her surgically repaired knee is on her kicking limb or support limb (during kicking) and to integrate sport-specific drills to accommodate this performance characteristic. Typical prevention programs will last approximately six weeks and include one to three sessions per week.

Chapter 22

Condition	Exercise contraindications	Safety concerns
SCI	■ Exercising within 2 to 3 h after a meal ■ Exercising while ill	■ Overuse injuries at the shoulders, wrists, and elbows ■ Heat- and cold-related injuries ■ Poor venous return ■ Spasticity ■ Exercise-induced hypotension ■ Extra padding on equipment
MS	■ Possibly muscular strength testing ■ Rapidly advancing resistance training loads ■ Vigorous/high aerobic exercise intensities (i.e., exercise to exhaustion) ■ Complex skill-oriented exercises ■ Exercising through an exacerbation	■ Heat sensitivity and intolerance ■ Fatigue ■ Dehydration ■ Hip abductor-adductor spasticity ■ Sensory loss, poor balance ■ Muscle imbalance across joints (agonist vs. antagonist) ■ Depression

Epilepsy	■ Possibly vigorous exercise	■ Effects of weight loss on the side effects of medication ■ Seizures
CP	■ Short or nonexistent aerobic warm-up and stretching	■ Seizures ■ Contractures ■ Poor coordination, balance ■ Joint pain ■ Spasticity

Chapter 23

Phase	Week	Goal reps	Tuesday Heavy day	Thursday Light day	Saturday Medium day
Hypertrophy/ Endurance	1	12	130 lb	100 lb	115 lb
	2	10	145 lb	115 lb	130 lb
	3	8	155 lb	120 lb	140 lb
Strength	4	6	165 lb	130 lb	145 lb
	5	6	165 lb	130 lb	145 lb
	6	5	170 lb	135 lb	150 lb
Strength/ Power	7	4	175 lb	140 lb	155 lb
	8	4	175 lb	140 lb	155 lb
	9	3	180 lb	140 lb	160 lb
Competition	10	2	185 lb	145 lb	165 lb
	11	2	185 lb	145 lb	165 lb
	12	1	195 lb	155 lb	175 lb

Chapter 24

A. (4 feet + 3 feet + 3 feet) × (3 feet + 3 feet + 3 feet) = 90 square feet

B. (4 feet + 3 feet + 3 feet) × (5 feet + 3 feet + 3 feet) = 110 square feet

C. (5 feet + 3 feet + 3 feet) × (4 feet + 3 feet + 3 feet) = 110 square feet

D. (8 feet + 3 feet + 3 feet) × (8 feet + 3 feet + 3 feet) = 196 square feet

E. (4.5 feet + 3 feet + 3 feet) × (7 feet + 3 feet + 3 feet) = 136.5 square feet

F. (5 feet + 3 feet + 3 feet) × (3 feet + 3 feet + 3 feet) = 99 square feet

G. (7 feet) × (7 feet) = 49 square feet

Chapter 25

According to the prevailing standards of practice, if the individual refuses to complete a PAR-Q or to otherwise provide any information for screening, a prospectively executed waiver/release of liability or at least an assumption of risk form should be secured before service is provided. The personal trainer should not examine the client or recommend a program to treat the client's medical condition. The personal trainer should not develop a program to rehabilitate the client's knee.

Glossary

1-repetition maximum (1RM)—The greatest amount of weight that can be lifted with proper technique for only one repetition.

2-for-2 rule—A guideline that can be used to increase the load when two or more repetitions above the repetition goal are completed in the final set of an exercise for two consecutive training sessions.

acceleration—An increase in velocity.

action potential—A temporary change (reversal) in the electrical charge of a muscle or nerve cell when it is stimulated.

actin—One of the two primary myofilaments; binds with myosin to cause a muscle action.

adenosine triphosphate (ATP)—The universal energy-carrying molecule manufactured in all living cells as a means of capturing and storing energy.

adenosine triphosphatase (ATPase)—An enzyme that hydrolyzes, or breaks down, ATP and causes the release of energy.

aerobic capacity—*See* maximal oxygen uptake.

age-predicted maximal heart rate (APMHR)—The estimated maximum heart rate as influenced by age (i.e., 220 − age).

agonist—A muscle that is shortening to perform a concentric action.

alpha blocker—A drug that opposes the excitatory effects of norepinephrine released from sympathetic nerve endings at alpha-receptors and that causes vasodilation and a decrease in blood pressure.

alternated grip—A grip in which one hand is pronated and the other hand is supinated.

amenorrhea—Loss of menses for at least three consecutive menstrual cycles.

amortization phase—The time between the eccentric and concentric phases.

anabolic—Referring to the synthesis of larger molecules from smaller molecules.

anatomical position—Position in which a person stands erect with arms down at the sides and palms forward.

angina—A pain in the chest related to reduced coronary circulation that may or may not involve heart or artery disease.

angular motion—Motion in which a body rotates about an axis.

angular velocity—An object's rotational speed.

antagonist—A muscle, typically anatomically opposite to the agonist, that can stop or slow down a muscle action caused by the agonist.

anthropometry—The science of measurement applied to the human body; generally includes measurements of height, weight, and selected body girths.

aortic stenosis—Narrowing of the aorta.

appendicular skeleton—Skeletal subdivision that consists of the shoulder girdle, arms, legs, and pelvis.

arteriovenous oxygen difference (a–$\bar{v}$O$_2$ difference)—The difference in the oxygen content of arterial blood versus venous blood expressed in milliliters of oxygen per 100 milliliters of blood.

assistance exercises—Exercises that involve movement at only one primary joint and recruit a smaller muscle group or only one large muscle group or area.

assumption of risk—A defense for the personal trainer whereby the client knows that there are inherent risks with participation in an activity but still voluntarily decides to participate.

atherosclerosis—A progressive degenerative process through which the interior lining of the arterial walls becomes hardened and inelastic.

atrium—An upper chamber of the heart that functions to pump blood to the lower chamber of the heart (i.e., ventricle).

auscultate—To listen to the sounds of the body by using a stethoscope.

automated external defibrillator (AED)—A portable device that identifies heart rhythms; uses audio or visual prompts, or both, to direct the correct response; and delivers the appropriate shock only when needed.

autonomic dysreflexia—Manifestation of a spinal cord injury that disrupts normal regulation of arterial blood pressure.

axial skeleton—Skeletal subdivision that consists of the skull, vertebral column, and thorax (rib cage).

axis of rotation—Imaginary line about which joint rotation occurs.

ballistic stretching—A rapid, jerky movement in which the body part is put into motion and momentum carries it through the range of motion until the muscles are stretched to the limits.

beta blocker—A drug that opposes the excitatory effects of norepinephrine released from sympathetic nerve endings at beta-receptors; used for the treatment of angina, hypertension, arrhythmia, and migraine.

beta oxidation—A series of reactions that modify fatty acids into acetyl-CoA, which can then enter the Krebs cycle to produce ATP.

bioelectrical impedance analysis (BIA)—A body composition test that measures the amount of impedance or resistance to a small, painless electrical current.

bioenergetics—The energy pathways of metabolism.

body weight exercises—Resistance training in which the client uses his own body weight as the form of resistance.

bradycardia—A resting heart rate of less than 60 beats/min.

breach of duty—Conduct of a personal trainer that is not consistent with the standard of care.

calcium channel blocker—Calcium antagonist that acts directly on the smooth muscle cells of blood vessels to cause vasodilation; for the treatment of angina and hypertension.

cardiac output ($\dot{Q}$)—The quantity of blood pumped by the heart per minute expressed in liters or milliliters (i.e., SV × HR).

catabolic—The breakdown of larger molecules into smaller molecules.

cerebral palsy—A group of chronic musculoskeletal deficits causing impaired body movement and muscle coordination.

chronic obstructive pulmonary disease (COPD)—A condition or dysfunction of the pulmonary system (e.g., chronic bronchitis, emphysema, asthma).

civil system—The judicial system that applies to one's private rights and therefore to personal responsibilities or obligations that individuals must recognize and observe when dealing with others.

closed grip—A grip in which the thumb is wrapped around the bar so that the bar is fully held in the palm of the hand.

closed kinetic chain—Referring to a movement during which the most distal body part's motion is significantly restricted or fixed; often occurs with lower (or upper) body movements with the feet (or hands) on the floor.

complex training—A combination of resistance and plyometric training.

compound set—Two different exercises for the same primary muscle group that are completed in succession without an intervening rest period.

concentric muscle action—A muscle action in which the muscle is able to overcome the resistance, leading to muscle shortening.

construct—A neural process that cannot be directly observed but must be indirectly inferred through the observation of behavior.

contract—A legally binding promise or performance given in exchange for another promise or performance supported by adequate consideration—something of value.

contraindication—An activity or practice that is inadvisable or prohibited because of a given injury.

core exercise—Exercises that involve movement at two or more primary joints and recruit one or more large muscle groups or areas.

Cori cycle—A gluconeogenic process, taking place in the liver, in which lactate is converted to glucose.

coronary artery disease (CAD)—A condition or dysfunction of the cardiovascular system (e.g., atherosclerosis, myocardial infarction, angina).

coronary risk factor—A characteristic, trait, or behavior that affects the probability of developing cardiovascular disease.

criterion-referenced standard—A method to compare data that involves a combination of normative data and experts' judgment to identify a specific level of achievement.

cross-training—A method of combining several exercise modes within one exercise program.

curvilinear motion—Motion along a curved line.

damages—Economic or noneconomic losses due to an injury; when there is a breach of contract, the amount of money owed by the breaching party.

deceleration—A decrease in velocity.

defendant—The person being sued or accused in a court of law.

diastolic blood pressure—The pressure exerted against the arterial walls between beats when no blood is ejected from the heart or through the vessels (diastole).

Dietary Reference Intakes (DRIs)—Current recommendations for the intake of vitamins and minerals; replaced the *Recommended Dietary Allowances*.

duration—Measure of the length of time an exercise session lasts.

duty of care—Obligation to demonstrate an appropriate standard of care.

dynamic stretching—Similar to ballistic stretching in that it utilizes speed of movement, but dynamic stretching avoids bouncing and includes movements specific to a sport or movement pattern.

dyslipidemia—Abnormal lipid (fat) levels in the blood, lipoprotein composition, or both.

dystonic spasm—Brief recurring muscle contractions that result in twisting and repetitive movements or abnormal posture.

eccentric muscle action—Action that occurs when a muscle cannot develop sufficient tension and is overcome by an external load, and thus progressively lengthens.

efficiency—Amount of mechanical output produced for a given amount of metabolic input.

elasticity—The ability of a muscle fiber to return to original resting length after a passive stretch.

electron transport chain (ETC)—A series of oxidative reactions that rephosphorylate ADP to ATP.

end-diastolic volume—The volume of blood from the left atrium that is available to be pumped by the left ventricle.

endomysium—The connective tissue encasing individual muscle fibers.

epilepsy—Two or more unprovoked, recurring seizures.

epimysium—The connective tissue encasing the entire muscle body.

excess postexercise oxygen consumption (EPOC)—The oxygen uptake above resting values used to restore the body to the preexercise condition; also termed *oxygen debt*.

false grip—A grip in which the thumb is not wrapped around the bar but instead is placed next to the index finger.

fasciculus or **fascicle**—Bundle of muscle fibers; plural of fasciculus is fasciculi.

feedback—The knowledge of results or awareness of success or failure.

Fick equation—$\dot{Q} = \dot{V}O_2 \div a\text{–}\bar{v}O_2$ difference.

field test—An assessment that is performed away from the laboratory and does not require extensive training or expensive equipment.

first-class lever—A lever for which the applied and resistive forces act on opposite sides of the fulcrum.

five-point body contact position—Proper body positioning to maximize stability and spinal support in supine and seated exercises.

flexibility—The ability of a joint to move through an optimum range of motion (ROM).

fluid ball—The abdominal fluids and tissue that are kept under pressure by the diaphragm and abdominal muscles to support the vertebral column from the inside out.

force—Mechanical action applied to a body that tends to produce acceleration.

forced repetitions—Repetitions that are successfully completed with assistance from a spotter.

forced vital capacity—The volume of air moved that results from maximal inspiration and maximal expiration.

Frank-Starling mechanism—The mechanism by which the stroke volume of the heart increases proportionally to the volume of blood filling the heart (the end-diastolic volume).

freestyle (front crawl)—A swimming stroke with a straight and prone body position, an overhand arm motion, and a flutter kick.

frequency—The number of workouts performed in a given time period (typically one week).

friction—The resistance to motion of two objects or surfaces that touch.

frontal plane—A vertical plane that divides the body or organs into front and back portions.

fulcrum—The point about which a lever pivots.

functional anatomy—The relation between body structures and their function, particularly with respect to movement.

functional capacity—*See* maximal oxygen uptake.

general warm-up—A type of warm-up that involves performing basic activities requiring movement of the major muscle groups (e.g., jogging, cycling, or jumping rope).

gestational diabetes mellitus—The onset of a diabetic condition that occurs only during pregnancy.

gluconeogenesis—The formation of glucose from lactate and noncarbohydrate sources.

glycogen—The stored form of glucose.

glycogenolysis—The breakdown of glycogen.

glycolysis—A series of reactions used to produce ATP that utilize only glucose or glycogen as the energy source.

goal repetitions—The number of repetitions a client is assigned to perform for an exercise.

goal setting—A strategy for increasing the level of participation or causing a behavioral change.

Golgi tendon organ—Sensory organ lying within the tendons of the musculotendinous region that recognizes changes in tension in the muscle.

grip width—The distance between the hands when placed on a bar.

ground-fault circuit interrupter (GFCI)—A device to protect against electrocution that cuts off an electric current when there is a difference between the amount of electricity passing through the device and returning through the device, or when there is a leakage of current from the circuit.

health appraisal—Process to screen a client for risk factors and symptoms of chronic cardiovascular, pulmonary, metabolic, and orthopedic diseases in order to optimize safety during exercise testing and participation.

heart rate reserve (HRR)—The difference between a client's maximal heart rate and his or her resting heart rate (i.e., APMHR − RHR).

high-density lipoproteins (HDLs)—Proteins produced in the liver that contain the largest amount of protein and the smallest amount of cholesterol; when elevated, these contribute to a decreased incidence of coronary artery disease.

hyperinsulinemia—High levels of insulin in the blood.

hyperlaxity—Condition that allows the joints of the body to achieve a range of motion that exceeds the normal range of motion.

hyperlipidemia—Elevated concentrations of cholesterol, triglycerides, lipoproteins, or a combination of these.

hyperplasia—An increase in the number of muscle fibers.

hypertension—A systolic blood pressure of ≥140 mmHg or a diastolic blood pressure of ≥90 mmHg (or both).

hypertrophic cardiomyopathy—Condition of unknown cause resulting in thickening in a part of the muscle of the heart.

hypertrophy—An increase in cross-sectional area of the muscle fiber.

hypoglycemia—Blood glucose level of ≤65 mg/dl.

indication—An indication is an activity that will benefit an injured client.

informed consent—A protective legal document that informs the client of any inherent risks associated with fitness testing and participation in an exercise program.

innervation—Stimulation of a muscle cell by a motor nerve.

intensity—The demand or difficulty of an exercise session that determines exercise duration and training frequency.

intermittent exercise—Several shorter bouts of exercise interspersed with rest periods.

isokinetic—Dynamic muscle activity in which a joint moves through a range of motion at a constant velocity.

isometric muscle action—Action that occurs when a muscle generates a force against a resistance but does not overcome it, so that no movement takes place.

Karvonen formula—A method to determine exercise heart rate that takes into consideration a client's age and resting heart rate.

Kegels—Exercises for the muscles of the pelvic floor that involve alternately tightening and relaxing the pelvic region muscle groups.

ketosis—High levels of ketones in the bloodstream caused by incomplete breakdown of fatty acids.

kinematics—Description of motion with respect to space and time, and without regard to the forces or torques involved.

kinetics—Assessment of motion with regard to forces and force-related measures.

Korotkoff sounds—Vibrations that are heard, through the use of a stethoscope, as a result of blood flow through a constricted artery.

Krebs cycle—A series of reactions used to produce ATP, indirectly, that utilize carbohydrate, fat, or protein as an energy source after their modification to acetyl-CoA.

lactate—An end product of glycolysis; most common marker of increased anaerobic metabolism during exercise.

lactate threshold (LT)—The exercise intensity at which blood lactate begins an abrupt increase above the baseline concentration.

legal duty—An obligation recognized by the law requiring a person to conform to certain conduct that reflects the standard of care.

licensure—A formal process by which a state-sanctioned licensing body grants permission to certain professionals the right to offer specified services.

liftoff—The movement of the bar from the supports of a bench or rack to a position in which the client can begin the exercise.

line of force action—The line along which the force acts, passing through the force's point of application.

linear motion—Motion along a straight or curved line.

load—The amount of weight assigned to an exercise set.

long-term goal—A strategy of sequencing and combining short-term goals to reach the client's primary outcome.

low-calorie diet (LCD)—A calorie-reduced yet nutrient-dense diet to achieve a caloric deficit.

low-density lipoproteins (LDLs)—Proteins that transport primarily cholesterol; when elevated, these contribute to an increased incidence of coronary artery disease.

macrocycle—The largest periodization division, typically composed of two or more mesocycles.

Marfan syndrome—Genetic disorder of the connective tissue; symptoms include irregular and unsteady gait, tall lean body type with long extremities including fingers and toes, abnormal joint flexibility, flat feet, stooped shoulders, and dislocation of the optic lens. Complications include a weakened aorta, which may rupture if not treated.

maximal heart rate (MHR)—The actual maximum heart rate.

maximal oxygen uptake ($\dot{V}O_2max$)—The highest capacity for oxygen consumption or utilization by the body during maximal physical exertion; also referred to as *aerobic capacity, maximal aerobic power, maximal oxygen consumption,* or $\dot{V}O_2max$ and sometimes *functional capacity.*

mean arterial pressure—The average blood pressure throughout the cardiac cycle (i.e., [(SBP – DBP) ÷ 3] + DBP).

mechanical advantage—The ratio of the length of the moment arm through which a muscular force acts to the length of a moment arm through which a resistive force acts.

mechanical energy—Capacity or ability to do mechanical work.

medical clearance—Approval by a physician indicating that the client is fit for exercise.

mesocycle—A division of a periodized program that lasts several weeks to a few months.

metabolic equivalent (MET)—Resting oxygen uptake, generally estimated to be 3.5 ml $O_2 \cdot kg^{-1} \cdot min^{-1}$.

metabolic syndrome—Any combination of three or more of the following unhealthy conditions: abdominal obesity, high triglycerides, low HDLs, hypertension, and high fasting glucose.

microcycle—A division of a periodized program that lasts from one to four weeks and can include daily and weekly training variations.

mitochondria—Specialized cellular organelles where the reactions of aerobic metabolism occur.

mitral valve prolapse—Valvular heart disease characterized by the displacement of an abnormally thickened mitral valve leaflet into the left atrium during systole.

mode—The specific type of exercise or activity that will be performed during an exercise session.

moment arm—Perpendicular distance from the axis of rotation to the line of force action.

moment of force—*See* torque.

momentum—Property of a moving body that is determine by the product of its mass and velocity.

motivation—A psychological construct that influences behavior, commitment, attitude, and the desire to exercise.

motor unit—A motor nerve and all the muscle fibers it innervates.

multijoint exercise—An exercise that involves movement at two or more primary joints.

multiple sclerosis—An immune-mediated (autoimmune) disorder that is characterized by inflammation and progressive degeneration of nervous tissue.

muscle fiber—The structural unit of muscle. Also referred to as a muscle cell.

muscle spindle—Sensory organ within muscle fibers that relays sensory information about length and speed of stretch to the central nervous system.

muscular endurance training—A resistance training program designed to target the ability of a muscle or muscle group to contract repeatedly over an extended time period. Also called strength endurance training.

MyPlate—A visual depiction that displays the USDA's recommended types and amounts of food to eat daily.

myocardial infarction—A result of the death of heart tissue due to an occluded blood supply; also referred to as a heart attack.

myocarditis—Inflammation of the heart muscle.

myofibrils—The elements of a muscle fiber that primarily consist of actin and myosin.

myofilaments—The two primary proteins in a myofibril (i.e., actin and myosin).

myoglobin—Iron-containing protein in muscle cells that stores oxygen for use in cell respiration.

myosin—One of the two primary myofilaments; binds with actin to cause a muscle action.

myotatic (stretch) reflex—An activation of previously stretched extrafusal muscle fibers that occurs in response to their being stretched.

near-infrared interactance (NIR)—A body composition test that measures changes in the absorption of light at various anatomical sites; sometimes referred to as *near-infrared reactance*.

negligence—The failure to conform one's conduct to a generally accepted standard or the failure to act as a reasonably prudent person would act under the circumstances.

neutral grip—A grip in which the palm faces in and the knuckles point out to the side, as in a handshake.

normotensive—Having normal blood pressure.

norm-referenced standard—A method to compare data that involves comparing the performance of a client against the performance of others in the same category (e.g., percentile scores).

onset of blood lactate accumulation (OBLA)—The point at which blood lactate concentrations reach 4 mmol/L during exercise of increasing intensity.

open grip—*See* false grip.

open kinetic chain—A movement during which the most distal body part is free to move; often occurs with lower (or upper) body movements with the feet (or hands) off the floor and typically involves pushing or pulling against a machine.

osteoporosis—A disorder characterized by the demineralization of bone tissue that results in a decreased bone mineral density.

outcome goal—A goal that is gauged by social comparison (e.g., the desire to beat an opponent).

overhand grip—A grip in which the hand grasps the bar with the palm down and the knuckles up.

overload—A training stress or intensity greater than what a client is used to.

overreaching—Short-term exercise training, without sufficient recuperation, that exceeds an individual's capacity.

overstriding—A walking or running gait in which the foot hits too far in front of the body's center of gravity, causing a braking effect.

overtraining—A condition in which a client trains too much or rests too little, or both, resulting in diminished exercise capacity, injury, or illness.

oxidative system—The group of chemical reactions used to produce ATP via aerobic means with a variety of energy sources.

oxygen debt—*See* excess postexercise oxygen consumption (EPOC).

oxygen deficit—The difference between the amount of oxygen required for exercise and the amount of oxygen actually consumed during exercise.

pace/tempo training—A type of training program that involves an exercise intensity at the lactate threshold.

paraplegia—Injury to thoracic segments T-2 to T-12 causing impairment in the trunk, legs, pelvic organs, or a combination of these.

PAR-Q (Physical Activity Readiness Questionnaire)—An assessment tool to initially screen apparently healthy clients who want to engage in low-intensity exercise and identify clients who require additional medical screening.

passive warm-up—A type of warm-up that involves receiving external warmth or tissue manipulation (e.g., hot shower, heating pad, or massage).

pennation angle—The angle between the direction of the muscle fibers and an imaginary line between the muscle's origin and its insertion.

percent of APMHR method—A method to determine exercise heart rate that takes into consideration a client's age.

percentile—Percentage of scorers at or below the client's score.

performance goal—A goal that is gauged by a self-referenced personal performance standard (e.g., client's desire to beat his own record).

perimysium—The connective tissue encasing groups of muscle fibers (fascicles).

periodization—The systematic process of planned variations in a resistance training program over a training cycle.

phosphagen system—The simplest set of chemical reactions needed to produce ATP.

pivot—*See* fulcrum.

plaintiff—The "injured" person who brings a suit or complaint into a court of law.

plasticity—The tendency of a muscle to assume a new and greater length after a passive stretch even after the load is removed.

postictal state—The period immediately following a seizure.

potentiation—The increase in activity of the agonist muscle caused by the reflexive response of the muscle spindles and the release of stored elastic energy.

power—The rate of performing work, often expressed as either work divided by time or force times velocity.

power (or explosive) exercise—A structural core exercise that is purposely performed very quickly.

preadolescence—Period of time before the development of secondary sex characteristics, corresponding roughly to the ages 6 to 11 years in girls and 6 to 13 years in boys.

preeclampsia—Hypertension that is induced by pregnancy.

precaution—An activity that an injured client can perform under the supervision of a qualified personal trainer and according to client limitations and symptom reproduction

process goal—A goal that is gauged by the amount or quality of effort during an activity (e.g., the desire to demonstrate perfect exercise technique).

program design variable—An aspect of an exercise program that, when manipulated properly, leads to a safe, effective, and goal-specific outcome.

progression—The gradual and consistent increase in the intensity of an exercise program.

progressive overload—A process by which training stress is altered as a client becomes better trained, allowing her to continue advancing toward a specific training goal.

pronated grip—*See* overhand grip.

prone—Lying facedown.

proprioceptive neuromuscular facilitation (PNF)—A type of stretching that involves a partner and both passive movement and active (concentric and isometric) muscle actions.

proximate cause—A cause that immediately precedes and produces an effect.

punishment—Any act, object, or event that *decreases* the likelihood of future target behavior (when the punishment follows that behavior).

pyruvate—A precursor of lactate during the final steps of glycolysis.

quadriplegia—Injury between the highest thoracic (T-1) and highest cervical (C-1) segments of the spine resulting in impairment of the arms, trunk, legs, and pelvic organs.

rate coding—The control of the motor unit firing rate (i.e., the number of action potentials per unit of time).

rate-limiting step—The slowest reaction in a series of reactions.

rate–pressure product—An estimation of the work of the heart (i.e., double product; HR × SBP).

rating of perceived exertion (RPE)—A self-rating system that accounts for all of the body's responses to a particular exercise intensity.

recruitment—The process in which tasks that require more force involve the activation of more motor units.

rectilinear motion—Motion along a straight line.

reinforcement—Any act, object, or event that *increases* the likelihood of future target behavior (when the reinforcement follows the target behavior).

reliability—An expression of the repeatability of a test or the consistency of repeated tests.

repetition maximum (RM)—The greatest amount of weight that can be lifted with proper technique for a specific number of repetitions.

repetition maximum zone (RM target zone)—A range of repetitions that the client attempts to perform using the heaviest weight he can.

repetitions (or reps)—The number of times a movement or an exercise is completed.

resisted sprinting—A method to increase stride length and speed-strength by increasing the client's ground force production during the support phase.

respiratory exchange ratio (RER)—The ratio of the volume of carbon dioxide expired to the volume of oxygen consumed as measured at the mouth.

resting heart rate (RHR)—The heart rate associated with the client's resting metabolic rate. *See also* resting metabolic rate.

rest interval—The time interval between two sets.

resting metabolic rate (RMR)—A measure of the calories required for maintaining normal metabolism.

risk management—A facet of the emergency plan designed to decrease and control the risk of injury from client participation and, therefore, the risk of liability exposure. Risk management may involve internal or external audits to identify potential problems, as well as actions taken to improve the safe delivery of services and reduce the chances of untoward events and potential lawsuits.

risk stratification—A method to initially classify clients as being at low, moderate, or high risk for coronary, peripheral vascular, or metabolic disease.

rotational motion—The product of the force exerted on an object and the distance the object rotates.

safety space cushion—The recommended area between each piece of equipment to enhances traffic flow in, out of, and around the exercise facility.

sagittal plane—A vertical plane that divides the body or organs into left and right portions.

sarcomere—The segment of a myofibril between two adjacent Z-lines (bands), representing the functional unit of skeletal muscle.

sarcopenia—Muscle loss due to aging.

sarcoplasmic reticulum—Highly specialized network system in a muscle fiber that stores calcium ions.

scope of practice—Legal boundaries that determine the extent of a personal trainer's professional duties.

second-class lever—A lever in which the applied and resistive forces act on the same side of the fulcrum, but with the applied force acting through a moment arm that is longer than that of the resistive force.

seizure—An uncontrolled electrical discharge within any part of the brain, causing physical or mental symptoms that may or may not be associated with convulsions.

self-determination—A desire to participate in an activity for self-fulfillment as opposed to a desire to meet the expectations of others.

self-efficacy—A perceived self-confidence in one's own ability to perform specific actions (e.g., reach a short-term goal) that lead to a successful outcome.

self-talk—A client's "internal voice."

series elastic component (SEC)—The structures that, when stretched, have the ability to store energy that may be released upon an immediate concentric muscle action.

set—A group of repetitions that are performed consecutively.

short-term goal—An attainable step that brings the client closer to reaching a long-term goal.

single-joint exercise—An exercise that involves movement at only one primary joint.

size principle—The recruitment of larger and more motor units as a response to an increased force requirement.

spasticity—A state of increased tonus of a muscle characterized by heightened deep tendon reflexes.

specificity—A strategy to train a client in a certain way to produce a particular change or result.

specific warm-up—A type of warm-up in which movements are performed that mimic the sport or activity (e.g., slow jogging before running or lifting light loads on the bench press before lifting training loads).

speed-endurance—The ability to maintain running speed over an extended duration (typically longer than 6 seconds).

speed-strength—The application or development of maximum force at high velocities.

sphygmomanometry—Measurement of blood pressure using an inflatable air bladder–containing cuff and a stethoscope to auscultate the Korotkoff sounds.

split routine—An exercise routine in which different muscle groups are trained on different days or training sessions.

sprain—Injury to a ligament.

sprint-assisted training—A method to increase stride frequency by having the client run at speeds greater than he is able to independently achieve.

stage of readiness—The degree or extent to which a client is ready to begin an exercise program.

standard error of measurement—The difference between a person's observed score—what the result was—and that person's true score, a theoretically errorless score.

standard of care—A set of criteria for the appropriate duties of a personal trainer. *See also* scope of practice.

state anxiety—The actual experience of anxiety, characterized by feelings of apprehension or nervousness, that is accompanied by an increased physiological arousal.

static stretching—Stretching performed at a slow constant speed, with the end position held for 30 seconds. A static stretch includes the relaxation and simultaneous lengthening of the stretched muscle.

status epilepticus—A seizure lasting more than 30 minutes or a seizure that occurs so frequently that consciousness is not restored.

sticking point—The most difficult part of the exercise that typically occurs soon after the transition from the eccentric to the concentric phase.

strain—Injury to a muscle.

stretch reflex—The immediate contraction of a muscle caused by a rapid stretch of that muscle.

stretch–shortening cycle (SSC)—The series of three phases that explains the mechanical and neurophysiological reactions to a plyometric movement.

stride frequency—The number of steps per minute.

stride length—The distance covered with each step.

stroke volume—The quantity of blood ejected by the left ventricle expressed in milliliters of blood per beat.

structural exercise—An exercise that loads the trunk (vertebral column) and places stress on the lower back.

subluxation—Partial displacement of the joint surfaces.

sudden cardiac death—Death occurring unexpectedly and instantaneously or within 1 hour of the onset of symptoms in a patient with or without known preexisting heart disease.

supinated grip—A grip in which the hand grasps the bar with the palm up and the knuckles down.

supine—Lying down on the back, facing up.

SWOT analysis—A strategic method of analysis consisting of strengths, weaknesses, opportunities, and threats.

sympathetic nervous system—A part of the nervous system that, when stimulated, speeds up various systems of the body (increases heart rate).

systolic blood pressure—The pressure exerted against the arterial walls as blood is forcefully ejected during ventricular contraction (systole).

tachycardia—A resting heart rate of more than 100 beats/min.

target behavior—A behavior that is the focus for change or improvement; also called an *operant*.

target heart rate range (THRR)—The minimum and maximum heart rates per unit of time that are assigned for an aerobic exercise session.

tendinitis—Inflammation of a tendon.

test protocol—Procedures required for administering a reliable test.

test–retest method—A strategy to promote reliability by repeating a test with the same individual or group.

tetraplegia—*See* quadriplegia.

therapeutic lifestyle change (TLC)—A lifestyle modification that includes diet, physical activity, and weight loss.

thermic effect of food—An increase in energy expenditure above resting metabolic rate, caused by the digestion and assimilation of food.

third-class lever—A lever in which the applied and resistive forces act on the same side of the fulcrum, but with the resistive force acting through a moment arm that is longer than that of the applied force.

thrombotic occlusion—Blockage due to a blood clot.

tidal volume—The amount of air moved during inhalation or exhalation with each breath.

torque—The tendency of a force to rotate an object about a fulcrum.

tort—A breach of legal duty other than a breach of contract that results in a civil wrong or injury; may be the foundation for a civil suit to collect damages.

total peripheral resistance—The impedance of blood flow caused by exercise, nervous stimulation, metabolism, and environmental stress.

trait anxiety—The potential perception or probability that a certain situation will cause anxiety.

transverse plane—A horizontal plane that divides the body or organs into upper and lower portions.

trial load—An estimated load that is based on a percent of the client's body weight.

triglycerides—A group of fatty compounds that circulate in the bloodstream; the predominate storage form of fat.

tropomyosin—A protein, attached to actin, that prevents actin from binding to the myosin cross-bridges.

troponin—A protein, attached to tropomyosin, that when activated shifts the tropomyosin to allow the actin to bind to the myosin cross-bridges.

type 1 diabetes mellitus—A disease in which the pancreatic beta cells are destroyed by an autoimmune process leading to absolute insulin deficiency; formerly known as *insulin-dependent diabetes mellitus (IDDM)*.

type 2 diabetes mellitus—A disease resulting in insulin resistance in peripheral tissues and an insulin production deficit of the pancreatic beta cells; formerly referred to as *non-insulin-dependent diabetes mellitus (NIDDM)*.

type I muscle fiber—A type of muscle fiber characterized by a slow rate of action and relaxation, high aerobic metabolic activity, and high fatigue resistance. Also known as a *slow oxidative* or *slow-twitch fiber*.

type IIa muscle fiber—A type of muscle fiber characterized by a fast rate of action and relaxation, moderate aerobic and high glycolytic metabolic activity, and moderate fatigue resistance. Also known as a *fast oxidative glycolytic fiber*.

type IIx muscle fiber—A type of muscle fiber characterized by a fast rate of action and relaxation, high glycolytic metabolic activity, and low fatigue resistance. Also known as a *fast glycolytic fiber*.

underhand grip—*See* supinated grip.

understriding—A walking or running gait in which the foot takes too short a stride, causing wasted energy.

undulating—Referring to a type of periodized training program that involves within-the-week or microcycle vacillations of training load and volume.

user space—The recommended area that a client needs to perform an exercise safely.

validity—The degree to which a test or test item measures what it is supposed to measure.

Valsalva maneuver—The act of breath-holding that contributes to maintaining intra-abdominal pressure; the client tries to exhale against a "closed throat."

variation—A purposeful change of the program design variable assignments to expose a client to new or different training stressors.

venous return—The return of the blood to the right atrium from the body (periphery).

ventricle—A lower chamber of the heart that functions to pump blood from the heart (right ventricle pumps to the lungs, left ventricle pumps to the body).

very low-density lipoproteins (VLDLs)—Proteins that transport primarily triglycerides; when elevated, these contribute to an increased incidence of coronary artery disease.

visualization—The ability of the brain to draw and recall mental images that can create positive emotional responses and improve motivation.

volume—The total amount of weight lifted in a training session (i.e., total repetitions × the weight lifted per repetition) *or* the total number of repetitions completed in a training session (i.e., the number of repetitions performed in each set × the number of sets).

waiver—A contract that serves as evidence that the injured client waived her right to sue for negligence.

Wolff's law—Law stating that bone density will increase in response to mechanical stress.

work—The product of the force exerted on an object and the distance the object moves (i.e., force × distance).

work-to-rest ratio—The relationship between the duration of the exercise interval and that of the recovery interval.

Index

Note: The italicized *f* and *t* following page numbers refer to figures and tables, respectively.

About the Editors

Jared W. Coburn, PhD, CSCS,*D, FNSCA, FACSM, is a professor of kinesiology at California State University at Fullerton, where he has earned numerous awards for teaching and research excellence. Before entering the world of academia, Coburn worked as a personal trainer, strength and conditioning coach, and director of physical therapy clinics and fitness and wellness centers. His interest in applying scientific principles to the training of clients and athletes is based largely on his experience as a practitioner.

Coburn has published widely and frequently lectures on topics related to exercise training. He is particularly interested in studying muscle function during strength, power, and endurance exercises and has presented his work in peer-reviewed journals and textbook chapters. Coburn is an active member of the National Strength and Conditioning Association, where he has held membership since 1984. He holds bachelor's and master's degrees from California State University at Fullerton and a PhD from the University of Nebraska at Lincoln.

Coburn lives with his wife, Tamara, and their two children in Norco, California.

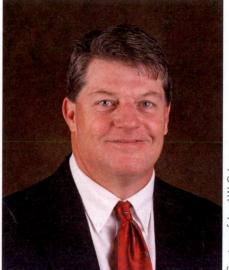

Courtesy of Jared W. Coburn.

Jared W. Coburn

Moh H. Malek, PhD, CSCS,*D, NSCA-CPT,*D, FNSCA, FACSM, is an associate professor in the College of Pharmacy and Health Sciences and director of the Integrative Physiology of Exercise Laboratory at Wayne State University in Detroit, Michigan.

Malek conducts research in both human and animal models examining the underlying mechanisms of muscle fatigue. In 2010, Malek received the NSCA's Terry J. Housh Outstanding Young Investigator of the Year Award. Malek has published over 60 peer-reviewed papers related to exercise physiology and has presented his research at the NSCA National Conference since 2004. Since 2007, he has served as associate editor of *Journal of Strength and Conditioning Research*. He also serves on the editorial board of *Medicine & Science in Sport & Exercise*. Malek received his bachelor's degrees in biology and psychology from Pitzer College, his master's degree in kinesiology from California State University at Fullerton, and a PhD in exercise physiology from the University of Nebraska at Lincoln.

Malek and his wife, Bridget, reside in Northville, Michigan. In his free time, Malek enjoys watching football, fitness training, and reading.

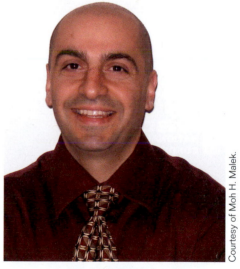

Courtesy of Moh H. Malek.

Moh H. Malek

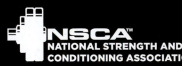
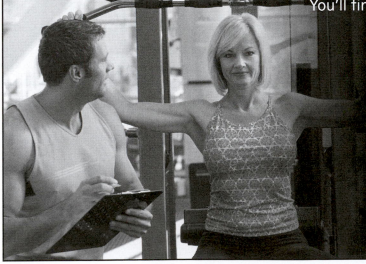
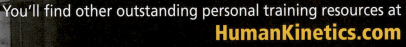